Family
NURSING
RESEARCH, THEORY, & PRACTICE

FIFTH EDITION

MARILYN M. FRIEDMAN, PHD, MS, MA, RN

Professor Emeritus
School of Nursing
California State University, Los Angeles
Los Angeles, California

VICKY R. BOWDEN, DNSc, RN

Associate Professor
School of Nursing
Azusa Pacific University
Azusa, California

ELAINE G. JONES, PHD, MS, RN

Associate Professor
College of Nursing
The University of Arizona
Tucson, Arizona

Prentice
Hall

Upper Saddle River, New Jersey 07458

Library of Congress Cataloging-in-Publication Data

Friedman, Marilyn M.
  Family nursing : research, theory, & practice / Marilyn
M. Friedman, Vicky R. Bowden, Elaine Jones.—5th ed.
    p. ; cm.
  Includes bibliographical references and index.
  ISBN 0-13-060824-6
  1. Family nursing. I. Bowden, Vicky R. II. Jones, Elaine,
Ph.D.   III. Title.
  [DNLM: 1. Family Nursing—Programmed
  Instruction. WY 18.2 F911f 2003]
RT120.F34 F75 2003
610.73—dc21
                                        2002025198

Publisher: Julie Levin Alexander
Executive Assistant: Regina Bruno
Executive Editor: Maura Connor
Acquisitions Editor: Nancy Anselment
Marketing Manager: Nicole Benson
Editorial Assistant: Sarah Caffrey/Aaron Reisner
Director of Manufacturing and Production: Bruce Johnson
Managing Production Editor: Patrick Walsh
Production Editor: Rhonda Peters, Rainbow Graphics
Production Liaison: Cathy O'Connell
Manufacturing Buyer: Pat Brown
Manufacturing Manager: Ilene Sanford
Design Director: Cheryl Asherman
Senior Design Coordinator: Maria Guglielmo Walsh
Interior and Cover Design: Judy Allan/Top Desk Publisher's Group
Illustration Studio: ElectraGraphics
Composition: Rainbow Graphics
Printing and Binding: RR Donnelley

Pearson Education LTD.
Pearson Education Australia PTY, Limited
Pearson Education Singapore, Pte. Ltd
Pearson Education North Asia Ltd
Pearson Education, Canada, Ltd.
Pearson Educación de Mexico, S.A. de C.V.
Pearson Education—Japan
Pearson Education Malaysia, Pte. Ltd
Pearson Education, Upper Saddle River, New Jersey

Notice: Care has been taken to confirm the accuracy of the information presented in this book. The authors, editors, and the publisher, however, cannot accept any responsibility for errors or omissions or for consequences from application of the information in this book and make no warranty, express or implied, with respect to its contents.

The authors and the publisher have exerted every effort to ensure that drug selections and dosages set forth in this text are in accord with current recommendations and practice at time of publication. However, in view of ongoing research, changes in government regulations, and the constant flow of information relating to drug therapy and drug reactions, the reader is urged to check the package inserts of all drugs for any change in indications of dosage and for added warnings and precautions. This is particularly important when the recommended agent is a new and/or infrequently employed drug.

21   17

ISBN 0-13-060824-6

To my husband, Amnon, who for the last six months has been battling a malignant brain tumor. I will always remember his bravery and support of me, while struggling with his devastating illness and the myriad of treatments and complications.

—*Marilyn M. Friedman*

To Greg, Christian, and Matthew—your love and support, so freely given, continue to bring me peace, joy, and strength.

—*Vicky R. Bowden*

To my own family from whom I learned how to sustain family connections, through many changes; and to the families who shared their lives with me in nursing, and taught me how nurses might best be helpful to diverse families.

—*Elaine G. Jones*

CONTENTS

PREFACE

As readers of the fifth edition, we think you will be pleased with the changes and additions that have been made. Much of this is due to the fact that two new co-authors have been added to the text. As the first author, I feel profoundly blessed to have two gifted and caring family nurses join me in updating and enriching the fifth edition's content and presentation. Dr. Vicky Bowden is a well-known nursing author, practitioner, and educator. Dr. Elaine Jones is also very experienced and expert in family nursing education, practice, and research with families with deaf members. Their positive contributions have made revising this text an exciting and very positive endeavor. We each revised about one third of the chapters, but carefully reviewed and made suggestions to the primary revisor on the other chapters to make them more comprehensive and relevant.

Great strides have been made in the field of family nursing since this text's inception in 1980 and the additions and changes in this text parallel family nursing's growth. There has been a proliferation of texts in family nursing that contain in-depth discussions of theories, research, and practice. The increase in publications about family nursing; the inception of the *Journal of Family Nursing* in 1995; the growing incorporation of family nursing into ANA Standards of Nursing Practice, NANDA nursing diagnoses, and the Nursing Intervention Classification (NIC); the holding of national and international family nursing conferences; the continuing activity of the family and health section of the National Council for Family Relations; and the increase in family nursing courses and content in both undergraduate and graduate nursing programs present strong evidence of the development of family nursing as both an integral part of generalist practice and as a specialty area in advanced practice nursing. Moreover, there is a growing consensus that family nursing is conceptually and empirically distinct from nursing of family members. And due to the profound influence of family therapy and the application of systems theory, family nurses are increasingly "thinking interactionally" in their writings and conversations about families and family nursing practice.

The text's focus in the fifth edition includes nursing diagnoses and interventions. In this edition, as previous editions, the same basic comprehensive family assessment tool is presented, with some modification. The family assessment model is based primarily on three theoretical perspectives: a systems perspective, a structural–functional perspective, and a family developmental perspective. A multicultural perspective is also integrated throughout.

This text is intended for undergraduate and graduate family nursing students and practitioners who are not practicing advanced family therapy or family systems nursing. Advanced family nursing practice requires the completion of a specialized program at the master's level. Hence, we included family nursing interventions that are basic and straightforward; these suggested interventions, although certainly necessary within family nursing practice, are insufficient for working with the very complex family in which more sophisticated, indirect interviewing and advanced counseling skills are required.

NEW FEATURES IN THE FIFTH EDITION

In the fifth edition of this text, the following new features have been added:

- Content outlines have been added at the beginning of each chapter.
- A bulleted summary at the end of each chapter highlights the key ideas within the chapter.
- A glossary containing the major terms used in each of the chapters augments comprehension.
- More tables and figures have been added to graphically depict key points.
- As part of the review questions at the end of each chapter, a family vignette has been added, which addresses chapter content and augments critical thinking skills.
- Chapters addressing practice areas include family assessment, family diagnoses, and family nursing interventions.
- In the family nursing practice chapters, three variables are considered: gender differences, sociocultural variation, and differences created by health alterations.
- Statistics and references have been carefully updated.
- The latest NANDA (North American Nursing Diagnosis Association) and NIC (Nursing Interventions Classification) descriptions are incorporated.

CONTENT NEW TO THE FIFTH EDITION

This book is subdivided into four broad sections. Part I includes two introductory chapters that discuss the family's importance and family definitions (Chapter 1) and family nursing's evolution, focus, and goals (Chapter 2). In Chapter 1, the sections outlining demographic trends impacting the family and the varied family forms have been updated and enlarged. The chapter on family nursing (Chapter 2) covers the gamut of emerging goals and roles of the family nurse from health promotion through rehabilitation. The rising costs of medical care; the implementation of managed care; the rising proportion of older, chronically ill individuals; and the recognition that many chronic illnesses can be prevented or ameliorated with lifestyle changes are prominent trends that have greatly expanded the role of the family nurse in both health promotion and acute and long-term care. Several major current issues facing family nursing facilitate our understanding of the status of family nursing today.

Part II addresses the basic theoretical foundations of family nursing (Chapters 3 through 6). Chapter 3, "Theoretical Foundations of Family Nursing," reviews the various theories used in family nursing practice, with much better coverage of nursing theories than in the previous edition. Integrated family nursing theories are also described and advocated. Chapter 4 is a short chapter describing structural–functional theory and how it has been applied in this text. Chapter 5, "Family Developmental Theory," has been revised and updated to include a broader range of developmental theories. In this chapter, family developmental theory is applied to single-parent and stepparent families, in addition to the two-parent nuclear family. Chapter 6, "Systems Theory," contains greater coverage of holism, cybernetics, and communication theory as more focused, midrange theories subsumed under general systems theory.

Part III introduces the reader to the family nursing process as well as the actual family assessment model or tool (located within each of the individual chapters), family nursing diagnoses, and family nursing interventions. Chapter 7, "The Family Nursing Process," has been updated and revised, combining two chapters from the previous edition of the text into one chapter that is more comprehensive and includes a very thorough discussion of family nursing interventions. Chapter 7 covers the new literature appearing in the counseling, education, case management, and family nursing process areas. Chapter 8, "Family Identifying Data: Sociocultural Assessment and Intervention," discusses family nursing in the context of sociocultural diversity. Updating of statistical data and literature on the significant demographic changes taking place in America provide a greater understanding about the urgency of practicing competently with families from diverse backgrounds.

In the remainder of the practice chapters (Chapters 9 through 16) pertinent research, theory, and practice implications have been incorporated. These chapters address family structural dimensions; family functions; and family stress, coping, and adaptation. Family structural dimensions are crucial to family nursing practice, since they cover family dynamics as seen in family communication patterns and processes (Chapter 10), family power and decision making (Chapter 11), the family role structure (Chapter 12), and family values (Chapter 13). The affective function (Chapter 14), family socialization function (Chapter 15), and the health care function (Chapter 16) are the three most relevant family functions to assess in family nursing. Family stress, coping processes, and adaptation (Chapter 17) are also essential components within family nursing assessment and intervention.

Chapter 9, "Family Environmental Data," has new sections on resources in the home (such as Internet access), discussion of differences in rural versus urban family environment, an updated section on the effects of homelessness on family health, and a new section focusing on the sociopolitical environment as an important factor in family health.

Chapter 10, "Family Communication Patterns and Processes," contains both classic and recent research and theoretical content related to functional and dysfunctional family communication patterns. This chapter also discusses the influence of cultural beliefs, family life cycle stage, gender, family form, and family mini-culture on family communication patterns.

Chapter 11, "Family Power and Decision Making," presents foundational concepts in family power. Discussion of family violence is now included in this chapter, with specific sections addressing intimate partner abuse, child and adolescent abuse, sibling abuse, parent abuse, and elder abuse.

Chapter 12, "Family Role Structure," focuses on research on family role changes during illness, with an expanded discussion about the family caregiver role, and the role of the father in contemporary families. A particular strength is the expanded section about grandparents' roles in families, especially grandmothers who are involved in raising grandchildren.

Chapter 13, "Family Values," contains new information regarding changes in family values that have emerged in recent years as a result of societal changes. Disparities in value systems are discussed, especially those that exist between the family and the health care professional.

Chapter 14, "The Family Affective Function," reviews essential components of the affective function. The chapter covers the process of family bereavement more thoroughly than in the previous editions.

In Chapter 15, "The Family Socialization Function," findings are incorporated from the latest socialization research. There is also broadened coverage of multicultural aspects of parenting, and unique socialization issues for single-parent families, stepparent families, and families with gay or lesbian parents.

In Chapter 16, "The Family Health Care Function," the critical thrust of family health promotion is clearly evident, with Pender's revised Health Promotion Model providing the theoretical foundation for identifying the multiple factors influencing family health promotion. Recent research findings on health care practices among families, such as lifestyle practices and the use of medically based and alternative/complementary health care, have also been incorporated.

A major revamping of the content within Chapter 17, now titled "Family Stress, Coping, and Adaptation" occurred. The Resiliency Model of Family Stress, Adjustment, and Adaptation is fully described, and other research and theoretical developments in the area of family stress and coping have been updated. Family resiliency, family coherence, and factors influencing coping are emphasized. In addition, social support research, theory, and clinical application have been added to this chapter.

In Part IV (Chapters 18, 19, and 20), cultural differences among families from the three largest minority groups in the United States, Latino, African-American, and Asian-American, are addressed. Current literature about each of these families, coupled with an expanded description of family nursing assessment and interventions that are culturally sensitive and appropriate, make these chapters quite useful for working with culturally diverse clients. Chapter 20, "The Asian-American Family," was a new chapter in the fourth edition, and is a reflection of the growing presence of Asian-Americans in the United States today. Their Eastern legacy is so disparate from our Western tradition that family nurses who work with traditional Asian-Americans need to be sensitive to these profound cultural differences.

The Appendices contain the Friedman Family Assessment Model (long form and short form), a family case description and the use of the family nursing process in the case example, as well as answers to the family vignettes and study questions. The family nursing example is included to give students a concrete model of family nursing practice and also an opportunity to retest themselves on the use of the Friedman Family Assessment Model and application of the family nursing process. Chapters in Part III describe the knowledge base needed to complete the family assessment and to develop family nursing diagnoses and intervention guidelines.

THE NEW EDITION: A REFLECTION OF EXPANDED VISTAS IN FAMILY NURSING

Our ardent belief is that health professionals, regardless of the setting, must broaden their commitment so that they serve families as units, as well as family subsystems (e.g., parental subsystems) and individual family members. It is well recognized that a considerable gap exists between the ideal (what ought to be) and the real (the actual practice of nursing today). In spite of nursing's and health care's shortcomings, family nursing continues to be a very exciting and rewarding dimension of professional nursing, as well as an emerging, vital, advanced practice nursing area. We hope this text is able to convey some of our excitement about family nursing to you, as well as give you the foundations to practice more comfortably and effectively with families. Happy reading!

—*Marilyn M. Friedman, Vicky Bowden, and Elaine Jones*

ACKNOWLEDGMENTS

We would like to thank our friends, family members, and colleagues for their support, encouragement, and understanding during the many months it took to complete the revision of this text. We would also like to acknowledge the assistance, support, and prodding of Nancy Anselment, nursing editor at Prentice Hall Health. Without Nancy's continual leadership and coaching us on, this text would still be a work in progress. We are also grateful for the ideas and suggestions we received from the several reviewers of the fourth edition of this text. And finally, we would like to acknowledge the chapter authors of previous editions—those ideas and contributions laid the foundations for this revision—as well as the contributors of this fifth edition.

CONTRIBUTORS

Terry A. Badger PhD, RN
Professor
College of Nursing
University of Arizona
Tucson, AZ
Re: Family Social Science Theories and Family Therapy Theories

Marilyn Morris McEwen, PhD(C), MS, BC, APRN
Doctoral Candidate
University of Arizona
Re: Rural Health, Housing

Gale Manke, MSN, RN
Clinical Associate Professor
College of Nursing
University of Arizona
Re: Homeless Families

❧ REVIEWERS

Wendy C. Booth, MSN, RN
Clinical Nurse Specialist, Community Health
University of Alabama at Birmingham
Birmingham, Alabama

Gail Hanscom, MS, MA, RN
Advisor, School Nurse Services Credential Program
San Diego State University School of Nursing
San Diego, California

Pamela Martin, PhD, RN
Assistant Dean for Nursing Undergraduate Programs
The University of Texas at Tyler
College of Nursing and Health Services
Tyler, Texas

Ann L. Bianchi, MSN, RN
Classroom and Clinical Instructor of Nursing
Calhoun Community College
Department of Nursing
Huntsville, Alabama

Barbara Larson, BA, MEd, RNC
Education Coordinator
UIC and Lode Star Enterprises
Illinois

MMF

I would also like to extend my thanks to my neighbors who because of my husband's illness and my writing of this text baked and cooked many dinners and other goodies for us over the last six months. I am also very grateful to my husband Amnon's two brothers, Leib and Ben-Ami, for they have continually visited and helped with my husband, making it possible for me to do my part of the revision.

VRB

I would like to thank Marilyn for this extraordinary opportunity to work with her on the fifth edition of *Family Nursing*. I was introduced to the first edition of the text while in my master's program in nursing. Never in my wildest dreams could I imagine I would have the occasion to collaborate with her on a text that I have used repeatedly as a resource in my clinical practice, my writing, and my work in academia. Marilyn is a pioneer in family nursing, who through her accomplishments as an author and educator, has imprinted an indispensable love and appreciation for family nursing on the heart of so many nurses. Thank you for continuing to share your passion for family nursing with Elaine and I.

EGJ

I would like to first thank Dr. Marilyn Friedman for affording me this marvelous opportunity to participate as a co-editor with her for the fifth edition of this stellar textbook. She was an exceptional mentor throughout the process, despite her very difficult personal situation. I am very grateful. Second, I would like to thank Dr. Vicky Bowden for her amazing organizational ability and energy. I have learned a great deal from her, as well. Third, I'd like to thank my friends and colleagues at the University of Arizona for their encouragement and material support throughout this undertaking. Three agreed to serve as contributors on short notice (Terry Badger, Gale Manke, and Marilyn McEwen, PhD(C), and their work added wonderful, contemporary perspectives to the text. Other colleagues provided me with key resources for other sections that I may not have discovered without them: Linda Phillips (elder abuse), and Amy Barnard (lesbian/gay parents). Many thanks!

one

INTRODUCTORY CONCEPTS

Part I includes foundational knowledge for family nursing practice. Chapter 1 presents basic information about the family, its importance, and family definitions. Chapter 2 covers family nursing's evolution, prime goals, and the roles of the family nurse.

1

INTRODUCTION TO THE FAMILY

❧ LEARNING OBJECTIVES

1. Describe the basic purposes the family serves for society and the individual family members.
2. Explain why it is important for nurses to work with families.
3. Describe how family and society mutually affect each other.

4. Explain how the family interacts with health/illness issues during six stages of family's interaction with health/illness.
5. Define family, nuclear (conjugal) family, extended family, and family of orientation or origin.

6. Explain the difference between the meaning of health and family health.
7. Identify characteristics of healthy families.
8. Discuss several societal trends that have had a major impact on the American family, as well as changes in the American family.
9. Discuss some of the factors associated with the growth of childless families, single-parent families, cohabiting families, and unmarried teenage mothers.

10. Define variant family forms and give examples of several diverse family forms.
11. Identify several stressors commonly found in single-parent, gay/lesbian, and stepparent families.
12. Present the arguments for a pessimistic and an optimistic view in regard to the future of the American family.
13. Name one key implication for family nursing practice relative to diverse family forms.

One of the most important aspects of nursing is the emphasis placed on the family unit. The family—along with the individual, group, and community—is nursing's client or recipient of care.

Empirically, we realize that the health of family members and the quality of family life are closely related. Until the last decade, however, remarkably little attention has been paid to the family as an object of systematic study in nursing. Apart from simple evaluative labeling of families with terms such as *good, problem, multiproblem,* or *dysfunctional,* nurses in the past were generally unable to describe the families they were caring for. This situation is changing. Today the study of families in both undergraduate and graduate programs has grown significantly.

This chapter will set the stage for systematic study of family theories and research and family nursing practice. Basic purposes of the family, the rationale for nurses working with families, how the society and family mutually influence each other, and most importantly, the salient interrelationship between the health status of family and the health status of its individual members will be described. The chapter also discusses the state of the American family and its future, basic family definitions, the family's various forms, and characteristics of healthy families.

❧TWO BASIC PURPOSES OF THE FAMILY

Because the family forms the basic unit of our society, it is the social institution that has the most marked effect on its members. This basic unit so strongly influences the development of an individual that it may determine the success or failure of that person's life.

The family unit occupies a position between the individual and society (Bronfenbrenner, 1979). Its basic purposes are twofold: (1) to meet the needs of the society of which it is a part, and (2) to meet the needs of the individuals in it. These functions, which are fundamental to human adaptation, cannot be fulfilled separately. They must be joined in the family.

For society, the family, through its procreation and socialization of new members, functions to fill a vital need. It forms a grouping of individuals that society treats as an entity; it creates a network of kinship systems that help stabilize a society, even in its industrialized state; it generates new members in order to assure the survival of the community; and it provides new "recruits" for society, preparing children to assume productive roles in society (Cherlin, 1996).

The family serves as the critical intervening variable (or as some authors term it, *buffer* or *bargaining agent*) between society and the individual. In other words, a basic purpose of the family is *mediation*—taking the basic societal expectations and obligations and molding and modifying them to fit the needs and interests of its individual family members.

The family also functions to meet the *needs of its members.* For the spouse or adult members it serves to stabilize their lives—meeting their affective, socioeconomic, and sexual needs. For the children, the family provides physical and emotional care, and concomitantly directs their personality development (Minuchin, 1974; Sitelman & Sitelman, 2001). The family system is the main learning context for an individual's behavior, thoughts, and feelings.

Parents are the primary "teachers," because parents interpret the world and society to children. The environment—outside forces—is important, particularly as it affects parents when children are young, because parents are the ones who translate to their children the major meanings these outside forces have. The interpretation parents give of the world and society is naturally based on their experiences and their "reality." If they have been discriminated against or lived in a crime-ridden community, they may see the world as being dangerous, hostile, a place to avoid, and thereby impart these perceptions to their children. If, on the other hand, the world has provided stability and security for them, this perspective will be transmitted to their children.

The family has long been seen as the most vital context for healthy growth and development. It has a crucial influence on the formation of an individual's identity and feelings of self-esteem. Minuchin (1974), a noted family therapist, so beautifully summarizes the dual role that the family plays:

> The family, then, is the matrix of its members' sense of identity—of belonging and of being different. Its chief task is to foster their psychosocial growth and well-being throughout their life in common. . . . The family also forms the smallest social unit which transmits a society's demands and values, and thus, preserves them. The family must adapt to society's needs while it fosters its members' growth, all the while maintaining enough continuity to fulfill its function as the individual's reference group. (p. 3)

An individual is the repository of group (especially primary group or family) experience. His or her identity is both individual (intrapersonal experiences) and social (interpersonal experiences). A person's intrapsychic experiences are largely developed from his or her interpersonal experiences, as through the parent–child relationship (Mead, 1934). A meaningful conception of an individual's mental health status can be achieved only when we relate the functioning of the individual to the human relation patterns of that person's primary group or family.

WHY WORK WITH THE FAMILY?

The family provides the critical resource for delivering efficacious health services to people. The follow-ing summary highlights the most cogent reasons why the family unit must be a central focus of our care.

1. The family is a critical resource for delivering health care to both individuals and families. When a family focus to care is provided, health care effectiveness has been found to improve (Gilliss & Davis, 1993). For instance, significant inroads can be made to curtail risks that lifestyle and environmental hazards create. A primary health promotion goal is to raise the level of wellness of the whole family, which should then significantly raise the wellness level of each of its members.

2. In a family unit, any dysfunction (illness, injury, separation) that affects one or more family members may, and frequently will, in some way affect other members as well as the unit as a whole. The family is a closely knit, interdependent network whose members mutually influence each other. The problems of one family member "seep in" and affect the other family members and the whole system (this is called the "ripple effect"). If a nurse assesses only the individual and not the family, he or she may be missing the gestalt needed to gain a holistic assessment of the situation. Although recent research in biology and genetics might disagree, one of the important tenets of family therapy is that the symptoms of the identified patient (the family member with the overt behavioral problems or psychosomatic illness) are indices of the family's level of adaptation, or in this case, maladaptation.

3. There is such a strong interrelationship between the family and the health status of its members that the role of the family is crucial during every facet of health care of its individual family members—from the health promotion stage through the rehabilitative stage. Assessing and rendering family health care is critical for assisting each family member to achieve an optimum level of wellness (Gilliss & Davis, 1993).

4. Case finding is another good reason for providing family health care. The presence of health problems in one member, which provides an entrée into the family, may lead to discovery of disease or risk factors in other family

members; this is often the case when visiting families with chronic health problems or communicable disease at home. The family-centered nurse often works through one family member to reach its other members.

5. One can achieve a clearer and more holistic understanding of the individuals and their functioning when they are viewed within their family context.

THE FAMILY–SOCIETY INTERFACE

As the basic unit in society, the family shapes and is shaped by the external forces (community and larger social systems) surrounding it. Most sociologists would agree that the influence of society on the family is greater than that of the family on society, although the family also exerts an effect on the society.

The pace of social change in recent decades has accelerated, with the family especially feeling its impact. Throughout history, however, the family has demonstrated tremendous resiliency and adaptiveness, just as political, educational, and other societal institutions have shown their ability to change as need dictates. Moreover, the forces operating in society and in the family are continually intervening, interacting, and changing (Berardo, 1988).

Society, with its beliefs, values, and customs, pervades every facet of family life, such as the age at which children may go to work and the age when they are legally given adult status. Society also sanctions illness definitions, sick-role behaviors, and the appropriateness of treatments and child-rearing practices. The adulation of youth by society, the participation of women in the labor force, and health care entitlement programs such as Medicare have altered the functions of the family relative to its role in assisting parents and grandparents.

On the other hand, the family influences society, which in turn may alter social norms. For instance, the egalitarian roles that women have assumed in family life have made drastic changes in the way society now views women and their roles and capacities. The ongoing controversies over family planning ser-

vices and abortion laws further exemplify the way in which the family exerts political pressure on society to change. With rising expectations for accessibility to comprehensive health services, families also continue to push for health reform legislation.

INTERACTION OF HEALTH/ILLNESS AND THE FAMILY

Family members' health/illness status and the family mutually influence each other. An illness within the family affects the whole family and its interactions, while the family in turn affects the course of an illness and members' health status. Hence, the impact of the health/illness status on the family and the family's impact on the health/illness status are reciprocal or highly interdependent (Gilliss, Rose, Hallburg, & Martinson, 1989; Wright & Leahey, 2000). Families tend to be both a reactor to family members' health problems and an actor in determining their health problems.

Turning to the interaction between the family and its members' health status, the family is the primary source for health and illness notions and health behavior. Research in the family health area has clearly demonstrated that families have a powerful impact on family members' physical health (Campbell, 2000). In one way or another, the family tends to be involved in the decision-making and therapeutic process at every stage of a family member's health and illness, from the state of being well (when promotion of health and preventive strategies are taught) to diagnosis, treatment, and recuperation (Doherty, 1992). The process of becoming a "patient" and receiving health services encompasses a series of decisions and events involving the interaction of a number of persons, including family, friends, and professional providers of care. Moreover, the role the family plays in this process varies over time depending on an individual's health, the type of health problem (e.g., whether it is acute, chronic, severe), and the degree of familial concern and involvement.

Six stages of health/illness and family interaction are presented (Table 1–1) to further illustrate the

TABLE 1—1

SIX STAGES OF HEALTH/ILLNESS AND FAMILY INTERACTIONS

Stage 1	Family Efforts at Health Promotion
Stage 2	Family Appraisal of Symptoms
Stage 3	Care Seeking
Stage 4	Referral and Obtaining Care
Stage 5	Acute Response to Illness by Client and Family
Stage 6	Adaptation to Illness and Recovery

Partially adapted from Doherty (1992); Suchman (1965); and Campbell (2000).

interdependency of the family and its members' health status. The following six stages represent an adaptation of Suchman's (1965) five stages of illness and medical care and Doherty and Campbell's (1988) five stages of the family health and illness cycle. These stages also present a temporal sequencing of a family's experience with illness/disability.

STAGE 1: FAMILY EFFORTS AT HEALTH PROMOTION

The family typically plays a vital role in all forms of health promotion and risk reduction (Campbell, 2000; Doherty, 1992). It is also true that the family may expose its members to health hazards. Many forms of health promotion, prevention, and risk reduction involve lifestyle issues such as the cessation of smoking and engaging in regular exercise. Whether a child gets a particular immunization, a father is encouraged to get more exercise and eat a more nutritious diet, or a mother receives proper prenatal care, all involve, to a great degree, family decisions and participation. Health promotion begins in the family. Wellness strategies, to be successful, usually require improvements in the lifestyle of an entire family. Moreover, within a family, members learn about their own health status and body image—such as whether they are frail and sickly or healthy and resilient.

Families unfortunately may also be the *genesis* of illness among family members. Family social disorganization often has negative health consequences for family members. A variety of specific health problems have been found more frequently in troubled families, among them tuberculosis, mental disorders (Bemak, Chung, & Bornemann, 1996), anorexia and bulimia (Campbell, 2000), hypertension (Harburg, Erfurt, Chape, & Havenstein, 1973), coronary heart disease (Knutsen & Knutsen, 1991; Syme, Hyman, & Enterline, 1964), and stroke fatalities. Many studies, as illustrated in a decade literature review (Ross, Mirowsky, & Goldstein, 1990), demonstrate the pervasive influence of family on health. These reviewers found that three family factors provided explanations for a causal relationship between family and illness: marital relationship, parenthood, and the family's social support system. A couple's type of marital relationship can affect family health status according to a well-documented study, the California Health Project (Fisher & Ransom, 1995). These researchers found that husbands and wives from "balanced" and "traditional" families reported higher health scores than marital partners from "disconnected" and "emotionally strained" families.

STAGE 2: FAMILY APPRAISAL OF SYMPTOMS

This stage begins when an individuals' symptoms are (1) recognized; (2) interpreted as to their seriousness, possible cause, and importance or meaning; and (3) met with varying degrees of concern by the symptomatic individual and his or her family. The stage consists of the family's beliefs about the symptoms or illness of a family member and how to deal with the illness (Doherty & Campbell, 1988; Campbell, 2000).

Because the family serves as the basic point of reference for assessing health behavior and provides basic definitions of health and illness, it influences the individual's perceptions. In North America and many other regions of the world, the mother is usually the major interpreter of the meaning of particular symptoms, the decision maker on what action should be taken, and the informal health caregiver (de Souza & Gualda, 2000; McGoldrick, 1989). The central family member (usually the mother) who influences health appraisal is called in some of the literature the "family health expert" (Doherty & Baird, 1987).

Families influence recognition and interpretation of symptoms of illness. Poor or recent immigrant families are often slower to respond to initial symptoms because of lack of access to health services or because they may not recognize some symptoms as signs of serious disease (Brown, Ponce, & Rice, 2001; Koos, 1954).

STAGE 3: CARE SEEKING

The care-seeking stage begins when the family decides that the ailing member is really sick and needs help. The ill person and family start to seek alleviation, information, advice, and professional validation from extended family, friends, neighbors, other nonprofessionals (the lay referral structure), and the Internet. The decisions as to whether a member's illness should be treated at home or in a medical clinic or hospital tends to be negotiated within the family (Doherty, 1992). For example, Richardson (1970), in a study of low-income, urban households, found that about one-half of those with illnesses reported consulting another family member concerning what they should do about the situation. Knapp and associates (1966) also found that the family was the most frequently mentioned source of information concerning home remedies and self-medication.

Not only does the family provide the basic definitions of health, but family members may press a family member into this stage if they believe he or she is failing to react favorably. This process may be extremely difficult for the family, particularly when a psychiatric disorder is the major problem (Pederson, Draguns, Lonner, & Trimble, 1996). This may be because in some cultures mental illness is seen as a stigmatized condition, bringing shame on the whole family. Moreover, the family has to label the person as mentally ill and make the problem public and/or acknowledge their own feelings of guilt and shame. The problem is compounded when the affected person denies the disorder or blames the family (Gavazzi & Schock, 2000).

STAGE 4: REFERRAL AND OBTAINING CARE

This stage commences when contact is made with a health agency or professional and/or with an indigenous or folk practitioner. Studies have clearly shown that the family is again instrumental in deciding where the treatment should be given and by whom (de Souza & Gualda, 2000; Pratt, 1976). The family serves as primary health referral agent and will refer a family member to whatever types of service or practitioner is deemed appropriate. Of course, decisions about what services to use are also determined by the availability and accessibility of health care to the family.

Most health care utilization data show that while the more affluent families use primary care physicians and medical specialists for their care, the most common resource for initial medical care for poor families is the emergency room (Center for Health Economics Research, 1993). Among working and middle-class families with health insurance, there has also been a growth in the use of prepaid group practice (health maintenance organization) and other managed care systems.

The type of health care sought varies tremendously. The folk or Eastern practitioner, the unorthodox "healer," the holistic health practitioner (using sometimes alternative modalities such as acupressure and acupuncture), the superspecialist (such as a neurosurgeon), the nurse practitioner, the primary care physician, and the family or individual therapist, should all be considered as possible sources of health care (thus broadening antiquated definitions of medical care providers).

How do families decide what clinic or health provider to contact? Although such variables as acceptability, appropriateness, perceived adequacy of service, and seriousness of condition are important, the accessibility to a primary care facility seems to also be a prime determinant of whom families contact (Campbell, 2000).

STAGE 5: ACUTE RESPONSE TO ILLNESS BY CLIENT AND FAMILY

As the client accepts care of health practitioners, he or she surrenders certain prerogatives and decisions, and is expected to assume the patient role, characterized by a dependence on the health professional's advice, the willingness to comply with health care advice, and a striving to recover. Parsons (1951) coined this social status "the sick role." How this role is further defined and enacted at home will be influenced by the family's sociocultural and idiosyncratic background. Some families exclude the sick member from all responsibilities and "serve and assist" to the fullest extent. Other families expect little change in the ill member's behavior, hoping that he or she can carry on as usual; this approach is seen frequently when it is the mother or the central caregiver who is sick.

Thus, the family unit plays a pivotal role in determining the sick member's patient role behaviors. The family is also instrumental in deciding where the treatment should be given—hospital, clinic, or home (Doherty, 1992). Efforts by health professionals to treat illness and promote good health may often conflict with family values and attitudes about treatment and what matters to them.

During the acute response stage, the family must make an adjustment to the family member's illness, diagnosis, and treatment. For serious or life-threatening illness, a family crisis may ensue, wherein the family undergoes a period of disorganization in response to the powerful health stressor event (Hill, 1940; Murray, 2000). "Most research on the spouses of acutely ill patients has shown that they experience levels of stress as high as or higher than that of the patients themselves" (Campbell, 2000, p. 165).

STAGE 6: ADAPTATION TO ILLNESS AND RECOVERY

The process of a family member's adaptation to illness as well as the family's adaptation and coping as a unit has been studied extensively by family scientists and family nurse researchers. The adaptation stage is a period when family nurses are called upon to assist families to cope with health stressors.

The presence of a serious, chronic illness in one family member usually has a profound impact on the family system, especially on its role structure and the carrying out of family functions. Families are the primary caregivers of patients with chronic illness (Campbell, 2000).

A crucial issue is whether the patient can resume his or her prior (pre-illness) role responsibilities or is able to establish a new, "workable" role in the family. When either the nature of the person's condition is serious (greatly disabling or progressively deteriorating) and the family member is a pivotal, crucial person to the family's functioning, the impact on family is much more pronounced (Murray, 2000; Sussman & Slater, 1963).

Families then play an important supportive role during the course of a client's convalescence and rehabilitation. In the absence of this support, the success of convalescence/rehabilitation decreases significantly.

DEFINITION OF FAMILY

The family has been defined in various ways. Definitions of the family differ depending on the theoretical orientation of the "definer"—that is, by the kind of explanation the professional seeks to make concerning the family. For instance, writers who follow the interactionist theoretical orientation of the family see the family as an arena of interacting personalities, thus emphasizing the family's dynamic transactional characteristics. Writers who espouse a general systems perspective define the family as a small open social system composed of a set of highly interdependent parts and affected by both its internal structure and external environment. Writers who espouse a postmodernist perspective of the family view that each succeeding generation of persons redefines the family anew; even the most basic family function of reproduction is seen as being disconnected from the family, with "choice" being the prime context within which the postmodern family exists (Dunphy, 2001). Therefore, there are multiple definitions, with theories shaping these definitions and our expectations of family life (Smith, 1995).

The U.S. Bureau of the Census uses a traditionally oriented definition of the family, which is as follows: The family is composed of persons joined together by bonds of marriage, blood, or adoption and residing in the same household. This traditional definition of the family is limiting today, both in terms of its applicability and inclusiveness. Any definition of the family must cover the wide array of family forms present today, which traditional definitions do not. Some family scholars have argued that we have defined the family according to a middle-class, white, nuclear family model and have tended to view families that do not conform to this model as "deviant" (Smith, 1995).

Whall (1986b), in her concept analysis of the family as the unit of care in nursing, defines family as "a self-identified group of two or more individuals whose association is characterized by special terms, who may or may not be related by blood lines or law, but who function in such a way that they consider themselves to be family" (p. 241). Taking into account who individuals identify as family members is a crucial component of this definition. Bozett (1987) incorporates the individual's definition by referring to family as "who the patient says it is" (p. 4). Family Service America (1984) also defines family in a comprehensive manner—as "two or more people joined together by bonds of sharing and intimacy" (p. 7). And Allen, Fine and Demo (2000) define a family as characterized by birth, marriage, adoption, or *choice*.

Incorporating the central notions from the above nontraditional definitions, **family** in this text refers to **two or more persons who are joined together by bonds of sharing and emotional closeness and who identify themselves as being part of the family.**

Because this definition is purposefully broad, it then encompasses the variety of relationships that are outside the legal perspective, including families not related by blood, marriage, or adoption and not restricted to household membership. This includes extended family living in two or more households, cohabiting couples, childless families, gay and lesbian families, and single-parent families, as well as the two-parent nuclear family.

It's clear that the only "sure" way of determining who the individual client's family is, is to ask him or her. This information can then be used in delivering health care (Hanson, 2001a).

The following additional family definitions are presented to facilitate an understanding of family literature.

- **Nuclear (conjugal) family**—The family of marriage, parenthood, or procreation; it is composed of a husband, wife, and their immediate children—natural, adopted, or both.

- **Family of orientation (family of origin)**—The family unit into which a person is born.

- **Extended family**—The nuclear family and other related (by blood) persons, who are most commonly members from the family of orientation of one of the nuclear family mates. These are "kin" and may include grandparents, aunts, uncles, nephews, nieces, and cousins.

FAMILY HEALTH

Given that family nursing is ultimately concerned with the health of the family, the concept of family health—or as Dunn (1961) called it, family wellness—needs to be clarified. In reviewing the literature in this area, it is clear that this concept is probably even less consistently and clearly defined than the concept of health (Anderson and Tomlinson, 1992). In both cases the concepts are defined so broadly and abstractly that to fully operationalize them becomes a most diffcult task.

Using systems theory as a starting point, we first need to assume that family health is more than just a sum of its parts (the health status of each of the family members). It is greater than and different from its parts. Yet, in the literature we see that the term *family health* or *familial health* is used ambiguously (Johnson, 1984), sometimes referring to the health of the individual family members and sometimes to the health of the family unit itself. Medical diseases are sometimes listed under "family health." Because only individuals can have medical diseases, it is obvious that the former usage of the term is flawed.

In family research, family health is most often conceptualized as family functioning or family adaptation (McCubbin & Patterson, 1983a), although variations within this broad definition exist. The World Health Organization (1974) proposed a similar definition to this latter definition. They state that familial health "connotes the relative functioning of the family as the primary social agent in the promotion of health and well-being" (p. 17).

The meaning of family health also differs depending on the discipline of the author or the theoretical perspective he or she adopts. For instance, in family mental health where an interactional perspective is taken, family health is referred to as the state of the family's internal processes or dynamics such as their interpersonal relationships. The focus is on relationships between the family and its subsystems, such as the parental or parent–child subsystem, or between the family and its members.

If a systems perspective is adopted, the outcome of internal interactions and exchange between the family and its environment are emphasized. One of the outcomes is a balance between growth or change and stability or equilibrium in the family (Wright & Leahey, 2000). Both tendencies are needed in the proper balance for a family to be functional or healthy.

In the family stress literature, family adaptation is defined as a measure of family health. It refers to "an ongoing family systems process identified by the use of multiple coping strategies used to address the stresses and demands the family is faced with" (Clawson, 1996).

Public health and community welfare authors use biostatistical indicators of family health. These address the relationships of family to the community and its stability as a unit. They include poverty and divorce rates among families, presence of criminal and juvenile problems, and high school dropout and unemployment rates as indicators of family health.

Family nursing authors tend to use a family interactional or systems perspective in defining family health. Hanson (2001b), a family nursing author, defines family health holistically as: "a dynamic changing relative state of well-being which includes the biological, psychological, spiritual, sociological, and cultural factors of the family system" (p. 6).

There is also growing interest in using nursing theories in family nursing to address family health. One example of the application of a nursing theory to working with families comes from Tadych (1985). Applying Orem's self-care theory, family health refers to the extent to which the family assists its members to meet their selfcare requisites, as well as the extent to which it fulfills its family functions and accomplishes the tasks appropriate to the family's developmental level (p. 52).

❧ CHARACTERISTICS OF HEALTHY FAMILIES

The characteristics of healthy families are described in various ways by several widely cited authors. Even the terms these authors use to describe healthy families varies. For example, Pratt (1976) called healthy families "energized families." Beavers (1977) and Beavers and Hampson (1993) describe healthy families as "competent" or "optimally functioning" families, while McCubbin and associates (1999) and Walsh (1998) call families who are functioning well, "resilient families."

The Beavers Systems Model is perhaps best known for including an observational rating scale of families in terms of their level of competence in six areas: (1) family structure—power, parental coalition, and closeness; (2) mythology; (3) goal-directed negotiations; (4) autonomy; (5) family affect; and (6) a global appraisal of health pathology, which ranges from optimal/adaptive to severely dysfunctional. The model incorporates clinical observations of families in treatment and research settings over a 30-year period and emphasizes family competence, i.e., "how well the family performs the necessary and nurturing tasks of organizing and managing itself" (Beavers & Hampson, 1993, p. 74).

The following is a summary of Beavers and Hampson's (1993) description of optimally functioning families. They are characterized as:

- Consistently demonstrating high degrees of capable negotiation skills in dealing with their problems.

- Being clear, open, and spontaneous in their expression of a wide range of feelings, beliefs, and differences.

- Being respectful of members' feelings.

- Encouraging autonomy of their members.

- Expecting members to take personal responsibility for their actions.

- Demonstrating affiliative attitudes (closeness and warmth) towards each other. The parents in these families are clearly the leaders and care for each other. Family leadership is egalitarian and flows from the marital/parental dyad. The parents form a strong parental coalition and provide models of respect and affection/closeness for the children. The family is optimistic and enjoys each other (Beavers & Hampson, 1993).

Some limitations to Beavers's portrayal of optimally healthy families have been noted. The most cogent of these criticisms is that the families about which observational ratings have been made are largely white, middle-class, two-parent families (Gershwin & Nilsen, 1989). Thus, we must consider that families from diverse socioeconomic and cultural backgrounds, as well as families with differing structures, may not "fit" well into Beavers's attributes of a competent family.

Pratt (1976) and McCubbin and McCubbin (1993) stress how important the family's interaction with the community is in facilitating high-level family health. According to McCubbin, McCubbin, Thompson, and Thompson (1998), family functioning is being redefined to include the degree to which families are able to adapt to the social context in which they live. That is, when families fit well into the cultural and general community in which they live, they are generally considered to be well-functioning. Pratt (1976) concurs when she says that energized families have varied and active contacts with a wide range of other groups and organizations, so as to enhance, support, and fulfill the interests and needs of family members.

Goldenberg and Goldenberg (2000), family therapists, emphasize that well-functioning families encourage individuals in the family to reach their own potential. Healthy families allow family members the freedom necessary for exploration and self-discovery while at the same time providing the protection and security they need to reach their own potential.

❧SOCIETAL CHANGES AFFECTING FAMILIES

Recent and ongoing societal changes have greatly influenced family life. Evidence of the profound changes and enormous diversity within American families comes from demographic data primarily compiled by the U.S. Bureau of the Census. Almost 20 years ago Naisbitt in *Megatrends* (1984) colorfully described the changes in the 1980s as a "decade of unprecedented diversity," and this trend has continued and perhaps even accelerated. Economic trends and changes are believed to have exerted the greatest impact on the family, but in addition to this factor, technological advances and demographic, sociocultural, and political trends are important factors that have influenced the family (Clark, 1984; Coates, 1996; Toffler, 1990).

ECONOMIC TRENDS

The most obvious economic trend today is the rising costs in all areas of family life. This is particularly true

in terms of the cost of health care (Brown, Ponce, & Rice, 2001; Nelson & Roark, 1985), particularly burdensome for poor families, older families (who are living on preinflationary dollars) and beginning families.

Another major economic trend is the growing disparity between rich and poor families in the United States today. Between 1990 and 2000, affluent families enjoyed rising incomes while the very poor remained at the same level of relative poverty (Arax, Curtius, & Nelson, 2000). The poverty rate for most groups actually decreased somewhat—to 11.8 percent in 1999. Hispanic and black poverty rates, however, are still three times higher than among non-Hispanic whites (Teachman, Tedrow, & Crowder, 2001; U.S. Bureau of the Census, 1999a). (See Figure 1–1.)

Who are these poor families? In addition to poverty being much higher among black and Hispanic families, it is also much higher among immigrant families, children, and working class families. Kozol (2000) in his report *Kids Count* states that since 1990 the number of children in working-poor families has increased by nearly one third. Whereas in the past, the concern has been focused on the nonworking poor—families on welfare—the concern today should also be on families that do work but whose wages are too meager to provide for a decent life (Brownstein, 1999). Single-parent, mother-headed families are also much more likely to be poor than two-parent families. In 1999, 37.4 percent of mother-headed families with children under age 18 were living below the poverty level (U.S. Bureau of the Census, 1999b). Homeless populations, of which families with children are a growing number, are also living in poverty (Schraneveldt & Young, 1992).

TECHNOLOGICAL ADVANCES

Under the rubric of technological advances is included the knowledge explosion (Toffler, 1970); the increased ability to prolong life (Clark, 1984); environmental pollution (air, water, food, and noise) and environmental protests; the use of nuclear energy, electronics, and automation (Clark, 1984); birth control advances; and the revolution in biotechnology (Isaacson, 2000). Automation has made a great differ-

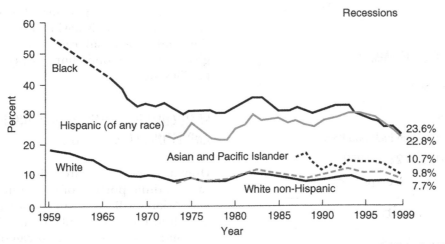

Figure 1–1. U.S. poverty rates by race and Hispanic origin: 1959 to 1999. *(Source: U.S. Census Bureau. Current Population Survey, March 1960 to 2000.)*
Note: Statistically significant decrease for all groups from 1998 to 1999.

ence in the home. The majority of women are now working and have had to reallocate their time; automation has allowed working women to spend less time working in the home. Birth control represents major technological advance. Having better control over reproduction has literally transformed the family, in particular the life cycles of families. Women are no longer having as many children and, equally important, are having their children in a shorter period of time, making the child-rearing period of the family's life shorter. Couples now have more time alone—before the advent of children and after they have been launched (Duvall, 1977; Teachman, Tedrow, & Crowder, 2001).

DEMOGRAPHIC TRENDS

Major demographic and prevailing characteristics of the population influence the type of family services required and to whom these services should be targeted. (See Table 1–2.)

ACCELERATED POPULATION GROWTH.   The population of the United States has steadily grown—by 89 million persons in 35 years (1965–2000). Current population rate of growth has accelerated from 1990 to 2000. Growth, however, has been unequal. The Western states increased by 19 percent. (U.S. Bureau of the Census, 2000c) versus the nation as a whole which grew by 13 percent. It is predicted that U.S. population growth will decline, but that is not expected until well into the twenty-first century. The size of the postwar (1945–1964) baby boomer generation and large inflows of immigrants are primary causes for the present rate of growth. The 2000 Census documented the substantial growth in the largest cities and the steady growth in the suburbs.

AGING OF THE POPULATION.   Probably the most important trend in demography is the increased general life expectancy and the fact that the majority of the population now survives into old age (U.S. Bureau of the Census, 2000c). Because of this, the United States is in the midst of a demographic revolution, the inexorable aging of our population (Figure 1–2). The aging of America is particularly pronounced after 2000, when baby boomers begin to reach age 55. There is a concomitant decrease in the number of younger children in the home. Senior citizen growth is particularly rapid in the group over 75 years of age (Figure 1–3).

TABLE 1–2

SOCIETAL CHANGES AFFECTING FAMILIES

ECONOMIC TRENDS

- Rising Cost of Living
- Growing Disparity between Rich and Poor
- Poverty Rate in the U.S.: 12% in 1999

TECHNOLOGICAL ADVANCES

DEMOGRAPHIC TRENDS

- Accelerated Population Growth
- Aging of the Population

SOCIOCULTURAL TRENDS

- Changing Racial and Ethnic Composition

CHANGES IN THE FAMILY

- Decline in Household Size
- Delayed Marriages and Decline in Marriage Rate
- Higher Divorce Rate and Lower Remarriage Rate
- Increase in Childhood Living Arrangements and Single-Parent Families
- Changing Gender Norms
- Growth in Women's Employment
- Increase in Family Heterogeneity

The aging population will have an enormous impact on the family and on health care. For instance, because women live 7 to 8 years longer than men, on average, most older persons, especially over 75, are women who live alone and are poor. In terms of health care, with over 13 percent of the U.S. population in 1995 being over 65 years of age (and the proportion expected to rise steadily to 24 percent in 2050), the nation's health care will be critically strained. The rapid growth of the very old, who are the biggest users of health care services as well as caregiver assistance, will have a profound effect on family life (Pifer & Bronte, 1986; U.S. Bureau of the Census, 2000c).

The number of persons who are disabled and chronically ill also is having a significant impact on the family. The health care function, because of caregiving and economic burdens, is strained in many families today.

SOCIOCULTURAL TRENDS: CHANGING RACIAL AND ETHNIC COMPOSITION

Dramatic changes are also occurring in the racial/ethnic portrait of the United States. Latinos and Asians will constitute more than half of the growth in the U.S. population for the next half century and beyond, the U.S. Bureau of the Census predicts (U.S. Bureau of the Census, 2000). The population of non-Latino whites, now at 69 percent, will shrink to 53 percent by the year 2050. Latinos will increase from 11 percent to 25 percent, African Americans from 12 to 14 percent, Asians/Pacific Islanders from 4 to 8 percent, and Native Americans from 0.8 to 0.9 percent according to census projections. Latino growth is due to both immigration and higher fertility rates (two thirds higher than non-Latino whites). A modest growth in African Americans is due to a somewhat higher fertility rate, while the growth in Asians is due to immigration (Pew Health Professions Commission, 1991; U.S. Bureau of the Census, 2000c).

In 2000 it was estimated that the foreign-born population was 30 million in the United States. This is about 10 percent of the U.S. population. Immigrants are, however, concentrated in big cities and cosmopolitan regions such as Los Angeles and New York City (U.S. Bureau of the Census, 2000c).

Although the United States population remains predominantly white, with minorities concentrated around major cities, pockets of racial and ethnic diversity are increasingly appearing across the country. Regions such as the Upper Midwest are ethnically changing due to technological and economic changes in various areas (U.S. Bureau of the Census, 2000).

CHANGES IN THE FAMILY

DECLINE IN HOUSEHOLD SIZE.   The decrease in family and household size is a major long-term demographic

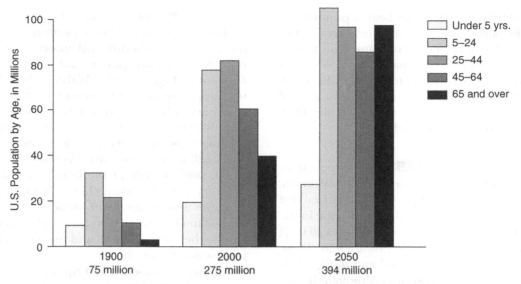

Figure 1-2. The U.S. population is getting older. *(Source: Wingert, Springen, Angell, & Meyer, 1988.)*

trend. Concomitantly, women also have experienced a shortened childbearing period, this period referring to the years they have raising children, from the youngest to the oldest child. These recent decreases in family size reflect the cumulative impact of a recent decline in fertility and the increases in age of first marriage and rates of out-of-wedlock births (Santi, 1987; Teachman, Tedrow, & Crowder, 2001).

DELAYED MARRIAGE AND DECLINE IN MARRIAGE RATE.   Americans have retreated from early marriage according to Teachman (Teachman, Tedrow, & Crowder, 2001), a leading demographer. The percentage of ever-married women aged 20 to 24 declined by approximately 32 percent between 1975 and 1998 for both Whites and

Figure 1-3. Increase in the very old population (percent of population 75 years and older). *(Source: U.S. Bureau of the Census, 1978, 1992, 2000.)*

African Americans. Changes among Latino women have been more modest.

Since the mid-1950s, marriages have been increasingly delayed (about 3 to 4 years on the average), as more young adults are attending school longer, more women are working, and more young couples are living together before marriage (Glick, 1994; Marshall, 1991). There has been a steady decline in first marriages since the end of World War II, but by the middle of the 1990s the rate had declined even further (Teachman, Tedrow, & Crowder, 2001).

HIGHER DIVORCE RATES.   The rate of divorce in the United States has slowly but steadily increased from 1940 to 1998. The increase in the divorce rate was especially great in the 1970s, but has leveled off since the mid-1980s (Glick, 1994; Teachman, Tedrow, & Crowder, 2001). At the current rate of divorce, about 50 percent of recent marriages will end in divorce.

Inasmuch as men remarry more than women, many divorced women live in a state of poverty or near poverty because of their disadvantaged economic position. The prominence of no-fault divorce has enhanced the disadvantageous economic position of the divorced woman by effectively removing legal support for the husband's long-term commitment to support the mother of his children (White, 1988).

LOWER REMARRIAGE RATES.   There has been a pronounced decline in the percentage of women remarrying after their divorce. The same is not true for men; that is, they remarry at a higher rate than women. About 70 percent of white women remarry by age 40 to 44, while 50 to 54 percent of African American and Hispanic women, respectively, remarry by age 40 to 44 (Teachman, Tedrow, & Crowder, 2001).

INCREASE IN FIRST BIRTHS TO OLDER MOTHERS.   In a report from the National Center for Health Statistics (Ventura, 1989), national data from 1988 were summarized that indicated there has been a significant increase in the numbers of first births to older mothers, ages 30 to 34 and particularly ages 35 to 39 (Ventura, 1989). These women tend to be better educated and during their pregnancy to receive prenatal care. Although the typical ages of childbearing continue to be 15 to 29 years, women in their early 30s accounted for 12 percent of all first births in 1986 compared with just 3 percent in 1970.

The dramatic rise in first births among older women is the result of several other demographic trends. First, marriage has been postponed by a sizable proportion of young people; second, there has been a sharp decline and then a leveling off of first births for women in their 20s, leaving larger numbers of women still childless at age 30 and older. In addition, there was a substantial growth in the number of women age 25 to 39 from 1970 to 1986. These are the children born during the baby boom years following World War II. Finally, national surveys show that most women intend to have at least one child, with only about 10 percent of women in their early 30s expecting to remain childless (Ventura, 1989).

INCREASE IN CHILDHOOD LIVING ARRANGEMENTS AND SINGLE-PARENT FAMILIES.   An increasing percentage of children (about 25 percent) are experiencing changes in their living arrangements—a situation that in the literature suggests detrimental effects to the well-being of children. These changes include a wide range of different living arrangements such as living with both parents, a parent and stepparent, a single parent, and so on (Teachman, Tedrow, & Crowder, 2001). Single-parent families have also significantly increased in number. Discussion of these trends is found in the next section.

CHANGING GENDER NORMS.   Since the 1980s, numerous studies and extensive feminist writing have addressed the issue of femininity and masculinity and their impact on family power and role relationships (Ellman & Taggart, 1993; Walsh, 1998). Because of traditional notions of "women's work," women's roles, and what was considered feminine, women have had diminished power in the family. Gender relationships are based on power, and power differences still greatly favor men. As women become educated, work outside of the home, and share in the provider role, however, their power in the family increases and norms about women's and men's roles in the family change. Women are also much freer to choose their own lifestyles and the type of family they wish or need to live in.

Among middle-class and upper-middle-class educated families and immigrant families in which wives work, changing gender norms have made major differences in the family. No longer does the man automatically make all the major decisions. We are in an era of transition with respect to gender (Goldenberg & Goldenberg, 2000). Nevertheless, many women and men do not feel comfortable with the past, gender habits die hard (Coltrane, 1997; Ellman & Taggart, 1993). Further discussion of changing gender roles is found in Chapters 10 through 17.

GROWTH IN WOMEN'S EMPLOYMENT.   In the aftermath of World War II, the labor force participation of women, particularly married women, rose steadily. Sixty-five percent of women with children under the age of 18 are in the workforce and now constitute almost half of the U.S. workforce. They continue to enter the labor market in increasing numbers (Coates, 1996; Teachman, Tedrow, & Crowder, 2001). Women working has had mixed effects on the family (Schraneveldt & Young, 1992). On the one hand, it provides the family with a higher standard of living (many families cannot survive unless both parents work). On the other hand, there is less shared time with family members. There is a greater need for marital sharing of family responsibilities, which often happens only partially (see Chapter 12).

INCREASE IN FAMILY HETEROGENEITY.   Never in recorded history has a society been composed of a greater multiplicity of attitudes, values, behaviors, and lifestyles.

These social, behavioral, and cultural differences are reflected in a variety of family forms (Teachman, Tedrow, & Crowder, 2001). There no longer is a "typical" family. Hence, families using health services come from all walks of life and represent all types of lifestyles. Most of our clients are not part of the idealized traditional nuclear family. It is imperative for health care professionals to understand and appreciate the wide varieties of family forms, as well as some of the reasons for their existence.

The *postmodern family,* the term sociological literature uses to refer to today's families, reflects the "ascendence of diversity over uniformity—persons throughout their life course creating living arrangements in response to ever-shifting situations, some of their own choosing, others imposed on them" (Scanzoni & Marsiglio, 1993, p. 125). Each family form has its own particular strengths and vulnerabilities. Nonetheless, it is probably true that certain family arrangements are probably more suitable for fulfilling certain basic functions than other forms. In studies that compare different family forms with each other, it has been very difficult to sort out the effect of the family form from the many other variables that also influence the outcomes being studied, such as socioeconomic factors, family developmental stage, and child care arrangements (Macklin, 1988).

Controversy exists between the effects on children of one family form versus another. Gottfried and Gottfried (1994) conclude from their review of numerous studies that the different family forms in themselves are not detrimental to children's development. However, Bronstein and colleagues (1993), Bianchi (1995), Popenoe (1995) and Teachman, Tedrow, and Crowder, (2001), in summarizing numerous studies, assert that children from two-biological-parent families show better psychological, social, and educational adjustment than children from other family forms.

❧VARIED FAMILY FORMS

There is no "typical" American family today. The various family forms are often classified as *traditional* and *nontraditional* **family forms.** A diverse reshaping of contemporary life encompasses a hodgepodge of multiples, evolving family cultures and structures: working mothers and two-earner households; divorced, single-parent, and remarried families; and domestic partners, both gay and straight (Walsh, 1998, p. 28). Table 1–3 presents a series of nine questions the reader can use to evaluate his or her definitions of and beliefs about families and who they encompass. As can be seen in Table 1–4, a multitude of different family forms exist. Because of their significance for family nursing, the major types of family forms will be described.

THE NUCLEAR FAMILY

The "vanishing" yet idealized nuclear family constitutes one of the most significant demographic and social transformations in recent history. With the acceleration of the divorce rate, remarriages, births to single women, and cohabitation from 1965 to the present, family forms other than the nuclear family have rapidly proliferated. According to the 2000 U.S. Census, the nuclear family, consisting of a husband provider, a wife homemaker, and children that was the norm in the 1950s and 1960s accounts for only 8 percent of all households (Fields, 2001a). Only 52 percent of American children live in a traditional nuclear family today. The percentage of children living in nuclear families varies significantly by race and ethnicity. Seventy-four percent of white children lived in "traditional nuclear families," while 36 percent of African American and 64 percent of Latino children did in 2000 (U.S. Bureau of the Census, 2000).

Although it is recognized that the traditional nuclear family is no longer modal, family scientists have asked "to what extent is the traditional family the norm?" This type of family still appears to be the "ideal" norm, but not the "real" norm. Surveys suggest the majority of Americans still wish for traditional family life but have a greater tolerance for nontraditional living arrangements than in the past. Although at any one point in time the majority of adults are not living in traditional nuclear households, over the course of their lives, most will do so. Yet increasing numbers, as previously described, are living in nontraditional family forms.

Two growing variations within nuclear families are dual-earner/dual-career and the childless family. Adoptive and foster families are other types of nuclear family noted in the literature as having special circumstances and needs.

TABLE 1—3

WHAT ARE YOUR ATTITUDES ABOUT FAMILIES?

1. Do you consider a two-parent nuclear family the *ideal and best* type of family?

   ☐ Yes ☐ Usually ☐ It depends . . . ☐ No

2. Do you consider your own family traditional?

   ☐ Yes ☐ No, because ☐ Don't know
   _____

3. Do you believe fathers can raise children on their own?

   ☐ Yes ☐ No, because ☐ Usually not ☐ No
   _____

4. Who determines whether a unit is a "family"?

   ☐ Society's legal definition ☐ Religious doctrine ☐ The family members ☐ Other

5. Do you think that the definition of the family is changing today?

   ☐ Yes ☐ To some extent ☐ No ☐ Don't know

6. Could a person living alone be a family?

   ☐ Yes ☐ Maybe ☐ No ☐ Don't know

7. Do you think a childless couple is a family?

   ☐ Yes ☐ No ☐ Don't know

8. Should gay and lesbian couples be allowed to marry?

   ☐ Yes ☐ No ☐ Perhaps ☐ Don't know

9. Do you believe that the American family is in serious trouble today?

   ☐ Yes ☐ Probably ☐ No ☐ Difficult to say

THE DUAL-EARNER FAMILY. With the striking increase in employment among married women, 68 percent of two-parent families are now dual-earners (Barnett & Rivers, 1996). In fact, the most numerous family form today is the dual-earner family with or without children. In 1995 a national survey conducted by Louis Harris showed that 55 percent of working women contribute half or more of their family income (Walters, 1995). In most dual-earner families, where both spouses are employed either part or full time, the majority of women have jobs that are undertaken because of economic necessity. Yet, despite wives' need to work, Harris's survey found that many women (48 percent) want to work part or full time regardless of whether they need to or not (Walters, 1995).

In dual-earner families, the major challenges focus on: (1) managing housework and child care; (2) having two paid jobs; and (3) family relationships (Piotrkowski & Hughes, 1993). "Family work" represents the household chores and child care tasks, the first-noted challenge above. Despite women's changing roles outside the family, within the family traditional sex-role attitudes often shape family life. Women, according to numerous studies, still do the "lion's share" of family work (Ehrenberg, Gearing-Small, Hunter, & Small, 2001). In turn, this workload imbalance frequently leads to role overload and sometimes marital conflict (Goldenberg and Goldenberg, 2002; Piotrkowski & Hughes, 1993). When children are young, the greatest challenge to dual-earner families is in arranging and coordinating the care of children while parents are at work. Child care arrangements are difficult to find and are often transient.

The challenge of managing two jobs is influenced by the types of jobs the couple have and the stress these jobs produce. Excessive job demands coupled with a lack of control over job demands generally produces high stress levels. Occupational stress is not just a personal problem but also a family problem. For example, job stress may have an adverse effect on parent–child relationships.

The third challenge, managing family relationships, is influenced by the previous two challenges. If "family work" and/or managing two jobs is stressful, then family relationships are negatively impacted.

A crucial concern in the dual-earner family literature revolves around possible effects on the couple's children of having two parents who work. There is no

TABLE 1—4

DIFFERENT FAMILY FORMS IN THE UNITED STATES

TRADITIONAL FAMILY FORMS	NONTRADITIONAL FAMILY FORMS

The most common traditional family forms now existing are:

1. Nuclear family—one parent working, living in same household.
   a. First marriage families
   b. Stepparent families
   c. Adoptive families

2. Nuclear family—dual-earner/dual-career, husband, wife, and children living in same household.
   a. First marriage families
   b. Blended or stepparent families
   c. Adoptive families

3. Nuclear dyad—husband and wife alone; childless, or no children living at home.
   a. Single career
   b. Dual career

4. Single-parent family—one head (female- or male-headed) as a consequence of divorce, abandonment, or separation.
   a. Working/career
   b. Unemployed

5. Single adult living alone.

6. Three-generation extended family—may characterize any of above family forms (1 through 4 above) living in a common household.

7. Middle-aged or elderly couple—husband as provider, wife at home (children have been launched into college, career, and/or marriage).

8. Extended kin network. Two or more nuclear households of primary kin or unmarried members living in close geographical proximity and operating within a reciprocal system of exchange of goods and services.

The most common nontraditional family forms are:

1. Unmarried parent and child family—usually mother and child.

2. Unmarried couple and child family—usually a common-law type of marriage.

3. Cohabiting couple—unmarried couple living together.

4. Gay/lesbian family—persons of the same sex living together as "marital partners."

5. Augmented family—household composed of nuclear or single-parent family with one or more unrelated persons.

6. Commune family—household of more than one monogamous couple with children, sharing common facilities, resources, and experiences; socialization of the child is a group activity.

7. Foster family—household of single or two parents with foster children and perhaps the parent(s) own children.

Adapted partially from Sussman (1974) and Macklin (1988).

evidence to date, however, to suggest that the dual-earner lifestyle, in and of itself, is stressful for children.

In a growing minority of dual-earner families, both husband and wife pursue careers while maintaining a family. Career-oriented people tend to view their positions as a primary source of personal satisfaction and identity. Both Skinner (1984) and Goldenberg and Goldenberg (2002) note that a significant feature of the dual-career lifestyle is that it is associated with considerable stress and strain, with more stress and strain reported by the wife than her husband. The basis of this stress is primarily the competing demands of the occupational structure and those associated with the family—child care, homemaking, and marital responsibilities. Two-career couples tend to do more sharing of traditionally female tasks than do one-career or dual-worker families, particularly in the area of child care (Barnett & Baruch, 1987; Goldenberg & Goldenberg, 2002; Macklin, 1988). But it appears that in many families, the wife still assumes the major responsibility for domestic tasks (Piotrkoski & Hughes, 1993).

There is also growing research interest in family dynamics about the dual-career families—particularly commuter families, in which spouses voluntarily live in separate residences for at least a majority of each week because of geographically separated jobs. Although usually a temporary pattern, research findings point to the difficulties that this lifestyle imposes (Goldenberg & Goldenberg, 2002; Macklin, 1988).

THE CHILDLESS FAMILY.   One type of traditional variant nuclear family is the family without children. About 5 percent or more of all ever-married women in the United States are voluntarily childless. The rate is expected to go up to 10 percent in the near future not only because of delayed marriage and childbearing patterns but because of the many career and educational options now available to women (Houseknecht, 1987; Kantrowitz & Wingert, 2001; Macklin, 1988).

THE ADOPTIVE FAMILY

Adoption is another way to form a family. By legally transferring ongoing parental responsibilities from birth to adoptive parents, there is typically a "win–win" situation for both parents and children. Adoptive parents are able to share their nurturance and love with their adopted child, while adopted children are given a family who very much wants them. With a more "futuristic" lens in mind, another type of adoption is or will be via technology. New adoptive families will be created when adopted children are matched for similar genetic inheritance, children are born of surrogate parents, and eventually children are born from cloned embryos. This broadened, futuristic definition of adoptive families is only beginning to be discussed in the literature (Coates, 1996).

Adults choose adoption for many reasons. Often, parents are couples who are unable to conceive biological children together, but still want to be parents. More common today than in the past are preferential adoptions. These take place when a couple or single adult decides to adopt a child for a variety of religious, moral, family, or personal reasons. Declining social and legal barriers and the increased need to place children with special needs into permanent homes have led to a rise in the number of unmarried men and women adopting children (Bowden, Dickey, & Greenberg, 1998; Finley, 2000). Forty-eight percent of adoptive parents are relatives of the child, implying that the types of children who are being adopted today have substantially changed. The availability of healthy infants for adoption has decreased due to contraception, abortion, more single women keeping their infants, and increased rates of infertility. At the same time the number of children with special needs has increased due to maternal drug abuse, neglect, abandonment or death (Finley, 2000). Special needs children are those children who are older at the time of adoption and/or who have complex medical, emotional, developmental, and behavioral needs (Kramer & Houston, 1998). Transracial and international adoptions are also more common today, as is the commercialization of adoption (i.e., making adoption placement a for-profit business).

Family nurses in pediatric and community-based settings often care for more adoptive families with special needs children. In adoptive families where the child was adopted as a healthy infant, the difference between biological families and adoptive families in terms of the prevalence of child or parental negative outcomes is generally negligible, although there is some disagreement in studies as to this conclusion (Borders, Black, & Pasley, 1998). In adoptive families where the child has special needs, many and diverse challenges are associated with parenting these children. Families who adopt children with a history of abuse or neglect often face serious problems that can threaten the stability of the adoptive family. For these adoptive families, there is an enhanced need for supportive services (Kramer & Houston, 1998). In one study, successful parenting of an adoptive child with special needs was described as being based on a partnership between the family, the adoption/child welfare agency, auxiliary health and welfare professionals, and members of the families' informal support network, as well as support from other families who also had children with special needs (Kramer & Houston, 1998).

THE FOSTER FAMILY

Foster care is a child welfare service in which children are placed in homes apart from their birth parent(s) so as to ensure their safety and emotional and physical well-being. Children are placed in foster homes when parents are unable to care for their chldren or are deemed unfit. In many cases, the placement is temporary and the children are returned to the biological parents eventually. Increasingly, however, children are being placed in foster homes on a more long-term basis or as an interlude to adoption because the biological parents have serious, long-term mental health or substance abuse problems. For many older and special needs children, adoption is probably not a realistic or appropriate option, and these children may remain in foster or other substitute care arrangements until they are 18 and able to live on their own.

Foster care placement has grown considerably in the last two decades, and the new millennium finds a record number of children in foster care (Lindsey, 2001). This trend is projected to continue and perhaps even accelerate.

There is widespread concern in the clinical and research literature about the quality of care children receive in foster homes. Several studies have found that about one sixth of all foster homes were unsafe and not developmentally adequate (Barth, 2001). The quality of care in foster homes varies considerably, from very poor to very good, in spite of the monitoring by child welfare workers. Children provided kinship foster care appear to be at higher risk for being placed in poor physical and socioemotional home environments than children provided nonkinship foster care (Lindsey, 2001). Kinship care placements have grown rapidly—they constituted 46 percent of all foster home placements in one large county in California in 1997—and are the predominant placement setting for children needing foster care (Barrick, 1997). Many of these kinship foster families are grandparent or grandmother families—here the grandparents have taken over the raising of their children's children. Grandparents may apply to be foster parents to their grandchildren and, if the situation warrants foster care, to receive reimbursement for doing so.

A serious problem with regard to foster families is the difficulty in finding good foster homes. Inadequate reimbursement of foster parents for child care and health services and a lack of Social Security insurance for foster parents are cited as problems creating a critical shortage of foster home placements (Barth, 2001).

In addition to concerns about the quality of care given by foster parents, there are also concerns about the health status of foster children. Research literature confirms that many foster children experience psychological difficulties such as depression, posttraumatic stress disorder, and separation and attachment problems (Kramer & Houston, 1998). Children who live in many different foster homes are found to have difficulty in attaching to each new set of foster parents (Rushton, 1989). It is also agreed upon that adoption is better for the well-being of children than having them remain in foster care.

Assessment of foster children who are at higher risk for health problems and provision of supportive services are needed. Parents need assistance in parenting and with their children's problems, particularly in accessing needed counseling and other services.

THE EXTENDED FAMILY

The traditional extended family is one in which the couple shares household arrangements and expenses with parents, siblings, or other close relatives. The children are then reared by several generations and have a choice of models after which to pattern their behavior. This type of family is more frequent in working-class and recent immigrant families. Extended families, more broadly defined by the U.S. Bureau of the Census are households in which a child lives with at least one parent and someone outside the nuclear family, either relatives or nonrelatives (U.S. Bureau of the Census, 1996). As people live longer, and divorces, teenage pregnancies, and out-of-wedlock births increase, houses also have become home to several generations, usually on a temporary basis. Affordability and availability of housing and employment force some families to double-up to conserve on housing and child care costs (U.S. Bureau of the Census, 1996). Demographers also have found that because of increased longevity, four- and five-generation families are becoming commonplace among poor and working-class families (Otten, 1989). In 1996, 14 percent of all children lived in extended families, according to the Bureau of the Census.

There is also another form of extended family—the extended kin network family. Here two or more nuclear households of primary kin or unmarried kin live in close proximity and operate within a reciprocal system of social support, including the exchange of goods and services. This type of family form is modal in the Latino community (see Chapter 18 for greater detail).

Although the great majority of Americans do not live in the two types of extended families mentioned, greater extended family ties are possible and widespread today due to advances in transportation and communication. The nuclear American family is not as isolated as it once was. The many ways in which families rely on one another create an extended family context that has been verified in several important studies.

The myth that the nuclear family is isolated from family supports is not borne out by this research, the evidence showing that a modified extended family usually exists within a rich network of generational interaction (Hill, 1970; Kingson, Hirshorn, & Cornman, 1986). Primary kin—parents and siblings of spouses—form the most important network of extended kinship relations.

THE SINGLE-PARENT FAMILY

The single-parent family is one in which there is one head of household, mother (83 percent of families) or father (17 percent of families) (U.S. Bureau of the Census, 1998). The traditional single-parent family is one in which the head is widowed, divorced, abandoned, or separated. The nontraditional single-parent family is one in which the head has never been married (see Table 1–4).

DEMOGRAPHIC TRENDS. One of the most dramatic demographic changes taking place in the United States is the radical shift in the modal household from one headed by a marital pair rearing their dependent-age

children to a household headed by a single adult (Bianchi, 1995; U.S. Bureau of the Census, 1996). Since 1940, the number of single-parent families has increased in the United States, from 8 percent in 1950 to 26 percent in 1996 (Figures 1–4 and 1–5). Breaking these statistics down by race and ethnicity, significant differences are apparent (Figures 1–4 and 1–5). According to U.S. census data (U.S. Bureau of the Census, 1996) in 1996, about 54 percent of all African American families were single-parent families, while 20 percent of all white non-Hispanic families were single-parent families. The growth of father–child families has increased since 1980, accounting for more than one third of the overall growth in the number of one-parent families (Bianchi, 1995). Eighty percent of this growth is among white father–child families.

The proportion of children nationally who are under the age of 18 and are cared for by a single parent, however, has skyrocketed, from 9 percent of all children in 1960 to 24 percent of all children in 1991. Among black children, the proportion is much greater, from 22 percent in 1960 to 51 percent in 1991 (Figure 1–6). Sixty percent of all children will spend about a year or longer in a single-parent home before they reach the age of 18.

Factors associated with the rapid increase in the numbers of one-parent families are (1) the high rate of divorce, (2) the large amount of financial aid to one-parent families with dependent children, (3) the loss of stigma associated with unwed motherhood, and (4) the tremendous growth in the number and proportion of births that occurred to never-married mothers.

Among never-married mothers, a significant number of unmarried older women have opted to have children. The major increase, however, is within the teenage mother group. From 1970 to 1995, there was a 25 percent increase in births among unmarried

Figure 1–4. Children living in two-parent households. *(Source: U.S. Bureau of the Census, 2000.)*

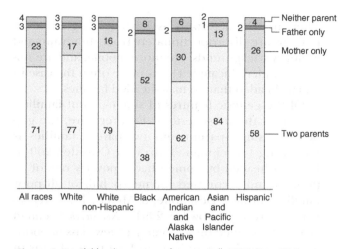

Figure 1–5. Children by presence of parents: Fall, 1996 (*Source: U.S. Census Bureau, 1996.*)

¹ People of Hispanic origin may be of any race.

women ages 15 to 17. Ninety percent of these teenage mothers had not completed high school and were on welfare (U.S. Bureau of the Census, 1996).

Of all single-parent families, the largest group is headed by divorced and separated mothers. These families have a different set of problems and challenges than never-married families. They are generally better off economically, which gives them a considerable edge over never-married families with largely young mothers. Seventy percent of divorced mothers work, as compared to only 38 percent of never-married mothers, and many more proportionally receive child support payments in comparison to never-married families (Bianchi, 1995).

Father-headed families have more than doubled since 1970, from 393,000 in 1970 to 2 million in 2000 (U.S. Bureau of the Census, 2000c). Although courts still favor mothers as custodial parents, men are making more vigorous claims to custody rights. Single fathers experience the same role change and role overload problems as single mothers. They are on average, however, much better off financially.

Goldenberg and Goldenberg (2002) and Mendes (1988), in reviewing the research on single-parent families, emphasize the fact that single-parent families are not homogeneous. They are, in fact, very diverse in terms of their resources, opportunities, and limitations. Mendes (1988) identifies five common lifestyles of the single parent:

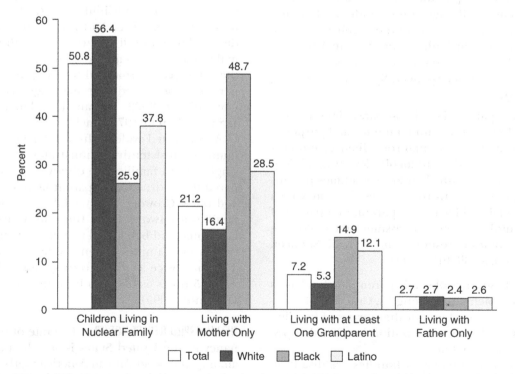

Figure 1–6. Percentage of children in various household structures broken down by race/ethnicity. One out of two children live in a nuclear family, which is defined as composed solely of both biological parents and full brothers and sisters. (*Source: Census Bureau's Survey of Income and Program Participation, 1991b.*)

1. Sole executive lifestyle. Here the single parent is the only parent actually involved in the lives and care of the children. In some cases, he or she attempts to fulfill both father and mother roles and is very much prone to stress, fatigue, and role overload. In other families, the sole executive handles what he or she can do without undue stress, and then coordinates the allocation of some of the other functions by assigning them to competent persons within or outside the family.

2. Auxiliary parent. In this lifestyle the custodial parent shares one or more of the parental responsibilities with an auxiliary parent, usually the father of one or more of the children.

3. Unrelated substitute. In this lifestyle the custodial parent shares one or more parental functions with a person who is not related to the family, such as a live-in housekeeper who is "like a mother" to the children.

4. Related substitute. Here the related substitute is a blood or legal relative who assumes a parental role. These persons are often grandmothers, but could also be aunts, uncles, cousins, or siblings of the children. There has been a large increase in the number of grandmothers, particularly in African-American families, who care for their teenage children's children (Kalil, Spencer, Spleker, & Gilchrist, 1998).

5. Titular parent. The titular parent lives with the children, but has, for all intents and purposes, abdicated the parental role. Teenage mothers or mothers who are alcoholics, drug addicts, or mentally disturbed are sometimes parents in name only. In these cases there may be a parental child acting as parent, or a parent of the titular parent who assumes the child care and domestic responsibilities (Kalil, Spencer, Spleker, & Gilchrist, 1998).

Each of these types of single-parent families has its own set of problems and strengths. Crucial to the successful functioning of any of these types of families, however, is the family's integration into a viable psychosocial support system.

As a group, single-parent families are disadvantaged when compared to other forms of families. They are characterized as having a high rate of poverty, are disproportionately from disadvantaged minority backgrounds, are more mobile, and are relatively undereducated. This is more often the case in female-headed than in male-headed families.

Of the generic features of single-parent families, poverty is the most serious. Furthermore, the gap between single-parent and two-parent families is increasing (Teachman, Tedrow, & Crowder, 2001). Families headed by women had a poverty rate of 36 percent and accounted for nearly half of all poor families (Bowen, Desimone, & McKay, 1995; Teachman, Tedrow, & Crowder, 2001). *Newsweek* (Gelman et al., 1985) called these women a "new class of poor." Single parenthood appears to be a major factor in "the feminization of poverty." Several variables are cited as causative factors: the minimal to nonexistent child support from fathers; the inequities of the workplace for women; cutbacks in social welfare programs; and the lack of education and work skills of young, never-married mothers.

Role changes, role overload, and role conflicts are other generic features of single parents. Role problems revolve around playing both mother and father roles; and the role overload of working, raising a family, domestic responsibilities, and of attempting to have a personal life. And lastly, since many single divorced parents will remarry, there is the necessity of making another major role change—relinquishing the other parent role and forming new marital and parental roles based on remarriage (Goldenberg & Goldenberg, 2002; Hogan, Buchler, & Robinson, 1984; LeMasters, 1974; Macklin, 1988).

Accumulated evidence from studies of single-parent families consistently demonstrates that children in single-parent families are disadvantaged when compared to children in two-parent families (Teachman, Tedrow, & Crowder, 2001). Children in single-parent families are two to three times more likely to have emotional and behavioral problems than children in two-parent families, when family income is equal. They are twice as likely to drop out of high school and 2.5 times as likely to become teenage mothers (Popenoe, 1995).

THE UNMARRIED TEENAGE MOTHER. The rate of teenage pregnancy in the United States is very high, particularly among adolescent African American girls. Fortunately, however, there was a dramatic drop of 20 percent in the birth rates for all female teenagers, especially for African American teenage girls, between the years 1991 and 1998 (Centers for Disease Control & Prevention, 2001). Births to unmarried teenagers are also high, and would be even higher if not for abortion. The causes for the prevalence of unmarried teenage families are multiple. The major factors cited in the literature are early sexual activity, no use or ineffective use of contraceptives, poverty, failing to marry before the child's birth, and relatively greater acceptance of unwed adolescent motherhood among lower-class African Americans (Chilman, 1988; Prater, 1995). The fact that over 50 percent of urban male African American youths are unemployed is one reason for the low marriage rate in the African American teenage group. The shortage of young African American men as compared to young women may also help explain why so many young African American teenage mothers do not marry.

Services to adolescent single parents to date are sorely inadequate. A continuum of services is needed. They range from primary preventive services in sex education and birth control to outreach programs, support networks, counseling, and school-based clinics and parenting classes, as well as services to the extended families of unmarried teenage mothers.

Single parents as a whole also have special needs. In addition to providing parenting classes and peer support networks, social policy changes are required so that adequate child care facilities and institutional supports such as flexible working hours are established.

THE SINGLE ADULT LIVING ALONE

The number of people living alone has also grown. According to Census 2000, the number of Americans living alone grew almost twice as swiftly as the population, accounting for 26 percent of all living arrangements. A preponderance of elderly women live alone, but the large increase in lone living is among adults in their 20s and 30s (Glick, 1988b; U.S. Bureau of the Census, 2000c).

Many home health clients, especially older chronically ill or disabled individuals, are single people living alone. Although these solitary people do not appear to fit into the text's definition of family, they probably have extended family members, siblings, or children whom they identify as their family. Most solitary people are part of some loosely formed family network. If this network is not made up of relatives, then it may be composed of friends such as those residing in the same retirement home, nursing home, or neighborhood. Pets can also be important family members.

Then there are those individuals who are truly "loners." They have a greater need for health and psychosocial services, because they have no support system and sometimes are not interested in developing one. Long-term and home care nurses can help these types of clients by developing a supportive relationship with them, thereby reducing the clients' social isolation.

THE STEPPARENT FAMILY

Although divorce is increasingly common, this trend has been accompanied by high rates of remarriage. Remarriage is used to include several different types of relationships—both partners may be in a second marriage or higher-order marriage or the marriage may be a remarriage for only one of the partners (Coleman, Ganong, & Fine, 2001). Seventy-five percent of divorced persons eventually remarry (Glick, 1994). Men remarry at higher rates than women, and African Americans and Hispanics remarry at lower rates than whites. Most remarriages tend to take place rapidly after the prior marriages end.

The high rate of remarriage has produced a dramatic growth in stepparent or blended families. These families are also known as "remarried families," in which there may or may not be children, and "reconstituted families." Usually, these types of families are composed of a mother, her biological children, and a stepfather. About one third of children in the United States will live in a remarried or stepparent family before they reach adulthood (Bumpass, Raley, & Sweet, 1995).

This family form typically is one that initially is a complex and stressful merger. Many adjustments need to be made, and different individuals and subgroups of the newly created family often move toward adaptation at different rates (Visher & Visher, 1996). Although all family members must adjust to the new family situation, children often have greater problems coping because of their age and concomitant developmental tasks, as well as their "dual citizenship" (membership in two households and cultures) (Hetherington & Stanley-Hagen, 2000; Visher & Visher, 1993).

Coleman, Ganong, and Goodwin (1994) reviewed 26 marriage and family textbooks and summarized both the strengths and stressors identified in stepparent families within these texts. They first mention that stressors and a deficit-comparison model are prevalently used in texts when discussing stepparent families—evidence perhaps of society's negative stereotyping. Three strengths are identified:

1. Remarriage is another opportunity to form new, gratifying, supportive relationships that promote the well-being of children and the remarried adults.

2. For stepchildren, stepparents can serve as additional positive role models, providing them with care, knowledge, and interests that the biological parent may not have been able to supply.

3. An escape from poverty and improved finances may also be a significant benefit of forming a stepparent family, particularly for divorced women and their children.

Six sources of stress are mentioned by Coleman and associates (1994), Visher and Visher (1993 & 1996; and Coleman, Ganong, and Fine (2001):

1. The relationship between stepparents and stepchildren is a primary source of many family difficulties. Discipline problems and the stepchildren's difficulty in accepting a stepparent as parent because of "divided loyalties" typically strain relationships in remarried families. Marital power issues may also be evident. Divorced women who during their divorced period become the primary decision maker and authority figure often have no interest in having anything but an egalitarian relationship with their new spouse. The new spouse may, however, have different expectations. In stepfamilies, children may also vie for power with the "conquer and divide" strategy—pitting their two biological parents against each other. Greater conflict is present.

2. The increased complexity of stepparent families is a significant feature that impedes adjustment. Complex and multiple roles and relationships can be a major source of difficulties for both parents and children, as they attempt to maintain previous and existing kin relationships and to cope with new kin relationships.

Children especially, feel divided loyalties as mentioned previously.

3. Role ambiguity is often a major stepparent family stressor. Stepparents often have little idea how to act as a stepparent and clear norms on how to enact the parenting role are lacking. Their marital partners may have high, unrealistic expectations for them in this role, and the stepchildren may not accept the new member in the stepparent role. Additionally, there are few societal guidelines to help stepparents learn their new roles.

4. Financial pressures may be present. Stepparents may have to provide financial support to two sets of children, placing a financial strain on both families.

5. Former spouse relationships may be strained and a source of tension and conflict, particularly when tied to child support, visitation issues, and how children should be raised.

6. Unrealistic expectations about what family life should be like create another primary source of dissatisfaction and disagreements in stepparent families, especially in the early months of the new family.

Stepparent development as a family system differs from the traditional two-parent nuclear family development. In Chapter 5 (Table 5–15), Carter and McGoldrick's (1989) Model of Stepparent Development is outlined as consisting of three phases or steps along with concomitant developmental issues to be addressed.

Only a few authors have discussed factors that help stepparent families adjust positively. A most helpful discussion of characteristics of successful stepparent families comes from Visher and Visher (1996) and Goldenberg and Goldenberg (2002). They list five characteristics found in large part in healthy stepparent families. These are:

1. Expectations for the stepparent family are realistic. The adults realize that initially things will be rocky, that it takes time to adapt, and that adaptation cannot be forced. Losses have to be mourned. Stepfamilies are "born of loss," being formed following either divorce or death. Adults support and assist their children in coping with the losses accompanying the creation of a new family.

2. Satisfactory step-relationships have been formed. This not only includes the marital relationship, but the relationship between marital partners and their respective extended families.

3. A strong, unified couple relationship exists.

4. The separate households have learned to cooperate—to make satisfactory arrangements involving the children.

5. Satisfying rituals, roles, and rules are established. The step-family members are able to decide what rituals and ways of doing things they would like to adopt in their newly created family.

6. Because there is a different balance of power in a stepparent family, discipline issues are handled by the biological parent.

THE BINUCLEAR FAMILY

The binuclear family refers to the postdivorced family in which the child is a member of a family system composed of two nuclear households, maternal and paternal, with varying degrees of cooperation between and time spent in each household (Ahrons & Perlmutter, 1982). With the movement toward sex-role equity, increased participation by some fathers in parenting, and the growing awareness of the loss of being a noncustodial parent and the negative consequences to children when there is no father contact, various ways of active coparenting have emerged. The most widely discussed form of active coparenting is joint custody, where both parents have equal legal rights and responsibilities to the minor child irrespective of residential arrangements.

There has been increased attention given to coparenting and joint custody. Nevertheless, these family arrangements are only seen among a small fraction of divorced families. A case in point: In a nationally representative sample of children in single-parent and stepparent families, almost half of the children had not seen their nonresidential parent in the past year. The residential parent assumed a disproportionately large amount of the child care (Furstenberg & Nord, 1985). Yet a father's continued involvement with his children is important for their well-being. Where possible and appropriate, coparenting should be encouraged and supported.

THE NONMARITAL HETEROSEXUAL COHABITING FAMILY

There is a substantial growth in the number of U.S. couples living together unmarried (U.S. Bureau of the Census, 2000; Koeninn, 1997). This wave of cohabitation appeared in the 1960s and has continued, with over a 100 percent increase nationally in the number of cohabiting household units from 1970 to 2000 (from nearly 523,000 to 3.8 million households). This trend has continued. In an earlier era, cohabitation was limited to the very rich, those in the theater, and the very poor. But today, cohabitation has become a much more acceptable nontraditional family form for young adults before and in between marriages (Koeninn, 1997; Weiss, 1988).

It is estimated that over one half of all couples live together before marriage (Popenoe & Whitehead, 1999). "What makes cohabitation so significant is not only its prevalence but also its widespread popular acceptance" (Popenoe & Whitehead, 1999, p. 3). In fact, increasingly cohabitation has come to be looked upon as a normative process leading to marriage. It is not only young people who are living together without being married; older persons and widowed or divorced persons also have begun to live together, often for companionship and to share limited financial resources (Goldenberg & Goldenberg, 2002). Underlying this trend toward cohabitation is the broad cultural shift from a more religious society to a more secular society focused on individual freedom and autonomy (Popenoe & Whitehead, 1999).

THE GAY AND LESBIAN FAMILY

There is no consensus as to what constitutes a gay and lesbian family. Allen and Demo's (1995) definition is presented here as it is broad and inclusionary of the rich diversity of gay and lesbian families. They suggest that gay and lesbian families refer to "the presence of two or more people who share a same-sex orientation (e.g., a couple), or the presence of at least one lesbian or gay adult rearing a child" (p. 13). Although there are no official estimates of the number of gay and lesbian families, this family form represents a significant minority of U.S. households (Allen & Demo, 1995; Eliason, 1996). Very little research has been presented or published about gay and lesbian families according to Allen and Demo (1995), who conducted an extensive literature review in this area. Allen and Demo (1995) and Laird (1993) concluded that very little is known of family relationships and what is presented or published is based on small samples of predominantly white, urban, middle-class, highly educated respondents.

Gay and lesbian families are richly diverse in their form and composition. First of all, they are families formed from lovers, friends, biological and adopted children, blood relatives, stepchildren, and even ex-lovers. In addition, families do not necessarily reside in the same household (Laird, 1993). Therefore, there is no normative or uniform family form among gay and lesbian families. Usually gay and lesbian families are same-sex couples, but they could also be headed by singly gay or lesbian parents or multiple parenting figures.

According to Goldenberg and Goldenberg (2002), who counsel gay and lesbian families, cohabiting homosexual couples have much in common with heterosexual cohabiting couples. There are, however, notable differences. One strikingly apparent difference is the pervasive homophobia in society and the probable stigmatization that gay and lesbian families face or potentially face if they disclose their homosexuality and nontraditional living arrangements (Laird, 1993). Efforts at concealment, self-condemnation because of their gayness, the negative self-labeling that occurs as a result of society's negative labeling, and, for gay men, fear of disenfranchisement as a result of the AIDS crisis are also stresses particular to gay and lesbian families (Goldenberg & Goldenberg, 2002). "Coming out" is a vital and ongoing stressful process that gay, lesbian, bisexual, and transgendered individuals experience throughout their lives (Wilcox & Allen, 2000).

In marked contrast to heterosexual marriages, there is no legal sanction for homosexual marriages in the United States with the exception of Vermont, where homosexual couples may form "civil unions." In Western Europe, however, four countries permit same-sex unions—France, Iceland, Belgium, and Sweden (Sussman, 2000; Times Wire Services, 1999). Homosexual unions are not "institutionalized," meaning that rules, standards, practices, and social sanctions for continuance are not present. Thus, lack of legal basis is a problem today in terms of inheritance and parental rights. For instance, the "lesbian baby boom" has brought to light some perplexing problems for lesbian couples who separate. In these cases, the lesbian partner who is not the biological parent, has no legal relationship with her child. In other cases, children have been legally removed from a lesbian family home because the lesbian parent has been deemed an "unfit mother" due to her sexual orientation alone (Eliason, 1996). Although the vast majority of studies have found no differences in child-rearing and child's adjustment by lesbian/gay parents versus heterosexual parents, legal barriers still exist in adoption and child custody matters.

According to recent national polls, the majority of Americans believe gay and lesbian parents are equal to heterosexual parents in their parenting abilities, indicating a greater acceptance of gay and lesbian families today (Savin-Williams & Esterberg, 2000).

LOOKING AT THE FUTURE OF THE AMERICAN FAMILY

With the family evidencing increasing complexities in household and family patterns, family members now have more options to pursue lifestyles that reflect their differences and preferences. Nevertheless, many family social scientists and family health professionals are concerned about the state of the American family.

In reviewing the many articles and chapters that discuss the state of families and their future, we agree with Hunter (1994), who comments that the family appears as the most conspicuous field of conflict in society—or as an institution under siege. A case in point was the heated political debate over "family values" in 1992. Hunter (1994) and Rodman and Sidden (1992) identify the following battleground family issues that so prominently fill our newspapers today: the concerns over "latchkey" children; the status and role of women, particularly those who have children (i.e., the debate about whether mothers who work "hurt" their children); the moral legitimacy of abortion; the appropriate pace of children's development; the legal and social status of homosexuals; the increase in family violence; the growth of cohabitation among young adults; and the growing demand for adequate day care.

The controversy over these family issues and the future of the family as an institution has been interpreted by some as one between optimists and pessimists. Although both sides acknowledge that the family is undergoing profound changes, they disagree sharply over the extent, meaning, and consequences of those changes (Hunter, 1994). The pessimists have deep-seated anxiety over the decline of the American family. They see the previously mentioned issues (and more) as having detrimental effects on the family and as cause for their gloomy outlook (Rodman & Sidden, 1992). Often, their concerns focus on the negative effects various family forms have on the children (Scelfo, Springen, Figueroa, Brant, & Abrahms, 2001). The optimists, on the other hand, view change as positive and mention such changes as rising egalitarianism and shared gender roles, the ability for women to work and have a family; the technological advances that give the family members more leisure time together, greater tolerance and respect of gays and lesbians. They point to the age-old adage that the family, being resilient and adaptive to new social conditions, is "here to stay" (Hunter, 1994).

A major problem with most pessimists is that they have a rather narrow time frame within which they analyze the family. History teaches us a lesson here. Attacks on the family and its status and future are *not* new. Coontz (1996), a family historian, impressively argues that "American families have been under siege more often than not during the past 300 years" (p. 38) and somehow have been able to adapt to social and economic changes. Coontz (1996) also remarks that "we can take comfort from the fact that American families have always been in flux and that a wide variety of family forms and values have worked well for different groups at different times. Our challenge is to grapple with sweeping transformations we are currently undergoing" (p. 43).

❦ FAMILY NURSING IMPLICATIONS

The preceding description of family forms illustrates the broad array of structures prevalent in families today. There is no "right," "wrong," "proper," or "improper" form of family. Families must be understood within their own context. Labels and types serve only as a reference to the family's living arrangements and primary group network. Every effort must be made to understand the uniqueness and strengths of each particular family. Society places complex and often conflicting demands on people; hence, the need for a range of family forms to coexist. Health professionals serving families must be tolerant and sensitive to the diversity of family lifestyles and should abandon the traditional model of the "ideal family." What is important in families is the quality of family relationships, not the structure within which the relationships exist (Dunphy, 2001).

We need, as a society and through our public policy and health care programs, to promote and strengthen the family and seek ways to make communities more supportive (especially in the area of child care) to children and parents who live in diverse family forms. In short, in our roles as family nurse and informed citizen, we need to make our programs and community "family friendly."

We also must recognize that many families are in trouble. It is only by recognizing the stressed state of these families that social action, broadened family-focused health services, and urgently needed domestic policy changes will occur.

❦ SUMMARY

Within this chapter the following family content is highlighted:

- Families serve two basic purposes—to meet the needs of society and to meet the needs of its individual family members.

- There are several important reasons nurses should work with families, including to provide more effi-

cacious care to family members and to gain a more holistic assessment of the individual client.

- During the six stages of the family's interaction with health issues, the family plays an ongoing, vital role.

- The key family definitions, include the definition of family, the nuclear family, the extended family, the family of origin, and family health.

- Healthy families can be described in various ways, depending on the theoretical orientation and clinical focus of authors. Critical attributes of healthy families include good interpersonal, communication and negotiating skills of family members, family members being respectful and affiliative towards each other, and the family encouraging autonomy and fulfillment of family members' potential as individuals.

- Societal changes which have had a major impact on the American family include: (a) economic trends (rising costs and growing disparity between the rich and poor); (b) technological advances; and (c) demographic trends (accelerated population growth and the aging of the population) and sociocultural trends (the changing racial and ethnic composition of society).

- The family has changed considerably in recent years, with these major changes: (a) a decline in household size; (b) delayed marriage and decline in marriage rate; (c) higher divorce rates; (d) lower remarriage rates; (e) an increase in first births to older mothers; (f) an increase in childhood living arrangements and single par-

ent families; (g) changing gender norms; (h) growth in women's employment; and (i) an increase in family heterogeneity.

- Various family forms have reshaped what the family looks like today. These family types include: the nuclear family (the sole provider, dual-earner), the adoptive family, the foster family, the childless family, the extended family, the single-parent family, the single adult living alone, the stepparent family, the binuclear family, the nonmarital heterosexual cohabiting family, and the gay and lesbian family.

- The debate regarding the future of the American family is summarized as a controversy between the pessimists—who interpret many of the family changes as having detrimental effects on the family and the children and the optimists—who see the family as resilient and adaptable to societal and internal changes and demands.

- Family nurses need to understand and accept families within their own context. Efforts must be made to appreciate the uniqueness, adaptability, and strengths of the families with whom we work.

✎ FAMILY VIGNETTE: THE STANLEY FAMILY

Doris Stanley, a clerk in a hardware store, was divorced two years ago from her husband of eight years. Their two children, ages 6 and 7, live with the mother although John Brown, who is also remarried, cares for the children every other weekend as part of the couple's joint custody agreement. This agreement is often violated, however, as John calls Doris and cancels his child care plans when other "important" matters come up in his life. Doris has Type II diabetes and is being seen in a health maintenance organization (HMO) by a nurse practitioner. She recently married Dick Stanley, a friend from work with whom she had much in common. They were both divorced and came from similar ethnic and regional roots—both had English parents and grew up in small towns in Ohio. Dick has never had children, but expressed his pleasure in marrying into a "ready-made" family.

Doris and Dick have been married three months now. They expected that the marriage and family life together would be smooth sailing, as they were both so excited and positive about creating a new family together. The children, however, appear very strained when relating to their new stepfather and seem resentful about the new marriage. The first time Dick disciplined the children for misbehaving at the dinner table, Doris yelled at Dick that disciplining was her responsibility—after all, she was the children's mother!

■ STUDY QUESTIONS

Review the Family Vignette and answer the related questions.

1. What type of family form does this family represent?
2. From the children's perspective, what other type of family are they in?
3. What benefits does Doris probably see in remarrying?
4. What are some primary issues that this new family is facing?
5. If you were working with this family as a nurse practitioner (seeing the mother for her diabetes management) what kind of supportive counseling could you provide to assist the family with their adaptation?

Answer the following questions.

6. Which of these characteristics belong in a broadened, inclusionary definition of "family"?
   a. Composed of one or more persons
   b. Geographic dispersion
   c. Emotional involvement and commitment
   d. Sense of identity as a family

7. Which statement is correct?
   a. The family of parenthood/procreation is the family into which you were born.
   b. The family of orientation/origin is the family of marriage.
   c. The extended family includes the family's close family and friends.
   d. None of the above.

8. The family functions to meet the *needs of society* by (select best answer):
   a. Mediating between society's expectations and the needs of the individual
   b. Providing recruits for society's job market
   c. Rearing of children

9. The family functions to meet the *needs of its members* by (select best answer):
   a. Providing recruits for society
   b. Serving as a "buffer" between society and the individual
   c. Facilitating the personality development of the individual

10. Which of these is (are) the main reason(s) for nurses to work with the family?
    a. The entire family is affected by the health problem of a family member.
    b. Promotion of healthy functioning of the whole family will positively affect each family member and his or her health status.
    c. By working with the whole family, the nurse may be able to discover health problems that other family members are having.

11. Which of these is (are) an example(s) of how the ill family member can adversely affect the family?

    a. Birth of handicapped child disrupts the marital relationship.
    b. Emotional disturbance of the husband disrupts the economic and emotional stability of the family.
    c. Family is brought together in a common effort to help the ill member get well.

How does the family affect the health of its family members in each of the following six stages of health/illness?

12. Stage 1: Family efforts at health promotion

13. Stage 2: Family appraisal of symptoms

14. Stage 3: Care seeking

15. Stage 4: Referral and obtaining care

16. Stage 5: Acute response by client and family to illness

17. Stage 6: Adaptation to illness and recovery

18. Some ways in which society has been able to influence/change family values, attitudes, or sanctions are:

    a. Judicial rulings on constitutional rights of people
    b. Postponement of marriage and childbearing
    c. Health legislation
    d. Advances in technology

19. How does the meaning of family health differ from the meaning of health?

Fill in the correct answers to the following questions.

20. Give three examples of traditional family forms.

21. Give three examples of nontraditional family forms.

22. Name three stressors that commonly affect single-parent families.

23. List two major recent general demographic trends and two family demographic changes in the United States today.

Choose the correct answer(s) to the following questions.

24. What are the usual ties between nuclear and extended family? (circle all accurate descriptions)

    a. A modified extended family exists within a network of generational interaction.
    b. Parents and siblings of spouses form the most important network of extended kinship relations.
    c. The extended family network provides significant support and continuing assistance to nuclear families.

25. Relative to the nuclear childless family, the cohabiting family, and the family with an unmarried teenage mother, which factor is associated with *all three of these family forms?*

    a. Need for birth contraception education

    b. Poverty

    c. High divorce rates

    d. Unavailability of males

    e. Postponement of marriage

    f. Early premarital coitus

26. Gay and lesbian families have much in common with cohabitating heterosexual couples, but also have major differences. These differences are:

    a. Among gay and lesbian families there is no uniform or normative family structure.

    b. Greater stigmatization of family among gay and lesbian families.

    c. The family developmental stages differ considerably between these two types of families.

27. Attributes of a healthy family include:

    a. An emphasis on traditional roles and decision making.

    b. Family members are optimistic about the future.

    c. Autonomy of family members is encouraged.

    d. Family members display capable negotiation skills in dealing with their problems.

    e. Family demonstrates resiliency in addressing their challenges.

28. The future of the American family continues to be a "hot" topic in public debate today, with the pessimists and optimists coming to opposite conclusions. Which of these viewpoints do you subscribe to and why?

29. With a steady, significant growth in diverse family forms, there are several important implications for family nursing practice. Name a key implication relative to this important demographic family trend.

2

FAMILY NURSING: FOCUS, EVOLUTION, AND GOALS

❧ LEARNING OBJECTIVES

1. Explain the differences in how the family is conceptualized in family nursing practice.

2. Compare how the family is incorporated into professional organizations' standards of practice.

3. Distinquish between family nursing and (a) community health nursing, (b) family therapy.

4. Identify the four specialty areas in nursing that historically have been most ardently involved in family health care.

5. Discuss several current issues in family nursing.

6. Briefly describe the three levels of prevention.

7. Explain why health promotion is a predominant thrust within family nursing.

8. Discuss the primary factors leading to increased interest in health promotion and health maintenance today.

9. Identify factors that have impeded the growth of primary prevention.

10. Explain the difference between health promotion and disease prevention.

11. Explain the purpose of the three risk appraisal tools.

12. Describe the family nurse's role in primary, secondary, and tertiary prevention.

This text is about family nursing and the basic knowledge base—consisting of theory, factual information, research, and clinical implications—needed to practice basic family nursing. The chapter begins the discussion of family nursing by addressing what family nursing encompasses, its evolution, and the incorporation of family into professional standards of care. Finally, the primary goal of family nursing, promotion and maintenance of family health, is analyzed by using Leavell and associates' (1965) levels-of-prevention framework as a vehicle for discussing the family nurse's role within the three levels of prevention. Particular emphasis is given to primary prevention, especially health promotion, because this focus is seen as the predominant thrust of family nursing. Discussions of family health, a healthy lifestyle, and risk appraisal and reduction are also elaborated upon as part of primary prevention. The family nurse's role in secondary and tertiary prevention completes the discussion of the family nurse's role in health and illness.

✤ FAMILY NURSING: DEFINING THE SPECIALTY

Family nursing is a specialty area that cuts across the various other specialty areas of nursing. Although as a distinct specialty it is still relatively young, there is strong evidence that family nursing is a growing, dynamic specialty area of focus in practice, education, and research. Significant progress is being made in broadening nursing's practice paradigm to include the family as client. Yet, a gap between conceptualization and practice still exists (Friedemann, 1989). Interestingly enough, there are several names of this specialty: family health care nursing (Bomar, 1996; Hanson, 2001); nursing of families or family systems nursing, depending on focus and the level of practice (Wright & Leahey, 2000); and system-focused or systemic family nursing (Friedemann, 1995).

When the first edition of this text was written in 1979 to 1980, there were no definitions of family nursing. Several texts discussed family nursing (Ford, 1979; Sobol & Robischon, 1975); family-centered community nursing (Reinhardt & Quinn, 1973); family-focused nursing (Janosik & Miller, 1980); and family health care (Hymovich & Barnard, 1979); but

notions about a specialty called family nursing were absent. Today, texts, articles, and professional presentations in the area of family nursing are extensive. The specialty even has its own journal, *The Journal of Family Nursing*. This journal, begun in 1995, has been vital to the advancement of family nursing as it has given family nurses a place to share their thoughts and research.

There is, however, disagreement over what family nursing actually encompasses (Hanson, 2001; Wright & Leahey, 2000), and how it differs from community health nursing (Friedman, 1986) and family therapy (Gilliss, Rose, Hallburg, & Martinson, 1989; Wright & Leahey, 1994). A review of the family nursing literature reveals that within the definition of family nursing family nursing practice is described in different ways. The way family nursing is practiced depends on how the family nurse conceptualizes the family and works with it. The degree of family-centeredness also is dependent on the philosophy of the system within which the nurse works. The work environment (what leadership rewards and negatively reinforces) is also a major determinant of behavior. Each of the following five ways of thinking about the family shape family nursing practice, education, research and theory development.

FAMILY AS CONTEXT

The first way family nursing is conceptualized is as a field where the family is viewed as context to the client or family member (Bozett, 1987; Robinson, 1995) (Figure 2–1). Nursing care is individually focused. The family, as typically the client's most important primary group, is visualized typically as a resource to the client although in some cases is viewed as a stressor. The family is the background or secondary focus and the individual, the foreground or primary focus relative to assessment and intervention.

The nurse may involve the family to varying degrees. In some cases the nurse may assess the family as part of the client's social support system, but with little incorporation of the family into the client's plan of care. In other cases, the nurse may extensively involve the family in the client's care. The family's tangible and socioemotional impact on the client is assessed and integrated into the treatment plan.

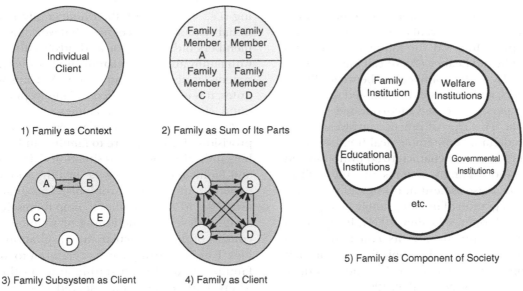

Figure 2–1. Five ways of viewing the family, all shaping family nursing.

Most nursing theories conceptualize the family's role in this light. Most specialty areas also view the family as a crucial social environment of the client and hence a primary social support resource. A case in point is the definition of family-centered care promulgated by the interdisciplinary Association for the Care of Children's Health (ACCH). They explain that family-centered care is a philosophy of pediatric health care that considers and treats the child in the context of the family and recognizes the family as the primary and continuing provider of care for the child. This organization stresses that the family is "the constant" in the child's life (Shelton & Stepanek, 1995).

FAMILY AS SUM OF ITS MEMBERS

In the second type of family nursing practice, the family is seen as an accumulation or sum of the individual family members. When care is made available to or provided for all the family members, family health care is seen as being provided. This is a model that is implicit to much of practice within family primary care and community health nursing. In this type of family nursing practice, the foreground is each of the clients, seen as separate rather than interacting units.

FAMILY SUBSYSTEM AS CLIENT

In the third type of family nursing practice, family subsystems are the focus and recipient of assessment and intervention. Friedemann (1993b) and Robinson (1995) refer to this model as being the basis for interpersonal family nursing. Family dyads, triads, and other family subsystems are the unit of analysis and care. Parent–child relationships, marital interactions, caregiving issues, and bonding–attachment concerns are examples of the nursing foci here.

FAMILY AS CLIENT

In the fourth type of family nursing conceptualization, the entire family is viewed as client or as the primary focus of assessment and care. The family is now in the foreground, with the individual family members in the background or context. The family is viewed as an interactional system. The focus is on internal family dynamics and relationships, the family's structure and functions, as well as the relationships of family subsystems with the whole and of the family with its outer environment. It is in this latter type of conceptualization of family that the unique contributions of family nursing are evident.

When systems theory and cybernetics, especially the notions of interaction, circularity, and reciprocity, become the prevailing way the family is viewed and analyzed, Wright and Leahey (2000) call this family systems nursing. Here the connections between illness, family members, and the family are assessed within this interactional perspective and incorporated into the treatment plan. This type of practice involves using a different paradigm or epistemological framework for assessment and care, one characterized by holism and circular causation. Family systems nursing utilizes advanced clinical assessment and intervention skills based on an integration of nursing, family therapy, and systems theory (Wright & Leahey, 1994). It represents advanced nursing practice, as its concentration is simultaneously on not only the whole family as the unit of care, but on multiple systems, such as the individual, the family, and larger systems (Bell, 1996).

Fortunately, there is a growing effort in family primary care to see the family unit as the focus of care (Doherty & Campbell, 1988; Campbell, 2000), but with cost-containment efforts and lack of reimbursement for family care, these efforts are not widespread.

FAMILY AS A COMPONENT OF SOCIETY

There is a fifth conceptualization of family described by Hanson (2001b), that is, *as a component of society.* Here, the family is visualized as one subsystem within a larger system—the community, society. The family is seen as one of basic societal institutions, such as the educational, welfare, or religious institutions are. This view of the family is discussed in the structural–functional theory chapter (Chapter 4), the systems theory chapter (Chapter 6), and the family environmental data chapter (Chapter 9).

DEFINING FAMILY NURSING

Family nursing encompasses all the five models described above, even though the fourth model is considered uniquely family nursing. In family nursing, nurses work simultaneously with individuals, subsystems, the whole family, and the family–society (other systems in the community) interface. In this text we emphasize the unique aspects of family nurs-ing (i.e., working with the whole family as an interactional system) but recognize that working with family members individually or as dyads/triads, or working with family and their relationship to other interacting systems, is also quite important. As Hanson (2001b) notes, it is important to keep all family perspectives in mind when working with families.

Family nursing practice is defined in this text as "the provision of nursing care to families and family members in health and illness situations." Hence, families and family members may be healthy and/or may be experiencing health problems. The goal of family nursing is to assist families to help themselves achieve a higher level of functioning or wellness within the context of their particular aims, aspirations, and abilities. Family nursing may be rendered to all forms of families in any health setting and in other settings where families are being served (e.g., educational and multipurpose service centers). The nursing process serves as the framework for providing care.

It is practice that is informed by nursing, family, social science, and family therapy theories. (Refer to Chapter 3 for more in-depth discussion of theoretical foundations.) The emphasis of family nursing practice should be health oriented, incorporating holistic, systemic, and interactional perspectives and drawing on and drawing forth family strengths (Bell, 1996; Friedemann, 1995; Wright & Leahey, 2000). (See Table 2–1.)

TABLE 2–1

FAMILY NURSING ENTAILS:

‹ Provision of nursing care to families

‹ Use of the nursing process applied to the family

‹ Working with families within a health and/or illness context

‹ Working with families in many settings—wherever families are being served

‹ Working with all forms of families

‹ Being guided by theories and research from family social science, family therapy, and nursing

‹ Emphasizing a health orientation, a holistic and an interactional perspective, and the importance of family strengths

DISTINGUISHING FAMILY NURSING FROM OTHER PRACTICE AREAS

Because family nursing historically has been aligned primarily with community health nursing (Whall, 1986a), some confusion exists between what is community health or public health nursing and family nursing. Whereas family nursing focuses on the family as its target or recipient of care, community health nursing's target of service is the community (Williams, 1996). The health of the community rather than the health of the family is the ultimate goal of community health nursing. It is through families that community health nurses improve and preserve the health of communities. The difference here is a matter of ultimate goals and priorities. The implications of this difference are that in rendering personal health services to a family—for example, a single-parent family of mother and young children—the "non–community-oriented" family nurse would be concerned with the family's unique problems first, and second with the community health problems common to young families (the first commitment being a client and family). In a community health setting, the nurse would be cognizant of the pressing maternal–child health problems in the community that were relevant to the client family, such as immunizations and family planning, and prioritize these needs along with the unique health needs of the family.

Another point of confusion is the difference between family nursing and family therapy (Gilliss et al., 1989) or family systems nursing. In Wright and Leahey's text, *Nurses and Families* (2000), they distinguish nursing of families from family therapy and family systems nursing. Wright and Leahey believe that advanced preparation is needed to practice as a family systems nurse clinician. However, nursing of families, consisting of basic family nursing assessment and intervention, should be part of baccalaureate nursing education. The nurse here is able to complete family assessments of healthy/functional and dysfunctional families. The family nurse or interviewer intervenes using educative–supportive strategies that are direct and straightforward. In family systems nursing or family therapy, the nursing interventions include more complex and indirect psychosocial interventions (Wright & Leahey) and the clinician works with multiple systems simultaneously (Bell, 1996).

Family nurse researchers working as a special interest group under the auspices of the Family Nursing Continuing Education Project, Oregon Health Sciences University (Kirschling et al., 1989), were also interested in clarifying what family nurses actually do. To address this question they conducted a national survey of 263 nurses who identified themselves as being family nurses, asking them about their practice and interaction with their clients. From this data, the researchers identified unique characteristics of family nursing practice. The following four major themes emerged when participants were queried as to what they did differently when they cared for families rather than individuals:

- Recognition and integration of family concepts
- Application of a broader perspective as identified in the nurses' approach to nursing care, primarily by assessing the family
- A focus on family interaction and family dynamics
- Involvement of family members in care, particularly in areas of decision making and caregiving

✺ INCORPORATION OF FAMILY INTO STANDARDS OF CARE

Ideally, family nursing should be a reality in all clinical areas of nursing practice. In some settings and specialty areas, however, incorporating the family as client is more difficult to achieve than in others. For instance, in episodic settings—especially in intensive care units and emergency departments, where immediate lifesaving measures are needed—a predominant patient focus is understandable.

Evidence of what specialty areas believe to be the appropriate standards and scope of their practice are found in publications from the American Nurses Association (ANA), which is responsible for defining and establishing the scope of nursing practice and standards in both the general field and in areas of specialization. The Association for the Care of Children's Health and the National Organization of Nurse Practitioner Faculties developed documents addressing standards of care in pediatrics and primary care, respectively.

We reviewed the ANA's *Social Policy Statements* (1980; 1995a) and *Standards of Clinical Nursing Practice* (general standards) (ANA, 1998), and standards/scope of practice statements in seven specialty areas to see the extent to which the family was incorporated into standards of care documents. Standards from psychiatric–mental health nursing (ANA, 2000), gerontological nursing (ANA, 1995b), public health nursing (ANA, 1999), and home health nursing (1999); pediatric clinical nursing (ANA, 1996); and rehabilitation nursing (ANA, 1988) and primary health care nurse practitioner (ANA, 1987) were reviewed. This survey revealed that the family as context was recognized, that is, as an important resource to the individual client in all standards documents. All these standards—with the exception of rehabilitation nursing—also stated that the client may be an individual, family, group, or community. However, when specific descriptions of standards and scope of practice were delineated, the family was clearly not considered as client in some of the specialties. The standards documents, with the exception of rehabilitation nursing, following the general *Standards of Clinical Nursing Practice* lead, used the nursing process framework to describe their standards of practice. Hence, the same basic framework, the nursing process, was used in all standards of care, but the description of practice varied widely with respect to family inclusion.

In the ANA's important social policy statements of 1980 and 1995, the association described the family, along with the individual client and community, as nursing's recipient of care. The family was also identified as a necessary unit of nursing services. The generic standards of clinical practice also stated that the family is a client along with individuals, groups, and communities.

In the psychiatric–mental health nursing standards (ANA, 2000), family psychotherapy was discussed as an intervention appropriate for a psychiatric–mental health nurse functioning at an advanced practice level (master's prepared advanced practice nurse).

In the *Standards of Public Health Nursing Practice* (ANA, 1999) and *Standards of Home Health Nursing Practice* (1999), the nursing process was utilized to assess, plan, diagnose, intervene, and evaluate *families*. Collaboration with families is stressed. Family nursing care was promulgated as a vital component of practice.

In the *Standards of Pediatric Clinical Nursing Practice* (ANA, 1996), family was heavily identified and integrated throughout the standards. For instance, the standards stated that nurses assist families to achieve health promotion and to cope with health problems and role transitions.

In the gerontology nursing practice standards (ANA, 1995b) and rehabilitation nursing standards (ANA, 1988), the family was clearly seen as a resource to the individual client. Finally, in the standards of practice for primary care nurse practitioners (ANA, 1987), there was no mention of family. The ANA 1985 scope of practice document mentioned family in the introductory section, stating primary care's orientation "to the family and/or broader systems of which the individual is a part" (p. 3). The National Organization of Nurse Practitioner Faculties (NONPF), in contrast to the ANA document on primary care nurse practitioner scope of practice, clearly described the nurse practitioner's role in working with families.

As seen in the *Standards of Pediatric Clinical Nursing Practice,* this specialty emphasizes a family-centered philosophy and approach in clinical practice. The best example of this "family-centerdness" is found in a document from the Association for the Care of Children's Health in which they list the following key elements of family-centered care:

- Incorporating into policy and practice the recognition that the family is the constant in a child's life, whereas the service systems and support personnel within those systems fluctuate

- Facilitating family/professional collaboration at all levels of hospital, home, and community care

- Exchanging complete and unbiased information between families and professionals in a supportive manner

- Incorporating into policy and practice the recognition and honoring of cultural diversity, strengths, and individuality within and across all families

- Recognizing and respecting different methods of coping and implementing comprehensive policies and programs that provide developmental, educational, emotional, environmental, and financial supports to meet the diverse needs of families

- Encouraging and facilitating family-to-family support and networking

- Ensuring that hospital, home, and community services and support systems for children needing special health and developmental care and their families are flexible, accessible, and comprehensive in responding to diverse family-identified needs

- Appreciating families as families and children as children, recognizing that they possess a wide range of strengths, concerns, emotions, and aspirations beyond their need for specialized health and developmental services and support (Shelton & Stepanek, 1995)

❧FAMILY NURSING'S HISTORICAL LEGACY

"The concept of family nursing has always been with us in nursing" (Ford, 1979, p. 4). It has, however, seen decline and regrowth.

In the preindustrialized, colonial era, when family members worked at home in cottage industries or farming, family care predominated. Then came industrialization, with family members moving into factories to work. Health care gradually moved from the home to the hospital.

In England, Florence Nightingale was aware of the importance of the family and home environment in the care of the sick. She mentions the needs of family members in military camps and the need "to keep whole families out of pauperism by nursing the breadwinner back to health" (Beard, 1915, as cited in Whall, 1986a, pp. 242–243).

During the 1800s and early 1900s in the United States, public health nurses and their equivalents in England served families in the home (initially the poor, but later also those with communicable diseases). With bureaucratization in society, specialization in medicine grew (obstetrics, pediatrics, surgery, etc.). Nursing also became specialized, and family medicine and family-oriented nursing practice fell into disuse. Insurance coverage limitations, private and public reimbursement policies and referrals, and lack of preventive funding also were policies that later mitigated against family-focused care (Ford, 1979).

Public health nursing, maternal–child health, and midwifery managed to bridge the gap in some instances and stand as examples of both family-centered and fractionalized care. For instance, obstetrics limits care to the mother, with care of baby left to a different provider, and little interest in other family members; and communicable disease public health nursing services typically include the family only with regard to case finding. An example of where family nursing continued was in the Frontier Nursing Service. Here, the Frontier Nursing Service provided both midwifery and public health nursing services to families.

The four specialty groups in nursing that have been the most ardent in focusing on the family have been community health nursing, which sees the family as client; parent–child nursing, which sees the family as context and client; psychiatric–mental health nursing, which sees extensive family involvement within the family therapy specialization; and the family primary care or nurse practitioner specialty, which sometimes sees the family as a sum of its members, but also views the family as context.

Each of these specialty groups has been informed by both specific developments in its own area of specialization and by more general developments within nursing, social science, and society. For instance, in community health nursing, the legacy was to consider the family as a focus of service. But not until the 1970s was there much substantive content within nursing programs that addressed family theory, assessment, and intervention. In the 1970s we saw texts focusing on family theory and its application to family-centered community health nursing. In community health nursing, sociological and cultural theories of family behavior (such as family socialization, poverty, roles, values, dynamics, and cultural diversity) were important in influencing the field.

Psychiatric–mental health nursing, in contrast, was more heavily influenced by the theories and clinical writings within the family therapy movement. Since these nurses work with troubled families, this knowledge base was more important to assist them in assessing and intervening with dysfunctional families. Family therapy theories and practice models, however, are only one psychotherapeutic modality in mental health. Hence, family nursing assessment and intervention are not widespread throughout the whole specialty area.

Maternal or parent–child nursing has a long history of family involvement—beginning with the early days of midwifery and visiting of mothers and children in the home. It has long been recognized that when caring for mothers and children, the family is crucial. Family-centered texts in pediatrics and maternity are the norm. Most texts primarily see the family as context. Parent–child family-focused nursing has been particularly influenced by growth and development, mother–child bonding, role, and socialization theories.

Family and pediatric nurse practitioners are the fourth specialty area identified as being family focused. In the 1960s it was recognized among health care planners and legislators that specialization in medicine was not meeting the primary health care needs of the whole population in the United States. Federal monies were granted to medical schools to open up family practice programs. The nurse-practitioner movement grew on the coattails of this larger movement concerned with cost-effective, accessible care to all sectors of society. Nurse-practitioner programs have also been heavily federally funded. Family nurse practitioners care for the whole family, but their predominant focus is to see the family as a sum of its members. Both pediatric and family nurse practitioners view the family as context to the individual client. This is changing, however, as some nurse-practitioner programs are incorporating advanced family nursing content into their curricula to attempt to broaden services and to help students "think family" (Wright & Leahey, 2000) or to "think interactionally" (Wright & Leahey).

In addition to the more specific influences each of these specialty areas experienced, certain more general factors have enhanced the growth of family nursing. These include:

1. The increased recognition in nursing and society of the need for health promotion and a health focus, rather than the practically exclusive disease orientation

2. Our aging population and the growth of chronic illness, which have brought self-care and the needs of family caregivers into prominence

3. The widespread awareness concerning the pervasiveness of troubled families in our communities

4. The promulgation and general acceptance of certain interpersonal and family-based theories, such as attachment and bonding theory,

general systems theory, and family stress and coping theories

5. The marriage and family therapy movements and the growth in child guidance, marriage, and family clinics and services

6. The growth of family research and the significance of its findings. Two cases in point are:

    (a) The extensive and influential family communication research in the 1950s and 1960s, which showed that troubled parents, particularly mothers and their communication patterns, were associated with troubled children

    (b) The growing number of family nursing research studies that demonstrate the impact of health stressors and coping on family health outcomes and the effectiveness of family-centered interventions

CURRENT ISSUES IN FAMILY NURSING

From our review of the literature and professional discussions with colleagues in family nursing, eight issues appear to be salient issues in family nursing today:

• **Practice Issue: The significant gap between theory and research and actual clinical practice.** The gap between extant knowledge and the application of this knowledge is clearly a problem in all fields and specialties in nursing, although this gap may be more striking in family nursing. Family-centered nursing also remains a stated ideal rather than prevailing practice. Wright and Leahey (2000) believe that the most important factor creating this gap is "how a nurse conceptualizes health and illness problems. It is the ability to 'think interactionally': from an individual to a family (interactional) level" (p. 15). Other authors point out that technology, economic trends such as downsizing services and staff, the greater diversity within the client population (Bowden, Dickey, & Greenberg, 1998), lack of good comprehensive family assessment tools and intervention strategies, nursing's ties to the medical model (individualistic and disease oriented), and our charting system and nursing diagnostic systems (Hanson, 2001) make incorporation of family-focused care difficult to realize.

- **Practice Issue: The need to make family nursing more feasible to incorporate into practice.** In recent years there has been a dramatic restructuring of health care, which includes the rapid growth of managed care systems wherein complex, multiunit, multilevel systems of health care delivery are being established. Part of this restructuring also involves the trend of patients going home "sicker and quicker" and the downsizing of hosptials, the downsizing of services and staff, and the growth of community-based services. These changes have led to increased job stress and a sense of work overload within the nursing profession. Nurses' time to work with their individual and family clients has been reduced. Thus, it is incumbent on family nurses to develop expedient and effective ways to incorporate family into nursing care. Wright and Leahey (2000) addressed this need by developing a 15-minute or less family interview. Development of realistic, time-saving ideas and strategies to practice family nursing are a key issue in practice today.

- **Practice Issue: Shifting of power and control from the health care provider to the family.** Based on conversations with nurses and writings by family nurses, there is a universal agreement that a shift in power and control from provider to patient/family is needed. This, we believe, still is a central issue in health care today. Wright and Leahey (2000) remind us that there needs to be a greater equality in the relationship between nurses and families, a better collaborative relationship, and more recognition of families' expertise. The consumer movement has influenced patients and families to see themselves as consumers, buying and receiving health care services just like any other service they purchase. The widespread use of the Internet and e-mail has provided many families with information they need to learn about their health problems and treatment options. In light of these trends, family members should be freed to decide what makes sense to them and what they should do on their own behalf (Robinson, 1994).

- **Practice Issue: How to work more effectively with culturally diverse families.** This issue probably receives more attention among health care providers, including nurses, than any other issue today. We live in a pluralistic society, one in which there are many ways to perceive and experience the world, particularly health and illness situations. In its broadest sense, culture (including ethnicity, religious background, social class, regional and political affiliations, sexual orientation, gender, generational differences) shapes our perceptions, values, beliefs, and practices. Other factors, such as experiences with health and illness, shape the way we see things. In spite of all the efforts made to work more effectively with diverse families, providing culturally competent care remains a continuing challenge. Chapter 8 addresses sociocultural aspects of family nursing care.

- **Practice Issue: The globalization of family nursing presents exciting, new opportunities for family nurses.** With the world becoming smaller and smaller due to the process known as *globalization,* family nurses are presented with new and exciting possibilities to learn about the interventions and programs other countries have established to provide better care to families. Globalization is the process by which people and societies become knit together through economic, political, and professional ties. Globalization has had a significant negative impact on health in that the threat of worldwide epidemics such as human immunodeficiency virus/acquired immune deficiency syndrome (HIV/AIDS) is much greater. But on the positive side, the exposure that family nurses in America have with nurses throughout the world via international conferences, travel, and reading of international health literature can be very enlightening. For example, in Japan, the growth of family nursing has been most impressive. There, nurses have developed family nursing curricula in schools of nursing and have generated nursing theory that is family focused and in keeping with Japanese values and context. Family nursing has gathered substantial momentum in nursing in Japan, as evidenced in their publications and research efforts (Sugishita, 1999). Other countries, such as Denmark, Sweden, Israel, Korea, Chile, Mexico, Scotland, and England have also made substantial progress in areas of family health and family nursing. We have much to share and learn from nurses in these countries.

- **Education Issue: What content should be taught in family nursing curricula and how should it be presented?** According to Hanson and Heims (1997) who reported a survey of U.S. nursing schools that they conducted relative to the school's inclusion of family nursing, there has been a growth in the incorporation of family nursing content and clinical skills into baccalaureate and graduate nursing programs. It is still unclear as to what content is appropriate for undergraduate and graduate programs and how clinical skills should be taught. There is no agreement as the foci of undergraduate and graduate programs relative to family nursing. However, there is some consensus that advanced nursing practice in family nursing involves learning the content and skills necessary to work with the whole family and individual family members simultaneously. The advanced practice family nurse is capable of working as a family therapist with troubled families. It is unclear, however, what content and skills are needed in family nursing for those nurses being prepared in other advanced practice programs (clinical nurse specialist and nurse practitioner programs). More discussion of the scope and leveling of content and clinical skills needs to take place.

- **Research Issue: The need to increase family nursing intervention research.** In the area of family nursing, nurse researchers have addressed normative and health-related family transitions and health outcomes. Developmental theory, stress, coping and adaptation theory, family therapy theories, and systems theory have largely guided the work of family nurse researchers. Research has been interdisciplinary, given that "no one discipline owns the family" (Gilliss & Knafl, 1999, p. 245). The real scarcity of nursing research lies in the area of intervention studies. The paucity of intervnetion studies in fam-

ily nursing is "startling," according to Knafl (1998). In her editorial "Wanted: Family Nursing Interventions," Janice Bell (1995), editor of the *Journal of Family Nursing*, laments about the shortage of nursing intervention research manuscripts she is receiving for review. With an inadequate number of intervention studies, we lack the scientific evidence needed to support the efficacy of family nursing strategies and programs. In addition, more true family research is needed; most family nursing research is actually family-related research (focusing on family members), rather than family research (focusing on the whole family as a unit) (Knafl).

- **Policy Issue: The need for family nurses to become more involved in the shaping of policy affecting families.** Hanson (2001a), in discussing the health care reform, urges family nurses to become involved at every level of the political system to advocate for family issues. We would agree with her. Practically all domestic issue legislation at the local, state, or national level has an impact on families. As family advocates we need individually and collectively to analyze the issues and policies being proposed, and to assist in formulating and implementing positive policies and regulations. Supporting candidates for office who are supportive of families and volunteering to serve on health and health-related commissions and organizational boards are other important avenues for "making a difference." We need to advocate for families to have the right to be informed, to understand their rights and options, and to become more skilled in advocating on their own behalf.

FAMILY NURSING GOALS: LEVELS OF PREVENTION

Leavell and associates (1965) developed a framework referred to as levels of prevention. This framework has served as the foundation for practice in public health and community health nursing (Allender & Spradley, 2001). This framework is used here to explain the goals of family nursing. The levels of prevention cover the entire spectrum of health and illness issues as well as the goals appropriate for each of the levels. The three levels are:

1. Primary prevention, which involves health promotion and specific preventive or health protective measures designed to keep people free of disease and injury. Specific preventive measures or health protective behaviors are also called health maintenance.

2. Secondary prevention, consisting of early detection, diagnosis, and treatment.

3. Tertiary prevention, which covers the stage of recovery and rehabilitation, is designed to minimize the client's disability and maximize his or her level of functioning (Figure 2–2) (Leavell et al., 1965; Williams & Torrens, 1999).

The three levels of prevention constitute the major goals of family nursing. They consist of health promotion and maintenance (primary prevention), detection and treatment, and restoration of health. Health promotion is a major thrust of family nursing. Certainly, however, early detection, diagnosis, and treatment (secondary prevention) are also important goals. In addition, tertiary prevention or rehabilitation and restoration of health are especially important goals in family nursing today, given the growth in home health care and the prevalence of chronic disease and disability among our rapidly increasing older population. Table 2–2 presents an example of the use of levels of prevention with one family health problem: family violence and abuse.

PRIMARY PREVENTION: FAMILY HEALTH PROMOTION AND DISEASE PREVENTION

FACTORS LEADING TO RENEWED INTEREST IN PRIMARY PREVENTION

Six important factors that have led to the renewed interest in primary prevention are briefly discussed below (Table 2–3). The first is probably the most important.

NEED FOR A CHANGE IN FOCUS AND NATIONAL INITIATIVES.
In today's health care system, most health resources go toward curative, acute care. Our present health care system spends most of its resources on crisis-oriented and high-tech curative health care, with the treatment given in many cases being too little, too late. In the case of chronic illness—our prevailing cause of morbidity and mortality—we are not treating and eradicating disease, but only minimizing its impact, repairing the damage as much as possible, and treating its complications. We are spending most of our money treating the end result of self-destructive lifestyles rather than focusing on the causative factors of ill health, such as lifestyle and environmental hazards (Ardell & Newman, 1977; Pender, 1996). Only 3 percent of all health care expenditures are for preventive services (Smith & Wesley, 1993).

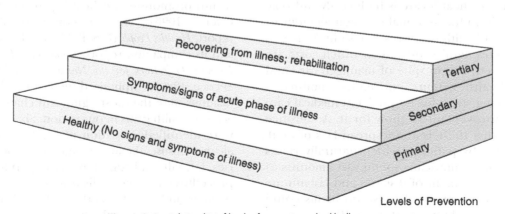

Figure 2–2. Relationship of levels of prevention to health–illness stages.

TABLE 2–2

LEVELS OF PREVENTION

FAMILY VIOLENCE AND ABUSE

Goal: To avoid family violence and abuse and enhance healthy family relationships.

PRIMARY PREVENTION:

Family Health Promotion:	Teaching and counseling family regarding healthy lifestyles including the use of good communication, problem-solving, and negotiating skills with each other. Assisting parents with their parenting skills and in understanding their childrens' growth and developmental needs.
Specific Preventive Measures and Risk Reduction:	Parenting education and support groups; assertiveness training for women; reducing economic strains in family (e.g., adequate employment).

SECONDARY PREVENTION:

Early Diagnosis:	Identifying high risk behaviors in individuals and families. Family nurses must be knowledgeable about the symptoms of abuse (spousal, elder, child).
Prompt Treatment:	Reporting the suspected abuse and encouraging the child, partner/spouse, or elder to go to the appropriate facility for care and documentation of the abuse. Referring the abused to shelters; referring the abuser to anger-management classes; helping the partner(s) to obtain individual, marriage, and/or family therapy, and to participate as needed in substance abuse treatment, AA meetings, or other support groups.

TERTIARY PREVENTION:

Rehabilitation:	The family unit may be changed in composition at this time (partners separated by choice, incarceration, or death). If the family stays together, long-term mental health intervention is needed for all the family. If the family is separated, the family that remains is typically highly emotionally stressed and also needs support and counseling.

There is widespread concern among laypersons, legislators, and health care professionals that the present system of health care is both costly and relatively ineffective. Only minimal cost containment or conservation of health resources is in sight. Managed care is the most significant way in which costs are being contained. Yet, in spite of managed care and integrated health systems, enormous amounts of money are being spent for hospital and medical care with little improvement to show for it. Adherence studies show that there is a widespread lack of medical adherence by patients, which naturally raises costs even more. Americans spend vast amounts of money on the treatment of diseases and last-minute miracles; however, many of these problems could have been prevented for free (Castro, 1991).

Within the last two decades the federal government has taken the leadership in making a shift toward health promotion and health protection (Loveland-Cherry, 1996). The Surgeon General's landmark report, *Healthy People* (U.S. Public Health Service, 1979), and its companion report, *Promoting Health/Preventing Disease: Objectives for the Nation* (U.S. Public Health Service, 1980), emphasized the fact that lifestyle modifications were the most significant changes needed to achieve health gains in our nation. Six lifestyle changes were identified: cessation of smoking; reduction of alcohol misuse; dietary changes to reduce excess calories, fat, salt, and sugar; exercise; periodic screening procedures for major disorders such as high blood pressure and diabetes; and use of seat belts and following speed limits on highways.

TABLE 2–3

FACTORS LEADING TO RENEWED INTEREST IN PRIMARY PREVENTION

1. Need for a change in focus
   - Most health resources are spent on acute care
   - Rising costs have produced minimal evidence of improvement
   - Growth in national efforts to encourage health promotion and disease prevention (e.g., *Healthy People 2000* and *Healthy People 2010* are national initiatives developed to improve the health of the nation).
   - There is greater recognition of the inseparability of mind and body and role of stress in illness and recovery

2. Consumerism and popular demand for increased self-control
3. The wellness movement
4. Growing acceptability of alternative health modalities by health professionals and the public
5. Lack of access to health services
6. Growing emphasis on health in advanced nursing practice
7. Growth in managed care including health maintenance organizations that emphasize providing quality care in a cost-efficient and effective manner

More recent publications such as *Healthy People 2000* (U.S. Department of Health and Human Services, 1991) and *Healthy People 2010* (U.S. Department of Health & Human Services, 2000) continue to influence health care in the direction of health promotion and maintenance activities. These publications represent national initiatives developed by the U.S. Department of Health and Human Services to establish goals and priorities to improve the health of the nation. Priorities are established in the areas of health promotion, risk reduction, and preventive services. Smoking, violence, physical fitness, mental health, occupational safety, environmental health, HIV/AIDS and other sexually transmitted diseases, cancer, and immunizations are major health issues addressed in these documents. In *Healthy People 2010,* the Department of Health and Human Services identifies the need to strengthen the scientific basis for health promotion and disease prevention, as well as increase the government's commitment and provision of services to provide universal quality care. (See Table 2–4.)

Another factor leading to an emphasis on health promotion is a growing realization that mind and boyd are inseparable—each mutually influencing the other—and that an integration of body and mind are needed for recovery and wellness to occur. This recognition has resulted in the incorporation of a holistic approach in both nursing and the mental health professions whereby the whole person is considered in assessment and care (ANA, 1995a).

Along with the awareness of mind–body interaction, the role that stress plays in illness is increasingly acknowledged. It is estimated that 80 percent of all illnesses are stress induced, with stress being responsible for aggravating all illnesses and illnesses aggravating existing stress. Multiple studies have shown the negative role stress plays on an individual's or family's health status (Campbell, 2000; Pelletier, 1979). Because of this, treatment of a client's medical problem alone is often insufficient.

CONSUMERISM AND POPULAR DEMAND FOR INCREASED SELF-CONTROL.

Consumers today are more assertive than in the past (Bomar & McNeely, 1996) and expect to be informed about their medical services and to be given more self-control over their lives. This usually translates into being given sufficient information to be reasonably informed about available options so that they can make their own choices and evaluate services (Zeliff, 2001). The need for greater self-control is

TABLE 2–4

ABOUT *HEALTHY PEOPLE 2010*

Healthy People 2010 is a national initiative that builds on similar initiatives pursued over the past two decades. Two overarching goals of *Healthy People 2010* are (1) to increase the quality and years of healthy life and (2) to eliminate health disparities. These two goals served as a guide for developing objectives in 28 focus areas, each representing an important public health problem. **Leading health indicators** have also been developed. They represent very central, broad public health issues. These are:

Physical Activity
Overweight and Obesity
Tobacco Use
Substance Abuse
Responsible Sexual Behavior
Mental Health
Injury and Violence
Environmental Quality
Immunizations
Access to Health Care

The objectives of this initiative are national, not solely federal, and thus the achievement of the objectives is dependent on widespread participation by citizens and all levels and types of organizations in order to assess progress. Another document, **Tracking Healthy People 2010,** has been developed for this purpose.

Source: U.S. Department of Health and Human Services (2000).

related to present societal values, anti-authority sentiments, and the growing professional value being given to client empowerment, that is, the shifting of decision-making power from the health provider to the client (Labonte, 1989; Zeliff, 2001).

Individuals and families should have control over their own actions. The responsbility for one's health lies not with the health care professional, but with the individual and/or his or her family. Wellness training, holistic health care, and self-care, all part of health promotion, share in the fundamental belief that taking responsibility for and being in control of one's own health are necessities.

There have been unprecedented public disclosures of the inadequacies and inequities of the health care system (Marsa, 2001), which have intensified consumer demand to be in control over one's own health care. The women's movement is an example of successful pressures being applied for participation in their own health care decisions. The women's movement has focused national attention on the infe-

rior or inappropriate health care received by women in a male-dominated system and the paucity of research using female samples. The women's movement has encouraged women to retain control over their health. In addition, the trend toward more primary health care being provided by nurse practitioners, who emphasize teaching and supportive counseling, enhanced the possibility that more control is being transferred from providers to individual and family clients.

THE WELLNESS MOVEMENT.   Since the mid-1970s, there has been increasing interest in and incorporation of healthy lifestyles into the lives of many middle-class and affluent Americans. The wellness movement of the 1970s evolved outside the traditional health system. It was a lay-initiated movement (Armentrout, 1993). Today, a greater value is being placed on health, personal fulfillment, and quality of life. Although the general level of health knowledge in our society is still relatively low, more educated persons, through reading of health-oriented articles and books and exposure to mass media and the Internet, have become well informed about general health promotional strategies and environmental hazards and risks. See Chapter 16 for greater detail on a healthy lifestyle.

GROWING ACCEPTABILITY OF ALTERNATIVE HEALTH MODALITIES BY HEALTH PROFESSIONALS AND THE PUBLIC.

Various alternative health promotion modalities have become respectable in most health care professional circles. As evidence of alternative medicine's growing acceptability, the National Institutes of Health (NIH) have recently created a new Office for Alternative Medicine. Even the most esoteric modalities for stress reduction and pain control are now being looked on as helpful by many health care practitioners. There is much more openness and acceptance of alternative modalities, including yoga, meditation, herbal medicine, massage, relaxation techniques, acupressure, acupuncture, guided imagery, visualization, and body therapies. Many of these approaches to health emphasize health promotion, holism, and client empowerment (Rodwell, 1996).

Many consumers—who are increasingly from cultures where alternative medicine is the convention—are turning to herbal medicine, Eastern medical modalities, and other holistic health approaches, which promote and restore health (Picker, 1996). The *New England Journal of Medicine*, for example, reported that one third of Americans visited at least one alternative practitioner in 1990 (McCall, 1996).

LACK OF ACCESS TO HEALTH SERVICES.

There is some evidence that as health services have become more inaccessible because of lack of insurance and high cost, consumers are turning more to health promotion and disease prevention self-care strategies. Thus, an impetus to self-care may arise from situations where professional health services are not readily available or accessible. Approximately 44.3 million persons lacked health insurance in 1998, a continual increase in the number of uninsured individuals in the United States (U.S. Department of Health and Human Services, 2000). It is unclear, however, how many of these uninsured individuals use self-care for health promotion and maintenance in addition to using self-care to treat common primary health care problems.

GROWING EMPHASIS ON HEALTH IN ADVANCED NURSING PRACTICE.

Health professionals, particularly advanced practice nurses, are being socialized to incorporate health promotion and disease prevention as integral and necessary parts of their nursing care. Nurse practitioners actively engage in a wide array of health promotion and maintenance activities. More nurses are assuming positions in community-based, primary care settings where health promotion and disease prevention can be addressed effectively in practice (Rodgers, 1993).

FAMILY HEALTH PROMOTION

A primary goal of family nursing is health promotion of the family as a whole and of each of its members (Bomar, 1996; Hartrick, Lindsey, & Hills, 1994). Health behaviors, values, and attitudes are learned in the family (Crooks, Iammarino, & Weinberg, 1987; Pender, 1996). One of the basic functions of the family is the health care function, the purpose of which is to meet family members' health needs. Because teaching of healthy behaviors in the family context is typically more effective than teaching individuals, it is perhaps a most important health promotion strategy (Rankin & Stallings, 2001).

Health promotion is one of the two components of primary prevention (Leavell et al., 1965). A clear distinction needs to be made between health promotion and disease prevention (preventive measures and risk appraisal/reduction) (Tripp & Stachowiak, 1992). Health promotion is not disease or health problem specific. It is designed to contribute to the growth, enlargement, or excellence of health. It is a positive, dynamic process that focuses on improving the quality of life and well-being, not merely avoiding disease (Pender, 1996). Health promotion involves "approach" behaviors consisting of a number of actions and activities whose end is high-level wellness (Dunn, 1961).

In contrast, disease prevention is disease or health problem specific and involves "avoidance" of risk behaviors as well as specific preventive or protective measures like immunizations. Both health promotion and disease prevention are important goals, and are complementary to each other (Duncan & Gold, 1986; Pender, 1996).

Family health promotion involves both promoting family members' health and promoting family system health (Loveland-Cherry, 1988, 1996). In the former case the emphasis is on the individual family members in the context of the family, while in the latter case the focus is health promotion of the family system both internally and in interaction with its external interaction systems, such as the social welfare or educational systems. Here the goals are the promotion of the health of the family unit.

Practically all the health-promotion literature deals with the individual rather than the family unit. Nevertheless, health promotion can be easily applied to the family as a whole. Because the family is a small interactional system, it means, however, that different areas need to be assessed (such as family functioning, family dynamics, communication patterns, parent–child relationships, and the family's interaction with the community) and different strategies applied. Refer to Chapter 1 for a review of the characteristics of healthy families. These characteristics are the behaviors and attitudes that we need to encourage families to acquire or maintain—given, of course, that they are mutually valued by and appropriate for the family in question. In the family assessment and intervention chapters that follow, health promotion of the family system is incorporated.

Health promotion and primary prevention of acute and chronic health problems pose the greatest health challenge to our society. Perhaps our most important goal should be to assist people (individuals and families) to learn how to be healthy in a natural, enjoyable way, rather than just focusing on assisting clients about how not to get sick, or worse yet, assisting clients only when they are sick. Harteck (1997) adds another significant idea about the role of the family nurse. She states that our practice should emphasize the capacity within families to promote their own health and healing.

IMPEDIMENTS TO PRIMARY PREVENTION

Although there has been a substantial growth in professional and public commitment to primary prevention, certain factors have created major impediments or obstacles to the incorporation of primary prevention, particularly family-focused health promotion, and health protection efforts in all sectors of society.

A major impediment is money or, more accurately, how we chose collectively to spend our money. Lack of third-party reimbursement for family assessments and interventions and for health promotion and preventive activities creates a situation whereby only the more affluent or the very needy can afford to obtain professional help or access to the needed health education and counseling.

A second obstacle is the attitudes and socialization of physicians and nurses in the United States. We are still very illness-oriented and often pay only lip service to the importance of disease prevention and health promotion. The medical model is still the dominant model for practice, policy making, and funding. The adherence of health professionals to the medical model—in which health and illness are looked on as discrete, separate entities and the client is seen as a set of physiological systems—has led us and society (the consumers) to view health care primarily in terms of curative medical care. Individuals, when ill, "turn themselves over" to health providers. There has been little encouragement or reward from health care professionals for assuming self-responsibility for staying well or striving to improve one's total functioning.

A third obstacle is the fact that many health care professionals act as poor role models for their clients. These professionals often are sedentary, overweight, and under apparent stress; thus, they are not in a position to speak effectively about improving anyone's lifestyle. They do not ask about the family, do not view their client as the family, and do not recognize the reciprocal impact of family and health/illness. Thus, the psychosocial and family factors involved in health care are given insufficient attention (Doherty & Campbell, 1988; Campbell, 2000).

Other obstacles to primary prevention are our materialistic value system; the presence of social problems such as inadequate health care, employment, and educational opportunities for stigmatized members of society (e.g., the poor, minorities, senior citizens); and widespread environmental hazards (e.g., air and water pollution and exposure to toxic substances) extant in our communities.

Primary prevention, in addition to health promotion, involves maintaining and improving the level of individual and family resistance to particular diseases. This is accomplished through the institution of specific preventive measures. Risk appraisal and risk reduction methods are also ways to decrease the possibility that a client will acquire specific illnesses or diseases.

SPECIFIC PREVENTIVE MEASURES

Increasing resistance to social, emotional, and biological forces that precipitate disease is a goal of primary prevention. A healthy lifestyle should enhance this resistance. (This is covered in more depth in Chapter 16.) Nevertheless, disease prevention is also needed. Prevention involves a defensive set of actions that ward off specific illness conditions or their sequelae (Pender, 1996). Specific preventive measures are part of disease prevention. Examples of specific preventive measures are immunizations and fluoride treatment.

RISK APPRAISAL/RISK REDUCTION

Because most people are concerned more with the threat of illness than with their health, the concept of risk has become part of our thinking about disease prevention. "Risk" implies that the probability of adverse consequences is increased by the presence of one or more characteristics or factors (Backett, Davies, & Petros-Barvazian, 1984). Risk, then, is a probability or statistical measure—the probability of a future occurrence. When the probability of the occurrence of an injury, disease, or death can be reduced or nullified if an anticipatory action is taken, then this action uses the risk approach at an individual or family level (Backett, Davies, & Petros-Barvazian, 1984).

Epidemiological studies have provided the empirical database for making predictions of risk to acquire certain health problems. Given these databases, one of the most popular ways in which primary prevention is practiced is by determining short- and long-term risks to which a client is exposed via a risk appraisal tool and then prescribing measures to reduce the client's risk factors. Determination of clients' risks is usually handled by use of one of three health risk appraisal approaches: (1) a health hazard appraisal tool (see Tables 2–5 and 2–6), (2) clinical guidelines and recommendations for preventive services, or (3) wellness appraisals or inventories (Stanhope & Lancaster, 2001).

Using a health hazard appraisal tool, as shown in Tables 2–5 and 2–6, the total personal risks to a client are estimated by identifying the average risk for the major causes of disease/death in the client's own age, sex, and racial group. From this the provider can (a) develop a prognosis for the well client; (b) estimate those causes most likely to bring about disease/death; and (c) recommend lifestyle changes, specific protective measure, and health treatments to reduce risk.

Clinical guidelines have grown in acceptance and are used widely by nurse pratitioners to delivering primary health promotion. The most widely used of clinical guidelines for health promotion is the U.S. Public Services Task Force publication, *A Guide to Clinical Preventive Services* (1989, 1995). The guidelines within this publication are based on sound scientific evidence and were the work of an expert panel. The guidelines direct primary care providers on what to do regarding health promotion and include specific preventive measures, such as immunizations, screening, physical examination, counseling, and teaching guidelines. To ensure that the above guidelines were widely and effectively used, the U.S. Public Health Service established the "Put Prevention into Practice" program and, as part of this initiative, developed a kit of materials designed to improve the delivery of preventive services. The *Put Prevention into Practice Education and Action Kit* (U.S. Public Health Service, 1994) is very valuable to health care providers, health care systems, and consumers.

Wellness appraisal or inventories, the third type of risk appraisal tool, differs from the other two types of risk appraisal tools in that they define risks more broadly (not specific to a particular disease/problem). They strongly advocate for client empowerment. A typical wellness inventory is that of Ardell (1982), which includes an inventory related to self-responsibility, nutritional awareness, physical fitness, stress management, and environmental sensitivity.

FAMILY'S ROLE IN PRIMARY PREVENTION

Families have been found to be the most important source of help for American adults who have changed their lifestyles to a more wellness-oriented one. A Gallup national survey in 1985 confirmed that when it comes to health matters, most people get more help from their family than any other source, even their doctor (Gurin, 1985). Moreover, the family plays a significant role as to the extent to which family members are exposed to risks (Campbell, 2000). The

TABLE 2–5

HEALTH HAZARD APPRAISAL TOOL: INDIVIDUAL CLIENT

Name: John Doe
Age: 43
Race and Gender: White male
Occupation: Small businessman

RANK— DISEASE/INJURY	PROGNOSTIC CRITERIA	CLIENT FINDINGS	RECOMMENDATIONS
1. Arteriosclerotic heart disease	Blood pressure	120/70	Reduce saturated fats, calories, and red meats; prescribe lovastatin 10 mg daily.
	Cholesterol level	280	
	Diabetes	No	
	Exercise	Sedentary—none	Initiate regular exercise program.
	Family history	None	
	Smoking	2 packs a day for 20 years	Referred to stop-smoking clinic.
	Weight	200 lb (5 ft 10 in)	Weight reduction diet. Reduce to 165 lb.
2. Auto accidents	Alcohol	Drinks occasionally (socially); no automobile accidents	
	Drugs	None	
	Mileage	30,000/year	
	Seat belts	Occasional use	Recommended to always use seat belts in car.
3. Suicide	Depression	None observed, client denies	
	Family history	Negative	
4. Cirrhosis of liver	Alcohol use	Social occasions only	

Adapted in part from Edelman & Mandle (1986); Robbins & Hall (1970).

family discourages or encourages risk behaviors such as smoking, alcohol use, seat belt use, good or poor nutrition and exercise, and so forth.

In summary, primary prevention—health promotion and disease prevention—is a primary thrust of family nursing. Family nurses should help families take responsibility for their own health and incorporate wellness lifestyle changes into both their family's lifestyle and their members' personal lives. The family continues to play a crucial role in helping its members learn new ways to live more healthy lives. By believing in families' abilities to provide their own self-health care and to act in their own best interests, we will provide positive support and more effectively become resource persons and facilitators to families. Thus, primary prevention is a most exciting and vital

role for family nurses. Primary care is an important instrument for achieving a stronger emphasis on primary prevention (Donaldson, Yordy, & Vanselow, 1994). Primary care providers (nurse practitioners and community-based nurses) are particularly well placed to provide family health promotion and health protection in their practice (Broering, 1993). Fortunately, the emphasis on this role is becoming more pronounced in practice (Venegoni, 1995), education, and research.

Primary prevention emphasis is particularly crucial in working with school-aged children and young families. Nurses in school settings have great occasion to teach primary prevention to their student clients and their families. Intervening with this population gives nurses the opportunity not only to help prevent the

TABLE 2—6

HEALTH HAZARD APPRAISAL TOOL: FAMILY CLIENT

Family Name:	Sawyer
Developmental Stage:	Family with preschool children
Race/Ethnicity:	African-American
Family Form:	Two-parent nuclear family
Family Composition:	Husband, 27; wife, 25; son, 3; daughter, 13 months
Parents' Occupation:	Both full-time high school teachers

COMMON HEALTH PROBLEMS	PROGNOSTIC CRITERIA	FAMILY FINDINGS	RECOMMENDATIONS
1. Marital relationship strains	Poverty Wife battering History of family instability Social isolation	Mother reports husband and she co-parent children and have active church and social network.	
2. Sibling rivalry	Sibling fighting Acting out by older sibling(s)	Older son occasionally resentful of parents' attention to baby sister.	Spend time alone with older son everyday. Encourage him to help care for his little sister.
3. Developmental lag(s)—Lack of growth and developmental information	Slowed development Parental expectations are incongruent with child's developmental age Poverty	Parents are well informed. Children's development is within normal limits.	

onset of health-damaging risk behaviors but to discourage health-compromising behaviors that may be less firmly established as part of a lifestyle. Early intervention provides an opportunity to introduce, reinforce, and help further establish healthy lifelong patterns.

SECONDARY PREVENTION

Secondary prevention involves early diagnosis and prompt treatment. Thus, detection of disease and case finding are keys to secondary prevention. If the nature of the disease precludes cure, then the goal is to control the progression of the disease and prevent or reduce disability. One important role of the nurse is to conduct screenings and assessments (histories, physicals, laboratory tests) of family members or to refer family members to providers to obtain these services.

Secondary prevention from a family standpoint, involves detection of family pathology or dysfunction. An obvious case is the case of family abuse, as seen in Table 2–2. Other examples of family "maladaptation" include the family's engaging in dysfunctional coping strategies (as discussed in Chapter 17), such as scapegoating of a family member or denial of a serious health problem in the family; and prolonged unclear communication problems in the family, leading family members to be estranged from each other. Some of these family problems may be successfully managed by a family nurse. In the case of more serious family problems, however, the treatment will probably need to be handled by a family therapist or advanced practice nurse specializing in family systems nursing.

Health teaching is often needed to enhance family members' understanding of the importance of certain screening tests, such as breast self-examinations or Papanicolaou (Pap) smears for women. Careful referral and follow-up are also part of secondary prevention.

TERTIARY PREVENTION

The goal of tertiary prevention is to "reduce the extent and severity of a health problem to its lowest possible level to minimize disability and restore or preserve function" (Allender & Spradley, 2001, p. 11) and well-being. Rehabilitation is the primary focus of tertiary prevention. Recovery and maintenance care for chronically ill people are also included under this rubric. Rehabilitation involves restoring individuals disabled by disease or injury to a level of functioning optimal for them—or to their highest level of functioning—physically, socially, emotionally, and vocationally.

Lorraine Wright (1997), the most outstanding family systems nurse and author of our time, asserts that her goal in her clinical work with families consists of alleviating or healing emotional, physical, or spiritual suffering (p. 7). Certainly, this goal is part of tertiary prevention even though it is expressed in a much more qualitative, phenomenological manner.

In learning to live with a permanent disability, the client and family need tremendous support and extensive teaching of self and dependent care. The nurse plays central roles in tertiary prevention, particularly in view of the growth of chronic illness and disability home health care. In addition to direct caregiving, the family nurse's most significant roles are that of coordinator or case manager, client/family advocate, teacher, and counselor.

SUMMARY

This chapter presents an overview of family nursing—its past, its present, and recommendations for its future. The following are key points made in the chapter.

- Family nursing is a growing, yet still relatively young, specialty area of nursing that cuts across various areas of nursing.

- The way family nursing is practiced depends on how the family nurse conceptualizes the family and works with it, as well as the philosophy of the system within which the nurse functions.

- There are five ways in which family nurses conceptualize and work with families. These are described as (a) the family as context; (b) the family as a sum of its members; (c) the family subsystem as client; (d) the family as client; and (e) the family as a component of society. Family as client is viewed as uniquely family nursing.

- Family nursing in this text is defined as the provision of care to families and family members in health and illness situations. It is distinguished from both family-centered community health nursing and family therapy or family systems nursing.

- The American Nurses Association in its numerous "standards of care" publications typically included family as context and client, although in this latter instance the emphasis varied. Pediatric clinical nursing practice and community-based practice standards (home health care and public health nursing) promulgated family nursing as a vital component of practice. The Association for the Care of Children's Health, in their standards, strongly endorsed a family-centered approach in care of children.

- The historical legacy of family nursing was briefly sketched, showing the decline and regrowth of family-focused care in the United States.

- Four specialty areas of nursing have had a long involvement with families—parent–child health, community health, psychiatric–mental health, and family and pediatric nurse practitioners.

- Family nursing has seen a regrowth due to increased attention on health promotion, our aging population, and increased prevalence of chronic illness; the growing awareness of the pervasiveness of troubled families; the marriage and family movement; and the growth and acceptance of family-based theories and research.

- Current issues in family nursing were discussed, including the significant gap between knowledge and practice; the need to make family nursing more practical to incorporate into practice; the shifting of power from provider to family; the challenge of how to work more effectively with culturally diverse families; the challenge of globalization in family nursing; what should be taught about family nursing in the various types of nursing programs; and the need for family nurses to become more involved in influencing policies impacting families.

- The goals of family nursing were described within the three levels of prevention framework. These levels of prevention are: primary prevention (health promotion and disease prevention), secondary prevention, and tertiary prevention. Definitions of these levels and application to family health are discussed.

- Factors that have led to renewed interest in primary prevention include the shift in focus toward health promotion that has been fostered by the development of national initiatives. *Healthy People 2010* is the most important and recent of these major health promotion and disease prevention publications. Six other factors that have encouraged the growing importance of health promotion are also discussed.

- A primary thrust and goal of family nursing is health promotion of the family as a whole and of each of its members. Family health promotion involves assisting families to develop healthy lifestyles and to improve the quality of their life and well-being, whereas disease prevention encourages families to curtail exposure to certain risks and to take specific action to avoid certain health problems.

- In addition to factors that favor the growth of primary prevention, there are also impediments to health promotion, such as how we as a society allocate our health dollars/resources; the socialization of health care providers toward disease rather than health, and poor role modeling by health care providers.

- Clients' risks are determined by three different types of approaches: (a) health hazard appraisal tools; (b) clinical guidelines and recommendations for preventive services; and (c) wellness inventories.

- Family members are found to be the most significant source of support and assistance in helping other family members change their lifestyles. Hence, health teaching is more effective when family centered.

- Secondary prevention, involving the early diagnosis and treatment of individual and family problems, and tertiary prevention, involving the rehabilitation of family members and the family, are also important goals of family nursing. With our aging population and the increased need for caregiving in the home, tertiary prevention, as a goal of family nursing, assumes greater importance.

❧ FAMILY VIGNETTE: THE BOWMAN FAMILY

Charlie Bowman, age 25, is being seen by the home health nurse who has been monitoring Charlie's recovery from pneumonia and his antiretroviral therapy for AIDS. Charlie has been hospitalized three times for pneumonia, his last hospitalization being very recent. According to his family he has been wrestling with the ups and downs of the disease since he was diagnosed five years ago. He has experienced many complications of AIDS and "side effects" of the drugs, such as nausea, vomiting, wasting, hives, and losing his sense of taste completely. Right now, still recovering from pneumonia, he is feeling very tired and hasn't been able to muster the energy to be totally compliant in regards to following his complex drug regime. When the home health nurse asked Charlie who his family is, he stated that it is his partner, Steve, with whom he has lived the last four years, and his mother. Steve and Charlie have a very stable and committed relationship, and Charlie's mother often comes over to help and offer support. No one in the family has participated in a support group, although Charlie knows of these groups from friends who had AIDS before him and are now gone.

▦ STUDY QUESTIONS

Review the Family Vignette and answer the related questions.

1. In this situation, what would be the role of the family-centered home health nurse?
2. What goals relative to the three levels of prevention are appropriate here?
3. What challenges does this family pose for the family nurse?

Answer the following questions.

4. One major difference between the five types of family nursing practice is:
   a. The setting in which family nursing is practiced
   b. The conceptualization of the family
   c. The specialty area of the nurse
   d. None of the above
5. What are the differences between family nursing and family systems nursing, as defined by Wright, Leahey, and Bell? (Select all correct answers.)
   a. Family systems nursing deals simultaneously with two or more systems.
   b. Family systems nursing is more concerned with cause-and-effect relationships.
   c. Family systems nursing represents advanced nursing practice in the family nursing specialty area.
   d. Family systems nursing is theoretically based in developmental theory and social learning theory.

6. What is the different mission of the family-centered community health nurse versus the family-centered nurse working in other settings?

7. Which of the following statements is/are true about the levels of prevention? The levels:

   a. Specifically identify the nurse's role only in the prevention of disease
   b. Cover the entire spectrum of health and disease
   c. Identify goals for each of the three levels of prevention
   d. Are generally synonymous with preventive, curative, and rehabilitative phases of health care

Match the correct level of prevention from the right-hand column (items 8–16) with the description in the left-hand column.

8. Case finding   a. Primary prevention

9. Health promotion   b. Secondary prevention

10. Specific preventive measures   c. Tertiary prevention

11. Early detection and treatment

12. Convalescence

13. Minimizing the complications of the disease

14. Rehabilitation

15. Disease prevention

16. Risk appraisal and reduction

17. The family as client is an integral part of the ANA standards of practice in *two* specialty areas in nursing. Which are these?

   a. Rehabilitation nursing
   b. Medical–surgical nursing
   c. Psychiatric–mental health nursing
   d. Community health nursing
   e. Pediatric clinical nursing practice
   f. Family nurse practitioners

18. Identify four factors that have led to increased interest and involvement in primary prevention.

19. Which of the following six factors is most important relative to impeding the growth of primary prevention?

   a. Society's materialistic value system
   b. The presence of social problems in communities (poor educational systems, etc.)
   c. The way in which resources are allocated
   d. Attitudes and socialization of health care providers
   e. Many health care professionals act as poor role models
   f. Widespread environmental hazards

20. What is the purpose of the three types of risk appraisal tools?

21. Why is the risk approach used in health care today?

22. How does the meaning of family health differ from the meaning of health? What factors would a family nurse assess related to health promotion?

23. Why is health promotion considered a primary thrust of family nursing?

24. Teaching and supportive counseling of the caregiver of a chronically ill spouse at home is an example of activities that are part of what level of prevention?

two

THEORETICAL FOUNDATIONS OF FAMILY NURSING

The theoretical foundations for family nursing practice are described in Part II. Theoretical perspectives used in family nursing are reviewed in Chapter 3. Although family social science and family therapy theories still form the basis for most of family nursing practice to date, notable progress is being made to reformulate family theories to fit a nursing perspective and to use nursing theories in family nursing practice. Chapters 4 through 6 present the three theories that are the primary basis for the Friedman Family Assessment Model (see Appendices A and B for the complete model). These three theoretical perspectives are structural–functional theory (Chapter 4), family developmental theory (Chapter 5), and systems theory (Chapter 6).

THEORETICAL FOUNDATIONS FOR FAMILY NURSING

CONTENT OUTLINE

LEARNING OBJECTIVES

1. Explain the conceptual sources and functions of theory in family nursing.
2. Describe selected nursing models and their application to family nursing practice.
3. Summarize the current state of the art for theory development in family nursing.
4. Describe selected family social science theories and how each contributes to family nursing practice.
5. Describe family therapy theories and how they contribute to family nursing practice.
6. Identify the theoretical legacy of three integrated family systems nursing models.

The purpose of this chapter is to provide a basic grounding in the major theoretical/conceptual foundations for family nursing theory, family nursing practice, and family nursing research (Table 3–1). Conceptual models and theories are necessary to guide family nursing practice and research. This background is even more critical with respect to family nursing because thinking interactionally and systematically in family nursing requires a paradigm shift from the individual-as-client approach to that of family as client.

CONCEPTUAL SOURCES AND FUNCTIONS OF THEORY IN FAMILY NURSING

The function of theory is to characterize, explain, or predict phenomena evident within nursing. Thus, nursing theories ideally represent logical and intelligible patterns for observations within nursing practice (Fawcett & Downs, 1992). The relationship of theory to practice constitutes a dynamic feedback loop rather than a static linear progression. That is, family nursing theory informs practice, and family practice, in turn, facilitates the development of family nursing theory. And, research questions in family nursing may be drawn from family nursing practice or derived from family nursing theory. Thus, theory, practice, and research in family nursing are related in synergistic patterns to advance the discipline of nursing.

The terms conceptual model and theory are often used interchangeably due, in part, to lack of consensus about what degree of specificity distinguishes a conceptual model or framework from a theory. A conceptual model "is a set of relatively abstract and general concepts and the propositions that describe or link those concepts" (Fawcett, 1999, p. 3). A *concept* is a "word or phrase that summarizes the essential characteristics or properties of a phenomenon" (Fawcett, p. 1) and a *proposition* is "a statement about a concept or the relations between concepts." The "family" is an example of a concept that should be in any conceptual model for family nursing. Propositions are state-

ments that describe or link concepts. For example, the statement "the family interacts with the community" is a proposition linking the concepts of "interaction," "family," and "community."

A theory is also composed of concepts with propositions explaining the relationships among the concepts. However, a theory is typically less abstract than a conceptual model or framework. Theories focus on more specific situations than conceptual models, and the relationships among the concepts in a theory are better developed than in conceptual models. For purposes of this chapter, however, the terms will be used interchangeably.

There has been a substantial amount of cross-fertilization among the theories used in family nursing practice. Many of the concepts incorporated in nursing models were borrowed or adapted from preexisting theories in sociology, anthropology, psychology, and physiology with new applications to nursing. Likewise, contemporary family social science and family therapy theories derive many of their key concepts and propositions from earlier work in developmental psychology, symbolic interactionism, and structural–functional theory. There is no singular theory/conceptual framework from nursing, family social science, or family therapy that fully describes the relationships and dynamics of family life and for family nursing. One theoretical perspective does not give nurses a sufficiently broad knowledge on which to assess and intervene with families. Hence, nurses must draw upon multiple theories to work effectively with families. Thus, an integrated approach is necessary for the theory, practice, research, and education of family nursing (Figure 3–1).

Of the three genres of theory, family social science theories are the most well developed and informative with respect to how families function, the environment–family interchange, interactions within the family, how the family changes over time, and the family's reaction to health and illness. One striking limitation in using the family social science theories in family nursing is that their clinical application is parsimonious, although recent work has made some strides toward greater application to family nursing practice.

Family therapy theories, although less developed than family social science theories, are more relevant to family nursing practice because they emanate from a professional/practice heritage rather than acade-

TABLE 3–1

THEORETICAL APPROACHES USED IN FAMILY NURSING PRACTICE

NURSING THEORIES/CONCEPTUAL MODELS

Systems orientation
- Neuman's health systems model

Developmental orientation
- Orem's self-care model

Systems and interactional orientations
- Roy's adaptation model

- King's interacting systems model

Systems and developmental orientations
- Rogers's science of unitary human beings model
- Newman's expanding consciousness model
- Nightingale's environmental model

FAMILY SOCIAL SCIENCE THEORIES

Developmental theory

Systems theory

Structural–functional theory

Interactional/Communications theory

Family Stress theory

Change theory

Others:
- Conflict theory
- Social exchange theory
- Multicultural theory

FAMILY THERAPY THEORIES

Structural family therapy theory

Family systems therapy theory

Interactional/Communications family therapy theory

Others:
- Psychodynamic therapy theory

- Experiential therapy theory
- Strategic therapy theory
- Behavioral therapy theory
- Solution-oriented therapy theory
- Narrative therapy theory

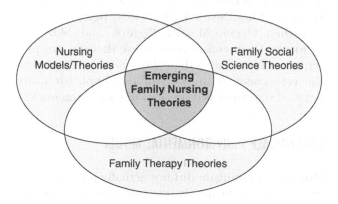

Figure 3–1. Conceptual source of family nursing theories.

mic disciplines, such as family social science. The foundation for many of the family therapy theories is family social science theories. Family nursing theory, practice, and research currently draw more from family therapy theories as the profession grows more sophisticated within the specialty of family nursing. Family therapy models are also more applicable to advanced nursing practice. Whall (1986b) urged family nurse therapists to reformulate existing family therapy theories to fit the nursing perspective in accordance with nursing theory.

Finally, of all three genres of theories, nursing models/theories are the least developed in regard to family nursing. (See Table 3–2 for differences between the three genres of theory.) The metaparadigm for the discipline of nursing consists of four concepts—person, environment, health, and nursing—together with three propositions, which explain the relationships among the four key concepts:

1. Nursing is concerned with the principles and laws that govern the life process, well-being, and optimal function of human beings, sick or well.

2. Nursing is concerned with the patterning of human behavior in interaction with the environment in normal life events and critical life situations.

3. Nursing is concerned with the processes by which positive changes in health status are effected (Whall & Fawcett, 1991b, p. 3).

The concept of person referred originally to the individual client. However, the concept of person or client can be redefined to include individual, family, and/or community as the client and the recipient of nursing care (American Nurses Association [ANA], 1995a). In fact, the concept of family as client has been accepted in the nursing discipline as is evidenced in the literature from 1950 (Whall & Fawcett, 1991a), in the ANA Social Policy Statement (1995a), and the various ANA's Standards of Clinical Nursing Practice (see Chapter 2 for details).

Whall and Fawcett (1991b) adapted the nursing metaparadigm propositions to address family:

1. Family [nursing] is concerned with the principles and laws that govern family process, family well-being, and optimum function of families in various states of illness and wellness.

2. Family [nursing] is concerned with the patterning of family behavior in interaction with the environment, in normal life events and critical life situations.

3. Family [nursing] is concerned with the processes by which positive changes in family health status may be affected (Donaldson & Crowley, 1978; Gordner, 1980, cited by Whall & Fawcett, 1991b, pp. 3–4).

Whall and Fawcett (1991a) suggested that family is articulated differently in the metaparadigm of nursing from other disciplines that address the family in terms of the following three aspects:

1. Considering environmental influences on family health and the effect of actions taken by nurses on behalf of or in conjunction with the family

2. Incorporating comprehensive biopsychosocial or holistic perspective of health

3. Focusing on family well-being, rather than pathology (p. 4)

Some nursing theorists have revised their original theories to accommodate nursing care for families and other aggregates (such as communities) as the nursing client. The remainder of this chapter presents each of the three genres of theories that are significant to evolving family nursing theories. First, nursing models applicable to family nursing are summarized, and then the dominant family social science theories central to family nursing are highlighted. Three significant family therapy theories informing family nursing are then presented, and finally, an overview of selected integrated models are discussed.

NURSING CONCEPTUAL MODELS APPLICABLE TO FAMILY NURSING

The development of nursing models and theories has profoundly influenced the discipline of nursing, beginning with Florence Nightingale's writings and continuing with the work of contemporary nursing theorists. Nursing models specifically suited to family nursing practice include those developed by Imogene King, Sister Callista Roy, Betty Neuman, Dorothea Orem, Martha Rogers, and Margaret Newman. Distinct aspects of these theories are presented in historical order. The reader is referred to the references at the end of this book for more detailed resources and specifics of each framework.

NIGHTINGALE'S ENVIRONMENTAL MODEL

Florence Nightingale did not actually present a theory of nursing or family nursing. Nevertheless, she acknowledged the family in many of her writings and

TABLE 3–2

DIFFERENCES AMONG NURSING THEORIES, FAMILY SOCIAL SCIENCE THEORIES, AND FAMILY THERAPY THEORIES

CRITERIA	NURSING THEORIES	FAMILY SOCIAL SCIENCE THEORIES	FAMILY THERAPY THEORIES
Purpose of theory	Descriptive and prescriptive (practice models); guide nursing assessment and intervention efforts	Descriptive and explanatory (academic models); explain family functioning and dynamics	Descriptive and prescriptive (practice models); explain fully dysfunction and guide therapeutic actions
Discipline focus	Nursing focus	Interdisciplinary (although primarily sociological)	Marriage and family therapy and family mental health
Target population	Primarily those families with health and illness problems	Primarily "normal" families (normality oriented)	Primarily "troubled" families (pathology oriented)

Adapted from Jones & Dimond (1982).

in much of her nursing practice (Nightingale, 1859). Lobo (1995) referred to Nightingale's approach to nursing as an environmental model, consistent with Nightingale's emphasis on the importance of environmental factors in health and illness. For example, she wrote (Nightingale, 1859/1992), "Badly constructed houses do for the healthy what badly constructed hospitals do for the sick. Once . . . the air in a house is stagnant, sickness is certain to follow" (p. 15) Nightingale promoted both nurse-midwifery and home-based health services and wrote "Notes on Nursing" for women charged with caring for ill family members and maintaining health of children at home. In a document entitled "Training Nurses for the Sick Poor"(Nightingale, 1949), she admonished nurses to engage in both sick nursing and health nursing in the home environment. She appeared to have given both home health nurses and maternal–child nurses the charge to carry out nursing practice with the whole family as the unit of service (1949). Nightingale made many efforts to encourage laywomen to provide good nursing care in their homes concurrently with her efforts to create training programs for "professional" nurses. She may have agreed with some contemporary writing distinguishing between nursing as an action and nursing as a profession and a distinct discipline. For example, Moules (2000) reflected on the loving nursing care given to a terminally ill woman in her home by lay caregivers: "These caregivers are not nurses, but they know how to nurse . . ." (p. 4) "These caregivers might not have had theory, they still had heart" (p. 6). Moules believes theory-based practice is important, but that family nurses "are obligated to look at families' lives, not simply to gaze at them in some removed way but to enter into their suffering, joys, deaths, and illnesses" (p. 6).

KING'S THEORY OF GOAL ATTAINMENT

Imogene King (1981, 1987) developed a transaction process model of interacting systems called the Theory of Goal Attainment. In King's (1981) model, the goal of nursing is to "help individuals maintain their health so they can function in their roles" (pp. 4–5). King's model focuses on the nurse–patient interaction, which is the forum for identifying the individual's goals, problems, and concerns. Throughout the process, the nurse and individual collaborate to achieve the goals they have set together. In her earliest works, King included a family-as-context approach. King's concept of individual client can be expanded to include family as her model includes concepts relevant to families, such as perception, interaction, communication, transaction, space, time, growth and development, and stress (Whall & Fawcett, 1991a). King broadly defined family as a small group of individuals bound together for the socialization of its members and to transmit values and norms of behavior across the life span (King, 1983; Frey & Sieloff, 1995). The family was viewed as both an interpersonal and a social system. King's model has been used to guide nursing practice focusing on family care. As early as 1989, nurses were utilizing King's model in care of families. King's model guided Sirles and Selleck (1989) in describing the impact of cardiac disease on the family social system. More recently, Norris and Hoyer (1993) used King's model to plan strategies for improving interactions between neonatal intensive care unit (NICU) nurses and parents, consistent with a philosophy of family-centered care.

ROY'S ADAPTATION MODEL

Sister Callista Roy's Adaptation Model (1976) conceptualized the individual as an adaptive system interacting with stimuli via four response modes: physiological, self-concept, role function, and interdependence. According to Roy, nursing care focuses on the person's response to interactions with the external environment and to internal and external stimuli affecting adaptation. In Roy's original work (1976), the family was viewed as the context for the individual. Later, Roy and Roberts (1981) altered this family-as-context conceptualization to the "family as an adaptive system that, like the individual, has inputs, internal control and feedback processes, and output" (Whall & Fawcett, 1991a, p. 23). Roy explained that the family, as well as the individual, group, social organization, and community, may be the unit of analysis and a focus of nursing practice. McCubbin and Figley (1983) suggested that the concept of coping in Roy's model could easily be broadened to the family unit, where ineffective family coping patterns lead to family functioning problems. Moreover, Roy's theory stressed health promotion and the importance of assisting clients in manipulating their environment, consistent with environmental–family interactions emphasized in family nursing.

The usefulness and popularity of Roy's model is evident in the Boston-Based Adaptation Research in Nursing Society (BBARNS), founded to promote collegiality and collaborative projects among nursing scholars who work from Roy's model (Pollack, Frederickson, Carson, Mawssey, & Roy, 1994). Examples of research framed with Roy's Adaptation Model include Zhan's (2000) study of cognitive adaptation and self-consistency in hearing-impaired older persons and Jones and Badger's (1991) study of internal body image among deaf and hearing children. Recently, Hanna and Roy (2001) discussed the continuing development of Roy's model in relation to family nursing and noted that family may be conceptualized as the context for the individual or the family may be conceptualized as relational persons or groups.

NEUMAN'S HEALTH SYSTEMS MODEL

The Neuman Health Care Systems Model views the client as an open system, which engages in reciprocal exchange with the environment. The open system may be an individual, group, family, community, or any aggregate (Neuman, 1982, 1995). Clearly, Neuman (1982) addressed the family as client from the beginning of the model's development. The major aspects of the model are the physiological, psychological, sociocultural, developmental, and spiritual variables; basic structure and energy resources; lines of resistance; normal line of defense; flexible line of defense; stressors; reaction; primary, secondary, and tertiary prevention; intra-, inter-, and extrapersonal factors; and reconstitution (George, 1995). Neuman (1983) defined the family as "a group of two or more persons who create and maintain a common culture; its most central goal is one of continuance" (p. 241). According to Neuman, the family may be viewed as a system composed of family member subsystems. The focus of Neuman's theory is primarily on relationships among individual family members. The family system is exposed to stressors that affect its stability and threaten its state of wellness. The family's goal is to maintain stability by preserving the integrity of its basic structure (Whall & Fawcett, 1991b).

Hanson and Mischke (1996) and Berkey and Hanson (1991) presented a Family Assessment Intervention Model that was adapted from Neuman's Health Care Systems Model, described in more detail in this chapter's section on integrated models. Tomlinson and Anderson (1995) further analyzed Neuman's model. They defined family health as "a holistic function of the family system and its health promotion capability" (p. 134). Anderson and Tomlinson (1992) presented a Family Health System paradigm that merged concepts of family health, nursing practice, and Neuman's Health Care Systems Model. Within five broad areas, these nursing scholars make specific statements that demonstrate ways in which Neuman's theory interfaces with the Family Health System paradigm (Tomlinson & Anderson, 1995). These address complexity of the system, the core of the family, the goal of family health, the nurse entry point in caring for families, and nursing interaction.

The Neuman conceptual nursing model may become even more important in the twenty-first century as the emphasis of health care continues to move toward community-based health care. (See Hanson, 2001b, for further development of this model to families.)

OREM'S SELF-CARE MODEL

Dorothea Orem's (1971) Model of Self-Care posits that nursing care is required when an adult is unable to perform self-care sufficiently to sustain life, maintain health, recover from disease or injury, or cope with the effects of disease or injury (Orem, 1991). Orem's model also accommodates circumstances when nursing care may be directed toward the caregivers of others. For example, nursing care may be directed toward a parent or guardian caring for an ill child. The six central concepts in Orem's model are self-care, self-care agency, therapeutic self-care demand, self-care deficit, nursing agency, and nursing systems. One secondary, but important, concept is the concept of basic conditioning factors that address the variable personal characteristics and circumstances of the client.

Orem's model can be extended beyond its original parameters of individual to family self-care. In the original work, Orem (1971) did not address family in the self-care theory other than to indicate that nurses would need to work with family members to help the family member achieve self-care. Orem (1983a, 1983b) described the family as a basic conditioning unit in which the individual learns culture, roles, and responsibilities. Later, Orem (1985) suggested that people receive health care as individuals and as members of a multiperson unit (i.e., a family). In Orem's theory, the family is viewed mostly as the context of the individual client and not as a recipient of care itself.

However, Orem's Self-Care Model can be expanded to include families as a unit of care (Taylor, 2001) even if the nurses' analysis begins with the persons who are members of the family. Gray (1996) proposed that each individual family member can be viewed as a self-care agent who makes a personal continuous contribution to his or her own health. Further, self-care relates to the personal values and health beliefs of the family. Gray wrote that the family's self-care behavior could evolve through a combination of social and cognitive experiences that have been learned through interpersonal relationships, communication, and culture that are unique to each family. The family members, either individually or collectively, can initiate or perform self-care requisites that include attitudes about their health and their ability to perform self-care behaviors. Self-care can be used to foster the promotion of health in families and to recognize and evaluate areas where diminished health may exist (Gray, 1996, p. 88).

ROGERS'S SCIENCE OF UNITARY HUMAN BEINGS

Martha Rogers (1970, 1986, 1990) viewed the human being as a unitary multidimensional energy field that is engaged in a continuous mutual process with the environment. Her conceptual framework is known as the Science of Unitary Human Beings. Much of Rogers's model reflects the influence of general systems theory. According to Rogers (1970, 1990) nursing is a humanistic and humanitarian science directed toward describing and explaining the human being in synergistic wholeness and in developing the hypothetical generalizations and predictive principles basic to knowledgeable practice. The science of nursing is a science of humanity—the study of irreducible human beings and their environments. Falco & Lobo (1995) wrote that Roger's principles of homeodynamics—integrality, resonancy, and helicy—were key concepts in Rogers's view of human beings in their wholeness: "Change proceeds by continuous repatterning of both human and environmental fields by resonating oscillations of longer waves of lower frequency to shorter waves of higher frequency. Change reflects the mutual simultaneous interaction between the two fields in pandimensionality" (Falco & Lobo, 1995, p. 234).

Fawcett (1991), in expanding Rogers's model, posited that the family is a constant open system energy field that is ever changing in response to its interaction with the environment. Casey (1996) applied Rogers's theory to family nursing, considering the family unit in terms of its wholeness. Casey conceptualized the family from a Rogerian perspective as an open system in constant interaction with the environment through exchange of matter and energy, evolving toward greater complexity. Casey explained that family subsystems are interdependent but together form a unity different than the sum of the family subsystems. Casey referred to Rogers's concepts in writing that families are continuously influenced by information within the environment, and depending on the degree of permeability of the boundaries, they are constantly responding to this input. From a Rogerian perspective, Casey saw the family system subject to change along a space–time axis, and moving through stages of development in a sequential, unidirectional manner. Winstead-Fry (2000) also provided a discussion of how Rogers's ideas could be used in family nursing, such as how "Rogers' ideas of continuous innovation, unpredictability, and increasing diversity of patterns manifested by non-repeating rhythms fill the picture presented by current family systems theory and offer potential answers to some of the questions [in family science]" (p. 278). Rogers's conceptual framework has been used by nurse researchers as a base for grounding nursing theory and as a base for family nursing practice.

NEWMAN'S EXPANDING CONSCIOUSNESS MODEL

Newman's (1994) Expanding Consciousness Model was inspired by her experiences with family illness when she was a youth, influenced by earlier nursing theorists, especially Martha Rogers's concepts of unitary human beings and the importance of patterns, and Newman also incorporated ideas from theorists in other disciplines (George, 1995; Newman, 1994, 1995). In Newman's model, health is defined as expanding consciousness and is not dichotomous with illness. Rather, health and disease are reflections of the larger whole of health patterning of unitary human beings. The four original key concepts of

Newman's model were movement, time, space, and consciousness (Newman, 1979). Movement was defined as an essential property of matter, and timing was related to the rhythm of living phenomena. Space and consciousness were not defined separately from their integration with movement and time. Newman's newer concepts include expanding consciousness, pattern, pattern recognition, and transformation.

According to Newman, humans move unidirectionally toward higher levels of consciousness. Movement, diversity, and rhythm characterize the pattern of the whole energy field. Transformation is change, which occurs at specific points in time. In Newman's model, the patterns of individual energy fields (persons) are embedded in the patterns of their families, communities, and wider societal energy fields (George, 1995). Newman contends that her model of expanding consciousness is well suited to family health nursing (Newman, 1995). As applied to families, movement addresses the freedom of individual movement within the family system as well as movement of family members outside the family. The concept of time relates to private time for individual family members, in contrast to coordinated or shared time within the family. Space focuses on tension between territoriality versus shared space or distancing among family members. Finally, consciousness may mean the diversity and quality of interaction time within the family, informational capacity of the family system, and the diversity and quality of interaction of the family with the community energy fields (Newman, 1994).

Newman (1995) wrote that

> The pattern that will emerge will be one of energy flow and will illustrate areas where energy is blocked, areas where energy is depleted or diffuse, or areas where there is buildup, or overload. As the overall pattern of family emerges, the informational capacity of the family will be increased by participation in this process of pattern identification. (p. 123)

Yamashita and Tall (1998) provided examples of how Newman's model could guide nursing praxis and social action research. They noted that Newman's conceptualizations were consistent with certain aspects of Eastern thought and alternative medicine, enhancing its use in selected cross-cultural nursing situations.

EVOLUTION OF FAMILY NURSING THEORIES

Only a few major nursing models with potential for family nursing were reviewed here in relation to family nursing research and practice. Family nursing theory continues to evolve along with nursing research and practice, and nursing scholars continue with lively debates about nursing theory development in all areas of nursing, including family nursing (Reed, 1995). Many of the debates focus on new conceptualizations of nursing's metaparadigm concepts and reflect the influence of postmodernist and neomodernist perspectives. Drevdahl (1999) expressed concerns about nursing's past conceptualization of a "generic person" from postmodernist and feminist perspectives. She advocated increased attention to the interactions between the individual's unique characteristics and institutional societal factors, and she believed the goal of nursing theories should be social justice. Certainly, societal issues are key factors in family resources and health status.

Thorne and colleagues (1998) argued that nursing theory development would benefit by unifying definitions of the metaparadigm concepts and decreased polarization among advocates of specific nursing theorists. Their explanation of nursing's core concepts is inclusive of families as clients, for family nursing practice emphasizing health promotion, and recognizes the context of care.

> Nursing is the study of human health and illness processes. Nursing practice is facilitating, supporting and assisting individuals, families, communities and/or societies to enhance, maintain and recover health, and to reduce and ameliorate the effects of illness. Nursing's relational practice and science are directed toward the explicit outcome of health related quality of life within the immediate and larger environmental contexts. (Thorne et al., 1998, p. 1265)

In addition, there has been a strong shift in family nursing toward a strength-based perspective in working with families (Feeley & Gottlieb, 2000), as opposed to the traditional deficits or problem-focused approach. Feeley and Gottlieb (2000) present the McGill Model of Nursing as an example of a model that focuses on the family's capacities, competencies, and resources.

American nursing theories have long been faulted for their implicit or explicit ethnocentrism. Nursing theorists from diverse cultural backgrounds have begun developing models reflective of their own cultural contexts and unique aspects of family life in their cultures. For example, Hisama (2000) presented four evolving nursing theories designed for Japanese nurses, and Tierney (1998) described British nursing models widely used to guide nursing practice in Scotland and England. American nursing theorists may draw from these new theories in care of American families of diverse cultures.

FAMILY SOCIAL SCIENCE THEORIES

The *second tradition* that contributes to our model of family nursing theory as depicted in Figure 3–1 comes from the family social sciences. These theories were developed from various family social science disciplines (largely sociology) and originally evolved with little conscious awareness of their potential use by clinicians (Jones & Dimond, 1982). These theories proliferated during the first half of the twentieth century so that by the early 1950s there was an attempt to organize the accumulated conceptual knowledge about the family.

Reviewing the literature on social science theoretical frameworks used to study families, it is clear that there has been little consensus as to what theories constitute the major theoretical frameworks. From 1960 to 1980 it was generally recognized that the following family conceptual approaches dominated the field of marriage and the family: (1) structural–functional, (2) systems, (3) developmental (Broderick, 1971; Nye & Berardo, 1981, pp. xxv–xxvi), (4) interactional, and (5) stress theories. Other frameworks emerging for studying the family have included conflict, exchange, psychoanalytic, social–psychological, developmental, systems, economic, and legal.

More recently, three new resources have tracked the state of family social science with more emphasis on their practice utility. In a source book of family theories and methods (Boss, Doherty, LaRossa, Schumm, & Steinmetz, 1993), scholars traced the development of family theory, from its origins in religion and philosophy, through the construction of theory and methodology in the mid-twentieth century, to emerging models emphasizing the interaction between theories and methods. Klein and White (1996) reviewed what they deemed major family social science frameworks of today: exchange, symbolic interaction, family development, conflict, systems, and ecological frameworks. Winton (1995) summarized the different frameworks for studying families. In essence, family social science theories continue to evolve, which has made the knowledge base more user friendly for practice disciplines such as family nursing. The following is a summary of three major theories from the family social science area that have been useful to the understanding of families and family nursing.

STRUCTURAL–FUNCTIONAL THEORY

The structural–functional framework defines the family as a social system and is considered by some family theorists as the earliest form of systems theory (Broderick, 1993a). Family analysis consists of examining the family in terms of its relationship with other major social structures (institutions) such as medicine, religion, education, government, and the economy. This perspective looks at the arrangement of members within the family, relationships between the members, and relationships of the members to the whole (Artinian, 1994; Friedman, 1992). A primary focus is on how family patterns are related to other societal institutions and to the overall structure of society (Nye & Berardo, 1981). Emphasis is placed on the basic functions of families (Hanson & Boyd, 1996b): economic, reproductive, protective, culture, socialization, status conferring, relationships, and health functions. A central issue of the structural–functional theorist is how well the family structure allows the family to perform its functions. This approach characterizes the family as open to outside influences, yet at the same time, is concerned with maintaining its boundaries. The family is seen as a passively adapting institution rather than an agent of change. The framework has tended to emphasize a static view of the societal structure and to neglect

change as a structural dynamic. Assumptions of this perspective include:

- A family is a social system with functional requirements.
- A family is a small group that has generic features common to all small groups.
- Social systems such as families accomplish functions that serve the individuals in addition to those that serve society.
- Individuals act in accordance with a set of internalized norms and values that are learned primarily in the family through socialization.

This perspective is useful for assessing families and health. Illness of a family member results in alteration of the family structure and function. For example, if a single mother is ill, she cannot carry out her various roles, so grandparents or siblings may have to assume child care responsibilities. The power structure and communication patterns of the family are affected with illness of parents. Assessment includes determining whether changes due to illness influence the family's ability to carry out its functions. Using this perspective, sample assessment questions could be: How did the illness alter the family structure? What family roles were changed with the onset of the chronic illness? Intervention becomes necessary when changes in family structure alter the family's ability to function. Examples of intervention using this model are assisting families to use existing support structures and assisting families to modify their organization so that role responsibilities can be distributed.

The major strength of the structural–functional approach to family nursing practice is that it is comprehensive and views families within the broader community context. The major weakness of this approach is its static view, which tends to view families at one moment in time rather than as a system that changes over time. The structural–functional approach is one of this text's three organizing and theoretical frameworks and as such is elaborated in Chapter 4.

SYSTEMS THEORY

Systems theory is one of the most influential and generative of all the family frameworks. This approach to understanding families was influenced by theory derived from physics and biology by von Bertalanffy (1950, 1968a, as cited in Mercer, 1989). A system is composed of a set of interacting elements; each system is identifiable as distinct from the environment in which it exists. An open system exchanges energy and matter with the environment (negentropy) while a closed system is isolated from its environment (entropy). Systems depend on both positive and negative feedback, in order to maintain a steady state (homeostasis). Assumptions of the systems perspective applied to the family system include:

- Family systems are greater than and different from the sum of their parts.

- There are hierarchies within family systems and between subsystems (i.e., mother–child) and the family and community.

- There are boundaries in the family system and they can be open, closed, or random.

- Family systems increase in complexity over time, evolving to allow greater adaptability, tolerance to change, and growth by differentiation.

- Family systems change constantly in response to stresses and strains from within as well as from outside environments. Change in one part of family systems affects the total system.

- Causality is modified by feedback; therefore, lineal causality never exists in the real world.

- Family systems patterns are circular rather than linear; therefore, change must be directed toward the cycle.

- Family systems are an organized whole, with individuals in the family being interdependent and interactive.

- Family systems have homeostasis features to maintain stable patterns, which can be adaptive or maladaptive.

The family system perspective encourages nurses to see clients as participating members of a family. Nurses using this perspective assess the effects of illness or injury upon the entire family system and the reciprocal effects of the family on the illness or injury (Wright & Leahey, 2000). Emphasis is on the whole rather than on individuals. Relevant concepts in family systems theory include subsystems, boundaries, open systems,

feedback loops, family interactions, adaptation, and change. A sample of assessment questions includes: Who makes up the family system? How has a family member's critical illness affected the family and its members? Interventions need to address subsystem and whole family processes and functioning.

Four major strengths of the general systems framework are that it is: (1) a grand theory that covers a large array of phenomena, (2) a contextually based theory in that it views the family within the context of its suprasystems (the large community in which it is embedded) and subsystems, (3) an interactionally focused theory, and (4) a holistic theory. It looks at processes in the family rather than content and at relationships between parts (the relationship between and within subsystems and the relationship between the family and its interacting and suprasystems). The family is viewed as a whole, not as merely a sum of its parts. Two limitations of using this theoretical orientation in family nursing practice are: (1) it is broad and very general, and more specific concepts and practice guidelines need to be developed outside the theory; and (2) this approach may not be as helpful as individually oriented theories for addressing individual client concerns.

General systems theory, because of its broad applicability and noted strengths, was selected in this text as one of the three theoretical perspectives foundational to the Friedman Family Assessment Model. Systems theory is discussed in detail in Chapter 6.

FAMILY DEVELOPMENTAL THEORY

Individual developmental theory has always been at the core of nursing. Developmental stages were introduced by Freud and expanded by Erikson, Piaget, and others. Basic assumptions of the developmental model include:

- Developmentally based tasks occur at a specific period.

- Successful achievement leads to happiness and success with later tasks.

- Failure to achieve tasks leads to unhappiness, disapproval, or difficulty in achieving later tasks.

Evelyn Duvall (1977) applied the principles of individual development to the family in her classic book *Marriage and Family Development*. Her stages of family development were based on the age of the eldest child. She identified overall family tasks that needed to be accomplished for each stage of development for heterosexual couples with children. The stages started with the marriage of couples and ended with death. Developmental concepts include movement to a higher level of functioning, implying unidirectional progression. Disequilibrium occurs during the transitional periods from one stage to the next. The intimate small group called the family has a predictable natural history designated by stages, beginning with the simple husband–wife pair. The group becomes more complex with the addition of each new position/member over time. The group again becomes simple and less complex as the younger generation leaves home for jobs or marriage. Finally, the group comes full circle to the original husband–wife pair. At each family life cycle stage, there are family developmental needs and tasks that must be performed (Duvall & Miller, 1985).

Developmental theory was an attempt to transcend the structural–functional (large-scale analysis) and interactional (small-scale analysis) frameworks: It addressed the passage of time. Its goals were to integrate the small- and large-scale analyses of the other two approaches while viewing the family as an open system in relation to other configurations in society (Jones & Dimond, 1982, p. 13). Developmental theory explains how and what developmentally based changes occur to human organisms or groups over time. Achievement of family developmental tasks assists individual members to accomplish their tasks.

The framework assists family nurses in anticipating clinical problems in families as well as in identifying family strengths. The framework serves as a guide for assessing the family's developmental stage, the extent to which families are fulfilling the tasks associated with their respective stage, the family's developmental history, and the availability of resources essential for performing developmental tasks.

In conducting an assessment of families using the developmental model, several questions can be asked, including: Where does this family place on the continuum of family life cycle stages? What are the developmental tasks that are and are not being accomplished? Typical kinds of nursing intervention strategies using this perspective would be helping families to understand individual and family growth and development

stages and helping families to deal with the normalcy of transition periods that fall between developmental periods (i.e., tasks of the school-aged family versus tasks of the adolescent family). Family nurses must recognize that in every family there are both individual and family developmental tasks that need to be accomplished for every stage of the individual/family life cycle. Basic assumptions include:

- Families change and develop in different ways because of internal and environmental stimulation/demands.
- Developmental tasks are goals worked toward rather than specific jobs completed at once.
- Each family is unique in its composition and in the complexity of its age–role expectations and positions.
- Individuals and families are a function of their historical milieu as well as the current social context.
- Families have enough in common despite their uniqueness to chart family development over the family life span.
- Families may arrive at similar developmental levels through quite different processes.

The major strength of the family developmental approach is that it provides a basis for forecasting what a family will be experiencing at any period in the family life cycle (e.g., role transitions and family constellation changes). The major weakness is the fact that the model was developed at a time in history when the traditional nuclear family was emphasized. The perfect linear progression of families, from marriage through death, is simply not a reality of our times. What happen to the stages of the individual/family life cycle when there is a divorce, death, adoption, and the other multiple forms that we now call family?

Developmental concepts have been adapted for use with a variety of family forms in recent years. Examples of five family life cycles described in the literature are: (1) middle-class North American, (2) divorce and postdivorce, (3) remarried family life cycle, (4) professional versus low-income, and (5) adoptive (Wright & Leahy, 2000). In each case, there are unique stages of development with specific developmental tasks or issues that challenge the family at each stage. Because there are important differences in stages and family developmental issues among diverse family forms, it is essential that family nurses employ the developmental model appropriate for specific families in evaluating family functioning.

Developmental theory was selected in this text as one of the foundational theories guiding the Friedman Family Assessment Model, and will be discussed in detail in Chapter 6.

FAMILY INTERACTIONAL THEORY

The family interactional approach stems from a grand theory in social psychology and sociology, that of symbolic interaction; today, the term *symbolic interaction* represents a diverse family of theories. Symbolic interaction stems from pragmatist philosopher and social psychologist George Herbert Mead. In his posthumous work, *Mind, Self and Society* (1934), Mead's students described his thinking from lecture notes. Central to Mead's thinking is the idea that by sharing common symbols, human beings adapt to and survive in their environments. Other scholars (e.g., Blumer, 1969; Kuhn, 1964) have contributed to the formulation of symbolic interaction theory. Blumer (1969, p. 2) lists three basic assumptions that are critical to symbolic interaction theory:

1. Human beings act toward things on the basis of the meanings that these things have for them.

2. The meaning of such things is derived from, and arises out of, the social interaction that one has with one's fellows.

3. These meanings are handled in, and modified through, an interpretive process used by the person in dealing with the things he encounters.

These assumptions together form the general focus of symbolic interaction, that of generating and acquiring meaning. Symbolic interaction theorists recognize the influence of culture and society on families as families formulate meanings (Crotty, 1998). What this means to the family is that family members create meaning to help them make sense of their world. Meanings are constructed by family members relevant to the situation in which the family is situated. For example, two families, each consisting of a single parent and two children, would form different meanings about whether they were a traditional family. One family may believe they are nontraditional because the family does not include two parents, whereas the other family may consider single-parent families traditional and two-parent families as nontraditional. Nurses cannot understand the family unless the nurse understands the meaning(s) that families attach to the situations they experience (i.e., their interpretations of events).

There are relevant concepts and propositions of this theoretical perspective for the family. Among the processes involving communication, roles, decision making, problem solving, and socialization, communication and roles are especially relevant (Burr, Leigh, Day, & Constantine, 1979; Klein & White, 1996; Rose, 1962). Several variants of symbolic interaction theory have evolved that focus on communication (see discussion later in this chapter) and roles. The structural approach emphasizes the concept of role. Roles are learned and enacted by individuals within a social structure. Family members enact their roles based on the expectations for those roles learned through the socialization process; thus, the metaphor often used to describe structuralist is that of "actors on a stage" (Turner, 1991). This approach equates role enactment with actors acting out a written script. In contrast, interactional approaches emphasize the fluidity and contingency of roles (Klein & White, 1996). Unlike structural theorists who emphasize that individuals perform the scripted role, interactional approaches posit that individuals not only take on a role but make the role their own through interaction with others (Turner, 1970). Turner emphasizes the creative and problem-solving processes of roles (Klein & White, 1996). Family members develop their roles through what they have learned are the expectations of the role and through interaction with others about role expectations. For example, how the caregiver role will be enacted will be determined not only by the expectations of the caregiver about how the caregiver role should be enacted, but the role will also be shaped by interactions with others (e.g., ill member, other family members, health care professionals). These interactions will determine what expectations make up the caregiving role and how the caregiver will enact the role.

Much of the clarity and power to explain family behavior and processes originates from the propositions of Burr and colleagues (1979) that focus on roles, discussed in more detail in Chapter 12. These propositions can be used to guide clinical practice with families. For example, one method to assist families during role transitions and to decrease role strain is to clarify role expectations through education. Nurses have been particularly proactive in developing educational programs, such as prenatal classes and caregiver classes, to name just a few, to assist families during role transitions.

These approaches to understanding families' internal dynamics are most relevant to family nursing. Hence, a major strength of its approach is its focus on internal processes within families and understanding these processes. The major limitation in using this approach is that interactional theorists generally fail to include the impact of social institutions. These interactionalists consider families to be comparatively closed units, with the external world having little effect on what occurs within the family.

Assessment of families within an interactional framework emphasizes assessment of interaction/communication between and among family members; family role and power analysis; family coping; relationships between marital/adult partners, siblings, parents, and children; and family socialization patterns. Interventions are then generated, based on the family's needs for health promotion, health maintenance, or health restoration in the above areas.

In this text, the family interactional approach is integrated into the family structural and functional focus. Six chapters address internal family dynamics, including assessment and intervention guidelines: Chapter 10, "Family Communication Patterns and Processes"; Chapter 11, "Family Power and Decision Making"; Chapter 12, "Family Role Structure"; Chapter 14, "The Family Affective Function"; Chapter 15, "The Family Socialization Function"; and Chapter 17, "Family Stress, Coping, and Adaptation."

FAMILY STRESS THEORY

The family stress model is especially germane to health care situations because of the pervasive illness-related stress the family experiences (Artinian, 1994). Reuben Hill (1949), who originally developed family stress theory, conducted research on war-induced separation and reunion within families to discover the factors that determine how families under stress adapted.

In Hill's model, the *A* variable is the provoking event or stressor with its associated hardships. This event may be of such magnitude as to cause change in the family system. The *B* variable refers to the family's strengths or resources available to assist it in dealing with stressor events. Family resources include religious faith, finances, social support, physical health, family flexibility, and/or family coping mechanisms. The *C* variable refers to the definition families make of the seriousness of stressor events or the subjective meaning the family attaches to the events. The family's definition of the events determines how it deals with them and how stressful the events will be for the family. This last point is critical, because sometimes nurses cannot understand from the reality of situations why families react in certain ways to events, when indeed they are reacting from their perceptions rather than the external reality. All three of these variables in combination influence the family's ability to prevent changes associated with stressor events. Changes created by stressful illness may lead to a crisis, the *X* variable. The *X* variable refers to the amount of disruption or incapacitation within the family system. Susceptibility to crisis is a function of both a deficiency in family resources and the tendency to define hardships as crisis producing. Assumptions of the family stress model include (Artinian, 1994):

- Unexpected or unplanned events are usually perceived as stressful.

- Events within families, such as serious illness, and events defined as stressful, are more disruptive than stressors that occur outside the family, such as war, flood, or depression.

- Lack of previous experience with stressor events leads to increased perceptions of stress.

- Ambiguous stressor events are more stressful than nonambiguous events.

Hill's theory was later expanded by McCubbin and Patterson (1983a) to cover the postcrisis period. Called the Double ABCX Model, each of Hill's variables was modified; the notion of coping was inserted as a central predictor of family adaptation. The latest family stress theory, the Resiliency Model (McCubbin

& McCubbin, 1993) builds on the former two models and is discussed in depth in Chapter 17.

Assessment areas should cover the prominent variables within the theory itself (i.e., stressors, perception of the stressor event, family resources, family coping, and how much the crisis has disrupted the family functioning). Questions nurses could ask include: Did the family have time to prepare for the event or was it unexpected (i.e., sudden unexpected death versus death after long-term fatal illness)? Has the family experienced similar stressor events? Interventions include helping families to enhance their resources and support systems and helping families to modify their subjective perceptions of the events. The major strengths of this framework are that it is fairly simple to understand (i.e., it makes sense), and it fits what nurses see and do in clinical settings. The model emphasizes that perception of stressor(s) is more important than objective reality and by identifying resources and strengths, family nursing approaches that empower families can be developed. The model is limited in its usefulness for addressing the needs of healthy families in terms of health promotion and disease prevention.

CHANGE THEORY

The process of change is important for family nursing theory and practice. The family nurse works with families in order to facilitate change and, therefore, needs to understand the application of change theory as it applies to families, both in terms of changes in the family structure and in terms of changes in the family's health behaviors.

Nurses are confronted with the paradoxical relationship between persistence (stability) and change in families. Maturana (1978) noted that change is an alteration in the family's structure that occurs as compensation for perturbations and has the purpose of maintaining structure (i.e., stability). According to Wright and Watson (1988), "the most profound and sustaining change [within a family] will be that which occurs within the family's belief system (cognition)" (p. 425).

Watzlawick, Weakland, and Fisch (1974) referred to first- and second-order changes. In first-order change, the system itself remains unchanged while its parts undergo some type of change. For example, in

learning a new behavioral strategy to discipline a child, the family remains the same but a new approach is used. It is like treating the symptom instead of the cause. In second-order change, a change occurs in the system itself, hence a "change of change." In second-order change, there are actual changes in the rules governing the system and, therefore, the system is transformed structurally and/or communicationally, sending the family to a different level of functioning. Second-order change is said to occur when parents begin to treat their teenager as a growing adult instead of as a young child.

Families do not change in smooth, linear progression, but rather in discontinuous leaps, a form of transformation in which new patterns appear that did not exit before. Bateson (1979) suggested that we are unaware of changes and that we become accustomed to a new way of being before our senses advise us. To effect change within a family system, nurses need to be able to maintain a metaposition to the family, observing the connections between systems (e.g., between the family and community). Wright and Leahey (2000) proffered a number of concepts relative to change theory that assist family nurses in their practice.

1. Change is dependent on the perception of the problem. Nurses must recognize that there are as many truths or realities as there are members of a given family. The nurse must accept all these perceptions and offer the family another view of their problems.

2. Change is determined by structure. Nurses must recognize that an individual's present structure will determine which interactions will trigger structural changes. Nurses cannot predict which nursing interventions will fit for a particular person and must think about interventions that are most likely to disturb the person's structure to facilitate change.

3. Change is dependent on context. Efforts to promote change in family systems must take into account the contextual constraints and resources. In the assessment of families, nurses must be cognizant of the family's relationship to larger or suprasystems.

4. Change is dependent on co-evolving goals for treatment. It is important that goals are mutu-

ally developed between nurses and families with a realistic time frame. Nurses often set one-sided, unrealistic goals for families. One of the primary goals in family nursing is to change or alter the family's view of the problem. Nurses can assist families to find alternative behavioral, cognitive, and affective responses to problems.

5. Understanding alone does not lead to change. Understanding problems does not bring about change but rather change occurs through alterations in belief and behavior. Nurses often search for the "why" answers with families rather than focusing energies into the "what" questions. Focusing on what is being done here, which perpetuates the problem, and what can be done to effect a change provides the family with alternative avenues for action.

6. Change does not occur equally in all family members. Change can lead to a variety of reactions, with some family members changing more dramatically and quickly than others.

7. Nurses are responsible for facilitating change. Nurses cannot make families change, as that responsibility belongs to the family. Nurses facilitate a context for change.

8. Change occurs by the "fit" between the therapeutic offerings (interventions) of the nurse and the biopsychosocial–spiritual structures of family members. Nurses operating from a therapeutic stance appreciative of fit look for ways to increase the fit for family members, and adopt a nonjudgmental, nonblaming attitude when fit does not occur. Those who operate from this stance do not use terms such as noncompliance or nonadherence.

9. Change can be due to a myriad of causes. Change is influenced by many different factors; thus, it is difficult to know what specifically precipitated the changes.

Many health behavior change theories indicate that families are key influences in both the health status and health behaviors of individual family members. The relationship between the quality of social ties (especially within families) and health has been documented in the literature since the 1970s (House, Landis, & Umberson, 1988; McEwen, 1998). Social integration refers to the extent to which a person has social ties or social connections, in contrast to social isolation (Seeman, 1996). This may be interpreted to mean that the quality of family life affects the health of family members, with positive family relationships serving as protective factors for the health of the family members.

In addition, many of the theories of health behavior change (Glanz, Lewis, & Rimer, 1997) posit that family support is a key element in the success of individual family members in initiating and maintaining new health behaviors, such as smoking cessation or improved eating patterns. Individuals with strong family support for the health behavior change are far more likely to successfully adopt and maintain new health behaviors than individuals who do not have family support for the health behavior change. For example, Wing and Jeffrey (1999) found that participants in a weight-loss program who engaged family and friends in home activities fared better than other groups in losing weight and maintaining the weight loss over six months. Family nurses may facilitate positive changes in health behaviors by talking with families about the importance of supporting one another in adopting or maintaining positive health behavior.

OTHER FAMILY SOCIAL SCIENCE THEORIES

Only the major frameworks that have historically been used in family social science and that are relevant for family nursing practice were presented. Other frameworks that inform family nursing include chaos theory, social exchange theory, conflict theory, the ecological framework, an anthropological/multicultural approach, and phenomenology theory (Nye & Berardo, 1981; Klein & White, 1996; Friedman, 1992). The multicultural approach to family nursing is presented in Chapter 8, while conflict theory is discussed in Chapter 10.

✖ FAMILY THERAPY THEORIES

Family therapy theories are a blend of family social science theories and practice theories. Both family social science theory and family therapy have a short history, with family therapy theories having a more recent vintage. Over the last 35 years there has been extensive theory development in the field of family therapy. Family therapy theories have been developed to work with troubled families and, therefore, are pathology oriented for the most part (see Table 3–2). Even so, these theories describe family system dynamics and patterns that exist in all families to some extent. Because this genre of theories are concerned with what can be done to facilitate change in "dysfunctional" families (Whall, 1983), they are both descriptive and prescriptive (suggesting treatment or intervention strategies).

Multiple family therapy theories exist; these all have been influenced by the multiple theories that are extant in the psychological and sociological disciplines. No single approach to family therapy can be put forth as the "right" or "wrong" approach; each is simply an alternative explanation of family phenomena and a specific approach to family assessment, diagnoses, and treatment. Over time, family therapy theories have been classified in various ways by a variety of theorists (Gladding, 1995; Becvar & Becvar, 1996).

The family therapy theories presented in this section all share common family systems concepts. All posit that the family system shares characteristics of open, ongoing, goal-seeking, self-regulating systems as well as the additional features of social systems (Broderick, 1993). Social systems such as families have component parts that are self-aware, self-directed, and independent unlike more mechanistic systems. For family members to form themselves into a system, they must share a common set of meanings. Meanings are developed through communication, and communication theory is the first family therapy theory discussed.

INTERACTIONAL/COMMUNICATION FAMILY THERAPY THEORY

The interactional/communication therapy approach was heavily influenced by ideas derived from general systems theory, cybernetics, and information processing theory (see Chapter 7 for description of these latter two theories) (Goldenberg & Goldenberg, 2000). The interactional/communication perspective has undergone major revisions over four decades, but much of the original theory development was done by the Mental Research Institute (MRI) in Palo Alto,

California (Don Jackson, John Weakland, and Paul Watzlawick), and Virginia Satir (Becvar & Becvar, 1996). According to Watzlawick and colleagues, the analysis of communication processes involves three separate aspects of syntactics, semantics, and pragmatics (Watzlawick, Beavin, & Jackson, 1967). Communication theorists have attached differential importance to these different aspects and have developed interventions based on these aspects. Syntactics is concerned with how accurately a message is conveyed from one party to another (Broderick, 1993). Therapists using this approach focus on how to assist family members to clearly communicate with each other so that the message sent is the message received. Semantics is concerned with meaning. Kantor and Lehr (1975) list pursuit of meaning as one of the most important goals of a family that family members hope to achieve through interaction. As a result, family theorists have written about family themes, family myths and legends, and family stories as ways to create and sustain shared meanings, and that through reframing or changing family meanings one can change the meaning of the interaction (Broderick, 1993). Symbolic interactionists also are concerned with meaning.

Finally, pragmatics concerns itself with the impact communication has on behavior, and it is this aspect of communication that has been most fully explored. The fundamental rules of communication theory developed by Watzlawick, Beavin, and Jackson (1967) in *Pragmatics of Human Communication* are as follows:

1. One cannot not behave, thus one cannot not communicate. All behavior is communication at some level. For example, a client who does not answer questions but sits quietly throughout the interview is still communicating, but the nurse must determine what meaning the behavior has to the client to determine what is being communicated.

2. All communication has a report (digital) level and a command (analog) level. The command level defines the nature of the relationship.

3. All behavior/communication must be examined in context. Without contextual awareness, complete understanding is not possible.

4. All systems are characterized by rules, which maintain homeostatic balance and preserve

the system. For example, among certain cultures (see McGoldrick, 1993), rules to preserve the system include not telling outsiders (read nurse) family problems. To do so would disturb the homeostatic balance of the family. Thus, among these families, the nurse must develop sufficient trust with the family before family problems can be discussed.

5. Relationships may be described as either symmetrical or complementary. Symmetrical implies equality, and complementary implies oppositeness (a dominant–submissive relationship).

6. Each person punctuates his or her reality according to his or her own reality. Behavioral sequences are understood and meaning is experienced relative to the epistemology of the observer.

7. Problems are maintained within recursive feedback loops of recurrent patterns of communication.

8. The functional or normal family is able to maintain its basic integrity even during periods of stress. Changes are accommodated as needed, and clear, congruent communication is present.

9. Dysfunctional families are said to be "stuck." Symptomatic behavior maintains the family's current equilibrium and needed change is avoided. A problem is a symptom of system dysfunction.

Satir (1982) built on the above communication ideas by adding four fundamental assumptions. First, the natural movement of all individuals is toward positive growth and development and a symptom indicates an impasse in the growth process. Second, all individuals possess the resources necessary for growth and development. Third, families possess mutual influence and shared responsibility. Therefore, no person in the family is to blame; there are only multiple stimuli and multiple effects. Fourth, therapy is a process involving interactions between both clients and therapists, with the therapeutic goal of moving the family toward positive growth. Although the therapist may take the lead in facilitating growth, each person is in charge of his or her own growth. A primary goal of family therapy is to understand the communication rules and processes that a troubled family uses and to teach the family functional communication rules and processes.

The unit of analysis in this approach was derived from the dynamics of interchange between individuals, thus the term *interactional* analysis. In this perspective, the assumption is that psychiatric problems result from the way people interact with each other in the context of the family. "Individual symptoms reflect family system dysfunction and these symptoms persist only if they are maintained by that family system" (Goldenberg & Goldenberg, 1996, p. 211). A breakdown in family functioning occurs when unclear family communication predominates and when the rules of family functioning become ambiguous. Key interventions focus on establishing clear, congruent communication as well as clarifying and changing family rules (Jackson, 1965b; Satir, 1967). The interactional/communication perspective has a strong emphasis on communication between members and the focus of the interactional perspective discussed earlier is on shared meanings. The strength of this approach is its focus on communication within the family environment. The weakness of this theory is that it looks primarily at internal family behavior and not at how the larger culture and environment impact the family.

The next two family therapy theories to be discussed focus on distance regulation of family members, of finding the balance in ongoing family systems between the bonding forces that connect families, and the buffering forces that insulate them from one another (Broderick, 1993, p. 50). Family therapists identified that when families were too tightly bonded or had too rigid boundaries, there was greater dysfunction within those families than among families who were more balanced. Family theorists focused on different aspects of distance regulation. For example, the classic work of Minuchin (1974) focused on maintenance of system boundaries, and the classic work of Bowen (1978) focused on differentiation of self. In the following sections, Minuchin's and Bowen's theories will be discussed in more depth.

STRUCTURAL FAMILY THERAPY THEORY

Minuchin and associates (Minuchin, 1974; Minuchin & Fishman, 1981; Minuchin, Rosman, & Baker, 1978) developed this systems-oriented approach to family therapy. It used spatial and organizational metaphors, both in describing the structural problems of the family and in identifying solutions to change the family structure (Goldenberg & Goldenberg, 2000). Minuchin's main structural concern was with maintaining the appropriate vertical distance between the generations and his intervention strategies were targeted at "restructuring the family."

Four major concepts central to understanding structural family therapy are (1) transactional patterns, (2) adaptation, (3) subsystems, and (4) boundaries. *Transactional patterns* refer to habitual, repeated transactions among family members that become fixed laws that govern the interactions and conduct of various family members. *Adaptation* refers to the family's ability to mobilize alternative transactional patterns to these fixed patterns to meet external and internal demands for change. Transactional patterns help the family to be stable or homeostatic. Family dysfunction occurs when transactional patterns no longer work for the family and, as a result, there is poor adaptation. *Subsystems* are the ways in which the family system differentiates and carries out its affective and socialization functions. These subsystems in families are usually individuals or relation/relational subsystems such as the marital, parent–child, or sibling subsystem. *Boundaries* ensure differentiation of the family subsystems. The clarity of these boundaries provides a prime barometer of how well the family functions. Minuchin introduced the idea of two pathological extremes in boundaries: the disengaged, in which boundaries are too rigid, to the point where there is little cohesiveness between family members; and the enmeshed, in which the boundaries are diffuse or porous to the point where subsystems do not function autonomously or independently at all. An example Minuchin (1974) used to illustrate the enmeshed family was that when one person sneezes, everyone runs for the Kleenex.

Olson (1993) has expanded Minuchin's early conceptualizations and for the past three decades has developed and tested the circumplex model, in which he categorizes families on their degree of cohesion (closeness or bonding) and adaptability (extent to which families can change roles and rules as necessary). Most families occupy a range along a continuum in which cohesion and adaptability are balanced rather than at the extreme points (enmeshed versus disengaged cohesion or rigid versus chaotic adaptability). His approach can incorporate changes in the balance that families experience over time. Olsen's approach has a broad range of applications from dating couples to elderly families, and his careful attention to developing instruments to measure concepts in his model have added enormously to the family literature.

The goal of structural family therapy is to facilitate a change in family structure. The clinician using this approach attempts to change family patterns through changing family interaction. Therapy is present centered, action oriented, and problem focused. For example, when caring for an ill child within a two-parent family, the nurse may help the family learn which rules are less important (i.e., it is okay not to continue all social obligations due to the demands of caring for the child) or may help the family understand the boundaries between generations (i.e., the parents are still the parents despite the ill child's often being allowed to dictate family rules). Assessment of families occurs through asking questions, observing family transactions, and having family members interact with each other about a particular situation in the interview itself. Intervention includes joining with the family by respecting the current family structure, intervening directly to restructure the family, and working with family success through praise and support (Minuchin & Fishman, 1981). The role of the therapist is active, directive, and action oriented.

The strengths of this approach are that the concepts are fairly clear, well integrated, developed, and tested. The present-centered, action-oriented, and problem-focused approach is very consistent with models of therapy used in today's health care. The limitation of the model is that the approach calls for a very directive and active role on the part of the therapist, which may be uncomfortable for some therapists and families.

FAMILY SYSTEMS THERAPY THEORY

Murray Bowen first developed family systems theory in the mid-1970s, and he is one of the prominent pioneers in family therapy. His family systems theory is one of the best developed and integrated of the family therapy theoretical frameworks (Goldenberg & Goldenberg, 2000). Since Bowen's death in 1990, his work has continued to evolve through the work of Michael Kerr (Kerr & Bowen, 1988) and David Freeman (1992). The underlying assumption or premise in this theory is that chronic anxiety is an inevitable, omnipresent part of life and is the underlying basis for dysfunction (Goldenberg & Goldenberg, 2000). Its only "antidote is resolution through differentiation," the key concept within Bowen's theory (Goldenberg & Goldenberg, 1996, p. 169). Bowen emphasized eight interlocking concepts in order to address chronic anxiety and emotional processes in families and society (Gladding, 1995) (see Table 3–3).

The key concept within his theory is *differentiation of self*. This refers to the ability of persons to distinguish themselves from their family of origin on an emotional and intellectual level. There are two counterbalancing life forces: togetherness and individuality. On one end of the continuum is autonomy, which signals an ability to think through a situation clearly and separate out feelings from rational thought. At the other end of the continuum is undifferentiated ego mass, which implies an emotional dependence on the family of origin even if living away from the family. Bowen believed that the greater the differentiation of self, the more individuals are able to adapt to change and stress from their surroundings and,

TABLE 3–3

BOWEN'S FAMILY SYSTEMS THEORY — EIGHT INTERLOCKING CONCEPTS

- Differentiation of self
- Nuclear family emotional system
- Multigenerational transmission process
- Family projection process
- Triangling
- Sibling position
- Emotional cutoff
- Societal regression

therefore, the less apt they are to run into emotional difficulty.

There are seven remaining interlocking concepts in Bowen's family systems theory (these concepts are indicated in italics). The nuclear family is defined as the *nuclear family emotional system*. Families pass on coping strategies and patterns from generation to generation, a phenomenon known as the *multigenerational transmission process*. Families who are not functioning well have carried the problematic behavior(s) over several generations. When people marry, they tend to partner with those at their own differentiation level and produce offspring at the same level of differentiation as themselves. The *family projection process* refers to the transfer of the parental anxiety and low level of differentiation to a susceptible child. *Triangulation* is another major concept. Triangles are seen as a basic building block of any emotional system and are the smallest stable relationship system. In triangulation, the anxiety and tension between two persons is projected onto another object/person in the family. In stressful situations, anxiety may spread from one central triangle within the family to triangles with a person(s) or object outside the family. *Sibling position* addresses the importance of birth order. In Bowen's theory, people are seen as developing fixed personality characteristics based on their functional birth order in their family of origin (Toman, 1961). The more closely a marriage replicates one's sibling position in the family of origin, the better chance that couple has of having a successful marriage. *Emotional cutoff* refers to emotional withdrawal from other family members due to unresolved attachments. Adult children who are emotionally fused to their parents and family of origin may attempt to regulate anxiety by living near or far from them. These children remain emotionally fused to their family of origin and often have dysfunctional relationships in their families of procreation. *Societal regression* is the analog on a societal level for differentiation of self. It refers to a society that is under so much stress that it regresses because excessive toxic forces counter the tendency to achieve differentiation.

The major focus of Bowen's family systems therapy is on promoting differentiation of self from family and of intellect from emotion (Becvar & Becvar, 1996). Family members gain insight and understanding into the past by examining the above processes, and are then freed to choose how they will behave in the present. Assessment using the Bowen model consists of having individuals or couples discuss their family tree with the therapist. The therapist, functioning as coach and teacher, asks about people's histories while constructing a multigenerational genogram. This genogram can be a useful tool for nurses in clinical practice. It can provide the practicing nurse with a clear picture of who is in the family, the relationships among family members, and the history of the family (see Chapter 8 for further information on family genograms). Bowenian therapists coach people on how to detriangulate, develop interpersonal relationships, and end cutoffs, and how to understand their intergenerational patterns, thus gaining insight into ways they currently interact.

The logic of Bowen's approach appeals to many people who lead with their intellect rather than their feelings; thus, it has been noted to appeal to male clients. A major weakness of this therapy is that most people are not inclined to stay in therapy long enough to see it to its completion. An emphasis on the past rather than on the present (i.e., the presenting problem) means that the presenting problem may not be addressed or resolved as soon as it is in other approaches.

OTHER FAMILY THERAPY THEORIES

Due to limitations of space, only three mainstream family therapy frameworks were presented. Other frameworks and approaches from family therapy that contribute to family nursing theories include psychodynamic (Ackerman, 1966), experiential/humanistic (Whitaker & Keith, 1981), strategic (Madanes, 1991), behavior/cognitive (Falloon, 1991), interpersonal (Segrin, 2001), narrative (White & Epston, 1990), and problem-focused or problem-centered (Pinsof, 1995).

🐾 FAMILY NURSING THEORIES: INTEGRATED MODELS

The integration of nursing models with family social science theories and family therapy theories will be essential as the subspecialty of family nursing becomes more clearly delineated. Cody (2000) noted that nursing theories specific to family nursing are limited, and that while we benefit from theoretical perspectives borrowed from other disciplines, family nurses need family theories that are distinctively nursing.

Thus, integrated approaches are needed to guide family nursing practice because no singular theory provides a comprehensive framework for the diversity of families with whom we work. Presently, three family nursing practice models are cited widely and used extensively in family nursing (Hanson & Boyd, 1996a). These are the Family Systems Stressor–Strength Model and Inventory (Berkey & Hanson, 1991), Calgary Family Assessment and Intervention Models (Wright & Leahey, 2000), and the Friedman Family Assessment Model (the model used in this text). Although there is much overlap in the content and processes involved in these three models, there are also substantial differences in approach.

FAMILY ASSESSMENT INTERVENTION MODEL (FAMILY SYSTEMS STRESSOR–STRENGTH MODEL)

Berkey and Hanson (1991) and Hanson and Mischke (1996) developed an integrated family nursing model by extending Neuman's Health Care System Model. Using family theory, Neuman's theoretical concepts were expanded to focus on the family as client. The Family Assessment Intervention Model (Berkey & Hanson, 1991; Hanson & Mischke, 1996) focuses on (a) wellness/promotion, (b) family reactions and the degree of instability, and (c) restoration of family stability and function. Hanson and Mischke (1996) stated that families are consistently exposed to stressors on a daily basis that challenge the stability of the family unit. Families develop coping strategies to maintain equilibrium and conserve energy resources. The family unit is influenced when any member experiences a stressor or the whole family experiences a stressor that threatens the ability of the family system. Working together, family nurses and families strive for the goal of family stability. Each family responds to stress events based on (a) the perception of the situation and (b) the family's ability to adjust and restore the impaired family function created by the stressor.

The Family Assessment Intervention Model and Family Systems Stressor–Strength Inventory (FSSI) are more focused than the other two models, in that they involve the appraisal of family stressors and strengths, as well as the restoration of family stability and family functioning by the application of primary, secondary, and tertiary preventive approaches. The FSSI can be used for assessment and intervention as well as a measurement tool for both practice and research. This model is an excellent example of an adaptation of the Neuman conceptual framework based on actual family nursing practice.

CALGARY FAMILY ASSESSMENT MODEL AND CALGARY FAMILY INTERVENTION MODEL

The second integrated family systems nursing model is the Calgary Family Assessment Model (CFAM) and the Calgary Family Intervention Model (CFIM), developed by Wright and Leahey and associates (Wright & Leahey, 2000; Wright, Watson, & Bell, 1996). The Calgary family systems nursing model integrates theories from general systems theory, cybernetics, communication theory, and change theory. Increasingly, the Calgary family systems nursing model is informed by family therapy theories and approaches, more specifically Maturana's and Varela's theory of the biology of knowing, Gregory Bateson's theory of mind, and constructivist and narrative approaches (White & Epston, 1990; Wright, Watson, & Bell, 1996).

These theories and ideas are incorporated into a nursing paradigm or perspective focusing on families experiencing health problems. The Calgary Family Assessment Model emphasizes identification of family strengths and resources. Intervention strategies are planned with the strong recognition that families should and must decide what is best for them. They are designed to assist families to empower themselves. The assessment and intervention models are grounded in solid clinical practice observations and qualitative clinical research. Chapter 7 highlights the Calgary model, particularly assessment and intervention strategies that are cornerstones of the Calgary family systems nursing model. The model's intervention strategies are used to assist families to have facilitative beliefs and modify their constraining beliefs.

THE FRIEDMAN FAMILY ASSESSMENT MODEL

The Friedman Family Assessment Model constitutes an integrated approach by utilizing general systems theory, family developmental theory, structural–functional theory, and cross-cultural theory as primary theoretical foundations for a family assessment model and tool. Other midrange theories are also incorporated into the various structural and functional dimensions assessed, such as communication theory, role theory, and family stress theory. Chapters 3 through 6 as well as Chapters 8 through 17 elaborate on these family assessment content and process areas. Family nursing diagnoses and intervention strategies are also discussed relative to each of the identifying data, sociocultural, developmental, structural, functional, and stress and coping assessment areas.

✺ SUMMARY

- The function of theory is to characterize, explain, or predict phenomena evident within nursing. Thus, nursing theories ideally represent logical and intelligible patterns for observations within nursing practice (Fawcett & Downs, 1992).

- Many of the concepts incorporated in nursing models were borrowed or adapted from preexisting theories in sociology, anthropology, psychology, and physiology with new applications to nursing. Likewise, contemporary family social science and family therapy theories derive many of their key concepts and propositions from family social science theories and general systems theory with new applications to the family.

- The development of nursing models and theories has profoundly influenced the discipline of nursing, beginning with Florence Nightingale's writings and continuing with the work of contemporary nursing theorists. Nursing models specifically suited to family nursing practice include those developed by Imogene King, Sister Callista Roy, Betty Neuman, Dorothea Orem, Martha Rogers, and Margaret Newman.

- Florence Nightingale did not actually present a theory of nursing or family nursing. Nevertheless, she acknowledged the family in many of her writings and in much of her nursing practice (Nightingale, 1859).

- King developed an interacting systems model and included a family-as-context approach.

- Neuman addressed the family as client from the beginning of the model's development, with family viewed as a system composed of family members as subsystems.

- Orem described the family as a basic conditioning unit and as the context for the individual client.

- Sister Callista Roy's Adaptation Model (1976) conceptualized the individual as an adaptive system interacting with stimuli via four response modes: physiological, self-concept, role function, and interdependence. The family could be context or the client, and care was directed at promoting positive adaptation to focal, contextual, and residual stimuli through regulator and cognator processes.

- Rogers viewed the family as an open system in constant interaction with the environment through exchange of matter and energy, ever evolving toward greater complexity.

- Newman focused on family patterns as energy fields and movement through time and space toward expanded consciousness.

- The second tradition that contributes to our model of family nursing theory comes from the family social sciences. Three family conceptual approaches dominated the field of marriage and the family: (1) structural–functional, (2) systems/interactional, and (3) developmental.

- The structural–functional framework defines the family as a social system. Family analysis consists of examining the family in terms of its relationship with other major social structures (institutions) such as medicine, religion, education, government, and the economy. The major strength of the structural–functional approach to family nursing practice is that it is comprehensive and views families within the broader community context. The major weakness of this approach is its static view, which tends to view families at one moment in time rather than as a system that changes over time.

- General systems theory concepts include subsystems, boundaries, open systems, feedback loops, family interactions, adaptation, and change. Major strengths are that it covers a large array of phenomena, views the family within the context of its suprasystems (the large community in which it is embedded), is an interactionally focused, holistic theory. Two limitations are that it is broad and very general and it may not be as helpful as individually oriented theories for addressing individual clients.

- Family developmental theory addresses the passage of time in the lives of families. It explains how and what developmentally based changes occur in families over time. Its major strength is that it provides a basis for forecasting what a family will be experiencing at any period in the family life cycle. The major weakness is the fact that the model was developed at a time in history when the traditional nuclear family was emphasized. Although the stages and tasks may differ somewhat with family forms, the developmental processes may be similar regardless of family form.

- The family interactional approach stems from symbolic interaction. From this approach, meanings are constructed by family members relevant to the situation in which the family is situated. A major strength is its focus on internal processes within families and understanding these processes. The major limitation is that interactional theorists generally fail to consider the impact of the family's outer environment.

- The family stress model is especially germane to health care situations because of the pervasive illness-related stress the family experiences. The major strength is its relative simplicity. The model emphasizes that perception of stressor(s) is more important than objective reality and by identifying resources, family coping, and strengths, family nursing approaches can be developed that empower families. The model is limited in its usefulness for addressing the needs of healthy families in terms of health promotion and disease prevention.

- In change theory, first-order change means the system itself remains unchanged while its parts undergo some type of change. In second-order change, a change occurs in the system itself, hence a "change of change"; actual changes in the rules governing the system so that the system is transformed structurally and/or communicationally, sending the family to a different level of functioning. Many health behavior change theories indicate that families are key influences in both the health status and health behaviors of individual family members.

- Other frameworks that inform family nursing include: chaos theory, social exchange theory, conflict theory, the ecological framework, an anthropological/multicultural approach, and phenomenology theory.

- Family therapy theories are a blend of family social science theories and practice theories. Both family social science theory and family therapy have a short history, with family therapy theories having a more recent vintage. The interactional/communication therapy approach was heavily influenced by ideas derived from general systems theory, cybernetics, and information processing theory. Therapists using this approach focus on how to assist family members to clearly communicate with each other so that the message sent is the message received.

- Minuchin and associates (Minuchin, 1974; Minuchin & Fishman, 1981; Minuchin, Rosman, & Baker, 1978) developed this systems-oriented approach to family therapy that used spatial and organizational metaphors, both in describing the structural problems of the family and in identifying solutions to change the family structure (Goldenberg & Goldenberg, 1996). Minuchin's (1974) main structural concern was with maintaining the appropriate vertical distance between the generations and his intervention strategies were targeted at "restructuring the family."

- Murray Bowen, a prominent pioneer in family therapy, first developed family systems theory in the mid-1970s. The major focus of Bowen's family systems therapy is on promoting differentiation of self from family and of intellect from emotion (Becvar & Becvar, 1996). Family members gain insight and understanding into the past by examining the above processes, and are then freed to choose how they will behave in the present.

- Three integrated family nursing practice models cited widely and used extensively in family nursing (Hanson & Boyd, 1996a) are the Family Systems Stressor–Strength Model and Inventory (Berkey & Hanson, 1991), Calgary Family Assessment and Intervention Models (Wright & Leahey, 2000), and the Friedman Family Assessment Model (the model used in this text). Although there is much overlap in the content and processes involved in these three models, there are also substantial differences in approach.

- Family nursing theory continues to evolve along with nursing research and practice, and nursing scholars continue with lively debates about nursing theory development in all areas of nursing, including family nursing. Many of the debates focus on new conceptualizations of nursings' metaparadigm concepts and reflect the influence of postmodernist and neomodernist perspectives.

✎ FAMILY VIGNETTE: THE KATZ FAMILY

The purpose of this activity is to contrast family assessments conducted from different theoretical perspectives. Read the following family vignette and answer study questions 1 through 4, first using family communication theory and then using concepts from Roy's Adaptation Model.

A home health nurse visited Mr. Herman Katz, a 68-year-old Jewish man who suffered his second myocardial infarction two weeks ago and returned home this morning. The purpose of the visit was to review Mr. Katz's diet and physical activity regimen with him. Mr. Katz lives with wife Sylvia in a nicely furnished three-bedroom home. Their single 40-year-old daughter is staying with them temporarily to help out when she gets home from work in the evening, and two grown sons live in the same city. Mr. Katz was a business manager before he retired three years ago. His recreational interests, prior to his first heart attack were heavy gardening and home remodeling.

The interagency referral form from the hospital states that Mr. Katz was alert and very conscientious about his care, but was quite reluctant to do any of activities—and thus was somewhat demanding and dependent on the nurses. He ate poorly and got up to go to the bathroom by himself. During the last week he has had no pain or dyspnea during self-care activities.

During the visit, Mrs. Katz and her daughter answer for Mr. Katz when the nurse asks questions. Mrs. Katz is very talkative and complains of being very tired herself. She has osteoarthritis, which makes it difficult for her to walk outside the home. Mr. Katz seems quite content to have his wife act as spokesperson and health leader in the family. Mrs. Katz is very solicitous of Mr. Katz's needs and requests. The sons have come over to visit and call on the phone often since their dad's illness, although they have not provided any care or help with errands or doctor's visits. Mrs. Katz appreciates their support, but feels very tired, as she tries to take care of Herman pretty much by herself (even though her daughter is some help). Mrs. Katz believes that Herman has to take it easy, eat his favorite foods so that he will not feel depressed and will get his strength back, and do as little as possible so that his heart will heal. Mr. Katz is not able or willing to try progressive physical activity. He has told his wife that he is "scared to death to move too much for fear of hurting his heart again." His wife seems to agree as she relates this conversation to the nurse. On the second visit a week later, the nurse observed the following: Mr. Katz continued to be unwilling and afraid to do things for himself and had not increased his level of activity. He appeared short of breath and uncomfortable (as though in pain) when talking about his illness and symptoms, but when distracted he appeared to have no dyspnea or pain. Mr. Katz has seen none of his social or work friends since he has been home, according to Mrs. Katz. He has not been getting dressed or taking care of his personal hygiene adequately.

■ STUDY QUESTIONS

From the family case example, answer questions 1 through 4, first using family communication theory and then using concepts from Roy's Adapatation Model.

1. Describe the family communication network.
2. What variables influence the family interactions?
3. State examples of family nursing diagnoses in communication and other areas.
4. Propose two family nursing interventions directed toward resolving the above family communication problem or other diagnoses.

Answer the following questions.

5. Explain the functions of theory in family nursing.
6. What are three genres of theories that contribute heavily to the theoretical foundations for family nursing?
7. Match the key concepts from seven nursing models relevant to family nursing with the theorists who authored the models:

Theorist	**Key Concepts**
a. ___Florence Nightingale	aa. Expanded consciousness, time, movement
b. ___Imogene King	bb. Open system energy field, evolving toward greater complexity
c. ___Sr. Callista Roy	cc. Family as basic conditioning unit
d. ___Betty Neuman	dd. Open system, stressors, lines of resistance
e. ___Dorothea Orem	ee. Family coping patterns, adaptation
f. ___Martha Rogers	ff. Family as context, interaction, perception
g. ___Margaret Newman	gg. Emphasis on environmental factors, home health nursing, clean air

8. Match the following family social science theoretical perspectives with the descriptions
    a. ___Structural–functional approach
    b. ___Systems approach
    c. ___Developmental approach
    d. ___Interactional approach
    e. ___Stress theory
    f. ___Change theory

Descriptions

   aa. Focus on family's response to crisis, resources, perceptions of the situation
   bb. Family viewed as an open social system and has a process orientation
   cc. Deals with internal family dynamics and roles of family members
   dd. Describes family's progression through its life cycle with predictable stages, tasks, and issues

ee. Family viewed as social system with emphasis on purposes the family achieves, its internal organization, and its relationship to the wider society

ff. Focuses on first-order and second-order transitions

9. What are the main advantages/strengths of these three genres of theoretical frameworks for family nursing?

a. Nursing theories
b. Family therapy theories
c. Social science theories

10. With respect to the three integrated family nursing models discussed in this chapter, which of these following statement(s) is/are accurate?

a. Berkey and Hanson's Family Stressor–Strengths Model/Inventory is an extension of Rogers's model.
b. The Friedman Family Assessment Model is based primarily on family interactional theory and Bowen's family systems theory.
c. The Calgary Family Assessment and Intervention Models integrate multiple theoretical approaches from both the social sciences and the family therapy genres of theories.

11. Describe some of the criticisms of family nursing theory, and discuss influences on the evolution of family nursing theory for the future.

4

STRUCTURAL–FUNCTIONAL THEORY

CONTENT OUTLINE

LEARNING OBJECTIVES

1. Identify the three primary theoretical perspectives used in this text for completing a family assessment.
2. Define the components and basic characteristics of the structural–functional approach as applied to the family.
3. Explain the usefulness of the structural–functional approach to family nursing.
4. Analyze the relationship of family structure to family functions and the system theory approach to the structural–functional approach.
5. List and briefly describe the five basic family functions.
6. Trace major alterations that occurred in family functions during the change from an agrarian, nonindustrialized society to present-day society.

A central assumption of this text is that clinical practice should be guided by theory. The decision regarding what theory or theories to use in one's practice—that is, in assessing, planning, intervening, and evaluating—should be based on practical grounds; in other words, what theory(ies) best/most powerfully explain(s) a situation and suggest(s) meaningful and effective nursing goals and actions. We agree with Blau (1977), a noted sociologist and theoretician, who advises us, "a choice between [theoretical] perspectives can only be made on pragmatic grounds: which theory is more useful for clarifying given problems" (p. 3). And to extend Blau's thought—and to guide nursing actions.

❧ THEORETICAL PERSPECTIVES USED IN THIS TEXT

Looking at the potpourri of theories presented in Chapter 3 (nursing theories, family therapy theories, and family social science theories), several family social science theories appear to be the best, most powerful theoretical perspectives to use in family nursing. These, we believe, are structural–functional theory, developmental theory, and general systems theory. Applying three general theoretical models in addition to some more middle range theories encourages family nurses to practice more holistic and comprehensive care of families.

The structural–functional perspective applied to the family is comprehensive and recognizes the important interaction between the family and its internal and external environment. The developmental approach is needed to provide the information of family development and life cycle tasks, to examine changes in a family's life over time, and to assess how a family is handling its developmental tasks. A general systems approach applied to the family is also needed to assess the adaptational and communications processes within the family. Family developmental and systems theories are needed to guide practice because structural–functional analysis tends to present a static view of the family, while both developmental and general systems theory handle change over time better. In addition, a structural–functional perspective minimizes the importance of growth, change, and disequilibrium in a family, while a general systems theory explains these processes more fully and convincingly. So while structural–functionalism has these apparent biases (and, in fact, has diminished explanatory power in research and practice today), we still need to understand its relevance as a theoretical perspective for family nursing practice.

❧ THE STRUCTURAL–FUNCTIONAL APPROACH

The structural–functional framework is a major theoretical frame of reference in sociology (Leslie & Korman, 1989; Smith, 1995), particularly in the areas of family and medical sociology. Applied to the family, the scope of the framework is very broad. The family is viewed as an open social system and as a subsystem within society for the reproduction and socialization of children as well as the stabilization of adult personalities (Doherty, Boss, LaRossa, Schumm, & Steinmetz, 1993). Relationships between the family and other social systems (e.g., the health care system, educational system) and the family within the larger social system are examined (Dickinson & Leming, 1995). A description of the family's structural (organizational dimensions) and family functions are emphasized in this text as an organizing framework for conducting a family nursing assessment.

According to Eshleman (1974), the structural–functional approach has its origin in the functionalist branch of psychology (particularly Gestalt psychology), in social anthropology (as exhibited in the writings of Malinowski and Radcliffe-Brown), and in sociology (particularly as described by social systems theorists such as Parsons). The Gestalt position emphasizes that one must view the whole and its parts, exploring the interrelationship between the whole and its parts. Along the same line of thinking, social anthropologists have concluded that one cannot understand a particular aspect of social life detached from its general environment (Eshleman, 1974).

Structural–functionalists see the family, one of the social institutions of a society, as being "functional" for or congruent with the society. In the 1950s, theorists (Parsons & Bales, 1955; Parsons, 1951) envisioned a good fit between society and the family, a basic institution functioning to meet society's needs. Today, with such a changing heterogeneous society, this harmonious, stable picture of the relationship between society and the family has changed. Nevertheless, stability and order in systems are viewed as natural and desirable in structural functionalism, whereas conflict and disorder are seen as deviant and dysfunctional in systems (Broderick, 1993). Neofunctionalists (those who have modified the Parsonian description of the theory) have incorporated into families the notions of conflict (struggles between family members) and "moving equilibrium" or change. By adding these notions to structural–functionalism, some of the obvious limitation of the theory are reduced (Kingsbury & Scanzoni, 1993).

Most of the sociological literature which applies to the structural–functional approach to the family makes use of a more macroscopic approach, looking at the family as a subsystem of the wider society. From this perspective, structural–functionalism can be considered the earliest form of systems theory (see Chapter 7) (Broderick, 1993). The general assumptions made include the following (Leslie & Korman, 1989; Parsons & Bales, 1955):

1. A family is a social system with functional requirements.

2. A family is a small group possessing certain generic features common to all small groups.

3. The family as a social system accomplishes functions that serve both the individual and society.

4. Individuals act in accordance with a set of internalized norms and values that are learned primarily in the family through socialization.

Family studies using a structural–functional perspective have demonstrated that the economy and technology are important determinants of family structure and function. In addition, ideological and cultural changes related to individualism, autonomy, and gender roles are vitally important in understanding family structural arrangements and dynamics (Smith, 1995).

The structural–functional perspective is a very useful framework for assessing family life because it enables the family system to be examined holistically (as a unit), in parts (as subsystems or dimensions), and interactionally (as a system interacting with other institutions, such as the educational and health systems, the family's reference group(s), and the wider society). Mancini and Orthner (1988), family educators, remind family professionals that both a micro- and macroscopic perspective is needed when working with families. They explain that "to understand families is to know about those internal dynamics, but also to know something about the common habitat, whether it be the values of society, current economic conditions, or government support for families" (p. 363). Structural–functional theory provides these two perspectives.

Structural–functional theory, then, has been selected, along with general systems theory and developmental theory, as an organizing framework for the text, because its use provides a comprehensive and holistic perspective for assessment purposes. The essence of family-centered nursing involves understanding the dynamics of the family and all the forces, both internal and external, that affect it. For this understanding, structural–functional theory serves as an organizing framework, particularly in guiding family assessment.

CONCEPT OF STRUCTURE

The structural–functional approach analyzes the family's structural characteristics—the arrangement of the parts that form the whole, and the functions it performs for both society and its subsystems. The structure of the family refers to how the family is organized, the manner in which units are arranged, and how these units relate to each other. The dimensions, or definitions, of this concept of family structure vary considerably. Some theorists base structure on the type of family form (e.g., nuclear versus extended); type of power structure (e.g., matriarchal versus patriarchal); or marital patterns (e.g., exogamy versus endogamy) (Eshleman, 1974). Another way of looking at the family structure is by describing the subsystems as the structural dimension (Minuchin, 1974).

Assuming that the family is a special kind of small group, the structural dimensions identified by small-group theory as being relevant for assessing such groups are used in this text. Parad and Caplan (1965), in analyzing a family under stress, have identified three structural dimensions, which they call the family lifestyle. Family lifestyle refers to "the reasonably stable patterning of family organization, subdivided into three interdependent elements of value system, communication network, and role systems" (Parad & Caplan, p. 55). In this text a fourth structural dimension has been added to Parad and Caplan's structural elements—the power and decision-making structure. To repeat, then, the four basic structural dimensions that are subsumed under family structure in this text and that will be elaborated on in separate chapters, are (1) role structure, (2) value structure, (3) communication processes, and (4) power and decision-making structure.

These elements are all intimately interrelated and interacting. When one aspect of the internal structure of the family is affected by input from the external environment, the processing of this input within the family system will also affect the other structural dimensions. The family's high degree of interrelatedness and interdependency is seen when a family health care professional observes how certain family behaviors often become indicators of strengths or dysfunction within several or all the structural elements in the family.

A case in point is the following. A husband, in an authoritarian way, is observed ordering his wife and children on when and what will be served for dinner. The mother is then seen directing the children to each prepare certain assigned parts of the meal. Mother and children carry out father's wishes with no comments or sign of feelings. No other communications are noted. We can see from this one vignette (and this would have to be verified by further observation of the family) that the power figure in this situation is the father; his role is one of a stern, commanding leader of the family, who probably needs and has much control over his family (because even details are controlled). The communication patterns here are one-way (father to mother and children, mother to children) and completely task centered. No feelings or sharing of thoughts are observed. Again speculating on this situation, the events are congruent with the family's value structure. One of the values central to this family probably would be male dominance, while another related value might be respect for and obedience to elders.

Family structure is ultimately evaluated by how well the family is able to fulfill its family functions—the goals important to its members and society. The family's structure serves to facilitate the achievement of family functions, because the conservation and allocation of resources is a prime task for the family structure. Because of this important relationship, functions should be viewed in tandem with family structures.

❧ CONCEPT OF FUNCTION

Family functions are commonly defined as outcomes or consequences of the family structure. Although some authors use "function" to mean "consequences of or results of," it is a little easier to think of family functions as being what the family does (Friedman, 1992; Ingoldsby, 1995a). Why does it exist? What purposes does it serve? "Social institutions exist because

they perform certain valuable functions for their members and for society of which they are a part" (Ingoldsby, 1995a, p. 84). As described in detail in Chapter 1, the family's basic functions meet the needs of both individual family members and wider society. The most vital of the purposes families fulfill are producing new members (the reproduction function) and training these individuals to become participating members of the society (the socialization function) (Kingsburg & Scanzoni, 1993).

Five family functions* are most germane when assessing and intervening with families. (See Figure 4–1.)

1. The affective function (personality maintenance function): for stabilization of adult personalities, meeting the psychological needs of family members. (See Chapter 14 for a detailed description of the family affective function.)

2. The socialization and social placement function: for the primary socialization of children aimed at making them productive members of their society, as well as the conferring of status on family members. (See Chapter 15 for a detailed description of the family socialization function.)

3. The reproductive function: for maintenance of family continuity over the generations as well as for societal survival.

4. The economic function: for the provision of sufficient economic resources and their effective allocation.

5. The health care function: for the provision of physical necessities—food, clothing, shelter, health care. (See Chapter 16 for a detailed description of the family health care function.)

AFFECTIVE FUNCTION

The affective function is a central basis for both the formation and the continuation of the individual family unit, and it thus constitutes one of the most vital functions of families. Today, when many societal tasks

---

* These functions represent an adaptation or modification of several theorists' descriptions of family functions, including those of Murdock (1949), Ogburn (1933), Parsons and Bales (1955), and Hill (1965).

Figure 4–1. The five basic family functions.

are performed outside the family unit, much of the family's effort is focused on meeting the needs of family members for affection and understanding. The ability to provide for these needs is a key determinant of whether a given family will persist or dissolve. As Duvall (1977) says, family happiness is gauged by the strength of family love. The family must meet the affectional needs of its members because the affectional responses of one family member to another provide the basic rewards of family life.

Primarily a role of adults in families, this function deals with the family's perception and care of the socioemotional needs of all its members. It involves tension reduction and morale maintenance.

The importance of this function within the family is found most strongly among middle-class and affluent families, where choice is more feasible. In middle- and upper-class families, personal happiness in the marital relationship based on companionship and love is critical. The salience of this function has a decreased emphasis in many working-class and lower-class families, largely because more basic functions such as providing the physical necessities of life predominate.

SOCIALIZATION AND SOCIAL PLACEMENT FUNCTION

Socialization of family members is a universal, cross-cultural functional requisite for societal survival

(Leslie & Korman, 1989). It refers to the myriad of learning experiences provided within the family aimed at teaching children how to function and assume adult social roles such as those of husband–father and wife–mother. The family has the primary responsibility of transforming an infant in a score of years into a social person capable of full participation in society. Furthermore, socialization should not be thought of as pertaining only to infant and child-rearing patterns, but rather as a lifelong process that includes internalizing the appropriate sets of norms and values for being a teenager, a spouse, a parent, an employee on a new job, a grandparent, and a retired person. In short, socialization involves learning the culture.

Because this function is increasingly shared with schools, recreational and child care facilities, and other extrafamilial institutions, the family plays a reduced, yet critical, role in socialization. Parents still provide the foundations and transmit their cultural heritage to their children.

An integral part of socialization in the family involves the inculcation of controls and values—giving the growing child (and adult) a sense of what is right and wrong. Kohlberg (1970) describes the process of moral development as having its foundations in the family. Moral development is seen as a process similar to the stages of emotional and cognitive development à la Erikson and Piaget, respectively. By identifying with parental figures and being consistently reinforced negatively and positively for their behavior, children develop a personal value system that is greatly influenced by the family's value system.

Gilligan (1982), a feminist who theorizes about moral development, also identifies the family's foundational influence in the inculcation of values. She challenged and extended developmental theorists' writing by explaining the gender differences in values. Men, she argues, value the ethic of justice, stemming from this premise of equal treatment to all, while women value the ethic of care, stemming from the premise of nonviolence—that no one should be hurt.

Social placement or status conferring is the other aspect of the socialization function. Conferring of status on children refers to passing on of the traditions, values, and privileges of the family, although today tradition no longer dictates the patterns of most adult Americans. At birth, a child automatically inherits his or her family's status—ethnic, racial, national, religious, economic, political, and educational. The family socializes the child into its social class, instilling in him or her relevant aspirations. Additionally, the family has the responsibility of providing necessary socialization and educational experiences that enable family members to assume a vocation and roles in groups that are consistent with status expectations.

Educating parents about child-rearing patterns and ways they may cope with family problems are major components of family health care, beginning with genetic and reproductive counseling, continuing through prenatal and child care, and extending throughout the life cycle of the family. The common health concerns and family problems with which the family nurse can assist families are described within the various stages of the family's life cycle in Chapter 5. Chapter 15 describes the family socialization function more extensively.

HEALTH CARE FUNCTION

The physical functions of the family are met by the parents providing food, clothing, shelter, health care, and protection against danger. Health care and health practices (which influence the individual family members' health status) are a most relevant family function for the family nurse. Chapter 16 is devoted entirely to an exploration of this significant function.

REPRODUCTIVE FUNCTION

One of the basic functions of the family is to insure continuity of the intergenerational family and of society—that is, provide recruits for society (Leslie & Korman, 1989). In the past, marriage and the family were designed to regulate and control sexual behavior as well as reproduction. These aspects (i.e., the control of sexual behavior, contraception and reproduction) are now less important functions of the family.

Until recent times, reproduction was largely the primary function of the family, its *raison d'etre*. But today, reproduction is being disconnected from the family. In the postmodern family, family is defined within the context of choice (i.e., "who you chose to be a part of your family") (Dunphy, 2001). Thus, once a child is born, a new family is born—with single-parent families becoming increasingly common. The number of births to unmarried mothers, for example, has risen in the United States in the last two decades, as greater acceptability and loosening of sexual mores has occurred (see Chapter 1 for demographic changes in the family).

Along with having children outside of the confines of the traditional family, greater use of contraception and reproductive technologies are other important trends, either within or outside the family context. Moreover, the move toward population control and family planning is affecting the importance of parenthood for both women and men. A shift of cultural priorities and personal values continues to diminish motherhood as a woman's central purpose in life and fatherhood as a man's chief reason to work. Increasingly, public expressions are heard against the bearing of more than two children per couple (as the couple's replacement quota), particularly in developing countries.

ECONOMIC FUNCTION

The economic function involves the family's provision of sufficient resources—financial, space, and material—and their appropriate allocation by decision-making processes.

An assessment of the family's economic resources provides the nurse with data relevant to the family's ability to allocate resources appropriately to meet family needs such as adequate clothing, food, shelter, and health care. By gaining an understanding of how a family distributes its resources, the family-centered nurse can also obtain a clearer perspective about the family's value system (what is important to the family) and what resources can be accessed to help it meet its needs.

Because this function is difficult for most poor families to fulfill satisfactorily, family nurses must accept the responsibility of assisting families to obtain appropriate community resources where they can secure needed information, employment, vocational counseling, and financial assistance.

CHANGES IN FAMILY FUNCTIONS

The functions that the family carries out for society and its members have changed over time, as depicted in Table 4–1. Certain functions have changed primarily in response to societal and economic changes. If one examines the American family as it existed before industrialization—when an agrarian lifestyle and culture predominated—and compares the family during that period with the family today, profound changes in family functions become apparent.

It is clear that industrialization, urbanization, and technological advances have intruded forcefully on the family, and social/public institutions have assumed many functions that were once the family's domain. In addition to changes in family functions, family values and the timing of family transitions have been markedly altered. Demos (1970), in describing the transfer of functions from the family to other social institutions, points out that the preindustrial family served as a workshop, church, reformatory, school, and asylum. Today, many older persons live apart in their own home or in residences for senior citizens. Rather than having to depend on the family for assistance, economic support is now provided to the old, unemployed, disabled, and dependent through Social Security and/or welfare programs. The young are no longer trained at home, but are educated in schools, and by the mass media, peers, and various other associations and groups.

Activities that traditionally took place within the home or involved the entire family now take place elsewhere and engage only certain family members. For instance, economic activity, which traditionally the family engaged in at home as a whole, has until recently been the father's responsibility—one that took him out of the home and away from family life. Today, with the growing number of dual worker families, both spouses are engaged in economic activities. One of the most interesting books in this area is by Christopher Lasch, a social historian. His brilliant book, *Haven in a Heartless World* (1977), expounds on the erosion of family in terms of the loss or partial loss of important family functions.

The affective function of the family is a central family function today. And kinship ties, thought at one time to be "weakened" or "practically absent" because of the demands created by industrialization and urbanization, continue to be "alive and well." Given the urbanized, impersonal character of much public life, people increasingly look to their families for more emotional solace and support than in earlier times.

SUMMARY

- Clinical practice should be guided by theory—a theory or theories that most powerfully explain clinical situations and offer guidelines for working with families.

- This text primarily uses three grand theories to organize and guide practice: structural–functional, family developmental, and general systems theories. Middle-range theories, in particular family stress and coping theories, also are used to guide practice.

- The structural–functional theory, a grand theory from sociology, is comprehensive and holistic, and recognizes the interaction between the family and its internal and external environments. There is notable overlap in the notions embedded in structural–functional theory and general systems theory, especially in their emphasis on the family's continual interaction with its external environment.

TABLE 4–1

CHANGES IN FAMILY FUNCTIONS: PRE- AND POSTINDUSTRIALIZATION PERIODS

FAMILY FUNCTION	FAMILY FUNCTIONS BEFORE INDUSTRIALIZATION (AGRARIAN SETTING)	PRESENT-DAY FAMILY FUNCTIONS (URBAN SETTING)
1. Economic	Work and family were not separate spheres. Family served as sole economic unit. It was a self-contained, self-sufficient unit; all family members helped. Family both produced and consumed its products. Family was supported by strong kinship associations (the extended family).	The family's economic function is much more limited. Food and clothes are bought outside of the home. Children are no longer economic assets. Single individuals survive well on their own. Family providers, who in many cases are both spouses, work outside of home, bringing home money to buy outside products and services.
2. Status conferring (Social placement)	Family conferred privilege, honor, and status on people. Family affiliation was crucial in locating and placing someone in society.	Function is still present but much decreased in importance except among upper-class families. People are seen primarily as individuals, not as family members.
3. Education	Education ("schooling") was done primarily in home. Father taught son his vocation. Mother taught daughter homemaking and child-rearing skills. Children taught vocation from parents/relatives at early age.	Education is carried on outside of home to a great extent; very formalized and institutionalized, which has a pervasive influence on children in both school and extracurricular activities (e.g., sports, music, school clubs). Economic activities require specialized training. Occupational skills and knowledge are learned outside of home.
4. Socialization of children	Child rearing occurred in the home and was the responsibility of mothers, grandmothers, aunts, and older female children when children were young. Parents were fully "in charge" of child rearing.	Socialization function remains as a major function, but is shared with outside institutions (e.g., nursery schools, baby sitters, child care centers, teachers, counselors). Parents' authority and control is diminished, especially after preschool period. .
5. Health care function (care of ill, disabled, and older family members)	Protection, supervision, and care of family members, especially of dependent, disabled, or aged individuals, was entirely family's responsibility. The aged, dependent, and infirm were cared for at home.	This function has decreased greatly, although still present. The family's ethnic background and degree of acculturation to white, middle-class culture influences the family functioning in this area. With older or disabled persons, society takes responsibility when family cannot or will not care for these dependent members. The high proportion of working women and the larger number of elderly in our society have also made home care by family members widespread, but more difficult.

TABLE 4–1 *(CONTINUED)*

CHANGES IN FAMILY FUNCTIONS: PRE- AND POSTINDUSTRIALIZATION PERIODS

FAMILY FUNCTION	FAMILY FUNCTIONS BEFORE INDUSTRIALIZATION (AGRARIAN SETTING)	PRESENT-DAY FAMILY FUNCTIONS (URBAN SETTING)
6. Religious	Religious training and practices were carried out in both the home and in religious institutions.	There is increasing secularization within society and religion has a declining influence on everyday behavior. Family religious involvement also declined. Religion is primarily taught in outside agencies.
7. Recreational	Because family was without commercial recreation, family-centered activities predominated.	Commercialization of recreation is ubiquitous. Family-centered activities are greatly curtailed after children are older.
8. Reproduction (procreation)	Marriage and family were necessary for survival.	Having a child creates a family, but marriage or having a family is not necessary. Nevertheless, reproduction remains the one *universal* family function.
9. Affective	Primary group relationships were not as strong; extended family was more important affectively.	This function not only remains, but has increased in importance. The typical American family has weakened extended family ties (although this varies across ethnic groups), whereas emotional relationships between the mates and parent–child are very intense. Historically, there existed an economic basis for marriage, which now is usually an affective basis, making divorce more of an acceptable alternative if the affective basis for the marriage fails.

- In structural–functional theory, the family is viewed as an open system, a subsystem within society, and a system with the following basic purposes or functions: the affective function, the socialization and social placement function, the economic function, the reproductive function, and the health care function. It is vital for the family to adequately fulfill each of these functions for the welfare of its family members, as well as for the welfare of society.

- The family is also viewed as having structural dimensions; these dimensions are interactive organizing characteristics that arrange the family system so that it functions as a whole. It is through these structural dimensions that the family functions are fulfilled.

- The family structural dimensions include: the family power structure, the family role structure, family communications, and the family value structure.

- Family structural and functional dimensions are highly interactive and interdependent on each other. Because of this, they are also consonant with each other. For example, if the family is husband dominant, then the communications would flow more heavily flow from father/husband to the rest of the family members and the family roles would reflect the differential power of family members.

- The family structural and functional dimensions form the organizing framework in this text for conducting a family nursing assessment.

- Each of the family structural and functional dimensions are defined and explicated in this chapter.

- Industrialization, urbanization, and technological advances have radically altered the extent to which and the way in which family functions are carried out today. Table 4–1 explains the changes that have taken place in the family—comparing the agrarian family to the family living in the industrialized and postindustrialized society.

✎ FAMILY VIGNETTE: THE RODRIQUEZ FAMILY

Family composition:

Name	Relationship	Age
Emma	Wife	40
Arthur	Husband	44
Danny	Son	17
Ronny	Son	14
Leonard	Son	11
Sammy	Son	7
Cindy	Daughter	5
Arlie	Son	4
Iris	Daughter	2

All the children appeared in good health and were dressed adequately. Arthur and Emma Rodriquez were rather short and obese.

The house was located in a suburban area, in a neighborhood full of children and pets. The house has three bedrooms, one-and-a-half bathrooms, attached garage, with small front and backyards. The interior is reasonably clean and orderly with bare floors and sparse furniture. The TV is in the living room where there are no pictures, books, or decorations.

This is a Mexican-American family. All the members are bilingual. Arthur completed the 10th grade and served in the army. He has since worked as a maintenance man on refrigeration units of food trucks. He has medical insurance through his company.

Emma has been a housewife since her marriage at 19. She has devoted most of her energies to the family and their care. She spends time cooking and provides hearty, nutritious meals, although overabundant in carbohydrates.

The children are in school with the exception of Iris. They do passable work. The older two boys are involved in athletics, which is a source of pride for the parents.

This is the only marriage for Arthur and Emma, who have been married for 21 years. There has been significant marital discord during the past 11 years.

From Emma's description of home life, she "wears the pants in the family." She describes her husband as a meek, passive man who takes no responsibility in the household. He brings home the check, eats, and sleeps there. She states she finds him "sexually unattractive" and difficult to be "close" to. Emma says she wants to be with her children but that she has no love for her husband.

Arthur says he works and makes a living. "The house is a woman's responsibility," which he has left to his wife.

Emma does all of the disciplining and is the parent that the children go to for permissions. Emma states that when Arthur tells the children to do something and they disobey, their excuse is they didn't think that he really meant it. The children verified that Emma does the greater part of the disciplining and that when she is home, they really watch their behavior.

Emma prefers her children to her husband. They are the apparent reason the marriage holds together. She seems very fond of all her children, but she mentions Leonard and Iris the most. She seems to favor Leonard because other children tease him for being fat. She tries to give him special attention. She talks about Iris as being her baby.

Arthur appears to love all the children, but makes extra comments about the oldest sons. Arthur says his wife is a wonderful mother and good housekeeper, but makes no comments about their personal relationship.

Danny and Ronny seem to pair off because of their ages. Leonard and Iris prefer mother's company, while Sammy cares for and plays with Arlie. Cindy, age 5, appears to be withdrawn and a loner.

■ STUDY QUESTIONS

From the above case study, list and describe how the Rodriquez family is fulfilling each of the five family functions.

1. Affective function
2. Health care function
3. Reproductive function
4. Socialization function
5. Economic function

✺ FAMILY VIGNETTE: THE KATZ FAMILY

A home health care nurse has been visiting Mr. Herman Katz several times to follow up on his dietary and progressive exercise regimen following a second heart attack. Here are her observations about the client and family. Mr. Katz, a Jewish male, age 68, suffered a myocardial infarction and just recently returned home after one week of hospitalization. From the hospital interagency referral form the home health nurse learned that Mr. Katz upon discharge was alert and feeling well, but very reluctant to do any of the activities suggested—and thus was somewhat demanding and dependent on the nurses and now on his wife. The nurse learned that Mr. Katz had been a certified accountant for many years and had

(continued)

retired three years ago. The family lives in a nicely furnished three-bedroom house. His first heart attack occurred six months after retirement. Past recreational interests had been heavy gardening and remodeling of his home prior to his first heart attack. Mrs. Sylvia Katz is 65 years old and also Jewish. She has been in fairly good health except for being overweight, sedentary, and bothered with osteoarthritis, which makes walking difficult for her. She prepares rich Jewish foods for herself, Herman, and their single daughter, Marion, age 40, who is temporarily living with them to help out during her father's recovery. Mrs. Katz constantly answers for her husband when questions about his health status or treatment are concerned. Mr. Katz seems quite content to have his wife act as spokesperson and health leader in the family. Mrs. Katz and Marion are very solicitous of Herman's needs and requests. Two sons live close by and have come over to visit and call on the phone often since their dad's illness, although they have not provided any care or help with errands or doctor's visits. Mrs. Katz appreciates their support but feels very tired, as she tries to take care of Herman pretty much by herself (even though the daughter is there to help). She believes that Herman has to take it easy, eat his favorite foods so that he will not feel depressed and will get his strength back, and do as little as possible so that his heart will heal. Mr. Katz is not able or willing to try to progressively exercise as the doctor recommended. He told his wife that he is "scared to death to move too much for fear of hurting his heart again." His wife seems to agree as she relates this conversation to the nurse. On the nurse's second visit, one week later, Mr. Katz was still lying around all day, not getting dressed, and only getting up to go to the bathroom.

■ STUDY QUESTIONS (Continued)

From the information provided in the above vignette, answer the following two questions:

6. Describe the family structure (the role, power, values, and communication structure).

7. Describe the family functions (affective, health care, economic, socialization and social class, and reproductive).

Answer the following questions:

8. The text's family assessment tool is based on three theoretical perspectives. These are:
    a. Orem's, Roy's, and Rogers's nursing theories
    b. Interactional, structural–functional, and institutional theories
    c. Structural–functional, developmental, and general systems theories
    d. Family coping, affective, and economic theories
    e. Role, communications, and power theories

9. The interactionist approach analyzes internal family dynamics. The structural–functional approach, which is broader in focus, analyzes what?

10. The following are reasons for using a structural–functional approach for assessing and working with families. Select the most accurate and inclusive reason.

   a. It is a microscopic approach, it centers on inner dynamics and provides information for transactional-based diagnoses.
   b. It consists of a comprehensive, holistic perspective by which not only the family can be assessed, but also the family's universe (its inner and outer environments).
   c. It provides the family health worker with an understanding of the forces from within and without that impinge on the family.
   d. Using this framework the common health problems are recognized as the family progresses through the life cycle.

11. The relationship of the family structure to family function is that (select one answer):

   a. The structure provides the organization for family functions to be accomplished
   b. The functions mandate the family structure
   c. Structure and function are separate entities and have no direct relationship to each other

12. The structural–functional approach differs from the systems approach in what way? (Select the correct answers.)

   a. They are two separate frameworks.
   b. The structural–functional approach is in opposition to the systems approach.
   c. The systems theory approach handles change over time better.
   d. The structural–functional approach emanated from theories in psychology (Gestalt), social anthropology (Malinowski), and social systems theory (Parsons).

13. Indicate whether the six descriptions in the left-hand column are structural dimensions or family functions.

   a. Roles of two adult family members
   b. Reproduction
   c. Communication patterns
   d. The provision of adequate economic support
   e. The family's priorities and value system
   f. Caregiving of family members

   1. Structure
   2. Function

14. Match each family function from the left-hand column with the appropriate description of it in the right-hand column showing how the function has changed (as society changed from an agrarian to industrialized state).

Function

a. Affective
b. Socializing
c. Economic
d. Religious
e. Care of disabled family members
f. Educational
g. Status conferring
h. Reproduction

Description

1. Continues to be crucial.
2. Decreased in importance or limited.
3. Increased in importance.
4. Function important; function shared with other institutions in society.

FAMILY DEVELOPMENTAL THEORY

✺ LEARNING OBJECTIVES

1. Discuss three basic assumptions of family developmental theory.
2. Define the meaning of family developmental tasks and the family life cycle or family career.
3. Identify and describe each of the developmental stages of the two-parent nuclear family.
4. Relative to the single-parent divorced family, describe the family life cycle stages.

5. Relative to the stepparent family, describe the family life cycle stages.
6. Relative to domestic partner relationships, describe variations that may be present when compared to the traditional family life cycles stages.
7. Discuss the factors that affect the extent to which family developmental tasks may be affected by the illness or disability of a family member.

8. Identify the primary assessment areas relative to family development and history.

9. Select nursing diagnoses that reflect potential or actual problems that impact family developmental stages.

10. Choose nursing interventions that will help families and their members move toward completion of individual and family developmental tasks.

One of the more recent frameworks generated for studying and working with families is that of family development. The framework focuses on the longitudinal career of the family, often called the **family career** or **family life cycle**. This theoretical approach seeks to explain change in the family system, including changes in interactions and relationships among family members that occur over time. It emphasizes members playing roles within and outside the family that affect family interaction. Family development does not cover nonfamily aspects of the life careers of individuals or events affecting them that do not impinge on the lives of other family members (Aldous, 1996).

🐝OVERVIEW OF FAMILY DEVELOPMENTAL THEORY

The family developmental approach is based on the observation that families are long-lived groups with a natural history that must be assessed if the dynamics of the group are to be fully and accurately interpreted (Duvall & Miller, 1985). Although each family goes through each stage of development in its own unique way, all families are considered as examples of an overall normative pattern (Rodgers, 1973).

Family development gives a temporal change perspective to the study of families. Time is measured in weeks and years. This theory describes family life over time as divided into a series of **stages.** A family stage is an interval of time in which the structure and interaction of role relationships in the family are qualitatively and quantitatively distinct from other periods (Klein & White, 1996). Family transitions are shifts from one stage to another and can be viewed over time as consisting of paths taken or not taken (Klein & White). Family stages cover sizable time spans and, although transitions link one stage to another, there are breaks that give each stage its distinctive character.

The notion of stages rests on the assumption that in families there is high family member interdependence. Families are forced to change each time members are added to or subtracted from the family, or each time the oldest child changes his or her developmental stage. For instance, changes in roles, marital adjustment, child rearing, and discipline have been found to change from stage to stage (Klein & White, 1996). The family takes one kind of structure when children are infants or preschool age; another structure when the parents enter into the prime of life and the children reach adolescence; and finally another when the children mature, marry, and go their own ways. Rodgers (1973) describes these changes further:

> The structure of the group changes during its history. As members interact with one another over a variety of matters happening in the group, a whole set of learned and shared experiences develop which become precedents for further interactions. Although many of these experiences are unique, a great many are related to the normal and inevitable issues that arise in living together. Recently married couples must work out a set of relationships that are mutually satisfactory concerning many matters. Once established, however, the relationships do not remain constant, but change subtly or perhaps dramatically because of later events, which may occur in the family or outside of it. . . . Many happenings are anticipated and prepared for, whereas many are unexpected—though not peculiar to that family alone. Thus, though each family's history is unique, it is also common. Furthermore, it has a certain quality of inevitability though not necessarily of predictability as to exact time or circumstance. The developmental approach does not seek to explain family dynamics in terms of its unique elements, but in terms of the common quality of its experience over its history. There exist many more events that are common than are unique. (p. 13)

The historical roots of family developmental theory can be traced to five theoretical legacies. Family developmental framework is eclectic, because it acquired concepts from individual growth and developmental theory and from different approaches to the study of the family. Contributions to family developmental theory were drawn from symbolic interactionism, structural functionalism, the sociology of work and professions, systems theory, and from family life stress and crisis theory (Mattessich & Hill, 1987). Evelyn Duvall and Reuben Hill, beginning in the 1940s, were the two family scholars who first developed this theoretical perspective (Burr, 1995).

The three basic assumptions of family developmental theory, as outlined by Aldous (1996), are:

1. Family behavior is the sum of the previous experiences of family members as incorporated in the present and in their expectations for the future.

2. Families develop and change over time in similar and consistent ways.

3. Families and their members perform certain time-specific tasks that are set by them and by the cultural and societal context.

A CRITIQUE OF FAMILY DEVELOPMENTAL THEORY

Family developmental theory is based on the common, general features of family life; it does not address situational or nonnormative stressors (unusual events), and can be criticized for its assumption of homogeneity (its lack of adequate attention to family diversity), its middle-class bias, its assumption of stability within each stage, and its lack of explanation of the processes that occur between stages that allow families to change. Yet the use of this framework for assessment and intervention is exceedingly helpful, because it provides family care health professionals with ways of anticipating what to expect and hence what kinds of teaching and counseling services may be needed. Family developmental theory increases our understanding of families at different points in their life cycle and generates "typical" or "modal" descriptions of family life during the various stages (Duvall & Miller, 1985). Moreover, by assessing the family's developmental stage and its performance of the tasks appropriate to that stage, family health

care professionals are provided with guidelines for analyzing family growth and health promotion needs. The family nurse is better able to provide the support needed for smooth progression from one stage to another.

THE FAMILY CAREER OR FAMILY LIFE CYCLE

Family career is the dynamic process of change that occurs during a family's existence. The concept of family career and family life cycle are used interchangeably (Aldous, 1996) and will be used as such throughout this chapter. The use of family life cycle, however, is somewhat misleading since a cycle is a repeated sequence of events (Klein & White, 1996). Existence over time does not constitute a cycle. For example, although the family members at the end of the family are the same couple who began the family's existence, the aging couple does not repeat the experiences of the newlywed couple.

A family career includes the diverse paths that unfold during a family's life. It is composed of all the events and periods of time (stages) between events transversed by a family, such as beginning a family, raising and launching children, and experiencing the loss of a partner. As the family progresses through different stages of development and situational events, a reorganization of family roles and tasks is required (Aldous, 1996).

In 1962, Duvall was among the first to divide the family life cycle into eight stages, with developmental tasks at each stage. These stages were based on the following criteria of (a) major change in family size, (b) the developmental stage of the oldest child (with the exception of the last two stages of family life, when children are no longer present in the family), and (c) the work status of the breadwinner. More recently, Carter and McGoldrick (1980, 1989) have conceptualized the family life cycle in a six-phase framework. In contrast to Duvall, the Carter and McGoldrick model formulated family life cycle stages that focus on the major points at which family members enter or exit the family, thus upsetting the family's equilibrium. Emphasis is placed on the altered relationships that are requisite so that the family can move from one life cycle stage to the next. Several other authors have delineated stages of the family life cycle, primarily adding stages to Duvall's model to account for the childless couple and more detailed transitions in the elderly couple (Table 5–1).

Each developmental stage is separated from the next by the amount of **family transition** that is required by a particular life event (Carter & McGoldrick, 1989; Nock, 1981; Rowe, 1981). These family transitions are considered "normal," and they carry implications for individual members who must critically assess their own well-being and alter their role functions and expectations to meet the changing developmental tasks of the family over the life course (Rankin, 1989). Just as the child, adolescent, and adult need to accomplish certain developmental tasks or milestones, the family must also move through predictable transitions for optimal family growth and development. Milestones of individual development, such as starting school, reaching adolescence, marriage, the birth of a new baby, and retirement, often serve as the normal transitions that affect the entire family (Gershwin & Nilsen, 1989). Unexpected events or paranormative transitions are those events that do not occur in every family, such as illness, disability, miscarriage, change in socioeconomic status, or divorce, which can result in crisis within the family (Carter & McGoldrick, 1989). These events or transitions can alter the developmental course for all the family members, therefore altering the natural movement of the family (Rolland, 1993).

FAMILY DEVELOPMENTAL TASKS

Just as individuals have developmental tasks* that they must achieve in order to feel satisfied during a stage of development and to be able to proceed successfully to the following stage, each stage of family development has its specific developmental tasks or role expectations. Family developmental tasks refer to growth responsibilities that must be achieved by a family during each stage of its development so as to meet (a) its biological requirements, (b) its cultural imperatives, and (c) its own aspirations and values (Duvall, 1977; Klein & White, 1996).

---

* Examples are the developmental tasks that are inherent within the following frames of reference: (1) Erikson's stages of psychosocial development, (2) Piaget's stages of cognitive development, (3) Kohlberg's stages of moral development, and (4) Freud's stages of psychosexual development.

How do the developmental tasks of the family differ from those of the individual family member? Although in reality many of them dovetail, family developmental tasks are generated when the family strives as a unit to meet the demands and needs of family members who in turn are striving to meet their individual developmental requisites. Family tasks are also created by community pressures for the family and its members to conform to the expectations of the family's reference group and of the wider society.

In addition, family developmental tasks include the tasks or role expectations specific to each stage inherent in accomplishing the five basic functions of the family, consisting of (1) affective function (personality maintenance function); (2) socialization and social placement function; (3) health care function—provision and allocation of physical necessities and health care; (4) reproductive function; and (5) economic function (see Chapter 4 for a fuller definition of these functions).

The real challenge for families is to meet each of the members' needs as well as to meet the general family functions. The meshing of individual developmental needs and family tasks is not always possible. For instance, the adolescent's task of developing autonomy includes changes in parental authority that may be in opposition to the family's social control task.

FAMILY CAREER OR LIFE CYCLE VARIATIONS

There are predictable stages within the life career of every family; however, they do not necessarily occur linearly. Families vary, as do the family stages. Stages of the family life cycle follow no rigid pattern (Duvall, 1977; Klein & White, 1996). It then goes without saying that many families today do not fit into the traditional two-parent nuclear family stages of Duvall or Carter and McGoldrick. Variations in the traditional family life cycle are seen among families in which couples do not marry, couples remain childless, and in which there are homosexual unions and single-parent and stepparent families. More people are choosing various family forms and hence the concept of the family career, covering the two-parent nuclear family, is obviously limited in applicability. For nontraditional families or families that are poor or from minorities, variations in the timing and sequencing of

TABLE 5—1

THEORISTS' VIEWS OF THE DEVELOPMENTAL STAGES OF THE FAMILY

DUVALL (1957)	FELDMAN (1961)	RODGERS (1964)	CARTER & McGOLDRICK (1980)
			1. Between families: The unattached young adult
Becoming Families 1. Couple without children	1. Early marriage (childless)	1. Childless couple	2. The joining of families through marriage: The new couple
Childbearing Families 2. Oldest child less than 30 months	2. Oldest child an infant	2. All children less than 36 months	3. Families with young children (infancy through school age)
Families with Preschool Children 3. Oldest child from 2½ to 5	3. Oldest child at preschool	3. Preschool children with oldest 3-6 and youngest under 3 4. All children 3–6	
Families with School-Aged Children 4. Oldest child from 5 to 13	4. All children school age	5. School-aged family with infants 6. School-aged family with preschoolers 7. All children 6–13	
5. Oldest child from 13 to 20	5. Oldest child a teenager, all others in school	8. Teenage family with infants 9. Teenage family with preschoolers 10. Teenage family with school-agers 11. All children 13–20	4. Families with adolescents
6. When first child leaves until last is gone	6. One or more children at home and one or more children out of the home	12. Young adult family with infants 13. Young adult family with preschoolers 14. Young adult family with school-agers 15. Young adult family with teenagers 16. All children over 20	5. Launching children and moving on
7. Empty nest to retirement	7. All children out of the home	17. Launching family with infants 18. Launching family with preschoolers 19. Launching family with school-agers 20. Launching family with teenagers 21. Youngest child over 20 22. When all children have been launched until retirement	
8. Retirement to death of one or both spouses	8. Elderly couple	23. Retirement until death of a spouse 24. Death of first spouse to death of survivor.	6. Families in later life

Source: Bowden V., Dickey, S., & Greenberg, C. (1998). Children and their families: The continuum of care (p. 105). Philadelphia: W. B. Saunders.

family events exist (Teachman, Polonko, & Scanzoni, 1987). Current research describes differing career stages and tasks for families not fitting the traditional two-parent nuclear family. The life stages of single-parent, stepparent, and lesbian/gay families are described later in the chapter.

Even within the traditional two-parent nuclear family there have been changes in the timing of life cycle stages. Increasingly, young adults are living with parents, living alone, or living with other young adults (the "between family life cycle stage" of Carter and McGoldrick). Couples are postponing marriage and childbearing, shortening the child-rearing period (largely the result of birth control and career and work demands), and are having fewer children. With these changes and with people living longer, there are a corresponding greater number of years within the last two stages of the family career—the middle years and retirement and old age stages.

CHANGING LIFE CYCLE

Rankin (1989) developed a developmental family framework that takes into consideration the changing life cycle of American families with respect to their expected transitions (Table 5–2). The *emerging family* is one concerned with the tasks of becoming a family unit. In the traditional life cycle, this would be the stage of beginning families and childbearing families (McGoldrick, Heiman, & Carter, 1993). In this framework, changing emerging families include opposite- or same-sex partners living together with a nonformalized bond. Common, expected transitions encountered by these families include changes in personal relationships, changes in family relationships, and change in role status. The new couple must establish new roles in both their relationship with each other and their relationship with their families of origin. They must also decide whether or not to move into a parental role. The transition to parenthood is often challenging for the traditional family as well as for the nontraditional family. In both situations, decisions need to be made defining the role each parent will play in the development of the child.

The *solidifying family* is the family whose primary tasks are to stabilize the bond between the parents and to socialize the children. This stage is consistent with the traditional life cycle of the progression of preschool, school-aged, and adolescent children. Common transitions that occur in these families require increasingly flexible boundaries to account for the developing independence of children and adolescents (Carter & McGoldrick, 1989).

The *reconstituting family* is one that occurs because of changes in the relationship of its members such as divorce, death, or separation (Rankin, 1989). The members need to adapt to the loss of the previous family form and adapt to a new type of family, whether it be a single-parent family or a new stepparent family.

The *contracting family* is similar to the traditional family life cycle of launching children and families in later life. Common transitions encountered in this family type are the changes in the relationships between the children and the new role that comes with that relationship if children are a part of the family. Adaptation to the loss of an adult partner through divorce or death, in addition to the changes that come with retirement such as decreased income and increased leisure time, are also common transitions.

FAMILY LIFE CYCLE FRAMEWORK

Zilbach (1989) developed a framework for the family life cycle that defines family development in terms of progress through certain predictable marker events or phases (Table 5–3). Each stage is precipitated by a particular life event (e.g., marriage, the birth of the first child) or by a **family stage marker.** These markers demand change and new adaptation. The change may be due to alterations in family composition (birth of new members) or as a result of a major shift in autonomy (starting kindergarten, retiring from the workforce). During each stage of the life cycle, families must achieve certain family tasks. If the carrying out of any task is incomplete, impeded, or disturbed, then family development may be delayed or suspended. Furthermore, the difficulties the family is experiencing will be carried on into subsequent stages of family development (Goldenberg & Goldenberg, 2000).

TABLE 5–2

CHANGING LIFE CYCLE: TASKS AND TRANSITIONS

FAMILY TYPE	TASKS	CHARACTERISTICS/ EXAMPLES	COMMON TRANSITIONS
Emerging	Finding suitable partners	Formalization of marital bond	Change in personal relationships, addition of spouse or significant other. Loss of friends, changes in family relationships
	Constitution of meaningful adult relationships	Decision to live with person of opposite or same sex with nonformalized bond	Changes in roles and status, unmarried to married status, addition of parental role. Possible changes in job, career, related to change in personal relationships
	Decisions related to child-bearing and infertility	Traditional or nontraditional family pattern; that is, opposite-sex partners obtain in vitro fertilization or same-sex partners adopt	
	Decision to remain childless	Opposite- or same-sex partners	Change in familiar environment, moving households
Solidifying or reconstituting	Solidification of adult partners' bonds. Child rearing and required interface with schools, health care institutions, and other societal institutions	Stable, nondivorcing families. Child-rearing tasks involve nurturance, education, socialization, and provision of climate suitable to development of responsible individuals. Characteristics of families with children are similar whether the family is traditional or not	Change in roles and status, loss or change in marital role through divorce and/or remarriage. Continued career changes. Changes in personal relationships' potential, loss of significant other, that is, mate, child. Loss of parents in family of origin. Changes in physical and mental capacities, major health change
	Reconstitution of family bonds with integration of new family members and loss of old ones	Divorced families and blended families	Changes in possessions; loss or acquisition of loved possessions necessitated by change in income or catastrophic occurrences
	Launching and release of children to environments separated from family	Traditional nuclear family releases young adult children to armed services, college, marriage, or work	Change in personal relationships, loss of spouse, children, siblings
	Adjusting to loss of adult partner	Death, late-in-life divorce	Change in roles and status retirement
	Adjusting to loss of work, parental roles	Forced retirement with consequences of lowered standard of living	Changes in physical and mental capacities, exacerbation of chronic problems, onset of acute episodes
Contracting	Integration of leisure time and adjustment to lack of responsibility for children and/or occupation. Development of avocation	Younger, healthy retired couples. Older, healthy workers who choose to continue employment	Changes in familiar environment; moves required by decreased income, loss of spouse, or health problems

Source: Rankin, S. (1986). Family transitions, expected and unexpected. In Gillis & Lynch (Eds.), Toward a science in family nursing. Reprinted by permission of Pearson Education, Inc., Upper Saddle River, NJ.

TABLE 5–3

FAMILY LIFE CYCLE FRAMEWORK: ZILBACH'S STAGES OF THE FAMILY

EARLY STAGES: FORMING AND NESTING

STAGE I: COUPLING

Family stage marker	The family begins at the establishment of a common household by two people; this may or may not include marriage.
Family task	Individual independence to couple/dyadic interdependence.

STAGE II: BECOMING THREE

Family stage marker	The second phase in family life is initiated by the arrival and subsequent inclusion/incorporation of the first child/dependent member.
Family task	Interdependence to incorporation of dependence.

MIDDLE STAGES: FAMILY SEPARATION PROCESSES

STAGE III: ENTRANCES

Family stage marker	The third phase is signaled by the exit of the first child/dependent member from the intrafamilial world to the larger world. This occurs at the point of entrance into school or other extrafamilial environment.
Family task	Dependence to facilitation of beginning separations–partial independence.

STAGE IV: EXPANSION

Family stage marker	This phase is marked by the entrance of the last child/dependent member of the family into the community.
Family task	Support of facilitation of continuing separations–independence.

STAGE V: EXITS

Family stage marker	This phase starts with the first complete exit of a dependent member from the family. This is achieved by the establishment of an independent household, which may include marriage or another form of independent household entity.
Family task	Partial separations to first complete independence.

LAST STAGES: FINISHING

STAGE VI: BECOMING SMALLER/EXTENDED

Family stage marker	Ultimately the moment comes for the exit of the last child/dependent member from the family.
Family task	Continuing expansion of independence.

STAGE VII: ENDINGS

Family stage marker	The final years start with the death of one spouse/partner and continue up to the death of the other partner.
Family task	Facilitation of family mourning; working through final separations.

Source: Zilbach, J.J. (1989). The family life cycle: A framework for understanding children in family therapy. In L. Combrinck-Graham (Ed.), Children in Family Contexts: Perspectives on Treatment (p. 65). New York: Guilford Press.

FAMILY LIFE SPIRAL

The *Family Life Spiral* is a developmental model devised by Combrinck-Graham (1985, 1990) that incorporates overlapping developmental tasks of the individual family member on the developmental tasks of each generation in the family. Erikson's (1963) stage of "generativity" of the adult leads to childbearing and to the raising of children. The midlife crisis of the adult usually occurs at the same period in time in which the family unit is also dealing with the turmoil of adolescence and the retirement of the grandparents (Figure 5–1). How a family member works through an individual developmental task will have a profound effect on the other family members who are also trying to move into the next stage of their development. Combrinck-Graham (1989) conceptualized that the family oscillates from periods of closeness or a *centripetal* family atmosphere to periods of differentiation or a *centrifugal* family atmosphere (Combrinck-Graham, 1990). Children require constant care and nurturing, whereas adolescents are moving toward independence. Centripetal forces lead to marriage, sexual intimacy, and childbearing. Centrifugal forces lead to adolescence, retirement, and preparation for death. The family moves between these two forces throughout the Family Life Spiral. The nurse can utilize this model in attempt to identify what life stages the family members are in and what impact that has on the family as a whole.

TWO-PARENT NUCLEAR FAMILY CAREER OR LIFE CYCLE STAGES

The following family life cycle stages have been described by Duvall and Miller (1985) and Carter and McGoldrick (1989). The nine stages include the eight stages of Duvall (Table 5–4) plus the addition of the "between stage" from the Carter and McGoldrick typology to give a more comprehensive depiction of changes in family life. These family life cycle stages portray the intact nuclear American family, but are limited in their applicability to single, divorced, and stepparent families. Common health concerns and health promotion needs are also discussed within each of the respective family life cycle stages.

TRANSITIONAL STAGE: BETWEEN FAMILIES (THE UNATTACHED YOUNG ADULT)

This stage refers to the period of time when individuals are in their 20s, are financially independent, and

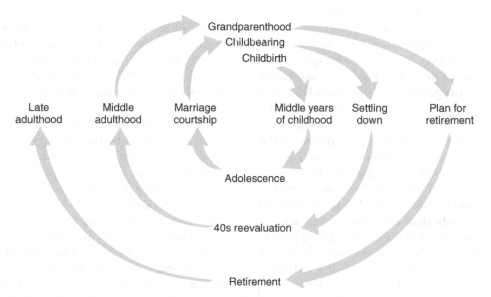

Figure 5–1. The Family Life Spiral shows the overlapping developmental tasks of family members from different generations. *(Redrawn from Combrinck-Graham, L. (1985) A developmental model for family systems. Family Process, 24(2), 139–150. Used with permission.)*

TABLE 5—4

DUVALL'S EIGHT-STAGE FAMILY LIFE CYCLE

Stage I	Beginning families (also referred to as married couples or the stage of marriage)
Stage II	Childbearing families (the oldest child is an infant through 30 months)
Stage III	Families with preschool children (oldest child is 2½ to 6 years of age)
Stage IV	Families with school children (oldest child is 6 to 13 years of age)
Stage V	Families with teenagers (oldest child is 13 to 20 years of age)
Stage VI	Families launching young adults (covering the first child who has left through the last child leaving home)
Stage VII	Middle-aged parents (empty nest through retirement)
Stage VIII	Family in retirement and old age (also referred to as aging family members or retirement to death of both spouses)

Adapted from Duvall (1977) and Duvall & Miller (1985).

have physically left their family of origin but have not begun their own family of marriage. Duvall and other sociologists do not consider the between-family stage a family life cycle stage or career. Yet, because this period is such a commonly experienced one (adolescents do not go directly from their family of origin to a family of marriage, as was more frequently seen in the past), and because this period is such a pivotal transition, the stage was added in this text. This stage has also been largely ignored by family health care professionals and family therapists (Aylmer, 1988).

Demographic data support the importance of this stage. Today in the United States more young adults delay marriage while they live in bachelor quarters or cohabitate outside of marriage. First marriage in the United States occurs generally three years later (for men) and five years later (for women) than it did a generation ago (U.S. Bureau of the Census, 2000a). Unmarried couples account for 3.8 million of the country's 104 million households, an increase of 1,000 percent from 1990 to the present (Popenoe & Whitehead, 2000; U.S. Bureau of the Census, 2000a). In 2000, 56 percent of men 18 to 24 years of age lived at home with one or both of their parents, 43 percent of women the same age followed suit. Among people 18 to 24 years of age, only 10 percent of men and 18 percent of women were married and living with their spouses (U.S. Bureau of the Census, 2000a)

The between-family stage is considered by Aylmer (1988) and other family therapists to be the cornerstone for all the successive stages to follow; how the young adult goes through this stage profoundly affects his or her choice of marriage partner as well as when and how marriage occurs. To complete this stage successfully, the young adult must separate from the family of origin without cutting off ties to the family members or without attaching reactively to an emotional surrogate.

DEVELOPMENTAL TASKS. This stage is "between families," meaning that the developmental tasks are individual in nature rather than family oriented. Carter and McGoldrick (1989) explain that the primary developmental task of the unattached young adult is "coming to terms with his or her family of origin" (p. 13). It is a time for the young adult to form personal life goals and a sense of self before joining with another in marriage. It is time for the development of intimate relationships and the time to independently establish oneself both financially and as a productive working member of society (Table 5–5). This is generally a difficult transitional stage, inasmuch as individuating from one's family of origin physically, financially, and emotionally is generally delayed in many families today.

This stage is typically experienced differently depending on one's gender. Carol Gilligan's seminal

TABLE 5–5

FAMILIES IN THE TRANSITION STAGE

DEVELOPMENTAL TASKS	HEALTH CARE CONCERNS
Separating from family of origin	Family planning
Developing intimate peer relationships	Birth control
Establishing work and financial independence	Preventing sexually transmitted diseases
	Safe sexual practices
	HIV
	Accidents
	Hepatitis C
	Suicide
	Mental health concerns
	Good health practices (e.g., sleep, nutrition, exercise)

work, *In a Different Voice* (1982), describes the contrasting orientation of males and females through their socialization. Men generally are taught to pursue their self-identification through self-expression while women pursue theirs through self-sacrifice. As young men and women go through the unattached young adult period, they have different identity issues to resolve. A balance of both autonomy and attachment is needed in relationships and work, but men generally struggle with issues of attachment and relationships, while women struggle with issues of autonomy.

Most of the above issues involve relationships between the young adult and his or her parents (Aylmer, 1988) and creating a new balance between separateness and connectedness. How the parents of the young adult interact with their young adult child during this period is therefore vitally important. From a family systems perspective, there are reciprocal or circular effects taking place between the parents and young adults (each mutually influence each other's actions), which enhance or inhibit the

process of separation and individuation of the young adult. If parents have an unsatisfying marriage and need the young adult to stay connected to meet their needs, this hinders the young adult's efforts at separating; in turn, if the young adult feels anxious and incompetent about managing independently, he or she will delay separation and attempt to keep the parents involved.

HEALTH CONCERNS. Health concerns are both personal and familial during this transitional stage (see Table 5–5). Family planning and birth control use is a major concern and need. Sexually transmitted diseases are more frequently seen in this group (venereal disease, AIDS, etc.). Accidents and suicides are leading causes of mortality. Mental health problems are also common, and as explained above, deal primarily with the issue of separating in a functional way from one's family of origin so that healthy, intimate relationships can be formed.

Health promotion needs are similar to subsequent stages. Because young adults are now on their own, their lifestyles typically do not incorporate the recommended health-protective practices such as avoidance of drugs, alcohol, and tobacco; engaging in safe sexual practices; and obtaining adequate sleep, nutrition, exercise, and preventive dental and medical examinations and care.

STAGE I: BEGINNING FAMILIES

The formation of the couple marks the beginning of a new family with the movement from the former family of origin to the new intimate relationship. This stage is also called the stage of marriage. Married couples today are making up a smaller portion of family households than in previous decades. The number of married-couple households was 45 million in 1970, and though the 2000 figures of 55 million married-couple households looks to be an increase, in truth the increase has been at a rate far slower than other family household types. The proportion of married-couple families with children declined from 87 percent in 1970 to 69 percent in 2000. Married-couple family groups are now more likely to live in the suburbs, own their own home, and have higher levels of education. They are less likely to be unemployed as compared to all other family groups (U.S. Bureau of the Census, 2000a).

FAMILY DEVELOPMENTAL TASKS. Establishing a mutually satisfying marriage, relating harmoniously to the kin network, and planning a family constitute the three critical tasks of this period (Table 5–6).

ESTABLISHING A MUTUALLY SATISFYING MARRIAGE. When two people become united in marriage, their initial concern is preparing for a new type of life together. The resources of the two people are combined, their roles altered, and new functions assumed. Learning to live together while providing for each other's basic personality needs becomes a crucial developmental task. The couple has to mutually accommodate to each other in many small ways. For example, they must develop routines for eating, sleeping, getting up in the morning, cleaning house, sharing the bathroom, recreational pursuits, and going places they both enjoy. In this process of mutual accommodation, a set of patterned transactions are formed and then maintained by the couple, with each spouse triggering and monitoring the behavior of the other.

The success of the evolving relationship depends on the mutual accommodation just discussed and on a complementarity, or the fitting together of the needs and interests of the mates. Just as important, individual differences need to be acknowledged. In healthy relationships, differences are seen to enrich the marital relationship. Achieving a satisfying relationship is dependent on the development of satisfactory ways to handle "differentness" (Satir, 1983) and conflicts. A healthy way of resolving problems is related to the mates' ability to empathize, to be mutually supportive, to be able to communicate openly and honestly, and to approach a conflict with feelings of mutual respect (Harley, 1994).

Moreover, how successful the evolving marital relationship will be depends on how well each of the partners has differentiated or separated from their respective families of origin (the previous developmental task) (Bowen, 1978). A mature person must separate/differentiate from his or her own parents in order to form his or her own self-identity and healthy intimate relationships. McGoldrick (1988) presents an excellent description of this process and of psychosocial problems during this period.

Many couples experience problems in sexual adjustment, often because of ignorance and misinformation leading to unrealistic expectations and disappointment. Moreover, many couples bring their own unresolved needs and desires into the relationship, and these can adversely affect the sexual relationship (Goldenberg & Goldenberg, 2000; Heinrich, 1996).

RELATING HARMONIOUSLY TO KIN NETWORK. A basic role shift occurs in the first marriage of a couple, as they move from their parental homes to their new setting. Concomitantly, they become members of three families—those of their respective families of origin in addition to the one they have recently created. The couple faces the tasks of separating themselves as a newly formed family from each of their families of origin and in working out different relationships with parents, siblings, and in-laws, since their primary loyalty must shift to their marital relationship. For the couple, this entails forming a new relationship with each set of parents, one that allows not only for mutual support and enjoyment but also for an autonomy that protects the newly formed family from outside intrusion that might undermine the building of a satisfying marriage.

PLANNING A FAMILY. Whether or not to have children and the timing of pregnancies becomes a significant family decision. McKinney and colleagues (2000) underscore the importance of considering the whole family pregnant when one is working in maternity

TABLE 5–6

TWO-PARENT NUCLEAR FAMILY LIFE CYCLE STAGE I: BEGINNING FAMILIES

DEVELOPMENTAL TASKS	HEALTH CARE CONCERNS
Establishing a mutually satisfying marriage	Family planning education and counseling
Relating harmoniously to the kin network	Prenatal education and counseling
Planning a family (decisions about parenthood)	

care. The type of health care the family as a unit receives during the prenatal period greatly influences the family's ability to cope effectively with the tremendous changes after the baby's birth.

HEALTH CONCERNS. Health concerns during this time include those related to sexual and marital role adjustment, family planning education and counseling, prenatal education and counseling, and communication. It becomes increasingly apparent that counseling should be provided premaritally. Lack of information often results in sexual and emotional problems, fear, guilt feelings, unplanned pregnancies, and venereal disease either before or after marriage. These unfortunate events do not allow the couple to plan their lives and begin their relationship with a stable foundation. Traditional marriage concepts are being challenged by love relationships, as well as cohabitating heterosexual and homosexual relationships. People entering into nonmarriage unions often need as much if not more counseling from health care workers who may be called on to assist such couples. It is perhaps at this point that family nurses may be caught between two "families," the family of orientation and the forming union. In such a situation, family health professionals need not make value judgments but attempt to help each of the two groups to understand themselves and each other.

STAGE II: CHILDBEARING FAMILIES

Stage II begins with the birth of the first child and continues through the infant's 30th month. The transition to parenthood is a key one in the family life cycle. With the birth of the first child, the family becomes a threesome, making it a permanent system for the first time (i.e., the system endures regardless of the outcome of the marriage) (McGoldrick, Heiman, & Carter, 1993).

Although parenthood represents an extremely important goal for most couples, most find it a very stressful life transition. A period of disequilibrium is inevitable as the family moves from one stage to another (Martell & Imle, 1996). Frequently, this disequilibrium requires so much change that some researchers find that it can lead to family crisis (Clark, 1966; Hobbs & Cole, 1976; LeMasters, 1957),

causing feelings of inadequacy in parenting and a disruption in marital relations.

Miller and Myers-Walls (1983), based on their review of studies of new parents, summarized the specific parenting stressors identified in the literature. The most commonly mentioned stressor appeared to be the loss of personal freedom due to parenting responsibilities; in addition, less time and companionship in marriage were frequently identified.

The adjustment to marriage is usually not as hard as the adjustment to parenthood. Although a very meaningful and gratifying experience to most parents, the advent of the baby calls for a sudden change to an incessantly demanding role. It is especially difficult in the beginning because of the feelings of inadequacy of new parents; the lack of help from family and friends; the conflicting advice of helpful friends, family, and health care professionals; and the frequent awakening of the baby at night—which usually continues for about three to four weeks. Also, the mother is fatigued psychologically and physiologically. She often feels the burdens of household duties and perhaps also employment responsibilities, in addition to caring for the baby. It is especially difficult if the new mother has been ill or has had a long, difficult labor and delivery or a cesarean section.

Two important factors contribute to the difficulty of assuming the parental role. Most persons today are not prepared to be parents, and many deleterious, unrealistic myths romanticizing the rearing of children exist in our society (Szafran, 1996). Parenthood is the only major role for which little preparation is given, and difficulties in role transition adversely affect the quality of the marital and parent–child relationships.

The arrival of a new baby into the home creates changes for every member of the family and for every set of relationships. A stranger has been admitted into a close-knit group, and suddenly the balance of the family shifts—each member takes on new roles and begins new relationships. In addition to a baby's being born, a mother, father, and grandparents are born. The wife must now relate to the husband as both a spouse and a father and vice versa. And in families with previous children, the impact of the new baby is as significant on the siblings as on the new parents.

Dramatic social changes in American society since the 1950s have also had a marked effect on new parents. The large proportion of women working outside the home and having careers, the rise in divorce and marital instability, the common use of contraception and abortion, and the large increase in costs of having and caring for children are all factors influencing the passage through the early childbearing life cycle stage (Bradt, 1988; Dobson, 2001; Miller & Myers-Walls, 1983).

FAMILY DEVELOPMENTAL TASKS.   After the coming of the first-born, the family has several important developmental tasks (Table 5–7). Husband, wife, and baby must all learn new roles, while the nuclear family unit expands in functions and responsibilities. This involves the simultaneous meshing of the developmental tasks of each family member and the family as a whole (Duvall & Miller, 1985).

The birth of a child makes radical changes in family organization. The functions of the couple must differentiate to meet the new demands of the infant for care and nurturance. How these responsibilities are fulfilled varies tremendously with the sociocultural position of the couple. Although most parents continue to assume traditional roles or division of responsibilities, it is not uncommon in contemporary society for both mother and father to share in infant care tasks (Tiller, 1995).

Relationships with the paternal and maternal extended family must also be realigned during this stage. New roles need to be established with respect to grandparenting and relationships between parents and grandparents (American Association of Retired Persons [AARP], 2000; Bradt, 1988).

One of the most important roles for family nurses to assess when working with the childbearing family is the parental role—how both parents interact with and care for the new infant and how the infant responds. Klaus and Kendall (1976), Kendall (1974), Rubin (1967a, b), and others verify the critical impact of early attachment and a beginning warm, positive parent–child relationship on the future parental relationship with the child. The parents' attitude about themselves as parents, their attitudes about the baby, and the characteristics of parental communication and stimulation of the infant (Davis, 1978) are related areas that need to be assessed.

Role changes and adaptation to new parental responsibilities are often more rapidly learned by the

TABLE 5–7

TWO-PARENT NUCLEAR FAMILY LIFE CYCLE STAGE II: CHILDBEARING FAMILIES

DEVELOPMENTAL TASKS	HEALTH CARE CONCERNS
Setting up the young family as a stable unit (integrating of new baby into family)	Preparation for birth experience
Reconciling conflicting developmental tasks and needs of various family members	Transition to parenthood
Maintaining a satisfying marital relationship	Infant care
Expanding relationships with extended family by adding parenting and grandparenting roles	Well-baby care
	Early recognition and appropriate handling of physical health problems with the children
	Immunizations
	Normal growth and development
	Safety measures
	Family planning
	Family interaction
	Good health practices (e.g., sleep, nutrition, exercise)

mother than by the father. The child is a reality to the expectant mother much earlier than for the father, who usually begins to feel like a father at the birth, but sometimes even later than that (Minuchin, 1974).

The way in which most fathers have traditionally been left out of the perinatal process has certainly delayed men from taking on this important role change and thereby hindered their emotional involvement. Fortunately, increased awareness of the important role fathers play in child care and the child's development has led to greater involvement of fathers in infant care among the middle class (Hanson & Bozett, 1985; Henderson & Brouse, 1991; Kaufman & Uhlenberg, 2000; Zimmerman, Northen, & Seng, 1999).

The mother and father grow and develop their parental roles in response to the continually changing demands and developmental tasks of the growing youngster, the family as a whole, and themselves. According to Friedman (1957), parents go through five successive stages of development. The first two stages fall into this phase of family life. First, during the child's infancy, parents learn the meaning of cues their baby expresses in making his or her needs known. With each successive child, parents will go through this same stage as they adjust to each infant's unique cues.

The second stage of parental development, learning to accept the child's growth and development, occurs in the toddler years. Just prior to and during this stage, parents—particularly parents with their first child—need guidance and support. Parents need to understand tasks the child is attempting to master and the child's needs for safety, limits, and toilet training. They need to understand the concept of developmental readiness, or "the teachable moment." At the same time, parents need guidance in understanding the tasks they themselves are mastering during this stage.

New marital communication patterns evolve with the coming of a child, with mates relating to each other both as mates and as parents. Spouse transactional patterns have been found to change drastically. Feldman (1961) observed that parents of infants talked less with each other and had less fun, less stimulating conversation, and a diminished quality of marital interaction. Some parents feel overwhelmed with the added responsibilities, particularly those in dual-worker families in which both parents work full time. Dalgas-Pelish (1993) found that marital happiness was lower for childbearing families compared to childless couples.

The reestablishment of satisfying communication patterns—including personal, marital, and parental feelings and concerns—is critical. Mates must continue to meet each other's personal adult psychological and sexual needs as well as share and interact with each other about parental responsibilities.

The sexual relationship of couples generally declines during pregnancy and through the six-week postpartum period. Sexual difficulties during the later period are common, arising from such factors as the mother's absorption in her new role, fatigue, and feelings of loss of sexual attractiveness, as well as the husband's feeling of being "left or pushed out" by the new baby.

Family communications now include a third member, making for a triad. Parents must learn to perceive and discern the communication cries of the infant. For instance, the baby's cries need to be differentiated into expressions of discomfort, hunger, overstimulation, sickness, or fatigue. And the baby begins responding to cuddles, fondling, and talking, which then are received and reinforced by the parents.

This life cycle stage also requires an adjustment of relationships within the extended family and with friends. When other family members try to support and assist the new parents, tensions may result. Although grandparents, for instance, can be of great help to the new family, the potential for conflict exists because of differences in values and expectations existing between the generations.

Despite the importance of having a social network or social support system for achieving satisfaction with, and positive feelings about, family life, the young family needs to know when it needs help and from whom to accept it as well as when to depend on its own inner resources and strengths (Duvall & Miller, 1985).

A strong, viable marital relationship contributes to the stability and morale of the family. A satisfying husband–wife relationship will give the mates the strength and energy to "give" to the infant and to each other. Conflicting pressures and demands, such as between the mother's loyalty both to her infant and to her husband, are problematic and can be agonizing. This type of conflict can become the central source of unhappiness during this life cycle stage.

HEALTH CONCERNS. Concerns of families in this stage begin with preparation for parenthood (see Table

5–7). Family planning counseling should begin during the prenatal or early postpartum period since many couples do not wait to resume intercourse until the traditional six-week postpartum examination. Parents should be encouraged to openly discuss family spacing and planning. Due to the increased personal and family demands new babies bring, parents need to realize that frequent, closely spaced pregnancies can be harmful to the mother, as well as to the father, siblings, and the family unit.

Family-centered maternity education with a wide variety of prenatal and postnatal classes is available to help prepare young parents for the birth experience and for the transition to parenthood (Szafran, 1996). Follow-up home visits after the birth are recommended for meeting the educational and support needs of the childbearing family in the early days of parenthood (Evans, 1991; Williams & Cooper, 1993). Infant care, well-baby care, early recognition and appropriate handling of physical health problems, immunizations, normal growth and development, safety measures, family interaction, and general health promotion (lifestyle) are all important areas for discussion.

Other concerns that contribute to the family's health during this period of a family's life are inaccessibility and inadequacy of child care facilities for working mothers, parent–child relationships, sibling relationships, parenting (including child abuse and neglect), and parent-role transition problems.

STAGE III: FAMILIES WITH PRESCHOOL CHILDREN

The third stage of the family life cycle commences when the firstborn child is about 2½ years old and terminates when he or she is 5 years of age. The family now may consist of three to five persons, with the paired positions of husband–father, wife–mother, son–brother, and daughter–sister. The family is becoming more complex and differentiated (Duvall & Miller, 1985).

Family life during this stage is busy and demanding for the parents. Both parents have greater demands on their time, as it is probable that the mother is working also, either part or full time. Nevertheless, realizing that parents are the "architects of the family," designing and directing family development (Satir, 1983), it is critical for them to

strengthen their partnership—in short, to keep the marriage alive and well. This is often a problem during this particular stage of family life (Olson et al., 1983).

Preschool children have much to learn at this stage, especially in the area of independence. They must achieve enough autonomy and self-sufficiency to be able to handle themselves without their parents in a variety of places. Experience in nursery school, kindergarten, Project Head Start, a day care center, or similar programs is a good way to foster this kind of development. Structured preschool programs are especially helpful in assisting parents from inner-city, low-income communities with their preschool children. Although multiple studies have shown the benefit of quality child care and preschool programs such as Head Start, access to these programs is generally difficult or nonexistent for working poor families. Obtaining adequate child care arrangements is a major concern for parents (Kelleher, 1996). Infant and preschool day care centers that are affordable and of good quality are difficult if not impossible to locate in most communities. Mothers with careers and adolescent mothers are particularly in need of better child care facilities and programs (Adams & Adams, 1990).

Many single-parent families exist within this particular life cycle stage. Demographers now predict that more than half of the children born in the 1990s will spend at least part of their childhood in a single-parent home (Kantrowitz & Wingert, 2001). Among single-parent families, the role strain of parenting the preschooler, coupled with other roles, is great.

FAMILY DEVELOPMENTAL TASKS. The family is now growing in both numbers and complexity. The need of preschoolers and other young children to explore the world around them, and the parents' needs for their own privacy, make housing and adequate space major problems. Equipment and facilities also need to be childproofed, for it is at this stage that accidents become the most common causes of childhood mortality and disability. Assessing the home for safety hazards is of prime importance for the community health nurse, and health education must then be included so that the parents and children are cognizant of the risks involved and of ways of preventing accidents (Table 5–8).

TABLE 5–8

TWO-PARENT NUCLEAR FAMILY LIFE CYCLE STAGE III: FAMILIES WITH PRESCHOOL CHILDREN

DEVELOPMENTAL TASKS	HEALTH CARE CONCERNS
Meeting family members' needs for adequate housing, space, privacy, and safety	Communicable diseases of children
Socializing the children	Accident prevention and home safety (e.g., falls, burns, poisoning)
Integrating new child members while still meeting needs of other children	Marital relationship
Maintaining healthy relationships within the family (marital and parent–child) and outside the family (extended family and community)	Sibling relations
	Family planning
	Growth and development needs
	Parenting issues
	Child abuse and neglect
	Good health practices (e.g., sleep, nutrition, exercise)

The husband–father generally assumes more involvement in the household responsibilities during this stage of family development than during any other stage, with the largest percentage of this stage being spent in child care activities. Although the evidence is mixed, some studies suggest that father–child contact has beneficial effects on children including higher psychosocial scores, greater self-esteem, fewer behavioral problems, higher academic achievement, and better peer relationships (Amato & Rezac, 1994; Healy, Malley, & Stewart, 1990; Hetherington, 1993; Lund, 1987; Peterson & Zill, 1986).

Contrary to expectations, research has shown that the advent of the second child into the family has a more deleterious effect on the marital relationship than does the first birth (La Rossa & La Rossa, 1981). Involvement in parental roles tends to make the carrying out of marital roles more difficult, as exhibited by the following clinical research observations: Couples perceive more negative personality changes in each other; they are less satisfied with their home; there is more task-oriented interaction and fewer personal and child-centered conversations; more warmth is exhibited toward the children and less toward each other; and there is a lower level of sexual satisfaction (Feldman, 1971). Compounding these clinical observations is the myth that more fathers are spending more time at home and less time at work. Kaufman & Uhlenberg (2000) have reported that gender differences in the effect of parenthood on work performance continue to persist. Fathers were found to be employed more often and to do more work than their counterparts who did not have children. In addition, women with children continue to be employed fewer hours than women without children and than the father–partner in the home.

Feldman's well-recognized study parallels reports and observations of family counselors—that the marital relationship is often troubled at this phase of family life. In fact, many divorces occur within these years due to weak or unsatisfactory marital ties. Privacy and time together are prime necessities. Marriage counseling and marriage encounter groups have become important resources among the middle class. For the family without economic resources, however, limited assistance is available for strengthening a salvageable marriage. There is a trend for clergy to become trained as marriage and family counselors and counsel couples who cannot afford private therapy.

A major task of the family is socializing the children. Preschoolers are developing critical self-attitudes (self-concepts) and rapidly learning to express themselves, as seen in their rapid grasp of language. A more mature role is assumed by the preschooler, who gradually takes on more responsibility for his or her own care, plus helping the mother or father with household jobs. It is not the productivity of the child that is important here, but the learning that is occurring.

Another task during this period deals with how to integrate a new family member (second or third child) into the family while still meeting the needs of the older child(ren). The displacement of a child by a newborn is psychologically a very traumatic event. Preparation of children for the arrival of a new baby helps ameliorate the situation, especially if the parents are sensitive to the older child's feelings and behavior. Sibling rivalry is often expressed by hitting or negatively relating to the new baby, regressive behaviors, and attention-getting activity. The best way to handle sibling rivalry is for the parents to spend a certain amount of time each day exclusively relating to an older child to give him or her the assurance that he or she is still loved and wanted.

About the time children become preschoolers, parents enter their third parenting stage, one of learning to separate from children as they toddle off to nursery school, a day care center, or kindergarten. This stage continues during the preschool and early school years. Separation is often difficult for parents, and they need support and an explanation of how the preschoolers' mastery of developmental tasks contributes to their child's growth in autonomy.

Separation from parents is also difficult for preschool children. Separation may occur as parents go to work, to the hospital, or on trips or vacations. Family preparation for separation is important in helping the children adjust to change.

Assisting parents to obtain family planning services after the arrival of a new baby, or to continue with contraception if there has been no intervening pregnancy, is also indicated. It is, for instance, not unusual for a woman to have stopped using contraceptives because of a missed period with the belief that she was pregnant, only to find out later that her eventual pregnancy resulted from sexual intercourse during the time she thought she was pregnant and was not using contraception.

Both parents need to have some outside interests and contacts to rejuvenate themselves to carry on the multitude of home tasks and responsibilities. Poor and single parents often do not have this opportunity. These families usually have the least satisfactory associations with the wider community due to their alienated position and the paucity of resources available to them.

HEALTH CONCERNS. The major physical health problems concern the frequent communicable diseases of the children and the common falls, burns, poisonings, and other accidents that occur during the preschool age (see Table 5–8). Due to both the lack of specific resistance to the many bacterial and viral diseases and to increased exposure to them, preschoolers are frequently sick with one minor infectious illness after another. Infectious diseases often "ping-pong" throughout the family. Frequent visits to the doctor, caring for sick kids, and running home from work to pick up an ill child from the nursery school are common weekly crises. Thus, children's contacts with infectious and communicable diseases and their general susceptibility to disease are prime health concerns (Shelov, 1991).

Accidents, falls, burns, and lacerations are also quite common occurrences. These injuries are seen even more frequently where there are large families, families in which an adult caretaker is not present (latchkey children), and in low-income families. Environmental safety and adequate child supervision are the keys to reducing accidents (Shelov, 1991).

The prime psychosocial family health concern is the marital relationship. Studies verify the diminished satisfaction many couples experience during these years and the need for working to strengthen and reinvigorate this vital unit (Olson et al., 1983). Other important health concerns involve sibling rivalry, family planning, growth and developmental needs, parenting problems such as setting limits (disciplining), child abuse and neglect, home safety, and family communication problems.

General health promotion strategies continue to be germane during this stage, as lifestyle behaviors learned during childhood can have both short- and long-term consequences. Family health education directed at prevention of major health problems is indicated in the areas of smoking, alcohol and drug misuse, human sexuality, safety, diet and nutrition, exercise, and social support/stress management. "The chief goals for nurses working with the child and family are to assist them in establishing healthy lifestyles and in facilitating the child's optimal physical, intellectual, emotional, and social growth" (Wilson, 1988, p. 177).

STAGE IV: FAMILIES WITH SCHOOL-AGED CHILDREN

This stage begins when the firstborn child enters school full time, usually at the age of 5 years, and concludes when he or she reaches puberty, around 13 years of age. Families usually reach their maximum number of members and family relationships at the end of this stage (Duvall & Miller, 1985). Again, these are busy years. Now children have their own activities and interests in addition to the mandatory activities of life and school, and the parents also have their own, different activities. Each person is working on his or her own developmental tasks, just as the family attempts to fulfill its tasks (Table 5–9). According to Erikson (1950), parents are struggling with the twin demands of finding fulfillment in rearing the next generation (the developmental task of generativity)

and being concerned in their own growth; at the same time, school-aged children are working at developing a sense of industry—the capacity for work enjoyment—and trying to eliminate or ward off a sense of inferiority.

The parental task at this time is that of learning to deal with the child's separation or, more simply, letting the child go. More and more, peer relationships and outside activities play larger roles in the life of the school-aged child. These years are filled with family activities, but there are also forces gradually pushing the child to separate from the family in preparation for adolescence. Parents who have interests outside of their children will find it much easier to make the gradual separation. In instances in which the mothering role is the central and only significant role in a woman's life, however, this separation process may be a very painful one and one that is strongly resisted.

During this stage parents feel intense pressure from the outside community via the school system and other extrafamilial associations to have their children conform to the community's standards for children. This tends to influence the middle-class family to stress more traditional values of achievement and productivity, and to cause some working-class families and many poor families to feel alienated from and at conflict with school and/or community values.

TABLE 5–9

TWO-PARENT NUCLEAR FAMILY LIFE CYCLE STAGE IV: FAMILIES WITH SCHOOL-AGED CHILDREN

DEVELOPMENTAL TASKS	HEALTH CARE CONCERNS
Socializing the children, including promoting school achievement and fostering of healthy peer relations of children	Health challenges to children (e.g., vision, hearing, speech)
Maintaining a satisfying marital relationship	Dental health
Meeting the physical health needs of family members	Child abuse and neglect
	Substance abuse
	Communicable diseases
	Chronic conditions
	Behavior problems
	Good health practices (e.g., sleep, nutrition, exercise)

FAMILY DEVELOPMENTAL TASKS. One of the critical tasks of parents in socializing their children at this time involves promoting school achievement. Another significant family task is maintaining a satisfying marital relationship. Again, it has been reported that marital satisfaction is diminished during this stage. Several large studies reinforced these observations (Burr, 1970; Olson et al., 1983; Rollins & Feldman, 1970). Promoting open communication and supporting the spousal relationship is vital in working with the school-aged family.

HEALTH CONCERNS. Children's handicaps may come to light during this period of a child's life. School nurses and teachers will detect many visual, hearing, and speech defects, in addition to learning problems, behavior disturbances, inadequate dental care, child abuse, substance abuse, and communicable diseases among the school population during this stage (Edelman & Mandle, 1986). Working with the family in the role of health educator and counselor, in addition to initiating appropriate referrals for follow-up screening, takes up much of a school nurse's energies. He or she also acts as a resource person to the schoolteacher, enabling the teacher to handle the common and more individualized health needs of her or his pupils more effectively (see Table 5–9).

There are a number of other handicapping conditions occasionally detected during the school years, including epilepsy, cerebral palsy, mental retardation, cancer, and orthopedic conditions. The family health nurse's primary function here—in addition to referral, teaching, and counseling parents regarding these conditions—would be to assist the family in coping so that any adverse impact of the handicap on the family is minimized.

For children with behavior problems, family nurses in schools, clinics, doctor's offices, and community agencies should seek active parental involvement and provide supportive counseling. Initiating a referral for family counseling/therapy is often very helpful in assisting a family to be aware of some of the family problems that may be adversely affecting the school-aged child. When parents are able to reframe the child's behavior problem as a family problem and work toward its resolution with that new focus, more healthy family functioning often results as well as healthier child behaviors (Bradt, 1988).

STAGE V: FAMILIES WITH TEENAGERS

When the firstborn turns 13 years of age, the fifth stage of the family's life cycle or career commences. It usually lasts about six or seven years, although it can be shorter if the child leaves the family early or longer if the child remains home later than 19 or 20 years of age. Other children in the home are usually of school age. The overarching family goal at the teenage stage is that of loosening family ties to allow greater responsibility and freedom for the teenager in preparation for becoming a young adult (Duvall & Miller, 1985).

Preto (1988), in discussing the transformation of the family system in adolescence, describes the family metamorphosis that takes place. It involves "profound shifts in relationship patterns across the generations, and while it may be signaled initially by the adolescent's physical maturity, it often parallels and coincides with changes in parents as they enter midlife and with major transformations faced by grandparents in old age" (p. 255).

This stage of the family's life is probably the most difficult, or certainly the most discussed and written about (Kidwell et al., 1983). The American family is affected by the tremendous developmental tasks of both the adolescent and parents and the inevitable conflicts and turmoil these create. The family faces new organizational challenges particularly with respect to autonomy and independence (Goldenberg & Goldenberg, 2000). Parents no longer maintain complete authority, nor can they abdicate authority either. Rule changing, limit setting, and role renegotiation are all necessary.

The major challenges in working with a family with teenagers revolve around the developmental changes adolescents undergo in terms of cognitive changes, identity formation, and biological growth (Kidwell, Fischer, Dunham, & Baranowski, 1983) and developmentally based conflicts and crises.

PARENTAL ROLES, RESPONSIBILITIES, AND PROBLEMS. Needless to say, parents find it a most difficult task to raise teenagers today. Nonetheless, parents need to stand firm against unreasonable testing of the limits that have been set in the family as they go through the process of gradually "letting go." Duvall (1977) also identifies the critical developmental task of this period to be the balancing of freedom with responsibility as teenagers mature and emancipate themselves. Friedman (1957) similarly defines the parental task during this stage as learning to accept rejection without deserting the child.

When the parents accept themselves as they are, with all their own weaknesses and strengths, and when they accept their several roles at this stage of development without undue conflict or sensitivity, they set the pattern for a similar sort of self-acceptance in their children. Relationships between parents and adolescents should be smoother when parents feel productive, satisfied, and in control of their own lives (Kidwell et al., 1983) and parents/families function flexibly (Preto, 1988).

Schultz (1972) and Elkind (1994) have expressed the view that the increasing complexity of American life has made the role of parents unclear. Parents may feel in competition with a variety of social forces and institutions—from school authorities and counselors to birth control and premarital sex and cohabitation options. Other factors add to their considerably diminished influence. Because of specialization of occupations and professions, parents are no longer able to help children with their vocational plans. The residential mobility and lack of continuing trustworthy adult relationships for both adolescents and parents, in addition to the inability of many parents to discuss personal, sexual, and drug-related concerns openly and nonjudgmentally with their children, has also contributed to parent–adolescent problems. Among immigrant families, generational clashes and value conflicts amplify the common communication problems between parents and children (see Chapter 20).

FAMILY DEVELOPMENTAL TASKS.   The first and central family developmental task at this stage is balancing freedom with responsibility as teenagers mature and become increasingly autonomous (Table 5–10). The parents must progressively change their relationship with their teenage son or daughter from the previously established dependent relationship to an increasingly independent one. This evolving shift in the parent–child relationship is typically one that is fraught with conflicts along the way.

In order for the family to adapt successfully during this stage, the family members, especially the parents, have to make a major "system change"—that is, set up new roles and norms and "let go" of the adolescent. Kidwell and associates (1983) summarize this needed

change: "Paradoxically, the [family] system which can let go of its members is the system which will endure and reproduce itself effectively in later generations" (p. 88).

Parents who, in order to meet their own needs, do not let go, often find a major "revolution" by the teenager when separation occurs later. Parents may also thrust the adolescent into independence prematurely, ignoring his or her dependency needs. In this case the teenager may fail in attempts to achieve independence (Wright & Leahey, 2000).

As with the last three stages, the marital relationship is also a focus of concern. The second family developmental task is for couples to refocus their marital relationship (Wilson, 1988). Many couples have become so preoccupied with their parental responsibilities that their marriage no longer plays a central role in their lives. The husband may spend much time away from home working and furthering his career, while the wife probably also works while trying to keep up with housework and parental responsibilities. Under these conditions, little time or energy is left for the marital relationship.

The other side of the coin, however, is that since the children are more responsible for themselves, the couple can more easily leave home to engage in their careers or establish individual and marital postparental interests. They can begin to build a foundation for the future stages of the family career.

A third pressing family developmental task is for family members, particularly the parents and teenager, to openly communicate with each other. Because of the generation gap, open communication is often an ideal rather than a reality. There is often mutual rejection by parents and adolescents of each other's values and lifestyles. Parents in multiproblem families have been found to frequently reject and then to disengage from their older children, thereby reducing whatever open communication channels there might have been.

Maintaining the family's ethical and moral standards is another family developmental task (Duvall & Miller, 1985). Although family rules need to change, family ethical and moral standards need to be maintained by parents. While adolescents are searching for their own beliefs and values, it is of paramount importance for parents to defend and adhere firmly to their own sound principles and standards. Adolescents are very sensitive to incongruities between what

TABLE 5–10

TWO-PARENT NUCLEAR FAMILY LIFE CYCLE STAGE V: FAMILIES WITH TEENAGERS

DEVELOPMENTAL TASKS	HEALTH CARE CONCERNS
Balancing of freedom with responsibility as teenagers mature and become increasingly autonomous	Accidents (e.g., driving)
	Sports injuries
Refocusing the marital relationship	Drug and alcohol misuse
Communicating openly between parents and children	Birth control
	Unexpected pregnancies
	Sex education
	Marital relationship
	Adolescent–Parent relations
	Good health practices (e.g., sleep, nutrition, exercise)

is "preached and practiced." Nonetheless, parents and children can learn from each other in the fast-changing and pluralistic society of today. Value transformations of youth are transforming families. The adoption of a freer and more casual lifestyle symbolizes a value transformation affecting every phase of family life (Aldous, 1996).

HEALTH CONCERNS.   At this stage the physical health of the family members is usually good, but health promotion remains an important concern (see Table 5–10). Risk factors should be identified and discussed with families, as should the importance of a healthy lifestyle. From age 35 on, the risk of coronary heart disease rises appreciably in males, and at this point both adult members are beginning to feel more vulnerable to ill health as part of their developmental changes and are usually more receptive to health promotion strategies. With teenagers, accidents—particularly automobile accidents—are a great hazard, and broken bones and athletic injuries are also common.

Drug and alcohol misuse, birth control, unwanted pregnancies, and sex education and counseling are relevant areas of concern. In discussing these topics with families, the nurse may get caught squarely in the middle of a parent–youth dispute or problem. Adolescents often seek health services for pregnancy testing, drug use, AIDS screening, birth control and abortion, and venereal disease diagnosis and care. There has been a legal trend to allow adolescents to receive health care without parental consent. Where parents are involved, separate interviews with the teenager and parents prior to bringing them together are often indicated (American Academy of Pediatrics, 1989).

Teenage pregnancy is a critical family problem in many families today. Teenage pregnancy prevention includes both family- and community-based interventions. Family nurses need to assist families with teenage pregnancy prevention. Referrals for family planning services, sexuality counseling and education, encouraging adolescents to participate in after-school leisure time activities, and educational opportunities are basic teenage pregnancy prevention strategies (The Family Connection, 1996).

Another health need is again in the area of support and assistance in strengthening the marital relationship and the adolescent–parent relationships. Direct supportive counseling or initiation of referral to community resources for counseling, as well as recreational, educational, and other services, may be needed.

STAGE VI: FAMILIES LAUNCHING YOUNG ADULTS

The beginning of this phase of family life is characterized by the first child's leaving the parental home and ends with "the empty nest," when the last child has left home. This stage could be quite short or fairly long, depending on how many children are in the family or if any unmarried children remain at home after finishing high school or college. Although the usual length of this stage is six or seven years, in recent years the stage is longer in some families due to more older children living at home after they have finished school and begun working. The motive is often economics—the high cost of living independently. The more widespread trend, however, has been for young adults, who generally delay marriage, to have a period of being unattached during which they live independently in their own households. In a large Canadian survey it was found that children who grow up in stepfamilies and single-parent families leave home earlier than those raised in families with two biological parents. This difference was not seen to be influenced by economic factors, but rather was caused by parent differences and family milieu (Mitchell, Wister, & Burch, 1989).

This phase of family life is marked by the culmination of years of preparation of and by the children for an independent adult life. Parents, as they let their children go, are relinquishing 20 years or so of the parenting role and returning to their original marital dyad. Family developmental tasks are critical while the family is shifting from a household with children to a husband–wife pair. The major family goal is the reorganization of the family into a continuing unit while releasing matured young people into lives of their own (Duvall & Miller, 1985). During this stage the marital pair may take on grandparent roles—another change in both roles and their self-image.

Early middle age, which is about the average age of parents during the launching of their oldest child, has been characterized as a "caught" period of life: caught between the demands of youth and the expectations of the elderly and caught between the world of work and the competing demands and involvement of the family, with the often seeming impossibility of meeting the demands of both realms. Studies indicate, however, that while the middle-aged adult may feel squeezed or "sandwiched" between the poles of youth and aging, at least for middle- and upper-class individuals, they can often appreciate their own importance and achievements: They often know that they are the nation's decision makers; they set the tone for life in this society.

FAMILY DEVELOPMENTAL TASKS.   As the family assists the oldest child in his or her launching, the parents are also involved with their younger children, helping them to become independent. And when the "released" son or daughter marries, the family task involves expanding the family circle to include new members by marriage and becoming accepting of the couple's own lifestyle and values (Table 5–11).

With the emptying of the nest, parents have more time to devote to other activities and relationships. Hopefully, they have not grown so far apart from each other that they cannot reinstitute or reestablish the wife and husband roles to the place of primary importance these roles once held. LeShan (1973) views this stage as a challenge to the marital relationship. When the children leave, marriage faces a moment of truth; is there strength enough to sustain it without the excuse of parenthood?

In the past, it was conventional to see this phase as a difficult time for women. The loss of roles related to child care left a feeling of emptiness. Today, far from feeling useless after their children grow up, the majority of women continue to be busy in their job and partner roles (Aldous, 1996). Most women feel satisfaction that their children have taken on adult responsibilities and are still in close contact with them. They now have the time and energy to devote to their own development and to couple intimacies and companionship.

This period has been associated with menopause, with women historically seen as past their prime, getting old, and unappealing. However, research over the years has documented that many women find this period not only not problematic, but also desirable (N. Woods, personal communications, 1996).

Men in middlescence (the name for middle age in the developmental literature) face potential developmental crises. One potential crisis is the drive to get "ahead" in their careers with the realization that they have not succeeded or have not reached their aspirations. Also, signs of diminished masculinity, such as lower energy levels and lessened potency and sexual excitation, as well as figure, hair, and skin aging signs, and financial worries, are stressors for men during

TABLE 5—11

TWO-PARENT NUCLEAR FAMILY LIFE CYCLE STAGE VI: FAMILIES LAUNCHING YOUNG ADULTS

DEVELOPMENTAL TASKS	HEALTH CARE CONCERNS
Expanding the family circle to young adults including new family members acquired by marriage of children	Communication issues between parents and young adult
Continuing to renew and readjust in the marital relationship	Role transitional problems for husband and wife
Assisting aging and ill parents of the husband and wife	Emergence of chronic health problems
	Family planning for young adult
	Menopausal concerns
	Effects associated with prolonged drinking, smoking, poor dietary practices
	Wellness lifestyle

this family life cycle stage. The frequency of extra-marital affairs, divorces, mental illness, alcoholism, and suicide all rise among adults of these age groups, underscoring the middle-age developmental crises that occur.

Friedman (1957) reiterates the significance of the marital relationship by characterizing the parental developmental stage at this point in the family as the building of a new life together. Both men and women are looking for married lives that are less hectic than in the child-dependent years (Aldous, 1996).

Another important developmental task of the middle-years family is that of assisting aging and ill parents of the husband and wife. Even though the actual care of aging and/or dependent parents is not an expected function of the American family with the exception of certain ethnic groups, the husband and wife are expected to assist and support elderly family members as much as they feel is feasible. Such activity takes all forms—from frequent telephoning and supportive calls to assisting financially, providing transportation, and visiting and caring for their parent(s) in the home.

In America, the family is seen as primarily responsible for the succeeding generation, the offspring, and only secondarily for the previous generation, the parents (Roth, 1996b). Currently, however, there is a political trend throughout the country for families to assume greater responsibility for all family members, including preceding generations.

Three-generation families, although not the usual pattern, are not uncommon, particularly in "traditional" Asian, Hispanic, Greek, Italian, Middle Eastern, and Armenian families. Most often in the United States the multigenerational family seems to develop primarily when the nuclear family is disrupted by death or divorce. Financial expediency or child care needs may also encourage such living arrangements.

Older parents typically desire to live independently so as not to impinge on their children's lives and, more importantly, to retain their own feelings of competence, independence, and privacy (Bengtson, Mangen, & Landry, 1987; Troll, 1971). Parents may also have to wrestle with the decision to place their parents in a nursing home or retirement or board-and-care facility during these years.

In summary, it can be seen that as children disperse, parents must again learn independence. In readjusting, the marriage must be viable if parents' needs are to continue to be fulfilled. Parents have to readjust their relationship—to relate to each other as marital partners rather than primarily as parents. For this stage to be complete, children must be autonomous, while at the same time maintaining ties and bonds with parents.

HEALTH CONCERNS. The primary health concerns involve communication problems between young adults and their parents; role-transitional problems for wife and husband; caretaker concerns (for aging parents); and the emergence of chronic health conditions or predisposing factors such as high cholesterol levels, obesity, and high blood pressure (see Table 5–11). Family planning for the adolescent and young adult members remains important. Menopausal concerns among women are common. The effects associated with prolonged drinking, smoking, and dietary practices become more obvious. Finally, the need for health-promotion strategies and a "wellness lifestyle" become more pressing for the adult members of the launching center family.

STAGE VII: MIDDLE-AGED PARENTS

The seventh stage of the family life cycle, the stage of the middle years for parents, begins when the last child departs from the home and ends with retirement or death of one of the spouses. This stage usually starts when parents are about 45 to 55 years of age and ends with the retirement of a spouse, usually 16 to 18 years later. Typically, the marital couple in their middle years constitutes a nuclear family, although still interacting with their aging parent(s) and other members of their own family of origin, as well as with the new families of marriage of their offspring. The postparental couple is not usually isolated today; more middle-aged couples are living out their full life span and spending a greater portion of it in a postparental phase, with extended kin relationships between four generations not being unusual (Roth, 1996a).

The middle years include changes in marital adjustment (often better), in the distribution of power between husband and wife (more shared), and in roles (increased marital role differentiation) (Leslie & Korman, 1989). To many families with increased satisfaction and economic status (Rollins & Feldman, 1970), these years are seen as the prime of life. For example, Olson and associates (1983), in a large, cross-sectional, national survey of predominantly white, middle-class, intact families, found that marital and family satisfaction and quality of life increased and peaked during the postparental phase. Middle-aged families, in general, are also better off economically than at other stages of the family career (McCullough & Rutenberg, 1988). Increased labor force participation by women and higher earning power than in previous periods by men account for the greater economic security experienced by most middle-aged families. Mutually enjoyable leisure activities and companionship are mentioned as the prime factors leading to marital happiness. Sexual satisfaction is also positively correlated with both good communication and marital satisfaction (Levin & Levin, 1975), even though middle-aged husbands may experience a decline in sexual adequacy. Intimate husband–wife communication is essential for maintaining understanding and interest in each other throughout these years (Heinrich, 1996).

For some couples, however, these years are generally difficult and onerous ones because of problems of aging, the loss of children, and a sense of themselves as failures in parenting and work efforts. Some marital satisfaction studies show that marital satisfaction drops soon after marriage and continues to decline through the middle years (Leslie & Korman, 1989).

FAMILY DEVELOPMENTAL TASKS. By the time the last child leaves home, many women have rechanneled their energies and lives in preparation for the empty nest. For some women, a middle-age crisis is experienced during the early period of this life cycle. Women work at encouraging their grown children to be independent by redefining their relationship with them (not intruding on their personal and family life). In order to maintain a sense of well-being and health, more women begin to live a healthier lifestyle of weight control, balanced diet, regular exercise program, and adequate rest, as well as to attain and enjoy a career, work, or creative accomplishments.

Occupationally, men may find the same frustrations and disappointments that were present in the previous stage. On the one hand, they may be at the peak of their career and not have to work as hard as previously; on the other hand, may find their job monotonous after 20 to 30 years at the same type of work. Many middle-class workers suffer from the "plateau phenomenon"—in which increased salaries and promotions are no longer available—leaving them to feel in a rut. Career discontent is said to reach alarming proportions under these conditions, with many persons making midlife job changes due to the feelings of discontentment, boredom, and stagnation. On the other hand, in the era of company "downsizing," unemployment during this peak in one's career is often most stressful. Because work has traditionally been a man's central role in life, work discontentment as well as the threat or occurrence of being laid off significantly influence a man's stress level and general health status.

The cultivation of leisure-time activities and interests is significant during this stage, since more time is now available and preparation for retirement must take place in a more planned fashion.

An important developmental task for this stage is the provision of a healthy environment (Table 5–12). It is in this period when taking on a healthier lifestyle becomes more prevalent for couples, despite the fact that they have probably been engaging in self-destructive habits for 45 to 65 years. Although not inadvisable to start now, since "better now than never" is always true, it is largely too late to significantly reverse many of the physiological changes that have already taken place, such as arthritic changes due to inactivity; moderate to severe weight gain; high blood pressure due to lack of exercise, prolonged stress, or poor dietary habits; and vital lung capacity diminution due to smoking.

The primary motivation of middle-aged persons to improve their lifestyle appears to be a feeling of susceptibility or vulnerability to illness and disease generated when a friend or family member of the same age group has a heart attack, stroke, or cancer. In addition to fear, a belief that regular checkups and healthful living habits are effective ways of reducing

susceptibility to various diseases are also powerful motivating forces. Heart disease, cancer, and stroke account for two thirds of all causes of mortality between the ages of 46 and 64 years of age, with accidents the fourth cause of death (National Center for Health Statistics, 1989).

A second developmental task for the middle-aged couple is to find satisfying and meaningful relationships with children as they mature to adulthood and with aging older parents. Studies indicate that adverse life changes for parents take a toll on how their children will view the relationship with their parents. These adverse changes are predominantly noted as a decline in the parent's health status and late-life disruption of the parent's marriage due to divorce. There is no evidence to support that disruption of the parent's marriage due to widowhood has negative repercussions on the relationship with the adult children (Kaufman & Uhlenberg, 1998).

Accepting and welcoming grandchildren into the family assists in promoting satisfying intergenerational relationships (Duvall & Miller, 1985; Kaufman & Uhlenberg, 1998). It allows the middle-aged couple to continue feeling like a family and brings the joys of grandparenthood without the 24-hour responsibilities of parenthood. With increased life expectancy, being a grandparent typically occurs during this stage (Sprey & Matthews, 1982). Grandparents provide a wide range of support to their children and grandchildren in times of crisis and assist their children in the parent role through their encouragement and support (Bengtson & Robertson, 1985).

TABLE 5–12

TWO-PARENT NUCLEAR FAMILY LIFE CYCLE STAGE VII: MIDDLE-AGED PARENTS

DEVELOPMENTAL TASKS	HEALTH CARE CONCERNS
Providing a health-promoting environment	Good health practices (e.g., sleep, nutrition, exercise)
Sustaining satisfying and meaningful relationships with aging parents and children	Marital relationship
Strengthening the marital relationship	Communication with and relating to children, in-laws, grandchildren, and aging parents
	Caregiver concerns
	Adjustment to physiological changes of aging

More recent research studies on grandparenting suggest that 11 percent of grandparents over 50 are providing primary caregiving for their grandchildren, and 8 percent are providing day care on a regular basis (AARP, 2000). Divorce, drugs, alcohol problems, incarceration, and unemployment within the parental generation are contributing to the increase in grandparents who are the primary caregiver (Burton, 1992; Calfie, 1994). Although the great majority of grandparents accept this grandparental responsibility willingly, such caregiving may take a significant toll on them. Minkler and Roe (1995) describe a number of problems experienced by grandparents—ranging from stress-related illness and social isolation to severe financial difficulties. In spite of these potential difficulties, the results of grandparenting are generally not all that negative. Burton and de Vries (1995) report that while providing full-time care for a grandchild may be stressful, grandparent caregivers are likely to obtain certain rewards and informal support from their generational family relations.

The more problematic role is that of relating to and assisting the aging parents and sometimes other older extended family members. Eighty-six percent of middle-aged couples have at least one parent each still alive (Hagestad, 1988). Thus, caregiving responsibilities for aging parents who are frail or ill are a frequent experience. While men are assuming greater caregiving responsibilities than in the past, women do the majority of caregiving. Therefore, more women find themselves in a "generational squeeze" in their attempt to balance the needs of their aging parents, their children, and grandchildren. Multiple intergenerational roles and relationships are likely to be more extensive among certain minorities, such as African-American, Asian, and Latino families.

Filial caregiving to disabled elderly parents may lead to physical, emotional, and financial strains for middle-aged persons, who are usually daughters (Brody, Litvin, Hoffman, & Kleban, 1992a). Prolonged caregiving may also cause marital relationship strains. According to Brody and associates (1992a), married daughters who had their husband's emotional support fared best in their filial caregiving. The same was true when unmarried daughters had a supportive "significant other," a special male friend whom unmarried daughters saw exclusively (Brody et al., 1992b).

The third developmental task to be discussed here is that of strengthening the marital relationship. Now the couple is really alone after many years of being surrounded by other family members and relationships. Although appearing as a welcome relief, for many mates it is a difficult experience to have to relate to each other as marital partners rather than as parents. Wright and Leahey (1994) describe this family developmental task as being "renegotiation of marital system as a dyad" (p. 69). The balance of dependency–independency between couples needs to be reexamined. Often couples develop different arrangements in marriage, such as having greater independent interests, as well as meaningful mutual interests. For couples who experience problems, the reduced pressure of life in postparental years may lead not to marital bliss, but to marital "blahs" and being in a "comfortable rut" (Kerckhoff, 1976).

HEALTH CONCERNS.   The health concerns mentioned throughout the description of the life cycle stage include the following (see Table 5–12):

1. Health promotion needs: Adequate rest, leisure activities, and sleep; good nutrition; regular exercise program; reduction of weight down to optimum weight; cessation of smoking; reduction or cessation in use of alcohol; and preventive health screening examination

2. Marital relationship concerns

3. Communication with and relating to children, in-laws, grandchildren, and aging parents

4. Caregiver concerns: Assisting in care of aging or disabled parents

5. Adjusting to physiological changes, such as the hormonal, menopausal changes in women

STAGE VIII: FAMILIES IN RETIREMENT AND OLD AGE

The last stage of the life cycle of the family begins with the retirement of one or both spouses, continues through the loss of one spouse, and ends with the death of the other spouse (Duvall & Miller, 1985). The number of aging individuals—people 65 and older—in our country has rapidly increased during the last two decades, twice as fast as the rest of the population. In 1900 elder adults comprised 1 in every

25 Americans. In 1994, these older citizens made up 1 in 8 Americans (33.2 million) (U.S. Bureau of the Census, 1995). By the year 2050, as the baby boom generation joins this age group, the population of older citizens is expected to reach 80 million, and as many as 1 in 5 Americans could be elderly (U.S. Bureau of the Census, 1995). Information on population aging suggest that the "oldest old"—the 85-plus population—is growing especially rapidly. The 85-plus population rose 274 percent between 1960 and 1994. It is projected that in the year 2050, this population will number 19 million Americans, or 5 percent of the entire American population (U.S. Bureau of the Census, 1995). As the result of improved disease prevention and health care, more people are also expected to survive into their tenth decade. Because of the increase in the very old population, it is increasingly possible that older people will themselves have at least one surviving parent.

Perceptions of this stage of the life cycle differ significantly among aging families. Some persons are miserable, while others feel these are the best years of their lives. Although much is dependent on the adequacy of financial resources and the ability to maintain a satisfactory home, one's health status has been identified as a primary predictor of the well-being of older persons (Brubaker, 1990; Quinn, 1993). The more health difficulties experienced, the more likely the presence of negative feelings toward old age. Those who have lost their independence due to ill health generally have low morale, and poor physical health is often an antecedent to behavioral and psychological problems in the elderly (Chilman, Nunnally, & Cox, 1988). Conversely, those elders who have maintained their health, who have kept active, and have adequate economic resources represent a substantial proportion of older people and usually feel positive about this stage of life.

SOCIETY'S ATTITUDE TOWARD THE ELDERLY. Our society emphasizes the achievements of those in the young adult years, glorifying the period of youth. Therefore, adults, through grooming, dress, and styles, try to maintain their youthful appearance as long as possible. Aging has been viewed as an abrupt decline, and the debilitating diseases that affect only a small percentage of the elderly are often viewed as the norm rather than the exception. Normal aging is frequently thought of as a period of sickness, senility,

and dependency. For both the community at large and individual families, dealing with the aged has had a negative connotation, one loaded with feelings of being burdened down with imposing problems. Additionally, society has not allowed most aged people to remain productive. Hence, society's negative appraisal of older people has negatively affected their self-image.

Yet today, many associations and much of the literature advocate and illustrate the strengths, resources, and other positive aspects of aging. This has begun to diminish the negativism and stereotypical thinking about the aged and help us recognize the assets of the older person and the great diversity of lifestyles among members of this age group.

Our attitudes toward aging and the aged, albeit still negative, appear to be changing. Recent studies conducted on society's attitude toward the elderly have validated that the elderly are being viewed more positively (Austin, 1985; Schonfield, 1982). McCubbin and Dahl (1985) report, "Many observers believe that age is regaining respect in the United States. A new generation of old people—better educated, more affluent, healthier and more active than previous elderly generations—is redefining the notion of 'being old'" (p. 276). This change in attitude enhances the elderly's image of themselves.

LOSSES COMMON TO AGING PEOPLE AND FAMILIES. As aging progresses and retirement becomes a reality, there is a variety of stressors or losses experienced by some older people and couples that confound their role transition. These may include the following:

- Economic—Adjusting to a substantially reduced income; later perhaps adjusting to economic dependency (depending on family or government for subsidy)

- Housing—Often moving to smaller quarters, assisted living facilities, and later perhaps being forced to move to an institutional setting

- Social—Loss (death) of siblings, friends, and spouse

- Work—Voluntary or involuntary retirement and loss of the work role and a sense of productivity

- Health—Declining physical, mental, and cognitive functions; caregiving for the less healthy spouse

Entry into full retirement is a main life cycle turning point. It typically means a moderate to significant loss of status and social support and, for many, lifestyle changes, including increased leisure time (Rubin & Neiswiadomy, 1995). This transition involves reorientation of values and goals and a redirection of energies. What such changes entail, however, is not entirely clear, because the roles and norms for the older person and couple are ambiguous. Clear boundaries may become vague as the retired spouse, especially the husband, is incorporated into domestic activities. This reintegration may not pose problems for some couples, whereas for others it may be difficult (Walsh, 1989).

The retirement years constitute up to a quarter or more of an average person's life. The median retirement ages of both men and women have declined from 66 years of age (1995 through 1990) to about 63 years of age (1985 through 1990) (Gendell & Siegel, 1996). The number of dual-retired couples has been growing steadily in the last two decades, and this trend is expected to continue. While some older persons may be fortunate to return to work after retiring from their former position, others may not or cannot, sometimes because of declining health.

Certainly, declining health affects adaptation to retirement. Haug, Belgrove, and Jones (1992) also report that the wife's education is a significant variable that influences the retirement transition. Other factors influencing a couple's ability to cope with retirement are their readiness to retire, spouse's expectations, planning for retirement, financial security, and the external support they have (Dorfman & Rubenstein, 1993; Honig, 1996; Knesek, 1992).

FAMILY DEVELOPMENTAL TASKS.   Maintaining satisfying living arrangements is a most important task of aging families (Table 5–13). Housing after retirement may become problematic. In the years immediately following retirement, couples usually remain in the family home until property taxes, neighborhood conditions, size or condition of house, or health forces them to find more modest accommodations. Although a majority of older people own their own homes, a substantial proportion of these are old and often run down; many are located in high-crime areas where older people are likely to be victims. The elderly often tend to "stay put" despite deteriorating neighborhood conditions (Lawton, 1985). Nonetheless, older persons living in their own homes are generally more well adjusted than those who live in their children's homes. According to a study by Day and Day (1993), women living with their spouses and women living alone demonstrated more successful aging than women living with relatives.

TABLE 5–13

TWO-PARENT NUCLEAR FAMILY LIFE CYCLE STAGE VIII: FAMILIES IN THE LATER YEARS

DEVELOPMENTAL TASKS	HEALTH CARE CONCERNS
Maintaining a satisfying living arrangement	Increasing functional disabilities
Adjusting to a reduced income	Mobility impairment
Maintaining marital relationships	Chronic illness
Adjusting to loss of spouse	Diminished physical vigor and function
Maintaining intergenerational family ties	Long-term care services
Continuing to make sense out of one's existence (life review and integration)	Caregiving
	Social isolation
	Grief/depression
	Cognitive impairment

A person's living arrangements are a powerful predictor of well-being among the elderly (Berriesi, Ferraro, & Hobey, 1984). Relocation is a traumatic experience for the elderly, whether it is a voluntary or involuntary move. It means leaving behind neighborhood ties and friendships that have provided the elderly with a sense of security and stability. Relocation means separation from one's heritage and the cues that bolster old memories (Lawton, 1980).

Relocation, however, does not affect all of the elderly in the same way. Given adequate preparation and careful planning for the change, the new environment may have a positive impact on the elderly. Nevertheless, some research findings suggest that when older people move, some deterioration of their health often results (Lawton, 1985).

The disabled elderly (functionally, physically, or cognitively impaired) are more likely to enter nursing homes because of the lack of assistance in the home. Only about 5 percent of older people live in institutions. This means 95 percent of older people live at home or in other community-based living facilities. Moreover, even among the older people who are disabled, 90 percent live at home with family members; with the care they receive being provided totally or partially by one of their family members.

According to the AARP Report (1993), the oldest old (age 85 and above) are more likely to be in nursing homes (25 percent). Moreover, more women than men will be in nursing homes. Among those not institutionalized, 9 percent of those age 65 to 69 and 50 percent aged 85 or older will need assistance performing everyday living activities.

The provision of full-time help in the home or, more feasibly, part-time health and homemaker services through a home health agency or homemaker agency is protective of the older person's need to remain in his or her own home and retain his or her independence as long as possible. In addition, it is less costly than institutionalization. Albeit difficult, one of the mates and/or grown children of the couple (or the remaining parent) often has to decide what is the best path to take—home health services, retirement home, nursing home, or living with grown children.

Adjusting to a reduced income is a second developmental task for the aging family. When men retire, there is an immediate drop in income, and usually as the years pass by, this income becomes less and less

adequate because of the steady rise in cost of living and the depletion of savings. Older people have substantially less cash income than those under 65. The elderly rely heavily on Social Security benefits and asset income. Elderly women (16 percent) have a higher poverty rate than elderly men (9 percent) (U.S. Bureau of the Census, 1995). Women are more likely to delay their career, to work part time, and to experience disruptions in the work cycle that may lead to lower pay and fewer benefits. They also tend to retire early to assume caregiving responsibilities for their aging parents or spouses (Brody, 1985; Minkler & Stone, 1985). Also due to divorce and death of spouse, women are more likely to be alone after retirement and may remain poor (Haywood & Liu, 1992). Black and Hispanic elderly have substantially lower money incomes as well as lower median incomes than their white counterparts (U.S. Bureau of the Census, 1995).

Because of the frequency of long-term health problems, health expenses are a major financial concern. The elderly spend more on health care—both in actual dollars and as a percentage of total expenditure—than the nonelderly. Medicare has certainly alleviated part of this problem, but there are still unpredictable, and many times substantial, out-of-pocket expenses to be paid. For instance, Part B of Medicare covers only 80 percent of "reasonable" costs for medical services. Medicaid is also available to those who are medically indigent and qualify for supplemental security income (SSI). This health insurance program then supplements Medicare coverage.

As average life expectancy increases, older people will spend more years with severely limiting medical problems. Even though women outlive men by an average of seven years and the gap in life expectancies between men and women is increasing, more married couples are surviving longer (U.S. Bureau of the Census, 1995). This means that wives are more likely to be caregivers to their husbands. Stone and colleagues (1987) confirmed this fact in a study they conducted. They found that more wives were caregivers than husbands (23 percent versus 13 percent of all caregiving). Furthermore, according to Montgomery (1989), spouses tend to provide a greater level of assistance for longer periods of time than do their adult children.

Although several studies document the fact that

caregiving is uniformly stressful, its impact on individuals who are caring for their ill spouses is not clear. While some researchers report that there are no differences in the level of burden between spouses and adult children (Montgomery, 1989; Montgomery & Kosloski, 1994), other researchers suggest higher levels of burden among spouse caregivers when compared to adult children (George & Gwyther, 1986). Spouse caregivers, as compared to spouses who are not involved with caregiving, tend to have a lower level of well-being (Sistler, 1989). Also, caregiving spouses are more likely than noncaregiving spouses to be lonely and to experience mild depression, financial worries, and low life satisfaction (Staight & Harvey, 1990). Some researchers report that the physical health of the caregivers suffers, with the negative consequences ranging from a compromised immune system function to undetected hypertension and cardiac problems (Kiecolt-Glaser & Glaser, 1989; Koin, 1989).

Some caregiving literature today describes "the caregiver career," referring to a process or trajectory of caregiving that occurs, particularly in long-term caregiving situations. For example, Lindgren (1993) describes the caregiver career of spouses who are caring for family members with dementia as a "fatalistic" career process. Here, Lindgren identifies three stages: (1) the encounter stage, (2) the middle enduring stage, and (3) the final, exit stage. During the encounter stage, the caregivers are adjusting to the impact of the diagnoses, learning new skills, and making lifestyles changes. The enduring stage is characterized by heavy work and disruption of routine work. In this stage of the caregiving career, Lindgren (1993) states that the caregivers are likely to feel hopeless and to have an overwhelming sense of frustration and loss. The third or exit stage is characterized by the caregiver's making decisions, taking on activities, and making adjustments associated with total or partial relinquishment of the caregiving role. The caregiving role is relinquished to some degree either through death or institutionalization of the ill spouse.

Maintaining marital relationships, a third developmental task, continues to be paramount to the family's happiness. Marriages perceived as satisfying in the later years usually have a long positive history and vice versa. Researchers have also shown that marriage contributes greatly to both morale and continued activity of both older spouses (Brubaker, 1985; Lee, 1978). Maintaining a satisfactory marital relationship after one or both spouses retire is also influenced by the support each spouse receives from the other and changes that occur in the health of either or both spouses (Brubaker, 1983; Gilford, 1984; Keating & Cole, 1980). This latter factor often creates caregiving challenges and burdens, which, in turn, influence a couple's marital adjustment (Fitting, Rabins, Lucas, & Eastham, 1986).

One of the myths of old age is that sex drives and sexual activities are no longer possible (or should not exist). Considerable research has shown just the reverse, however. Such studies have found that although there is a slowing down of sexual capacity, the pleasure in sexual activity and interest are consistent with interest and activity during early adulthood (AARP, 1999; Heinrich, 1996; Starr, 1985). Ill health sometimes diminishes the sex drive, but usually the lack of sexual activity is due to socioemotional problems.

Adjusting to the loss of spouse, the fourth developmental task, is in general the most traumatic developmental task. Older women suffer the loss of a spouse more than men. According to statistics for 2000, 67 percent of noninstitutionalized men 75 years and older were living with their spouses compared with only 29 percent of women of the same age (U.S. Bureau of the Census, 2000a). On the other hand, elderly women were more than three times as likely as elderly men to be widowed (48 percent versus 14 percent). Consequently, many elderly (8 in 10 noninstitutionalized elderly) live alone, and most of these are women (U.S. Bureau of the Census, 1995).

In comparison with young groups, the aged are aware that dying is part of the normal process of living. The majority of older persons fear death less than younger persons and are more concerned with the death of their loved ones than of themselves (Butler & Lewis, 1982; Neimeyer, 1988).

The awareness of death does not, however, mean that the spouse left behind will find adjustment to loss easier. Loss of spouse takes its toll—the widowed die earlier than their married counterparts, and the living are more likely to have a serious health problem (social isolation, being suicidal or mentally ill). In addition, the loss of a spouse demands a total reorganization of family functions. This is especially difficult to achieve satisfactorily, since the loss has depleted the emotional and economic resources needed to deal with the change. For women, this means a shift from mutual dependency and sharing activities of family living to being alone or associating with a group of unattached older women. For men, the loss of spouse means the loss of a companion, as well as of linkages to kin, family, and the social world in general. The aged widower often does not have the same interest in or the ability to perform the home-maker–housekeeper roles as his deceased wife and may need assistance in meal preparation, homemaking, and general care.

How difficult the adjustment is can be seen by the increase in suicides within individuals over 65. Even though there is some increase in suicides among women over 65, the preponderance of suicides is found within the older male population.

Elderly men who commit suicide tend to use more violent methods to kill themselves (Kaplan, Adamek, & Johnson, 1994). According to Kastenbaum (1994), the concerns of older persons that often lead to thoughts of suicide include poor health, loss of mobility and independence, loneliness, isolation, and loss of control. Regardless of the mode of death (a suicide or natural death), the loss of a loved one is a difficult and profound psychological trauma in which depression, confusion, and pervasive feelings of emptiness are often present (Farberow, Gallagher-Thompson, Gilewski, & Thompson, 1992).

Studies of the widowed have consistently verified the difficult living conditions and life of the widowed. The widowed have lower morale and fewer social roles and ties than the married of the same age group. Bild and Havighurst (1976), in a large study of the elderly in Chicago, reported that the loss of a spouse removed the strongest support of the elderly person, although children, when available, usually stepped in to fill the vacuum somewhat. They also found that the childless widowed were even more isolated.

Negative consequences in response to the death of a spouse are many. For instance, widowhood produces negative effects on eating behavior and specific nutrient quality of the elderly widowed person's diet (Rosenbloom & Whittington, 1993). Also, widowed individuals are more likely to have depressive symptoms or even experience a major depressive episode. Zisook and Shuchter (1993) reported that poor health, the use of psychotropic medications, and increased use of alcohol and other nonprescribed substances were associated with postbereavement depression. Fortunately, social support by families, relatives, friends, and/or professionals reduces the likelihood of depression. Mullins and Mushel (1992) suggested that friends, especially close friends, have a positive influence on the emotional well-being of older widowed persons.

A fifth developmental task deals with the maintenance of intergenerational family ties. Although there is a tendency for older persons to disengage from social relationships, the family remains the focus of aging persons' social interactions and their primary source of social support. As the older person withdraws from activities in the surrounding world, relationships with spouse, children, grandchildren, and siblings become more important. The majority of older Americans live close by their extended family members and have frequent contact with them (Harris et al., 1975; Shanas et al., 1968, 1980). Hence, family members are an important source of direct assistance and social interaction. Older families are found generally to reciprocate in the giving of help to the extent to which they are capable.

As people age they must continue to make sense out of their existence. Reminiscing about one's past life, called life review, is a common and vital activity because it represents a search for the central meaning of life. It is viewed as a sixth "cognitive-type" developmental task. Its importance lies in the fact that life review eases the adjustment to difficult situations and provides insight into past events. The elderly are concerned with the quality of their life and being able to live with respect, meaning, and dignity (Duvall, 1977; Roth, 1996a).

HEALTH CONCERNS. The elderly are the heaviest users of health services (U.S. Senate Special Committee on Aging, 1987–1988). More than four out of five elderly have at least one chronic condition, and multiple conditions are commonplace among the elderly. In 1990, the elderly made up 12.7 percent of the total population, but they accounted for 33 percent of health care expenditures in the United States.

Advancing age is also highly correlated with functional disability, though poor health is not as prevalent as many assume. In 1992, about three in every four noninstitutionalized persons aged 65 to 74 considered themselves to be in good health. Two in three aged 75 or older felt the same (U.S. Bureau of the Census, 1995). Older women tend to experience greater functional disability, mobility impairment, and chronic illness than older men (Penning & Strain, 1994; Santiago & Muschkin, 1996). Seven in ten elderly deaths can be attributed to either heart disease, cancer, or stroke (U.S. Bureau of the Census, 1995).

Factors such as diminishing physical vigor and function, inadequate financial resources, social isolation, loneliness, and the many other losses that the older person experiences demonstrate some of the psychophysiological vulnerabilities of human aging. Therefore, multiple chronic health concerns and long-term care needs exist (see Table 5–13).

FAMILY CAREER OR LIFE CYCLE STAGES IN DIVORCED FAMILIES

One of the major variations in the family life cycle or career is seen when parents divorce. As mentioned in Chapter 1, one of the most profound changes taking place over the past two decades has been the rise in divorces and female-headed households. Since 1970, the number of single-mother families has risen from 12 percent (3 million families) to 26 percent (10 million) in 2000. For single-father families, this increase has been from 1 percent (393,000 families) in 1970 to 5 percent (2 million) (U.S. Bureau of the Census, 2000a). The percentage of adults who are divorced has quadrupled since 1960 (Dobson, 1999). Divorces are so common today (almost 50 percent of all marriages end in divorce) that the event is being viewed as a normative transition. Thirty-seven percent of children in single-parent families are in families in which the parent is divorced. Thirty-five percent of children now live apart from their biological father (Dobson, 1999).

The single-parent, divorced family passes through the same life cycle stages, with most of the same responsibilities, as the two-parent nuclear family. The basic difference is the absence of the second parent to carry his or her (mostly his) share of the family tasks with respect to support, child rearing, companionship, and gender role modeling for the children.

Hill (1986) explains, "The differences in paths of development of single-parent and two-parent families are seen primarily, not in stages encountered, but in the number, timing and length of the critical transitions experienced" (p. 28).

Carter and McGoldrick (1989) conceptualize divorce as an interruption or dislocation of the traditional family life cycle. Divorce, with its losses and shifts in family membership, creates major family destabilization and disequilibrium. Peck and Manocharian (1988) underscore the emotional and physical impact of divorce on the family. "Divorce affects family members at every generational level throughout the nuclear and extended family, thus producing a crisis for the family as a whole as well as for each individual within the family" (p. 335).

As with the two-parent nuclear family, there are crucial changes in roles and relationships and important family developmental tasks to be completed in order for the divorced family to move forward developmentally (Carter & McGoldrick, 1989). As a major disruptive force, divorce compounds the complexity of the developmental tasks the family is experiencing. Each subsequent stage is also affected, so that each postdivorce stage must be viewed within the context of both the stage itself and the consequences of the divorce.

After the divorce, family systems research has found that it takes about one to three years for the family to restabilize itself. "If a family can negotiate the crisis and the accompanying transitions that must be experienced in order to restabilize, it will have established a more fluid system that will allow a continuation of the normal family developmental process" (Peck & Manocharian, 1988, p. 335). Carter and McGoldrick have summarized the research and writings of Ahrons (1980) on the process of adjustment that divorced families go through. Table 5–14 outlines the pre- and postdivorce adjustment process, including concomitant emotional processes and family developmental issues.

To describe the impact of the divorce on the family life cycle stages, it first should be said that the impact varies depending on what stage the family is in when the divorce occurs. Other factors also make a difference on impact, such as ethnic, social, and economic factors. Divorce is the least disruptive during the first stage of marriage, as there are fewer people involved, fewer traditions established, and fewer couple-based

TABLE 5–14

DISLOCATIONS OF THE FAMILY LIFE CYCLE BY DIVORCE, REQUIRING ADDITIONAL STEPS TO RESTABILIZE AND PROCEED DEVELOPMENTALLY

PHASE	EMOTIONAL PROCESS OF TRANSITION—PREREQUISITE ATTITUDE	DEVELOPMENTAL ISSUES
Divorce		
1. The decision to divorce	Acceptance of inability to resolve marital tensions sufficiently to continue relationship	Acceptance of one's own part in the failure of the marriage
2. Planning the breakup of the system	Supporting viable arrangements for all parts of the system	a. Working cooperatively on problems of custody, visitation, and finances
		b. Dealing with extended family about the divorce
3. Separation	a. Willingness to continue cooperative co-parental relationship and joint financial support of children	a. Mourning loss of intact family
	b. Work on resolution of attachment to spouse	b. Restructuring marital and parent–child relationships and finances; adaptation to living apart
		c. Realignment of relationships with extended family; staying connected with spouse's extended family
4. The divorce	More work on emotional divorce: Overcoming hurt, anger, guilt, etc.	a. Mourning loss of intact family; giving up fantasies of reunion
		b. Retrieval of hopes, dreams, expectations from the marriage
		c. Staying connected with extended families
Postdivorce family		
1. Single-parent (custodial household or primary residence)	Willingness to maintain financial responsibilities, continue parental contact with ex-spouse, and support contact of children with ex-spouse and his or her family	a. Making flexible visitation arrangements with ex-spouse and his or her family
		b. Rebuilding own financial resources
		c. Rebuilding own social network
2. Single-parent (noncustodial)	Willingness to maintain parental contact with ex-spouse and support custodial parent's relationship with children	a. Finding ways to continue effective parenting relationship with children
		b. Maintaining financial responsibilities to ex-spouse and children
		c. Rebuilding own social network

Source: Carter B., & McGoldrick, M. (Eds.). (1989). The changing family life cycle: A framework for family therapy (p. 22). New York: Gardner Press. Reprinted by permission.

social ties (Peck & Manocharian, 1988). The impact is much greater during the third and fourth stages in those families with preschool and school-aged children. Moreover, the family is most at risk for divorce during these periods.

Young children are initially most affected by parents' divorce. Children may regress developmentally, making child rearing and separation of parents and children difficult. Single parenthood is often very onerous for the mother, who usually struggles both emotionally and economically. The economic status of female-headed divorced families declines considerably following divorce. Two frequently seen problems are that the father loses his sense of connection to his children and, because of the mother's anger at the father; the mother leaves no room for him. Yet maintaining both the mother–child and father–child relationships is very important for both parents and children. Unfortunately for both father and children, a large proportion of children virtually lose contact with their fathers after the divorce (Hagestad, 1988).

When divorce occurs among families with school-aged children, the long-term impact of the divorce is even more profound on the school-aged child. In one study, children six to eight years of age were the age group that had the hardest time adjusting to divorce (Wallerstein & Kelly, 1980). Children are old enough at that time to realize what is happening, but not old enough to deal effectively with the divorce.

Families with adolescents are often already in turmoil, and divorce only compounds the problem. For the single parent, raising the adolescent alone is difficult. Co-parenting is also problematic when the adolescent is having behavior problems. Progressing through the developmental tasks of adolescence and the family life cycle is initially delayed.

In later stages of the family life cycle, children are likely to be affected less profoundly than in the previous family stages because they are older and better able to cope and function more autonomously. In the case of midlife divorce, however, older children may be propelled into filial maturity, accepting of the dependency of a parent, particularly the mother, when a parent turns to a child for support during the divorce crisis.

During these later family life cycle stages, divorce is typically profoundly traumatizing to the divorced partners. Years of shared possessions, memories, and habits have created "a couple identity." Divorce during later years is likened to a death of a partner in some of the divorce literature.

FAMILY CAREER OR LIFE CYCLE STAGES IN STEPPARENT FAMILIES

Divorce is commonly a transitional state, followed by remarriage. Remarriage has been so prevalent from the mid-1980s on that nearly one half of all marriages are remarriages (Teachman, Tedrow, & Crowder, 2001). Before age 40, both men and women remarry fairly equally, but after age 40, remarriage is disproportionately a male transition (Hagestad, 1988). Remarriages tend to take place rapidly after prior marriages end, with a mean length of time between divorce and remarriage of less than four years. Thirty percent marry within a year after divorce. Children lower the likelihood of remarriage for both men and women, though remarriage among women is impacted negatively more by this variable (Coleman, Ganong & Fine, 2000).

Not all stepfamilies incorporate a remarriage. That is, many adults in the stepfamily arrangement choose to not marry. Approximately 25 percent of cohabiting couples in the United States are households in which at least one adult brings children from prior relationships, thereby creating a new cohabiting stepfamily household (Coleman, Ganong, & Fine, 2000).

Carter and McGoldrick (1989) present a developmental outline of the remarried family formation—the steps involved in the remarriage process, the prerequisite attitudes, and the developmental issues (Table 5–15). The family's emotional process at the transition to remarriage is typically one that involves struggling with fears about investment in a new relationship and a new family; dealing with hostile or upset reactions of the children, extended families, and the ex-spouse; worrying about the ambiguous new family situation; feeling guilty and concerned over the welfare of the children; and renewing of attachments (negative or positive) to the ex-spouse. The stepparent–stepchild relationship is generally considered to be the most problematic and stressful relationship in stepfamilies, requiring considerable strategies to develop warm

TABLE 5—15

REMARRIED FAMILY FORMATION: A DEVELOPMENTAL OUTLINE

STEPS	PREREQUISITE ATTITUDE	DEVELOPMENTAL ISSUES
1. Entering the new relationship	Recovery from loss of first marriage (adequate "emotional divorce")	Recommitment to marriage and to forming a family with readiness to deal with the complexity and ambiguity
2. Conceptualizing and planning new marriage and family	Accepting one's own fears and those of new spouse and children about remarriage and forming a stepfamily	a. Work on openness in the new relationships to avoid pseudomutuality
		b. Plan for maintenance of cooperative financial and co-parental relationships with ex-spouses
	Accepting need for time and patience for adjustment to complexity and ambiguity of:	c. Plan to help children deal with fears, loyalty conflicts, and membership in two systems
	1. Multiple new roles	
	2. Boundaries: space, time, membership, and authority	d. Realignment of relationships with extended family to include new spouse and children
	3. Affective issues: guilt, loyalty conflicts, desire of mutuality, unresolvable past hurts	e. Plan maintenance of connections for children with extended family of ex-spouses(s)
3. Remarriage and reconstitution of family	Final resolution of attachment to previous spouse and ideal of "intact" family; acceptance of a different model of family with permeable boundaries	a. Restructuring family boundaries to allow for inclusion of new spouse/stepparent
		b. Realignment of relationships and arrangements throughout subsystems to permit interweaving of several systems
		c. Making room for relationships of all children with biological (noncustodial) parents, grandparents, and other extended family
		d. Sharing memories and histories to enhance stepfamily integration

Source: Carter B., & McGoldrick, M. (Eds.). (1989). The changing family life cycle: A framework for family therapy (p. 24). New York: Gardner Press. Reprinted by permission.

and affectionate bonds between family members (Ganong, Coleman, & Fine, 1995). Remarriage, again because it is a disruptive transitional process, impedes the family's movement through and completion of family developmental tasks. Stepparent adjustment and integration, as with divorce adjustment, seems to take a minimum of two to three years before a new structure allows the family to move on developmentally (Carter & McGoldrick, 1989; Coleman, Ganong, & Fine, 2000).

FAMILY CAREER OR LIFE CYCLE STAGES IN DOMESTIC PARTNER RELATIONSHIPS

Domestic partnerships refer to gay, lesbian, and heterosexual cohabitants who have an intimate relationship and are financially interdependent (Ames, 1992). In 2000, there were 3.8 million households that were classified as unmarried-partner households. The gay and lesbian couples who cohabitate are a large proportion of the numbers represented in this group (U.S. Bureau of the Census, 2000a).

LESBIAN/GAY FAMILY CAREER STAGES

There are estimated to be in the United States today 1 to 5 million lesbian mothers, 1 to 3 million gay fathers, and from 6 to 14 million children with homosexual parents (Ames, 1992). The discrimination against same-sex family life within the mainstream culture, however, may lead many families to keep their status secret. Lesbian/gay families, as with other families, change and grow over time.

Lesbians/gays form families based on personal selection of family members. Slater (1995) refers to the lesbian family as the family of creation. It consists of the couple alone or a lesbian/gay couple and their children. Outlining a lesbian/gay family career, however, is complicated by numerous simultaneous influences determining a couple's journey through the stages of their relationship (Slater, 1995). Competing influences of lesbian/gay identity formation, typical lesbian/gay stressors, coping mechanisms, other minority identity development, and the couple's lifelong voluntary and required social relationships shape the family career.

Slater's model of the lesbian/gay family career reflects the rich diversity and points of common experience among lesbian/gay families. Slater (1995) describes five stages, which are sequential and with limited duration, some stages enduring far longer than others. The couple's adaptations to the challenges of previous stages become incorporated into their relationship and strengthen or diminish their capacity to confront subsequent obstacles. The layers of partner chronological development, lesbian/gay identity formation, other minority identity formation, and the stage of the life career intersect continually. For an in-depth discussion of lesbian family careers, see Slater's book, *The Lesbian Family Life Cycle*. Table 5–16 outlines the lesbian/gay family career.

IMPACT OF ILLNESS AND DISABILITY ON FAMILY DEVELOPMENTAL STAGES

Serious illness or long-term disability of a family member significantly affects the family and its functioning, just as the behavior of the family and its members simultaneously affects the course and characteristics of the illness or disability (Bahnson, 1987). Given this widely accepted assumption of reciprocity, it is clear that serious illness or disability profoundly influences family development, as well as individual family member development, especially of the sick or disabled member. Often, when a family is delayed in meeting its family developmental tasks, it is the interaction of the developmental demands/stressors and a situational demand/stressor that compounds and overloads the family. The added family stress created by the presence of both types of stressors often results in lowered family functioning, whereby mastering of family developmental tasks becomes impeded or retarded.

The extent to which family developmental tasks are affected depends on several factors. One is certainly the family life cycle stage that the family is in; second, which family member becomes seriously ill or disabled makes a difference. Some particular stages are already developmentally hazardous, and completing family developmental tasks of a particular stage are more crucial for certain family members. For instance, in a family with a teenager, if the adolescent sustains a serious injury and is left in a dependent state, this will greatly impede the adolescent's own mastery of the developmental task of becoming more independent from the family. Likewise, the family developmental task dealing with balancing freedom with responsibility so as to assist the teenager to become increasingly autonomous will also be impeded. The challenge for the family is to attempt to

TABLE 5–16

LESBIAN/GAY FAMILY CAREER

STAGE	TRANSITION PROCESS	DEVELOPMENTAL TASKS
I. Couple formation	Partners need to differentiate when they began to show interest from when they began an actual couple relationship	a. Building a beginning sense of themselves as a unit b. Relaxing boundaries around themselves as they tentatively blend aspects of their lives c. Developing trust between partners d. Increasing self-disclosure e. Engaging in empathic responses that encourage further risk f. Controlling who knows about their relationships
II. Ongoing couplehood	Couple moves from unbridled passion to beginning of stability, combining passion and dailiness	a. Recognizing and managing a range of differences that are becoming evident b. Negotiating conflict c. Developing relational security and sense of belonging
III. Middle years	Couple's movement into a permanent or long-range commitment	a. Diligent reworking of the rewards and disappointments within extended relational commitment b. Creating security and continuing newness within the relationship
IV. Generativity	Couple's desire to associate themselves with and provide a sense of identity that will endure beyond their own finite existence	a. Creating a personal legacy
V. Couple over 60	Couple facing imposed life changes, some occurring all at once and others emerging, such as retirement, physical illness, and widowhood	a. Partner renegotiation of interdependence and autonomy b. Each partner working to secure some power and unique identity for self within the relationship c. Balancing financial, physical, and emotional independence

Adapted from Slater (1995).

resume working on normal developmental family tasks as soon as possible.

Another major factor that makes a difference in regards to the impact of illness or disability on family development is the formal and informal resources the family is utilizing. A good social support system of extended family and friends, as well as competent, helpful health and psychosocial supports, will augment the family's ability to more quickly get back on track developmentally.

When working with a family with a serious illness or disability, it is useful to compare the "ideal" family developmental tasks within the appropriate family life cycle stage with the family's actual behavior (Friedman, 1987). This type of comparison is useful in evaluating the probable impact of the illness or disability on the family.

❧ FAMILY ASSESSMENT AREAS: DEVELOPMENTAL STAGE AND HISTORY OF THE FAMILY

Throughout the assessment process, a focus on the family career or family life cycle enhances the family health professional's understanding of the stresses that are impinging on a family and the actual or potential problems of a family. In completing the developmental part of a family assessment, the following areas are suggested:

1. The family's present developmental stage.

2. The extent to which the family is fulfilling the developmental tasks appropriate for the present developmental stage. It is important to note any significant deviations from the norm, as this may serve as an indication of impending or present problems.

3. The family's history from inception through present day, including developmental history and unique health and health-related events and experiences (e.g., divorce, deaths, losses) that happened in the family's life. Some of this information (divorces, marriages, deaths) can be included on the family genogram (see Chapter 8).

4. Both parents' families of origin (what life in family of origin was like; present and past relations with parents of parents). This assessment may or may not be helpful, depending on the family's concerns and the family nurse's role in working with the family.

As mentioned, both the family's common and unique experiences and perceptions as they progress through the family career should be assessed to make the developmental history more comprehensive. A description of each parent's family of origin is also useful to include in a family history because of how crucial intergenerational influences are on family life.

It may be more significant to elicit a developmental history from some families than from others. It is important to make sure the family you are working with is open to exploring their past and that your collection of historical data in any of the suggested areas is relevant for understanding and working with the family.

To reiterate, developmental or historical data on a family can be gleaned by (a) asking about common experiences and tasks and how these were accomplished and perceived and (b) asking about special or unique family problems or experiences. The latter include divorces, deaths in nuclear or extended family, separations due to illness or military service, unemployment, and so forth. Asking parents about their present and past relationships with their family of orientation and what life in the original family was like gives the family-centered nurse a better appreciation and understanding of the parents during their formative years.

In order to elicit a family history, Satir (1983) begins by having parents first talk about their own marital relationship, focusing on this relationship because the parents are the family architects. Satir and the parents, with the children present when appropriate, discuss the following areas:

- First meeting of the couple, their relationship before marriage, and how they decided to get married

- Any obstacles to their marriage; their responses to getting married

- Marriage without the children; how they established tasks and roles

- What life was like in both original family environments, including both parents' families of orientation
- Any other people who live or have lived with the family
- Relationships with in-laws
- Description of each mate's parents and their relationship with them.
- Plans for and arrival of each new child (Were children planned? What was the impact of the arrival of each child?)
- How much time the family spends together
- Daily routine of family life

Smoyak (1975), in her nursing practice as a family therapist, stresses the significance of assessing the parents' respective families of orientation:

> It is important to know how each present parent was reared and what lessons in childrearing were learned. How the two present parents put together their different backgrounds in childrearing is easier to understand when the background of each has been described. For instance, a German-Jew married to an English Protestant who live as a nuclear unit produce a very different set of mutual expectations than do two Catholic . . . Mexican-Americans living in an extended family. (p. 8)

Another point of inquiry related to the couple's families of origin involves the state of health and marriage of the mates' own parents. Are they still alive, well, married, living together, residing nearby, or geographically distant (Smoyak, 1975)? Satir (1983) also inquires into each parent's ordinal position among their siblings, quoting Toman's (1961) work on family constellation, which showed that siblings' ordinal position greatly influences the type of interactions and relationships one is likely to have with others, as well as one's personality development. For instance, Toman found that firstborn children were more apt to be leaders than followers, while the reverse was more common among last-born children.

One of the ways family nurses obtain a better idea of the progress of the family system over time, as well as the intergenerational family system, is to construct a genogram. The genogram is a type of genealogical table that traces the kinship history of families. It is widely used by family therapists and family nurses. The advantage to using family genograms is that one can organize a large, unwieldy amount of data in a way that makes it comprehensible and helps reveal important patterns and themes in families (Hartman & Laird, 1983; McGoldrick & Gerson, 1985). Chapter 8 contains both a genogram and instructions for completing this type of family tree.

FAMILY NURSING DIAGNOSIS

Nursing diagnosis can be formulated after a thorough assessment of the family's developmental history and a clear articulation of their current family developmental needs and concerns. The use of a North American Nursing Diagnosis Association (NANDA) nursing diagnosis related to development can, however, be misleading to the family nurse, in that the diagnoses identified in this classification system are directed toward the individual, not the family. With that caveat in mind, the following NANDA nursing diagnoses may be germane:

- Development, Risk for Altered
- Growth, Risk for Altered
- Growth and Development, Altered

Diagnosis selected for a family undergoing developmental challenges as a unit would need to reflect potential or real unmet family needs in relation to specific developmental tasks or actions needed to complete in order for the family to successfully transition from one developmental stage to another. Nursing diagnoses that may reflect some of these issues are included in Table 5–17.

FAMILY NURSING INTERVENTIONS

One important goal of family nursing is to help families and their members move toward completion of individual and family developmental tasks (Friedman, 1987). Mastery of one set of family developmental tasks allows the family to progress developmentally to the next stage of family development. Family devel-

TABLE 5-17

NURSING DIAGNOSES SPECIFIC TO DEVELOPMENTAL STAGES OF THE FAMILY LIFE CYCLE

STAGE I: BEGINNING FAMILIES

Decisional conflict related to choice of living arrangements, employment, and relationships

STAGE II: CHILDBEARING FAMILIES

Altered family processes related to marriage of adult children and establishment of new relationships through marriage, birth, and divorce

Altered parenting related to inability to promote optimum growth and development of the children

Risk for altered parent/infant/child attachment related to lack of parenting role models, parenting skills, or knowledge of child development issues

STAGE III: FAMILIES WITH PRESCHOOL CHILDREN

Ineffective, compromised (or disabling) family coping related to chronic or acute health care conditions of children

Family coping: Potential for growth related to health challenges of family members

Impaired home maintenance management related to lack of safe home environment

Altered parenting related to inability to promote optimum growth and development of the children

STAGE IV: FAMILIES WITH SCHOOLCHILDREN

Ineffective, compromised (or disabling) family coping related to chronic or acute health care conditions of children

Family coping: Potential for growth related to health challenges of family members

Impaired home maintenance management related to lack of safe home environment

Altered parenting related to inability to promote optimum growth and development of the children

STAGE V: FAMILIES WITH TEENAGERS

Impaired home maintenance management related to lack of supervision of adolescent children

Altered parenting related to inability to promote optimum growth and development of the children

STAGE VI: FAMILIES LAUNCHING YOUNG ADULTS

Risk for loneliness related to "empty nest" syndrome

Impaired social interaction related to family's inability to develop new relationships outside of family

STAGE VII: MIDDLE-AGED PARENTS

Impaired social interaction related to family's inability to develop new relationships outside of family

STAGE VIII: FAMILY IN RETIREMENT AND OLD AGE

Impaired adjustment related to changes in health status

Caregiver role strain related to ongoing care of ill family members or well grandchildren

Death anxiety related to potential death of life partner

Relocation stress syndrome related to move of elderly parent from own home to other living arrangements opmental tasks, if unfulfilled, produce dysfunctional families (Mattessich & Hill, 1987).

To accomplish this goal, the family nurse "assists families to achieve and maintain a balance between the personal growth needs of individual family members and optimum family functioning" (family developmental needs) (American Nurses Association, Division on Maternal and Child Health Nursing Practice, 1983). The balance between individual and group developmental needs is not easily achieved, particularly during certain stages, creating dissonance when an imbalance occurs.

When working with troubled families and individuals, family developmental theory helps family health professionals think about life cycle events that establish the context within which family and individual problems occur. Hence, it is important during both the diagnostic and planning phases that a developmental perspective is incorporated into family nursing practice.

It is also significant to incorporate a family developmental perspective into one's family nursing practice when working with healthy families. With healthy families, anticipatory guidance and teaching is often indicated in order to fulfill primary prevention goals (Bobak, Jensen, & Zalor, 1989). Family nursing diagnoses, plans, and interventions should cover potential problems families may encounter because of the need to transform family structures so that family developmental tasks be accomplished. Helping families anticipate and go through different normative transitions in family life is a most germane family nursing goal.

The family nurse and other family clinicians assist families by teaching and counseling modalities. Referral to social support groups, such as a group for parents of infants or older ill parents, is also very helpful. Chapter 7 discusses general family nursing interventions in detail.

❧SUMMARY

This chapter presents an overview of family developmental theory. The following are key points made in this chapter:

- The family developmental approach is based on the observation that families are long-lived groups with a natural history that must be assessed if the dynamics of the group are to be fully and accurately interpreted.

- The three basic assumptions of family developmental theory are:
  - Family behavior is the sum of the previous experiences of family members as incorporated in the present and in their expectations for the future.
  - Families develop and change over time in similar and consistent ways.
  - Families and their members perform certain time-specific tasks that are set by them and by the cultural and societal context.

- The theory has been criticized for its lack of adequate attention to family diversity, its middle-class bias, its assumption of stability within each stage, and its lack of explanation to describe the

processes that occur between stages that allow families to change.

- The family career or family cycle refers to the diverse paths (events and periods of time) that unfold during a family's life.

- Theorists have identified predictable developmental stages of the family. Duvall's eight-stage theory and Carter & McGoldrick's six-stage theory are most often cited in the literature.

- Rankin developed the Changing Life Cycle framework. This framework identifies the emerging family (one concerned with the tasks of becoming a family unit, the solidifying family (one whose primary tasks are to stabilize the bonds between the parents and socialize the children), the reconstituting family (one that occurs because of changes in the family such as death or divorce) and the contracting family (one in which children are being launched and parents are experiencing older age).

- Zilbach developed a family life cycle framework in which each stage is precipitated by a particular life event or family stage marker. These markers demand change and new adaptation.

- The Family Life Spiral is a developmental model that incorporates overlapping development tasks of each generation in the family.

- Family developmental tasks refer to growth responsibilities that must be achieved by a family during each stage of its development so as to meet its biological requirements, its cultural imperatives and its own aspirations and values.

- Developmental tasks associated with the Transitional Stage: Between Families are to differentiate self in relation to the family of origin, to develop intimate peer relationships and to establish self in relation to work and financial independence.

- Developmental tasks associated with Beginning Families are to establish a mutually satisfying marriage, to relate harmoniously to the kin network and to plan a family.

- Developmental tasks associated with Childbearing Families are to set up the young family as a stable unit, to reconcile conflicting developmental tasks and needs of family members, to maintain a mutually satisfying marital relationship, and to expand relationships with extended family.

- Developmental tasks associated with Families with Preschool Children are to meet basic family needs (housing, food, etc.), socialize the children, integrate new child members into the family, and maintain health relationships within the family.

- Developmental tasks associated with Families with School-Aged Children are to socialize the children, maintain a satisfying marital relationship, and meet physical health needs of family members.

- Developmental tasks associated with Families with Teenagers are to balance freedom with responsibility of teenagers as they mature, refocus the marital relationship, and communicate openly between parents and children.

- Developmental tasks associated with Families Launching Young Adults include expanding the family circle to accept new relationships acquired by marriage, continuing the renewing of the marital relationship, and assisting aging and ill parents of the husband and wife.

- Developmental tasks associated with Middle-Aged Parents are to provide a health-promoting environment, sustain satisfying relationships with aging parents and children, and to strengthen the marital relationship.

- Developmental tasks associated with Families in the Later Years are to maintain a satisfying living arrangement, adjust to a lower income, maintain the marital relationship, adjust to loss of a spouse, maintain intergenerational family ties, and continue to make sense out of one's existence.

- Variations in the family career have been identified for divorced and stepparent families as well as for those with domestic partner relationships. These frameworks account for critical changes in roles and relationships that differ from the two-parent nuclear family.

- Serious illness or long-term disability of a family member often impedes the family's ability to meet its family developmental tasks.

- A developmental assessment of the family should include:
  - The family's present developmental stage
  - The extent to which members are fulfilling the developmental tasks of that stage
  - The family history from inception through present day
  - A summary of the parents' families of origin

- During the family assessment, the nurse may identify potential problems that have occurred as a result of the changes in family relationships or function that family members have experienced as they transition through a specific stage in the family life cycle. Each family is unique, and while one stage in the family life cycle may require few adjustments in family adaptation, another stage may bring challenges with which the members do not feel prepared to cope at that time.

- Family nursing interventions should be aimed at assisting families to accomplish the developmental tasks associated with each stage in the family life cycle.

◆ FAMILY VIGNETTE: THE MAY FAMILY

Elizabeth May is participating in a support group for parents with teenagers. She and her husband, both in their early 50s, feel they are having a difficult time raising their third child Joshua, an active 16 year old. Joshua has two siblings—18-year-old Mary, who has just left for her first year of college, and 24-year-old Anthony, who will be married in six months. Elizabeth and her husband are feeling quite stressed by Anthony's wedding plans and the knowledge that he, a practicing Catholic, is marrying a Jewish woman. Anthony is living at home and has been even through his college years. Mary is the first child to leave the home, as she will be attending a college 100 miles away. Joshua has teamed with a group of friends who are known in the community for their rowdy behavior. Elizabeth is confused by his recent attachment to this group, as he has always been a compliant child and dedicated to his studies.

▬ STUDY QUESTIONS

Review the Family Vignette and answer the related questions.

1. Identify the developmental stage of this family and state your rationale.

2. State the developmental tasks this family must achieve during this stage and give your assessment of their current ability to meet these tasks.

3. Identify the role conflicts that may potentially exist in this case study.

4. List resources you would recommend to the family to assist them in meeting their current developmental tasks.

Answer the following questions.

5. Family developmental theory is built on some basic assumptions. What are these? (List at least two.)

6. Usually reliable predictions can be made regarding the common health concerns and forces that are at play within a family if the family nurse knows (select one answer):

   a. The developmental tasks of each member
   b. The family life cycle or family career stage
   c. Where the family lives and their social class
   d. The composition of the family

7. Which of the following illustrate(s) the value of the developmental approach when assessing and working with families? (Choose all correct responses.)

   a. Gives cues as to the families past problems and progress
   b. Forecasts a given family's future needs
   c. Views the common experiences of families during each of the family career stages
   d. Highlights critical periods of family and individual growth and development

    e. Helps to anticipate what to expect in terms of health concerns

    f. Better able to evaluate the family normatively

8. The best definition for the family life cycle or family career is:

    a. Predictable stages within the history of the family

    b. The growth and developmental stages of each family member as he or she progresses throughout life

    c. Successive stages and commonly experienced events of the family as a unit through its existence

9. Family developmental tasks have these characteristics (choose all correct answers):

    a. They change in response to cultural imperatives and the family's unique aspirations and values.

    b. They change in response to the developmental needs of their members.

    c. They remain constant throughout the family's existence.

    d. They adapt the family's broad functions to meet the specific tasks of each stage.

    e. They satisfy the biological requirements of the family as a whole.

    f. They avoid clashing with individual needs.

    g. They are growth requirements that must be achieved by the family during each life cycle or family career stage.

    h. Failure to achieve developmental tasks leads to difficulty in achieving later developmental tasks.

    i. Developmental tasks cover only aspects that directly influence psychosocial (interactional) components of family functioning.

10. The developmental approach seeks to explain family dynamics in terms of its:

    a. Unique elements

    b. Common elements in its history as a family

    c. Both common and unique elements of family history

11. The developmental tasks of the family result from a combination of (more than one answer):

    a. Individual developmental tasks of family members

    b. Sexual norms

    c. Chronological ages and school placement

    d. Community pressures for family to conform to societal norms

    e. General family functions adapted to specific life cycle stages

12. The stage of the family life cycles are defined by Duvall in terms of (select one answer):

    a. The age and school placement of the oldest child

    b. The ages of the parents

    c. The age of the middle child, if present

    d. Years of marriage

Complete the following outlines.

13. In the outline below, list the following:
   a. The eight phases in the family life cycle for the two-parent nuclear family (excluding the transition stage)
   b. A definition for each phase
   c. Three basic health concerns (biopsychosocial and health concerns) frequently present and appropriate for intervention by family nurse

Family Life Cycle Stage	Definition of Phase	Health Concerns or Needs
I.		1. 2. 3.
II.		1. 2. 3.
III.		1. 2. 3.

Family Life Cycle Stage	Definition of Phase	Health Concerns or Needs
IV.		1. 2. 3.
V.		1. 2. 3.
VI.		1. 2. 3.
VII.		1. 2. 3.
VIII.		1. 2. 3.

14. Within each of the eight life cycle stages of the family, identify the developmental tasks of parents as described by Friedman.

Life Cycle Stage	Developmental Task(s) of Parent
I.	1.
II.	1.
	2.
III.	1.
IV.	1.
V.	1.
	2.
VI.	1.
VII.	1.
VIII.	1.

Choose the correct answer(s) to the following question.

15. When does the marriage relationship, according to studies, appear to be the strongest and most satisfying?
    a. Stage of preschool children
    b. Stage of childbearing families
    c. Stage of marriage
    d. The postparental period (middle-aged parents)
    e. Stage of the contracting family (family in later years)
    f. Stage of families launching young adults

16. Give the three aspects of the adolescent process that explain the developmental tasks and problems faced in this stage.

17. What is the usual impact of adolescent family members on the family as a whole?

For each question from 17 through 25, select the lettered choice that applies to it. *

    a. Beginning families
    b. Childbearing families
    c. Families with preschool children
    d. Families with school-aged children
    e. Families with teenagers
    f. Families as launching centers
    g. Families in the middle years
    h. Families in the later years

---

* *These questions are adapted from Borlick M., et al. (1974). Nursing examination review book, vol. 9: Community health nursing (2nd ed.) Flushing, NY: Medical Examination Publishing Company.*

18. Beginning of loosening of family ties

19. Reaching maximum size in number of members and of interrelationships

20. Being totally responsible for the first time for another human being

21. Establishing a home base

22. Releasing members into lives of their own

23. Rediscovery of couple as husband and wife

24. Learning to supply adequate space, facilities, and equipment for a rapidly expanding family

25. Dealing with death of spouse

26. Which of the following descriptions apply to the single-parent or divorced family with respect to its development?
    a. The single-parent or divorced family passes through the same family life cycle stages.
    b. The characteristics of the family life cycle—after the divorce—differ because of the absence of a second parent in the family.
    c. The single-parent or divorced family skips one or two of the family life cycle stages, depending on when the divorce occurred.
    d. The timing of the family life cycle transitions will probably be delayed in the immediate postdivorce period.

27. In the stepparent family, remarriage creates initial crisis and destabilization. How does remarriage generally affect the family career stages?

28. What general areas (name three) would you assess to gather information about family development and the family's history?

SYSTEMS THEORY

LEARNING OBJECTIVES

1. Describe the characteristics of the paradigm associated with systems theory.
2. Define the following general systems theory terms: systems, social systems, open versus closed systems, differentiation, wholeness or nonsummativity, and feedback.
3. Relative to the family system, explain either narratively or diagrammatically the family system's relationship to its internal and external environment (the hierarchy of systems).
4. Using systems concepts, name four characteristics of a successfully functioning, healthy family.
5. Examine the impact of stress on the family system.
6. State the limitations in the use and application of systems approaches to the family.

Three grand theories—developmental theory, structural–functional theory, and general systems theory—are used in this text to formulate the family assessment areas and questions. These theories also suggest family strengths and problems upon which goals and implementation strategies can be formulated. Structural–functional and systems theory are not mutually exclusive perspectives. Structural–functionalism can be considered the earliest form of systems theory (Broderick, 1993).

Of the three above-mentioned theories, systems theory is clearly the most inclusive and powerful, as is so convincingly demonstrated by the wide number of fields and substantive areas (including nursing) that have adapted this perspective as the foundation for their organizing framework (Cox & Paley, 1997; Hawley & Geske, 2000). General systems theory has received wide usage in such diverse areas as educational systems, game theory, computer science, systems engineering, computer information systems, and communication fields. Growth in the use of systems theory in the health care fields has been especially impressive within the last 35 years, as evidenced by the proliferation of books and clinical investigations using this approach to study individuals, the family, nursing and other health care professionals, the health care delivery system, and the community.

Contemporary systems theories about families are derived from general systems theory (Whitchurch & Constantine, 1993). Systems theory forms the conceptual basis for "thinking systems" or for working with family systems as "the client" rather than just focusing on an individual person. Systems theory has probably stimulated most of the efforts made to achieve a systematic understanding of the normal and troubled family. As Broderick (1990), a leading family theorist, asserts, systems theory "is one of the most influential and generative of all of the family frameworks" (p. 172).

✎ GENERAL SYSTEMS THEORY: PARADIGM AND ASSOCIATED THEORIES

Von Bertalanffy (1950), an Austrian biologist, is credited with first delineating general systems theory in biology and physics, although sociologists and social anthropologists prior to and concurrent with von Bertalanffy's early publications were also describing systems—social systems (Parsons, 1951). In general systems theory, certain universal principles were applied to all kinds of groups of phenomena (e.g., amoebas, computer programs, families), which von Bertalanffy termed *systems*. Thus, systems theory can be applied across disciplines whereby universal laws are useful in working with various types of complex,

organized systems (Lee & Lancaster, 1988; Whitchurch & Constantine, 1993).

In looking at human behavior, be it of an individual, a family, or a whole community, general systems theory serves as a valuable "umbrella" under which various, more middle-range theoretical perspectives may be subsumed (such as the ecological perspective, family communication theory, cybernetics or information processing theory, and adaptation theory). Systems theory constitutes a way of explaining a unit such as the family as it relates to and interacts with other systems. It is an organizational theory that is concerned with studying and describing the way things interrelate together rather than with analyzing the things themselves (Braden, 1984). It explains how each discrete variable affects the whole and how the whole affects each part.

As part of a "systems" revolution (Hartman & Laird, 1983), we have witnessed a shift in thinking from mechanistic, outcome-oriented theories to holistic, process-oriented theories. General systems theory has allowed health care professionals to utilize this shift in their field as well. Systems theories provide us with the concepts and framework to think in terms of facts and events in the context of wholes, rather than in a vacuum: "Looking at the world in terms of sets of integrated relations constitutes the systems view" (Lazlo, 1972, p. 19, as cited in Hartman & Laird, 1983, p. 59). Using a systems framework—namely, the organization of knowledge concerning the specific phenomena of interest as a complex system—one focuses on the interaction among the various parts of the system rather than on the function of the parts themselves (Buckley, 1967; von Bertalanffy, 1966).

HOLISTIC PARADIGM

Some theorists consider general systems theory to be broader than just a theory, instead considering it to be a unique worldview in which "systems thinking" is a way of looking at the world in terms of how objects are interrelated with one another (Whitchurch & Constantine, 1993). Before general systems theory, the tendency was toward reduction and parts analysis (Young, 1982). Those in the holistic health movement labeled that way of looking at things as "the mechanistic paradigm."

The mechanistic paradigm, in seeking to analyze and explain phenomena, reduces them to their parts—in many cases to their smallest parts—to find cause-and-effect relationships. Medical science and most of the sciences tend to operate within this linear (straight-line cause-and-effect or "A leads to B"), atomistic, reductionistic, and highly analytic paradigm. For example, using the mechanistic paradigm and linear thinking, infections in humans are explained in terms of bacterial invasions of certain cells and organs.

In contrast to this traditional paradigm, the systems paradigm is holistic; it looks at whole systems such as individuals or families, with regard to their interconnectedness rather than separateness. The systems paradigm posits the concept of circular causality. For instance, from a systems perspective, infections in humans would be conceptualized as an imbalance in man's interaction with his environment—where factors in the host (the person) influence the infectious agent and the infectious agent likewise affects the host. Using a holistic approach then, a system must be understood as a whole and cannot be comprehended by examining its individual parts and interactions in isolation from each other (Whitchurch & Constantine, 1993, p. 328).

It was Bateson (1972, 1979), a cultural anthropologist who is considered to be the father of the family therapy movement, who stressed this new epistemology regarding how one should go about gaining knowledge and making conclusions about the world. He pointed out the limits of linear thinking with respect to living systems. He proposed that a shift in thinking was needed to look at ongoing processes, interrelationships, and circular causality in order to understand human behavior. For instance, applying the systems paradigm to the family, he asserted that there is no true victim and prosecutor in a troubled family. A particular entity (in this case, a family member) is examined in relation to the things he or she affects and is affected by rather than in relation to his or her individual characteristics. Since both the "victim" and "prosecutor" in a family are serially and simultaneously affecting each other's roles and responses, only circular causality can adequately begin to explain the complex dynamics of a situation such as family violence (Figure 6–1).

In the 1950s and 1960s, Parsons's (1951) social systems theory was used in the fields of sociology, social work, and nursing (Johnson's nursing theory grew out of Parsons's work) to explain personal and group behavior. Moreover, general systems theory, à la von Bertalanffy (1966), began to filter into nursing theorists' thinking and into the literature (Rogers's and Roy's nursing models and the family therapy systems models are examples of this influence). Today, the systems theoretical perspective and paradigm is widely accepted and is utilized in nursing education, particularly in family nursing (Richards & Lansberry, 1995).

A broad array of other health-related disciplines have found the general systems theory's perspective useful. In medicine, the general systems theory sparked the development of family medicine; in psychology, family psychology, and social work, the theory generated the ecological perspective. This latter perspective, derived from general systems theory, focuses primarily on the adaptive balance that exists between living systems and their environments (Hartman & Laird, 1983).

Figure 6–1. Comparison between linear and circular causality in a troubled family.

ASSOCIATED THEORIES: CYBERNETICS AND COMMUNICATION THEORY

Two other systems-derived theories, again more middle range in scope, have also revolutionized family-centered practice. These are the theories of cybernetics and family communication processes.

Cybernetics is a science that deals with communication and control theory. Cybernetics focuses on information processing and how feedback mechanisms operate in controlling both simple and complex systems (Goldenberg & Goldenberg, 2000). Cybernetics explains how systems maintain their stability through self-correcting feedback mechanisms. Systems can be self-correcting by reinserting the results of past performance into current functioning (Goldenberg & Goldenberg, 2000). With this focus, a way to change future performance may be generated by modifying feedback information (a strategy used in family counseling). Both parts and wholes are examined in cybernetics relative to their patterns of organization (Keeney, 1982; Weiner, 1948).

Cybernetics and general systems theory provided the legacy for family communication theories (Bateson, 1979; Jackson, 1969; Satir, 1983; Watzlawick, Beavin, & Jackson, 1967), the theoretical foundations that modern-day family therapists rely on most heavily both in terms of assessment and of intervention.

THE RELATIONSHIP BETWEEN THE STRUCTURAL–FUNCTIONAL AND SYSTEMS THEORIES

With regard to the family, apparent similarities between structural–functional and systems theory include the notion that the family (the focal system) interacts with its inner and outer environments and must be examined in context. Systems theory characterizes the family and other systems as containing a structure and functions. In structural–functionalism, however, these two concepts represent the central

TABLE 6–1

KEY CHARACTERISTICS OF SYSTEMS THEORY AND THE FAMILY

- Family systems do not exist in a vacuum—the context in which systems function is critical.
- All parts of the family system are interconnected or inter-related.
- The whole is greater than the sum of its parts (nonsummativity).
- Understanding is only possible by viewing the whole family.
- Whatever affects the system as a whole family affects each of its parts (the ripple effect).
- Causes and effects are interchangeable (circular causality notion).
- Family systems are self-reflexive and goal seeking.

thrust of the theory, certainly a much more important emphasis than found in systems theory. Both theories discuss adaptation, with structural–functionalism stressing the tendency toward equilibrium, while systems theory stresses the balance between equilibrium (stability) and change in its analysis.

Systems theory, as noted earlier, is derived from a holistic paradigm, where circular causation and feedback loops are essential elements. Structural–functionalism, counter to some of its assumptions, tends to resort to more "part analysis," linear notions of causation, and a more static view of the family.

Much foundational family theory has been generated within a structural–functional frame, and structural–functional theory, technically speaking, is the earliest form of systems theory (Broderick, 1993). Both theories converge and diverge at certain points, and both are useful in identifying and describing important content areas, explaining family behavior, and providing guidelines for family nursing practice.

CENTRAL CONCEPTS AND PROPOSITIONS OF GENERAL SYSTEMS THEORY

An overview of the following systems concepts and propositions were eclectically derived. Three main sources were used: general systems theory, Parsons's (1951) social systems theory, and family systems theory from the family therapy field. Table 6–1 summaries the main characteristics of systems theory. Only the basic concepts used in a systems analysis of the family are presented in the following discussion. Because these concepts are only briefly explained and systems theory is rather abstract, additional sources on this theory may be useful. The references in this chapter are suggested as supplementary reading to the discussion presented here.

SYSTEM

A system is defined as a goal-directed unit made up of interdependent, interacting parts that endure over a period of time. This system, together with its environment, makes up a "universe," that is, the totality of what should be studied in a given situation. Systems and their parts have both functional and structural components. Structure pertains to the arrangement and organization among the parts of the system, whereas function refers to the purposes or goals of the system, such as activities necessary to assure the survival, continuity, and growth of the system. Function in systems analysis also is defined as the result or outcome of the structure.

HOLISM OR NONSUMMATIVITY

Whitchurch and Constantine (1993) state that "no assumption is more fundamental to modern general systems theory than that of holism" (p. 328). Thus, a system is characterized by its property of wholeness (or *nonsummativity*). "The whole is greater than the sum of its parts" is a fundamental gestalt concept first asserted by Aristotle and subsequently embraced by systems theorists (Broderick, 1993). A system cannot be understood by examining its individual parts in isolation from each other. "Understanding only is possible by viewing the whole" (Klein & White, 1996, p. 156).

INTERCONNECTEDNESS

A vital characteristic of a system is the interconnectedness or interrelatedness of its parts (Klein & White, 1996). This foundational assumption of general systems theory is a basic epistemological statement asserting that systems theory does not believe in isolating behaviors from the environment in which they occur.

SOCIAL SYSTEM

A social system is a model of social organization; it is a living system possessing a total unit distinctive from its component parts and distinguishable from its environment by a clearly defined boundary. Parsons and Bales (1955) define a social system as composed of two or more persons or social roles tied together by mutual interaction and interdependence (Anderson & Carter, 1974).

OPEN SYSTEM

Systems are characterized on the basis of their degree of interaction with the surrounding environment. An open system exists in an environment with which it interacts—from which it derives its inputs and to which it gives its outputs. This environmental interaction is necessary for its survival (Buckley, 1967). By definition, all living systems are open systems.

CLOSED SYSTEM

Theoretically, a closed system, in contrast to the open system, does not interact with the environment. A closed system would then be a self-contained unit, not dependent on continual environmental interchange for its survival. Because no totally closed system has yet been demonstrated in reality, "closed" denotes a relative lack of energy exchange across a system's boundaries (Parsons & Bales, 1955).

HIERARCHY OF SYSTEMS

No system functions in a vacuum. The system's universe, therefore, needs to be examined to determine its effect on the system under study. The universe—the system and its environment—contains a hierarchy of systems. Each higher-level unit contains lower-level systems. For instance, a hierarchy of systems from higher to lower levels might be as follows: community → family and other interacting systems → parental and other subsystems → individual organism → organ systems → tissues → cells.

When using system theory as a working framework, one must be clear and specific about what system is being assessed. The system under study at a particular time is called the *target* or *focal system*. After specifying the target system as, for example, the family, one would assess that system and then its relationship to the interacting systems within its environment, and finally its relationship to suprasystems and subsystems.

In the case of the family focus, one would thus want to study the family and both its interacting, internal, and external environments. The *suprasystems* are larger environmental systems of which the focal or target system is a part. The *subsystems* are smaller subunits or subcomponents of the focal system. For example, if the family is the focal system, then one suprasystem would be the family's cultural reference group and the relational subsystems would consist of the sets of family relationships, such as the spousal, sibling, and parent–child subsystems (Figure 6–2).

BOUNDARIES

Each system has a boundary that defines the system and demarcates it from its environment. The boundary represents the interface or point of contact between the system and other systems; that is, between the system and its subsystems and suprasystems (Whitchurch & Constantine, 1993). Auger (1976) explains that

> A boundary may be defined as a more or less open line forming a circle around the system where there is greater interchange of energy within the circle than on the outside. It is helpful to visualize a boundary as a "filter" which permits the constant exchange of elements, information, or energy between the system and its environment. (p. 24)

The more porous or permeable the filter or boundary, the greater the degree of interaction is possible between the system and its environment. In contrast, the less porous or permeable the boundary, the more isolated the system is from its environment. The ability of a boundary to control the degree of exchange is of great significance because it regulates the amount and type of input from the environment at any time, enabling the system to maintain equilibrium or to adapt to new demands.

INPUT

As mentioned above, all open systems must receive input from their environment in order to survive. Input refers to such things as energy, matter, and information that the system receives and processes. When input is received in a system, it must be processed *(input processing)*. This can be done either by accepting or rejecting the incoming input without change (also called *assimilation*) or by transforming or accommodating, whereby the system modifies the input or alters its structure in response to incoming information. Systems have rules of transformation. For example, a rule of transformation for a marital subsystem might be the quid pro quo rule; that is, if one spouse behaves badly towards the other, the affected spouse reacts in the same manner (Klein & White, 1996). Whether unaltered or transformed, the processed input flows through the system and is released as output. It is by this process that adaptation occurs, whereby a social, open system adjusts to demands (inputs) from its outer and inner environments.

OUTPUT

The results of the system's processing of the input constitute the output. Output in the form of energy, matter, or information is released into the environment.

FEEDBACK

Feedback refers to the process by which a system monitors the internal and environmental responses

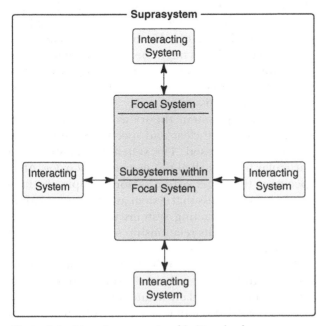

Figure 6–2. Schematic representation of the hierarchy of systems.

to its behavior (output) and accommodates or adjusts itself accordingly (Weiner, 1948). Feedback involves receiving and responding to the return of its own output. Information about how a system is functioning is looped back (feedback) from the output to the input, thus altering subsequent input (Goldenberg & Goldenberg, 2000). The system adjusts both internally, by modification of its subsystems, and externally, by controlling its boundaries. Thus, it is able to control and modify both input and output.

Feedback can be either negative or positive. Positive feedback refers to the system's output that is returned to the system as information that moves the system away from equilibrium and toward change. It involves amplifying feedback loops. Conversely, negative feedback is informational output that is returned to the system, promoting equilibrium and stability of the system (Casey, 1989). The use of attenuating feedback loops maintain aspects of the system's functioning within prescribed limits (Goldenberg & Goldenberg, 2000). Figure 6–3 diagrammatically describes these last four concepts.

SELF-REGULATION, HOMEOSTASIS, STEADY STATE, AND EQUILIBRIUM

All of these terms are used interchangeably in the literature, although there are fine distinctions between the terms. Here, only two distinctions will be pointed out. System self-regulation is a mechanism within a system that assists the system to balance and control input and output via feedback loops. When the system is in balance, the result is homeostasis, a steady state, or equi-

librium. This balance is not static, however, but is dynamic and is always changing within certain degrees of variation. Adaptation occurs through system self-regulatory mechanisms. The outcome of this regulation and adaptation is equilibrium, a steady state, or homeostasis (Hazzard, 1971; Klein & White, 1996).

Fishman (1985) asserts that when family members develop symptoms, these symptoms may serve to maintain family homeostasis. For instance, if a child in a family "acts out" (consistently or over some time period), the focus of attention may shift from solving the conflicts in the marital relationship to managing the rebellious child. With a focus on the child who is acting out, the couple may decrease their fighting—a situation the child prefers.

DIFFERENTIATION

General systems theory states that the growth and change toward a higher order of organization occur through differentiation. This concept, then, denotes a living system's capability and propensity to progressively and serially advance to a higher order of complexity and organization (referred to also as negentropy). A social system, if acting normally, has a tendency to "grow" (called morphogenesis). The propensity to grow or to change is counterbalanced by the tendency of a system to stabilize (return to a state of equilibrium or homeostasis). A balance between stability (called morphostasis) and change is needed for a system to grow or to differentiate. Figure 6–4 illustrates the tendency for a system to experience periods of both change and stability. Energy input flowing into the system is utilized by the system in order to grow in complexity and organization (Bowen, 1960).

ENERGY

"All dynamic, open systems require continuous supplies of energy in sufficient quantity so that demands for system integrity can be met" (Auger, 1976). The most important factor governing the amount of energy needed is the rate of utilization of energy within the system itself. Systems with high levels of activity utilize large quantities of energy, and therefore must receive greater amounts of input from the

Figure 6–3. Energy, matter, and information exchange and processing model. *(Adapted from Hazzard, 1971).*

Figure 6–4. A system's tendency toward stability and change.

environment in order to meet their energy demands. This, in turn, implies that the system's boundaries would have to be more open, or porous, to allow a greater input of energy.

FAMILY SYSTEMS: DEFINITION AND CONCEPTS

The basic general systems concepts and propositions will now be applied to the system that is the focus of the text: the family. The following family systems definitions have come primarily from family process or systems theorists who have applied general systems theory, as well as cybernetics and communication theory, to analysis of the family system.

FAMILY

The family is defined as a living social system that typically extends over at least three generations (Goldenberg & Goldenberg, 2000). It is a unique, small group of closely interrelated and interdependent individuals who are organized into a single unit in order to attain family functions or goals.

[It] has evolved a set of rules, is replete with assigned and ascribed roles for its members, has an organized power structure, has developed intricate overt and covert forms of communication, and has elaborated ways of negotiating and problem solving that permits various tasks to be performed effectively. The relationship between members of this micro culture is deep and multilayered, and is based largely on a shared history, shared internalized perceptions and assumptions about the world, and a shared sense of purpose. Within such a system, individuals are tied to one another by powerful, durable, reciprocal emotional attachments and loyalties that may fluctuate in intensity over time but nevertheless persist over the lifetime of the family. (Goldenberg & Goldenberg, 2000)

RECIPROCAL DETERMINISM OR THE RIPPLE EFFECT

The interrelationships found in a family system are so intricately tied together that a change in any one part inevitably results in changes in the entire system. This reverberating effect is referred to as *reciprocal determinism* by Goldenberg & Goldenberg (2000), or as a *ripple effect* by Boss (1988) and by other family theorists. Each family member and subsystem is affected by transitional and situational stressors that initially impact one or more family members—with the effects on each family member varying in intensity and quality. For example, family health professionals have observed a powerful collective family impact when there is a sick or disabled child in the family. Boss (1988) explains that

> There is a ripple effect when a parent over focuses on that child in the subsequent reaction of a sibling (or mate) who feels left out. The family member who feels neglected begins to distance him or herself or to act out for attention. A sibling may run away; a mate may indulge in self-destructive behavior or have an affair. (p. 16)

Forces in the family move in a *circular* fashion, that is, in many directions simultaneously, not in a linear cause-and-effect manner. An example of circular causality is the situation in which parents ask their children who are fighting with each other, "Who started this fight?" They usually get the same answer from both children, "He/she did!" Both children are right and wrong. From each child's perspective, the other started it, because it all depends on where in the communication loop the investigation begins— each child starting at the point where he or she felt the other one instituted the fight. Circular causality, the language used in systems thinking, suggests that any search for a "real or ultimate" cause of any interpersonal event is impossible and pointless.

NONSUMMATIVITY (WHOLENESS OR HOLISM)

An essential property of the family as an open system is nonsummativity (wholeness), which was defined earlier in the context of systems theory. Here it means that the family cannot be considered as merely the sum of its parts. The family viewed as a whole is greater than the sum of its parts. In other words, a family is something more than parent(s) plus child(ren). The assessment of the family unit cannot be based on knowledge about each of the family members or sets of relationships (Wright & Leahey, 1994). "Family systems have emergent properties," state Hartman and Laird (1983, p. 62). By this they mean that the interrelatedness of components in the family system gives rise to new qualities and characteristics that are a function of that interrelatedness.

SELF-REFLEXIVITY AND GOAL SEEKING

Family systems are self-reflexive and goal-seeking systems. All cybernetic systems (i.e., systems with feedback) are self-monitoring, although in nonhuman systems this does not require self-awareness. Human systems, including families, are self-reflexive, meaning that they possess the ability and tendency to make themselves and their own behavior the focus of examination and the target of explanation (Whitchurch & Constantine, 1993). Because families are self-reflexive, they examine their own systems and then set goals for themselves (Broderick, 1993). Communication allows for self-reflexivity because it facilitates persons' creation of meaning and their sending and receiving symbolic messages (Whitchurch & Constantine, 1993).

HIERARCHY OF SYSTEMS: FAMILY AS FOCAL SYSTEM

Hierarchy of systems means then that systems exist at multiple levels. The family is viewed as a hierarchical organized system that is comprised of smaller subsystems (e.g., spouse, parent, and sibling), but is also embedded within other larger systems or suprasystems (Cox & Paley, 1997). Figure 6–5 illustrates the relationship of the family to its subsystems, its interacting systems, such as the welfare and educational system, and its suprasystems, e.g., the family's reference group(s), the community, and wider society.

Relative to the family system's environment, generally speaking, the more immediate the environment is, the greater the influence on the system and the greater the input it has on the family. Conversely, more distant environments generally have less influence on the family. Thus, systems with which the family continually interacts, such as the school system, generally have a more potent impact on the family than a remote suprasystem does.

OPEN, CLOSED, AND RANDOM FAMILY SYSTEMS

All families are, strictly speaking, open systems because they must exchange materials, energy, and information with their environment in order to survive. Families are in constant interaction with their physical, social, and cultural environment.

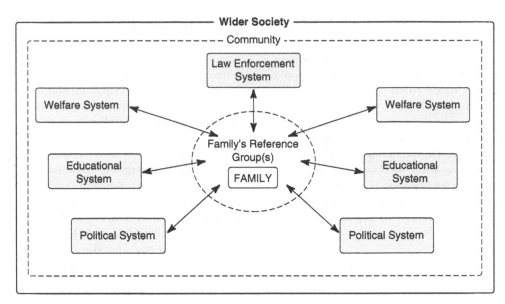

Figure 6-5. Schematic illustration of the family and its external environment.

From a clinical perspective, it is possible, however, to identify degrees of openness, closedness, and/or randomness in a family and thus to evaluate a family's ability to change and to maintain stability. Kantor and Lehr (1975), in an in-depth qualitative study of families, described three types of families: *open, closed,* and *random families.* In *open families* the exchange of information, friends, and activities is extensive. Open families welcome new ideas, information, techniques, opportunities, and resources. Moreover, open families take the initiative by actively seeking out new resources and by using these resources to solve their problems. Creative and flexible solutions to problems are sought and are utilized in response to changing and unique needs (Satir, 1972).

Open families are those that perceive change as normal and desirable and view people as inherently good and helpful and thus to be sought and needed. Open families reach out to the larger community and interact extensively with it. Family boundaries of the open family are much more permeable than in the closed family.

In contrast, *closed families* view change as threatening and are resistant to it. Strangers are perceived as being potentially harmful or at least not to be trusted. Closed families believe that a person's negative qualities are a basic fact of life and that people must therefore be under strict control; thus, relationships have

to be regulated by force. Within the family there is extensive social control. These types of families are rigid; as a result, things and events in the closed family remain as constant and predictable as possible. Stability and tradition are core purposes of closed families. Kantor and Lehr (1975) describe the situation existing in the closed family:

> Locked doors, careful scrutiny of strangers in the neighborhood, parental control over the media, supervised excursions, and unlisted telephones are all features of a closed-type family. Closed bounding (boundary) goals include the preservation of territoriality, self-protection, privacy, and, in some families, secretiveness. Perimeter traffic control is never relinquished to outsiders or even to anyone within the family not specifically assigned bounding responsibilities. (p. 120)

The third type of family described by Kantor and Lehr is the *random family.* It is easy to think of this type of family as being the polar opposite of the closed family in terms of family social control and rigidity to change. Whereas time, activities, and family routines are closely regulated and controlled in the closed family, just the reverse is true in the random type family. Individual family members establish their own boundaries, values, activities, routines, and schedules.

Traffic in and out of the family is loosely regulated even when strangers are involved. These are high-energy families that value spontaneity, free choice, very fluid norms, and challenge (Mercer, 1989). Here the core purpose of the family is exploration through use of members' sense of intuition (Kantor & Lehr, 1975). In the extreme, this type of family is chaotic and prone to dissolution.

FAMILY BOUNDARIES

Probably the most crucial means families have of facilitating adaptation to outside demands and internal needs is through their effective use of their semipermeable family boundaries. The function of metaphoric boundaries is to actively expand (or open) and retract (or close) according to need, thus regulating the amount of input from the environment and output to the environment (Reinhardt & Quinn, 1973). In other words, the key to successful family adaptation is selective permeability of family boundaries. In healthy family functioning, input is screened so that a family takes in what is needed from the environment and assimilates or modifies it to promote its own survival and growth.

When families have boundaries that are too rigid and impermeable, important resources are not forthcoming. These families are deprived of the necessary information and support, as well as, perhaps, the physical resources necessary for family wellness. Family boundary maintenance in information processing determines the openness of the system relative to exchanging information with the external environment. The amount of information a family can handle adequately is limited, and an excess of information or conflicting information from the outer environment amplifies and creates family disequilibrium. Conversely, too little information can also threaten family stability. In the healthy family, boundaries adequately screen information input and output. When an excessive amount of information flows into the family, the boundaries close, and when an underflow of information occurs, boundaries open (Reinhardt & Quinn, 1973).

The family with an underflow of information from the environment relies more heavily on inner familial resources. Relatively closed families may discharge more energy than is constructive, with eventual disorganization the result.

The abused child is frequently found in families that are isolated and have closed boundaries with society. In healthier isolated families, the members tend to believe that all or most of the needs of the members can be met either by the family itself or by its reference group. Family self-sufficiency may be overemphasized, however, causing family members to view wider society in a distorted or negative way. The children of such families often experience great strain when they are required to interact with the wider society.

On the other hand, families that are indiscriminately open to information tend to become disorganized and chaotic. In this case, ineffective boundary regulation allows information to flow constantly into the family system, with resultant distortion and high levels of anxiety manifested among family members. Children and adults of these families are often forced into the extra familial environment of neighbors, community organizations, and state agencies in order to get their needs met. In these cases, relationships within and outside of the family are generally shallow, nonrewarding, and frustrating to family members.

FAMILY ADAPTATION

Family adaptation refers to the capacity of the family and its members to modify their behavior to each other and to their outer world as the situation demands. In response to internal or external input, the family adapts by either accepting or rejecting incoming information, energy, or services, or by modifying input to meet its needs.

In an open system, the family balances input from the external and internal environments by the feedback process. Balanced adequately, this is called family homeostasis, steady state, or equilibrium. Homeostasis or its synonyms (steady state and equilibrium) should not imply stagnation, however, but should be seen as the degree of balance needed while continual change and growth are taking place. Healthy families are flexible, more spontaneous, open to growth and change, responsive to new stimulation, and not status quo oriented (Beavers & Hampson, 1993; Cox & Paley, 1997).

Because families must change in order to meet both internal and external demands, a sufficient range of behaviors and patterns, plus the flexibility to mobilize these when needed, is essential. Nevertheless, the family system has a tendency to offer resistance to change beyond a certain range and to maintain preferred patterns as long as it possibly can. The family's threshold of tolerance for change stimulates self-regulatory mechanisms that reestablish the accustomed range even though there may be feasible alternatives available. An example of this phenomenon is one when a family member begins to distance him- or herself from the family, it is common for other family members to feel the distancing member is not doing his or her part. Guilt-producing techniques may then be used to return the family member to his or her usual family roles.

A steady state is achieved internally by balancing family members' roles. Family members help to maintain this internal balance either covertly or overtly. The family's repetitious, circular, and predictable communication patterns will reveal this balancing act.

FAMILY SUBSYSTEMS

The family is a system of interacting personalities intricately organized into positions, roles, and norms, which are further organized into subsystems within the family. These subsystems become the basis for the family structure or organization. The family system differentiates and carries out its functions through personal and interpersonal or relational subsystems (Kantor & Lehr, 1975). *Interpersonal subsystems* are made up of sets of relationships involving two or more family members. Each individual within the family is also a personal subsystem—the smallest of the subsystems in the family. Family subsystems, however, primarily refer to the interpersonal subsystems discussed here. Family members belong to different interpersonal subsystems, where they have different levels of power and learn differentiated roles. An adult female, for example, can be a daughter, wife, or older sister. Each of these roles involves different complementary relationships and the use of a different cluster of behaviors (Minuchin, 1974).

A family contains at least one it *control subsystem* that sets the rules for processing input, and compares output with family goals (a cybernetic description). In a two-parent nuclear family, the primary control subsystem is the spouse subsystem.

The two-parent nuclear family has at least three interpersonal subsystems, each of which serves some unique function in addition to common objectives. (see Table 6–2).

Minuchin (1974), a family therapist and the author of several important books in his field, has worked extensively with families using a systems-based approach in family counseling. He stresses the need to work with and through the several subsystems of the family to effect positive change within the whole family. His approach is to assist in the strengthening of the subsystems so that they function in an effective manner and do not lose their identity or unique contribution to the whole.

Minuchin suggests that in the same way that the family system has a boundary, so does each subsystem, the purpose of which is to protect the differentiation

TABLE 6–2

FAMILY SUBSYSTEMS BASED ON SETS OF RELATIONSHIPS IN THE NUCLEAR, TWO-PARENT FAMILY

1. *The Spouse Subsystem:* Here two adult members relate to each other as (a) marital partners and (b) parents of their offspring.
2. *The Parent–Child Subsystem:* This subsystem is composed of the parents and their children. The subsystem has parenting functions (socialization) involving the mother–father roles and the children's roles.
3. *The Sibling Subsystem:* This subsystem is composed of the children and is characterized by the children's relationships with each other.
4. *Other Subsystems:* There may also exist, for example, a grandparent–grandchild subsystem or uncle–nephew subsystems in an extended family.

of the system; that is, it is through the growth and evolution of subsystems that the whole family differentiates. Each subsystem has specific functions, which in turn lead to special demands on its members. Thus in the spouse system, the parent is given the child-rearing function. Clear and intact boundaries are required to deter any interference by other subsystems. For example, the spouse subsystem often becomes usurped by the parent–child subsystem because of the overwhelming demands on the adult members (parents) of the parenting role. In another case, the parent–child subsystem cannot function effectively if siblings interfere in the parent–child relationship and compromise the parents' capacity to parent one of their offspring. Minuchin refers to this blurring of subsystem boundaries as "diffuse" boundaries.

A brief explanation of each of the three subsystems will help illuminate their critical functions.

THE SPOUSE SUBSYSTEM.   The traditional spouse subsystem is formed when two adults of the opposite sex agree to join together for the primary purposes of mutual support and the meeting of each other's affectional and sexual needs. The couple needs to mutually accommodate and complement each other. The spouse subsystem is vital to the couple, because it acts as a refuge from external stresses and constitutes an avenue for contacting other social systems. It is also the most important subsystem of the family (Goldenberg & Goldenberg, 2000). Utilizing the systems framework, the spouse subsystem boundary needs to be intact and protected from the demands and needs of other systems. Children especially have a tendency to intrude on the spouse subsystem, creating a situation wherein husband and wife have a relationship based not on their own personal relationship with each other but on their parenting functions (Minuchin, 1974).

THE PARENT–CHILD SUBSYSTEM.   With the birth or adoption of a child by the couple, the original dyadic family grows in complexity as the new subsystem is created. The spouse subsystem now must differentiate itself to perform both mutual support (marital roles) and child-rearing (parental) functions. The parent–child subsystem involves parents and their relationship with each of their children (Minuchin, 1974).

THE SIBLING SUBSYSTEM.   With the advent of additional children, the sibling subsystem comes into being. As only children will attest, having a sister or brother is important. These relationships serve as the first social skills laboratory for children. Here they learn to relate in the peer world. They learn to support, become angry, express feelings, negotiate, cooperate, and imitate each other. In relating to their siblings, children learn to play different roles, which then serve them when they go out into the extrafamilial world. Within these relationships there is an openness and honesty unmatched in outer society; that is, the child obtains constant feedback from siblings concerning his or her behavior.

The significance of the sibling subsystem is underscored by frequent observations made by only children. Only children accommodate in the adult world rather than their peer world, often exhibiting precocious development because of extensive parental exposure. Concurrently, they may have difficulty sharing, cooperating, and competing with children of their own age, and are usually more dependent in their behavior (Minuchin, 1974; Toman, 1961).

DIFFERENTIATION

Differentiation refers to the family's propensity to evolve and grow so that as growth takes place the system becomes more complex, articulate, and discriminate. Developmental studies—studies of families throughout their life cycle—have demonstrated this tendency. Families are dynamic systems that are continually differentiating themselves both functionally and structurally. Because of the family's evolution and growth, there is also a concomitant need for increased numbers of specialized roles. This specialization and increased complexity are direct outcomes of differentiation (Minuchin, 1974).

🐾 A SYSTEMS THEORY PERSPECTIVE ON HEALTHY FAMILIES

In concluding an exploration of the basic concepts and definition of systems theory and how these are applied and illustrated within the family system, it is fitting to draw a "composite picture" of the healthy family. According to systems theory, the healthy family is a maximally viable system characterized by complexity of structure; highly flexible organization capable and tolerant of internal changes; highly autonomous subsystems and considerable internal determination; and openness with the outer environment that results in a continual flow of a wide variety of information, experience, and input into the family (Beavers & Hampson, 1993; Lewis, Beavers, Gossett, & Phillips, 1976). Constantine (1986) adds that healthy family systems succeed at balancing family system needs simultaneously with individual family members' needs. In a well-functioning family, all the family subsystems operate in an integrated way to maintain the differentiation and integrity of the family system (Goldenberg & Goldenberg, 2000).

IMPACT OF STRESS AND CRISES ON THE FAMILY SYSTEM

As with individuals, the presence of stress in a family initially aids the family to mobilize its resources and to work at solving its problems. Stress causes family homeostasis or its steady state to become precarious, in which case family members initially exert considerable effort to regain its balance. However, when initial attempts to resolve problems or to meet demands fail, stress increases. Often, a stressor originally affects one individual, followed by one and then the other subsystems—until finally all family subsystems are involved (the ripple effect). For instance, problems in the spouse subsystem can be localized for a while. Then, as they continue and intensify, other subsystems, especially the parent–child subsystem, becomes affected. Although stress is experienced by all the subsystems, each subsystem may tolerate and handle the stress differently, as discussed under the ripple effect earlier.

In time, if no solution is found to reduce the stress, the system eventually reaches its limits to respond adaptively, reaching a point of exhaustion. When important familial resources are depleted, family functioning deteriorates, and symptoms of family disorganization set in, such as overt symptoms of an individual family member's distress, economic difficulties, intrafamilial conflicts, or parenting problems. At this point, a family crisis is present. If no outside assistance is received, the end result may be the family adapting at a lower level of functioning or perhaps the separation or loss of a family member. In contrast, a stable system under stress will move in the direction that tends to minimize the stress; for example, it will seek help from external sources when its internal resources are inadequate.

When health care professionals intervene to help a family experiencing stress, a systems approach would suggest that interventions aimed at the individual alone will be less effective than those aimed at the relationship systems in which the individuals behavior is regulated (Cox & Paley, 1997). Thus, interventions should be directed toward the multiple levels of the system rather than at individual behavior in order to assist the family in their adaptive processes (Cowan & Cowan, 1995).

LIMITATIONS OF FAMILY SYSTEMS THEORY

The complexity of studying the family as a system has made it difficult to understand and to operationalize all of the terms and concepts associated with general systems theory. The fact is, we know very little about the family as a system. Little is known about control in the family, maintenance of boundaries, how family input is converted to family output and about the timing and determiners of the use of negative feedback within the family (Mercer, 1989; Whitchurch & Constantine, 1993). Simply put, the family and its processes are much more complex to analyze than is a single-cell amoebae. Thus, as family scientists attempt to study multiple dimensions of the family system simultaneously, many variables can arise that create methodological ambiguities and increase the opportunity for error in analysis of the data. In addition, systems theory does not have explanatory power. That is, it is used as a way to conceptualize events, but cannot be used for eventually delineating the relationship of phenomena to each other (Whitchurch & Constantine, 1993, p. 346).

Family systems theory has received some criticism from feminist theorists. First, there is criticism that, because of the pervasive patriarchy evident in the resources and power distributed in society, those who use systems theorists are therefore subtly biased in their approach to analysis of the family. Second, it is perceived that systems theory trivializes women's experience through the terminology used to describe those experiences (e.g., terms such as enmeshment and fusion contain hidden bias against women). Finally, the complaint exists that systems theories suggest that all parts of the system contribute equally to the dysfunction. It can be argued that in cases such as abuse and incest, systems theory, when applied, minimizes the man's accountability and the woman's experience by ignoring the power differences between male and female family members. Proponents of systems theory argue that feminist theorists are misinterpreting the theory, and that the theory does allow one to attribute different levels of control over, or contributing to, the family members' behavior (Whitchurch & Constantine, 1993). Thus, it is argued that systems theory is sensitive to the issues of women, children, and minority groups in society. The nurse who adopts a systems paradigm in his or her practice is likely to ensure that interventions are not focused on a single entity or family subsystem, and that interventions are viewed within the context of how they impact on, or are influenced by, corresponding environmental systems (e.g., the family's friends, cultural reference group, religious groups, etc.).

⚜ SUMMARY

This chapter presents an overview of family systems theory. The following are key points made in this chapter:

- Family systems theory has evolved as "one of the most influential and generative of all family conceptual frameworks" (Broderick, 1990, p. 172). Certainly from a nursing perspective, the theory "makes sense" as we witness the influence of a single injury to one family member and of its reverberating (ripple effect) on all other family members.

- Family systems theory is derived from general systems theory as developed by von Bertalanffy in 1950. As the theory has developed, it has been influenced by the holistic paradigm (the whole is greater than the sum of its parts) and by cybernetic and communication theories.

- Technically, structural–functional theory is the earliest form of systems theory. Both theories converge and diverge at certain points and both are useful in identifying and describing important family behaviors.

- A system is a goal directed unit made up of interdependent, interacting parts that endure over a period of time. The family is a living system that typically extends over at least three generations.

- An open family system welcomes new ideas, information, techniques, and resources as it creatively works through day-to-day issues. Open family systems perceive change as normal and desirable.

- A closed family system views change as threatening and is resistant to it. These types of families are rigid, and do not seek exchange with other environmental systems in order to change, adapt, and grow.

- The family utilizes semipermeable family boundaries to facilitate adaptation to outside demands and internal needs. The function of these metaphoric boundaries is to actively expand (or open) and retract (or close) according to need, thus regulating the amount of input from the environment and output to the environment.

- Family adaptation is the capacity of the family and its members to modify their behavior to the changing demands of the family's inner and outer world.

- The family consists of subsystems, which can be either the individual family members or relational subsystems. These relational subsystems include the spouse subsystem, the parent–child subsystem, and the sibling subsystem.

- According to systems theory, the healthy family is characterized as being highly flexible and tolerant of internal changes and highly autonomous; it has an open exchange of resources, energy, and information with the outer environment.

- Stress causes family homeostasis or its steady state to become precarious, in which case family members initially exert considerable effort to regain the family unit's balance. However, when initial attempts to resolve problems or to meet demands fail, stress increases. In time, if no solution is found to reduce the stress, the system eventually reaches its limits to respond adaptively and reaches a point of exhaustion. If no outside assistance is received, the end result may be the family's adapting at a lower level of functioning or perhaps the separation or loss of a family member. In contrast, a stable system under stress will move in the direction that tends to minimize the stress; for example, it will seek help from external sources when its internal resources are inadequate.

FAMILY VIGNETTE: THE RODRIQUEZ FAMILY

Allie and Marty Rodriquez are a Hispanic couple who married when they were in their early twenties, and who are now celebrating 15 years of marriage. They have two sons, Daniel, age 13, and Joseph, age 11. Allie works full time as a teacher at the school her children attend. Marty is employed as an architect. Allie had difficult pregnancies with both her children due to severe gynecological complications, and she had to have a hysterectomy 10 years ago. The Rodriquezes always wanted to have more children, and especially desired to have a girl added to their family. After many years of discussion, they decided to seek the adoption of a female child, preferably Hispanic. One month ago, Allie and Marty were notified that they would become adoptive parents. Previously, the boys agreed to the adoption plan; however, now that it has actually taken place, they have shown little enthusiasm or interest in their new baby sister. In fact, Joseph has shown a dramatic decline in his school grades, and Daniel has taken to spending a great deal of time at a friend's house. Allie is on a short-term maternity leave to care for her daughter. She feels tired and overwhelmed as she again involves herself in the many tasks of caring for a newborn child who appears to have colic. Marty adores his new daughter and is equally frustrated that his sons are not as enchanted as he is with the baby. He finds he is spending a lot of time disciplining his sons and coercing them to assist their mother in the care needs of their sister. Marty is also very tired from the night feedings and from trying to carry extra responsibilities at home, while maintaining his daily work schedule.

■ STUDY QUESTIONS

Review the family vignette and answer the related questions.

1. What factors have led to a change or disruption of homeostasis in this family?

2. Select two nursing diagnoses you think would be appropriate for this family.

3. Describe the real and potential changes in the family subsystems that occur with the addition of an adopted child to the family.
4. Describe ways the family can reduce stress and reestablish equilibrium.

Are the following six statements true or false?

5. A system is defined as a unit with distinct parts and boundaries, extending over a period of time and with some identified purpose(s).
6. A social system is either an animate or inanimate system.
7. Open systems depend on the environment for exchange of information, matter, and energy, whereas closed systems do not interact with the environment.
8. Family differentiation occurs when a system bifurcates or splits into smaller subunits or systems.
9. With greater energy use, system boundaries need to be more open.
10. Differentiation, particularly as it applies to the family system, describes the family's tendency to grow and evolve (as time progresses) into a more complex and specialized system.

Answer the following questions.

11. Relative to the family system and its internal and external environments, supply the following information:
    a. Name a focal or target system.
    b. Name a suprasystem.
    c. Give three examples of interacting systems.
    d. Give three examples of family subsystems.
12. Draw a diagram of the energy, matter, and information exchange and process model and show a specific example of this energy exchange and processing pertinent to the family system.
13. Match the correct term from the left-hand column with a characteristic from the right-hand column.

    a. Equilibrium
    b. Adaptation
    c. Homeostasis
    d. Steady state
    e. Feedback loop
    f. Self-regulation
    g. Nonsummativity

    1. Synonymous with balancing (used interchangeably)
    2. The result of balancing
    3. A survival mechanism
    4. The whole is greater than its parts

14. Identify which of the following adjectives or terms accurately describe the paradigm used in systems theory.
    a. Reductionistic
    b. Objective
    c. Partial analysis
    d. Atomistic
    e. Linear causality
    f. None of these

15. The following elements and characteristics are true of the family system. It is a (an):

    a. Open social system
    b. Highly organized system
    c. Highly interdependent system
    d. System with specified purposes
    e. System with necessary processes (e.g., integration, adaptation, and decision making)
    f. Independent system
    g. Undifferentiated system
    h. Suprasystem to the spouse, parent–child, and sibling systems
    i. Dynamic system but with little capacity for change

16. What is the significance of the boundaries of the family system and subsystems?

17. Using the systems approach, explain how family boundaries function to maintain family homeostasis.

18. Match the proper function(s) in the left-hand column with each of the family subsystems in the right-hand column.

    a. A social skills laboratory   1. Spouse subsystem
    b. Mutual support   2. Parent–child subsystem
    c. Meeting of adult needs for affection 3. Sibling subsystem
    d. Learning to relate to peers
    e. Socialization function
    f. Disciplining—control and
       guidance function

19. Give four characteristics of a successfully functioning, healthy family according to systems theory.

20. Match the advantages/disadvantages and/or characteristics with "open," "closed," or "random" families.

    a. Open families   1. Provide for change
    b. Closed families   2. Are stagnated, rigid
    c. Random families   3. Offer choices and flexibility
    d. Does not apply   4. View change as threatening
                              5. Employ greater structuring
                                 and control mechanisms
                              6. Stress privacy and territoriality
                              7. See people as good, helpful,
                                 and needed
                              8. Seek out new resources
                              9. Family members set their own
                                 rules and schedules

21. Sequentially number the events below in terms of their order when a family crisis occurs.

    a. No solution is found to reduce stress—that is, failure of adaptive strategies exists.
    b. Stress and strain are experienced.
    c. A change occurs as stressor presents itself.
    d. Family homeostasis or its steady state becomes precarious and the family exerts additional efforts to maintain balance and reduce stress.
    e. Stress spreads from one individual or subsystem to all subsystems of family.
    f. System reaches point of exhaustion.
    g. Family disorganization results.

three

FAMILY NURSING PRACTICE

In Part Three, we now move into more specific applications for working with families. There are six basic areas subsumed under the comprehensive assessment approach used in this text: (1) family nursing process, (2) identifying data, (3) environmental data, (4) family structural dimensions, (5) family functions, and (6) family stress, coping, and adaptation.

Chapter 7 presents a discussion of each of the basic processes integral to family nursing practice: family assessment, identification of problems/needs, planning, intervention and evaluation and modification of plans of care. Chapter 8 covers the identifying and sociocultural data and Chapter 9 the environmental data regarding the family. The four dimensions of family structure (communication, power and decision making, role, and values) are discussed in Chapters 10 through 13. Three of the critical family functions (affective, socialization, and the health care function) are elaborated on in Chapters 14 through 16. Chapter 17 addresses family stress, coping, and adaptation. In each of the chapters, assessment areas specific to the focus of the chapter are described relative to families in a multitude of settings and throughout the family's life cycle. Family nursing diagnoses and interventions and a family vignette appropriate for the area being addressed are also presented. The actual family assessment tool and a suggested care plan form are included as Appendices A and B. Appendix C presents a hypothetical family situation, which is followed by an analysis of the family in Appendix D.

THE FAMILY NURSING PROCESS

✎ LEARNING OBJECTIVES

1. Explain the difference between using the nursing process in family nursing and using the nursing process in working with individuals.

2. Identify several sources of family assessment data.

3. Explain the advantages of examining the problem, etiology or contributing factors, and defining characteristics when making a family nursing diagnosis.

4. Describe several variables that the family nurse would consider when determining priorities for the nursing plan of care.

5. Describe factors that influence the particular family nursing intervention selected.

6. Explain how active family participation can be accomplished during the intervention phase of the family nursing process.

7. Explain the family nursing interventions of teaching, counseling, contracting, case management, and collaboration.

8. Describe the family nurse's role relative to consultation, client advocacy, and coordination.

9. State the desired outcomes of the evaluation and modification component of the family nursing process.

10. Describe the therapeutic actions that should be taken by the nurse when terminating the nurse–family relationship.

Comprehensive family nursing is a complex process, making it necessary to have a logical, systematic approach for working with families and with individual family members; this approach is the nursing process. According to Yura and Walsh (1988), "The nursing process is the core and essence of nursing; it is central to all nursing actions, applicable in any setting and within any theoretical–conceptual frame of reference" (p. 1). "Process" refers to a deliberate and conscious act of moving from one point to another toward goal fulfillment. The steps of the nursing process—assessment, diagnosis (problem identification), planning, implementation, and evaluation—"are interrelated forming a continuous circle of thought and action that is both dynamic and cyclic" (Doenges, Moorhouse, & Burley, 2000, p. 4). It is basically a systematic problem-solving process that is utilized when working with individuals, families, groups, or communities.

OVERVIEW OF THE FAMILY NURSING PROCESS

The family nursing process will differ depending on who is the focus of care. This difference in focus depends on the nurse's conceptualization of the family in his or her practice. If he or she sees the family as the background or context of the individual patient, then the individual family members become the focus and the nursing process is individually oriented, as is the traditional way of proceeding. If, however, the nurse conceptualizes the family as the unit of care, then the family as a unit or system is the focus even though the process itself does not vary.

Most family nurses in practice work simultaneously with both individual family members and with the family and its subsystems. This means the family nurse will utilize the nursing process on two levels—on the individual and on the family and family subsystem level. In this case, assessment, diagnosis, planning, intervention, and evaluation will be more extensive and complex.

If feasible, it is important to assess and focus on both levels of analysis. Nursing services in the United States are typically very specialized if nurses only assess and work with the family as a system. Conversely, an adequate understanding of each family member cannot be gained without viewing that member within the context of the primary group—the family.

This two-level approach to assessing and carrying out family nursing care is illustrated in Figure 7–1. In reality, the steps in the diagram are interdependent and not strictly sequential or linear in organization. In practice, one or more steps or phases may overlap or may take place simultaneously, with movement back and forth among the various steps.

FAMILY ASSESSMENT

In order to work effectively with family clients, to conduct assessments and to provide care, the family nurse must "think interactionally" (Wright & Leahey, 2000). Wright and Leahey explain that perhaps the most significant variable that promotes or impedes family nursing is how the nurse conceptualizes problems. A knowledge of family theory and research as well as utilizing a systematic framework for assessing

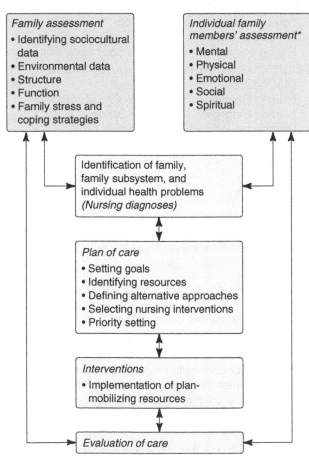

Figure 7-1. Steps in the individual and family nursing process.
*Individual client nursing process is not covered in this text.

and working with families greatly help the nurse to make the transition from an individualistic to a familistic perspective.

The process of family assessment is highlighted by continuous information gathering and professional judgments that attach meaning to the information being gathered. In other words, data are collected in a systematic fashion using a family assessment tool, and are then classified and analyzed to interpret their meaning. Often, cursory data are collected on each of the major areas. When the assessor then finds significant probable or potential problems, he or she then probes those areas more deeply. Additionally, family strengths should be explored in the assessment process. The amount and type of information is also dependent on the client, who may wish to convey more information in one area than another. Although assessment is the first step of the nursing process, data continue to be gathered throughout the provision of services, showing the dynamic, interactive, and flexible nature of this process.

SOURCES OF FAMILY ASSESSMENT DATA

Family data collection comes from many sources: client interviews relative to past and present events, objective findings (e.g., observations of the family home and its facilities); subjective appraisals (e.g., reported experiences of family members); and written and oral information from referrals, various agencies who are working with the family, and other health team members (Table 7–1).

The **interview** is a face-to-face meeting with one or more family members. Whenever possible, it is desirable to interview the whole family during the initial assessment phase rather than waiting until a later date. This gives everyone a chance to share their perceptions, and gives the nurse an opportunity to see the interactions of family members (Holman, 1983). The interview should be focused, but, according to the purpose of the interview, should vary in its degree of structure.

There may be times when the nurse conducts an interview with only one family member. In these cases, it is essential to "think family" by asking questions that include other family members. For instance, a question such as "What do you think your husband would say if he were here?" could shift an individually focused interview toward one that draws forth family data.

One of the important roles of the family health nurse is that of an **active participant observer** in the family. While the nurse is working with families, he or she must also have the ability to "stand back" and

TABLE 7–1

SOURCES OF FAMILY ASSESSMENT DATA

Client interviews relative to past and present events

    Questioning and listening

    Genogram

    Ecomap

Objective data

    Observations of the home

    Observations of family interactions

Subjective data

    Reported experiences of family members

    Reported observations of significant others

    Assessment instruments completed by family members

Written and oral information from referrals

Reports from agencies working with the family

Reports from other health team members

---

observe the conditions and situations existing in the home and in the "dance" between family members (i.e., their interactive patterns).

Two family system tools are used to gather information during a family interview. The **genogram** and the **ecomap** are commonly used for this purpose (see Chapter 8 and Chapter 17 for descriptions of these tools). The Friedman Family Assessment Tool used in this text can be used to structure interview questions and foci (Appendices A and B).

More **structured checklists, inventories,** and **questionnaires** may also be used in data collection (Holman, 1983). They may be especially useful when a great deal of information is needed to be gleaned or recorded. When a nurse is seeing a family over an extended period of time, or when more than one nurse is working with the family, checklists and other structured, easily completed tools may be useful.

One of the most frequent uses of structured family assessment tools is in the area of family research. There are over 100 family assessment instruments that have been developed for clinical and research purposes (Table 7–2). Many of these tools focus on

TABLE 7–2

FAMILY ASSESSMENT TOOLS

TOOLS	SUPPORTING THEORIES OR MODELS	CONCEPTS MEASURED	ADMINISTRATION & SCORING	ADVANTAGES	LIMITATIONS
FACES III/FACES IV Family Adaptation and Cohesion Scale (Olson et al., 1982; Olson, 1994)	Circumplex model	• Cohesion • Adaptability/flexibility • Communication	• 20 items in 4-point scale • Likert-type scale • Easy to administer	• Measures relevant for nursing • Measures real and ideal perceptions of the family	• Family members may be unwilling to assess themselves • Assumes family has children
FAD McMaster Family Assessment Device (Epstein, Baldwin, & Bishop, 1983)	McMaster model of Family Functioning	• Problem solving • Communication • Roles • Affective responsiveness • Behavior control • Affective involvement • General functioning	• 60 items • Likert scale • Easy to administer	• Measures areas nurses could change through care plans	• Requires family members to speak for family • Not clear if useful with clients of different social and cultural backgrounds, or in different life stages
Family APGAR Family Adaptability, Partnership, Growth, Affection, and Resolve Test (Smilkstein, 1978)	Family structure, function, and social support	• Adaptability • Partnership • Growth • Affection • Resolve	• 5 items • Quick to administer	• Measures relevant factors • Can be completed by adults and children age 10 years and older	• Not to be used to evaluate a family problem in depth • Has screening function
Family Satisfaction (Olson & Wilson, 1982)	Circumplex model	• Family satisfaction • Cohesion	• 14-item Likert scale • Easily administered • Norms obtained	• Directly measures family satisfaction	• None identified
FES Family Environment Scale (Fuhr, Moos, & Dishotsky, 1981; Moos & Moos, 1976, 1984)	Interactionist perspective	• Relationships • Personal growth • System maintenance	• 90 items—true/false • Scoring is complex • Standardized scores; two categories	• Short form available • Useful to measure change after interventions • Measures real and ideal	• A research-oriented tool that does not have a clinical model associated with it, thus clinical utility is unclear

Tool	Theoretical Basis	Content	Administration/Scoring	Uses	Limitations
FFI Family Functioning Index (Pless & Satterwhite, 1975)	Family functioning	• Communication • Togetherness • Decision making • Child orientation • Marital satisfaction	• 19 items • Likert scale • Quickly administered • Complicated scoring	• Identifies families at risk, distinguishes between well-functioning or troubled families	• Not for families without children, or with adult children • Not sensitive to short- or long-term change, thus will not measure change after a nursing intervention
FFFS Feetham Family Functioning Survey (Roberts & Feetham, 1982)	Ecological Systems Approach	Three major areas of family relationships: • Between family and broader social units such as school and work • Between family and subsystems within the family • Between family and individuals within the family	Somewhat complicated scoring	Differences between what is and what should be are measured • Identifies factors nurses could focus on • Evidence of class-bias	• Somewhat difficult to understand • Developed with families with handicapped children
FILE Family Inventory of Life Events and Changes (McCubbin, Patterson, & Wilson, 1981)	Double ABCX model	• Pile up of stressors or life events	• 85 items • Can be hand scored • Evaluates life changes on 9 different subscales	• Assesses stress in a family presently and over past year • Examines the multiple stressors a family is experiencing	• May be difficult for family members to remember events within the past year
IFF Inventory of Family Feelings (Lowman, 1980)	• Families Affective Structure • Patterns of agreement and conflict in dyadic relationships and alliances	• Positive/negative feeling toward each member	• 38 items • 3-point Likert-type scale • Easily scored	• Focuses on a single dimension of interpersonal and family relationship	• Limited clinical usefulness because of narrow focus
SFIS Structural Family Interaction Scale (Perosa, Hansen, & Perosa, 1981)	Minuchin's Family Functioning Theory	• Enmeshment and disengagement • Neglect/overprotection • Rigidity/flexibility • Conflict/avoidance • Patient management • Triangulation of parent–child coalition • Detouring	• 85 items on 4-point agreement scale • Easy to administer	• Useful for family counseling and assessment	• Length and complexity of tool make it difficult for clinical use

Sources: Partially adapted from Bowden, Dickey, & Greenberg (1998); Touliatos, Perrimutter, & Strauss (1990); Filsinger (1983); Jacob & Tennenbaum (1988).

family functioning/adaptation and family coping. All of the tools have been tested empirically and can be administered and scored by the health care provider. Some tools are more clinically relevant, while others are more appropriate for family research.

BUILDING A TRUSTING RELATIONSHIP

Establishing a trusting relationship in which there is mutual respect and open, honest communication goes hand in hand with the assessment process and orientation phase of working with a family. Reciprocal trust (Thorne & Robinson, 1989; Robinson, 1996) in the nurse–family relationship sets the stage for, and is the cornerstone of effective family nursing care. By promoting trust, the nurse is also creating a context for the family to be open to implementing future family nursing interventions.

Trust is developed when the nurse conveys an acceptance of the family and acknowledges the family's abilities, rights, and beliefs irrespective of the nurse's goals, values, or expectations. Wright and Leahey (2000) maintain that families should be encouraged to explicitly state their expectations for health care at the outset. This clarification of goals between nurse and family at the beginning of the therapeutic relationship promotes trust in the nurse–family relationship and may prevent family disappointment with services later on. Embedded in this conversation is a message of caring and an acknowledgment that the nurse respects the family's perspective and their expertise in managing their lives. The nurse's acknowledgment of family strengths serves to increase the family's own problem-solving abilities and to decrease potential dependency. A positive nurse–family relationship is enhanced when the nurse assumes an active, confident approach; builds on family strengths; cultivates a context of racial, ethnic, and class sensitivity; maintains a nonjudgmental stance; and takes an equal interest in all family members (Levac, Wright, & Leahy, 1997).

The orientation phase in working with families is seen as the time for assisting the family members to begin to express their present concerns so that the nurse may more fully understand the family and the meaning of its experience. The family members may deepen their understanding of their own concerns during this phase. The family may begin to solve their problems at this time, and family members may feel some sense of relief from sharing their concerns.

PREPARATION FOR FAMILY INTERVIEWS AND HOME VISITS

Before interviewing the family, the nurse must be prepared both conceptually and practically to conduct a family assessment. In terms of conceptual preparation, Wright and Leahey (2000) state that the nurse needs to be clear about the purpose of the meeting and should consult with the family about where the meeting will be held. Before interviewing the family, the nurse can read available records, should discuss the family with health care team members who know the family well, and should anticipate the family needs (both common developmental and unique situational needs). The nurse should then formulate some beginning ideas about the family system and should develop purposeful assessment questions to ask family members. When interviewing the family in the home, the anticipation of family needs is even more critical because home visits are quite costly in terms of both time and money for both the nurse and the family.

In order to be practically prepared for a home visit, the nurse should gather the information, the assessment, and the intervention tools (e.g., tongue blades, developmental screening kit, dressings) that are needed before leaving the agency. Flexibility, of course, is essential, because unanticipated or priority needs often become apparent during the home visit, and part of the preparation may not be needed—or at least not on the particular visit. When the family has a telephone, it is preferable for the nurse to call ahead of time to introduce him- or herself, stating the reason for the visit and making arrangements during the phone call.

After collecting data using a systematic family assessment tool, the nurse's next step is analyzing the data. The data need to be summarized and collated by grouping similar data together and by arranging it in an orderly form so that accurate conclusions and problems can be identified. It is also at this time that gaps in information become obvious, indicating where further probing and detailing of information are needed.

When analyzing the data, we advocate that **family strengths** be identified first as a vital part of an assessment. The family's strengths can be used as resources to draw upon when planning nursing interventions. Several authors have identified specific family strengths, most notably Otto (1973), Pratt (1976), Curran (1983), Beavers and Hampson (1990), and Power and Dell Orto (1988). They deal with the family atmosphere, flexibility and adaptability, and the extent of autonomy of members, as well as cohesiveness, the relationship of the family to the community, and communication skills. Table 7–3 gives the family strengths identified by Power and Dell Orto. Characteristics of healthy families discussed in Chapter 1 are also family strengths. To solicit strengths, the nurse might ask, "What are the strengths in your family?" or "What family qualities would you not want to change?" (Wright & Levac, 1993). Otto has successfully used a family-strength method in counseling of families. He explains that family strengths are first identified and then progressively shared with family members in order to increase their awareness of their resources and to take inventory of further potentials or strengths they have. Family members are encouraged to discover latent strengths and unfulfilled potentials as part of their problem-solving efforts.

✤IDENTIFYING FAMILY PROBLEMS: FAMILY NURSING DIAGNOSES

The family assessment culminates in an identification of actual or potential family problems. Many family health problems are within the nurse's scope of practice and are called family nursing diagnoses. Other family problems, however, fall under the scope of practice of other professions and fields, such as medicine, law, education, recreation, or social welfare. In these cases, the family's problems still need to be identified and discussed with the family, which serves to verify that the need or problem is mutually perceived. Often, the nursing role in this situation is to refer the family to appropriate resources and to provide the necessary coordination, teaching, and sup-

TABLE 7–3

FAMILY STRENGTHS

COMMUNICATION SKILLS

- The ability to listen
- The ability of the family members to discuss their concerns (family expressiveness)

SHARED FAMILY PARADIGM

- Shared common perceptions of reality within the family
- Family's willingness to have hope and appreciate that change is possible

INTRAFAMILY SUPPORT

- The ability to provide reinforcements to each other
- The ability of family members to provide an atmosphere of belonging

SELF-CARE ABILITIES

- The ability of family members to take responsibility for health problems
- Family members' willingness to take good care of themselves

PROBLEM-SOLVING SKILLS

- The ability of family members to use negotiation in family problem solving
- The ability to focus on the present, rather than on past events or disappointments
- The ability of family members to use everyday experiences as resources

Source: Adapted from Power & Dell Orto (1988).

port related to the problem and referral. Other family problems are the concern of several health care professionals, with each having a different way of assessing and working with the family. In these instances, collaboration and coordination with the other team members is imperative to avoid unnecessary client confusion and lack of efficient, effective services. These problems are called collaborative problems (Carpenito, 2000).

Family nursing diagnoses are an extension of nursing diagnoses to the family system and its subsystems and are the outcome of the nursing assessment. Family nursing diagnoses include actual or potential health problems that nurses are capable and licensed to treat by virtue of their education and experience (Gordon, 1994, 2000). They are used as a basis for projecting outcomes, planning intervention, and evaluating outcome attainment (Gordon).

At the family level, the nursing diagnosis can be derived from using one of the family or nursing theories or from using North American Nursing Diagnosis Association (NANDA) diagnoses. For instance, if a structural–functional or interactional framework is utilized, family nursing diagnoses might include role conflicts or transitions, child-rearing problems, value conflicts, or communication problems. If a systems framework is utilized, then the family's closed boundaries relative to interactions with the community, lack of an intact parental subsystem, or excessive separation of family members from each other are possible nursing diagnoses. In the discussions of each of the assessment and intervention areas that follow (Chapters 8 through 17), the reader will be able to gain insight into the types of family nursing diagnoses and other problems that may result from unmet needs in the family system and its structure or functions.

Rather than using a nursing diagnosis, some authors propose developing a more generic problem identification and family needs list. Wright and Leahey (2000) propose the formulation of a list of both problems and strengths in such a way that a balanced view of the family is identified. The notion of "hypothesizing" about family problems and strengths (Watson, 1992; Wright & Leahey) allows the nurse to offer speculations about family structure, development, and functioning in a "spirit of wondering" rather than in a hierarchical stance of certainty. Hypothesizing may guide the continuous assessment process and may also form the basis for nursing interventions.

NURSING DIAGNOSIS: THE NANDA CLASSIFICATION

The nursing diagnosis movement represents a very significant effort on behalf of nurse leaders to system-atize nursing practice and promote the use of a standardized list of diagnoses in practice. The North American Nursing Diagnosis Association (NANDA) (2001) defines nursing diagnosis as a clinical judgment about individual, family, or community responses to actual or potential health problems/life processes. A nursing diagnosis provides the basis for selection of nursing interventions to achieve outcomes for which the nurse is accountable.

Although family is included in NANDA's definition of nursing diagnosis, the list of diagnoses applicable to the family remains limited, and thus has been criticized by nurses concerned about family-centered care (Table 7–4) (Donnelly, 1990; Maturana & Varela, 1992; Wright & Levac, 1993). In examining a recent list of accepted NANDA nursing diagnoses, some diagnoses address family system and subsystem health problems. Moreover, the number of family diagnoses continues to increase over the years. Table 7–5 lists these selected nursing diagnoses. Gordon's (1994, 2000) and the NANDA format for stating nursing diagnoses consists of the statement of the diagnosis, signs and symptoms (defining characteristics), and etiologic or contributing factors. This formatting provides a rich and broadened resource for goal setting and formulating treatment plans.

NURSING DIAGNOSIS: THE OMAHA SYSTEM

The Omaha system is another classification system of client problems that has received favorable evaluation from home health agencies. It was developed by the Visiting Nurses Association (VNA) of Omaha (1986). An orderly, comprehensive list of client problems has been generated and studied as part of a larger operationalization of the nursing process.

Martin and Scheet (1992) described three components of the Omaha system: problem classification scheme, intervention scheme, and problem rating scale for outcomes. The problem classification scheme consists of 40 problems that fall into one of the four domains (environmental, psychosocial, physiological, and health-related behaviors). Modifiers appear at the third level of the problem classification scheme. One set of modifiers includes "family" and "individual," enabling the nurse "to clarify ownership and acknowledge involvement of one or more significant others" (Martin & Scheet, p. 67). An implemen-

TABLE 7–4

LIMITATIONS OF NURSING DIAGNOSIS WHEN APPLIED TO FAMILY NURSING

- They are individually oriented.
- They are atheoretical, which can be both a strength and a weakness, depending on one's viewpoint.
- The family-oriented nursing diagnoses are very broad and may not be sufficiently specific to guide nursing interventions.
- They are essentially illness oriented.
- The present list is incomplete and does not cover the array of family nursing actual or potential problems/diagnoses that clinicians see.
- There is an absence of standardized diagnostic categories that address family health promotion.
- Diagnostic categories do not fully address the family-as-client throughout the broad spectrum of health–illness concerns and over the entire scope of the family life cycle.
- Diagnostic labels use pathologizing language such as *dysfunctional* and *ineffective* as descriptors of families or family behavior.
- They do not account for variations in family behaviors related to their cultural context.

tation manual is available (VNA of Omaha, 1986) as well as a comprehensive textbook (Martin & Scheet) describing its application to community health nursing.

DETERMINING THE FAMILY PROBLEMS

Active family participation through the nursing process should be of central concern. In terms of identifying problems and strengths, the family nurse and the family are jointly responsible for this part of the process. This process of mutually determining problems and strengths will also enhance the nurse–family relationship. The nurse needs to indicate at what family system level the problem lies—at the family unit level or at the level of one of the family subsystems or sets of relationships such as the marital dyad, the parent–child subsystem, or the sibling subsystem.

Diagnosis involves the process of putting information together with the family to formulate the problem(s) and to explore a possible course of action. A case in point: It is not enough for the nurse working with a family to observe that the family is under stress and is not following its plan for bringing in family or friends to help. Together with the family, the nurse

needs to generate a diagnosis as to what is happening and why the family is not able to follow through with its intended action. If the nurse has collected adequate information and verified it with the family, the diagnosis will be reasonably accurate. His or her diagnosis should then lead to goals and interventions aimed at assisting the family to cope more effectively.

INTERRELATIONSHIP OF DATA AND PROBLEMS. One of the problems in determining health needs or problems of families is that all the information gathered is interrelated, and there are almost insurmountable difficulties involved in sorting out the cause-and-effect relationships. This is because, according to systems theory, there is circular causality. Feedback loops exist (which will be discussed in Chapter 6) wherein one person's behavior (A) sets off another person's behavior (B) causing A to act in response to his or her (A's) previous behavior plus B's response. Also, there is an overlapping of family problems such as role and power conflicts, and certain problems are not of the same type or level of generality or specificity as others.

POTENTIAL PROBLEMS. The problems identified in family nursing often focus on the family's ability to cope

TABLE 7–5

NANDA NURSING DIAGNOSES RELEVANT TO FAMILY NURSING

Anticipatory Grieving

Caregiver Role Strain

Chronic Sorrow

Compromised Family Coping

Decisional Conflict (specify)

Deficient Knowledge (specify)

Disabled Family Coping

Dysfunctional Family Processes: Alcoholism

Dysfunctional Grieving

Health-Seeking Behaviors (specify)

Imbalanced Nutrition: Less than Body Requirements

Imbalanced Nutrition: More than Body Requirements

Impaired Adjustment

Impaired Home Maintenance

Impaired Parenting

Impaired Social Interaction

Ineffective Role Performance

Ineffective Family Therapeutic Regimen Management

Interrupted Family Processes

Noncompliance (specify)

Parental Role Conflict

Post-Trauma Syndrome

Powerlessness

Readiness for Enhanced Family Coping

Readiness for Enhanced Spiritual Well-Being

Risk for Caregiver Role Strain

Risk for Imbalanced Nutrition: More than Body Requirements

Risk for Impaired Parenting

Risk for Impaired Parent/Infant/Child Attachment

Risk for Loneliness

Risk for Other Directed Violence

Risk for Powerlessness

Sexual Dysfunction

Social Isolation

Spiritual Distress

Source: NANDA diagnoses are described in McFarland & McFarland (1997) and NANDA (2001).

with a health or environmental problem. In many situations there will be no present medical illness or disability. In these cases the most frequent diagnoses are preventive, such as reduction of risks (nutritional modification—salt, caloric, sugar, and fat reduction; lowering stress levels); and lifestyle improvements (regular exercise, more rest and relaxation, better communication). By definition, a nursing diagnosis may involve potential health problems that originate from existing or anticipated conditions. Because of anticipated periods of unusual demand on the family and its members, anticipatory guidance or health teaching, health counseling, and the initiation of referrals to community resources are often indicated. Examples of foreseeable stressors are pregnancy, movement into a new community, retirement, adolescence, a wife beginning full-time employment, and the progressive deterioration of an aging parent.

WELLNESS DIAGNOSES.   Families may also come to a point where they desire to achieve a higher level of functioning in a specific area (Alfaro-LeFevre, 2001). In these cases, a wellness or health promotion diagnosis would be selected. This indicates the family is already in a healthy state, yet wishes to focus their plan of care on further enhancing their strengths and assets.

DETERMINING PRIORITY NEEDS.   The problems we should be assisting families to alleviate or ameliorate are the needs for which family health nurses can affect change or on which we can make a discernible, positive health impact in an efficient manner. Of low priority and hierarchy relative to providing services are those needs that are impossible to do anything about, because of either client or agency constraints. Other needs or problems will resolve themselves or can be handled by the family's support system or by someone who is less costly and more available to the family, such as a homemaker–home health aide. There are also needs and problems that are beyond the control of the client or the control and/or level of expertise of the nurse. These limitations must be recognized. If a problem is not within our area of expertise, the family may need a referral to the appropriate source of help.

Once family and individual health problems have been identified, they should be listed in order of priority, according to their importance to the family. There is often a disjuncture between how the professional views client needs and how the client (or members within the family) views his or her own problems. In these cases, it is essential that the nurse explore and listen to each family member's perspective in a nonjudgmental way. Then nurse and family may co-determine the direction for nursing care. This process enhances collaboration, and it demonstrates respect for the family's abilities to be active decision makers in their health care.

Only by ranking needs and priorities from the client's perspective can plans for intervention have any chance of success. Some nurses assign low-, medium-, and high-priority ratings, with high-priority needs being those that must be addressed immediately or very soon. In addition to client safety or life-threatening situations, two important factors to consider in assigning priorities are (1) the client's sense of urgency (this is important in building rapport), and (2) actions that will, or might have, therapeutic effects on future client and family health behaviors. These problems will then form the basis for setting goals and planning interventions.

PLANNING

During this stage of the nursing process the family nurse is engaged in developing a plan of care, in collaboration with the family, that prescribes interventions to attain the expected outcomes. The plan is communicated to all members of the health care team to promote a consistent approach toward working with the family in assisting them to meet their desired outcomes.

MUTUAL GOAL SETTING

Mutual goal setting with families is the cornerstone of effective planning. One of the basic premises of family nursing is that clients have the ultimate responsibility for managing their own lives (the principle of self-determination) and that we respect others' beliefs (Carey, 1989). The nurse can help families determine their own health goals by providing them with relevant information about themselves and/or their concerns. This allows families to make sounder decisions about what goals and services they wish to plan. Thus, the main determinant of what goals are set is the family, not the nurse (Otto, 1973).

Mutual goal setting with family members is consistently superior to unilateral goal setting for several reasons:

- The process of mutual goal setting has a positive effect on interactions with families.
- People tend to resist being told what to do, but are likely to work toward goals that they themselves choose and support.
- People who make decisions tend to feel accountable for them (Carey, 1989).

Goal setting has been increasingly recognized as a highly important component in planning. The development of clear-cut, specific, and acceptable goals is crucial. If family goals are not clear, it does not make much difference what activities are carried out because the end point is not known. To the extent that the stated objectives are defined and accepted as valid by the family, the desired action is likely to follow. In addition to the acceptability, clarity, and specificity of goals, goals also need to be stated in behavioral terms so that they can be measured (evaluated). Goals need to be specified as short term, that is, specific, immediate, and measurable; intermediate-level goals; or at the other end of the continuum as long-term, more general, ultimate goals that indicate the broad purposes the nurse and family hope to achieve. Short-term goals are necessary to motivate and give confidence to the family and individuals that progress is being made, as well as to guide the family toward the larger, more comprehensive goal. This process is consistent with the major contemporary theorists related to health behavior change (Glanz, Lewis, & Rimer, 1997).

In goal setting it is desirable to work with the family in differentiating problems that need to be resolved by nursing intervention, problems the family as the self-care agent can handle by itself, and problems that need to be referred to other members of the health care team or handled on a collaborative basis. A case in point is an elderly couple that needs (a) assistance in obtaining Medicaid, (b) diet counseling, and (c) basic nursing care for the nonambulatory husband. The nurse may decide to handle diet counseling herself, refer the couple to a social worker for Medicaid assistance, and suggest a home health aide to provide the routine nursing care needed for the husband. As a member of the health care team serving families, the family-centered nurse must also be continually alert to situations in which team conferences (formal or informal) might be beneficial to the clients. Collaborative planning and goal setting with other team members helps foster a better understanding of client's needs, in addition to mapping out who will do what.

NURSING OUTCOMES CLASSIFICATION (NOC). During the planning stage specific outcomes are formed. These outcomes are identified as client responses that are achievable and desirable by the family (Doenges, Moorhouse, & Burley, 2000). A classification of outcomes associated with nursing diagnoses and nursing interventions has been researched and developed (Johnson, Maas, & Moorhead, 2001). The Nursing Outcomes Classification (NOC) is designed to describe the desired status of the patient/family following the implementation of nursing interventions. Each outcome was developed with an associated list of indicators that are measured by a variety of specific Likert scales. Using this standardized means to evaluate patient/family outcomes can be an effective method to critically measure and analyze the effect of specific nursing interventions. In collaboration with the use of NANDA Diagnosis, and Nursing Interventions Classification (NIC) (discussed later) and the Omaha Classification system, nursing is making great strides in delineating how the nursing process is to be put into action.

GENERATING ALTERNATIVE APPROACHES AND IDENTIFYING RESOURCES

After setting goals, the health care professional and family need to generate alternative ways for reaching the stated goals. As these needs are delineated, possible resources for handling those needs are identified. Such resources include use of family inner strengths, including their self-care resources, the family's support system, and physical and community sources of assistance. Limitations to the plan of care may include factors such as agency policies and time and money constraints. Limitations on the availability of personnel and other resources may also influence selection of approaches and the identification of resources.

Specific actions or approaches facilitated by the nurse are selected by family members from the available alternatives and resources. These are approaches that both the family and the nurse feel are appropriate and, hopefully, have a high probability of success. One strategy for increasing the family's confidence in their ability to succeed with planned actions is to discuss their successes in other situations. Some of the strategies may involve some or all of the family members, other health care team members, or extended family and friends, as well as the nurse.

In thinking through the planning of nursing approaches, the nurse needs to ask the following questions:

- Is this plan being developed in collaboration with the family?
- Will the proposed approaches enhance family strengths and increase family member independence?
- Is this action within the information and skill level of the family members or their own resources? Do they have prior experience with similar actions?
- On a scale of 1 to 10 (with 10 being highest), how committed and motivated are family members in regards to adhering to the plan?
- Are there adequate resources available to carry out the plan?
- How would family members respond to these questions?

Families have the right and responsibility to make their own health decisions. Because of this premise of family nursing, there will be certain actions that fully informed families choose that we may personally and professionally disagree with. So important is the issue of client information and understanding of possible consequences of action (so that families can make an informed decision) that there are strong laws requiring informed consent and clear patient rights documents that affirm the need for patients and their families to be involved in all aspects of their health care decisions. Some of the approaches we plan with families may be less than ideal, but are intended to improve the client's (family's) present situation.

Seeking obtainable ways to reach goals is both realistic and pragmatic. Barriers may include suprasystem (sociopolitical) factors, which cannot be addressed with individual families; however, nurses may consider interventions designed to promote community action in some cases, or may act through professional organizations in nursing to advocate for health-promoting neighborhood and sociopolitical environments for families (see Chapter 9).

The operationalization of the nursing care plan follows the mutual selection of approaches designed to reach each of the stated goals. Once that is done, the implementation of the plan involves setting the priority and sequence of interventions and a phasing in and coordinating of the plan.

FAMILY NURSING INTERVENTIONS

Family nursing intervention builds on family assessment, family nursing diagnoses, statements of family strength(s), and planning, wherein goals are formulated, alternative intervention strategies and resources are identified, and priorities are set. Interventions are not routine, random, or standardized, but tailor-made to the particular family with whom the family nurse is working.

There are several different definitions for nursing interventions in the literature. The American Nurses Association (ANA) Social Policy Statement (1995a) defines them as "the actions nurses take on behalf of patients, families or communities" with an aim "to assist patients, families and communities to improve, correct or adjust to physical, emotional, psychosocial, spiritual, cultural and environmental conditions for which they seek help" (p. 9). Bulechek and McCloskey (2000) define nursing interventions as "any treatment, based upon clinical judgement, that a nurse performs to enhance patient/client outcomes. Nursing interventions include both direct and indirect care; those aimed at individuals, families, and the community; include nurse-initiated, physician-initiated, and other provider-initiated treatments" (p. xix). As defined by Wright and Bell (1994), nursing interventions are: "action(s) or response(s) of the nurse, which include the nurse's overt therapeutic actions, that occur in the context of a nurse–client relationship to affect individual, family or community functioning for which nurses are accountable" (p. 3). In collaboration and/or consultation with the nurse, implementation may be directly carried out by a number of people: the client (individual or family), health care team members, the extended family, and other persons in the family's social network.

During the time that nursing interventions are being offered, new data will continue to evolve and surface. As this information (client's responses, changes in situation, etc.) is collected, the nurse needs to be sufficiently flexible and adaptable in order to reassess the situation with the family and to extemporaneously make modifications to the plan.

There are different levels of family nursing interventions with respect to the complexity of the interventions themselves. Wright and Leahey (2000) define two levels of expertise in the nursing of families—generalists and specialists. According to Wright and Leahey, generalists conceptualize the entire family as the context for working with an individual patient. They are prepared at a baccalaureate level. Specialists conceptualize family as the unit of care with competency in clinical interviewing skills and knowledge of family systems theory, family research, and models of family assessment and intervention; they are prepared at the master's or doctoral level. In contrast to Wright and Leahey's belief that baccalaureate graduates function as generalists (according to their definition), we believe that baccalaureate graduates, in completing family system coursework, are usually effective in working with families as units. More complex families would, nevertheless, need to be referred to specialists with advanced preparation.

INDICATIONS FOR FAMILY NURSING INTERVENTIONS

Subsequent to the family assessment and a joint discussion of family concerns and problems, the family nurse and the family members need to decide whether family intervention is indicated. Criteria for making this decision includes the family's interest and motivation in receiving help and working on its problems, the family's level of functioning, the nurse's own skill level, and the availability of resources (Wright & Leahey, 2000). In addition to routine health promotional and preventive care,

Wright and Leahey suggest that family nursing intervention may be indicated when:

- A family member presents with an illness that is having an obvious detrimental impact on the other family members.
- The family members are contributing to the symptoms or problems of an individual.
- One family member's improvement leads to symptoms or deterioration in another family member.
- A family member is first diagnosed with an illness.
- A family member's condition deteriorates markedly.
- A child or adolescent develops an emotional, behavioral, or physical problem in the context of a family member's illness.
- A chronically ill family member moves from a hospital or rehabilitation center back into the community.
- A chronically ill patient dies (pp. 22–23).

NURSING INTERVENTIONS SYSTEMS/MODELS

The classification and description of more specific nursing interventions continues to be developed. This is a necessary accomplishment if nurses are to provide evidence for the effectiveness of their interventions on the health of families.

NURSING INTERVENTION CLASSIFICATION.
To date, commendable progress has been made by Bulechek and McCloskey and their research associates from the University of Iowa (2000) to develop a standardized language that covers 486 nursing interventions. A major strength of the NIC is that it provides a broad range of interventions for both generalists and specialists. It also includes interventions for high-acuity patients (Moorhead, McCloskey, & Bulechek, 1985).

CALGARY FAMILY INTERVENTION MODEL.
Another milestone in developing and describing nursing interventions is the Calgary Family Intervention Model (CFIM) by Wright and Leahey (2000). CFIM is "an organizing

framework for conceptualizing the relationship between families and nurses that helps change occur and healing to begin. Specifically, the model highlights the family–nurse relationship by focusing on the intersection between family member functioning and interventions offered by the nurse" (p. 26). CFIM focuses on promoting, improving, and/or sustaining effective family functioning in three domains: cognitive (thoughts), affective (emotions), and behavioral (actions) (Table 7–6).

Using this model, the nurse needs to determine which domain of family functioning needs to change and then determine the most appropriate intervention(s) that would target that domain. In a collaborative manner, the nurse seeks input from the family about which interventions may be most useful. For example, if a problem were identified as a lack of information, the nurse may determine that the domain of family functioning that needs to be changed is the cognitive domain. By offering an intervention (such as providing information), the nurse may assist the family to learn better ways of managing a problem. If the problem is that of inadequate exercise, the nurse may determine that the behavioral domain of family functioning needs to change and may offer an intervention that will change the family's exercise (behavioral) patterns. However, there will be situations in which more than one domain needs changing or when one intervention could effect change in more than one domain of family functioning. This is not surprising since a change in one part (of family functioning) will likely effect change in another.

In order to determine the fit between the domain that needs changing and the intervention of choice, the nurse may need to experiment with different interventions. Continuous evaluation of the effectiveness of the interventions is necessary. Table 7–7 illustrates application of CFIM to the problem: an elderly parent is requesting more visits from his adult children; the adult children do not enjoy visiting their parent, who is always complaining. Note specific skills the nurse can use to operationalize the intervention of "caregiver support."

GUIDELINES FOR FAMILY NURSING INTERVENTIONS

Recently, several useful principles to keep in mind while intervening with families have been described.

TABLE 7–6

CALGARY FAMILY INTERVENTION MODEL: THREE DOMAINS OF FAMILY FUNCTIONING

Cognitive: Interventions directed at the cognitive domain of family functioning provide new ideas, opinions, information, or education on a particular health problem or risk. Some examples are: offering information/opinions, reframing, offering education, and externalizing the problem. Additionally, interventive questions may be formulated to trigger change within the cognitive domain of family functioning.

Affective: Nursing actions directed at the affective domain of family functioning are intended to assist families with intense emotional responses that may be blocking their problem-solving efforts. Some examples are: validating/normalizing emotional responses, storying the illness experience, and drawing forth family support. Interventive questions may be developed to effect change within the affective domain of family functioning.

Behavioral: Nursing strategies directed at assisting family members to interact/behave differently with each other and with those outside of the family are included here. Some examples are: encouraging family members as caregivers, encouraging respite, and devising rituals. Interventive questions may be devised to invite change within the behavioral domain of family functioning.

Source: Adapted from Wright & Leahey (2000).

A foundational concept is that interventions can only be offered to families and that the best work that the nurse can do is create a context for the family to discover solutions (Wright & Leahey, 2000). In other words, the nurse applies his or her experience and knowledge to devise interventions in collaboration with the family but cannot force or direct change (Maturana & Varela, 1992; Wright & Levac, 1993). It is important that the nurse not blame himor herself or the family should the family choose not to implement a particular intervention or idea. Thus, rather than reacting negatively toward oneself or the family, the nurse could become more curious about the family's functioning and could collaborate with them to develop new ideas or to readjust prior interventions with the family to meet the goals. Vosburgh and Simpson (1993) maintain that "a focus for intervention becomes searching for strengths, welcoming differences in families and being respectfully curious about their uniqueness" (p. 232). Interventions need to be devised with sensitivity to the family's language and ethnic and religious preferences.

Robinson (1996) found that interventions that made a difference to families were those that promoted and enhanced relationships between the family and the nurse. Robinson stressed that "these relationships are not central to care, they are care" (p.

153). Thus, the nature of the nurse–family relationship is not a prerequisite to effective interventions, but rather may be considered an intervention in and of itself.

In keeping with the premise that families have the right and responsibility to make their own health decisions, families and nurses need to form a partnership to promote health and address families' health concerns. This partnership between health professionals and families is at the core of all good health care systems (Green, 1994). Active family participation is an essential approach to incorporate into each of the subsequent family nursing intervention strategies. Family involvement in the implementation phase often means engaging the family in mutual problem solving, as well as creating a context for change through therapeutic conversations in which family strengths are drawn forth. Family members are then freed to decide what makes sense to them and what they should do on their own behalf (Robinson, 1994; Wright & Leahey, 2000).

Inclusion of as many family members as possible in planned educational and counseling/supportive sessions is very helpful (Doherty & Campbell, 1988; Rolland, 1994). It allows family members to express themselves and support each other. It also stimulates much-needed group discussion and feedback and assures that all attending members obtain the needed information. One family member may ask novel ques-

TABLE 7–7

APPLICATION OF THE CALGARY FAMILY INTERVENTION MODEL: CAREGIVER SUPPORT

Parent–Child System Problem: Aging parent requests more visits from his adult children; adult children do not enjoy visiting their father because he frequently complains about their lack of visits.

DOMAINS OF FAMILY FUNCTIONING

1. Cognitive

2. Affective

3. Behavioral

INTERVENTIONS (ENCOURAGING FAMILY MEMBERS TO BE CAREGIVERS AND CAREGIVER SUPPORT)

Teach adult children that their aging parent is having difficulty remembering their visits (short-term memory deficits), which is a common phenomenon of aging. Therefore, it is not useful to remind their aging parent of when they last visited him.

Empathize with the aging parent; say that you understand that it must be lonely at times being a resident in a geriatric care center. The adult children would appreciate knowing that their parent is lonely so that they can respond appropriately. Therefore, advise the elderly parent to avoid complaining to the children that they do not visit enough and instead, to tell them when they come that "sometimes, I feel lonely here. I'm really glad you came to visit me."

Advise the adult children to stop giving excuses and explanations as to why they cannot come more often. Instead, obtain a guest book or calendar and write down each visit. Write down who visited and on what day, and perhaps any interesting news, so that the aging parent may read this between visits.

Source: Wright, L. M., & Leahey, M. (2000). Nurses and families: A guide to family assessment and intervention (3rd ed.). Philadelphia: Davis.

tions, which then exposes the rest of the participating members to the discussion that follows.

In families with a chronically ill child, it often happens that only the mother is involved in managing the child's illness, so including the father in family visits/interviews can be particularly important. This most common constraining arrangement leads to the father and healthy siblings feeling "left out" (Drotar, Crawford, & Bush, 1984; Rolland, 1994), and it progressively distances them from the mother–sick child dyad. It also keeps them from having firsthand information about the health problem and treatment and from having opportunities to share concerns and support each other.

In caring for a sick family member in the hospital or home, especially if the illness is life threatening, the family members often feel helpless, powerless, and stressed. Wright and Leahey (2000) provide several intervention suggestions aimed at involving the

entire family and at reducing its stress. These include teaching caregiving techniques to the family members such as how to touch and hold the patient without disrupting treatments, as well as encouraging family members to take on particular caregiving roles. Involvements such as these provide the family with a sense of competency (Power & Dell Orto, 1988).

PROMOTING CHANGE. As the definitions outlined above imply, the primary aim of intervening with families is to invite change such that suffering may be alleviated and/or a higher level of family wellness may be achieved. For the nurse working with a family over a period of time, change may seem slow or even nonexistent. It must be remembered that change in families comes about "over time through a sequence of interventive moves, each one growing out of information gained, in part, through observing the outcomes of the previous interventions" (Hartman & Laird, 1983, p. 306). Thus, the astute nurse pays particular attention to differences that, over time, even though they are subtle, punctuate progress regularly. Wright and Leahey (2000) have highlighted some important concepts of change that they have found critical in assisting families with health problems:

- Change is dependent on the perception of the problem.
- Change is determined by structure.
- Change is dependent on context.
- Change is dependent on co-evolving goals for treatment.
- Understanding alone does not lead to change.
- Change does not necessarily occur equally in all family members.
- Facilitating change is the nurse's responsibility.
- Change occurs by means of a "fit" or meshing between the therapeutic offerings (interventions) of the nurse and the biopsychosocial–spiritual structures of family members.
- The family's readiness for change may increase over time due to a variety of factors (e.g., media campaigns, personal experiences, increased confidence due to incremental, small successes, and new information).
- Change can be due to a myriad of causes (pp. 51–59).

SPECIFIC FAMILY NURSING INTERVENTIONS

A myriad of family nursing interventions exist that may be used in working with families (Table 7–8). Which interventions are selected is often influenced by the level of nurse competency, the theoretical model the family nurse utilizes in the care of a particular family, as well as the family nursing diagnoses made and the goals formulated. Two examples of how the theoretical model makes a difference in what interventions are selected are the following: anticipatory guidance (a type of teaching strategy) is emphasized in the developmental model, while crisis intervention strategies are used frequently when

TABLE 7–8

FAMILY NURSING INTERVENTIONS

Behavior modification

Contracting

Case management, including coordination and advocacy

Collaboration

Consultation

Counseling, including support, cognitive reappraisal (reframing), crisis intervention, and group work

Empowerment strategies

Environmental modification

Family advocacy

Lifestyle modification, including stress management

Networking, including use of self-help groups and social support

Referring

Role modeling

Role supplementation

Teaching strategies

Values clarification

a family stress and coping model is applied in practice.

Moreover, the specific intervention strategies health care professionals utilize with families may depend on the level of functioning of the family. Leavitt (1982) classifies families into highly functional, moderately dysfunctional, highly dysfunctional, acute and highly dysfunctional, and chronic. Nursing interventions vary depending on the nurse's perspective about the family's degree of functionality. For instance, with a highly functional family, the family nursing actions are largely preventive and health promotive (teaching, providing information). In contrast, with the highly dysfunctional, acute family, short-term and long-term therapeutic, supportive, and preventive actions are advised (Leavitt). The particular interventions implemented also depend on the families, as they are active participants in goal setting and selection of interventions. In any case, educative (teaching) and supportive strategies are core intervention strategies regardless of all the other factors involved.

Just as the vast majority of nursing diagnosis nomenclature is individually focused, a similar situation exists when searching for family-oriented interventions. As previously mentioned, interventions classifications tend to be individual oriented, though some significant family nursing interventions are also identified. Nevertheless, as Bell (1995) reminds us, "further work is needed to articulate specifically what the nurse does when he or she intervenes with families" (p. 356).

One of the reasons that family nursing interventions have been difficult to identify is suggested by Beavers and Hampson (1990). They maintain that family assessment and intervention are inseparable elements in clinical practice. Moreover, they assert that for some family's assessment (the questions that the clinician asks and resultant feedback) constitutes intervention. They mention that the families who typically make positive changes based on the assessment process and associated feedback are more competent families who are able to constructively use information provided in the assessment process.

Several family nursing intervention strategies are explored in this chapter: teaching strategies, counseling, contracting, case management, collaboration, and consultation. In addition, family nursing interventions are found in the concluding sections of Chapter 5 and Chapters 7 through 17. More specific family nursing interventions are described within these chapters, interventions that are most germane to the particular foci of each of the respective chapters (Table 7–9).

TEACHING. Including the family in patient education is vitally important. Educating the patient without including the family will frequently result in poor self-care and poor recovery outcomes (Rankin & Stallings, 2001). Teaching or health education is one of the major family nursing intervention approaches. It may cover many areas of content and focus, including health promotion and disease prevention, illness/disability concerns and impact, and family dynamics. Teaching strategies are processes that facilitate learning. The aims of learning are to support healthy behaviors or to change unhealthy behaviors,

albeit alterations of behavior are not always immediate or observable. For learning to occur, family nurses need to utilize principles of teaching/learning (Table 7–10). Four specific goals of family health teaching are presented in Table 7–11.

Watson (1985) stresses that education provides information to clients, thereby assisting them to cope more effectively with life changes and stressful events. Gaining meaningful information helps family members feel a greater sense of control and less stress. It also enables them to more clearly define their own options and more successfully solve their problem.

In the era of managed care and the emphasis on self-care and self-responsibility, the need for client education is greater than ever before. Hence, health teaching needs to be geared toward assisting patients and families to engage in self- and family care and self-/family responsibility. As early as possible, adults and children need to feel that they have the capacity to care for themselves and their family members and the right to obtain pertinent information so that they can make their own informed decisions. If this philosophy is established early in family–nurse relationships, then the traditional hierarchical model, with superordinate–subordinate positions, is no longer appropriate. As health educators, nurses need to play the role of facilitator and resource person to clients, who will decide which options are best for them. There are numerous factors that can positively or negatively influence the efficacy of the teaching intervention. Client and contextual variables that affect teaching effectiveness are listed in Table 7–12.

Teaching interventions today increasingly involve teaching skills to family caregivers. With the advent of diagnostic-related groups (DRGs), managed care, and other cost-saving policies, growing numbers of hospitalized patients are being discharged early. Both inpatient nurses and home health nurses are assuming much greater responsibility for teaching family caregivers how to care for their recovering family member in the hospital and at home.

Types of Learning Learning involves acquiring new thoughts and ideas (cognitive learning), attitudes (affective learning), and behaviors (psychomotor skill acquisition) (Bloom, 1956). Recognition of these three kinds of learning is needed when planning teaching interventions because all three types of learning are important (Lester, 1986). Moreover, the

TABLE 7–9

NURSING INTERVENTIONS SUMMARIZED IN OTHER PARTS OF THE TEXT

FAMILY NURSING INTERVENTION	CHAPTER LOCATION
Calgary Family Intervention Model (CFIM)	7, 10
Sociocultural interventions	8
Financial interventions	8
Social support and social networking, including use of self-help groups	8
Interventions to promote family recreation and leisure-time activities	16
Environmental health promotion	9
Environmental modification strategies	9
Interventions to assist the homeless	9
Conflict management techniques	10
Referral to parenting programs	10, 15
The empowerment model (family power area)	11
Role supplementation/Role enhancement strategies to role transitions	12
Interventions for role strain	12
Interventions for caregiver role fatigue	12
Interventions for role distance or role inadequacy	12
Interventions for role failure	12
Values clarification	13
Cross-cultural counseling approaches in area of family values	13
Interventions promoting healthy need–response patterns	14
Interventions promoting mutual nurturance among family members	14
Assisting families with closeness–separateness issues	14
Assisting families with grieving	14
Supporting parents in childrearing area	15
Making interventions socioculturally appropriate for single-parent and stepparent families	15
Specific interventions for childrearing area: Teaching and anticipatory guidance, behavior modification, initiating referrals to parenting and early intervention programs	15
Lifestyle modification: Self-confrontation, cognitive restructuring, modeling, operant conditioning, and stimulus control techniques	16
Assisting families at risk to cope	17
Family crisis intervention principles	17
Empowering families (family coping area)	17
Protecting family members at risk for violence	17
Referring families with complex coping problems	17
Intervention guidelines for working with culturally diverse families	18, 19, 20

TABLE 7–10

PRINCIPLES OF TEACHING–LEARNING

- Start where the learner is.
- Proceed from simple to complex.
- Proceed from the familiar to the unfamiliar.
- Use terminology that is appropriate for the learner.
- Set both short-term and long-term goals.
- Apply knowledge to enhance learning.
- Provide positive reinforcement to enhance learning.
- Incorporate the "four Cs" into teaching (display confidence, act competent, communicate clearly, and demonstrate caring).
- Use teaching materials that are suitable for the literacy skills of the learner.
- Model the desired role behaviors
- Provide opportunity to practice
- Give feedback on performance
- Planning support available from others

Sources: Partially adapted from Doak, Doak, & Root (1996); Rankin & Stallings (2001); and Sparks (1995).

TABLE 7–11

GOALS OF FAMILY HEALTH TEACHING

- To provide information so that clients are able to make informed decisions with regard to health and illness
- To assist clients to participate effectively in their care
- To assist clients to adapt to the realities of an illness and its treatment, trajectory, and prognosis
- To assist clients to experience the satisfaction of seeing their own efforts contribute toward improvement of health

Sources: Adapted partially from Rankin & Stallings (2001); and Steiger & Lipson (1985).

- Attentively listening to family members' questions and concerns
- Informing the family of relevant Web sites or other sources of information (books, videotapes at the library)
- Advising families how to handle the health and rehabilitation needs of the patient (p. 132)

The breadth or depth of health information provided may vary depending on the family members with whom one speaks. Accuracy of information is paramount, however, and who provides what information should be coordinated when teaching efforts are interdisciplinary.

Clinical practice and family research indicate that in health care settings families desire more information than they currently obtain from health professionals (Wright, Watson, & Bell, 1996). This need for information is heightened when family members are hospitalized and are critically ill (Wright & Leahey, 2000). Families want to be informed regularly about their loved one's condition, treatments, and progress. One important informal teaching strategy suggested for the hospital nurse is to make regular telephone contact with the family (Bozett & Gibbons, 1983). This strategy has benefits for both the nurse, who now controls the dissemination of information, and the family, who feel that they do not have to be constantly at the hospital now that they are receiving ongoing progress reports. Family members will be less anxious because of the supportive information that regular telephone calls provide.

three types of learning are interdependent. For example, sufficient knowledge (cognitive learning) is foundational, but is insufficient alone, to the other two types of learning. When our attitudes about food and nutrition change positively, then behavioral changes often follow. Acquiring self-care skills can also lead to more positive attitudes about self-care.

INFORMAL TEACHING: PROVISION OF INFORMATION. Where sharing of information occurs in spontaneous encounters between nurse and family members, or information is communicated to family members in an unstructured manner, informal teaching is involved. Doherty and Campbell (1988) detail the skills that health care professionals need when providing ongoing medical information and advice to families:

- Regularly and clearly communicating health findings and treatment options to family members

TABLE 7–12

VARIABLES AFFECTING TEACHING EFFECTIVENESS

CLIENT FACTORS

- Motivation of family members: Motivation is the critical force or drive that activates persons to change
- Ages of family members
- Members' psychological state (e.g., anxiety, depression level)
- Family members' perception of health problem(s)
- Self-efficacy related to proposed behavior
- Perceived risk or benefits versus barriers

COMMUNICATION FACTORS

Communication involves the exchange of information between the sender and the receiver. Barriers to communication include those due to:

- Lack of comprehension of subject matter
- Cultural and language barriers
- Socioeconomic barriers
- Inability of family members to communicate clearly with teacher and with each other

SITUATIONAL FACTORS

- The environment in which the teaching/learning takes place
- The timing of the teaching
- The teaching modalities used

ROLE MODELING. In addition to informal teaching strategies, role modeling is a powerful modality for teaching family members how to modify their behaviors. Bandura, a social learning theorist, points out how central role modeling is in learning. He contends that "learning through observing complex behaviors and then modeling such patterns is the source by which the most important learning of the social world takes place" (Jacob & Tennenbaum, 1988, p. 9). This approach is particularly important for pediatric family-centered nurses, who serve as important role models when teaching parents; for primary care and community-based nurses when they teach positive health behaviors; and for family mental health nurses when they teach family members how to communicate and interact more functionally.

ANTICIPATORY GUIDANCE. Anticipatory guidance is an important facet of health teaching. It provides the family with information on what to expect with respect to a future event, a potential problem/issue, or a child's next developmental phase. Discussing probable events, feelings, and situations with the family provides for clarification of ideas, reduction of anxiety, and future role change adaptability. Anticipation of, and preparation for, a coming event, a subsequent developmental phase, or a probable trajectory or prognosis of an illness will make the event less traumatic for the family and will allow family members to better handle the situation (Green, 1994).

An example of the benefits of anticipatory guidance is the success that childbirth preparation classes such as Lamaze enjoy. When labor begins, both parents trained in the Lamaze technique are fully prepared and usually go through the labor and delivery with excitement and positive feelings. A positive birthing experience gives parents positive feedback about their ability to handle future parenting challenges.

In conclusion, teaching interventions are one of the most essential types of family nursing interventions. Family health professionals need to keep in mind, however, that knowledge in and of itself does not necessarily lead to needed changes in behavior. As Health Belief Models describe (Rosenstock, 1974; Pender, 1996), changes in health behaviors are due to multiple factors with knowledge alone not being sufficient. A meta-analysis (a synthesis of multiple studies) of patient teaching research demonstrated that presentation of knowledge alone is not the most effective option. Approaches that combine information with emotional support to relieve anxiety and practice opportunities were reported to be superior to the provision of information alone (Mumford, Schlesinger, & Glass, 1982). In another study of patient teaching methods, it was found that both individual and group education improves patient outcomes, although group education (such as family) teaching in some studies was more effective (Rankin & Stallings, 2001).

COUNSELING. Until recently, counseling has been thought by most nurses to be appropriate only for those in psychiatric–mental health nursing. It is now widely accepted, however, that there are levels of sophistication and complexity in counseling and that basic family counseling (called family interviewing by Wright and Leahey, 2000) is a core family nursing intervention. Family therapy and family systems nursing, advanced forms of family counseling, are viewed by these authors as well as by the American Nurses Association Council of Psychiatric–Mental Health Nurses as requiring advanced practice nursing education.

Although it is not called counseling, nursing theorists and educators have long been concerned with the profession's therapeutic interpersonal process (Peplau, 1952). In their description of humanistic nursing, Patterson and Zderad (1976) assert that the crux of nursing is the existence of an authentic dialogue between nurse and patient and that the goal of this dialogue is the promotion of growth and nurturance of the human potential. Counseling and supportive intervention strategies are congruent with these ideas about nursing's role and goals.

Defining Counseling Although there are numerous approaches in counseling, all connote an interpersonal intervention process. Banks (1992) offers the following broad definition of counseling:

> Counseling is an interactive helping process between a counselor and a client characterized by the core elements of acceptance, empathy, genuineness, and congruency. This relationship consists of a series of interactions over time in which the counselor, through a variety of active and passive techniques, focuses on the needs, problems, or feelings of the client which have interfered with the client's usual adaptive behavior. (p. 281)

The core elements of counseling, then, are empathy, or the experiencing or sensing of another's feelings and behaviors; acceptance or positive regard for the client; and congruency or genuineness, being unpretentious and honest in the client–nurse relationship (Pedersen, Draguns, Lonner, & Trimble, 1996; Rogers, 1951; Truax & Carkhuff, 1967). Underlying these attributes is a respect for others that is free of authoritarian judgments and coercive pressure (Banks, 1992), as well as caring for and about the family.

Counseling is a process that seeks to help families and their members address, resolve, and effectively cope with their problems, and to utilize their competencies and other resources more fully. Encouraging family members to express and share their concerns, perceptions, and feelings with other family members is an essential part of this process. Assisting family members to positively reframe or cognitively restructure their thoughts and perceptions about events—in order to bring about healthier behavior—is also a major counseling intervention approach (Goldenberg & Goldenberg, 2000; Minuchin & Fishman, 1981). Working with individual family members, family subsystems, whole families, and groups of families are ways to provide family counseling services (Greiner & Demi, 1995).

Family counseling strategies are very broad, covering a wide array of more specific techniques and foci. These strategies also range in complexity from very basic supportive counseling interventions to family therapy or family systems nursing in which advanced practice preparation is needed. At a basic level of counseling, it is difficult to distinguish when teaching ends and when counseling begins. It is also difficult to identify the conceptual differences between teaching and counseling. Doherty (1995) addresses these two issues by suggesting that teaching and family therapy (an advanced form of family counseling) are part of a continuum in which educational approaches are the focus at one end of the continuum and therapeutic approaches are the focus at the other end of the continuum. To demonstrate his idea about this issue, he devised Levels of Family Involvement, guidelines for family professionals working with families. Table 7–13 outlines these five levels of family involvement, which start with very minimal involvement (i.e., level I, patient teaching) to an intensive level of involvement (i.e., level V, family therapy). Family nurses—without advanced family nursing practice preparation—should be able to work with families at levels I through IV.

As with teaching, counseling interventions can be used in addressing many different types of family nursing diagnoses and problems. Of the NANDA

TABLE 7–13

THE TEACHING–COUNSELING CONTINUUM AS SEEN IN HEALTH PROVIDERS' LEVEL OF FAMILY INVOLVEMENT

LEVEL OF FAMILY INVOLVEMENT	DESCRIPTION OF INVOLVEMENT	TEACHING OR COUNSELING
I	Minimal emphasis on family. Individually oriented education/teaching.	Patient teaching
II	Collaborative educational activities with members; providing information and advice.	Family teaching
III	Adds to level II involvement by the eliciting of feelings and experiences of family members.	Combination of supportive teaching and educationally focused counseling
IV	Brief focused family assessment and interventions. Particularly suited for work with families with health promotion and health problems, as well as families in high-risk situations. Basic family assessment and interventions included here.	Basic family counseling
V	Family therapy aimed at treating serious psychological and family problems. Advanced skills needed to deal with treatment of intense personal and family distress, conflict, and resistance to needed change.	Advanced family counseling (family therapy)

Sources: Partially adapted from Doherty (1995); and Doherty & Campbell (1988).

diagnoses relevant for family nursing (see Table 7–5), counseling could be an appropriate type of intervention for all these diagnoses. A nice example of the use of family counseling interventions is presented by Follen, Johnson, and Kronenwetter (1994). They describe the family counseling approaches they used in the critical care setting: interventive questioning, empowering family members to translate the meaning of their experience, facilitating patient–family discussion about patients' preferences for care and about care outcomes, and redefining the context of relationships.

The barriers to counseling effectiveness are similar to those associated with teaching. Socioeconomic and cultural differences between the nurse and the family can pose a particularly troublesome barrier if the nurse is not competent in modifying his or her approach to be socioculturally appropriate (Pedersen et al., 1996). Family client motivational problems are also critical barriers to successfully assisting families.

Four additional limitations often curtail what nursing can do in counseling families. First, if the organization for which the family nurse works is not supportive of family nursing counseling interventions (Wright & Leahey, 2000), and hence does not allocate time for this type of intervention or reward the nurse for counseling families, this serves as a major barrier. Second, if the families themselves do not see a nurse as competent to fulfill this role, they may be resistant to counseling, unless the nurse can clarify his or her role and gain the participation of the family. A third basic limitation to counseling by family nurses is the reality of today's cost-containment practice milieu. With time and efficiency highly valued to keep costs contained, family supportive counseling activities are often neglected or are not feasible. A fourth barrier to counseling effectiveness is the nurse's preparation. If the family has complex problems, advanced nursing preparation is often necessary to adequately address these more difficult family needs.

The decision as to whether to counsel a family is ultimately based on several primary factors. The first of these is the family's level of functioning, which then implies the extensiveness of the family's problems—or the reverse, the family's strengths or competencies. The family nurse's competence to counsel a particular family is a second consideration. A third consideration is the feasibility of counseling within the work context. If counseling is indicated, and it is possible within the work environment and is mutually agreed upon, then the key considerations are: which areas to focus on, who to see, and how long to work with the family (Wright & Leahey, 2000).

Family Counseling of Families in Crisis Family counseling is often used to help a family deal with a crisis (Hartman & Laird, 1983; Walsh, 1998). The most widely used model of working with families in crisis is the family crisis intervention model (Ell & Northen, 1990). Kus (1992) defines the crisis intervention model that may be used with individual or family clients:

> Crisis intervention is the systematic application of problem-solving techniques, based on crisis theory, designed to help the client in crisis move through the crisis process as swiftly and painlessly as possible and thereby achieve at least the same level of psychological comfort [or family functioning in the case of families] as experienced before the crisis. (p. 181)

The major goals of family crisis intervention are to decrease the immediate negative effects of stress felt by family members and the family as a whole, as well as to mobilize their coping capabilities in adaptive ways (Ell & Northen, 1990; Walsh, 1998). Reframing family members' view of their problem(s) is often used to assist them to search for alternative behavioral, cognitive, and affective responses to their problem (Hartman & Laird, 1983; Minuchin & Fishman, 1981; Goldenberg & Goldenberg, 2000).

The family nurse's functions using this model are to initially and quickly provide access to needed services and then, after the initial stress level is reduced and immediate problems are addressed, to assist the family in problem solving and coping, with the aim being to have the family and its members to regain homeostasis or to move to a higher level of functioning. Helping families develop their own methods for coming up with solutions to their problems is congruent with a self-care approach and represents an empowering counseling intervention.

CONTRACTING. An effective means by which a family-centered nurse can realistically assist individuals and families to make behavioral changes is through the use of contracts. Contracting is also an excellent way to involve a family in a collaborative process.

Client contracting has been used in nursing since the 1970s and has been particularly efficacious when working with certain types of families such as families with substance abuse, pain control, or problems with self-management, as well as families with marital and child behavioral problems (Goldenberg & Goldenberg, 2000; Jensen, 1985).

A contract is a working agreement made between two or more parties, such as between a family and a nurse or between parents and a child. To be timely and relevant, contracts are continuously renegotiable and should cover the following areas: goals, length of the contract, client responsibilities (commitments) and health care team members' responsibilities, steps toward meeting the goals, and rewards for meeting goals (Sloan & Schommer, 1975; Steiger & Lipson, 1985). A contract may be written (Table 7–14) or verbal. One of the advantages of making a contract is

TABLE 7–14

BASIC COMPONENTS OF WRITTEN CLIENT CONTRACTS

- Purpose or goals of the contract: Short term and/or long term
- Implementation: Activities taken to reach goals and by whom
- Priorities in terms of goals or activities
- Reward when goals are met
- Time parameters: When activities are to be accomplished
- Reevaluation date to determine progress
- Co-signers and date

that at the end of the contract period, progress is evaluated and either a new contract is made or the relationship is terminated (Boehm, 1992; Wright & Leahey, 2000).

Usually, the contract is written, straightforward, simple to construct, and noncoercive (Goldenberg & Goldenberg, 2000). It also clarifies expectations for the parties involved (Boehm, 1992). The philosophy underlying the use of contracts is that of client involvement and the encouragement of self-care and self-responsibility. The contract draws clients in as the chief partners in their own health care. In fact, effective use of contracts is dependent on family involvement. For contracts involving family health problems, it is essential that the contract be made with the responsible and appropriate family members. Otherwise, family system problems cannot be properly addressed.

According to Jensen (1985), client contracting is particularly appropriate for clients with the following types of nursing diagnoses: noncompliance (treatment plan failure), knowledge deficit, ineffective coping, alterations in parenting, and self-care deficit diagnoses. Contracting has also been useful in addressing parenting problems or problems created by parent–child differences (Goldenberg & Goldenberg, 2000). Loveland-Cherry (1988, 1996) encourages family-centered nurses to also use contracting with family health-promotion diagnoses.

In client contracting, the clients must first and foremost be actively involved in the development, goal setting, and implementation of the contract. Because of this requirement, certain types of clients are automatically not appropriate candidates. Families in which the adult members are very dependent, disturbed, cognitively impaired, developmentally disabled, or not responsible are poor candidates because of their inability to help develop and carry out their part of the agreement. Very young children within the family, unless the parent(s) is involved, are also not able to develop or carry through on their commitment.

It is also pointed out in the literature that client contracting takes time and effort. Because the majority of the responsibility for implementation shifts to the family client, the nurse may feel some loss of control.

CASE MANAGEMENT.   Although nursing case management of the family as client is not directly discussed in the

nursing literature, recently nursing case management of the individual client has received extensive attention and interest. Case management has a long history of being part of public health nurses' role; more recently, its prominence in the acute care setting has emerged (Cary, 1996). The growth in managed care has been a prime force behind the emergence of case management (Cary). Managed care's emphasis on controlling costs and improving efficiency of care, while maintaining quality of care and client satisfaction, has definitely shaped the way case managers are functioning (Jones, 1994; MacPhee & Hoffenberg, 1996).

Defining Case Management   Case management is seen as a system, a clinical decision-making process, a technology, a role, and a service (Bower, 1992). Many definitions of case management appear in the literature. Nevertheless, there is a consensus that the process involves five essential steps: client assessment, planning, linking (referring, coordinating, and advocacy), monitoring, and evaluating (ANA Task Force on Case Management, 1988; Joint Commission for Accreditation of Community Mental Health Service Programs, 1976; Weil et al., 1985). As a process of determining, integrating, and monitoring complex client needs, it seeks to balance quality of care outcomes with efficient use of existing resources (Bower). Specific characteristics of case management identified in the literature include (a) its emphasis on active client participation; (b) its holistic orientation; (c) its self-care, self-deterministic orientation; and (d) the coordination and efficient use of a wide range of human services (Bower; White, 1986).

As can be seen from the preceding definition, the case management process and the process used in nursing practice (the nursing process) appear very similar. The crucial difference lies in the breadth and scope of the client assessment (the case management assessment is more comprehensive relative to assessment of psychosocial, environmental, and health-related variables) and the planning and resource identification with clients and members of the service network. This entails greater service coordination (Martin & Scheet, 1992; Weil et al., 1985).

Zander (1995), a nursing expert on case management in the acute care setting, states that case management builds on nurses' existing professional roles by adding three new dimensions to their job: (1)

authority—the heightened authority to coordinate client services; (2) accountability—for favorable financial and clinical outcomes; and (3) time—a greater time commitment. Many parents and families require sequencing or organizing multidisciplinary services across settings—hospital, clinics, home, and hospice. Managing these transitions is a crucial role for family-oriented case managers.

Limitations and Barriers to Nursing Case Management There are three primary limitations or barriers to using a case management approach in family nursing. The first of these is the reimbursement policies that exist in health care. Nurses, except for those in specialized positions in which case management is identified as one of their functions, are not paid for providing case management to individuals, let alone to families. Completing a more comprehensive assessment, actively involving the family, and linking, coordinating, and monitoring services takes time. Adequate funding must be available for case management services to be effectively provided.

Second, nurses are often not sufficiently educated to function as case managers using the broadened definition of case management described above. "Few basic nursing education programs today, regardless of their level of preparation, provide nurses with the knowledge and skills to function efficiently as case managers" (ANA Task Force on Case Management, 1988, p. 8). Nursing programs typically do not emphasize the assessment of social, economic, and environmental areas, or the initiating linkages and coordinating services to families. For instance, referral for assistance with financial problems resulting from health care expenditures involves the family health professional's being knowledgeable about available services and programs, agency referral procedures, and how best to refer the family.

Special programs that teach case management skills to nurses have been recently developed and implemented. These programs have been evaluated as increasing nurses' documentation of case management services to clients, particularly nurses' patient counseling, education, and health promotion interventions (Connors, 1988; Winder, 1988). Because case management is being seen in nursing schools as an advanced nursing practice role, the number of master's-level nursing case management programs is growing.

A third limitation, which is related to the first two barriers, is that some health care agencies do not see nurses as operating as case managers (in these cases social workers are generally seen in this role), or the agencies do not see this broadened responsibility as being within their scope of provided services. In spite of social workers' being better educated in some aspects of case management, when clients have complex health problems, nursing case managers often are more appropriate. The consequences of a complex and life-threatening disease demands a case manager who is well educated in both health and psychosocial/environmental areas.

CLIENT ADVOCACY.   A major component of case management is client advocacy (Smith, 1993). An advocate is one who speaks for and on behalf of some other person or group. It is also someone who vindicates or espouses a cause by argument, a defender or intercessor, such as the position that a defense attorney assumes. Kosik's (1972) definition relative to client advocacy by nurses extends the above definitions, incorporating a deeper commitment to the client. She explains:

> For me, patient advocacy is seeing that the patient knows what to expect and what is his right to have, and then displaying the willingness and courage to see that our system does not prevent his getting it. The goals of patient advocacy are, first, making a person more independent because he knows the what, why, and how of the system and, second, changing the system to make it more sensitive and relevant by revealing injustices and inadequacies, thereby making complacent continuation of the status quo impossible. The nurse may have to make waves. She may have to see that workers and agencies do their jobs and expose the indifference and inhumanity of caregivers. (p. 694)

The role of being a client advocate involves informing clients and then supporting them in whatever decision they make (Bramlett, Gueldener, & Sowell, 1990; Kohnke, 1982). Although a goal of client advocacy is client independence, the advocate may have to accept and perhaps even foster dependency temporarily. Thus, we need to start where the person or family is and encourage growth.

Although there are multiple ways of defining what advocacy means, in all cases there is a basis in ethical principles—using the principle(s) of self-determination (autonomy), justice (fairness and equality), beneficence (doing good), and nonmaleficence (doing no harm)—to guide each of the varied definitions of advocacy. Some nurses see advocacy as the philosophical foundation of nursing (Curtin, 1979; Gadow, 1980).

Community-based family nurses are in a strong position to act as advocates. They are in the community working with families that are often poor and feeling powerless and hopeless. Not only is there a great need for these nurses to assume this role because of client needs, but, unless the advocacy role is assumed, the rendering of other essential services may not be obtainable. Nurses in hospitals also have an important opportunity to act as family advocates—making sure that families and their members receive needed services and that the services they are receiving are appropriate and of good quality.

Thus, the family nurse can be a client advocate in at least four ways:

1. By assisting clients to obtain services they need and are entitled to

2. By taking action to create health care systems that are more responsive to client needs

3. By advocating for the inclusion of more socio-culturally appropriate services

4. By advocating for more responsive social policy (Canino & Spurlock, 1994)

Family advocacy can range from calling the welfare department before referring a family, in an effort to pave the way for them, to testifying in court on behalf of a client, calling a meeting with representatives from several agencies to coordinate and improve services to the community, or acting as a political activist working in the political and legislative policy areas to create needed changes in health and human services for families.

Clark (1984) points out that "advocacy necessitates involvement and commitment" (p. 53). The effective community health nurse cannot be content with the attitude, "I'd like to help you, but my hands are tied." Advocacy is not a popular concept, because it often means standing up to other health care and social service professionals and health care agencies for the rights of families. Advocacy also means assisting families to learn how to speak up for themselves—to be their own best advocates.

Rafael (1995) examines the various meanings of advocacy and how advocacy and empowerment have similar, yet different features. She concludes that existential or human advocacy (where the client is viewed as subject rather than object, and the nurse as a caring, valuing person) and empowerment are synchronous.

COORDINATION. One of the most widely accepted roles of the client advocate is the coordinator (Leddy & Pepper, 1985). Because the essence of case management is also coordination, the notions of advocacy and coordination substantially overlap. In fact, case management is often referred to as service coordination (particularly in the social work field), designed to provide multiple services to clients with complex needs within a single locus of control (Seltzer, Litchfield, Lowy, & Levin, 1989).

The family nurse in community and home health, as well as in primary care, is often a key person in the provision of comprehensive, continuous family health care. In addition to the particular functions the nurse is implementing, he or she supports other team members and interprets the nursing objectives and service, as well as coordinating health services with the various other agencies from which the family is receiving assistance.

Without coordination, the client may receive a duplication of some services from different agencies or, even more distressing, a gap in essential areas of need. An illustration of this problem from home health care follows. A rehabilitation clinic patient once remarked to various members of the health care team that she was having difficulty getting out of the bathtub and had no shower facilities to use. Each time she mentioned this to the team members they noted her response, but no one made any suggestions of what to do. A social worker, sanitarian, homemaker–home health aide, and visiting nurse were all visiting the family concurrently. In this type of situation it was the nurse's responsibility to make sure that collaboration was taking place and coordinated efforts being achieved. With a greater number of more acutely and seriously ill patients discharged early from hospital to home and followed by multiservice home health agencies, the nurse's role as case manager or coordinator of services is being expanded. Hospice home care programs are examples of interdisciplinary programs in which the nurse plays a vital coordination function.

DISCHARGE PLANNING. Promoting continuity of care for hospitalized and long-term, chronically ill clients and their families is a particularly significant need. Discharge planning from one level of care to another within a hospital or from the hospital to home or another health care facility is one example of continuity of care (Kelly, McClelland, & Day, 1992). Effective discharge planning is a central component of case management/coordination. It is essential to the individual patient and family that an appropriate plan and transition be made. From a health care agency's fiscal perspective, it is also critically important to have effective discharge planning to expedite the earliest possible appropriate discharge. Because discharge planning addresses health care access, quality, and cost, this component of case management is receiving wide attention (Kelly et al.).

In this role, the nurse must make continuing efforts to improve referral systems between the various health care and social service agencies in the community, and must be willing to share information with referring agencies, given the client's approval. Referral is a two-way street, and communication must flow in both directions for the system to be functional.

COLLABORATION. Another intervention of growing importance to family nursing is collaboration. It is vital to the provision of comprehensive health care to families. As members of a health care team, nurses collaborate and plan comprehensive family-centered care with other team members, as well as with their family clients. Collaboration, according to Lamb and Napadano (1984), is "a process of shared planning and action over time with joint responsibility for the outcomes and the ability to work together for common goals using problem-solving techniques" (p. 26). Collaboration is a synergistic alliance, in which the outcomes are different and better than any of the collaborators could generate on their own (Kyle, 1995). The end result should be the enhancement of client care and greater professional satisfaction (King, Parrinelo, & Baggs, 1996). The positive impact of collaboration is being increasingly recognized and advocated by nursing and other professional organizations, as well as by accreditation agencies (Lee & Cohen, 1995).

Collaboration can be considered both as a separate family nurse intervention strategy and as an important strategy used in case management. In the various ANA standards of practice, one standard of practice focuses specifically on the nurse's involvement in collaboration. Collaboration in most of the ANA standards of practice includes the client (individual and family) as part of the collaborative process also.

Ability to communicate clearly and negotiate effectively are interpersonal skills necessary for successful collaboration. "Collaboration involves the mutual give and take of cooperativeness and an active participation of all parties . . ." (Kyle, 1995, p. 174).

Collaboration implies a professional, collegial relationship in which there is mutual respect, egalitarianism, and joint decision making (Clark, 1984). An authoritarian type of relationship, in which the leadership and direction flow from the physician to nurse to nurse's aide to patient, cannot be considered a team or collaborative relationship. With a hierarchical model (in which one person is in charge), communication is not open, direct, or truly two way, and team members' contributions and effective functioning are seriously stifled. The composition of the health team (or health and welfare team) may vary depending on an agency's available resources, the health care professionals' practices, and a family's needs. Doherty (1988), a family therapist, identifies the therapeutic triangle composed of family, family professional, and medical team as being the treatment context within which collaborative health care should take place when families have chronically ill family members.

In a home health agency, the team is commonly composed of a community health nurse, a licensed vocational nurse, a homemaker–home health aide, a social worker, and a physical therapist. The occupational therapist and nutritionist may also be members of the team, or may act as consultants to the team. The family physician acts only partially and indirectly as a team member, because he or she is not present, is often difficult to reach, and is typically involved in the medical aspects of care only. Many independent health goals need to be formulated by the home health team based on medical information, on physician's orders, and on client assessments of patient and family. The patient and family themselves are also central members of the team. In dealing with chronic illness and long-term care, effective collaboration is essential to address the many-faceted interdependent needs of clients (Marosy, 1994).

In primary health care, the health care team usually involves the physician, nurse practitioner, and clinical nurse. A social worker, nurse's aide/vocational nurse, clinical psychologist, and other physician specialists may also be members of the team. Because nurse practitioners often work very closely with physician colleagues, the ability to collaborate effectively is vital to delivering care.

In the official public health agency, the team may be broader or smaller in size depending on the family's particular health, welfare, and educational needs. The community health nurse working in an official health care agency may be a member of a community-based team working with a young, child-rearing family wherein the school nurse, teacher, probation officer, caseworker, and psychologist are a part of the team. School nurses routinely function as collaborative members of teams that assess and plan educational programs for students with disabilities.

In an acute care setting, physician, nurse, social worker, patient, and family usually make up the team. Family professionals (nurse, social worker, and/or psychologist) need to maintain access and collaboration with the patient's physician, as the disease process and its treatment are affected by the family context.

Kindig (1975) points out that the structure of each health care system and the mix of people working on a health care team depend on the needs of the patient population and on available resources. For the team to function effectively, all members must have a common understanding of their respective roles and responsibilities, as well as clients' needs and the goals of treatment plan. Moreover, when a health care team continually works together, there is a great need for members to work out the process by which decisions are made, communications channeled, and procedures adopted. If a team runs smoothly, this frees more energy for client care, as less energy will be needed for team maintenance and coping with members' interpersonal concerns.

The need for an interdisciplinary process, whereby the efforts and skills of different professionals are coordinated, is clear when one adopts a family systems perspective and focuses on ways in which the family both affects and is affected by the health or illness of its members (Glenn, 1987). Moreover, in research studies, collaboration has been shown to be both therapeutic and cost effective (ANA, 1992; Koerner & Armstrong, 1984).

Glenn (1987), a family physician and advocate of collaborative health care, writes about common barriers to collaboration. He addresses the problem of power conflicts between health care professionals. "The main conflicts that emerge involve turf and money, authority and power" (p. 160). The problem of physician dominance and nurse deference is widely cited as a collaborative barrier (Kyle, 1995). Trust and mutual respect among the collaborators are crucial to successful collaboration (Kyle, 1995).

In conclusion, collaboration is an increasingly exciting, promising, and vital role in the nursing of families because it facilitates a holistic approach and the achievement of shared goals. For the family nurse, collaborative health practice can be energizing, rewarding, and both therapeutic and cost effective (Daka-Mulwanda, Thornburg, Filbert, & Klein, 1995).

CONSULTATION. Consultation is included as a general family nursing intervention because family nurses often serve as consultants to other nurses and other professionals and paraprofessionals when individual and family client information and assistance are needed. Most of the literature indicates that consultation requires both expert clinical practice skills and knowledge and advanced nursing practice preparation (ANA, 1992; Fraley, 1992; Kearney & Yurick, 1996).

Consultation is defined by Caplan (1970) as "a process of interaction between two professional persons—the consultant, who is a specialist, and the consultee, who invokes the consultant's help" (p. 19). The consultant's role is often to provide problem-solving assistance with clinical issues. In the consultation process the consultee is free to accept or reject the consultant's recommendations and remains directly responsible for implementing action and outcomes of care.

In nursing, consultation may take the form of deliberating together about a particular case or client and giving suggestions/information about clients with particular health problems. Or it may entail interviewing a family and providing another assessment of the family and its needs. Lewis and Levy (1982) classify the consultation process into two types. The first type in the above description is an example of indirect consultation, where a case-centered meeting is held and the family is not interviewed by the consultant. The second type of consultation is the latter example, where family members are directly interviewed by the consultant and a second opinion is given. This particular model is used extensively in medicine and substantially in psychiatric nursing where psychiatric clinical nurse specialists act as consultants to hospital nurses when patients are experiencing psychological and behavioral problems (Kearney & Yurick, 1996).

Family-oriented nurses who function as clinical nurse specialists, school nurses, family counselors, community health nurses, and occupational health nurses include consultation as one important component of their practice. Many family nurses develop special areas of expertise—such as family and child abuse, family crisis intervention, genetic counseling, family health promotion and diabetes education programs, and parenting—and provide assistance to other professionals in these special areas.

FAMILY EMPOWERMENT INTERVENTIONS.   Empowerment is a popular "buzz word" in many helping professions today, particularly nursing. The literature on empowerment has grown exponentially in the last decade. Rodwell analyzes the various meanings of empowerment in a 1996 concept analysis article. She identifies four defining attributes of empowerment:

- It consists of a helping process.
- It involves a partnership that values self and others.
- It is characterized by mutual decision making.
- It includes freedom to make choices and accept responsibility.

From Rodwell's (1996) literature review and analytic process, she generates the following inclusive definition of empowerment. "In a helping partnership, it is a process of enabling people to choose to take control over and make decisions about their lives. It is also a process which values all those involved" (p. 309).

An empowerment philosophy underlies all the interventions described in this chapter. They are designed to increase families' knowledge, skills, and capacity so that they can take effective action on their own behalf. The ultimate goal is to assist families to become their own best advocates and resource. Table 7–15 identifies key family empowering interventions.

BARRIERS TO IMPLEMENTING FAMILY INTERVENTIONS

FAMILY-RELATED BARRIERS: APATHY AND INDECISION.   Barriers to implementing interventions may be either family behaviors and/or nurse behaviors. Dyer (1973) in his work with culturally diverse and poor families in the community identified problematic family behaviors that confront nurses. The first of these behaviors is apathy. It is manifested when the family responds to nursing actions with an apparent "so what" attitude and gives no sign of action or concern. Does the family really not care? Usually, they do care. Often, however, there are differences in values or beliefs that influence the family's responses, particularly if the family is of a different socioeconomic or ethnic background than the nurse. Behaviors that may be related to apathy include hopelessness (the belief that "whatever the family does, it won't matter anyway") and fatalism (the feeling that "what will be, will be"). Fatalism is a central theme among many poor and powerless families. Apathetic behavior also may be related to a sense of futility about the effectiveness or availability of services. Without a perception that effective and accessible treatment exists, clients are not going to seek health services.

Dyer (1973) also describes family indecision as a problem. In this instance, family members have difficulty making decisions or tend to use a "de facto style" when making decisions (letting things just happen). Such families often need the nurse to explore their feelings with them and to review the pros and cons of various options. Rather than assuming responsibility for making the family's decisions and inadvertently encouraging dependency, it is recommended that the nurse assume the role of a supportive resource person to the family.

TABLE 7–15

FAMILY EMPOWERING INTERVENTIONS

- Encouraging active family and family member participation
- Acting on and carefully listening to family members' concerns and starting where they want
- Recognizing families as equal partners or team members in the health care system
- Expanding families' visions of what options and possibilities exist
- Encouraging family self-help
- Enabling clients to exercise their autonomy and self-determination in deciding which options to choose
- Appreciating that families and nurses each have their own specialized expertise in maintaining health and managing health problems
- Recognizing that both families and nurses each bring strengths and resources into their relationship
- Discovering and affirming the strengths and resources of families, which becomes a foundation for trust
- Advocating on behalf of families at the client, health care system, and health policy levels
- Helping families develop more social supportiveness within their own families through the development of family relations skills
- Giving families the credit for positive changes and accomplishments that occur

In both of these situations, it is important for the nurse to probe into what is happening within the family and to be curious about the root of the problem so that it can be identified and subsequently addressed.

NURSE-RELATED BARRIERS.   Often, we think of barriers to implementing interventions as behaviors separate and apart from ourselves. However, some barriers to effective implementation of interventions may be related to the nurse's ideas or behaviors. Professional nurses must routinely reflect on their own beliefs and behaviors as they work with families to ensure that they are not inadvertently closing down options for families. Some common barriers are presented in Table 7–16 with an example of a self-reflective question that the nurse may routinely ask himself or herself to avoid such barriers.

EVALUATION AND MODIFICATION OF THE PLAN OF CARE

EVALUATION

The fifth component of the nursing process is evaluation. The evaluation is based on how effective the interventions were that the family, nurse, and others instituted. Effectiveness is determined by looking at family system and family member outcomes (how the family responded), rather than the interventions implemented. The evaluation, again, is a joint endeavor between the nurse and the family.

Although a client-centered approach to evaluation is most relevant, it is often frustrating because of the

TABLE 7–16

NURSE-RELATED BARRIERS TO IMPLEMENTING FAMILY INTERVENTIONS

BARRIER 1: IMPOSING IDEAS

The nurse assumes, and thus engages, in a noncollaborative relationship (a "one up" stance) with the family. Here the nurse may fall into the trap of imposing her or his ideas on the family without fully considering the family's expertise and ideas. The nurse assumes full responsibility for the nursing plan and its implementation (as opposed to an equal, nonhierarchical approach in which both nurse input and family input are respected and encouraged).

Self-Reflective Question: How frequently are decisions about the patient's health care made mutually by the patient, family, myself, and other members of the health care team?

BARRIER 2: NEGATIVE LABELING

The nurse may negatively label the family (or himself or herself) when interventions appear unsuccessful. For example, if a family returns for a clinic visit and has not implemented the nurse's ideas, the nurse may refer to this family as "resistant" or view his or her actions as "ineffective."

Self-Reflective Question: When interventions are not successful, what might I do differently? What might the family do differently? The treatment plan was ineffective—can I explain why?

BARRIER 3: OVERLOOKING STRENGTHS

Instead of paying attention to the strengths and resources that exist in the family, or to the family's previous success in other situations, the nurse highlights weaknesses and problems in the family.

Self-Reflective Question: What assessment or intervention activities can I use to further enhance this family's strengths?

BARRIER 4: NEGLECTING CULTURAL OR GENDER IMPLICATIONS

The nurse does not sufficiently take into account ethnic or cultural diversity or gender issues when planning interventions with the family.

Self-Reflective Question: In what ways does my plan of care reflect the cultural needs of this family? What, if any, are my own cultural or gender biases that may be constraining my work with this family?

Partially adapted from Leahey & Harper-Jaques, 1996.

difficulties in establishing objective criteria for desired outcomes and because of factors other than planned interventions that intervene and affect family/client outcomes. Because of such factors, one never gets a clear-cut, "pure" look at the efficacy of a nursing intervention.

The nursing care plan contains the framework for evaluation. If clear, specific behavioral goals have been delineated, these can then serve as the criteria for evaluating the degree of effectiveness achieved. In some instances there may be a need to develop even more specific criteria for evaluation of goals. For example, the goal, "The family will seek medical services for their sick baby," may need more specific criteria to judge whether the goal has been attained. Criteria for evaluation might include the fact that the family has been seen by a pediatrician and has received treatment for the baby's illness. In many cases, however, the goal is written in more specific terms to avoid further criteria development, such as, "The child will obtain diagnostic and treatment services from pediatrician within 1 to 3 days."

Evaluation is an ongoing process that occurs each time a nurse updates the nursing care plan. Before care plans are expanded or modified, certain nursing actions need to be reviewed by the nurse and family together to decide if they are really helpful. Unless family responses to nursing intervention are jointly evaluated, ineffective nursing action may persist.

The following questions should be contemplated when evaluating family responses:

- Is there a consensus between the family and other health care team members on the evaluation?

- What additional data need to be collected to evaluate progress?

- Were there any unforeseen outcomes that need to be considered?

- If the family's behavior and perceptions indicate that the problem has not been satisfactorily resolved, what are the reasons?

- Were the nursing diagnoses, goals, and approaches realistic and accurate?

Various methods of evaluation are used in nursing. Martin (1994) discussed some methods for measuring the quality of nursing practice. To this end, she recommended the use of case conferences; shared evaluation visits and observations, record audits, peer reviews, and utilization reviews; client satisfaction surveys; and external audits. The most important factor is that the method needs to be tailored to the goals and interventions being evaluated.

MODIFICATION

Modification follows the evaluation plan and begins the cyclical process of returning to the original assessment and reassessing it—feeding in the new information obtained from previous encounters, and then continuing to revise each phase in the cycle as needed. Modification is often difficult to do, as it can be frustrating and ego deflating to admit that a plan and/or an implementation was ineffective. So often in working with families on a long-term basis nurses see only very slow results or perhaps no movement of a family at all—at least not when they are

working with them. At this point, nurses need to make sure that if they continue the search for a more accurate diagnosis or a more effective plan, their efforts have some chance of success and the resources to be expended will be commensurate with the gain achieved. It is most important, however, to remember and work from the principle of self-determination—that families have a right to decide what is best for them and to make their own health decisions.

TERMINATING THE NURSE–FAMILY RELATIONSHIP

In working with a family over time, it is difficult to know when the time is right to bring closure to the nurse–family relationship. Wright and Leahey (2000) indicate that the most important indicator of termination is the family's ability to master or live with problems, not to eliminate them. Discussion about termination should occur early in the therapeutic process, so that both nurse and family are clear about expectations. Regular review of goals and progress helps to prevent problems with termination. Final termination may be initiated by the nurse, the family, or by another professional or agency (Wright & Leahey, 2000). Ideally, termination is mutually agreed upon by both the family and the nurse and when time is set aside for it, there is a final conversation about the work completed. Nurses need to be cautious about continuing to work with families when they are showing an ability to live with their problems; otherwise, continuing to work with the family may encourage unnecessary family dependency and may deplete system resources. Wright and Leahey (2000) provide a list of nursing actions that can be used in the therapeutic termination of the nurse–family relationship: review contracts, decrease the frequency of sessions, give credit to the family for changes it has made, evaluate family interviews, and offer follow-up services or referrals. These actions help to place a closure on the relationship and are intended to assist the family to sustain positive gains.

❧ SUMMARY

- The family nursing process will differ depending on the focus of care. If the nurse sees the family as the background or context of the individual patient, then the individual family members become the focus and the nursing process is individually oriented. If the nurse conceptualizes the family as the unit of care, then, even though the process itself does not vary, the family as a unit or system is the focus.

- Most family nurses in practice work simultaneously with both individual family members and with the family and its subsystems. This means the family nurse will utilize the nursing process on two levels—the individual level and the family and family subsystem level.

- Family assessment data should be collected in a systematic fashion using a family assessment tool, classified and analyzed for its meaning. Often, cursory data are collected on each of the major areas. When the assessor then finds significant probable or potential problems, the nurse then probes those areas more deeply.

- Family strengths should be identified in the assessment process.

- Family data collection comes from many sources: client interviews relative to past and present events, objective findings (e.g., observations of the home and its facilities), subjective appraisals (e.g., reported experiences of family members), written and oral information from referrals, various agencies working with the family, and other health team members.

- The establishment of a trusting relationship in which there is mutual respect and open, honest communication goes hand in hand with the assessment process and orientation phase of working with a family. By promoting trust, the nurse is also creating a context for the family to be open to implementing future family nursing interventions.

- After the assessment is completed, the data need to be summarized and collated, grouping similar data together and arranging them in orderly form so that accurate conclusions and problems can be identified.

- In this text, a comprehensive family assessment tool is presented in Chapters 8 through 17 and Appendices A and B.

- At the family level, the nursing diagnosis can be derived from using one of the family or nursing theories or from using North American Nursing Diagnosis Association (NANDA) diagnoses or the Omaha System.

- Although family is included in NANDA's definition of nursing diagnoses, the list of diagnoses applicable to the family remains limited, and thus has gained criticism from nurses concerned about family-centered care.

- The Omaha system is a widely used tool in community-based nursing. It consists of a problem classification scheme, an intervention scheme, and a problem rating scale for outcomes.

- In stating a family nursing diagnosis, the nurse needs to indicate at what family system level the problem lies—at the family unit level or at the level of one of the family subsystems or sets of relationships such as the marital dyad, the parent–child subsystem, or the sibling subsystem.

- One of the problems in determining health needs or problems of families is that all the information gathered is interrelated, and there are almost insurmountable difficulties involved in sorting out cause-and-effect relationships.

- Problems identified in family nursing often focus on the family's ability to cope with a health or environmental problem. In many situations there will be no present medical illness or disability. In these cases the most frequent diagnoses are preventive or health promotional.

- The needs for which family health nurses can affect change or on which we can make a discernible, positive health impact in an efficient manner are the problems we should be assisting families to alleviate or ameliorate.

- In goal setting, it is desirable to work with the family in differentiating problems that need to be resolved by nursing intervention, problems the family as the self-care agent can handle by itself, and problems that need to be referred to other members of the health care team or handled on a collaborative basis.

- Families have the right and responsibility to make their own health decisions. Because of this premise of family nursing, there will be certain actions that fully informed families choose with which we may personally and professionally disagree.

- Nursing interventions are any treatment, based on clinical judgment, that a nurse performs to enhance patient/client outcomes. Nursing interventions include both direct and indirect care; those aimed at individuals, families, and the community; and nurse-initiated, physician-initiated, and other provider-initiated treatments.

- Nursing Intervention Classification (NIC) and the Calgary Family Intervention Model (CFIM) are two systems developed to date to systematically organize and describe nursing interventions.

- CFIM focuses on promoting, improving, and/or sustaining effective family functioning in three domains: cognitive (thoughts), affective (emotions), and behavioral (actions).

- The aims of teaching are to support healthy behaviors and to change unhealthy behaviors, albeit alterations of behavior are not always immediate or observable.

- The skills that health care professionals need when providing ongoing medical information and advice to families consist of regularly and clearly communicating health findings and treatment options to family members, attentively listening to family members' questions and concerns, and advising families how to handle the health and rehabilitation needs of the patient.

- Role modeling is a powerful modality for teaching family members how to modify their behaviors.

- Anticipatory guidance provides the family with information as to what to expect with respect to a future event, a potential problem/issue, or a child's next developmental phase.

- Counseling is a process that seeks to help families and their members address, resolve, and effectively cope with their problems, and to utilize their competencies and other resources more fully.

- A contract is a working agreement made between two or more parties, such as between a family and a nurse or between parents and a child. To be timely and relevant, contracts are continuously renegotiable and cover the following areas: goals, length of the contract, client responsibilities (commitments) and health care team members' responsibilities, steps toward meeting the goals, and rewards for meeting goals.

- Case management is seen as a system, a clinical decision-making process, a technology, a role, and a service. Barriers to using this approach with families include the lack of funding to provide these services to families, the dearth of nurses educated to serve in this role, and the perception that the role need not be filled by a nurse.

- Patient advocacy is seeing that the patient knows what to expect and what he or she is entitled to have, and then displaying the willingness and courage to see that our system does not prevent him or her from getting it.

- Acting as a coordinator, the nurse ensures that the client does not receive a duplication of some services from different agencies or, even more distressing, a gap in essential areas of need.

- Collaboration is a process of shared planning and action over time with joint responsibility for the outcomes and the ability to work together for common goals using problem-solving techniques.

- The consultant's role is often to provide problem-solving assistance with clinical issues. In the consultation process, the consultee is free to accept or reject the consultant's recommendations and remains directly responsible for implementing action and outcomes of care.

- Barriers to implementing interventions include family apathy, family indecision, and possibly the nurse's own behaviors and beliefs that may be in discord with the family's values and goals.

- Evaluation is based on how effective the interventions were that the family, nurse, and others instituted. Effectiveness is determined by looking at family member outcomes (how the family responded), rather than the interventions implemented.

- Modification follows the evaluation plan and begins the cyclical process of returning to the assessment and reassessing—feeding in the new information obtained from previous encoun-

ters, and then continuing to revise each phase in the cycle as needed.

- It is ideal, when termination is mutually agreed upon by family and nurse and when time is set aside, to have a final conversation about the work completed.

❧ FAMILY VIGNETTE: THE PAUL FAMILY

The visiting nurse has made her first home visit to an elderly couple. Mr. Paul, age 80, has severe emphysema and has just been discharged from a local general hospital. His sister is also 80 and has assumed the caretaker role. Both siblings lost their spouses within the past year and have now taken up residence together. In completing a nursing assessment, one of the observations the visiting nurse made is that Mr. Paul is seeing three doctors (a pulmonary specialist, an internist for his "heart condition," and a general practitioner who is a lifelong friend and sees Mr. Paul for immediate problems or "anything else"). Mr. Paul's bathroom is filled with prescriptions—new, old, same drugs with different doses, and several drugs that have similar actions—prescribed by the different physicians. The patient, being quite concerned regarding his health, is complying by taking all of these. The sister is confused and finds caring for her bedridden brother alone a real burden. She complains of a continual backache and fatigue.

▪ STUDY QUESTIONS

Review the Family Vignette and answer the related questions.

1. Select a nursing diagnosis that summarizes a primary need of this family.
2. Identify the family strengths that exist within this family.
3. Propose four nursing interventions to implement with this family.

Answer the following questions about the nursing process.

4. The primary difference between the nursing process when working with families versus working solely with individual clients is:
   a. The community setting must be assessed.
   b. The level of assessment, diagnosis, planning, implementation, and evaluation is broadened to include the family, its subsystems, and its members.
   c. The level of assessment, diagnosis, planning, implementation, and evaluation is the family system.
   d. Prevention and health promotion are the aim versus cure and rehabilitation when working with individuals.

5. Match the correct process characteristics in the left-hand column with the nursing phase/component on the right.

Process Characteristics

a. Continuous data collection
b. Approaches based on identified goals
c. Client outcome appraisal
d. Anticipated behaviorally stated client responses
e. Setting of priorities
f. Nursing action, therapy, or approaches
g. Execution of the nursing care plan
h. Existing or potential family and individual health problem
i. Mobilizing community resources
j. Identification of resources
k. Refinement and revision efforts
l. Defining alternative approaches

Phase/Components of Nursing Process

1. Assessment
2. Diagnosis
3. Goal setting
4. Plan of care
5. Intervention
6. Evaluation
7. Modification

6. The nursing assessment is:

a. Based on initial gathering of data
b. Done by all persons involved in providing client care
c. A sensitive and continuing process conducted by all involved health providers

Match the nurse's statements (questions 7 through 11) with the appropriate step in the nursing process.

a. Establishing a relationship
b. Obtaining information
c. Clarification of focal problem
d. Assessment of strengths and resources
e. Formulation of a therapeutic plan and mobilization of client's and others' resources

7. "How have things been with your family?"

8. "I'm concerned about your problem and would like to know more."

9. "Can you tell me about the fight with your wife?"

10. "How can I be most helpful to you and your family at this time?"

11. "When you discuss your worries with your sister, what is her response?"

Answer the following questions.

12. List three activities the family health nurse could carry out in preparation for a home visit.

13. In planning nursing intervention, priorities need to be established. These variables are significant when establishing priorities:

a. Family/individual interests and perceptions
b. Degree of urgency or acuteness of problem
c. Availability of resources
d. Agency policies
e. Actions that are prerequisite to other actions

14. Active family involvement in the nursing process should occur during phase(s) of the nursing process.

15. List two situations when family nursing intervention may be indicated according to Wright and Leahey (2000).

16. From the list below, select two major concepts of change that are important to consider when assisting families to make changes.
    a. Change depends on the nature of the stressors families face.
    b. Change only occurs if both parents are in agreement.
    c. Gaining the right information leads to change.
    d. Change is situationally determined.
    e. The client's perception of the problem is critical in considering change.

17. What are three sources of data for family assessment?

18. List the three domains of family functioning discussed in the Calgary Family Intervention Model and one possible intervention that could be directed at each domain.

19. According to Wright and Leahey (2000), the most important indicator of therapeutic termination with a family is _____.

20. Ways to actively involve families include (check the appropriate choices):
    a. Asking them questions about how they have solved similar problems in the past.
    b. Advising them to follow prescribed recommendations.
    c. Encouraging them to discuss the various options available to them to meet their needs.
    d. Bringing all the family members together to discuss what might be done and who could do it.
    e. Recognizing that clients often lack the competency to make their own health decisions and, hence, need advice on what decisions to make.

21. Match the specific family interventions (from the left-hand column) with the descriptions of the interventions (in the right-hand column). More than one answer is correct for each intervention.

___ Teaching	a. Role modeling
___ Case management	b. Involves intraagency and/or extraagency linkages
___ Coordination	c. A working agreement between two or more parties
___ Advocacy	d. Processes that facilitate learning
___ Collaboration	e. An interpersonal, interventive process
___ Consultation	f. Assist families to use their own problem-solving skills and strengths
___ Contracting	g. Giving professional advice to another helping person.
___ Counseling	h. Speaking for or on behalf of a client.
	i. Working closely with another professional to provide health services.

22. Match the types of limitations/barriers in the right-hand column with the interventions in the left-hand column. More than one limitation/barrier can be associated with each of the interventions.

___ Case management   a. Decreased client motivation to change health behaviors.

___ Teaching   b. Cultural and language barriers between involved parties.

___ Collaboration   c. Families do not see nurses fulfilling this interventive role.

___ Contracting   d. Organization for which nurse works is not supportive of nursing intervention.

___ Counseling   e. Setting for sustained or sufficient interaction inadequate.

   f. Working relationships are often hierarchical or stratified.

   g. Families are leaderless, chaotic, or very dependent.

   h. Inhibiting economic factors (lack of reimbursement, payment for intervention).

23. Identify three NANDA nursing diagnoses for which teaching would be an appropriate intervention.

24. Identify three NANDA family nursing diagnoses for which counseling would be an appropriate intervention.

25. For what types of families would basic supportive family counseling versus family therapy be more appropriate?

26. For what type of health problems would family case management be most indicated?

Are the following statements true or false?

27. The steps in the nursing process and the teaching/learning process are the same.

28. In the assessment phase of the teaching/learning process, the sole focus is assessing the learner's readiness to learn.

29. Learning needs are analogous to assessment in the nursing process.

30. Determining the particular teaching strategies to be employed is part of the implementation phase.

31. Contracts can be unwritten or written.

32. Contracts are legal agreements between two sets of individuals.

33. Contracts encourage self-responsibility and self-care.

34. Using contracts greatly aids in the evaluation process.

35. A contract must contain time limitations.

36. A contract is made by the nurse and signed by the patient.

37. A contract spells out goals to be achieved and the respective responsibilities of the involved parties.

Answer the following short-answer question.

38. There are many factors that serve to promote or inhibit learning in families. Identify several important inhibiting factors.

FAMILY IDENTIFYING DATA: SOCIOCULTURAL ASSESSMENT AND INTERVENTION

❧ CONTENT OUTLINE

❧ LEARNING OBJECTIVES

1. Explain why an understanding of a family's ethnic background is crucial for family health practice.

2. Discuss several of the major problems that result when cultural insensitivity and ignorance exist on the part of a health care professional.

3. Define these basic concepts: culture, ethnicity, stereotyping, acculturation, assimilation, biculturalism, cultural relativism, ethnocentrism, cultural imposition, cultural conflicts, cultural shock, indigenous health care system, self-fulfilling prophecy, cultural empathy, and ethclass.

4. Discuss the importance of the cross-cultural/transcultural approach to family health care.

5. Define the difference between cultural variation and cultural deviance models with respect to ethnic families.

6. Identify some of the differences in values and norms among the social classes.

7. With respect to health disparities among the poor, name two particular health problems that are positively correlated with poverty.

8. Define and describe the following family identifying data, applying content to a family vignette:

a. Family composition
b. Type of family form
c. Cultural (ethnic) and religious orientation
d. Social class status

9. Based on the family vignette, assess the family's sociocultural background.

10. Present two reasons why retaining ethnic identity can be a positive resource for family members.

11. Describe broad sociocultural intervention strategies that are effective in working with ethnic families.

12. Identify two strategies for assisting families with their health-related financial difficulties.

This chapter presents content about the sociocultural context in which the family is embedded. A crucial key to unlock our understanding of a family and why and how it behaves is the family's sociocultural background. The chapter begins by discussing the family's cultural orientation—its importance, the role of pluralism in our society, and the cross-cultural or transcultural approach to family health care. Basic sociocultural concepts and minority families are described. The concept of social class and its significance in understanding families' lifestyles and values includes a discussion of the social class structure in the United States, with particular emphasis on the lower class, poverty in America, and the impact of poverty on health. Family's economic status and social class mobility are also addressed. The chapter ends with a discussion of family assessment areas (identifying data, culture, socioeconomic status, and social class mobility), family nursing diagnoses, and family nursing interventions in the sociocultural and financial areas.

THE FAMILY'S CULTURAL ORIENTATION

A family's cultural orientation or background may well be the most pertinent variable in understanding a family's behavior, its value system, and functions. Because culture permeates and circumscribes our individual, familial, and social actions, its consequences are pervasive and its implication for practice broad.

Given that understanding the family's cultural background is so critical in working with families, familial differences among three major ethnic groups in the United States are explored in Chapters 18 through 20. Chapter 13 on the family's value system will also help the family nurse look at cultural patterns, because family values and beliefs are often a reflection of the value and belief systems of the family's reference groups, such as the ethnic and religious subcultures with which the family identifies.

IMPORTANCE OF CULTURE FOR PRACTICE

In a culturally diverse society such as ours, we need to develop cohesiveness as a society and community, while at the same time recognize and celebrate the uniqueness of our diverse parts (Marks, 2000). Bringing this notion down to the level of practice, to understand and to be able to work efficaciously with families from cultures different from their own, health care professionals must be aware of the unique, distinctive qualities and the variety of lifestyles, values, and structures in families' cultures. Hence the importance of culture lies in its vital, unique character. Because cultural differences are often at the root of poor communication, interpersonal tensions, avoidance in working effectively with others, and poor assessment of health problems and their remedies, successful nursing care of clients of various ethnic backgrounds is dependent on the nurse's knowledge of and sensitivity to the clients' culture (Canino & Spurlock, 1994; Lipson, 1996; Ridley & Lingle, 1996).

In counseling and teaching families, the importance of culture is paramount. Without knowledge of the differences in cultural norms and patterns, behavior that differs from normative patterns is usually labeled as noncompliant, deviant, crazy, immoral, or illegal (depending on the type of prescribed behavior violated). In the absence of cultural data and understanding, it becomes impossible for the health care worker to recognize the possible cultural meaning of the client's behavior or actions. Four important areas where cultural dissimilarity may permeate and disrupt counseling and teaching are: (1) goal expectations, (2) the establishment of rapport, (3) communication, and (4) client's acceptance of ideas or recommendations (Coddy, 1975; Pedersen, Draguns, Lonner, & Trimble, 1996; Rankin & Stallings, 2001).

The benefit of nurse–client cultural congruence is well documented. Several noted authors have pointed to the greater ease and efficacy of client and the health care professionals when they have similar ethnic and religious backgrounds (Flaskerud, 1984; Leppa, 1999). When similar frames of references exist in a relationship, the possibilities of greater freedom of expression, deeper identification, and increased empathy present themselves. However, having a health care worker and client of the same ethnic background is an ideal but usually not a practical situation. In reality ethnic congruency is not often possible, and not even socially desirable. Otherwise, how are we, as citizens in a multicultural society, to learn to live and relate well to one another?

Language is a fundamental aspect of culture/ethnicity. The critical nature of language barriers also deserves mention (Lipson & Meleis, 1999). In some regions, where a majority or plurality of one's clients are from a different culture and speak a different language, learning the culture's language will not only result in dramatically improved communication but also in a much greater understanding and appreciation of the culture (Giger & Davidhizar, 1999). Padilla (1976) verifies this assertion in his study of lower-class Mexican-Americans who were being seen in therapy in a counseling center in East Los Angeles. He states that it has generally been assumed by therapists that lower-class persons have difficulty benefiting from psychotherapy because of their nonverbalness, inarticulateness, and lack of ability to think abstractly. Padilla reports, however, that in counseling

Latino clients, this generalization does not hold true when clients were given the opportunity and encouraged to communicate in Spanish, English, or a combination of both in order to enhance the meaningfulness of their communication. He concludes that, "It now seems clear that the Chicano poor are quite capable of verbally expressing themselves in the most intensive 'insight' therapy situation, if they are not forced to communicate in English, a language that may be partly or completely foreign to these individuals" (p. 289).

CULTURAL–ETHNIC PLURALISM

Our country is truly a matrix of many ethnic groups or subcultures. The United States is experiencing the greatest growth in immigration in 100 years. A massive surge of immigration in the 1990s makes one in every three U.S. residents a minority (U.S. Bureau of the Census, 2000). Three quarters of immigrants are from Mexico and Asia. Almost 44 percent of the nation's foreign-born arrived in the last 10 years, compared to a previous peak in immigration of 32 percent in 1910 (Fields, 2001).

Although various geographical regions felt this influx of immigrants differentially during the 1990s, there was a major dispersal of immigrants to all regions of the nation. Cities that have experienced high rates of immigration are Los Angeles and New York. In Los Angeles, 4 out of 10 immigrants are foreign born, while in New York 3 out of 10 are foreign born. The U.S. Census figures (U.S. Bureau of the Census, 1990, 2000) illustrate this trend (Table 8–1).

In the largest state in the Union, California, it is projected that by 2030, non-Hispanic whites will be an aging minority within the state's population, while ethnic minority people (Latinos, African-Americans, and Asians/Pacific islanders) will be "the emergent majority" (Fields, 2001; Hayes-Battista, 1990).

Massive waves of immigration have continued to mold and revolutionize the character of the United States throughout the last two centuries. The myth of the American melting pot has been intellectually recognized, although its implications not completely dissipated. This myth encouraged all diverse ethnic groups immigrating to the United States to succeed in American society by becoming part of the one predominant group. Any differences were typically seen as

TABLE 8–1

PERCENT OF ACTUAL AND PROJECTED U.S. POPULATION OF ETHNIC MINORITIES ACCORDING TO 1980, 1990, AND 2000 CENSUS DATA

| | PERCENT OF U.S. POPULATION | | | | |
ETHNIC GROUP	1980	1990	1996	2000	2050 PROJECTION
Blacks	11.7%	12.1%	12.2%	12.1%	14%
Hispanics[a]	6.4%	9.0%	10.2%	11.3%	25%
Asians and Pacific Islanders	1.5%	3.0%	3.3%	3.7%	8%
Native Americans	0.6%	0.8%	0.8%	0.8%	0.9%

[a] Hispanics will become the nation's largest minority group by 2009, based on U.S. Census projections.

Sources: Baringer (1991); Rosenblatt (1996); and U.S. Bureau of the Census (1991a & 2000)

deviant and inferior. Ethnic variation was perceived as an element of the lower social class and of recent immigrant groups. Moving up the social class ladder to success meant discarding one's ethnic traditions and values and assimilating into the mainstream of society.

The social protests of the 1960s brought about the harsh realization that the society had not, and did not wish to, move toward one homogeneous entity. The civil rights movement and the rise of black consciousness and identity set the model for all other ethnic groups. This model stressed a reaffirmation of cultural differences, a greater demand for equal treatment, and an acceptance of the value of ethnic or cultural diversity in society. Stemming from this push for cultural pluralism and the growing demographic imperative, American values have changed, reflecting a greater tolerance for diversity.

McGoldrick and Giordano (1996) point out that a ". . . positive sense of ethnic and racial identity is essential for developing a healthy personal and group identity" (p. 4). Trying to assimilate and forget one's heritage may be hazardous to one's health. Several studies agree that "when people are secure in their identity, they act with greater flexibility and openness to those of other cultural backgrounds" (McGoldrick & Giordano, p. 9). Ethnic identification provides for many persons and families an alternative link to the broader society, partially compensating for the cold, impersonal, and bureaucratic qualities of society today. Moreover, ethnicity can be seen as enriching family life and strengthening the bonds of intergenerational continuity.

The reality of the new millennium is that the United States is truly multicultural. A demographic imperative exists for practicing transcultural family nursing.

THE CROSS-CULTURAL OR TRANSCULTURAL APPROACH

The cross-cultural approach used in anthropology provides a broad comparative picture of human nature and human behavior and is the basis for transcultural nursing (Leininger, 1970, 2001). This approach to family nursing care is both a practical necessity and a social reality, due to the pervasive part culture plays and the growing number of people in the United States from different cultural backgrounds. As we become familiar with other cultures and learn to appreciate why certain values and norms are effective through time in those cultures, it is hoped that health care workers will become more sensitive and effective in providing family health care.

Leininger (1970, 1995, 2001) asserts that it is not only sound for nursing to use a cross-cultural or transcultural approach, it is mandatory: Clients have a *right* to have their sociocultural backgrounds understood in the same way that they expect their physical and psychological needs to be recognized and understood. The cultural and the social aspects of care has been, until only recently, largely ignored. We often pay only lip service to assessing clients' sociocultural factors. Transcultural nursing practice, with a theoretical and research knowledge base, is essential for providing quality care to people and families from diverse cultures (2001).

The following concepts or terms are of fundamental importance for understanding cross-cultural principles and practice.

CULTURE.   Foremost among these concepts is that of **culture.** Culture is usually viewed as a blueprint for our way of living, thinking, behaving, and feeling. It circumscribes and guides the ways in which societies and ethnic groups solve their problems and derive meaning from their lives. From a systems perspective, culture is defined as systems of socially transmitted behavioral patterns that link human groups to their environmental settings, as well as systems of social change and organization that act to mediate societal adaptation (Leininger, 1976). Culture denotes patterns of learned behavior and values that are transmitted from one generation to the next (Giger & Davidhizar, 1999).

In other words, culture is a mold from which we all are cast. It constrains and regulates our daily behavior, attitudes, and values in many latent and manifest ways. Because people rely on learned behavior or culture for survival, it is the prime source of our adaptability.

When defining culture, a broad, comprehensive, inclusive definition is needed. With this in mind, culture includes:

1. Ethnographic variables (e.g., nationality, ethnicity, language, and religion)

2. Demographic variables (e.g., age, gender, place of residence, and generation)

3. Status variables (e.g., social, economic, and education)

4. Affiliation variables (e.g., formal and informal group memberships) (Falicov, 1988; Locke, 1992).

The following definition of culture by Falicov (1988) incorporates these components:

Those sets of shared world views and adaptive behaviors derived from simultaneous member-

ship in a variety of contexts, such as ecological setting (rural, urban, suburban), religious background, nationality and ethnicity, social class, gender-related experiences, minority status, occupation, political leanings, migratory patterns, stages of acculturation or values derived from belonging to the same generation partaking of a single historical moment, or particular ideologies. (p. 336)

ETHNICITY.   **Ethnicity** is a key facet of culture and refers to a common ancestry, a sense of "peoplehood" and group identity. From a common ancestry and a shared social and cultural history and national origin have evolved shared values and customs (Giger & Davidhizer, 1999; McGoldrick, 1993; McGoldrick & Giordano, 1996). Our ethnic background significantly influences our thnking, behaving, feelings, perceptions, rituals and celebrations, diet, values, and health and illness beliefs and practices (Huff & Kline, 1999).

Ethnicity is deeply tied to the family as it is the family that transmits this legacy. "A group's sense of commonality is transmitted over generations by the family and reinforced by the surrounding community" (McGoldrick & Giordano, 1996, p. 1).

Race and ethnicity should not be confused with each other. Race denotes biological variation, distinguishing people based on physical characteristics such as skin color, facial features, and hair texture (Huff & Kline, 1999). People of one race can vary in terms of their ethnicity and culture. For example, in the white race there are perhaps a hundred or more different ethnic groups. With the exception of the Census Bureau, race is not considered a correct or useful means of classifying people. Because there has been substantial genetic inbreeding of world populations, there are no distinct, pure races today (Henderson, 2000). In addition, the growth in intermarriage reinforces the need to eliminate the old notion of race. The Census Bureau, in face of this new reality, permits residents to indicate more than one ethnic/racial category (Meacham, 2000).

Ethnicity is often used interchangeably with culture or subculture, even though ethnicity is defined more narrowly; that is, the term culture includes many more dimensions than just ethnicity. Using the two terms interchangeably leads to confusion.

However, when we speak of a person's or families' "cultural background," we most often are referring to their ethnic background. Therefore, in this text, ethnicity will be used primarily to discuss persons or families from different national origins and different group identities.

Religion is very much intertwined with ethnicity. In some families, the family's religion is a vital shaper of health values, beliefs, and practices (Andrews & Boyle, 1995). But in secular families, religion's influence is generally more muted.

INTRAETHNIC VARIATION (VARIATION WITHIN ETHNIC GROUPS). Just as there are enormous differences in people between ethnic groups, there is also a great variation in people *within* the same ethnic group. Much of the variation we see *in* families with the same ethnic background is a function of the degree to which the family subscribes to the American culture, as well as regional differences in the native culture, social class differences, histories of intermarriage, or simply idiosyncratic variation. It is of utmost importance to take into account the diversity among families within the various ethnic groups (Goldenberg & Goldenberg, 2000).

THE IMMIGRATION EXPERIENCE. Many ethnic minority families are recent immigrants. These immigrant families have experienced the complex stress of immigration and migration and perhaps the even greater stress associated with being a refugee. Although these stressful experiences are often "buried," they subtly continue to shape a family's outlook and its adjustment (Bullrich, 1989).

Being a refugee is particularly stressful, as most refugees leave their countries of origin involuntarily. They usually enter the United States and other countries to escape from intolerable and chaotic conditions. Leaving one's own country of origin under these conditions causes loss of family ties, identity, and culture; a lowered socioeconomic and employment status; language problems; dramatic shifts in social, familial, and gender roles; acculturation problems in the new country; and mental health issues (Bemak, Chung, & Bornemann, 1996; Lipson & Meleis, 1999).

STEREOTYPING. Lack of recognition of individual differences or labeling is termed **stereotyping.** Cultural

stereotyping involves the nonacceptance or disallowance of individual or group diversity; everyone from a particular culture is viewed as the same and perceived of as fixed in their characteristics. And usually these characteristics are negative. Stereotyping often leads to discrimination such as the widespread "isms" prevalent in our society, that is, racism, sexism, classism, ethnocentrism, ageism, and heterosexualism (homophobia). Moreover, recent research has shown that when people are reminded of a negative stereotype that pertains to themselves, such as "women can't do math," it can adversely affect performance (Begley, 2000).

Unfortunately, the tendency is to simplify things by stereotyping people. Kay (1978) discusses the perennial problem of generalizing about a group of people in anthropological–ethnographic descriptions:

> Most ethnographies, or accounts of the life style of people who participate in a specific culture, are like still photographs. They describe people staggered in time and space. We call such fixed images stereotypes. Modal personalities are frozen in a changeless place, and subsequently are supposed to represent millions. But if we try to qualify groups by describing certain differences (e.g., 72 percent of *barrio* women make their own tortillas as compared with 12 percent who buy Rainbo bread), we end up by describing no one. (p. 89)

We need to be able to generalize about an ethnic group in order to learn about and discuss that group of people; but at the same time, remember that cultural characteristics refer to group characteristics only.

Hence the knowledge that the father typically holds primary power in the traditional Mexican-American home, or that the Jewish mother often is "the power behind the throne" in the Jewish family, serves as a clue about a family's background. However, these culturally derived patterns need to be verified with the particular family the nurse is assessing.

Tripp-Reimer and Lauer (1987) caution family nurses who plan nursing care on the basis of a family's ethnicity. They explain that

> clients may not want traditional beliefs and customs incorporated into their care if alternative approaches are acceptable. Ethnic clients may not wish to remain unassimilated; indeed, it may sim-

ply perpetuate another form of stereotype to assume that all members of an ethnic group sub- scribe to the culture's most conservative position. (p. 96)

Tripp-Reimer and Lauer call this problem the "tra- ditionalist fallacy." We cannot assume we know what a family and its members want simply because we know the family's ethnic background. A cultural assessment of each individual family is essential before delivering care.

ACCULTURATION.   Exposure of persons from one cultural group to another culture leads to a sociocultural process called **acculturation.** As one of the major causative factors of variation within an ethnic group, acculturation comprises those gradual changes pro- duced when an individual from one culture adopts the traits of the dominant/host culture (Huff & Kline, 1999). When ethnic groups immigrate to the United States, the American culture exerts great influence on the ethnic group to conform to its cul- tural patterns. The resultant **assimilation** may pro- ceed so far as to practically extinguish the ethnic cul- ture (as occurred with the African culture during slavery) or factors may intervene to counterbalance the forces of assimilation and keep the two cultures isolated from one another. For example, historically language and religious, economic, and geographic barriers kept Mexican-Americans and Native Americans fairly separate from American society. The strong cul- tural traditions of Jews and Armenians have to a large extent limited their assimilation. Assimilation denotes the more complete and one-way process of one culture being absorbed into the other. There are degrees of acculturation, ranging from the bicultural person to the traditional person, who has held on to all or most of his or her traits from the mother country.

The rate and degree of acculturation of any ethnic group into the dominant culture depends primarily on the degree of congruency between a group's own basic value orientations and those of the dominant (American) culture. Also, certain groups within a par- ticular ethnic subculture are more receptive to social and cultural change. For instance, among urban resi- dents, the more educated, occupationally successful, or socioeconomically advantaged are more likely to experience greater assimilation. Hence, socioeco-

nomic and class factors are crucial elements to con- sider in learning about a family's ethnicity.

Acculturation, then, implies that members of cul- tures other than the dominant culture of the society have internalized to a great extent the norms and val- ues of the dominant, mainstream culture. Moreover, the wider society has been influenced to varying degrees by its exposure to ethnic or subcultural groups immigrating to a host country. Examples of regions where immigrating ethnic groups have greatly influenced the local culture include the bor- der states with Mexico, where the influence of the Latino culture is pervasively seen in many spheres of life (e.g., food, the visual and performing arts, the job/occupational structure, mass media, and neigh- borhood businesses).

The level of acculturation of family members is often mediated by generation. Older generations, particularly those who emigrate late in life, tend to cling to values and traditions from the old country. In contrast, first-generation persons born in the United States and those who emigrate while young are found to acculturate, even while claiming to retain their own cultural heritage (McCallion, Janicki, & Grant- Griffin, 1997).

Thus, acculturation does not necessarily suggest the loss of ethnic identity—of a detaching of oneself from an ethnic community—nor does it imply the loss of many of the customs related to that culture. Customs that continue, more or less unscathed, are those that are not stigmatizing or illegal, customs such as those involving food, religion, music, and dance. Many times these become the major tangible cultural difference, remnants of cultures quite differ- ent. As elements of the old and new culture inter- twine, a unique subculture is formed.

Members of ethnic minorities are inevitably part of two cultures to some extent. Most ethnic minority families are then bicultural. **Biculturalism** signifies participation in two cultural systems and often requires two sets of behavior and ways of thinking (Ho, 1987). All ethnic groups have expressed bicul- turalism as an important adaptive strategy (Harrison et al., 1994).

REAL VERSUS THE IDEAL.   To understand a family's cultural background we need to understand both its values (what family members say is important or *the ideal*) and its actual behavior (*the real*). Often the variance between the two is striking. It is typically due to the pragmatic adaptation of a family to a particular social and historical context (Friedman, 1990). Sheer practical necessity can often distort one's values in everyday life, so that they become unrecognizable (Graedon, 1985). Numerous examples of the distinction between the real and ideal can be seen in the adaptations ethnic families make to poverty and discrimination.

CULTURAL RELATIVISM. In working with clients from various cultural backgrounds the aim in the health care professions is to eliminate ethnocentric beliefs and substitute instead a relativistic cultural perspective. **Cultural relativism** refers to the perspective that holds that "cultures are neither inferior nor superior to one another and that there is no single scale for measuring the value of a culture. Therefore, customs, beliefs, and practices must be judged or understood relative to the context in which they appear" (Aamodt, 1978, p. 9). To do this, the health care worker must be flexible enough to understand and accept the cultural perspective of those with whom he or she works.

ETHNOCENTRISM. **Ethnocentrism** implies the lack of cultural relativism. There is the assumption that one's way of believing and behaving is the most preferable and correct one (Huff & Kline, 1999). Health care professionals may be ethnocentric when working with families from different sociocultural backgrounds. It is then important to become informed about families from other ethnicities to counter the tendency of believing that the way our own family or health system culture operates is the way in which all (normal) families do and should operate.

CULTURAL IMPOSITION. A result of ethnocentrism is the problem of **cultural imposition.** When health workers feel either consciously or unconsciously that their beliefs and practices are superior and proper, they use subtle and/or apparent ways to force their own values, beliefs, and practices on individuals from different ethnic orientations (Leininger, 1974).

Cultural imposition may then lead to cultural conflicts—situations in which health care professionals covertly or overtly try to impose their health practices on their clients and the clients react negatively. As nurses, we can think of many ways in which clients

"fight back," many times to their own detriment, because of the health system's lack of recognition of their culturally patterned beliefs and practices. The commonly seen reticence of Hispanic families to place one of their members in a hospital because of being forced to separate from the family member is a case in point. When family visiting and participation rights are relaxed to allow for a flexible consideration of client and family attitudes and patterns, both the client and the health care system benefit.

To counter the frequently experienced problems of cultural imposition and cultural conflicts, Leininger (1976) suggests that "the nurse must truly understand a culture before imposing any changes on the people. Sensitivity and foresight are essential to work in diverse cultural contexts" (p. 40). In order to understand a client's culture and provide *culturally competent* care, one must first be aware of one's own value orientation and the health care patterns in one's own culture (McGoldrick & Giordano, 1996; Spector, 2000). The family nurse must also discover— through questions we ask and observations of responses we make—the family member's beliefs about health and illness, particularly of the family's perception of the health problems family members are having. We must assume nothing until adequate validation takes place.

CULTURAL SHOCK. Family nurses and students commonly experience feelings of cultural shock when visiting with or interacting with families whose culture is (a) at great variance with their own, (b) one about which they are uninformed, and/or (c) one to which they have had little exposure. **Cultural shock** refers to a condition in which a person, in response to an environment so altered that meaningful objects and experiences have been replaced by those from a different culture, feels confused, immobilized, and "lost" (Aamodt, 1978). Feelings and sensations of discomfort are more pronounced or noticeable when visiting in the home environment, because the family's differences are much more obvious than when the nurse–client encounter is in a health care setting. Discomfort is also more intense because of the fact that the health care worker is in the client's "territory."

Lifestyle and value differences are not easy to deal with. Our own values and attitudes will greatly influence our perceptions and nursing assessments and interventions. Therefore, personal feelings, beliefs, and attitudes must be identified, discussed, and accepted before we can effectively help families seeking assistance.

INDIGENOUS HEALTH CARE SYSTEMS.   The last of the more general cultural concepts has to do more specifically with health care practices. Every culture has devised its own **indigenous,** or **lay health care system** as opposed to the Western *scientific or professional health care system.* Some of these systems are well-developed and have been used effectively for centuries to treat certain conditions, such as the Eastern system of health care. The indigenous health care system uses traditional folk care modalities. Practitioners of an indigenous system are often the first-line, primary care practitioners—the first healers to be consulted by unacculturated ethnic families. They also may be contacted for certain "folk" illnesses or when Western medicine fails to be effective. As part of the cross-cultural approach proposed earlier, it is recommended that professional systems need to become more culturally attuned to these systems and to learn how to work cooperatively with non-Western health care practitioners, rather than in opposition to them (Bushy, 1990; Engebretson, 1994; Germain, 1992). Health care professionals tend to downplay the significance and value of folk-health care and practices. These feelings are both inaccurate and detrimental, however, because much folk medicine is effective (Leininger, 1976).

In fact, in most cases the merits of any indigenous treatment depend on whether the sick client recovers or not, and indigenous health care does work in many instances. This is particularly true in illnesses where psychogenic factors are prominent and where effective treatment of the disease depends on a knowledge of the context of the person's cultural belief system. Given this, who knows or appreciates the psychogenic and the cultural context better than the folk practitioner?

ETHNIC FAMILIES

Ethnic families are those families that are classified as belonging to ethnic or cultural groups other than white ethnic groups, such as the Irish, Poles, and Jews. They also are called "ethnic people of color,"

this group comprised about 29 percent of our population in 1996 (U.S. Bureau of the Census, 2000). Minority families, then, in contrast to *all* ethnic families (both white and people of color), have certain common attributes and problems. One common experience they share is that while facing all of the same stressors faced by all other families, they have the added burdens of the effects of discrimination and racism (McAdoo, 1978, 1993). Being an ethnic individual in America lowers one's social status. Sociologists note that ethnic groups vary in their status, with some groups, such as black-Americans and Latinos, suffering more status inequality than white ethnics or Asian-Americans (Dilworth-Anderson, Burton, & Johnson, 1993; Vincent & Ransford, 1980).

CULTURAL VARIATION OR DEVIANCE?   Families are not isolated groups that exist independently from the society of which they are a part. Thus if a disproportionately large number of families of a particular minority or ethnic group are poor, unemployed, and "dysfunctional to the whole society," a comprehension of their status can be achieved only through an examination of the role played by the larger society in shaping family life.

If we live in a society in which ethnic families and their members are devalued and seen as inferior, this message and perception very effectively becomes the perception and beliefs of those people (Dilworth-Anderson, Burton, & Johnson, 1993). It is a well-known tenet of social psychology that people develop their identities and perceptions of their worth in interactions with others (Mead, 1934). As the minority family and individual interacts in a white majority world that encourages feelings of inferiority and degrades self-esteem, they begin to believe what the outer world is saying about them. This trap is termed the **self-fulfilling prophecy:** People will conform to other's expectations and perceptions of them by internalizing their beliefs, even negative ones, and thus seem to fulfill the "prophecies" that were made about them.

Problems within society set up conditions to which ethnic families and individuals must adapt (Dilworth-Anderson, Burton, & Johnson, 1993). Some of these adaptations—such as going on welfare, dropping out of school, "babies having babies," joining gangs, or selling drugs—are viewed as "dysfunctional." The tendency becomes one of blaming the victim—the welfare mother, the unskilled, unemployed African-American male, the African-American family, the Chicano gangs—instead of looking more broadly at the problem. By seeing the ways in which the entire system is involved (the institutions of society and the individual's interactions within this larger environment), contextual solutions may be identified (Edelman, 1987). This approach is termed the *cultural variation* or *cultural relativity model,* whereas "blaming the victim" is termed a *cultural deviance approach.*

CONTROVERSIES ABOUT ETHNIC FAMILY STRUCTURES. One way in which social scientists have unwittingly stereotyped and stigmatized whole ethnic groups is by attempting to describe a particular ethnic group in toto by data actually derived from, and thus only reflective of, *poor* segments of that group (Dilworth-Anderson, Burton, & Johnson, 1993). In many of these instances, the particular segment of the ethnic group being described is not clearly identified, thereby giving readers an erroneous notion of what that ethnic group is like as a whole.

This overgeneralization has certainly been true within the social science studies of Mexican-Americans in the period between 1950 and 1970. "The net result of this extraordinary scientific oversight is the perpetuation of very damaging stereotypes of Mexican-Americans" (Casavantes, 1970, p. 22). Willie (1976) and Billingsley (1968) have pointed out the same criticism of studies about the African-American family and conscientiously differentiate lifestyles and values of the African-American family by the family's social class position. Research has concentrated predominantly on the most oppressed families with findings then generalized to all minority families. In this process, biased attitudes are perpetuated and reinforced. As part of this bias, the majority of stable ethnic families, and the processes by which they have become economically mobile, have largely been ignored (McAdoo, 1978, 1993).

THE FAMILY'S SOCIAL CLASS

Socioeconomic status, social status, or social class (the terms are used interchangeably) refers to a grouping of persons with relatively similar income, amounts of wealth, life conditions, life changes, and lifestyles (Ropers, 1991). Curran and Renzetti (2000) explain that social class is a "measure of individual or family economic stratification that includes three elements: wealth (the material element); status (the prestige element); and political power (the decision-making element)" (p. 134). Socioeconomic status, because it has a pervasive effect on families and family members' lives, especially within complex, heterogeneous societies, produces significant differences in a family's culture and lifestyle. Its influence is so pervasive that Oscar Lewis, a noted anthropologist, in 1966 conceptualized poor families as living within a common "culture of poverty." Family lifestyle, structural and functional characteristics, and associations with the external environment of home, neighborhood, and community vary tremendously from social class to social class.

Social class, along with ethnic background, exerts the greatest overall influence on family life, influencing family values and priorities, family behavioral patterns, socialization practices, family role expectations, and world experiences. The crucial difference between classes is simply economic resources (Teachman, 2000). Due to differences in resources, there is also a positive association between socioeconomic status and physical and mental health (Grzywacz, 2000; Ross, Mirowsky, & Goldstein, 1991), meaning that individuals from families who are poor are more likely to have poorer physical and mental health than those who are socioeconomically better off. Education is the aspect of social status that is the most important correlate to health status because education is important in shaping knowledge and behavioral patterns.

Occupational position, formal educational attainment, and household income of adult members of the family are used as indicators of social class in American society, with the husband's occupational status continuing to be the most used and probably the most powerful indicator of social class (Smith & Graham, 1995). Currently, however, it is being acknowledged that the wife's occupational level and income also have a major impact on the lifestyle and social class of a family. In fact, it is usually the wife's income (added to the husband's) that elevates the family to a higher social class (Teachman, 2000). Most occupationally based social class scales, however, leave women's occupations out (Smith & Graham)—given there is a man in the family. Generally the work deemed to have the greatest value to the society receives the greatest rewards, which include not only money, but power, prestige, privilege, and autonomy. Wealth (the accumulated stock of goods and money) and family background can also be a factor for determining social class status, especially among the affluent classes (Stewart, 1998).

Social class or socioeconomic status pertains not only to the family's educational level, occupation status, and income, but also to the intricate interplay of these variables. Persons with different basic conditions of life, by virtue of their varied experience and exposure, come to see the world differently, to develop different conceptions of social reality as well as different aspirations, fears, and values.

Every society differentiates and ranks people, styles of life, automobiles, dress, and work in accordance with what it views as most valuable and important. No society, including American society, is classless. Although Americans like to believe theirs is an open society with equal opportunity, where people can pull themselves up by their own bootstraps, American society is stratified into classes. Status consciousness is present even among children who begin very early to recognize their "place" and also the "place" of others in their little world.

By identifying a family's social class, family nurses can better anticipate a family's lifestyle characteristics and some of its stressors. A family's structure and functions, moreover, are better understood in the light of its social class background.

SOCIAL CLASSES IN THE UNITED STATES

Six discrete classes were described by Warner (1953) in a pioneering study of U.S. social structure as the upper-upper, lower-upper, upper-middle, lower-middle, working class, and lower class. Gilbert and Kahl (1993) presented another taxonomy of social class and their estimates of what percentage of the population is situated in each of these classes. Their taxonomy is similar to the previous taxonomy but differs in that there are only four classes identified (upper, middle, working, and lower or poor). They also divide the social structure up into the capitalist class, the upper-middle class, the middle class, the working class, the working poor class, and the underclass (see Table 8–2).

In the American class structure it is the family, not merely the individual, that is ranked. The family is the keystone of the stratification system, the social mechanism by which the social class structure is maintained. Presently, there is much blurring between the social classes; moreover, within each of the groupings relative to their values and status there

TABLE 8–2

TAXONOMY OF SOCIAL CLASSES IN THE UNITED STATES

SOCIAL CLASS	OCCUPATION AND ESTIMATED PERCENT IN POPULATION
Capitalist class	Heirs, top executives, and investors (3% of population)
Upper-middle class	University educated, professionals, and managers (14% of population)
Middle class	White-collar, lower-level professionals, managers and skilled blue-collar workers (both upper-middle and middle class are 40%–45% of population)
Working class	Semiskilled blue collar and low-level white collar (30%–35% of population)
Working poor	Laborers and service workers (20% of population)
Underclass	Chronically unemployed, underemployed, or erratically employed (5% of population)

Source: Adapted from Gilbert & Kahl (1993).

is certainly not homogeneity (Curran & Renzetti, 2000).

INTERACTION BETWEEN SOCIAL CLASS AND ETHNICITY.

Other factors are also significant in creating diversity within a social class grouping—religion, ethnicity, family form, and gender (for the individual) being prime examples (Teachman, 2000). Intra-ethnic variation, created as a result of the interplay of the family's cultural and social class backgrounds, is called in sociology **ethclass** (Gordon, 1964). Gordon uses this concept to explain the significant role that both the social class membership and ethnicity play in defining the basic conditions of life and simultaneously accounting for differences between ethnic groups situated in the same social class.

Ethnic middle-class families are closer to the dominant culture in lifestyles, values, and beliefs than families from other social classes; however, they are still distinctive from the white middle-class family because of their ethnic identity and sense of peoplehood. Families of the same social class, but of a different ethnic group show behavioral and value similarities, but not the same sense of historial identification of peoplehood. And conversely, those of the same ethnic group but of a different social class manifest a sense of peoplehood, but dissimilar lifestyles.

Using Gilbert and Kahl's (1993) typology of social class in North America, the subsequent section of this chapter will briefly describe some characteristics of each of the four primary social classes, with an emphasis on value differences. Again, these classes are not precise explanations of reality, but are constructs designed to show the patterned relationships and lifestyle differences between classes.

UPPER-CLASS FAMILIES.

These are the families who have wealth (either "old" wealth that they inherited or "new" wealth that they acquired themselves). They represent only about 3 percent of the U.S. population (Curran and Renzetti, 2000). The United States has great class inequality, with income, wealth, prestige and power being heavily concentrated in this small segment of society (Scarpitti, Anderson, & O'Toole, 1997). Most upper-class families are Anglo-Saxon and Protestant.

Newly affluent families are, however, more likely to have a greater cultural diversity. The upper class is considered to be "capitalists" according to Gilbert and Kahl (1993).

MIDDLE-CLASS FAMILIES.

The middle class is considered *dominant* numerically (estimated at 40 to 45 percent and shrinking) and socially, in the sense that they are most able to disseminate their views on what is right, proper, and expected behavior—whether in the family, school, or health agency. This dominance is due primarily to the key positions of the upper-middle class in government, education, and mass communications. The middle class may be divided into two groups, which demonstrate some of the important differences within this class.

The Upper-Middle-Class Family. This class is comprised of professionals in law, accounting, and medicine; higher-level businesspeople; middle management in corporations; successful entrepreneurs; service professionals, particularly at the university level; mental health workers; and administrators of social service and governmental organizations (Langman, 1987). Being the career-oriented bearers of the "American success syndrome," most in this class are college graduates and comprise the "solid highly respectable" people in the community. Most are white Americans, although there is more ethnic diversity than seen among the upper class (Curran & Renzetti, 2000). Individualism, rationality, personal achievement, and the other secular Protestant ethnic values (mastery, future orientation, work, etc.) are stressed (Adams, 1980; Schultz, 1972).

The number of dual-career, upper-middle-class families has recently increased. In dual-career families, patterns of traditional sex differentiation have blurred and more egalitarianism is seen between spouses (Perry-Jenkins & Folk, 1994).

Upper-middle-class families are often geographically mobile in pursuit of career goals. But in spite of their mobility, extensive visiting, communication, and aid between generations occur.

The Lower-Middle-Class Family. The lower-middle class is composed of people who work primarily in white-collar occupations, such as small businessmen, clerical workers, other low-level white-collar workers, bureaucratic functionaries, and salespersons. This class repesents a wide variety of national and ethnic backgrounds. Because of recent economic changes, the ability of middle-income families to maintain a middle-class lifestyle has become more difficult. Both parents need to work and even then there has been a decline in the percentage of middle class in America (Scarpitti, Anderson, & O'Toole, 1997).

Like those in the upper-middle class, the families are relatively stable in spite of problems connected with their economic security and the education of their children. Frequently, students report that conflicts exist between themselves and their parents. The parents work to provide an education for their children, which in turn introduces the children to a set of values that is often in conflict with those of the parents.

The major distinguishing values of the members of this status group are respectability and achievement. Hard work and honesty are also highly valued.

In the lower-middle-class family today, the power structure is usually egalitarian or mildly husband dominated. The wife defers to the husband's authority, yet maintains control over personal and familial household realms. Socially, the kinship group is close, and major social activities often take place with relatives from the husband's or wife's family. Families are generally child-oriented (Langman, 1987).

WORKING-CLASS FAMILIES. About 30 to 35 percent of the U.S. population is working class (Curran & Renzetti, 2000). The blue-collar or working class is made up of skilled workers, semiskilled workers in factories, service workers, and workers in the construction trades. The elite of the working class—electricians, plumbers, and other highly skilled operators—frequently earn more than members of the middle classes and are now in some classifications viewed as part of the lower-middle-class or middle-class group. For members of this class who are in trades that depend on the swings of the business cycle, economic stability is lacking.

The working class is especially vulnerable to economic downturns and financial crisis. Most wives are employed outside of the home and typically take a job out of economic necessity (Curran & Renzetti, 2000). Family strains are often associated with economic uncertainties.

It is within the less educated blue-collar family more than any other class that one still sees many husbands and wives conforming to the traditional husband and wife roles. The husband is often seen as dominant and is generally not very involved in child-care activities (Rubin, 1994). Both of the sexes tend to think that friendship and companionship are more likely to exist between members of the same sex than among marital partners, and see the principal

marital ties as involving the sexual union, complementary tasks, and mutual devotion. Obedience and stricter traditional child-rearing patterns are typically seen in this class (Peterson & Rollins, 1987).

When there is need for assistance, relatives are likely to be called on before turning to a public agency. The extended family, the neighborhood peer group, and the informal work group provide much social interaction as well as actual assistance for blue-collar families.

LOWER-CLASS FAMILIES. Lower-class families (the poor) are at the impoverished level of existence, although their degree of impoverishment varies. Gilbert and Kahl (1993) divide the lower class into the working poor and the underclass, estimating that 25 percent of the population fits into this class: 20 percent into the working poor and 5 percent into the underclass. The federal government, however, classifies 11.9 percent of the population as officially poor (U.S. Bureau of the Census, 2000). This is the lowest reported poverty rate since 1979, but social scientists generally believe that the official counts underestimate the number of poor people in this country (Curran & Renzetti, 2000). See Table 8–3 for federal guidelines on family poverty levels. Wide variations exist in lifestyle, as seen in rural versus urban areas, and in different regional and ethic/social lower-class communities.

TABLE 8–3

FAMILY INCOME GUIDELINES: FEDERAL POVERTY LEVELS

- Federal poverty levels or poverty thresholds were developed by the Social Security Administration and updated annually by the Census Bureau.

- A person's level in the poverty depends on total family income and the number of persons in the family.

- In 1999, the poverty level was $8,667 for one person under age 65, $11,214 for a family of two under age 65, $13,290 for a family of three, and $17,029 for a family of four.

Source: Census Bureau at http://www.census.gov/hhse/poverty/threshld.

POVERTY IN AMERICA

A widening gulf between the rich and the poor continues to be documented by the press and social scientists (Arax, Curtius, & Nelson, 2000). The 1980s and 1990s were decades in which the rich got richer and the poor got poorer (Brownstein, 2000; Silverstein, 1996). During the 1980s a significant change in the distribution of income and wealth occurred in the United States. This shift is due to the reduction of social programs designed to aid the poor and working and middle classes and certain economic and technological trends such as the competitive globalization of markets and the shift in jobs from goods-producing industries to service-producing industries, which generate many minimally paying jobs (Seccombe, 2001). Winnick (1988), a sociologist, calls this a movement toward "two societies, separate and unequal." The gulf in income and resources between rich and poor Americans is wider than at any time since figures were recorded, starting in the 1940s (Kozol, 1990; Stewart, 1998). There is s shrinking of the middle class, with an increasing proportion of the population located in the upper and lower classes (Hong, Dickerson, & Cleeland, 2002; Leeds, 1996).

The effects of certain economic and technological trends, and the last decade of declining domestic and social programs, have had an indelibly harsh impact on poor families. Research findings since the 1930s consistently indicate that economic distress is associated with shorter longevity and poorer health (Carney, 1992; Monmaney, 1997), along with lower levels of family stability, marital adjustment, family coping, family cohesion, marital communication, and harmonious family relationships (Voydanoff & Donnelly, 1988).

The nature of poverty is changing in America (Brown-Stein, 1999). More and more the lower class is composed of working poor families—families in which one or both parents are working full or part time in minimum-wage jobs, which are not enough to lift them and their families out of poverty. In addition, the lower class is disproportionately composed of ethnic minorities and recent legal immigrants, undocumented workers and families, female-headed households, children, and those with certain personally disorganizing problems: chronic mental illness, alcoholism, and drug abuse.

Minority status contributes substantially to poverty (see Figure 8–1). Among families, the incidence of poverty is almost three times higher for African-Americans and Hispanics than for whites (Fulwood, 1996). Among children, poverty is widespread (see Table 8–4). The average poor African-American and Hispanic child today appears to be in the middle of a prolonged poverty period in the United States because of cutbacks in social and health benefits and declining family wages (Ehrenreich, 2001; Wright, 1996).

Forty-nine percent of female-headed families with children are poor (Annie E. Casey Foundation, 1999). This disproportionate representation of poor single mother families largely contributes to what is called "the feminization of poverty" (Rodgers, 1990; Starrels, Bould, & Nicholas, 1994).

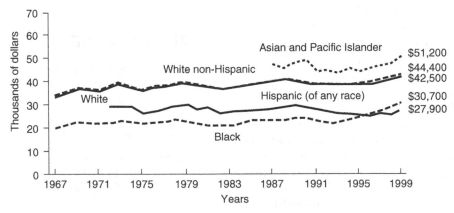

Figure 8–1. Median Household Income by Race and Hispanic Origin: 1967 to 1999. *(Source: U.S. Census Bureau, March 1968 to 2000.)* Note: Income rounded to the nearest $100. Income in 1999 dollars.

TABLE 8—4

FACTS ABOUT CHILDREN AND POVERTY

About 40% of the nation's poor are children.

29% of American families with young children live below the poverty line.

Among the world's developed countries, U.S. children have the highest poverty rate and greatest likelihood of living in single-parent homes.

A child in the United States living in a mother-headed home is five times more likely to be poor than a child living in a two-parent home.

65% of poor children live in households that do not have a biological father present.

65% of African-American mother-headed families with children are poor.

67% of Hispanic mother-headed families with children are poor.

The number of children living in working poor families rose 33% between 1989 and 1999.

African-American and Hispanic children are three times more likely to live in poverty than are white children.

Study after study documents the negative effects of poverty on children—on their physical growth, cognitive development, academic achievement, socioemotional functioning, and productivity in later life.

Sources: Annie E. Casey Foundation (1996); Ellis (1995); Ehrenreich (2001); Dadds (1995); Fulwood (1996); Grimes (1996); Leeds (1996); U.S. Bureau of the Census (1991a); and Wright (1996).

In summary, current problems of poor families are profound and almost intractable, according to recent national reports and surveys. Families are weakened by joblessness, poor and crowded schools, loss of family support systems, family breakdowns, drug and alcohol abuse, crime-ridden neighborhoods, and depression (Ellis, 1995; Family Service America, 1984).

It is difficult for most students and teachers to describe the lifestyle of the lower class without imposing middle-class evaluations. Even the use of the term "lower class" imposes a negative connotation and interpretation to people who occupy this class level. What Rodman (1965) stated over 35 years ago still applies, "It is little wonder that if we describe the lower-class family in terms of illegitimate children, deserting men, and unmarried mothers, we are going to see the situation as disorganized and chock-full of problems" (p. 223).

In observing social conditions of lower-class life from a middle-class perspective, we should not become so engrossed in looking at the victims that we fail to understand the reasons for the problems.

Perhaps it is more realistic to think of these conditions as consequences of, or in some instances solutions to, other issues faced by lower-class people as they experience all the social, economic, political, and legal realities of life.

In contrast with the working class, the lower class does not have the respect of the larger community. Its existence often becomes a "political football" such as the conflict seen over "family values." Its members are likely to be stigmatized and characterized as being lazy, unmotivated, dependent, and "those people." Tacit in public rhetoric is also the assumption that many poor persons "have only themselves to blame" (Grimes, 1996; Seccombe, 2001).

POVERTY IN THE FAMILY

Directly related to the poverty of the lower class is the irregularity of employment or low wages. Because income is low or irregular, a considerable amount of insecurity exists in regard to food, clothing, shelter, transportation, health care, and other family essentials. Children may be forced or encouraged to contribute to the financial needs of the family, and many drop out of high school.

Lower-class family life, adapting to scarce resources, is based on assumptions and norms that are different from those of the middle class. The poor cannot "afford" such values of the middle class as productivity, achievement, work, and long-range planning. The *Chicago Tribune* staff (1986) did a nice job of describing the impact of poverty on family life:

> Poor parents have the same job to do with their children that middle-class parents do; the difference is that poor parents have less money, less education, and less access to resources and alternatives. Most live under extraordinary stress, facing constant crises centered around food, shelter, and physical illness; these lead to feelings of helplessness, hopelessness and powerlessness. These feelings are based in reality and relate to forces largely beyond the control of the poor family. Much of the time the energy of the poor is focused on getting through a day. Yet tomorrow they expect to have to do more of the same. (p. 95)

It is interesting to note, however, that parents' aspirations for their children are often very "middle class," despite their inability to provide the ways and means for achieving such goals.

As noted in Table 8–4, many poor families are headed by minority group women who are unemployed or underemployed and dependent on welfare. A growing number today, however, are working poor families.

THE AMERICAN UNDERCLASS

A large portion (about 25 percent) of the poor is now being termed "the American underclass" (Gilbert & Kahl, 1993). These are the poor who are in persistent, as compared to temporary, poverty. These are the people who remain more or less permanently at the bottom of the social ladder. The underclass is isolated socially from mainstream patterns and norms of behavior (Wilson, 1987). Although its members come from all races and live throughout the United States, the underclass is made up primarily of (a) impoverished urban African-Americans, who suffer from the

heritage of slavery and discrimination as well as the changing economy; (b) Hispanics, primarily Mexican-Americans and Puerto Ricans, who have recently immigrated into cities and rural areas (as migrant workers); and (c) Appalachian migrants who live in dilapidated neighborhoods of some cities (Russell, 1977; Gilbert & Kahl, 1993).

The underclasses' long-term poverty and welfare dependency, plus their bleak environment, nurture values that are often at radical odds with those of the majority—even the majority of the poor. For instance, stable marriages and legal divorces tend to be luxuries in this class. Toughness is a desirable interpersonal trait. Children are frequently taught to defend themselves physically rather than with mental or psychological tactics. Thus, the underclass minority is disproportionately represented among the nation's juvenile delinquents, gang members, drug addicts, physically disabled people, homeless persons, and single parents on welfare. They are "responsible," therefore, for a considerable amount of the adult crime, family disruption, urban decay, and need for social expenditures. The underclass remains a nucleus of psychological and material destitution despite some two decades of civil rights gains in the 1960s and 1970s. Federal reductions in domestic social programs, beginning in 1980 and continuing into the 1990s, have only magnified the problem.

The underclass is made up of people who lack the necessary education, skills, discipline, and self-esteem to succeed (Curran & Renzetti, 2000). Long-term unemployment is a common factor here, and large numbers of the underclass are single parents on welfare. The 1996 welfare reform legislation is targeted at the underclass. The goal is to enhance self-sufficiency through work. This is all well and good, but there needs to be safeguards to make certain that working will actually enable families to meet the minimum needs of their children (Leeds, 1996).

More jobs with living wages and better education are clearly two pressing needs. In our achievement-oriented society, work is more than a source of income. It is also a source of feeling productive, which brings self-esteem, status, a point of identification with the system, and a satisfying social environment. Affordable housing, safety in neighborhoods, and educational and health care reform (universal access to care) must also be addressed if families are to escape from poverty (Allen, 1994).

People from the underclass subculture within our communities, especially our cities, are in the greatest need of our health and social services. In official health agencies, much of the nurse's effort is necessarily concentrated on the very poor. It is only through understanding and appreciation of some of the major problems and daily realities of the poor that families can be assisted with a resolution to their health needs.

IMPACT OF POVERTY ON HEALTH

Health disparities between poor people and those with higher incomes are almost universal for all dimensions of health, according to the U.S. Public Health Service in their influential and far-reaching publication, *Healthy People 2010* (2000). The following list indicates the areas where national survey data show a significant relationship between the poor (versus the middle class) and particular health problems.

- Poorer self-rated health
- Increased restricted activity days
- Increased chronic activity limitations
- Increased disability
- Increased work and school absences
- Increased risk of leading chronic diseases and injuries
- Increased infant mortality and infectious disease rates
- Shortened longevity (increased mortality)

There is mounting evidence that a family's neighborhood impacts on the health status of its residents. Research in the 1990s examined the role that the broader social context (neighborhoods, schools, day care centers, and peer groups), played relative to the consequences of poverty (Seccombe, 2001).

Although socioeconomic factors are probably a more powerful determinant of health than medical treatments (Nelson, 1994), no interventions aimed at families' economic status have been proposed by the health community. Furthermore, health disparities by social class will persist as long as inequalities in the fundamental social, economic, and political structure of society remain. Thus, argues Nelson, "socioeconomic conditions that constitute or contribute to health risks must also be targeted in policies and pro-

grams to improve the health of populations" (p. 2). Assisting families' economic impoverishment is most essential in working with the disadvantaged and is well within nursing's scope of practice (Nelson; Seccombe, 2001).

⚘ FAMILY'S ECONOMIC STATUS

Family's economic status, a component of social class, refers to the family's income level and source of income. Income that is sufficient to meet a family's needs is generally derived from the work of family members or from private sources such as pensions and support payments (nonpublic), while income derived partially from welfare or unemployment insurance is generally marginal, unstable, or barely adequate. The family that has inadequate economic resources exhibits these characteristics: (a) income derived entirely from welfare because of failure or inability of adult(s) in the family to work; (b) income derived from welfare by fraudulent means; and (c) amount of income so low or unstable that basic necessities are lacking. Families receiving income from programs such as Aid to the Totally Disabled, Aid to the Blind, Aid to Families of Dependent Children, Old Age Assistance, and Social Security (alone) would fall under the marginal or inadequate category, because the level of funding is so low that basic necessities are barely or inadequately provided for.

One basic family function is the provision of adequate economic support and allocation of resources. Hence, in order to assess economic adequacy, not only income level should be estimated but also expenditures, focusing on the allocation of resources. Assessing expenditures, again a sensitive subject that should be discussed specifically only when needed, consists of asking about regular financial obligations: rent or mortgage payments, insurance, transportation costs or car payments, phone and utility bills, food expenses, and any special bills the family may have incurred.

⚘ SOCIAL CLASS MOBILITY

Another family assessment area related to social class is social class mobility. This refers to vertical mobility upward or downward through the social class strata and is included here because a change in either direction produces considerable stress. Holmes and Rahe (1967), in their social readjustment scale, identified changes of position, status, or prestige, whether positive or negative, as stress producing. Although upward mobility is seen as desirable by most persons, and often results in new recognition and social prestige, it may also result in rejection and social isolation, such as the cohesiveness of the extended family may decrease. In addition, lower levels of family participation are found in upwardly mobile families. Interpersonal relationships and the degree of personal comfort may also be compromised.

In America, people have expected a move upward as a natural state of affairs. The majority of the vertical mobility has been upward, as evidenced by our large middle class. This is no longer true. Due to structural changes in the economy, frequent recessions, and widespread employment instability, more and more families will not move up the social class ladder as in previous decades, but will remain stationary or move downward (Stewart, 1998; Voydanoff, 1991). Social mobility was probably never as widespread as generally believed. About 70 percent of families remain in the same social class, and this stability of social class placement can be seen through a number of generations. Examples of the stability of social class status are found among upper-class families, where their wealth or prestige has continued through several generations. A similar continuity is also observed in the lower classes. In the well-known classic social class study by Hollingshead (1949), he showed that the lower-lower social class of "Elmstown" had retained this position since before the Civil War. Mobility occurs most frequently in the lower-middle, working, and upper-lower classes.

Downward social mobility is more commonplace today. Downward social mobility of whole communities may occur because of prolonged economic recession. Retirement and becoming disabled also often bring downward social class mobility because of the marked reduction in income.

🐝 FAMILY ASSESSMENT AREAS

As with all assessment tools, it is important to begin by obtaining broad identifying information about the family client. As discussed in Chapter 7, during the initial visit or client contact, the focus is typically on getting to know the family and all its members, as well as attempting to meet their immediate health needs. To learn about the family, a family genogram is an excellent assessment strategy.

ASSESSMENT OF FAMILY COMPOSITION: THE FAMILY GENOGRAM

Family composition refers to who the family members identify as being part of their family. This may include not only the household inhabitants, but also other extended family or fictive family members who are part of "the family," but do not live in the same household. Obtaining data on the family composition lets family members know of your interest in the whole family rather than solely on an individual client.

To get to know the family and identify the family composition, completing a family genogram is recommended. The family genogram is a diagram that delineates the family constellation or family tree. It is an informative assessment tool used to get to know the family and the family's history and resources.

A genogram interview is seen as one part of a comprehensive clinical assessment of a family (McGoldrick & Gerson, 1985; Wright & Leahey, 2000). The diagram maps relationships vertically (across generations) and horizontally (within the same generation) and often helps family nurses think systemically about how events and relationships in the nuclear family members' lives are related to family patterns of health and illness within and across generations, as well as to generate tentative hypotheses about what's going on in the family.

Based on the conventions used in diagraming family trees or genealogical charts and genetics, the family genogram incorporates information about three generations of the family (the two generations within the nuclear family and the family of origin of each parent). Not only are the nuclear and extended family members included on the genogram, but also significant nonfamily members who have lived with or played a major role in the family's life. This visual representation of the family consists of information about members' age; gender; significant life events (e.g., birth, marriage, divorce); health/illness status;

death; and selected identifying features such as race, social class, ethnicity, religion, occupation, and place of residence.

There has been widespread use of family genograms by family health practitioners and therapists, and much variety in the way genograms are diagrammed. McGoldrick and Gerson have written an entire book on genograms, *Genograms in Family Assessment* (1985). If a more thorough description of genograms and their application is needed, this excellent reference is suggested.

CONSTRUCTING GENOGRAMS.   Figure 8–2 shows an example of how a genogram is constructed. Symbols used in diagraming are also presented. The example given is relatively uncomplicated, given the number of families that have experienced multiple significant family transitions and events. Wright and Leahey (2000) explain the basic method involved in recording family data on the family genogram.

Family members are placed on horizontal rows that signify generational lines. For example, a

Figure 8–2. Example of family genogram with accompanying legend (symbols used in genograms).

marriage or common-law relationship is denoted by a hortizontal line. Children are denoted by vertical lines. Children are rank-ordered from left to right beginning with the eldest child. Each individual is represented. (p. 87)

Males are designated by squares, females by circles. Horizontal lines that are broken denote a separation or divorce. Household members are identified by encircling all the members of the household with a broken line.

Usually the family genogram is completed on the first visit or interview and revised later as new information becomes available. Letting the family know that background information is needed to more fully understand the specific problems the family is experiencing, coupled with an explanation of the family tree method, usually suffice as explanations to gain family members' participation. It is suggested that questions about the immediate family are asked first (names, ages, sex of household members). Recent life cycle transitions as well as changes in the family situation (additions or deletions of members) may also be inquired about at this time (McGoldrick & Gerson, 1985).

Generally a brief two-generational genogram is most useful in the first interview, particularly if the family has minor health problems or preventive health needs (Wright & Leahey, 2000). When constructing a three-generation genogram, it is suggested to first address the immediate family and then ask about the parents' families of origin. Inquiring about the two extended families brings to focus the wider family context. Querying the marital partners about each of their families of origin is a way to obtain this information. Moreover, questions should be asked about friends, clergy, caregivers, health care professionals, and others important to the family's functioning; this information may be included on the genogram or used to assess the family's social support system/network. At this point, nonfamily members may also be added as either household members or "family."

Begin the interview by asking "easy" questions. Difficult questions about family members' functioning and subsystem relationships are often saved to later in the interview, when greater trust and rapport has been built. Areas family nurses should ask about include serious medical or psychological problems, work or school changes/problems, drug and alcohol problems, and trouble with the law (McGoldrick & Gerson, 1985).

ASSESSMENT OF FAMILY'S CULTURAL BACKGROUND

A cultural assessment of clients (individuals and families) is an essential facet of assessment in the provision of culturally congruent care (Kelley, 1997). Just as a family nurse would not intervene without an assessment of the biopsychosocial aspects of a family and its members, he or she should also not proceed until a cultural assessment has been completed (Leininger, 1976; Tripp-Reimer et al., 1984).

Cultural assessment "requires an acceptance of multiple realities, an understanding of differences and an open, sensitive, inquiring manner" (Kelley, 1997, p. 32).

As part of the broader assessment of families from ethnic groups different than the nurses, we need to become informed about the cultures of the families with whom we interact (Lipson, 1996). It is extremely important that family nurses try to obtain the perceptions, views, values, and practices of people from the particular ethnic group with which they are working. "It is significant to remember that the ability to work with cultural groups is dependent upon the ability to understand the group in terms of their background as they view it and not in terms of our interpretations of their background" (Clemen, 1977, p. 192).

Ridley and Lingle (1996), cross-cultural counselors, agree that the ability to understand clients in terms of their cultural backgrounds and from their own perspective is essential in assessing and working with the family. They assert that practitioners working with families from cultures different from their own must develop **cultural empathy** in order to be effective. Having cultural empathy should lead to an understanding of clients' culture, which includes the culture's assumptions, values, and patterns of thinking. "Cultural empathy involves the ability of counselors to communicate this understanding effectively with an attitude of concern for culturally different clients" (Ridley & Lingle, p. 32). Ridley and Lingle believe that before beginning to work with ethnic families, practitioners must understand their own culture, and only after this self-examination can they effectively examine the clients' "cultural self."

When assessing ethnic families, it is also important to bring out family strengths, positive adaptations that families have made in dealing with their constraints, and vulnerabilities (McAdoo, 1993). Attention to family strengths facilitates positive opinions of families and leads to family nursing approaches that tend to raise a family's sense of competency and empowerment.

ETHNIC AND RELIGIOUS ASSESSMENT AREAS

For many families a thorough cultural or ethnic assessment is not possible, and yet assessing the family's ethnic background (as identified by the family) and the degree to which they identify with the dominant American culture or their traditional culture (if different from the dominant culture) is basic identifying information needed in any family assessment. Complicating matters, ethnic backgrounds of parents or spouses may differ, and if this is so, it is important to assess how this difference is handled and how it affects family life.

Information on the family's religious beliefs and practices is intimately tied to ethnicity and thus should also be included as part of the assessment (Tripp-Reimer et al., 1984). Religious beliefs often influence a family's conceptions of health and illness and how sick family members are treated. Family roles, rituals, values, and coping patterns are also affected by the family's religious orientation or legacy.

The following specific areas are suggested as part of the identifying ethnic and religious data about the family:

1. *The family's ethnic background (self-identified).*

2. *The family's degree of acculturation.* The assessment question posed here is, "To what extent has the family retained its ethnicity or cultural heritage?" Or posed in the reverse fashion, "To what extent has the family assimilated American culture?" Table 8–5 presents overall cultural assessment questions that, when answered, give pertinent information on the family's degree of acculturation. Some of the behavioral clues that indicate that the family still retains traditional (ethnic) practices, values, and beliefs follow:

    a. Family members' English language proficiency and native language literacy (reading and writing skills) are limited.

    b. Recent migration from another country (first generation).

    c. Native culture is very different from American culture.

    d. The family's friends and associations are of the same ethnic group (strong ethnic ties).

    e. Family lives in an ethnically homogeneous neighborhood.

    f. Strong political and religious ties to the ethnic group.

    g. Social, cultural, recreational, and/or educational activities are within the family's cultural group.

    h. Dietary habits and dress are traditional.

    i. Traditional family roles are carried out.

    j. Home decorations, art, and other visual representations are congruent with the cultural background.

    k. Native language is spoken exclusively or frequently in the home.

    l. The territorial complex—the wider community the family frequents—is primarily within the ethnic community.

    m. The family uses folk medicine or traditional practitioners, or perhaps a community health worker in whom the ethnic neighborhood has confidence.

    n. Family members' beliefs about illnesses and treatments are culturally based and differ significantly from Western health care beliefs and practices (McSweeney, Allen, & Mayo, 1997).

    o. Community discrimination (encouraging segregation) against the identified ethnic group of the family exists.

    p. Family members are nonwhite (creating obvious racial difference making acculturation more difficult).

Not all members of the family may have the same emotional ties to their ethnic background or religion. Older persons and parents who are in or beyond the life cycle stages of raising children are usually more traditional than the children and young adults without children. Those members of the family who work outside the home are more acculturated than those members who work in the home. Those who speak and read English in the fam-

TABLE 8–5

ETHNIC ASSESSMENT GUIDELINES

ASSESSMENT CRITERIA	QUESTIONS
Ethnic/racial identity	How does the family identify itself in terms of ethnicity and racial group? Are the parents both from the same ethnic background?
Language	What language(s) is/are spoken in the home? And by whom? What language is preferred when speaking to outsiders? What is the level of English language proficiency of family members? Are family members literate in their own native language—in terms of writing and reading skills?
Place of birth and immigration history	Where were the parents and children born? If they immigrated from another country, when did they immigrate to the United States and what was their reason for immigrating?
Geographic mobility	Where have the parents lived? When did they move to their present residence?
Family's religion	What is the family's religion? Are both parents from the same religious background? How actively involved is the family in religiously based activities and practices?
Ethnic group affiliation	What are the characteristics of the family's friends and associations? Are they all from the family's ethnic group? Are recreational, political, educational, and other social activities within the ethnic reference group, the wider community, or both? To what extent does the family use services and shop within the family's neighborhood or within the wider community?
Neighborhood affiliation	What are the characteristics of the family's neighborhood? Is it ethnically heterogeneous or homogeneous?
Dietary habits, dress	What are the family's dietary preferences and prohibitions? Do the family members dress in traditional clothing?
Household appearance	Are the family's home decorations, art, and religious objects culturally derived?
Use of folk & alternative health systems	To what extent does the family use folk healing practices or practitioners or alternative health modalities? What are the family's health and illness beliefs and practices?
Cultural health beliefs	What are the family members' beliefs about the etiology, effects, course, and treatment of the health problem(s) of family member(s)?
Family life transitions	What are the customs and beliefs about family life transitions such as births, illness, mourning and death, pregnancy and well-baby care?
Acceptance by community	To what extent is the family affected by discrimination?

Sources: Adapted partially from Ferguson-Marshalleck & Miller (2001); Friedman (1990); Kleinman (1980); and Lipson (1996).

ily are typically more acculturated. And the poor are generally less acculturated than the more affluent classes.

Within immigrant groups the degree of acculturation into the new culture has gener- ally increased with each succeeding generation. An illustration of this phenomenon is the Japanese acculturation pattern (Matsui, 1996). The first-generation Japanese-Americans, the Issei, who came here from Japan between 1890 and 1920, retained almost all of their former traditions. The second-generation Japanese-Americans, the Nisei, occupied an intermediate position on the acculturation continuum, while the third generation, the Sansei, are quite westernized. Interestingly enough, an opposing trend among the Yonsei, the fourth generation, is also being seen. As with other groups, there is a resurgence of interest in ethnic "roots," particularly among the Yonsei, with whom the learning of Japanese language and culture has become increasingly popular.

In spite of the tendency for persons from immigrant families to become more acculturated over time and in succeeding generations, some values, practices, and beliefs are retained. In the Mexican-American family the importance of the extended family has not waned over time; in fact, research shows that the extended family has grown in structure and functions when studied across generations (Baca-Zinn, 1981).

3. *The family's religious preference and practices.* The family's religious background should be noted, taking into account how individuals within the family differ in their religious beliefs and practices. How actively involved is the family in a particular church, temple, mosque, or other religious organization? As we learned from looking at families historically, the function of religion in family life has diminished in many families (D'Antonio & Aldous, 1983). Nevertheless, we have great cultural diversity in our country and are currently seeing a resurgence of fundamental religion among some sectors of society. Hence, the role and importance of religion in families varies tremendously. In addition, it is suggested that an assessment be made of what religious practices the family engages in and what religiously based beliefs appear centrally important to the family.

In addition to the above general assessment areas, cultural assessment questions/areas are integrated throughout the entire family assessment guidelines. By completing the entire family assessment, one should have culled comprehensive data on cultural influences pertaining to the family organization (role, power, values, and communication facets),

child-rearing practices, affective responses, health care practices and beliefs, and coping strategies.

CRITICAL QUESTIONS FOR NURSES IN AMBULATORY CARE. In ambulatory settings where community-based nurses and nurse practitioners may only see a client or family for a short period of time, a shorter list of critical assessment questions may be needed. Key assessment areas are: (a) the family's self-identified ethnic and religious background; (b) their immigration status (from where and how long they have been here); (c) the language(s) they speak at home and the language they prefer to communicate in; (d) what they believe about their present health problem, such as symptoms and causes, and the appropriate treatment; and (e) the client's use of traditional healing methods (Jiang, 1995).

ASSESSMENT OF SOCIOECONOMIC STATUS AND SOCIAL CLASS MOBILITY

SOCIAL CLASS STATUS. Based on the family's income level and source of income, and the adult members' occupation and education, identify the family's social class status.

ECONOMIC STATUS. Asking how much the adults earn can be an invasive question, as income is considered a private matter among most families. A question should be asked only if there is an important reason to do so, such as in determining eligibility for assistance, services, or community resources. Questions relevant to this area include the following:

- Who is (are) the wage-earner(s) of the family?
- Does the family receive any supplementary funds or assistance? If so, what are they and from where (e.g., retirement fund, Social Security, food stamps, family)?
- What major expenditures does the family have?

From this information, plus information on occupations, one can often estimate weekly or monthly income or ask a question regarding approximate income.

- Does the family consider its income adequate? How does it see itself managing financially?
- What financial resources does the family or could the family have (for example, medical insurance, disability insurance, dental insur-

ance, workmen's compensation, food stamps, unemployment insurance, crippled children's services, reduced transportation fares)?

SOCIAL CLASS MOBILITY. Describe the family's social class mobility—the change(s) that occurred to produce downward or upward mobility, when these changes occurred, and how the family has adjusted to the changes.

FAMILY NURSING DIAGNOSES

The foundation for developing family nursing diagnoses is an accurate, thorough cultural assessment of the family. There are no sociocultural family diagnoses per se. Nevertheless, the family's cultural heritage influences the diagnoses nurses develop for their clients. This is particularly true in the nonphysiologic, family areas. Smith in the text *Transcultural Communication in Nursing* (1999) discusses developing culturally appropriate nursing diagnoses (See Table 8–6 for tips on developing culturally appropriate nursing diagnoses). She states that one major controversy in using NANDA diagnoses (or any other diagnostic clas-

TABLE 8–6

TIPS ON DEVELOPING CULTURALLY APPROPRIATE NURSING DIAGNOSES

- Nursing diagnoses cannot be indiscriminately applied to all clients. They must be individualized, taking into account the family's cultural heritage.

- Remember to elicit family members' explanations for why an illness developed. Encourage family members to discuss their beliefs and viewpoints concerning health and illness.

- Validate your nursing diagnoses with the family and continually reevaluate and update diagnoses as the family and family members change.

- How family nurses formulate nursing diagnoses impacts client interventions and outcomes.

Source: Adapted from Smith (1999, pp. 223–224).

sification system) is that some nursing diagnoses are more sensitive to cultural bias. For example, the diagnosis of noncompliance can be judgmental when applied to culturally diverse families. Families may wish to use their own indigenous health care practices rather than Western health care (Smith, 1999). Leininger (1990), a leader in transcultural nursing, agrees with Smith relative to the inappropriate, culturally biased use of some nursing diagnoses. She critiques the NANDA system by stating that: the NANDA taxonomy is based on Anglo-American Western cultural standards and values; the NANDA categories seem to be ethnocentric and focus on medically oriented conditions; the NANDA categories do not account for transcultural variations; and the NANDA diagnoses present ethical issues when used internationally. Hence, we as family nurses must very carefully take into consideration a family's cultural background, individualizing family nursing diagnoses within the family's cultural context. To do otherwise impairs the nurse–family relationship and our effectiveness in delivering culturally appropriate care.

FAMILY NURSING INTERVENTIONS

All nursing interventions occur in a sociocultural context. This cultural context has been described as silent and invisible, yet ever present (Pedersen et al., 1996). Thus, a central goal of family nursing is to provide culturally appropriate and competent care to families. Culturally competent care involves a "continuous process of awareness, knowledge, skill, interaction, and sensitivity among those who render care . . ." (Smith, 1998). It also involves the adaptation of care in a matter that is congruent with the client's culture (Purnell & Paulanka, 1998). This section discusses intervention guidelines associated with the several aspects covered in this chapter—guidelines for working with ethnically diverse families and for assisting families with economic difficulties.

SOCIOCULTURAL FAMILY INTERVENTIONS

Guidelines for providing culturally competent family health care to ethnic families are necessarily broad, because more specific intervention strategies are limited to only certain ethnic groups. Davis and Voegtle (1994) and Ridley and Lingle (1996) outline six key aspects involved in providing culturally competent health care. These are:

1. Awareness and acceptance of cultural differences, including ethnic/religious and social class differences

2. Self-awareness of one's own culture

3. Understanding the dynamics of cultural differences. Seeing the family within its own cultural context

4. Knowledge of the client's family culture

5. Adaptation of services to support the client's culture

6. Responding to families/family members in an empathic manner

The first four elements are necessary to the culturally sensitive, but it is the fifth and sixth aspects that make our services "culturally competent."

Seven basic strategies for working with culturally diverse families that are suggested in the cross-cultural literature include: (1) selecting the appropriate system to work with, (2) providing more time to work with unacculturated families, (3) dealing with language differences, (4) taking into account the family's interactional norms, (5) focusing on family strengths and families' positive adaptation, (6) promoting positive change, and (7) being aware of and utilizing the family's social support system. Each of these strategies are subsequently discussed.

Selecting the appropriate family system to work with is a crucial consideration. Which system to work with (a family subsystem such as the marital or parent–child subsystem, the nuclear family, the extended family, or the individual client's self-identified family, which may be composed of unrelated persons) can determine the outcome. Understanding and respecting an ethnic minority family's cultural norms and present social context are perhaps the most important skills in selecting a system for counseling and teaching (Dilworth-Anderson & McAdoo, 1988; Ho, 1987). Ho gives us a good example of this guideline:

Considering the intense involvement that ethnic minority families have with their extended family, some family problems can be resolved simply by

involving the extended family members, especially the spokesperson, who normally is the grandfather (Asian/Hispanic) or grandmother (black and Indian). (p. 258)

Family nurses should be aware of extended kinship networks and should search out significant others to be included in the family assessment and intervention, given, or course, this is mutually agreeable with the family.

A second general intervention guideline deals with the time needed to provide care to ethnic families. If the family is unacculturated, Harwood (1981) stresses the importance of allowing more time for health care interventions. More time is typically required for translation and using an interpreter (Lipson & Meleis, 1999) for assessing relevant health beliefs and practices, for discussion and clarification of health information, for explanation of diagnosis and treatment plans, and for socializing the family members to the health care system.

Language use in clinical encounters with members of ethnic families is a third general consideration. When the language ability of the individual is not apparent, asking what language he or she prefers to use is indicated. The health practitioner should not assume that a foreign-born client and his or her family wish to carry on an interview in their native language. Having translators is not without its problems, but usually is preferable to attempting to use a phrase book or a very limited vocabulary to communicate (Harwood, 1981).

Harwood (1981) and Kelley (1997) give three recommendations to clinicians working with ethnic families that address interactional norms. First, in ethnic families that are kin-based or from peasant societies, the elderly are accorded more respect than they are in our society. Moreover, social interaction between sexes is more limited, and standards of modesty more strictly prescribed. As a result, the style of interaction between the family nurse and family members should reflect these interactional norm differences. For example, a younger health care professional should show greater respect and deference to an older Asian family member. Certain potentially embarrassing topics should be discussed only with certain members of the family present. Because the health care professional is usually seen as an authority figure in Asian, Hispanic, and Middle Eastern Muslim families, he or she needs to assume an active, more directive role in the beginning interviews/visits (Ho, 1987).

Second, due to professional and class status differences, members of ethnic families are often reticent to ask questions or discuss their concerns. Active encouragement to ask questions and bring up concerns is needed to break down this barrier.

A third related approach is to listen actively and carefully to what family members have to say. The family nurse should convey an interest and concern in the client and family, personalizing the encounter such as the folk healer might do.

The fifth general strategy for working with ethnic families is to recognize and reinforce family strengths and families' positive adaptation. This focus facilitates a more positive opinion about ethnic families and their cultural differences (McAdoo, 1993; Walsh, 1998). It also leads to family nursing approaches that tend to raise a family's sense of competency and empowerment. Moreover, focusing on strengths tends to minimize the clinician's tendency to compare an ethnic family to mainstream notions of families and how families should look and act.

The sixth general intervention guideline for working with ethnic families is to promote positive change (Spector, 2000). This can be done by building on cultural practices. Cultural health practices that are positive should be reinforced and, if possible and practical, incorporated into the plan for care. Promoting changes in health practices should only occur when self-care and health practices are harmful or when additions to a family's self-care or folk remedies are called for. After making recommendations, there is a need to check for client understanding and acceptance. If the recommendation is not accepted, it may be at a later date. For the fit between the family's need and the recommendation may not have been good at that particular time for that particular family.

The seventh general intervention strategy addresses social support systems. Informal social support systems are probably more important for ethnic families to call upon than for Anglo-American families (Delgado, 1997). Thus, family nurses need to be aware and help families to utilize their natural support systems (McGoldrick & Giordano, 1996). Important social support systems such as extended family, friends, and social and religious groups may not be available or relationships may be strained. In these cases, assisting family members to strengthen

clients' connections to family and community resources is indicated.

Ho (1987), a family therapist, discusses culturally relevant techniques and skills in the phases of family therapy. Due to cultural barriers to family mental health services, he stresses the cruciality of developing trust with the family in the beginning phase of family counseling. During the early engagement phase, he suggests that the clinician may need to explore with the family ethnic/cultural differences between the clinician and family.

Family nursing interventions that are culturally appropriate during health care treatment include facilitating access to needed health knowledge (Rankin & Stallings, 2001), consideration of dietary practices and beliefs, family visiting and participation practices, and understanding preferences for home care versus inpatient and long-term care.

Unacculturated ethnic families generally have poor access to health knowledge. Especially if they do not speak English, are poorly educated, and have a social network composed of families from the same socioeconomic and ethnic background, they have limited access to accurate, up-to-date health knowledge. As a consequence, these families are much more in need of health education than more advantaged majority families. Health knowledge deficits need to be carefully addressed here.

As part of medical regimens, therapeutic diets must incorporate ethnic/religious preferences if they are to be followed; hence, the importance of getting a dietary history before intervening. Ethnically acceptable therapeutic diets should reflect both ethnic food preferences and ethnic food beliefs.

Family visiting and participation in a family member's care while he or she is in the hospital varies from ethnic group to ethnic group. In many cultures, the family plays a major role in patient care. In ethnic groups with strong familistic orientations, such as in Armenian, Jewish, Muslim, Asian, and Hispanic families, sickness is a time when relatives display their support and solidarity. Hence, visiting the hospital and fully participating in care are important family activities for the psychological state of not only the patient but also the family.

There may be a difference in preferences of ethnic minority groups to home care versus hospital care or long-term care. "Many ethnic groups strongly prefer home care over institutionalized care for the

TABLE 8–7

ECONOMIC/FINANCIAL ASSESSMENT AND INTERVENTION STRATEGIES

- ### ASSESSMENT STRATEGIES

  Establishing trust and rapport with family.

  Assessing family's financial costs, resources, and allocation of resources for health care.

  Assessing family's coping efforts and resources.

- ### INTERVENTION STRATEGIES

  Teaching family ways to reduce health care costs by presenting available alternatives/options.

  Teaching family to understand and evaluate insurance coverage.

  Informing family about community services and programs available, such as bus passes, transportation for the disabled, governmental programs like W.I.C. and "Healthy Children," public health immunization, and school-based clinics.

  Referring family to appropriate services within and outside health care agency.

  Helping family cope with financial stress.

  Thinking about ways to help families being discharged from hospital, e.g., in pediatrics, encouraging immunizations to be given prior to discharge and encouraging physicians to order generic medications when possible.

incapacitated and terminally ill. . . . Chinese, Haitians, Italians, Mexicans, and Puerto Ricans all manifest this preference, while urban blacks and Navajos do not" (Harwood, 1981, p. 503). Harwood explains that the reasons for this preference among the former groups has to do with their strong extended family ties.

ECONOMIC INTERVENTIONS

Interventions that assist families in ameliorating the financial strain of health and illness problems are often overlooked in family nursing. If family nurses are aware of the financial impact of health problems on families, there is often much they can do to help (Millington & Zieball, 1986), particularly if the nurse is in the primary care or community setting. A family that is at high risk medically is also a family that is at high risk financially, given the need for expensive, specialized diagnostic and treatment procedures, personnel, and long-term care.

Financial stress often permeates the family system and results in family disruption. For example, the medical bills may necessitate that the mother work outside the home, the father take on a second job, and vacation and leisure-time activities be eliminated. Strains in the marriage that then "ripple" into the other sets of family relationships are commonplace. Divorce, separation, acting-out children, psychosomatic problems, and substance abuse are symptomatic of the long-term disruptive effects that financial stress may induce (Millington & Zieball, 1986).

For the most part, nurses have tended to leave financial concerns up to the social worker to handle. Yet in many settings there is no available social worker and the nurse is the appropriate health care professional to intervene. Even if there is a social worker available, only when the nurse assesses for financial problems can he or she then become aware of the problem and make the appropriate referral.

Usually, nursing interventions in this area center around providing information to families on health care costs, health insurance, and community resources, as well as making referrals—a case management intervention (see Table 8–7).

Nurses need to be aware of the costs to families when complex problems arise, as well as the family's financial resources and how the family is paying and/or will pay for the needed services, supplies, equipment, and so forth. He or she should be familiar with the types of medical care programs available for the medically needy within the particular target population as well as the community services available free or at reduced costs for all regardless of their ability to pay. Immunizations and screening clinics are examples of these latter types of community resources.

Teaching in the financial area, according to Millington and Zieball (1986) includes teaching families about ways to reduce health care costs, to evaluate their insurance coverage, to determine how their health resources are being allocated, and where costs could safely be reduced. Teaching families how to look at their financial situation objectively and problem solve effectively is also suggested. Table 8–7 summarizes assessment and intervention strategies for assisting families at high risk for financial stress.

❧SUMMARY

- A crucial key to unlock our understanding of a family and how it behaves is the family's sociocultural background.

- To work effaciously with families, health care professionals must be aware of the unique, distinctive qualities and the variety of lifestyles, values, and structures in families' cultures.

- Cultural differences between client and provider are often at the root of poor communication, interpersonal tensions, and inadequate assessment and care.

- Because language is a fundamental aspect of culture, language barriers present major obstacles to effective family nursing care.

- Demographically, the United States is substantially changing. A massive surge of immigration in the 1990s, largely from Mexico and Asia, makes one in every three U.S. residents an ethnic minority.

- The American melting pot notion (the push toward homogeneity), has been replaced by the idea of an American stew (the push for cultural pluralism or heterogeneity). Moveover, retaining one's ethnic identity typically enriches family life and personal life satisfaction.

- A cross-cultural or transcultural approach to delivering family health care is mandatory in today's society.

- Fundamental concepts important for understanding cross-cultural principles and practice are described. These include the concepts of:

culture, ethnicity, intra-ethnic variation (variation within ethnic groups), the immigration experience, stereotyping, acculturation, biculturalism, the real versus the ideal, cultural relativism ethnocentrism, cultural imposition, cultural shock, and indigenous health care systems.

- Ethnic families are discussed in terms of how we view them. Do we see in their family structures and lifestyles cultural variation or deviance? The broader societal context must be examined to understand its role in shaping ethnic family life.

- In the past social scientists, when studying ethnic families, have gathered data from certain segments of those subcultures (i.e., the poor), often presenting an erroneous notion of the ethnic group.

- Socioeconomic status or social class in addition to ethnic background, exerts the greatest overall influence on family life, influencing family values and priorities, family behavioral patterns, socialization practices, family roles, and world experiences.

- There are four basic social classes in America: upper, middle, working, and lower class. Each social class is described. The foremost difference between the classes is simply economic resources.

- Due to differences in resources, there is a positive association between socioeconomic status and physical and mental health.

- Diversity within social classes is created because of the effects of the interaction of social class with ethnicity, religion, gender, and family form.

- The United States has great class inequality, with income, wealth, prestige, and power being heavily concentrated within the upper class.

- Middle-class families are numerically dominant in the United States and are subdivided into upper-middle- and lower-middle-class families. Although important commonalities exist, distinctive personal and family attributes are present within these two groups.

- The lower class constitutes 25 percent of the U.S. population. This class is subdivided into the working poor (20 percent) and the underclass (5 percent).

- Poverty in America is described in terms of its persistence and prevalence, the plight of working poor families today, the greater rates of poverty among ethnic and female-headed families, and the impact of poverty on family life.

- The underclass is composed of people who remain more or less permanently at the bottom of the social ladder. Their long-term poverty, welfare dependency, and bleak environmental living conditions nurture values and lifestyles that are at radical odds with the majority of Americans. Their lifestyle, values, and social and health needs are described.

- The family's economic status is a key indicator of social class. Income level, sources of income, and expenditures need to be considered when assessing a family's economic status.

- Social class mobility may be an important consideration in a family's life, as both upward and downward movement can produce major changes in the family and considerable stress.

- It is recommended that family identifying data be collected via the use of a family genogram. How to construct a family genogram is explained.

- A listing and explanation of areas to assess when conducting a cultural assessment of a family are presented. Table 8–6 summarizes ethnic assessment guidelines.

- In regards to family nursing diagnoses in the sociocultural area, there are no nursing diagnoses per say. Nevertheless, culture shapes values and family health behaviors. Some nursing diagnoses (in NANDA and other taxonomies) may be culturally biased and inappropriate to use with culturally diverse families.

- Assessment of family social class covers the family's income, adult members' occupations, and their educational attainment. Further discussion is included on how to assess family's economic status and social class mobility.

- A central goal of family nursing is to provide culturally appropriate and competent care to families.

- Guidelines for providing culturally competent health care to ethnic families are necessarily broad and varied.

- Seven basic strategies suggested in the cross-cultural literature are outlined and described.

- In those instances in which an economic (financial) assessment and interventions are needed, recommendations are made.

⚓ FAMILY VIGNETTE: THE GOMEZ FAMILY

There are four ethnic family case studies in this text (the following case, plus one in Chapters 18, 19, and 20). Please refer to those later chapters for more application of cultural content.

Nine-year-old Maria was initially seen in the emergency room by Mrs. Gomez, the emergency room nurse practitioner. Maria was brought to the ER by her parents and maternal grandmother. The family, according to the father, consists of the grandmother and his nuclear family (he, his wife, four school-aged daughters, and one teenager son). The family recently migrated here from El Salvador, and the parents speak some English but prefer to speak in Spanish when possible. The grandmother speaks only Spanish.

The parents stated that the crisis occurred because a young teenage cousin who was "high on some type of dope" had sexually abused Maria. In the first encounter with Maria and the family, the family nurse practitioner noticed that the Spanish-speaking grandmother had a very supportive impact on her granddaughter, who was very anxious and withdrawn, and on the parents, who were quiet and tense. It was the grandmother who was able to get the family members to explain clearly and fairly calmly what had happened and why they decided to come to the emergency room. She was able to provide comfort and support to Maria and persuade her to allow the nurse practitioner to examine her and ask her some questions about what happened. (Vignette adapted from Canino & Spurlock, 1994, p. 137).

■ STUDY QUESTIONS

1. From the data presented in the family vignette, assess the family's cultural background and social class status.

2. Identify what sociocultural data are missing and therefore needed to complete a sociocultural assessment.

3. Discuss sociocultural interventions that would be appropriate to incorporate into the care of this family and child.

Answer the following questions.

4. Briefly describe why it is essential to understand a family's ethnic background when providing family health care.

5. One of the assumptions made in dealing with families from different cultures is that we become less judgmental of other people's behavior as we attempt to (select the one best answer):
   a. Give up our values and learn to accept people as they are.
   b. Recognize the origins of our own values and understand why we hold them.
   c. Work purposefully to overlook other people's values that are contrary to our own.
   d. Gradually work to change other's values when we consider them detrimental.

6. Cultural ignorance and insensitivity lead to the following problems (choose all the correct answers):
   a. Poor communication
   b. Interpersonal tensions
   c. Stigmatization
   d. Inadequate assessments
   e. Professional objectivity

7. According to the U.S. Public Health Service (and other researchers), poverty is associated with which of the following health problems (select all correct answers)?

   a. Leading chronic illnesses
   b. Increased disability
   c. Increased infant mortality
   d. Teenage pregnancy
   e. Reduced longevity

8. Ethnicity is an important resource for individuals and families because (choose all the correct answers):

   a. It guides them in occupational choices.
   b. It compensates for the cold impersonality of modern society.
   c. Its traditions enrich family life and strengthen its continuity.
   d. It facilitates upward mobility.

9. Match the proper definition with the corresponding concept.

Concept	Definition
1. Cultural conflict	a. Blueprint for a person's way of living.
2. Acculturation	b. Common ancestry and shared cultural history.
3. Assimilation	c. Nonacceptance of diversity within cultural group.
4. Ethnic identity	d. Gradual changes created as one culture is influenced by another.
5. Ethnocentrism	e. The way individuals see themselves relative to their cultural identity.
6. Stereotyping	f. Denotes the more complete one-way process of acculturation.
7. Cultural relativism	g. Culture is viewed nonjudgmentally and understood within its own context.
8. Ethclass	h. Lack of cultural relativity (seeing one's own culture as superior to others).
9. Cultural imposition	i. Local professional health care system.
10. Culture shock	j. Lay or folk health care system.
11. Indigenous health care system	k. Primary tactic used in cultural anthropology to analyze cultures.
12. Self-fulfilling prophecy	l. Discomfort and confusion created by experiencing cultural differences.
13. Culture	m. The interaction of ethnicity and social class.
14. Ethnicity	n. Forcing one's values and practices on another person because of ethnocentricity.
	o. A degraded person's tendency to conform to the beliefs and expectations others have about him or her.
	p. Negative responses of clients to culturally unacceptable practices of health agencies and health workers.

10. The use of a cross-cultural or transcultural approach is vital when providing for family health care because it (select the one best answer):

  a. Provides information about different cultures.
  b. Predicts ethnic minority family behavior.
  c. Provides a broad comparative picture of individual and group behavior.
  d. Assumes a cultural deviant perspective in assessment.

11. Social class is based generally on three criteria: income, education, and occupational status. Identify which of these is the most important determinant.

  a. Income level
  b. Occupational status
  c. Educational level

12. The primary difference between a cultural variation versus a cultural deviance perspective with respect to ethnic families is:

  a. Feelings of evaluators
  b. Historical legacy
  c. Perception of etiology of differences.
  d. Objective reality of demography

13. Lower-middle-class families, in contrast with upper-middle-class families, tend to (choose all correct answers):

  a. Value education highly.
  b. Be more racially and ethnically mixed.
  c. Have closer kinship relations.
  d. Put more emphasis on individualism and productivity values.

14. The blue-collar or working class is often difficult to distinguish from the lower-middle class, especially because there may be little income difference. Nevertheless, the most obvious differences between the two groups are (choose all correct answers):

  a. Wife's employment.
  b. Emphasis on family background.
  c. Spending patterns.
  d. Husband's type of employment—manual versus nonmanual labor.
  e. Education.

15. The lower class consists of the poor. In this social class the following characteristics are prevalent (choose all correct answers):

  a. Most often families live in rural or suburban areas.
  b. Adult members have minimally paying jobs.
  c. The family may receive welfare.
  d. Family aspirations and behavior are very similar.

16. The poor family's value system is substantially different from the dominant culture values. Identify three examples of these contrasting values.

17. Family nursing interventions appropriate for promoting better family financial health include the following (complete the sentence):

    a. Health teaching addressing health-related financial problems of families may be in the area of _____.

    b. Initiating referrals addressing health-related financial problems of families may be to _____.

18. Broad intervention guidelines for working with families who are ethnically different from the family nurse include (choose all correct answers):

    a. Working with extended family system.

    b. Providing more time to work with unacculturated families.

    c. Using an interpreter to deal with language differences.

    d. Modifying communication after considering family's interaction norms.

    e. Focusing on family strengths and adaptation to adversity.

    f. Promoting positive change by negatively reinforcing families' unscientific health care practices.

FAMILY ENVIRONMENTAL DATA

❧ THE FAMILY ENVIRONMENT AND FAMILY HEALTH

This chapter begins with an overview of how nursing theorists have conceptualized the relationship between environmental factors and human health. Next, an ecological perspective guides discussion of environmental subsystems and assessment areas for family health related to the home environment, the neighborhood and community environments, and the sociopolitical environment. The final two sections address nursing diagnoses related to the family's environment and nursing interventions targeting family environmental factors. In family nursing practice, the nurse must assess the fit between the family's needs and environmental factors affecting family health (Holman, 1983; Killien, 1985; McCubbin & McCubbin, 1993).

Nurses have been concerned with the effects of the environment on the health of families throughout the history of Nursing. Florence Nightingale (1859/1946) wrote a guide for women caring for ill family members in 1859, emphasizing the importance of a healthy environment for the family member's recovery:

> In watching disease, both in private houses and in public hospitals, the thing which strikes the experienced observer most forcibly is this, that the symptoms or the sufferings generally considered to be inevitable and incident to the disease are very often not symptoms of the disease at all, but of something quite different—of the want of fresh air, or of light, or of warmth, or of quiet, or of cleanliness, or of punctuality and care in the administration of diet, of each or of all of these. (p. 5)

Environment continued as a central concept in nursing into the twentieth century (Fawcett, 1989; Meleis, 1997). Environment was clearly identified as one of nursing's four metaparadigm concepts—environment, nursing, health, and person—in the 1970s (Fawcett, 1984). The main proposition about the relationship of the four concepts was that "Nursing studies the wholeness or health of humans, recognizing that humans are in continuous interactions with their environments" (Donaldson & Crowley, 1978, p. 119). The concept of environment has been integrated within most nursing conceptual models.

However, definitions of *environment* sometimes have reflected a relatively narrow view of environmental factors affecting the health of individuals and families, with emphasis on the immediate social and physical surroundings of the person or family. For example, Steiger and Lipson (1985) pointed out that health hazards in the home, on the road, in the workplace, and in the broader environment have striking, if sometimes subtle, effects on health (p. 276). Chopoorian (1986) was influential in changing how nurses conceptualized environmental factors related to health. She wrote, "In an effort to reconceptualize environment, I suggest here that nurses develop a consciousness of environment as social, economic, and political structures" (p. 47).

Models of environmental factors affecting family health have been drawn primarily from epidemiological and ecological literature (Kleffel, 1991). Public health professionals focus on epidemiological data in developing strategies to promote improved health among aggregates of people both nationally and globally. This is significant data but insufficient for nursing practice.

An ecological perspective guides discussion of key environmental factors related to family health with attention to the family microsystems, macrosystems, and suprasystems. Bronfenbrenner (1979) called the specific places where individuals and families engage in specific activities and roles microsystems or behavior settings. These are the immediate physical contexts in which face-to-face encounters between family members and others occur. At a broader level, the family is situated in environmental macrosystems. For instance, the macrosystems of a family could be the educational system, work system, and social service systems (Wiley, 1996). Suprasystems include the national and global sociopolitical context for macrosystem and microsystems functioning. Critical theory has great relevance for nurses assessing the effects of oppressive environmental effects on health, including the effects of sociopolitical power structures on health policy and, ultimately, family health (Meleis, 1997; Kleffel, 1991).

For purposes of this chapter, the family microsystem environment of interest is the family's home, the family macrosystems are addressed in terms of the family neighborhood and community, and the suprasystem is considered in terms of relevant sociopolitical and economic factors in the society where the family lives. The physical characteristics of the family's home environment are addressed in this chapter while social aspects of the home environment are addressed in separate chapters. Sociopolitical, economic, and physical dimensions of the family's environmental macrosystems and suprasystems are addressed in this chapter. Both systems and structural–functional theory, two of the text's organizing theoretical frameworks, stress the vital nature of the family's interaction with its external physical and cultural and sociopolitical environments.

Environmental demands and environmental stress (where the demands exceed the family's resources) can exist both within the family's micro- and macrosystems (Melson, 1983). For example, a microsystem stressor may be the lead-based paint in the home, while the macrosystem stressor may relate to child injuries or deaths sustained in pedestrian–motor vehicle collisions within the neighborhood. Additionally, the suprasystem (sociopolitical, economic environment) may pose the greatest challenge to resolving environmental stressors. Examples of suprasystem stressors are lack of funding for an elevated crosswalk through a busy intersection or refusal of elected officials to allocate funds for the crosswalk. Hence, the environment (micro-, macro-, suprasystems) directly and indirectly influence family health.

❧CHARACTERISTICS OF THE HOME ENVIRONMENT

This section focuses on selected characteristics of the family home environment, which can affect family health. The first section describes aspects of the family's housing in terms of structure, safety, and other health hazards. The second section addresses resources in the home related to the health of family members. The third section focuses on the circumstances for increasing numbers of families who are homeless and environmental factors affecting the health of homeless family members.

HOUSING: STRUCTURE, SAFETY, AND HEALTH HAZARDS

Provision of a healthy environment in the form of adequate shelter is an aspect of family functioning that is of special concern to family nurses. A family's home is extraordinarily significant for its members because the home environment has a significant impact on both the physical and mental health of the family and its members. Psychologically, one's home becomes part of the family identity. "Home is that place where things are familiar and unchanging and where people maintain some sense of autonomy and control" (Rauckhorst, Stokes, & Mezey, 1982, p. 159). A home provides a sense of origin and continuity with one's ethnic roots, a sense of privacy, a sense of safety and security, a sense of familiarity, and a sense of behavioral consistency, referring to family rules, and rituals (Taylor, 1995).

Through home visits, nurses are able to observe the physical setting of the home and the particular arrangement of family life space, observations that otherwise would be impossible. Direct assessment of the home environment provides a valuable aid in understanding the family and its lifestyle. Because the home is its territory, the family behaves more naturally and comfortably at home than in other settings, providing the visitor with a clearer picture of family life. In fact, many aspects on family life, such as sanitary and safety conditions, can be accurately assessed only during home visits (Daniel, 1986; Martin & Scheet, 1992). Before describing actual assessment areas relative to the home environment, the following section reviews salient literature on housing and its effect on families, the concept of territoriality, the impact of crowding and safety in the home.

The effects of housing can be seen in two major areas. First, there are psychological aspects that affect self-perception and life satisfaction; if these are negative, they can serve as stressors and illness-producing factors. Second are the effects of possible physical hazards—due to the house's state of repair, its facilities, and its arrangement (Schorr, 1970; Wiley, 1996). Such physical conditions may influence privacy, child-rearing practices, housekeeping, study habits, as well as contribute to the transmission or exposure to disease and the possibility of accidents and poisonings (Wiley). Moreover, the placement of houses and apartments in relation to one another and to the larger urban environment clearly influences family and social relationships.

Housing may affect behavior by contributing to or dissipating stress, albeit some people have more effective adjustive mechanisms than others. Almost any characteristic of housing that negatively affects individuals may be interpreted as stressful—crowding, dilapidation, vermin infestations, or high noise levels are examples. Two further stressful factors are social isolation and inadequate space. There is some evidence that aged people who live alone are more likely to require psychiatric hospitalization than those living with families. Findings from an interdisciplinary case management program along the United States–Mexico border indicated that 44 percent of the clients served had problems related to social contact; 71 percent of the clients had limited social contact, while 58 percent had minimal outside activities (Slack & McEwen, 1999). Any environment that tends to isolate an individual from others represents a stress that will lead to distinguishable personality changes. The amount of space per person and the way space is arranged to promote or interfere with privacy have also been related to stress (Schorr, 1970).

Home environments need to be suitable for the development and health of family members as well as for the family as a whole. One of the most difficult problems poor and working-class families face is that their home, neighborhood, and community environments are not conducive to wellness, and yet they do not have the option to move. For example, the neighborhood may not have sidewalks or adequate lighting, both of which represent barriers to families walking for exercise.

Substantial evidence links poor housing with poor health. It is well understood that certain diseases are correlated with poor housing (see Table 9–1 for examples).

Healthy People 2010 builds on earlier national initiatives and identifies health improvement goals and objectives to improve health for all Americans. This document targets objectives to reduce indoor allergen levels including dust mite and cockroach allergens (U.S. Department of Health and Human Services, 2000) both known to adversely affect health (Ricchini, 1997). Even though family pets provide tremendous psychosocial benefits, they also can cause health problems, either directly from animal bites or through animal-transmitted infections (*Salmonella* from dogs, psittacosis from pet birds, fleas from dogs and cats, allergies—eczema and asthma—from the fur of hairy pets).

Individuals and family groups have a sense of territoriality, also referred to as spatial behavior (Giger & Davidhizar, 1995). Animals, as part of their innate repertoire of behaviors, lay claim to a specific area and defend this area against intruders, while other animals, in turn, tend to respect their claims. A similar type of instinctual characteristic applies to people and families. The human desire to possess and occupy specified areas is pervasive, even though overt expression of infringement by others is attenuated by socialization. Space also refers to the distance between individuals in the context of interaction (Davidhizar & Bechtel, 1999). An individual's personal space expands, shrinks, and changes in openness depending on the social situation, the physical context, the culture of the person, and the other persons present (Meisenhelder, 1982;

TABLE 9–1

EXAMPLES OF DISEASES ASSOCIATED WITH POOR HOUSING

- Acute respiratory infections related to the multiple use of toilet and water facilities, inadequate heating or ventilation, and inadequate and crowded sleeping arrangements.

- Minor digestive diseases and enteritis related to poor facilities for the cold storage of food and to inadequate washing of hands and toilet facilities and sharing of food and drink and towels.

- Injuries resulting from home accidents related to crowded physical space in home, inadequate kitchens, poor electrical wiring, poorly lighted and unstable stairs, and slippery floors.

- Infectious and noninfectious diseases of the skin related to crowding, shared towels, and inadequate facilities for washing.

- Lead poisoning in children who eat scaling paint from typically poor, older homes.

- Repiratory diseases related to asbestos and radon exposure in the home.

Davidhizar & Bechtel). A person's level of comfort is very much related to his or her personal space, and if a person's personal space is invaded, discomfort results (Giger & Davidhizar).

Home territory is an area where the family has relatively more freedom of behavior and a sense of control and power over both the area and its members. The home visit represents a shift in the nurse–client relationship—that is, the nurse is now a guest in the client's home rather than the client being a visitor in the nurse's professional territory (e.g., a clinic). At home, the client controls the nurse's entrance into the home and what happens following the encounter. Consequently, nurses may feel uncomfortable during the first home visits due to the feeling that they are intruding into someone else's home territory. Families may also feel uncomfortable about this intrusion, especially when health care workers come unannounced or uninvited. To increase the success of the initial home visit and the likelihood of being invited back, the nurse should keep the first encounter brief and not overly structured (Martin & Scheet, 1992). It is essential that the nurse clarify her or his role and purpose for the first and subsequent home visits. For example, the nurse might explain that because the client is enrolled in the Health Start Program, the nurse would be providing education related to fetal growth and development and maternal body changes during weekly home visits. It is important to engage family members in the home visits through the process of collaboration and mutual goal setting to work on issues that are of priority to both the identified client and the family.

Within families there are both spatial (physical) and behavioral dimensions of territoriality. The feelings of belonging and cohesiveness among family members make up the behavioral component, while the actual physical space of home, yard, family name and address, and frequently visited community systems—school, work, shopping centers, churches, and community agencies with which the family interacts—are the spatial aspects of territoriality (Anderson & Carter, 1974).

Some families may be at ease moving in a wider geographic complex. The territory that the family feels comfortable in and moves in may in part be a function of economics, citizenship status, physical mobility, cultural or personal values, or socialization. For example, a survey administered at a health fair in south Los Angeles County (approximately 140 miles from the Mexican border) revealed that 14 percent of the survey respondents had crossed the border for health care within the past year. Interestingly, almost 80 percent of the respondents crossing the border for health care were uninsured, which also reveals the function of economics in their decision making (Macia & Morales, 2001). Moreover, for many Hispanics, accessing health care in Mexico is driven by the cultural values of personalismo and collectivism or a preference for health care providers with similar backgrounds (Caudle, 1993).

During the 1970s, well over 200 studies researched some facet of crowding (Epstein, 1981). Schorr (1970), in summarizing the results of "crowding studies," commented that fatigue and too little sleep may be consequences of seriously inadequate, crowded housing. School nurses can certainly corroborate these findings, as they observe fatigued children come into their school health offices. The effect of crowding on intrafamily friction has also been observed. One of the results of seriously inadequate space in the home is that family members spend much of their time outside the home. This tendency may be a particularly serious matter in relation to children and adolescents. It has been observed that poor children from crowded, inadequate homes do not study sufficiently and are not within reach of parental control. "Street life" takes on increasing importance for many of these children during grammar school years and by the time the adolescent years begin, peer associations "on the street" are frequently very influential.

There appears to be inconclusive findings with respect to the effects of crowding on family members' actual physical health status. Crowding does, however, make sufficient privacy difficult to achieve. Privacy functions to protect and maintain an individual's need for personal autonomy, to serve as an emotional release, and to provide an opportunity for self-appraisal and protected communication. Having one's own room, bed, possessions, clothes, toys, and pets are assets. Privacy for an adolescent is especially significant in assisting him or her to achieve the developmental needs of independence. Marital privacy is also critical in most families.

Epstein (1981) found that a person's perceived sense of control influenced how individuals adjusted to crowded conditions. If an individual perceived that he or she was able to maintain adequate personal control over his or her environment, this fostered more favorable adaptation to crowding in the home.

Crowding is very strongly associated with socioeconomic status and ethnic background and is relative to what a person has experienced in the past. If a family has never known anything but "crowded living," then this situation does not seem so intolerable. For example, because of their cultural background and economic conditions, many family residents of Colonias (housing developments in rural and unincorporated areas along the United States–Mexico border) are comfortable living in one-room dwellings, and it is common for neighbors to drop in uninvited (Davidhizar & Bechtel, 1999).

Two of the most valuable assessment areas for community health and home health nurses relative to the home are the assessment of safety conditions and of potential or real hazards, both inside and outside the home. Especially within the home, accidents are a major threat to a family's health status. Each family member is exposed to certain threats from accidents related to his or her developmental stage (Kandzari & Howard, 1981). For example, in Arizona during the period from 1988 to 1998, suffocation (aspiration of food or other foreign object or mechanical suffocation) was the leading cause of unintentional injury deaths among infants and children 5 to 9 years of age, burning by fire among preschoolers 1 to 4 years old, firearms among children ages 10 to 14, and poisoning/drug misuse among adolescents 15 to 19 years old (Arizona Department of Health Services [ADHS], 2000). "Increasing the family's awareness of the chief accident problems, providing factual information, and suggesting ways for the family to improve its level of safety wellness are the goals" (Kandzari & Howard, p. 223).

Nationwide injury is the leading cause of death among children (except infants under 1 year) and adolescents (ADHS, 2000). Unintentional injuries, many occurring in homes, are the leading cause of death in the United States for people aged 1 to 34 (Centers for Disease Control and Prevention [CDC], 1998). In the state of Arizona, injury surpasses all major diseases as the cause of premature mortality among preschoolers 1 to 4 years old, children 5 to 14 years old, and adolescents 15 to 19 years of age. Unintentional injuries include motor vehicle–related, drowning, poisoning, suffocation, and fire/flames

(ADHS, 2000). Each year, more than 90,000 people die in the United States as a result of unintentional injuries. During an average year in the United States, unintentional injuries account for nearly 31 million emergency room visits (Burt & Fingerhut, 1998).

Potential or actual hazards in the home include the possible presence of lead, which adversely affects children's intellectual and emotional growth, and is found in older plumbing and household dust as old paint deteriorates or is chipped away. Approximately 74 percent of dwellings built before 1980 contain lead-based paint (which has been prohibited since 1978). Exposure to lead "poses the nation's number 1 environmental health threat to children . . . an enormous number of young Americans will not realize their full potential because of their exposure to lead in their environments" (Lum, 1995, p. 27). Young children who are poor and African-American are disproportionally affected by this health threat.

Other hazardous substances that may be found in homes are indoor air pollution, substances found in some building materials, and radon. Indoor contaminants, especially, may present a widespread pollution threat. Concentrations of some airborne pollutants have been found to be as high as 100 times greater indoors than outdoors (U.S. Environmental Protection Agency, 1988).

One major source of indoor air pollution is tobacco smoke. The long-term secondary effects of tobacco smoke are clearly acknowledged as a serious health hazard. The pollutants in smoke caused by improperly maintained or vented wood stoves can be another air pollution hazard in homes. A wide variety of organic compounds from common household products may contribute to the threat of indoor pollution.

Commonly used household products such as air fresheners, shoe polish, paints, cleaners, mothballs, and dry-cleaned clothing contain low levels of chemicals that are known animal carcinogens. Cleaning solutions and powders containing chemicals that are toxic, abrasive, or caustic to eyes and mucous membranes are labeled by most manufacturers with warnings about potential dangers. Families should be encouraged to store such substances properly and out of reach of young children.

Noxious by-products of cigarette, pipe, and cigar smoking such as carbon monoxide and nitrogen dioxide may predispose household occupants, especially children, to pneumonia, other respiratory ailments, and cancer. Formaldehyde, widely used in newer building materials and furnishings, can cause eye, nose, and throat irritation; coughing; skin rashes; headaches; dizziness; nausea; vomiting; and nosebleeds. Products sold to kill household pests may leave pesticide residues, with many of these chemicals having never been tested to determine their health effects.

Building materials in older homes may be a hazard, particularly building materials containing asbestos. Asbestos was used in many types of building materials from about 1950 through the early 1970s to make materials sturdier. Asbestos exposure leads to serious respiratory disease.

Radon, an odorless, colorless gas is another home hazard. It is emitted through cracks in basement walls and floors and enters the body through ingestion of contaminated water supplies or in the home, through inhalation of air. Long-term exposure to radon is one cause of lung cancer (Lum, Hibbs, Phillips, & Narkunas, 1996). *Healthy People 2010* includes objectives to increase the proportion of persons who live in homes tested for radon concentrations and increase the number of new homes constructed to be radon resistant (U.S. Department of Health and Human Services, 2000).

RESOURCES IN THE HOME ENVIRONMENT

An important part of assessing the home environment in relation to family health is evaluation of resources to support optimal health of individual family members and the family unit. The assessment may be related to family members of any age and may focus on varied types of resources such as assistive devices or access to information. For example, the nurse may assess whether there are age-appropriate reading and play materials (Barnard, 1986) and other "IQ-boosting" (Begley & Springen, 2001) environmental resources to enhance children's cognitive development and academic success. Home resources could include simple assistive devices such as a telephone amplifier to enable a hearing-impaired elder to make phone calls or a sound-to-light intercom system ("crying light") to alert a deaf mother that her baby has awakened from her nap in the next room. Approximately 54 million Americans have some type of disability (Meadows, 1999) and so millions of families have family members of all ages with a range of physical and mental disabilities. Many of these families could benefit from assistive devices designed to promote optimal development and functioning for the individuals with disabilities and for their families.

Access to Internet and e-mail are key factors in accessing information and can enhance family communication. Because information is crucial to empowering families to participate in health-related decisions, nurses must assess whether a family has ready access to informational resources, especially through the Internet. Families without Internet access will be at a distinct disadvantage in terms of informational resources and communication with family and friends in other locations. Begley and Springen (2001) painted a picture of teen's use of technology: "Teen multitaskers—simultaneously IM'ing [using the instant message feature], downloading and channel surfing—may be exercising their memory (a component of intelligence) and training their attention to switch focus in the blink of an eye" (p. 2). Many families have at least one computer with Internet access at home, which is often used by family members of all ages: School children search for information for reports, parents access Web sites for direct health-related information, and grandparents exchange messages and photos with grandchildren in other states. Computer skills are necessary for school performance and are frequently part of required job skills for adults. In fact, the escalating use of technology has effectively widened the financial disparities among poor versus affluent groups. Hillary Clinton (1996) wrote about the expanding technological environment of families:

> The horizons of the contemporary village extend well beyond the town line. From the moment we are born, we are exposed to vast numbers of other people and influences through radio, television, newspapers, books, movies, computers, compact discs, cellular phones, and fax machines. Technology connects us to the impersonal global village it has created. (p. 13)

While it is rare to find a home without a telephone and television, there are still many families who cannot afford computers or do not have the skills to use home computers. Many public libraries offer classes in computer use, and families who do not have computers at home can access the Internet and e-mail through the computers at public schools and libraries. However, technological resources such as television and Internet are not without problems. Along with nearly immediate access to informational resources come problems of children accessing inappropriate sites (such as pornography), viewing age-inappropriate programming, or engaging in chat-room conversations with strangers. Nurses may discuss the importance of monitoring children's use of the Internet and security measures available on request. Assessment for home resources, such as assistive devices and Internet access, is consistent with a strengths-based approach to enhance the home resources to support family health.

HOMELESS FAMILIES

Homelessness as a societal problem has risen sharply in the United States since 1980. Particularly in cities and temperate regions, homelessness has been a major community health concern (Taylor, 1995). Among the most alarming characteristics of this growing population is the rising number of families with children, which constitute the fastest growing segment of the homeless population (Bassuk, 1990, cited in Taylor, 1995; Jackson & McSwane, 1996). The Children's Defense Fund estimated that 500,000 children in the United States are homeless (Kozol, 1990). Families with children constitute approximately 40 percent of people who become homeless (National Coalition for the Homeless [NCH], 1999). Nine out of 10 homeless families with children are female-headed households.

Poverty and the lack of affordable housing are the principal causes of family homelessness. Other contributing factors are domestic violence, substance abuse, and mental illness. Having experienced disruptive family events such as divorce, illness, physical abuse, and sexual abuse is common among homeless mothers (Anderson & Koblinsky, 1995).

Homelessness is an overwhelming and disruptive experience for families. It affects all aspects of family functioning and has an impact on the physical and emotional health of family members. Cramped living space, loss of privacy, and the rigid rules imposed in shelters affect the quality of family relationships and the ability of parents to parent their children (Lindsey, 1998). Family homelessness has an impact on the health and well-being of all family members. Homeless parents experience high rates of depression and chronic health conditions. Homeless children are ill more often than domiciled children and suffer from both acute and chronic illnesses, especially asthma, gastrointestinal problems, and infestations of lice. In addition, they often experience more developmental delays, anxiety, behavioral problems, and lower educational achievement (NCH, 1999; Choi & Snyder, 1999). However, even homeless families are not a homogeneous group. Danseco and Holden (1998) identified a typology of homeless families with three clusters: at risk, resilient, and "getting by" groups of homeless families. The clusters differed mainly in terms of whether they had been homeless previously, the degree of parenting stress, and major life stressors. Danseco and Holden suggested that the effects of homelessness on children differ, depending on the family's history, parental stress, and specific circumstances. Results of Lindsey's study of the impact of homelessness and shelter life on family relationships indicated that in addition to the negative experiences often described for families living in shelters, some mothers reported "increased closeness and heightened quality and quantity of interaction with their children" while living in shelters.

In response to the continuing family homelessness crisis, communities have built shelters and initiated transitional housing programs. Often, however, little attention has been paid to the unique issues presented by families. Assessment must address the immediate shelter environment (if the family is sheltered), accessing health care for family members, strategies for assisting families to achieve and maintain stable housing and to develop support networks (Letiecq, Anderson, & Koblinsky, 1998).

✎CHARACTERISTICS OF THE NEIGHBORHOOD AND COMMUNITY ENVIRONMENTS

The neighborhood and community in which the family lives exerts a tremendous influence on the health of the family. Using systems and structural–

functional frameworks for assessing families, the family nurse needs to examine the family microsystem within the context of its macro- and suprasystems or universe. The microsystem includes family's neighborhood and community. The neighborhood and adjoining community can be described relative to their physical and their psychosocial impact on families.

PHYSICAL AND GEOGRAPHIC CHARACTERISTICS OF THE NEIGHBORHOOD

The neighborhood and wider community that the family lives in have definite effects on family health. Wiley (1996) provides an extensive discussion of environmental issues, which may affect physical characteristics of neighborhoods and noted that "the macroecosystem is enormous, and yet it is shrinking with every passing day. Problems that once affected only small populations in distant corners of the globe are now important to townships, states and nations" (p. 347). Noise, traffic, air, and garbage pollution, of course, produce continual, probably low-level stress. For instance, living near a toxic dump or near stagnant water may adversely affect health. Chronic, low-level exposures to toxic substances in the air, water, and food can produce physical diseases and conditions that have a latency period, an insidious onset, or a diffuse set of symptoms (Wiley, 1996). Examples of environmental problems listed in the Omaha family assessment system at the neighborhood or community level include high crime rate, uncontrolled animals (e.g., stray dogs), and unsafe play areas (Martin & Scheet, 1992). **Rural communities** have drastically different effects on individuals and families than do urban areas. Recently, there has been extensive interest and concern about the health and other needs of rural families (Bushy, 1990; Weinert & Long, 1987). It seems that the rural environment, in spite of its more personalized social environment and tranquil setting, has some unique, special problems. The primary economic resources of a region, such as farming, ranching, lumbering, or mining directly affect the rural community. Inasmuch as farming, lumbering, and mining (three major industries) have experienced recent crises, stressors that rural communities and families face also have amplified. Rural people are described as being self-reliant and traditional in their values and as having a strong work ethic. Increased economic hardships, however, have markedly eroded the ability of families to uphold these values (DeFrain, LeMasters & Schroff, 1991). Accessibility to health care and other needed services has declined due to geographic remoteness as well as economic hardship (Bushy, 1990).

SOCIAL AND DEMOGRAPHIC CHARACTERISTICS OF THE NEIGHBORHOOD

In describing the psychosocial effects of the neighborhood on families, the type of social interaction that occurs in different types of neighborhoods has been studied. Substantial social and economic homogeneity has existed in most of the communities that have been studied. In homogeneous neighborhoods, because the families' behavior patterns, values, and interests are alike, neighborhood-based friendships tend to be formed. Homogeneity is found to be more significant in creating a large number of friendships and associations than is proximity (Schorr, 1970).

In stable working-class neighborhoods, family membership is concentrated in the locality, and the most active ties are with other members of the family. Proximity makes for frequent contacts with relatives and other neighbors, casually in passing and less casually on the sidewalk or in the local shops. There is considerable attachment to the place itself. Relationships are identified with locality.

Many middle-class Americans have few neighborhood and/or community roots and move from city to city and region to region as their jobs and personal preferences dictate. Mobility is highest among young adults, those in middle-income levels, and those in the military or migrant labor jobs. Hence, their support systems within the community may be lacking.

Another effect of neighborhood and community is its effect on life satisfaction. Satisfaction with neighborhood and community have been found to be closely associated with satisfaction with life in general (Chilman, 1978). It is also true that people's expectations of neighborhoods and communities by people differ, depending on social class status: The higher the social class, the greater the expectations of the community (Rainwater, 1972). These same differences in expectations are observed in community agencies. Low-income families may expect little assistance, while affluent families may have high demands and expectations. The lower expectations are correlated with and result from feelings of powerlessness and learned helplessness.

Neighborhood schools are important macrosystems with which many families interact. While the schools may provide valuable support for family members' health, such as school-based family clinics, there are often health hazards connected with school attendance. Recent reports indicate that up to 30 percent of U.S. school children do not feel safe at school. Bullying is rampant, and teenage suicide attempts are at epidemic levels. There has been a significant growth of violence among girls and now among younger children. One objective of *Healthy People 2010* is to increase the proportion of the nation's primary and secondary schools that have official school policies ensuring the safety of students and staff from environmental hazards, such as chemicals in special classrooms, poor indoor air quality, asbestos, and exposure to pesticides (U.S. Department of Health and Human Services, 2000). Consistent with an ecological perspective, problems originating with troubled schools affect both the individual students and their entire families. School safety impacts all members of the community who live there and so must be aware and involved in improving school environments (Wiley, 1996).

❧ SOCIOPOLITICAL ENVIRONMENT AND FAMILY HEALTH

The conceptualization of environment in nursing theory has changed from a focus on individuals' adaptation to the immediate environment to an ecological perspective describing interacting systems, and finally to incorporation of critical theory in evaluating the effects of the sociopolitical environment on family health. The sociopolitical environment encompasses an enormous arena with complex factors interacting to create circumstances, which may enable or limit families' health-related opportunities. Examples of how the political decisions about health policy and legal decisions can impact family life are abundant. Gebbie and Gebbie (2001) recite numerous examples of how legal definitions of family relationships can create situations in conflict with the social definitions of family and be detrimental to family health. Wiley (1996) gives numerous examples of laws about environmental hazards and occupational safety, which can effectively safeguard or endanger the health of families and communities across the country. A recent popular film, *Traffic*, portrays the conflict between public policy in favor of a war on drugs versus the actual human face of drug addiction in family life (Alter, 2001). The Bush administration nearly dismantled the Office of National AIDS Policy, which had the potential for serious consequences for families with a member with HIV/AIDS (Spencer, 2001).

This section presents three examples of specific sociopolitical forces related to family health: the Americans with Disabilities Act (ADA) and family income, access to health care for undocumented immigrants, and transition programs for homeless families.

Title I of the ADA prohibits most employers from discriminating against qualified individuals with disabilities in job application procedures, hiring, firing, advancement, compensation, job training, and other aspects of employment (McCrone, 1990). Nevertheless, employment and consequently family income for adults with disabilities continues to be significantly lower than for people who are not considered disabled. For example, deaf adults are more often unemployed or underemployed and have a lower mean educational level than their hearing counterparts, which result in a lower average income. McCrone (1990) estimated that deaf adults earned between $356,000–$609,000 less than their comparably educated hearing counterparts over the course of a lifetime. Deaf people are over-represented in blue-collar occupations, enjoy less job mobility, and are often underemployed (McCrone, 1990). This disparity is likely to be even larger now as the estimates are more than a decade old. For instance, Jones (1995) found that the income for 20 deaf-parented families was consistently lower than the income for a matched group of hearing-parented families, despite similarities in the parents' educational level across groups. These disparities translate directly into fewer family resources and lesser ability to fulfill family functions satisfactorily. The ADA has provided legal recourse for parents with disabilities to remedy job discrimination and seek to end disparities in potential family incomes.

The second example focuses on access to health care for families who are undocumented immigrants. These families may be constricted in their movement due to feelings of fear, discomfort, and/or poverty; and yet may be uncomfortable moving from their neighborhood. For example, a person who enters or remains in the United States without following established immigration procedures is considered an undocumented alien (Messias, 1997). Restricted mobility is one of the consequences of being undocumented due to the lack of legal documents that allow for mobility. Fear of immigration-related legal trouble keeps many undocumented immigrants socially isolated in their homes. In addition, undocumented immigrants' mobility problems are compounded by cultural, financial, and linguistic barriers resulting in low use of preventive health services and a delay in curative care (Messias; Asch, Leake, & Gelberg, 1994). In one study about the use of health services by Mexican immigrants, it was reported that women who were undocumented had less prenatal care utilization and worse follow-through on postnatal care for themselves and their newborns compared to both documented immigrants and U.S. citizens (Geltman & Meyers, 1999). Recent changes in immigration procedures and more liberal guest worker laws may decrease fears of deportation and result in increased use of health resources by families who were previously considered undocumented immigrants.

The third example relates to transition programs available for homeless families. An earlier section described the circumstances of homeless families, health problems associated with homelessness, the difficulties encountered in their efforts to gain stable housing, job skills, and employment necessary to sustain home residences. Successful transition from homelessness to having permanent housing and a more stable family life depend on favorable public opinion and political action for funding of transition programs for homeless people. Public policies directed toward family homelessness need to address the creation of jobs that pay livable wages, access to affordable child care, and provision of affordable decent housing. In addition, educational, health, and social services need to be available for children from homeless families to alleviate the negative educa-

tional, developmental, health, and psychosocial effects of poverty and homelessness (Choi & Snyder, 1999). What is called for is a unified preventive plan that focuses on definitive proactive prevention while maintaining intervention preparedness and crisis management. Many shelters for women and children are funded by private religious organizations. With a new president and a new party structure at the national level, there have been changes in policy to allow government funding for faith-based organizations. This policy change may increase funding levels for many existing shelters. These changes at the national level may well result in more and better transition programs for homeless families.

Political action toward humane health policy is not new in nursing. However, deliberate critical assessment of the sociopolitical environment and its impact on family health is strengthened by incorporating critical theory into family nursing theory. Nurses cannot fully address family health without considering the full environmental context of the family, including its sociopolitical environment.

AREAS OF ASSESSMENT

This section first presents questions designed to assess the home environment; both Kandzari and Howard (1981) and Rauckhorst, Stokes, and Mezey (1982) provide more detailed coverage of this area. Second, questions are presented for assessing the community and neighborhood environments.

ASSESSING THE HOME ENVIRONMENT

1. Describe the dwelling type (home, apartment, or rooming house). Does family own or rent its home?

2. Describe the home's condition (both the interior and exterior of house). House interior would include number of rooms and types of rooms (living room, bedrooms, etc.), their use, and how they are furnished. What is the condition and adequacy of the furniture? Is there adequate heating, cooling, ventilation, and lighting? Are the floors, stairs, railings,

and other structures in good repair? Is the water supply adequate? Is there a telephone in the home or accessibility to a phone? What is the condition of the yard?

3. In the kitchen, assess the water supply, sanitation, and the adequacy of refrigeration and cooking facilities.

4. In the bathrooms, observe sanitation, water supply, toilet facilities, and presence of towels and soap. Does everyone have his or her own towels or are towels shared? In bathtubs, are there grab bars (important to older persons' homes)?

5. Assess the sleeping arrangements in the house. Are they adequate for family members, considering their age, relationships, and special needs?

6. Observe the home's general state of cleanliness and sanitation. What are the family's hygiene and cleanliness practices? Are there any infestations of vermin (interior especially)? If there are pets, are there any sanitation problems related to their presence?

7. Are there signs of flaking, old paint (possible lead poisoning hazard), which young children might be exposed to?

8. Identify the family's territorial unit. Are family members comfortable driving out of their neighborhood to use resources/services in other parts of the community?

9. Evaluate the privacy arrangements and how the family feels about the adequacy of its privacy.

10. Evaluate the presence or absence of safety hazards in other areas of the home. Ask about the storage of medicines and substances containing toxic substances. Are they stored safely away from children and pets and clearly marked? If family members use poisonous or potentially harmful substances (e.g., cleaning fluids, glues, etc.), do they carefully follow directions on their use? Observe for dangerous objects that might cause safety hazards to children or elderly family members. Are the entrances and exits of the house barrier free, and is there adequate space and lighting to move safely through the house (Daniel,

1986)? Are there any exposed or frayed electrical cords, or loose rugs on the floor? Are there provisions for emergencies (smoke detector, emergency numbers by the phone)? Is there a swimming pool, and if so, is it adequately fenced in and locked if small children are in the home?

11. Evaluate the adequacy of waste and garbage disposal.

12. Assess the family members' overall feelings and satisfaction with their housing arrangements. Does the family consider its home adequate for its needs? Are there adequate resources for all family members?

Another listing of home environment hazards comes from the Omaha System, designed by the Visiting Nurse Association of Omaha. This system includes a problem classification scheme for the environmental domain, which consists of the client's home, neighborhood, and broader community (Martin & Scheet, 1992). The environmental domain is defined as "the material resources, physical surroundings, and substances both internal and external to the client, home, neighborhood, and broader community" (Martin & Scheet, p. 67). There are 12 items listed on the Omaha problem rating scale related to the home (see Table 9–2). The Omaha system also includes assessment of family financial resources, which may be related to the sociopolitical environment. For example, family problems of low/no income and difficulty buying necessities may be related to the difficulty experienced by a parent with a physical disability in finding work. The Omaha System is discussed in more detail in Chapter 7.

AREAS OF ASSESSMENT: NEIGHBORHOOD AND COMMUNITY

Healthy families are those that are active and reach out in self-initiating ways to relate to various community groups (Lewis & associates, 1976; McCubbin & McCubbin, 1993). Families who are functioning in a healthy way perceive themselves as being related to and part of the larger community. Part of families' successful coping is their ability to secure compliance from the environment or to maintain a good family–environment fit (Hall & Weaver, 1974; McCubbin & McCubbin,

TABLE 9–2

OMAHA SYTEM: PROBLEMS DESCRIBED IN ENVIRONMENTAL DOMAIN: RESIDENCE (FAMILY HOME)

Structurally unsound

Inadequate heating and/or cooling

Steep stairs

Inadequate and/or obstructed exits or entries

Cluttered living space

Unsafe storage of dangerous objects/substances

Unsafe mats or throw rugs

Inadequate safety devices

Presence of lead-based paint

Unsafe gas and/or electrical appliances

Inadequate or crowded living space

Homeless

Source: Adapted from the Omaha System's Data Base/Problem List in Martin & Scheet, 1992, p. 343.

1993), meaning that within the community the family is able to seek out, receive, and/or accept the appropriate resources to meet its needs for food, services, and information. Passive acceptance of community services, however delivered, may be an indication of an isolated, estranged family or a dependent family that is functioning on a much lower level of health. Completing a family ecomap (see Figures 17–4 and 17–5) is quite useful for obtaining information about family members' associations and transactions with their social network and community. These specific questions are suggested to assess the community.

1. What are the characteristics of the immediate neighborhood and the larger community?

    Type of neighborhood and community (rural, suburban, urban, inner city)

    Types of dwellings in neighborhood (residential, industrial, combined residential and light industry, agrarian)

    Condition of dwellings and streets (well kept up, deteriorating, dilapidated, being revitalized)

    Sanitation of streets and homes (clean, trash and garbage collected, etc.)

    Problems with traffic congestion

    Presence and types of industry in neighborhood

2. How exposed are family members to environmental hazards found in the soil, air, and water? Are family members subjected to high levels of noise on a regular basis?

3. What are the demographic characteristics of the neighborhood and community?

    Social class and ethnic characteristics of residents

    Occupations and interests of families

    Density of population

4. What changes have occurred in the neighborhood and community? Is the neighborhood and community in a state of transition or is it economically and demographically stable?

5. What health and other basic services and facilities are available in neighborhood and community?

    Marketing facilities (food, clothing, drug stores, etc.)

    Health agencies (clinics, hospitals, emergency facilities)

    Social service agencies (welfare, counseling, employment)

    Family's affiliation with religious organization (church, temple, mosque?)

    Schools. What is the accessibility and condition of the neighborhood school? Are there problems within the school (e.g., crowdedness, poor quality of education, gangs, racial/ethnic tensions) that affect children's education?

    Recreational facilities (playgrounds, parks)

    Public transportation. How accessible (in terms of distance, suitability, and hours) are these services and facilities to family?

6. How long has the family lived in the neighborhood and/or community? What has been the family's history of geographic mobility? From where did they move or migrate?

7. What is the incidence of crime in the neighborhood and community? Are there other safety problems?

8. Who in the family uses what community services or is known to which agencies? For example, the family with school-age children might be involved with the public school system, a church group, the welfare department, and/or a scouting organization.

9. How frequently or to what extent do they use these services or facilities (the area they frequent)?

10. What does the family consider to be their community (what area)?

11. Is the family aware of community services relevant to its needs, such as transportation? Is the family aware of availability of lower transportation fees and transportation services for the disabled, children, and senior citizens, as well as direct routes to health clinics and community resources?

12. How does the family feel about groups/organizations from which it receives assistance? Assess the family's perceptions and feelings regarding association with above community groups and agencies. If the experiences in using community or neighborhood agencies have been positive, these are resources that can be used again and perhaps with even greater success.

13. How does the family view the community? For example, is it a community where the family is worried about having children play outside during the day because of high crime and personal attack rate in the neighborhood? Or is it a neighborhood that is perceived as safe and rich in a sense of common ancestry and cohesion?

FAMILY NURSING DIAGNOSES

According to Killien (1985), nursing diagnoses related to an environmental perspective focus on the family–environment fit, "the balance of demands and resources between the client and the environment" (p. 270). The environmental demands can be either actual or potential, making room for preventive, curative, and rehabilitative types of nursing diagnoses. The

North American Nursing Diagnosis Association (NANDA) lists a number of nursing diagnoses related to environmental micro-, macro-, and suprasystems. The diagnosis of Home Maintenance Management, Impaired, is characterized by difficulty in maintaining home hygiene, inability to keep home up, difficulty in maintaining a safe home, or lack of sufficient finances (Carpenito, 2000). This diagnosis may include situations of overcrowding or infestations. Another diagnosis related to family residence could be Environmental Interpretation Syndrome, Impaired, related to the chronic confusion of persons with Alzheimer's. The family will need to provide a protective environment for such a family member.

Diagnoses related to environmental macrosystems include Risk for Altered Respiratory Function related to environmental allergens. For example, a family may live in an area with spring pollens that trigger respiratory distress for some family members. Another macrosystem diagnosis is the Potential for Enhanced Community Coping, related to availability of community programs to augment [family functioning]. This diagnosis is consistent with an ecological, systems view of families' relationship to their communities. There are no nursing diagnoses related specifically to the sociopolitical environment. However, there is a diagnosis for Coping, Ineffective Community, related to such factors as inadequate law enforcement services or natural disasters. This type of diagnosis suggests interventions targeting suprasystems interacting with family and community systems.

Nursing diagnoses are used to describe the array of environmental problems that result from an individual or family being unable or potentially unable to independently maintain a safe, hygienic, and/or growth-promoting home, neighborhood, or sociopolitical environment (Johnson, Bulechek, Dochterman, Maas, & Moorhead, 2001; McCloskey & Bulechek, 1996).

FAMILY NURSING INTERVENTIONS

McCloskey and Bulechek (1996) in Nursing Interventions Classification (NIC), the University of Iowa classification project, identify numerous nursing interventions that could assist families with environment safety problems, problems within the family–health care system, and family–formal social support system. Safety risk identification, environmental management, and home maintenance assistance are probably the most central of these interventions with respect to family microenvironment (home) environmental issues.

Many of the strategies for intervention related to environmental health are preventive in nature. Primary prevention should be a primary emphasis here. For instance, working with families to prevent falls in the elderly, poisoning of children in the home, or skin rashes due to vermin infestations, are significant goals of the community-based family nurse.

Family nurses working with family members with disabilities should be familiar with the common types of adaptive equipment and assistive technology needed for home safety and optimal functioning and independence of that family member. Moreover, the home health family nurse should understand the extent to which Medicaid, Medicare, and other third-party reimbursement sources cover these special adaptive devices so that this information can be shared with families.

Homeless families are in need of a wide variety of services and types of assistance. A comprehensive case management approach (see Chapter 7 for elaboration of this intervention strategy) is suggested due to the complex needs of homeless families. Homeless families need help not only with their multiple primary care needs, but also with subsistence services (shelter, food, and clothing), access to entitlements (welfare, Social Security, etc.), crisis intervention, ongoing mental health services, transportation, and child care. Assisting families to obtain these services, or initiating and monitoring referrals are suggested interventions. Taylor (1995) lists a broad array of intervention roles that are appropriate for family nurses working with homeless families. These include being a health educator, an interventionist (providing outreach and noninvasive emergency and supportive care for illness/ injuries), an advocate, a counselor, a case manager, a group leader, and a consultant.

Clinicians working with homeless families stress the importance of showing respect toward these clients, being nonthreatening, assuming a low profile, and minimizing reporting and paperwork requirements (Vernez, Burnam, McGlynn, Trude, & Mittman, 1988). Political advocacy is urged by nurses who work with homeless people—to exert pressure on government to expand available housing or housing subsidies to poor families.

There are interventions designed to initiate community action for improved environments related to community coping. For example, community-level interventions that could affect families' community and sociopolitical environments are providing opportunities for community members to meet and discuss the situation, promote community competence in coping, and establish methods to access information and support for the targeted issue (Carpenito, 2000).

❧ SUMMARY

- The concept of environment has been integrated within most nursing conceptual models. However, definitions of *environment* sometimes reflected a relatively narrow view of environmental factors affecting the health of individuals and families, with emphasis only on the immediate social and physical surroundings of the person or family. An ecological perspective guides discussion of key environmental factors related to family health with attention to the family microsystems, macrosystems, and suprasystems.

- Individuals and family groups have a sense of territoriality, also referred to as spatial behavior. Within families there are both spatial (physical) and behavioral dimensions of territoriality. The feelings of belonging and cohesiveness among family members make up the behavioral component, while the actual physical space of home, yard, family name and address, and frequently visited community systems—school, work, shopping centers, churches, and community agencies with which the family interacts—are the spatial aspects of territoriality

- The effects of housing can be seen in two major areas. First, there are psychological aspects that affect self-perception and life satisfaction; if these are negative, they can serve as stressors and illness-producing factors. Second there are effects of possible physical hazards—due to the house's state of repair, materials used in its construction, its facilities, and its arrangements.

- An important part of assessing the home environment in relation to family health is evaluation of resources to support optimal health of individual family members and the family unit. The assessment may be related to family members of any age and may focus on varied types of resources such as assistive devices or access to information such as the Internet.

- Homelessness is an overwhelming and disruptive experience for families. It affects all aspects of family functioning and has an impact on the physical and emotional health of family members.

- The neighborhood and community in which the family lives exerts a tremendous influence on the health of the family. Satisfaction with neighborhood and community have been found to be closely associated with satisfaction with life in general. Neighborhood schools are important macrosystems interacting with many families.

While the schools may provide valuable support for family members' health, such as school-based family clinics, there are often health hazards connected with school attendance.

- Rural communities have drastically different effects on individuals and families than do urban areas. Recently there has been extensive interest and concern about the health and other needs of rural families. Accessibility to health care and other needed services is generally limited due to geographic remoteness as well as economic hardship.

- The sociopolitical environment encompasses an enormous arena with complex factors interacting to create circumstances, which may enable or limit families health-related opportunities. Examples of how the political decisions about health policy and legal decisions can impact family life are abundant, including the effect of the Americans with Disabilities Act to functionally improve employment opportunities for disabled adults thus increasing family economic resources, the effect of immigration laws on family mobility, family stress and health care, and federal funding decisions on transition programs for homeless families.

- Guidelines for assessment of the home, neighborhood, and community are outlined, as well as guidelines for nursing diagnoses and interventions in environmental areas.

✒ FAMILY VIGNETTE: THE GARCIA FAMILY

Two years ago, the Garcia family moved to Texas searching for a better life for themselves and their two children. Mr. Garcia, age 24, and Mrs. Garcia, age 22, had grown up in migrant families who moved frequently to find work in the agricultural areas of New Mexico and Texas. Mr. and Mrs. Garcia both graduated from high school (the first in their families to do so). Their first language is Spanish, but they are fluent in English as well.

Both of their families were against their move and had severed all contact with them. Although they didn't have any family or friends in their community, Mr. and Mrs. Garcia were certain they had made the right decision. As parents, they wanted to provide a more stable home for their children, Rosita, age 3, and Carlos, age 1. Mr. Garcia soon found a job with a janitorial service, which included health insurance benefits. Mrs. Garcia provided day care for three other children in their home. The family was able to purchase an old, used car and began attending mass regularly at the neighborhood Catholic church. Many of the neighborhood residents were Mexican-American and Spanish speaking and, like Mr. and Mrs. Garcia, observed the traditional holidays, foods, and religious practices of their Mexican heritage.

One year after moving to their new community, Mr. Garcia was diagnosed with a brain tumor. Because of the advanced stage of the tumor, he never returned to work and after six months of treatment and suffering he died. Mr. Garcia's illness had forced Mrs. Garcia to use all of the money from their small savings account to meet expenses. After his death, Mrs. Garcia found employment at a local restaurant at minimum wage with no health insurance benefits. While she liked her job and the people she worked with, she found her wages were not enough to pay for child care, rent, car insurance, and all of the other expenses associated with providing for the needs of a family. Initially, her church and a few friends provided some help with her finances and child care.

Then, unexpectedly, the restaurant closed and Mrs. Garcia lost her job. By this time, she was behind in her rent payments, had sold the car, and she was evicted from her apartment. Her friends were not able to provide temporary housing for her and the children, and she was still estranged from her family. Mrs. Garcia was forced to seek assistance from a local homeless shelter.

Mrs. Garcia has now moved into the shelter with her two children who are now 5 and 3 years old. She and the children share one room, with a twin bed for Mrs. Garcia and bunkbeds for the children. All of Mrs. Garcia's belongings are piled in cardboard boxes in the room. There is a window evaporative cooler, which is noisy and keeps the room temperature at about 84 during the day. Mrs. Garcia and her children share a bathroom with another family and use a common kitchen and laundry facilities on site. There is a central play area for the children. Mrs. Garcia is embarrassed and depressed because she isn't able to meet the basic needs of her children and she still misses her husband very much. She feels isolated and anxious about her future and the future of her children. In addition, the cramped living quarters and rigid rules of the shelter make it difficult for her to parent her children. The children are reluctant to be away from her and sleep with her at night, making it difficult for any of them to sleep soundly through the night.

Tomorrow, she will be talking to her caseworker regarding the opportunity to learn new job skills and enroll Rosita in school. She also has many concerns about her eligibility for health care and the availability of transitional housing.

■ STUDY QUESTIONS

Review the Family Vignette and answer the related questions. (Questions are asked here that also relate to Chapters 6 and 8.)

1. Assess family identifying data
   1.1. Composition of family
   1.2. Type of family form
   1.3. Religious and ethnic orientation
   1.4. Social class status

     1.5. Social class mobility

     1.6. Developmental stage and history of family

     1.7. Social support/social network

2. Assess family environmental data

     2.1. Home

     2.2. Neighborhood and community, including geographic mobility

     2.3. Associations and transactions of family with community

     2.4. Family's perceptions and feelings about neighborhood and community

3. State a family nursing diagnosis related to the family's environment.

4. Propose two family nursing interventions aimed at promoting the family's environment.

Answer the following questions.

5. Housing may affect behavior by contributing to or dissipating stress. Several aspects of housing have been identified as frequently stress producing. Name three.

6. Substantial evidence of linkage between extremely poor housing and physical health exists. Identify three health problems associated with poor housing.

7. Discuss how technological advances such as widespread use of the Internet have widened the disparities in family resources available to low-income and higher income families.

8. Describe three health alterations commonly found among homeless families.

9. Provide examples of the relationships between neighborhood/community characteristics and family health.

10. The text provided three specific examples of how the sociopolitical environment is related to family health, especially family resources. Identify an example from your own experience.

FAMILY COMMUNICATION PATTERNS AND PROCESSES

❧ LEARNING OBJECTIVES

1. Define the key terms in communications theory and literature.
2. Identify the content and instruction levels of messages and compare the effects of negative and positive feedback.
3. Explain the meaning of the six principles of communication.
4. Explain how channels of communication reflect family relationships.

5. Name two characteristics of both the functional and dysfunctional sender and receiver.

6. Name two characteristics of both functional and dysfunctional communication patterns in families.

7. Give examples of how family communication patterns may vary in relation to the family ethnicity or cultural background, stage in the family life cycle, gender of family members, family form, and family mini-culture.

8. Provide examples of how communication patterns may vary in families with health alterations of family members.

9. Apply the nursing process to a hypothetical family vignette, using the communication area in Friedman's assessment tool.

10. Identify major ways in which family communication patterns differ across cultures.

Family communication is conceptualized as one of the four structural dimensions of the family system, along with the power, decision making, and role structure and the family norms and values (Figure 10–1). These dimensions are intimately interrelated and interdependent. Because the family is a social system, there is continual interaction and feedback between its internal and external environments. A change in one part of the family system is generally followed by a compensatory change in the other internal structural dimensions. Although these dimensions are not separable in real life, they will be dealt with individually in the text for heuristic purposes.

Family structure is ultimately evaluated by how well the family is able to fulfill its general functions (the goals important to its members and society). The family's structure and related communication processes facilitate the achievement of family functions. For example, adequate family communication is essential in order to socialize children, a basic family function (see Chapter 15). Moreover, the communication patterns within the family system reflect the roles and relationships of family members. Communication in the family can be considered as patterned content and described as a structural component. Concurrently, the communication in the family may be considered as sequential interactions over time and assessed as processes. Applying this perspective, behavior is seen as synonymous with communication. In keeping with dominant perspectives in family nursing literature, this chapter emphasizes a systems, process-oriented perspective in discussing family communication.

The emphasis in nursing on behavioral dimensions of communication, however, has come under fire recently as overly mechanistic. Hartrick (1997) suggests an alternative approach, derived from humanistic values and focusing on relational capacity of nurses and their clients. Hartrick describes five relational capacities relevant to communication experiences of nurses with clients: (1) initiative, authenticity, and responsiveness; (2) mutuality and synchrony; (3) honoring complexity and ambiguity; (4) intentionality in relating, and (5) reimaging. Hartrick believes that an overmechanistic, behavioral approach to communication may limit spontaneity and ultimately "hinder the expression of the human caring values that the discipline of nursing is attempting to move toward" (p. 524). While this chapter does indeed focus heavily on classic behavioral dimensions of family communication, family nurses must not lose sight of the essential human caring that must inform relationships and communication between nurses and the families they work with (Watson, 1988) as well as within families themselves.

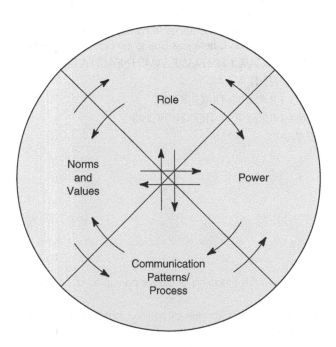

Figure 10–1. The structural dimensions of the family.

DEFINING COMMUNICATION

Communication refers to the process of exchanging feelings, desires, needs, information, and opinions (McCubbin & Dahl, 1985). Galvin and Brommel (1986) defined *family communication* as a symbolic, transactional process of creating and sharing meanings in the family. Just as each person has his or her distinct style of communication, so too does each family have a unique communication style or pattern.

Clear and functional communication among family members is the crucial vehicle for maintaining a nurturing environment through which the necessary feelings regarding self-worth and self-esteem develop and become internalized. Conversely, unclear communications are believed to be a major contributor of poor family functioning (Holman, 1983; Satir, 1983; Satir, Banmen, Gerber, & Gomori, 1991). The problem of flawed or problematic communication in families is ubiquitous. Watzlawick and associates (1967), researchers in family communication, estimated that 85 percent of all messages sent in families are misunderstood.

Ten sections are included in this chapter: elements of communication; communication principles; channels of communication; functional and dysfunctional communication processes; functional and dysfunctional family communication patterns; factors influencing family communication patterns; communication in families with health alterations; and applying the nursing process to family communication.

ELEMENTS OF COMMUNICATION

Family communication patterns and processes will be defined in this chapter as the processing of information within the family or its subsystems, consistent with a general systems framework. Communication requires a sender of a message, a form/channel of the message, a receiver, and interaction between the sender and the receiver. The sender is the person who is attempting to transmit a message to another person; the receiver is the target of the sender's message; forms/channels are the routes of the message. Communication extends from the cognitions (thoughts) of the sender, through space, to the cognitions of the receiver. Communication modalities named in the broader communication literature include spoken, written, and media such as television or the Internet. The communication modality commonly addressed in interpersonal or family communication literature is spoken language. However, there are many families with members who cannot (or choose not to) fully participate in oral/aural communication modalities (e.g., hearing mothers with deaf infants, Deaf parents with hearing children, hearing impaired elders with grandchildren). (*Note:* The word *deaf* is capitalized to indicate adults who are part of a sociocultural Deaf community, and not capitalized when it refers to an audiological condition alone). In families with hearing impaired, Deaf or hard-of-hearing members, adequate family communication requires use of modalities other than speech and hearing (Koester, 1992). For example, signed language is the most usual modality for communication of families with Deaf parents and hearing children (Jones, 1995). Late deafened elders may benefit from communication modalities using real-time captioning in group meetings or speechreading, which integrates more visual cues with the limited auditory input (Tye-Murray & Witt, 1997; Hallberg, 1996).

Interaction is a broader term referring to the sending and receiving of messages, including the response that the message elicits in the receiver and the sender. Interaction encompasses the dynamic, constantly changing process of communication between people (Watzlawick, Beavin, & Jackson, 1967).

Messages initiated by the sender are always somewhat distorted—either by the sender, through the interaction between sender and receiver, or by the receiver. One primary cause of distortion is anxiety of either interactant; the greater the level of anxiety, the greater the possibility of misunderstanding. Another common cause of message distortion is a difference in the frames of reference of the interactants, due to dissimilarities, such as those created by differences in ages, ethnic background, or gender. In their daily interactions, family members usually assume that other family members have a similar frame of reference; since this is untrue in many cases, misunderstandings inevitably arise.

✳ COMMUNICATION PRINCIPLES

Watzlawick and co-workers (1967), in their seminal text on family communication, *Pragmatics of Human Communication*, delineated six principles of communication that are basic for understanding family communication processes. *First and foremost was the dictum that it is impossible to not communicate, as all behavior is communication.* In any situation in which two or more persons are present, the individuals may or may not communicate verbally, but they cannot avoid communicating nonverbally. In this context, reference to nonverbal communication refers to nonlanguage expressions such as turning away or frowning, but does not refer to signed language.

A second principle of communication is that communication has two levels: information (content) and command (instruction). Content is what actually is being said (verbal message)while instruction conveys the intent of the message(Goldenberg & Goldenberg, 2000). The content of a message may be a simple statement, but the metamessage or instruction depends on variables such as emotion, intent, and context, and may be expressed nonverbally by the rate and flow of speech, gestures, body position, and tone of voice. For example, if "I am bored" is whispered in a theater to another member of the family, it may be a comment on the quality of the movie. However, if the "I am bored" message is sent in an emphatic manner during prolonged family discussion, the metamessage probably signifies anger, frustration, and heightened emotionality. In this example, emotion, intent, and context have produced very different meanings in a message containing identical content. In the presence of disparity between the two levels of communication, the family member receiver usually "tunes in" more to the instructional level.

A third principle of communication (Watzlawick et al., 1967) *relates to the "punctuations"* (Bateson, 1979) or the sequences of communication. Communications involve a transactional process, and in the interchange each response contains the preceding communication, in addition to the preceding history of the relationship (Hartman & Laird, 1983). Members of the family will each explain interactional events and sequences differently because they impose their own punctuation into explaining the situation. Goldenberg and Goldenberg (2000) give a graphic example of this tendency:

> Each [in this case a mother and daughter] arbitrarily believes that what she says is caused by what the other person says. In a sense, such serial punctuation between family members resembles the dialogue of children quarreling: "You started it first!" and so on. . . . It is meaningless to search for a starting point to a conflict between two people because it is a complex repetitive interaction. . . . (p. 210)

In effect there is no beginning (cause) or end (effect) in communication transactions, because a circularity of responses occurs. Family members' interpersonal behaviors (communications) are therefore best understood by taking a circular rather than a linear view of causality.

A discussion of **feedback loops** will further clarify the idea of punctuation in communication sequences. Communication serves as an organizing, purposeful, and self-regulating process in families. Self-regulating processes in a system are dependent on two-way communication, termed *feedback loops*. According to von Bertalanffy (1966), feedback loops are "circular, causal chains." As Figure 10–2 indicates, feedback loops in communication trigger necessary change in the family system that keeps the system "on track." A family member can alter his or her communications (output) based on the information he or she receives regarding the effects of his or her previous outputs of other members. Through feedback mechanisms, a portion of any system's output is reintroduced into the system as input information about the original output (Goldenberg & Goldenberg, 2000). A continual exchange of communication occurs in families—involving introducing new information, correcting misinformation, problem solving, having and resolving misunderstandings and conflicts, and so forth. The feedback loops entailed in these transactions may be negative or positive. Paradoxically, *negative feedback* is considered "positive" because it is corrective; it regulates or modulates communications or information flow so that the system may adjust homeostatically or maintain stability. *Negative* is not a judgmental term, but is simply a reference to the direction in which

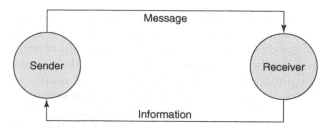

Figure 10–2. Negative feedback loop. *(Adapted from von Bertalanffy, 1968.)*

the information flows. Self-regulating negative feedback is present when a sender initiates an interaction by sending a message and then, because of a new input received from the sender, modifies his or her message before a reply is possible or expected. The problem-solving and decision-making process depends on negative feedback. This process begins when a problem arises and is identified. In the family problem-solving situation, the sender or initiator of the interaction usually identifies the problem, family members then explore the problem, various solutions are discussed, and a decision is finally made.

Positive feedback increases instability or deviation from a homeostatic state. Theoretically, if positive feedback continues it has the potential of amplifying deviation from homeostasis or stability, to the point that the system self-destructs or no longer functions (Steinglass, 1978, cited in Goldenberg & Goldenberg, 2000). An argument between parent and child that continues to escalate is an example of a common type of family positive feedback interaction. Positive feedback does not always have adverse consequences. In fact, positive feedback needs to occur in families for change and growth to take place. There may be immediate instability and tension created in the family system, but in the long run, selective use of positive feedback is necessary for change and growth to take place.

A fourth principle of communication described by Watzlawick and co-workers (1967) is that there are two types of communication: digital and analogic. Digital communication is essentially verbal (or signed) communication using words with commonly understood meanings. The second kind of communication, analogic, is where the idea or thing being communicated is transmitted nonverbally in a representational manner (Hartman & Laird, 1983). Analogic

communication, known commonly as body language, sends messages by means of posture, facial expressions, the rhythm and cadence of the spoken (or signed) words, "or any other nonverbal [non-language] manifestation of which the person is capable" (Watzlawick et al., p. 62). Analogic communication, which conveys the metacommunication, although often ambiguous and imprecise, tends to be a more powerful way to communicate about relationships (Hartman & Laird).

A fifth communication principle described by the same group of family communication theorists (Watzlawick, Beavin, & Jackson, 1967) *is called the redundancy principle.* It has been consistently observed that a family interacts within a limited range of repetitive behavioral sequences. Hence, if a family observer misses one instance of a behavioral sequence or pattern, according to the redundancy principle, this sequence will soon manifest itself again. This principle is the basis for the contention that family research, using limited observations of family interactions, can provide valid insights into the general patterns of family communications.

Watzlawick and associates (1967) point out that the repetitive behavioral sequences are circular communication patterns. Repetitive circular communication patterns occur in every family. An example of a repetitive communication pattern in a family is the following scenario. In the Lopez family, when the youngest child is angry and has a temper tantrum, the mother rushes to his side to console him. The child then responds by demanding his way and the mother gives in. Wright and Leahey (1984) suggest diagramming circular communication patterns, as the diagrams tend to "concretize and simplify repetitive sequences noted in a relationship" (p. 56). The basic elements of a circular pattern diagram are shown in Figure 10–3, and an example of a diagram is given in Figure 10–4.

The repetitive interaction patterns in families are evidence that communication rules operate in families. They naturally emerge as a consequence of the multiple interactions among family members, as they come to know what is expected of each family member. Knapp (1984) asserted that covert and overt rules exist to inform family members when and what communication is required, preferred, and/or prohibited.

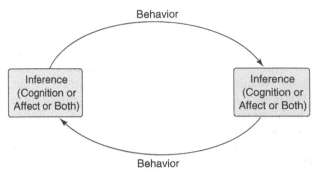

Figure 10–3. Basic elements of a circular communication pattern diagram. *(Wright & Leahey, 1994.)*

The sixth communication principle described by Bateson and associates (1963) is that all communicational interactions are either symmetrical or complementary. In symmetrical communication, one interactant's behavior mirrors the behavior of the other interactant (e.g., both mates would equally contribute to the decision about where to go for vacation). In complementary communication, one interactant's behavior supplements the other interactant's behavior (e.g., the husband says he has selected a particular place to go for vacation and the wife nods that she has heard him). When one of these two types of communication is used consistently in family relationships, the communication type is reflective of family values and role and power arrangements.

For example, researchers have studied family communication and role relationships in Deaf parented families, with an eye toward discovering whether the hearing children assumed inappropriate roles and

Figure 10–4. Example of circular communication pattern diagram.

power in the family decisions. Jones and Dumas (1996) reported that, during an activity to plan an imaginary vacation together, Deaf parents were more inclusive in their discussions with the child about the (hypothetical) vacation (i.e., there was more evidence of symmetry in the communication patterns). These findings are consistent with Rienza's (1990) position that Deaf parents were more democratic and less authoritarian with their children than hearing parents, as reflected in the differences in communication patterns. Rienza found that hearing fathers frequently excluded their children from the meal planning discussion, while Deaf fathers generally included their children in the conversation, and negotiated compromises about disagreements. These examples illustrate how differences in communication patterns reflect role relationships.

CHANNELS OF COMMUNICATION

Channels of information flow are the routes that information may take to reach a receiver. Family communication networks also refer to the flow of messages back and forth among family members (Jenkins, 1995). In the family, these involve the flow of information between the various sets of relationships or members. An example in a patriarchal family would be that a command-type communication would go from father to mother to children. This is called a vertical communication network. Families have usual channels of information flow, which reveal the family power structure (the example just described), the closeness of relationships, family roles, and the popularity of individuals within the family. The popularity or centrality of individual members is indicated by a convergence of many channels of information to one person. This person serves as intermediary or "go-between" in families. In contrast, a relative absence of channels to a family member may reveal unpopularity, fear, rejection, or the member's outsider position. For example, children of new immigrant families may become bilingual more quickly than their parents, become the interpreter for the family, and so assume a position as intermediary between the family and other systems.

Chapter 11 (Family Power and Decision Making) further explains this process.

FUNCTIONAL COMMUNICATION PROCESSES

According to many in family therapy, functional communication is viewed as the cornerstone of a successful, healthy family (Goldenberg & Goldenberg, 2000) and as such is defined as the clear, direct transmission and reception of both the content and instruction level of any message (Sells, 1973), as well as the congruency between the content and the instruction levels (Satir, 1983; Satir et al., 1991) (see Table 10–1). In other words, functional or healthy communication in the family requires that the intention or meaning of the sender be sent through relatively clear channels and that the receiver of the message has an understanding of its meaning that is similar to what the sender intended (Sells). Effective communication means matching meaning and attaining consistency and congruence between the intended and the received message. Thus, effective communication in the family is a process of constant definition and redefinition that will achieve a matching of the content and instructional levels of messages. Both the sender and the receiver must be actively involved and capable of interchanging positions by becoming either sender or receiver during the process.

In the following two sections, descriptions of the specific verbal behaviors the functional sender and functional receiver use when communicating are reviewed. Table 10–1 summarizes these processes.

THE FUNCTIONAL SENDER

Satir (1967) states that the sender who communicates in a functional way can (a) firmly and clearly state his or her case, (b) clarify and qualify what he or she says, (c) ask for feedback, and (d) be receptive to feedback when he or she gets it.

FIRMLY AND CLEARLY STATING CASE.   One of the foundations for firmly stating one's case is the use of communication that is congruent on both the content and instruction

TABLE 10–1

SPECIFIC FUNCTIONAL AND DYSFUNCTIONAL COMMUNICATION PROCESSES

FUNCTIONAL COMMUNICATION PROCESSES

SENDER

Firmly and clearly states case

Clarifies and qualifies messages

Invites feedback

Is receptive to feedback

RECEIVER

Actively and effectively listens

Gives feedback

Validates the merit or worth of the message

DYSFUNCTIONAL COMMUNICATION PROCESSES

SENDER

Makes assumptions

Expresses feelings unclearly

Makes judgmental responses

Is unable to define own needs

Exhibits incongruent communication

RECEIVER

Fails to listen

Uses disqualification

Responds offensively and negatively

Fails to explore sender's message

Fails to validate messages

BOTH SENDER AND RECEIVER

Communicate on different wavelengths (parallel talk)

Are unable to focus on one issue

levels (Satir, 1975). For example, in the case of a person who is angry, the literal message is consistent with the tone of voice, body position, and gestures.

INTENSITY AND EXPLICITNESS. When a person communicates, the sender is asking something of the receiver. Such requests include various degrees of intensity and explicitness, both of which involve how firmly the sender states his or her case. Intensity refers to the ability of the sender to effectively communicate internal perceptions of feelings, desires, and needs at the same intensity as he or she is experiencing these perceptions internally. To be explicit, the functional sender informs the receiver of how serious the message is by stating how the receiver should respond to the message. An example illustrating a high degree of explicitness is: "I want to go home now. I am very tired."

CLARIFYING AND QUALIFYING MESSAGES. Satir's second essential characteristic of functional communication is the use of clarifying and qualifying statements. These statements enable the sender to be specific and to check out his or her perception of reality against that of the other person. Examples of specific types of clarifying and qualifying statements include "I want" statements (Strayhorn, 1977) such as "Stop contradicting me when I'm disciplining the children"or "I feel" statements such as "I sometimes feel frustrated when my hands ache and I'm unable to do the chores around the house" (a man with arthritis).

INVITES FEEDBACK. A third element of a functional sender is asking for feedback, which enables him or her to verify whether the message was received accurately, as well as enabling the sender to gain information needed to clarify his or her intent. In the following examples, the sender seeks feedback to obtain the receiver's perception or reaction to what the sender has communicated: "I keep asking myself, should we tell the children that I have cancer? What do you think?" or "Since you're still on limited activities because of your heart condition, I think your parents should visit at another time. What's your reaction?"

RECEPTIVE TO FEEDBACK. The sender who is receptive to feedback will exhibit a willingness to listen, react nondefensively, and attempt to understand. In order to understand, the sender must recognize the validity of the receiver's point of view. Thus by asking for more specific criticism or "checking out" statements, the sender demonstrates his or her receptivity and interest in feedback (Strayhorn, 1977).

THE FUNCTIONAL RECEIVER

Functional receivers try to make an accurate assessment of the intent of a message. By doing this they are better able to correctly weigh the message's meaning and can more precisely assess the sender's attitudes, intentions, and feelings as expressed in the metacommunication. According to Anderson (1972), the functional receiver tries to understand the message fully before attempting to evaluate. This means that motivations and metacommunication, as well as content, are analyzed. The new information is checked with that which is already known, and the decision to act is carefully weighed. Listening effectively, giving feedback, and validating are three communication techniques that enable the receiver to comprehend and respond more fully to the sender's message (see Table 10–1).

LISTENING. The ability to listen effectively is perhaps the most important quality of a functional receiver. Listening effectively means focusing one's full attention on what is being communicated and blocking out extraneous distractions. The receiver attends to the sender's complete message rather than prejudging the meaning of the communication. Passive listeners respond with blank expressions and a seeming indifference while active listeners respond with gestures that communicate actively listening. Asking questions is a vital part of active listening (Gottman, Notarius, Gonso, & Markman, 1977). To listen actively means to be empathetic, to think of the other person's needs and desires, and to avoid disrupting the sender's flow of communication.

GIVING FEEDBACK. The second major characteristic of the functional receiver is feeding information back to the sender that tells the sender how the receiver interpreted the message. These statements encourage the sender to elaborate more fully. For example, "What do you mean when you say I get frustrated too easily with my sister?"

Feedback might also be through the process of associating. That is, the receiver makes a relationship between previous personal experiences (Gottman et al., 1977) or past related incidents and the sender's communication. For example, in her last trimester of pregnancy, Maria comments to the family nurse, "I have been getting upset quite easily and I never felt this way before I was pregnant." The nurse may respond by saying, "My wife had a similar experience when she was pregnant" or "Many of the women I see have shared these same types of feelings with me."

Paraphrasing and checking perceptions are other forms of feedback and can be accomplished with either questions or statements summarizing the sender's message (Gotman et al., 1977). The receiver does this by restating the senders' message in his or her own words. The central purpose of paraphrasing is to clarify the sender's message (e.g., "So you're saying . . ." or "What I understand is. . . .").

PROVIDING VALIDATION. The third major technique the functional receiver uses is validation. In utilizing validation, the receiver conveys understanding of the sender's thoughts and feelings (e.g., "I can see how you think and feel that way" or "It makes sense and is reasonable to feel that way"). Validation does not imply that the receiver agrees with the sender's communication, but demonstrates an acceptance of the merit and/or worth of the message (Gottman et al., 1977).

🌾 DYSFUNCTIONAL COMMUNICATION PROCESSES

Just as there are functional ways to communicate, there are also dysfunctional ways used to various degrees and at various times by most people (Table 10–1). The following sections provide overviews of dysfunctional communication of senders and receivers and of dysfunctional communication involving both the sender and receiver.

THE DYSFUNCTIONAL SENDER

The dysfunctional sender's communication is often ineffective in one or more of the basic characteristics of the functional sender: in stating case, in clarifying and qualifying, in eliciting, and/or in being receptive to feedback. The receiver is often left confused and has to guess what the sender is thinking or feeling. The communication of the dysfunctional sender is either actively or passively defensive and often negates the possibility of seeking any clear feedback from the receiver. "Unhealthy" sender communication is discussed under five major categories: assumptions, the unclear expression of feelings, judgmental expressions, inability to define needs, and incongruent communication.

MAKES ASSUMPTIONS. When assumptions are made, the sender takes for granted what the receiver is feeling or thinking about an event or person without validating his or her perceptions. The dysfunctional sender is usually not aware of the assumptions he or she is making. He or she rarely clarifies content or intent, thus obscuring and distorting meaning. When this occurs, it may elicit anger in the receiver, who is being given the message that his or her own opinions and feelings do not matter much. Another example of making assumptions is when the sender acts as a spokesperson for another by telling someone else what the person is thinking or feeling (Gottman et al., 1977). For example, a brother, without checking with his sister, comments that "It is quite clear that she isn't interested in going to the movies with us" Or a sender may take for granted that other people share his or her perceptions, thoughts, and feelings (Satir, 1983) (e.g., "I dislike going to the clinic, just like everyone else").

EXPRESSES FEELINGS UNCLEARLY Another type of dysfunctional communication by the sender is unclear expression of feelings. Due to fear of rejection, the sender's expressions of feelings must go underground or be uttered in such a covert manner that the feelings are not recognizable. In another instance, the sender may express his or her feelings but does so without the same intensity as the feelings were perceived internally, the usual situation being that feelings are understated. Sarcasm is often unclear and enables the sender to avoid taking responsibility for his or her hostile feelings. If confronted, the sender can always reply that he or she was just being humorous, for example, a mother's comment that "Of course, fathers were made to play with their sons while mothers were made to do all the work of raising them." Another example of unclear communication is "super-reasonableness" (Satir et al., 1991) when the sender's words bear no relationship to how he or she feels. Messages are stated in an unemotional way. Silent resentment is yet another case of unclear expression of feeling; the sender feels irritated with the receiver but does not express the anger overtly and/or may displace the resentment onto another person or thing (Satir, 1983). Or the sender expresses anger as a defensive maneuver to cover up feelings of hurt, rather than expressing the more basic emotion of hurt. This communication technique is extensively used. When hurt (the underlying emotion) is expressed, rather than the cover-up emotion, anger, the receiver then usually reacts in a more appropriate and positive fashion.

MAKING JUDGMENTAL RESPONSES. Judgmental responses are dysfunctional communication characterized by a tendency to constantly evaluate messages in terms of the sender's own value system. Judgmental statements always carry moral overtones where it is clear to the receiver that the sender is evaluating the worth of the other person's message as being "right" or "wrong," "good" or "bad," "normal" or "abnormal." It is not only a message that is being evaluated or judged, but also the sender of a message who is being indirectly evaluated or judged. Two types of judgmental expression are put-down statements or questions and "you should" statements. Insults ("put-downs") and blaming carry a negative connotation and value judgment. Judgmental expressions may also involve a covert unmet need or an unexpressed dissatisfaction with the other interactant, for example, "You are really clumsy" (as opposed to, "I want you to be more careful when carrying a glass of milk"). Blaming occurs in families in which the blamer wants to let the receiver(s) know who is boss. In families, blamers are often called "tyrants" (Satir, 1975; Satir et al., 1991). The words "should" or "ought to" imply that the sender is an authority figure who may judge others because he or she knows what is "good" or "bad."

INABILITY TO DEFINE OWN NEEDS. The dysfunctional sender is not only unable to express his or her needs, but due to fear of rejection is incapable of defining the behaviors he or she expects from the receiver to ful-

fill them. Often, the dysfunctional sender unconsciously feels unworthy, with no right to express needs or expect that personal needs will be met. The silent need for nurturance is defined as an unexpressed need for help, empathy, or some aspect of "being taken care of." This may also include an expectation that others should be able to anticipate the sender's needs and that asking for nurturance or assistance renders the response to such requests inauthentic and unsatisfying (Strayhorn, 1977). For example, after her radiation therapy, Jane sometimes experiences nausea. Her partner, Margaret, not realizing Jane's discomfort, does not offer to prepare dinner. When Jane finally asks Margaret for assistance, she feels angry even though Margaret quickly agrees to prepare dinner. Covert requests are made without acknowledging "ownership" (the sender does not overtly admit his or her wishes) (Strayhorn) (e.g., "It would do you good to spend more time with the dog") (the sender does not directly ask the other to spend time with the pet). Complaints may be indirect messages about the sender's needs or desires, expressed in terms of dissatisfaction. For example, the Smiths, a couple in their 70s, typically complain to their children, "You never visit us." (As opposed to, "Please come over for dinner Wednesday evening.")

INCONGRUENT COMMUNICATION. Exhibiting incongruent communication is a type of dysfunctional communication that occurs when two or more simultaneous and contradictory messages are sent (Goldenberg & Goldenberg, 2000). The receiver is left with the enigma of how to respond. In the case of verbal–verbal incongruency, two or more literal messages sent simultaneously oppose each other (e.g., "Jimmy's such a well-behaved child" followed immediately by "Did I tell you last week he had another fight at school?"). In verbal–nonverbal incongruency, the sender communicates a message verbally, but the accompanying nonverbal metacommunication contradicts the verbal message (Satir, 1983). This is commonly known as giving "mixed messages," for example, "I'm not angry with you!" spoken in a loud, gruff tone of voice with fists clenched.

THE DYSFUNCTIONAL RECEIVER

When the receiver is dysfunctional, a breakdown in communication occurs because the message is not received as intended due to the receiver's failure to listen, or the use of disqualification. Responding offensively, failing to explore the sender's message, and failing to validate the message are other dysfunctional characteristics.

FAILING TO LISTEN. In the case of failure to listen, a message is sent, but the receiver does not attend to or hear the message. There may be many reasons for failure to listen, ranging from willful inattention to an inability to listen. This is commonly due to concomitant distraction, such as noise, improper timing, or high anxiety (Sells, 1973) or simply due to a hearing impairment. A frequently used way in which individuals do not listen is by ignoring messages. Failure to listen causes distortion and misinterpretation of the message. A disqualification is an indirect response that allows the receiver to disagree with a message without really disagreeing sometimes referred to as "Yes-butting." The dysfunctional receiver partially agrees with the intent of the message, yet at the same time finds something wrong with the sender's opinion, feeling, or suggestions (Gottman et al., 1977).

USING DISQUALIFICATION. A dysfunctional receiver may employ evasion to disqualify the message by avoiding the crucial issue. A disqualification is an indirect response that allows the receiver to disagree with a message without really disagreeing. For example, the receiver may partially agree while simultaneously disagreeing. This tactic has been labeled "Yes-butting." For example, a mother may respond to one of the nurses suggestions by saying, "Yes, that's a fine idea, but I don't think it'll work with him." Or the receiver may "go off into a tangent." Here the receiver responds to a peripheral aspect of a message and ignores the central intention or content of the message. He or she "distracts" by responding with words and behavior that are irrelevant or unrelated to the message sent or what is going on (Satir, 1975).

INSULTING. Offensiveness in communication denotes that the receiver of a message reacts negatively, as if being threatened. The receiver seems to react defensively to the message by assuming an oppositional posture and an attacking position. Statements and requests are consistently made in a negative manner or with a negative expectation (Harris, 1975). The

family member receiving the consistently negative communication learns to respond with similar statements or behavior. Habitually conflicted couples behave this way (Sabatelli & Chadwick, 2000). A dysfunctional receiver may attack with a different issue, before any progress is made on a threatening issue introduced by the sender. The person receiving the message responds with an extraneous issue that hurts or threatens the sender—that is, the receiver uses a "counterattack."

Wife: I very rarely see you set any limits on the children.
Husband: After 5 years I keep wondering when you're going to learn to cook a decent meal.

A dysfunctional receiver may attribute a negative or insulting characteristic to the sender. In other words, the receiver attacks the sender through insults, rather than addressing the issue at hand (Gottman et al., 1977).

FAILING TO EXPLORE SENDER'S MESSAGE. In order to clarify the intent or meaning of a message, the functional responder seeks further explanation. In contrast, the dysfunctional receiver uses responses that negate exploration, such as making assumptions (as discussed previously), giving premature advice, or cutting off communication. When the dysfunctional receiver does not want to continue discussing the issue at hand, he or she makes a statement or uses an action that curtails any further discussion of that issue. This technique is often used to avoid dealing with unpleasant or negative feelings (Strayhorn, 1977), for example, "Let's just forget it" and "It's not that important." In addition, physical actions are another way of cutting off communication. For example, the receiver could leave the room, engage in busywork, or turn away from the sender. As stated previously, the receiver in an interaction often has the difficult task of attempting to correctly interpret both the content and the intent of the message.

FAILING TO VALIDATE MESSAGES. Validation, as previously defined, refers to the receiver's conveyance of acceptance. Therefore, lack of validation implies that the receiver either responds neutrally (shows neither acceptance nor nonacceptance) or distorts and misinterprets the message. Assuming rather than clarifying the thoughts of the sender is one example of a lack of validation.

DYSFUNCTIONAL SENDERS AND RECEIVERS

Two types of unhealthy communication interactional sequences, involving both senders and receivers, are also widely discussed in the communication literature. These are communications that reflect *"parallel" talk* and that demonstrate the *inability to focus on one issue.*

In parallel talk, each individual in the interaction constantly restates his or her own issues without really listening to the other's point of view or acknowledging the other's needs. Dysfunctional interactants may be unable to stay focused on one issue. Each individual rambles from one issue to another instead of resolving any one problem discussed or obtaining closure. An example from a cohabiting gay couple:

Mark: I'm tired of your mother visiting without calling first.
Bill: When are you going to get a job?
Mark: Soon as you learn to balance the checkbook.

Notice how each partner introduces a new problem without any attempts of a discussion of one problem at a time. As distinguished from the discussion of functional and dysfunctional communication processes in general, the following section covers family communication.

ᘓFUNCTIONAL COMMUNICATION PATTERNS IN THE FAMILY

Family communication patterns are the characteristic, ongoing, circular interactional patterns of the family that produce the meaning of transactions between family members (Peters, 1974). Most importantly, it is through interaction that the affective needs of family members are fulfilled. The ability of family members to recognize and respond to nonverbal messages is an important attribute of healthy families. Most family communications take place within the subsystems (the parent–child, spousal–parental/ adult partners, and sibling subsystems), making analysis of subsystem communications in the family a primary locus of interest (Minuchin & Nichols, 1998).

Curran (1983), who studied healthy families, writes that the first trait of a healthy family is clear communication and the ability to listen to each other. Good communication is necessary for loving relationships to develop and be maintained.

COMMUNICATING CLEARLY AND CONGRUENTLY

Family members communicate congruently in most cases in healthy families. Congruence is a key construct in the Satir growth and communication model. Congruence "is a state of being and a way of communicating with ourselves and others" (Satir et al., 1991, p. 65). When family members communicate congruently there is consistency between the content (the literal message) and the instruction (the metamessage) levels of the communication. What is actually being said is compatible with what the intent of the message is. The words we speak, the affect we express, and the behaviors we display are all consistent with each other. With congruency, the receiver is able more clearly to comprehend the sender's message, making communication in the family much healthier. Satir explains the meaning of congruence further when she states that the self (the sender), the other (the receiver), and the context or situation in which the communication takes place all are in harmony with each other (Satir, 1975).

Satir (1967) emphasizes that in healthy interaction family members recognize each other's differentness. Acknowledging the individuality and uniqueness of each member is encouraged to the degree that is reciprocally beneficial to the family system and to each individual. A sufficient amount of overt openness and honesty exists to enable members to recognize the needs and emotions of one another. The communication patterns in a functional family demonstrate acceptance of differentness, as well as a minimum of judgments and unrealistic criticism of each other. Adjustments that one family member needs to make in his or her behavior (like a mother returning to school or the father becoming disabled) generate healthy adjustments in the whole family; one person is not expected to do all of the changing necessary for the family to continue in a stable manner, and sufficient cohesiveness and flexibility exist for the family to adapt effectively.

Communication in healthy families is an extremely dynamic, reciprocal process. Messages are not simply sent and received. For instance, as the sender begins a message, the receiver may show a facial expression that will, through "negative" feedback, change the sender's message before he or she is finished speaking. As a result, the sender might change the wording of a message in the middle of the sending action so that the receiver will have a similar frame of reference. This dynamic nature of functional communication, however, makes interaction complex and unpredictable. Communication, even in the healthiest of families, many times is still tenuous and problematic much of the time.

EMOTIONAL COMMUNICATION

Emotional communication deals with the expression of emotions or feelings—from the expression of anger, hurt, sadness, and jealousy to happiness, affection, and tenderness (Wright & Leahey, 2000). In functional families feelings of family members are allowed expression. Satir (1983) believes that the acknowledgment of feelings is vital to a family's healthy functioning. A case in point: Lewis and associates (1976) studied the differences between dysfunctional and functional white, non-Hispanic families and found that healthy families displayed a full spectrum of feelings, while more dysfunctional families were emotionally constricted and rigid in their expression of feelings. In more dysfunctional families anger was permitted from parents to children, but not from children to parents. Neither were overt expressions of tenderness and affection permitted in the more dysfunctional families. Emotional expression (by both parents and children) in one recent study confirmed the positive impact that emotional expressiveness had on children's social competency (Boyum & Parke, 1995).

Affective communication—the verbal messages of caring and nonverbal, physical gestures of touching, caressing, holding, and looking—is especially important. As Bowlby (1966) demonstrated, physical expressions of affection in early infancy and childhood are essential in the development of normal affectional responses. Later in life, verbal affectional communication patterns become more predominant in relaying affectional messages, although the patterns may vary with the cultural heritage of the individuals. However, there is general agreement that family members need to be able to communicate their

enjoyment of each other's company. When their responses to each other are fresh and spontaneous, rather than controlled, repetitious, and predictable, this enjoyment can be realized.

OPEN AREAS OF COMMUNICATION AND SELF-DISCLOSURE

Families with functional communication patterns value openness; a mutual respect for each other's feelings, thoughts, and concerns; spontaneity; authenticity; and self-disclosure. It follows that these families would also be able to discuss most areas of life—both personal and social issues and concerns and would not be afraid of conflict. These areas are referred to as "open areas of communication." With respect to self-disclosure, Satir (1972) asserts that family members who are candid and honest with each other are people who feel self-confident enough to risk meaningful interaction, and tend to value self-disclosure (revealing intimate thoughts and feelings).

Satir and other family therapists admit, however, that complete honesty/self-disclosure is ideal. Contrary to this notion, research in marital relationships demonstrates that total honesty and self-disclosure may not work for many couples. Many satisfied couples report that they do not tell one another everything, for fear it would jeopardize the relationship, hurt the partner's feelings, or create more interpersonal or personal stress (McCubbin & Dahl, 1985; Pearlin & Schooler, 1978; Sabatelli & Chadwick, 2000). Hawkins, Weisberg, and Ray (1980), family communication researchers, observe that very few marital partners have ideal functional communication styles. It is generally true, however, that the more functional the family, the fewer areas of closed communication exist, and vice versa.

Consideration of a family's culture is also crucial here. Cultural norms concerning modesty, privacy, and sexual roles play a very large part in influencing what areas of communication are open and closed in families.

POWER HIERARCHY AND FAMILY RULES

Family systems are based on power hierarchies in which communication containing "commands or imperatives" generally flows downward in family communication networks. Functional interaction in the power hierarchy occurs when power is distributed according to the developmental needs of the family members (Minuchin, 1974), or when power is assigned according to the abilities and resources of family members and is consonant with the family's cultural prescriptions of family power relationships. (See Chapter 11 for a more complete discussion of the family power structure.) Power communications have characteristics that are readily apparent. The communication, "Joan, I want you to go upstairs and clean your room now or I will not take you to the mall this afternoon" is typical of a coercive power communication. It is a command-type message, specifying the action the receiver is to carry out (Miller, 1969).

FAMILY CONFLICT AND FAMILY CONFLICT RESOLUTION

Verbal conflict is a routine part of normal family interaction. The literature on family conflict indicates that healthy families seem to be able "to strike a delicate balance between enough conflict to realize the positive benefits, but not too much conflict which would disrupt family relationships" (Vuchinich, 1987, p. 591). George Simmel (1858–1918), one of the founding fathers of sociology, was the first scientific observer of the role that conflict plays in human interactions. Simmel's central thesis in writing about human interactions was that conflict is a vital form of social interaction. He believed that social conflict is both ubiquitous and essential for group development and maintenance (Coser, 1956). Conflict functions to maintain family communications and interaction in several important ways (Table 10–2).

Conflict resolution is a vital task of interaction in the family (Sabatelli & Chadwick, 2000). Adults in the family need to learn to have constructive conflicts. Although how adults resolve conflict varies, functional conflict resolution occurs when the conflict is openly discussed and strategies to solve the conflict are employed, or (in families with children) when parents

TABLE 10–2

SUMMARY OF SIMMEL'S IDEAS ON CONFLICT

1. Conflict is designed to resolve divergent dualisms; it is a way of achieving some kind of unity.

2. Conflict is often necessary to keep an ongoing relationship going. Without ways of venting hostility toward each other and expressing dissent, family members may feel completely powerless and demoralized, with withdrawal as the usual outcome. By releasing pent-up feelings of hostility, conflicts serve to maintain a relationship.

3. Close, intimate family relationships are likely to contain both converging and diverging motivations, both "love and hatred." In relationships in which persons are deeply involved, where they are engaged with their total personalities rather than a segment of it (like their work role only), there arise feelings of both love and hate . . . both attraction and repulsion. This great involvement or investment in a relationship also leads interactants to be likely to suppress hostility to avoid risking their relationship.

4. When conflict does occur, the closer the relationship, the more intense the conflict. The more we have in common with another, as whole people, the more easily our totality will be involved. Therefore, if a quarrel arises between people in such an intimate relationship, it is often passionately expansive.

5. In marriage and family relationships, the absence of conflict is not functional—it is not an appropriate criterion for judging the vitality, strength, or stability of family interactions. In fact, the very absence of conflict may be an indicator of the existence of underlying strain and insecurity. Closeness in family relationships generates frequent occasions for conflict, but if family members do not feel secure in their relationships, they will avoid conflict, fearing its presence might threaten the continuance of their relationship. In this case, the couple's or family members' disagreements, differences, and hostilities go underground, and their communication becomes more covert and indirect.

Source: Adapted from Simmel (1955).

appropriately utilize their authority to close off conflicts. Parents and other adults in families need to act as role models for their children in terms of expressing conflict/differences and resolving these conflicts.

RESEARCH ON MARITAL INTERACTIONS

Since the late 1970s, John Gottman (1995) has been investigating marital interaction in happy and unhappy marriages using observational research methods. He has exploded the myth of earlier researchers who thought that exchange theory explained marital interaction (e.g., if husband sends a sarcastic message, wife responds likewise). The following are some major differences he has found in marital interaction between happy and unhappy couples (Gottman; Gottman & Levenson, 1999):

- Happy couples in their interactions maintain a higher proportion of positive responses (e.g., validation and agreement) and a lesser proportion of negative responses (e.g., blaming, conflicts).

- Happy couples tend to have compatible styles of conflict resolution.

- Happy couples reduce negativity in interactions by editing their negative responses to their partner's negativity. They attribute his or her negativity to ephemeral, transient factors. Attempts to repair the interaction are made. In these repair attempts, the "repairing" partner develops "sentiment override." He or she responds positively, turning toward, rather than away from, the mate displaying negativity.

- In long-term happy marriages, husbands respect their wives' influence. In fact, it is Gottman's contention that marriages work to the extent that men accept the positive influence of their wives.

- In happy long-term marriages, one partner is able to have a physiologically soothing effect on the other mate. In other words, he or she (primarily the wife) is able to deescalate tense interactions by calming down the mate.

Results of Ruesch and associates' (1974) study indicated that in those marriages where conflict was avoided and negative feelings buried, the negative feelings "poisoned" the relationship. They observed that avoidance of conflict may lead to "devitalized marriages"—marriages in which mates feel emotionally detached and indifferent to each other. The presence of extensive interspousal conflict has been found to have a negative effect on parenting and child outcomes. In this area, spouses' ability to handle disagreements constructively and communicate clearly is shown to contribute to children's well-being. The interconnections between marital conflict, troubled parenting, and problems in children tend to persist from toddler through adolescent periods (Gable, Ernic, & Belsky, 1994).

However, emotional withdrawal as well as open hostility can have negative effects on the marital relationship. For example, Roberts (2000) conducted a longitudinal study of conflict among married couples. She specifically asked about the spouses' perceptions about how both hostile and distancing behavioral responses affected their satisfaction with their marriage. She found that the spouses' satisfaction with their marriage depended not only on their conflicts, but also on how they responded to opportunities for emotional intimacy. She found different patterns for men and women, with men being more negatively affected by their wives' emotional withdrawal and women being more negatively affected by their husband's hostile responses. This work demonstrates the complexity of interaction patterns during and outside of conflict and the effects on couples' satisfaction with their relationship over time.

DYSFUNCTIONAL COMMUNICATION PATTERNS IN THE FAMILY

Satir (1967, 1983) and other family therapists who advocate the use of family communications theory in practice assert that the more dysfunctional the communication, the more dysfunctional the family. This is a primary theoretical proposition within family communication theory. In this chapter functional and dysfunctional communication have been separated for discussion purposes. In reality, however, this demarcation does not exist, and communication patterns in families are not all healthy or all unhealthy. Rather, they should be viewed on a continuum from functional to dysfunctional, with all but a small percentage of families falling somewhere in between these poles.

Dysfunctional communication is defined as the unclear and/or indirect transmission and reception of either or both the content and instruction (intent) of a message and/or the incongruency between the content and instruction level of the message. Indirect transmission of messages refers to the messages being deflected from their appropriate target(s) to other persons in the family. Direct transmission of messages means the messages "hit" the appropriate target.

In dysfunctional family interaction, two or more family members have established repetitive networks and strategies of dysfunctional communication that attempt to maintain homeostasis of the family unit. These dysfunctional processes are often subtle, and the intent of the communication is covert or hidden. Thus, accurate assessment of this type of unhealthy circular communication pattern becomes more difficult. One of the primary factors that generates dysfunctional communication patterns is the presence of low esteem of both the family and its members (Anderson, 1972; Satir, 1972, 1983). Three interrelated types of communication patterns that perpetuate low esteem are self-centeredness, need for total agreement, and lack of empathy. These communication patterns are discussed next.

SELF-CENTEREDNESS.

Individuals focusing on their own needs to the exclusion of the other person's needs, feelings, or perspectives characterize self-centered communications. In other words, self-centered family members seek to get something from others to meet their own needs. When these individuals must give, they do so reluctantly and then in a hostile, defensive, or self-sacrificing manner. Thus, bargaining or negotiating effectively is difficult, because self-centered persons believe they cannot afford to lose what little they have to give (Satir, 1983).

NEED FOR TOTAL AGREEMENT.

The family's value of maintaining total agreement and avoiding conflict begins when the adult or marital partners discover that each is different from the other, although what these exact differences are may be difficult to explain. Differentness—as expressed in opinions, habits, preferences, or expectations—may be seen as a threat because it can and does lead to disagreements and the awareness that they are both separate individuals. If marital partners have low self-esteem and feel that it is absolutely necessary to be loved and approved at all times, they try to constantly please their mate. This need to continually please prohibits them from communicating openly when displeased or acknowledging disagreement. The couple perceives that expressions of their own unique thoughts and feelings might lead to conflicts that could then result in a "catastrophe" (Gottman et al., 1977). Distracting and placating tactics are often used to avoid conflict and act as if there is agreement (Satir, 1972).

Thus, unwritten rules come into being that forbid open expression of one's own individuality and differentness as a means of staving off this threat. These rules are often rigid and elude conflict or negotiation, so that there is no consideration of alternatives that would enable each person to interact differently and yet be accepted. As part of the socialization process, children in the family learn these same values and ways of relating and thus have difficulty in recognizing and interpreting a variety of feelings and experiences. These values and resultant communication patterns constrict the growth of all family members.

LACK OF EMPATHY.

Family members who are self-centered and cannot tolerate differentness also cannot recognize the effect of their own thoughts, feelings, and behavior on other family members; neither can they understand other family members' thoughts, feelings, and behavior. They are so consumed with meeting their own needs that they do not have the ability to be empathetic. Underneath a façade of unconcern, these individuals may suffer feelings of powerlessness. Not only do they devalue themselves, they also devalue others. This leads to an atmosphere of tension, fearfulness, and/or blame. The stage is therefore set for a style of communication that is confusing, vague, indirect, and covert, with defensiveness rather than openness, clarity, and honesty prevailing.

CLOSED AREAS OF COMMUNICATION.

While more functional families have more open areas of communication, less functional families often demonstrate more closed areas of communication. Families have unwritten rules about what subjects are approved or disapproved for discussion. These unwritten rules are most overtly seen when a family member breaches the family's rules by bringing up unapproved subjects or expressing forbidden feelings.

Unwritten family rules about what communication is open and closed reveal much about other aspects of a family's structure (their values, norms, power, and roles in the family). Communication restrictions may be limited to certain family subsystems: for example, discussion of sexual habits in front of the children, or a parent's dependence on alcohol. Financial issues may be discussed only between spouses but not with the children. Moreover, an area may be closed in terms of expression of feelings but open in terms of expression of thoughts. Cultural norms of modesty, privacy, and sexual roles play a large part in influencing the areas where closed and open communication exists. Thus, communication patterns must be evaluated in their cultural context.

A common interactional pattern utilized in families for avoiding discussion of meaningful issues and/or expressing salient feelings is termed "chitchat" or "small talk." The family, in using "chitchat" consistently, talks about superficial daily occurrences and avoids the meaningful issues of family life. For example, a mother has been taking her child to a pediatric clinic because of recurrent convulsions. At the clinic the diagnosis of epilepsy was recently confirmed. Since hearing of the diagnosis, the family has never discussed their thoughts or feelings about the diagnosis; their only conversation in this area has dealt with the inconvenient hospital parking arrangements and the long travel time to the clinic.

❧ FACTORS INFLUENCING FAMILY COMMUNICATION PATTERNS

Family communication patterns are influenced by multiple factors—including the immediate context in which the interaction takes place. In this section, five key variables that influence family communication are briefly described including the ethnic/cultural background(s) of family members, family life cycle stage, gender of the family members, family form, and family mini-culture (see Table 10–3).

TABLE 10–3

FACTORS INFLUENCING FAMILY COMMUNICATION PATTERNS

The context/situation

The family's ethnic background

The family life cycle

Gender differences

Family form

Idiosyncratic factors: The family mini-culture

COMMUNICATION PATTERNS IN FAMILIES WITH DIFFERENT ETHNIC/CULTURAL BACKGROUNDS

Communication is embedded within a matrix of beliefs and behavior patterns, many of which are culturally derived. Yet in research and in the literature, communication in families is often discussed without consideration of the surrounding cultural context—a criticism of the literature that this chapter also reports. For example, Sillars (1995) points out that many studies have been conducted to examine communication and marital satisfaction, only a few take the mates' cultural orientation into account. And yet in traditionally oriented ethnic families "ethnicity represents a way of living that is fully integrated with individual and family identity. . . . [W]here this sort of ethnicity still persists, the cultural patterns have considerable force" (p. 391). Hence, in traditional ethnic families, family communication patterns vary considerably from the American middle-class, predominantly white family described in the communication sections prior to this section. Communication in families varies in conversation (extent, style, pacing), personal space, eye contact, touch, and time orientation (Lipson, 1996).

A fundamental value orientation that shapes family life and family communication is the prominence in the family of a collectivistic/familistic orientation versus an individualistic orientation value (Gudykunst, 1991). This value and orientation is culturally derived. As discussed in Chapter 13, a familistic orientation is associated with sharing and mutual assistance, high interdependency among family members, and family needs and identity taking precedence over individual needs and identity (Schwartz, 1990; Sillars, 1995). The centrality of the family is the fundamental orientation among many ethnic groups, whereas a more individualistic orientation is apparent in the dominant Euro-American (mainstream) population. Individual needs and pursuits generally compete on a more equal footing with family needs and obligations in families ascribing to the values of the dominant American cultural groups (Sillars; Wilkinson, 1987).

Three areas in which ethnicity particularly affects family communication are talk (the extent and explicitness of information sharing), emotional expression, and tolerance for the expression of conflict. In different ethnic groups, communication differs by the "presumed instrumentality of talk" (Sillars, 1995, p. 381). White, non-Hispanic Americans commonly believe that it is important to put thoughts into words. They expect individuals to think and behave uniquely and believe extensive communication is needed first to know the other person, and then to maintain a relationship and to coordinate actions. Messages are verbally explicit. "Mind reading" is considered ill advised, presumptuous, and harmful to use in family communications (Sillars).

In contrast, in cultural groups in which roles are "scripted" (very structured and predictable), and roles and messages collectively understood, words are sometimes considered unnecessary to achieve understanding. In fact, too much talking could be considered "transparent." Messages may appear to be succinct and sparse, with meaningful silences interspersed. For instance, Navajo-Americans, as well as traditional Chinese- and Japanese-Americans view silence as being valuable (Giger & Davidhizar, 1995). Knowledge of the other person's thoughts is taken for granted (Sillars, 1995) and self-disclosure is limited (Draguns, 1996). Adult family members who come from this type of cultural orientation will reflect this type of communication in their families.

Sillars (1995) states that the expression of emotion versus emotional restraint is the most striking communication difference across cultural groups. In the mental health literature the expression of feelings, both negative and positive, is considered to be vital for healthy family functioning. However, the extent to which emotional expression is tolerated and encouraged varies widely. For instance, in traditional Japanese- and Chinese-American families, emotional expression is muted in comparison to typical Euro-American families. However, the expression of conflict in families also varies across cultures. Tolerance for the expression of confrontation, dissent, and disharmony dramatically differs. Although in the mental health field the dominant belief is that conflict is ever present and important to acknowledge and address (resolve), in some traditional ethnic families, this belief may not exist. In family relationships that are homogeneous, structured, and predictable, there is less need for ongoing discussion to maintain coordination. Hence, family members may rely on more passive and indirect conflict strategies. Direct conflicts are much less tolerated and thus are infrequent. However, when they do occur, they are likely to be more explosive (Sillars). In intercultural marriages or families in the midst of cultural change, such as recent immigrant families, conflict is more evident because of the clash of values and acceptable behaviors between the two cultures.

COMMUNICATION DIFFERENCES OVER THE FAMILY LIFE CYCLE

Family communication varies over the course of the stage of family development or career and with concurrent changes in the ages and developmental issues of individual family members. One striking change is in the explicitness and extensiveness of talk over the family life cycle. Family communication patterns often progress "from a maximal reliance on explicit talk in courtship and early marriage to increasing reliance on unspoken understandings later on" (Sillars, 1995, p. 383). In the last family life cycle stage (the aging family), research consistently finds that couples in long-term relationships, such as marriage, typically move toward a "disengaged" style of communication, in which extent of talk, conflict, and involvement are relatively low (Mares, 1995). These typical communication patterns are altered, however, during periods of family instability and restructuring.

The communication patterns also change over time, as family members progress through their individual developmental stages and everyone gets older. The most abundant age/stage-related family communication literature focuses on the parent–child subsystem, especially during the times when the children are very young or when they are adolescents. The outcomes of usual interest in studies of parents' communication interaction with young children are the child's mental health or later academic achievement. Others focus on both the affective and functional dimensions of the parent–child interactions. For example, Jones and Topmiller (1996) used Barnard's (1986) Nursing Child Assessment Teaching Scale to compare interactions of Deaf father/hearing child dyads with interactions in hearing father/hearing child dyads, with children who were infants and toddlers. Characteristics of positive interactions with infants and toddlers included providing clear cues to one another, responding positively and affectionately, and (for the parent) adapting language and teaching strategies to the age and behavior of the child. There were no significant differences in the Deaf and hearing father's scores indicating similar overall interaction patterns. Deaf fathers effectively adapted their communication strategies to their unique circumstances. For example, the Deaf fathers signed in the child's visual field, so that the child could look at the play materials and see the signs at the same time.

A great deal of literature discusses changes in family communication with the advent of adolescence (Fenwick & Smith, 1994) and issues arising with childbirth to teen mothers. Fenwick and Smith encourage parents to keep an open mind as their adolescents strive for greater independence and power, to try new communication strategies in order to navigate this stage of the family life, and to preserve the relationship. They also write to the teen reader about understanding the parents' concerns, and encourage mutual respect and reasonable negotiations during this time.

Some families experience additional stressors during a child's adolescence, affecting family communication. For example, East (1999) investigated the affect of teen pregnancy on the teen's entire family, rather than focusing primarily on the teen mother and her baby. East found that the teens' own mothers reported decreased communication with other, younger children following the first teenage pregnancy in the family and more difficult communication with the teen mother herself.

Families with adolescents may face challenges in shepherding the adolescent through school and toward self-sufficiency in adulthood. And communi-

cation between parents and adolescents may be difficult as the adolescent demands greater independence and power in all areas, including school. Masselam and Marcus (1990) studied families with adolescents who had left public school systems and were in alternative high schools. Their families were compared with the families of students still attending public high school, on a number of variables. As predicted, there was better overall family functioning and more positive communication in the public school families. The researchers did not hypothesize a causal relationship between family functioning or communication and the adolescent's school achievement. They did present data supporting predictable differences in family functioning and communication between the two groups of families, with greater difficulties in the families of teens attending alternative schools.

Other communication literature addresses changed patterns in all stages of the family's life cycle, such as adult children's relationships with their aging parents. An important concept at each stage of the family life cycle is whether there is a fit between the developmental issues of individual family members, called cogwheeling by Erickson, or whether there is disharmony related to conflicting developmental issues of family members and the family as a whole. For example, there may be a good fit between an adult's developmental task of nurturing the next generation and birth of a child. There may be considerable disharmony between the developmental tasks of a teen mother to gain independence, her baby's need for nurturing, and the grandmother's task of preparing for retirement from her career.

GENDER DIFFERENCES IN COMMUNICATION

As the women's movement gained momentum, so did the interest in gender differences in communication. It is now widely acknowledged that major differences in interaction exist between the genders. Hence, communication patterns will differ depending on the gender of the family members. Research has demonstrated differences in mens' and womens' attitudes and patterns of conversation (Tannen, 1990), different decision-making approaches (Kollack, Blumstein, & Schwartz, 1985), different ways of responding to others' concerns (Kollack et al., 1985; Steen & Schwartz,

1995; Tannen), and differences in conflict recognition and resolution (Gottman & Levenson, 1999). For instance, women see conversation as a way of building connections and creating intimacy, whereas men see conversation as a way to demonstrate their status and knowledge (a competitive opportunity to relate information and discuss activities). Women seek consensus, while men seek to make decisions expeditiously (Steen & Schwartz; Tannen). When women discuss problems, they want understanding, whereas men want solutions. When working at resolving a conflict, women tend to take an affiliative, cooperative stance and want to talk about the disagreement whereas men tend to assume a more coercive, competitive stance and want to distance themselves from the conflict (Gottman & Levenson, 1999; White, 1989).

In general, the gender communication research on marital couples has shown that wives as compared to husbands are more expressive, send clearer messages, and are more sensitive and responsive to their spouses' messages during conversations and conflict (Thompson & Walker, 1991).

COMMUNICATION DIFFERENCES IN FAMILY FORMS

"The family" today is defined more broadly than in past decades to include the diverse forms of families that exist in society (see Chapter 1 for a discussion of the various family forms). Family form refers to the various family structural arrangements, from the traditional two-parent nuclear family to the single-parent and gay or lesbian families. Family communication is affected by the type of family form under consideration. Most research has been conducted on heterosexual couples and two-parent nuclear families, usually excluding single-parent, dual-career, stepparent, gay and lesbian families and extended families. There has been limited research about communication in less traditional family forms, such as in stepparent families.

In the stepparent family, conflict within the family is the most widely cited communication feature. Because two families are joined together, each with its own culture and history, with few guideposts to rely on as to what the stepparent and stepchild role should be, it is no wonder that conflict is a major concern. Stepfamily integration is a process that may take five to six years or may never fully occur (Burrell, 1995; Visher & Visher, 1990). Authority and bound-

ary issues (who is in and out of the family) are also mentioned by spouses in stepfamilies as pressing concerns (Burrell). Loyalty issues such as the conflict between divided loyalties (i.e., the conflict between loyalty to one's biological children versus loyalty to the new spouse) and role-oriented issues are other sources of communication conflicts.

COMMUNICATION DIFFERENCES DUE TO THE FAMILY MINI-CULTURE

Fitzpatrick and Ritchie (1993) refer to the family as "a private miniculture." A particular family's communication patterns are a coherent configuration of family traits (Sillars, 1995), which constitute a family's unique mini-culture or family identity. In traditional cultures, ethnicity represents a way of living and valuing, thus the family mini-culture and the larger culture closely resemble each other. However, within modern heterogeneous societies, individual family members may come from different ethnic or cultural backgrounds and may vary considerably as to the extent to which they are acculturated. In these situations, the family mini-culture might reflect the cultural influence or be almost completely devoid of its influence. In nontraditional, secular families, there is much more openness to becoming unique—creating very particular communication patterns. When couples marry or develop long-term domestic partnerships, one of their challenges is creating a shared relational culture, one with its own shared meaning (Jenkins, 1995) and its own family paradigm—the family's fundamental and enduring assumptions about the world in which it lives (Reiss, 1981).

COMMUNICATION IN FAMILIES WITH HEALTH ALTERATIONS

The term *health alterations* refers to any change affecting the client's life processes (physiologic, psychological, sociocultural, developmental, and spiritual) (Carpenito, 2000). The changes in health status often include chronic and life-threatening illnesses and acute or chronic physical or mental disabilities but may include changes in others areas of health as well.

Research findings from studies of family adaptation to chronic and life-threatening illness have consistently demonstrated that a central factor in healthy family functioning is the presence of open, honest, and clear communication in dealing with the stressful health experience and related issues (Kahn, 1990; Spinetta & Deasy-Spinetta, 1981). When families do not discuss the important issues they are faced with, emotional distancing in family relationships results, and family stress increases (Friedman, 1985; Walsh, 1998). Increased stress affects not only family relationships but also the health of the family and its members (Hoffer, 1989).

For example, Lewis et al. (2000) described problems with family communication when a mother is diagnosed with breast cancer. The mother typically became immersed in issues related to the breast cancer (chemotherapy, survival, and radiation) and tended to give her children limited information about the breast cancer. Her children often had fears about their future and misconceptions about the mother's breast cancer but didn't talk with other family members about those feelings. Lewis et al. developed an intervention for these families to enhance the connections between the mothers and children. By teaching improved communication and active listening skills mothers were able to encourage their children to express their feelings about the breast cancer.

ASSESSMENT AREAS

The following assessment questions should be considered when analyzing a family's communication patterns.

1. In observing the family as a whole and/or the family's set of relationships, how extensively are functional and dysfunctional communication patterns used? Diagram recurring interactional patterns or circular communication patterns. In addition to diagramming circular communication patterns, the following more specific behaviors may be assessed:
   a. How firmly and clearly do members state their needs and feelings?
   b. To what extent do members use clarification and qualification in interaction?
   c. Do members elicit and respond favorably to feedback, or do they generally discourage feedback and exploration of an issue?
   d. How well do members listen and attend when communicating?
   e. Do members seek validation from one another?
   f. To what degree do members use assumptions and judgmental statements in interaction?
   g. Do members interact in an offensive manner to messages?
   h. How frequently is disqualification utilized?

2. How are emotional messages conveyed in the family and within the family subsystems?
   a. How frequently are these emotional messages conveyed?
   b. What types of emotions are transmitted within the family subsystems? Are negative, positive, or both types of emotions transmitted?

3. What is the frequency and quality of communication within the communication network and familial sets of relationships?
   a. Who talks to whom and in what usual manner?
   b. What is the usual pattern of transmitting important messages? Does an intermediary exist?
   c. Are messages appropriate for the developmental age of the members?

4. Are the majority of messages of family members congruent in content and instruction (including observations of nonverbal messages)? If not, who manifests what kind of incongruency?

5. What types of dysfunctional processes are evident in the family communication patterns?

6. What important family/personal issues are open and closed to discussion?

7. How do the following factors influence family communication patterns?
   a. The context/situation
   b. The family's life cycle stage
   c. The family's ethnic background
   d. Gender differences in family
   e. Family form
   f. The family's socioeconomic status
   g. The family's unique mini-culture

FAMILY NURSING DIAGNOSES

Although family communication problems are frequent and very significant family nursing diagnoses, the North American Nursing Diagnosis Association (NANDA) has not identified any family-based communication diagnoses. NANDA does, however, use communication behaviors as part of defining characteristics in some of their diagnoses, such as dysfunctional grieving. The one nursing diagnosis listed by NANDA is "impaired verbal communication," which is focused on the individual client who is unable to verbally communicate (McFarland & McFarlane, 1993). Giger and Davidhizar (1995) assert that "impaired verbal communication" does not take into consideration the client's culture and is, therefore, not a culturally relevant nursing diagnosis.

Stepping outside the NANDA diagnoses, broad family nursing communication diagnoses may be generated, such as dysfunctional family communication or dysfunctional parent–child, sibling, adult partners, or marital communication (if the problem is primarily located in the subsystem). Other general family nursing diagnoses in this area are impaired family communication or family communication problems. If broad diagnoses are used, then defining characteristics and related factors should accompany the diagnosis, following the NANDA pattern. Some family nurses may identify a more specific family communication problem as the diagnosis, such as minimal affective communication or incongruent communication patterns.

FAMILY NURSING INTERVENTIONS

Family nursing interventions in the area of communication primarily involve teaching and counseling, and secondarily collaboration, contracting, and referrals to self-help groups, community organizations, and family therapy clinics or offices. Family counselors often remark that one of the major roles they enact in working with families is to teach the members about family dynamics and how to communicate in a more functional way with each other. Much of the teaching that takes place is informal—that which goes on in the spontaneous client–nurse interactions.

Role modeling is also a crucial type of teaching. It is through the family members' observation of the family health professional and how he or she communicates during different interactional situations that they learn to imitate healthy communication behaviors. In role modeling functional communication, the nurse should listen intently, deliberately, and empathetically, following up with clarifying questions and encouraging further expression of thoughts and feelings. Role modeling becomes a particularly potent teaching method when family members positively identify with the family nurse.

Counseling in the area of family communication involves encouraging and supporting families in their efforts at improving communication between themselves. The family nurse is a facilitator of group process and a resource person. His or her presence gives families implicit or explicit permission to try out new ways of communicating and the safety of having "a third person" there when they bring out previously closed areas of communication to discuss or break other unwritten communication rules.

Satir and associates (1991) provided tips for clinicians who work with families in a facilitator role (Satir et al.). These tips are equally relevant for family nurses to use when working with families in the communication area (see Table 10–4). More specific intervention strategies in the area of family communication reflect what is known about functional family communication and how to promote it.

Wright and Leahey's (2000) classification of three types of direct family interventions (those focused on the cognitive, affective, and behavioral levels of family functioning) aid in organizing specific communication strategies that can be applied. Intervention strategies within each of the three domains include both teaching and counseling.

Family nursing interventions with a cognitive focus provide new information or ideas about communication. The information is educational and is designed to encourage family problem solving. Whether family members change their communication behavior is first largely dependent on how they perceive the problem. Wright and Leahey (2000) affirm the crucial role of perception and beliefs. When there are problems, the nurse must help the family to obtain a different view of their problems.

TABLE 10—4

SATIR'S TIPS FOR BEING A FACILITATOR IN ASSISTING FAMILIES WITH THEIR COMMUNICATION

1. Promote congruent communication.
   Respond with "I" messages.
   Clearly convey ownership for what you say and do.
   Share in descriptive rather than evaluative language, your reactions to what is being said and done by family members.
   In interviews, pay attention to the physical distance or closeness between you and the family members. [If culturally acceptable] be at eye level and at a comfortable closeness.
2. Provide alternatives and options for coping.
3. Present opportunities for raising family members' feelings of self-worth.
   Make person-to-person connections with each individual in the family.
   Acknowledge and validate feelings and thoughts of each family member.
   Offer dignity, trust, and respect to family members.

Sources: Satir, Banmen, Gerber, & Gomori (1991); and Schwab (1990).

Hence, the goal here is to change the family members' perception and beliefs about a specific communication problem.

Helping family members reframe certain messages so that they view a particular situation more positively is very helpful. For instance, helping family members see that when a family member expresses anger, this usually means he or she is feeling hurt, pain, and possibly a sense of rejection. Hurt is a much more "acceptable" and positive emotion for family members to respond to than anger and hostility (Satir, 1967).

Another important topic for discussion with family members is the different perceptions or "multiple realities" that exist among individual family members about a particular situation or event. In order to deal with conflicts or situations requiring decision making, family members' perceptions (and feelings) about the situation should be understood and considered, avoiding efforts to agree on which perspective is correct.

Interventions in the affective area are directed toward changing the emotional expression of family members—by either increasing or decreasing the level of emotional communication or modifying the quality of the emotional communication. The specific nursing goals here are, within the cultural context of the family, to help the family members express and share their feelings with each other so that (a) their emotional needs can be better conveyed and responded to; (b) more congruent, clear family communication occurs; and (c) family problem-solving efforts are facilitated.

Direct interventions aimed at the affective level of family functioning include urging family adults/parents to share their feelings with their children (as appropriate to the ages of the children and the subject). Likewise, supporting parents' efforts at encouraging their children to share the full range of their feelings with their parents, so that children can be better communicators. (Children learn to express themselves as they see their parents expressing themselves.) In addition, family nurses can point out incongruencies in family members' levels of communication and encourage them to be more congruent in their content and metamessages (the metamessage or instruction consists of how words are said, including the feelings that accompany the words).

Understanding or having more positive perceptions about a family communication problem is not sufficient for change to occur. There also must be behavioral change (Wright & Leahey, 2000). Rather than search for underlying causes and "whys" to problems, Wright and Leahey suggest that family nurses ask about the "whats" of the problem. For example, when an older sister decides what movie she will attend with her younger brother, the nurse might ask the older sister what effect that has on the younger sibling. This question is more helpful than asking why she made that decision herself.

Behavioral changes stimulate changes in perceptions of a family member's "reality" and perceptions stimulate changes in behavior (a circular, recursive process). Hence, when the family nurse assists family members to learn new, healthier ways of communicating, he or she is also helping family members to change their perceptions or construction of reality about a situation.

Teaching and counseling interventions designed to change family communication include:

1. Identifying specific behavioral changes the family members wish to address and developing a collaborative plan for change.

2. Recognizing, supporting, and commending family members when they begin attempts to communicate clearly and congruently.

3. Monitoring behavioral changes that have been targeted at previous meetings. Ask how new communication behaviors have worked, and if any problems occurred and if they have questions or concerns about the changes.

McCubbin and Dahl (1985), family scholars and educators, recommend communication tactics for adult couples to use to manage conflict productively. A summary of their guidelines follows:

1. Try not to engage in "kitchen-sink fighting" (throwing all kinds of additional issues into the conflict).

2. Talk in terms of issues, not personalities.

3. Be an active listener (obtain feedback and ask for clarification).

4. Recognize that your partner's unhappiness is not always your responsibility.

5. Find a way for both sides to win (pp. 187–189).

Families may be referred to appropriate family counseling facilities, family mental health clinics, private clinicians, or self-help groups depending on the family's circumstances, degree of communication dysfunction, and interest. There are numerous community organizations and programs designed to improve family communication and relationships as well as parenting skills. Marriage Enrichment, Marriage Encounter, and Marriage Communication Lab programs also help spouses enhance their communication skills (Hoffer, 1996). And finally there are parent and child communication training programs that have assisted parents and children improve or strengthen their communications such as the Parent Effectiveness Training (PET) program and others focusing specifically on family communication during the adolescent years (Riesch et al., 1993). Information about many of these groups can be easily accessed on the Internet or by telephone. For example, Mertensmeyer and Fine (2000) describe efforts in Missouri to simplify parents' access to research-based information, services, and problem-solving support related to parenting. There is a ParentLink's WarmLine and a ParentLink Web site.

SUMMARY

- Family communication is conceptualized as one of the four structural dimensions of the family system, along with the power, role and decision making, and values structural dimensions. The family's structure and related communication processes facilitate the achievement of family functions. Moreover, the communication patterns within the family system reflect the roles and relationships of family members.

- Communication refers to the process of exchanging feelings, desires, needs, information, and opinions. Family communication is a symbolic, transactional process of creating and sharing meanings in the family.

- Communication requires a sender of a message, a form/channel of the message, a receiver, and interaction between the sender and the receiver.

The sender is the person who is attempting to transmit a message to another person; the receiver is the target of the sender's message; forms/channels are the routes of the message.

- The six principles of communication are that (1) it is impossible to not communicate; all behavior is communication; (2) communication has two levels: information (content) and command (instruction); (3) communication involves a transactional process and family members each have their own "punctuations" of interactional events; (4) there are two types of communication: digital and analogic; (5) family interactions are redundant, that is, a family interacts within a limited range of repetitive behavioral sequences; and (6) all communicational interactions are either symmetrical or complementary.

- Channels of information flow are the routes that information may take to reach a receiver.

- Functional communication is defined as the clear, direct transmission and reception of both the content and instruction level of any message as well as the congruency between the content and the instruction levels.

- Dysfunctional communication is defined as the unclear and/or indirect transmission and reception of either or both the content and instruction (intent) of a message and/or the incongruency between the content and instruction level of the message.

- A key characteristic of a healthy family is clear communication and the ability to listen to each other. Good communication is necessary for loving relationships to develop and be maintained.

- Five variables that influence family communication are the ethnic/cultural background(s) of family members, family life cycle stage, gender of the family members, family form, and family mini-culture.

- A central factor in healthy family functioning when someone has health alterations (such as chronic illness) is the presence of open, honest, and clear communication in dealing with the stressful health experience and related issues.

- Guidelines for assessment of family communication are outlined as well as guidelines for nursing diagnoses and interventions to facilitate healthy family communication patterns.

❧ FAMILY VIGNETTE: THE SIMON FAMILY

John and Mary Simon are married with two children—Mark, age 8, and Susan, age 14. John is a computer engineer and Mary works out of her home, selling handmade crafts at local venues. John and Mary met when they were students at Gallaudet University. John's parents are deaf, John is profoundly deaf, comes from a strong Deaf cultural background, and much prefers signed communication within the family. Mary is considered hard-of-hearing, her (hearing) parents sent her to an "oral" school as a child, which emphasized speechreading and speaking skills. Mary became fluent in sign when she attended Gallaudet University, and she also began to affiliate with Deaf culture during that time. She uses her voice and speechreading with hearing people (including her own parents), but all the personal communication between Mary and John is in American Sign Language (ASL). John and Mary say that they enjoy their conversations at the end of each day, and feel that they really "listen" (pay close attention) to what they each have to say. John has a close relationship with his parents, while Mary feels estranged from her own parents, who never learned sign and forbade Mary from using sign language throughout her childhood.

John and Mary married after John graduated from Gallaudet. Their children are both hearing, and bilingual in ASL and English. The children vary in their signing fluency. The oldest, Susan, is skilled in sign and has served as an interpreter for her parents in everyday situations involving communication with hearing people, such as asking a question about a dress at the department store. However, the parents say that they always arrange for a professional interpreter for more complex situations, such as visits to the doctor. Mark signs poorly, depends on Susan or his mother to interpret for him with his father, and prefers that his mother use speechreading and voice in conversation with him.

Susan has recently begun to argue with her parents when they have asked her to accompany the family on outings, saying she prefers to spend time with her friends. Susan's mother says/signs that she can understand Susan's feelings, as "my friends have teenagers and it seems natural that they want to spend a lot of time with their friends at this age."

Another source of conflict is Mark's poor signing skills, and the consequent difficulty he has in communicating directly with his father. This creates particular difficulties when John and Mark are by themselves someplace without Mary or Susan, such as when John takes Mark to soccer practice. John believes that Mark refuses to learn more sign language because he is ashamed that his parents are Deaf. Susan scolds Mark, saying he is too lazy to make the effort to learn sign, just like their hearing grandparents. John and Mark have never discussed how Mark feels about having Deaf parents. Whenever John and Mark become frustrated trying to have a conversation, Mary intervenes and simply interprets for them to smooth things over. Mark feels he cannot understand his father's signing because he signs too fast and becomes impatient with Mark's requests that he slow down. Typically, Mark just signs "forget it" when he has trouble reading his dad's signs, stops looking at his dad, and leaves the room.

The nurse is visiting the family to check on John's recovery following surgery for a work-related problem with carpal tunnel syndrome. She is accompanied by a professional sign language interpreter. During the family interview, the daughter sits closes to her mother, and they seem comfortable and affectionate with one another. The nurse notices that there is clear consistency between the words (content) and expressions (command) in the family's communication, and that the family is quite animated in their conversation. Toward the end of the meeting, Mark leaves for soccer practice. John asks Mary what time Mark is coming home; the mother interprets for the father and son, and answers that Mark will be home by 6 P.M. There is clearly tension between the father and son. The nurse notes that the mother and son sign "I love you" to one another as they say goodbye.

▦ STUDY QUESTIONS

Review the Family Vignette and answer the related questions.

1. In observing the family as a whole and/or the family's set of relationships, how extensively are functional and dysfunctional communication patterns used? Diagram recurring interactional patterns or circular communication patterns.

2. How are emotional messages conveyed in the family and within the family subsystems?

3. What is the frequency and quality of communication within the communication network and familial sets of relationships?

   a. Who talks to whom and in what usual manner?

   b. What is the usual pattern of transmitting important messages? Does an intermediary exist?

   c. Are messages appropriate for the developmental age of the members?

4. Are the majority of messages of family members congruent in content and instruction (including observations of nonverbal messages)? If not, who manifests what kind of incongruency?

5. What types of dysfunctional processes are evident in the family communication patterns?

6. State one family nursing diagnosis in the area of communication.

7. Propose two family nursing interventions directed toward resolving the above family communication problem.

Answer the following questions.

8. From the list below select the four primary characteristics that are not representative of a functional sender.
   a. Listens
   b. Receptive to feedback
   c. Elicits feedback
   d. Makes assumptions
   e. Firmly states case
   f. Validates
   g. Clarifies and qualifies
   h. Generalizes

9. Name two characteristics of both functional and dysfunctional sender and receiver.

10. Match the five major categories of dysfunctional communication in the left-hand column with the specific illustrations given at the right.

Category	Example
a. Assumptions	1. "I'm not mad at you" (spoken in loud, sharp tone).
b. Unclear expression of feelings	2. "I dislike patients who are constantly complaining."
c. Judgmental expressions	3. "I don't understand how you can be so dumb."
d. Inability to define needs	4. "I just love it when you don't come home for dinner, then I have only a few dishes to wash."
e. Incongruent communication	5. "If you would like to go out for dinner, so would I."

11. Which of the following situations best demonstrates that information has been received from a sender?
   a. A parent tells a child to stop playing with his food and the child continues to play.
   b. A parent tells a child to drink his milk and the child looks at the parent.
   c. A parent shows a child how to butter bread and the child states that she knows a better way to butter her bread.

12. Gender differences in communication are striking. Which of the following is not a gender research finding?
   a. Husbands are clearer in their communication than wives.

b. In decision making, men want expeditious decisions made, while women seek to develop consensus.

c. Women are more emotionally expressive than men.

d. Women see conversation as a way to build connections, whereas men do not.

13. In the following situations identify the content and the instructional level of the message.

a. A newlywed couple is watching a movie. The woman caresses the man's arm and hugs it to her while she whispers, "I'm really not interested in this movie."

b. A child starts to crawl on his parent's lap. The parent pushes the child away and says, "You know I love you, go play with your new toy."

c. A child is throwing cereal with a spoon. The mother grabs the spoon and cereal bowl and emphatically states, "Stop it! You may not play with your food!"

14. When a transaction between two family members is repeated over and over again, this tendency is referred to as the _____ principle.

15. A woman, finding that her partner has not helped with the dishes as she promised to do, expresses her anger at her. She, in turn, yells back that "I'll wash the dishes when I get good and ready." The woman continues to berate her partner. What kind of feedback loops are illustrated in this series of transactions?

16. Communication patterns in families very widely according to the family's ethnic background. Noted communication differences are present in which of these areas:

a. The extent and explicitness of information conveyed in conversation

b. The meaning of silence in conversation

c. The expression of emotion

d. The expression of conflict

e. The communication networks in families

11

FAMILY POWER
AND DECISION MAKING

CONTENT OUTLINE

LEARNING OBJECTIVES

1. Define the following concepts and domains: power, authority, decision making, power outcomes, power bases, and family power.

2. Explain variations in family power related to gender, members ages, and family life cycle stage, ethnicity/culture, interpersonal skills, and social class of family.

3. Describe commonly used typologies for classification of family power.

4. Using the family power continuum, identify where "healthy" families typically are situated on the continuum.

5. Explain the theoretical perspectives related to family and intimate partner violence.

6. Apply the nursing process to a hypothetical family vignette in terms of family power.

Numerous authors in the fields of family sociology and family counseling have written of the importance of the power dimension within the family (Balswick & Balswick, 1995; Quinn, 1995). For instance, Cromwell and Olson (1975), researchers of family power, wrote that "power is one of the most fundamental aspects of all social interaction" (p. 3). Haley (1976), a noted family therapist, believed that power is central to all human relations. He portrayed human relationships as an ongoing struggle for status and control.

The family, like all social systems, has structures that determine who wields power and what the family's hierarchy or "pecking order" is. Power, as viewed in this text, is one of the four interdependent structural dimensions of the family, and as such is a reflection of the family's unwritten family rules and underlying value system. In addition, it is significant in understanding the interpersonal dynamics within the family and between the family and other social systems. Power and status dimensions are crucial in establishing and maintaining family communication channels and networks. In fact, Blood and Wolfe (1960), who conducted the foundational research in family power, maintained that the most important aspect of the family structure is the power position of the members. Furthermore, the close interrelationship with family roles is apparent in that a person's roles and positions are basic to his or her capacity to exercise power and are reflected in family communication patterns (see Chapter 10).

Power structures vary greatly from family to family, with differences positively related to the overall functioning of the family. Some power arrangements are dysfunctional and thereby contribute to family maladaptation and ill health. Moreover, decision making, as one measure of family power, has been a central concern in family therapy. Satir (1972) notes that "there is probably nothing so vital to maintaining and developing a love relationship (or to killing it) as the decision-making process" (p. 131).

Contemporary changes in the family have created an even greater need for family health professionals to assess the power dimension in families. As part of the rapid changes in family life, families are not rigidly bound by tradition to relationships as they once were. Decision making and family power are generally more shared in families now than in earlier decades (Scanzoni & Szinovacz, 1980; Szinovacz, 1987). No change in the American family is men-tioned more often than the gradual shift from one-sided male authority to the sharing of family power by the husband and wife. Declining sex role traditionalism, like many social changes, correlates with increasing complexity and conflict in family decision making (Scanzoni & Szinovacz, 1980).

Understanding a family's power structure may be crucial in providing effective health care, especially when families have problems implementing health behaviors or obtaining needed health services. The family member who acts as health leader (being the recognized authority in the area of health or the overall family leader) must be identified, acknowledged, and consulted. For instance, the nurse may find that, contrary to his or her expectations, the father or grandparent has the final decision-making power in family health matters.

Following a presentation of basic definitions and concepts, this chapter addresses specific areas of assessment of family power: (1) the bases for power, (2) power outcomes, (3) family decision-making, and (4) variables affecting family power. A discussion then follows of the assessment of overall family power structure, family power in healthy families, and power dynamics in family violence. Last, practice guidelines in the area of family power are presented.

✷ FAMILY POWER: CONCEPTS AND DOMAINS

Power has numerous meanings, including the capacity to influence, control, dominate, and to make decisions. In other words, power is the ability—potential or actual—of an individual(s) to control, influence, or change another person's behavior. Power always involves asymmetrical interpersonal relationships—one interactant exerts greater influence/control in the relationship. Power is also multidimensional in nature, meaning that it includes sociostructural, interactional (process), and outcome components (McDonald, 1980). Power is an abstract, complex, and multidimensional phenomenon that is not directly observable. It must then be inferred from observable behaviors and/or from self-reports of family members, conducted through goal-directed interviews. What is observed by outsiders and what is reported by family members in terms of family power, however, are often at odds with each other (Szinovacz, 1987).

FAMILY POWER

Family power, as a characteristic of the family system, is the ability—potential or actual—of individual members to change the behavior of other family members (Olson & Cromwell, 1975). Major components of family power are influence and decision making. The term *influence* is practically synonymous with power, being defined as the degree to which formal and informal pressure exerted by one family member on the other(s) is successful in imposing that person's point of view, despite initial opposition (McDonald, 1977). Dominance is also used in the same context. In this chapter, power, dominance, and influence will be used interchangeably.

Power is a dimension of the family system or subsystem, in that it is not a characteristic of a family member apart from the family system. Thus, family power can be assessed only within the context of the system or subsystems, and more specifically within the context of the circular processes of family interaction. Communication patterns reveal family role and power dimensions. Family power can be seen in family processes ranging from daily routine exchanges to negotiation of complicated conflictual issues. Moreover, the power dimension is found in the various subsystems within families (e.g., the sibling subsystem, marital/adult partner subsystem, and parent–child subsystems); the family as a total system; and the family system's relationship with the external social systems (Olson, Cromwell, & Klein, 1975). There are five different units that can be analyzed in terms of their family power characteristics (McDonald, 1980). These are marital [or adult partner] power, parental power, offspring power, sibling power, and kinship power. Most research and theoretical writing about family power, however, have focused on marital power (Balswick & Balswick, 1995).

AUTHORITY

Authority is another closely associated term referring to the shared beliefs of family members, which are culturally and normatively based and which designate a family member as the rightful person to make decisions and assume the leadership position. In other words, authority is present when the individuals involved believe that it is proper for power to be held by a particular member of the group. Traditional beliefs, values, and roles are largely the basis for these beliefs.

Power and authority do not always go hand in hand. A family member who has the authority to decide or act may not exercise this power for a variety of reasons. Thus, there may be an incongruency between the power and authority elements in a family. Comparing the family to a larger social system, one could equate authority with the formal power structure and power with the informal power structure of a bureaucracy. It has long been recognized that within an organization the formal and informal power structures may be quite different from each other. The same situation applies to families. A family member who nominally holds the power may not be the actual power holder. Although family members might tell the health worker that the father is "in charge," he or she might on observation note that the oldest son is actually the informal power holder (Pasquali, Arnold, DeBasio, & Alesi, 1985).

POWER BASES

One salient aspect of family power concerns the bases for power within the family and its subsystems—that is, the source from which a family member's power is derived. This information often has to be inferred from observed behavior and by asking relevant questions. The importance of making this determination lies in the fact that the nature of the particular power base significantly affects interpersonal relationships, marital [adult partner] satisfaction, and family stability. Cromwell and Olson (1975) identified three domains of family power: power bases, power outcomes, and decision-making processes. These domains are described below and further articulated in the later discussion. Raven and associates (1975) and Safilios-Rothschild (1976a) identified various types of power bases commonly observed in families (Table 11–1).

Legitimate power (sometimes called primary authority) refers to the shared belief and perceptions of family members that one person has the right to con-

TABLE 11–1

FAMILY POWER BASES

- Legitimate power/authority
- Helpless or powerless power
- Referent power
- Resource power
- Expert power
- Reward power
- Coercive power
- Informational power
- Affective power
- Tension management power

---

trol another member's behavior. By virtue of the roles and positions a person occupies, certain rights and culturally derived privileges exist that are associated with these roles and positions. For example, parental control or dominance over children is based on traditional and/or legal authority. Primary authority of an adult family member has remained the traditional and significant base for power in many families. For authority to be effective, the whole family must accept and support this ideology.

The *"power of the powerless"* is a second form of legitimate power that is often overlooked. This type of power is based on the generally accepted right of those in need or of the helpless to expect assistance from those in a position to render it. Weeks and Jackson (1982) label the person with this kind of power the victim. They explain that the victim acquires a great deal of quasi-power in families. The victim is able to covertly acquire influence or power from others who often already feel drained of resources. Helpless power may be very effective in families where one member is chronically ill, disabled, or aged. For example, a chronically ill family member may control the family on the basis of his or her frailty or helplessness. This is a commonly seen base for power and, unfortunately, may lead to a situation that makes it difficult for other family members' needs to be adequately met. Children's dependency

and helplessness arouse feelings of responsibility in parents and make them susceptible to children's control attempts and use of "helpless power."

A third source for power, *referent power,* applies to the power persons have over others because of positive identification with them, such as in a child's positive identification with a parent. Children imitate behaviors of family members, usually the parents, who serve as their role models.

Resource power comes from having the greater number of valued resources in a relationship. Possessions are seen as primary determinants of the ability to influence or pressure others (Osmond, 1978). Resource power is the main alternative to traditionally based traditional legitimate/authority family power. (McDonald, 1977). For example, one adult family member may be dominant because she controls the finances or because she is more practical and goal directed than other adult family members.

One important source of power is the use of *interpersonal techniques.* It is not uncommon to find one family member who has few of the objective resources controlling much of family life through his or her masterful use of interpersonal techniques (Turner, 1970).

As early as 1938, Waller explained what he called *"the principle of less interest"* as a source of power. This principle explains that exploitation is likely to occur in a relationship where the differences in levels of involvement are great. For instance, the principle of less interest states that within a dyadic relationship, the person who cares least about whether the relationship continues or not has the greatest power over the relationship. He or she usually has less interest and involvement in maintaining the relationship because he or she has many more alternatives or resources. The person in a relationship who has the least interest in maintaining the relationship has a very important resource at his or her disposal. With decreased involvement, the less interested person can use manipulative or coercive techniques at the expense of the other. A commonly seen example may help elucidate this principle. In a marital situation, one member may be quite valued and independent, while the other individual feels dependent and inferior. The dominant partner then makes decisions, since he or she has many more options open and there is less interest or involvement in the relationship. In middle-class America (among heterosexual couples) this principle still operates in favor of the man because of his greater economic resources (Quinn, 1995) and may apply in other committed adult relationships when there is a significant disparity in financial resources between family members.

Expert power, a particular type of resource power, exists in a relationship when the person being "influenced" perceives that the other person (the "expert") has some special knowledge, skill, expertise, or experience (Safilios-Rothschild, 1976a). For example, when a family member is a nurse, other family members may defer to her/his decisions related to health care.

Reward power stems from the expectation that the influencing, dominant person will do something positive in response to the other person's compliance. Overt bargaining may accompany the use of reward power. Children, according to Szinovacz (1987), possess an important resource in their compliance. Children's "good" behavior is a source of pleasure and pride to parents, and thus constitutes a basis for power (i.e., children often use "good" behavior in order to obtain desired benefits).

The effective use of *coercive* or *dominance power* is based on the perception and belief that the person with power might or will punish other family members through threats, coercion, or violence if they do not comply. Coercive power is used with coercive decision making (to be discussed later). Results of research about families with adolescents demonstrated that the use of coercive power or reward power was not nearly as effective a base of parental power for adolescents as the parent's legitimate, referent, or expert power (Gecas & Seff, 1991).

An *informational power* base stems from the content of the persuasive message. An individual is convinced of the "rightness" of the sender's message due to a careful and successful explanation of the necessity for change (Raven, Center, & Rodrigues, 1975). This type of power is similar to but more limited in scope than expert power. A variation of this direct information power is "indirect" informational power. This occurs when hints, suggestions, and information influences a person to act without obvious efforts at persuasion (Raven et al.).

Affective power refers to the power derived through the manipulation of a family member by bestowing or withdrawing affection and warmth, and, in the case of intimate adults, sexual activity. Some couples may be fairly equal in family power because affective resources are valued; for example, one brings greater economic resources while the other brings affection, which is highly valued by the partner (Balswick & Balswick, 1995).

Tension management power is derived from the control that one family member achieves by managing the tensions and conflicts in the family. Using tears, pouting, endless debating, and disagreements to get a family member to "give in" are examples of tension management power, which either children or adult family members may use to obtain power.

POWER OUTCOMES

A second area of assessment relative to family power is the area of power outcomes. Here the focus is on who makes the final decisions or ultimately possesses control—in other words, "who wins" or "has the last say" (Cromwell & Olson, 1975; Szinovacz, 1987). Specific questions can be asked of the family to elicit this information. For instance, one might ask who is responsible for making decisions about the areas of major importance in family life. Power can vary in intimate partner relationships, with role definitions determining who has power in a given area. For example, a man might have more power in regard to social and kin relationships and household matters, while his partner has more control over the finances. In other families power may be more equally divided, with a pattern of shared power prevailing.

Specific areas of responsibility and of decision making, however, may not coincide with the more general and dominant power pattern in a family. A family nurse can easily be misled by the obvious responsibilities and decisions of one family member rather than realize that these are actually delegated, or relegated, to the weaker partner by the dominant member of the family. This is the usual case in authoritarian or patriarchal families. In these types of families, the man's power may derive not only from a traditional value structure but also from possessing more resources. Economic resources (money) are particularly important in determining marital power (Blumstein & Schwartz, 1983).

A second related question dealing with power outcomes is a more global or general question that can be posed to family members. This question entails asking about whose idea or suggestion is finally adopted when major decisions or choices must be made. In families in which decisions are shared and represent the outcome of mutual discussion and exploration, this kind of information is difficult to obtain. But despite the difficulty involved in getting family members to describe the outcome (people remember what decision was made but find it harder to remember who had the last say or made the ultimate decision), assessment of the outcome of an issue, conflict, or argument is helpful to discover in ascertaining the source of power and in whom this resides.

Komarovsky (1964) notes that "power is most visible in contested decisions ending in victory of one partner. But power exists irrespective of conflict, because the powerful partner may so influence the wishes and preferences of his mate that a contest of wills does not even arise" (p. 221). Power differentials, then, may function to suppress potential conflictual situations and cause "silent agreement" (McDonald, 1980; Scanzoni & Szinovacz, 1980).

Discerning what kinds of problems or issues are involved in decision outcomes and how important they are to the family is helpful. Does a decision cut across all the major areas of family life or is it limited to a specific area? Komarovsky (1964) underscores the significance of ascertaining the centrality of the issue by observing that "general decision making in one or two areas of family life may not be a good index of general power. It depends upon the importance of such areas for each partner" (p. 221).

FAMILY DECISION MAKING

Family power has primarily been researched by focusing on decision making (Scanzoni & Szinovacz, 1980; Szinovacz, 1987). Decision making refers to the process directed toward gaining the assent and commitment of family members to carry out a course of action or to maintain the status quo. In other words, it is the "means of getting things accomplished" (Scanzoni & Szinovacz, 1980). Power is manifested through decision making.

The decision-making process is a principal index of power (Blood & Wolfe, 1960). Family decision making refers to "the interactional techniques that family members employ in their attempts to gain control in the negotiation or decision-making process" (McDonald, 1980, p. 843). The central focus is how

decisions are made. By understanding the techniques used in family decision making, the assessor will be better able to identify the relative power of each family member and his or her participation in family decision making.

There are three types of decision-making processes discussed in the literature: consensus, accommodation, and de facto decision making. Families tend to make use of one particular method of decision making over another, although the secondary use of one or both of the other basic techniques of decision making may occur. Analysis of the family decision-making processes reveals the tremendous interrelationship of these features with the other structural dimensions of the family.

The first technique of decision making is termed *consensus*. According to American ideals, this is the healthy way to make decisions. Here, a particular course of action is mutually agreed on by all involved. There is equal commitment to the decision, as well as satisfaction with the decision by family members. Consensus decisions are agreed on through discussion and negotiation. Because a substantial degree of interdependence and egalitarianism among family members is needed as well as an ability to discuss and problem solve, this kind of decision making is more difficult, complex, and unpredictable than other kinds. When there is initial disagreement regarding an issue, negotiation is one of the major techniques used in families to handle a conflictual situation (Klein & White, 1996). Consensus occurs when negotiating members agree to a solution that is seen as meeting their personal or shared values (Turner, 1970). In families with unilateral authority patterns, there is little room for negotiation. Negotiation is more commonly used in democratic or egalitarian families (Klein & White, 1996).

A second type of decision making is termed *accommodation*. Here the family members' initial feelings about an issue are discordant. One or more family members then make concessions, either willingly or unwillingly. Some member(s) assent in order to allow a decision to be reached. Hence it may involve a voluntary compromise in which concessions are made by all persons concerned or a sacrifice, made by one family member so that others may have their own way. Privately or publicly the conceding member(s) will not be convinced, however, that the decision in question was best (Turner, 1970). Accommodative decisions are made somewhere on a continuum from coercion to compromising. Differences in the attitudes of participants toward their commitment, as well as differences in the relationship under which the forms of accommodation take place, determine whether the decision making is more coercive or more compromising. Accommodation is always an agreement to disagree when a decision is adopted in the face of irreconcilable differences (Turner, 1970).

The processes of accommodation—compromising, bargaining, or coercion—vary in terms of how functional they may be. *Compromising* refers to the making of concessions by all family members involved so that the decision reached is not reflective of any of the members' original choices, but has some acceptable elements for all concerned. In *bargaining*, one or more members make concessions to another/others and expect reciprocity, so that ultimately the sacrifices of each balance out. The use of bargaining in family negotiations demonstrates that a trust exists among the members, along with a belief that others will be fair and honest in keeping up their ends of the bargain. *Coercion* is the least functional technique along the accommodation continuum. It results in an unwilling agreement by one or more family members, whereby commitment is assured only by the continuance of coercive power. The existence of threat of punishment shows the dominance of one member over others.

De facto decision making occurs when things are allowed to "just happen" without planning. In the absence of active, voluntary, or effective decision making, decisions just occur. De facto decisions may also be made when arguments occur to which there was no discernible resolution or when issues were not brought up and discussed. These decisions, then, are made by inaction or default rather than by deliberate action. De facto decision making is seen in many disorganized, multiproblem families, many of whom believe in fate and feel powerless to control their own destiny. Moreover, de facto decision making may be situationally limited or occur when problems in communication exist, as when significant problems or issues are not discussed. Cultural norms are important to consider here, because obstacles to open communication and active decision making may also have a cultural or ethnic basis. For example, among traditional Latino couples, sexual relations and family planning may be an area of closed communication; pregnancies may therefore become the outcome of de facto decision making.

🐝 VARIABLES AFFECTING FAMILY POWER DYNAMICS

There are some important contingency variables that significantly influence family power dynamics and decision-making (Table 11–2).

FAMILY POWER HIERARCHY

Each family has a power hierarchy or "pecking order." In the traditional nuclear family and in most nuclear families today, the power structure is clearly hierarchical, meaning that the power structure is tiered and the "pecking occurs downward." Men often develop or maintain power over women, and parents almost always have more power than children (Hoffman, 1981). In the egalitarian family, however, a clear gender and age-based power hierarchy may be absent.

Minuchin (1974) and Haley (1976, 1980) place great importance on the lines of authority or hierarchically arranged power structures in families. Minuchin asserts that parents constitute the execu-

TABLE 11–2

VARIABLES AFFECTING FAMILY POWER STRUCTURE

1. Family power hierarchy
2. Type of family form (single parent, blended family, traditional two-parent nuclear family, etc.)
3. Formation of coalitions
4. Family communication network
5. Gender differences
6. Age and family life cycle factors
7. Cultural and interpersonal factors
8. Social class

tive subsystem and should not forfeit or diminish that responsibility in any way. However, Minuchin describes variations in the power hierarchy due to differing family forms. In large families, single-parent families, or families where both adults are employed, some allocation of parental power is usually given to an older child(ren). Children may be assigned more rights and responsibilities than is the case in the traditional two-parent nuclear family (Ganong, Coleman, & Fine, 1995). Having older children parent younger children may work well, as younger children are cared for and the parental child can develop responsibility, competence, and autonomy beyond his or her years. The family with a parental child structure may experience problems, however, when the delegation of authority is unclear or if the parents abdicate their authority, leaving the parental child to become the primary source of decision making, control, and guidance. In these situations, the child is given a task that exceeds his or her abilities and that interferes with meeting his or her childhood needs of support and dependency.

TYPE OF FAMILY FORM

Family form is another factor that affects family power dynamics. For instance, in newly formed stepparent families, remarriage puts pressure on the new family to change the power hierarchy that existed in the prior single-parent family. Conflict may occur when stepchildren perceive a loss of power and control within the new stepparent family. Mothers often have more decision-making power in their new family than they had in their first marriage, retaining some of the power they had when they headed the family before they remarried (Ganong, Coleman, & Fine, 1995).

FORMATION OF FAMILY COALITIONS

Another way the power structure of the family is altered is by the formation of coalitions. *Coalitions* are either temporary, issue-based alliances, or long-term alliances made to offset the dominance of one or more other family members. Family members form coalitions based on each person's relative power (Caplow, 1968, cited in Klein & White, 1996).

Subgroups within a family band together to support each other and to increase their power position relative to other members of the family (Stachowiak, 1975). Obviously, then, coalitions generate more power for the members who join together. Coalition formation most commonly occurs with democratic versus primary (traditional) authority patterns. In addition, over a family's life cycle, the relative power of family members changes and, in turn, potential coalitions change (Caplow, 1968).

Coalitions in families are most healthy when they exist within the appropriate power levels (Gorman, 1975). Family therapists (Lidz, 1963; Minuchin, 1974; Satir, 1972) point out that a sustaining parental coalition is a healthy and a virtually necessary phenomenon to effectively parent children. In contrast, long-term, extensively used parent–child coalitions are unhealthy, because they disrupt the intact functioning of the parent–child and spouse subsystems (Smoyak, 1975). Nevertheless, mother–child coalitions are especially common in patriarchal families, where the father's power is great. Frequently, the mother and an older child form a coalition to dilute his power to some degree. In this situation, the child may receive special favors from the mother but may become enmeshed with that parent, inhibiting or preventing the child from achieving age-appropriate individuation (Stachowiak, 1975). Sibling coalitions are also common, as children join forces to oppose or evade the rules parents establish (Turner, 1970).

One of the difficulties in a single-parent family is the obvious inability to form a parental coalition. Two-parent families tend to have significantly more resources and alternatives available to them than do one-parent families, because partners in the former can support each other and form a coalition. In one-parent families, the strength of primary authority (legitimate power) may be a dominant and necessary factor for the single parent to exercise to control the family situation (Jayaratne, 1978).

FAMILY COMMUNICATIONS NETWORK

Communication networks correlate with the power structure. The age, sex, and personalities of family members influence the nature of the family communication network and so communication is seldom of equal intensity within each of the pairs of relationships in the family. Two siblings may have a close, confidential type of relationship, while a third sibling communicates only tangentially with her two other siblings. When there is unequal communication between family members, intermediaries ("go-betweens") usually exist. The person in the family who serves as an intermediary in communications between others (in many instances the mother), but who interacts directly with all family members, holds a central position in the communication network. The greater the centrality of the family member, the greater his or her power, due to his or her control over the outcome of the decision-making process. Because the intermediary understands the attitudes and opinions of most of the family members, he or she can use this information to influence family members. The go-between is also able to censor or screen information from the sender to the other family members. This censorship function and ability to alter messages gives the intermediary extensive power, at least in some areas. In larger families one may find a secondary intermediary—such as an older son or daughter—who acts as a link between other children and the mother (Turner, 1970).

GENDER DIFFERENCES

There is wide consensus in the literature, particularly the feminist literature, that gender relations are based on power (Ellman & Taggart, 1993) and that women typically have less power in the family than men. Much of the power differential in the family is based on economic inequality. Women, if they work outside the home, are paid less and thus have fewer economic resources than men to bring into the marital relationship. If women work inside the home, their work is unpaid and often devalued (Goldner, 1985; Okin, 1989). Moreover, our societal notions of what constitutes "masculinity" and "femininity" maintain these gender-based power inequities. Even when women have considerable resources, they often are inhibited from using them fully because of cultural norms that support male superiority and power (Blumstein & Schwartz, 1991). Goldner (1985), a feminist, considers power to be a key to understanding family interactions. She explains that since the power of women is less than that of men, the way in which women exert

power with men is different than vice versa. For instance, men who lack material or personal resources are more likely to use manipulation and intimidation to gain control, whereas women who lack material or personal resources are more likely to "give in" or gain influence by acting weak, dependent, or manipulative (Balswick & Balswick, 1995).

Research carried out from 1950 through 1990 consistently demonstrates that family power is significantly related to men and women's marital satisfaction. Higher levels of satisfaction are found most frequently among egalitarian couples and couples in which the husband is dominant versus when the wife is dominant. Wife-dominated couples have generally been found to rate their marriages as less satisfying (McDonald, 1980; Szinovacz, 1987). It is curious that women who were dominant classified themselves as the least maritally satisfied, far below their husbands' satisfaction. One explanation offered is that the wife is dominant by default, not choice. Unilateral dominance of the wife is contrary to normative expectations, that is, the cultural prescriptions of either the traditional (husband-dominated) or the modern (egalitarian) marriage.

In comparison to feminist interpretations of gender and power inequalities, Kranichfield (1987) gives a more positive view of women's power in the family. She points out that in the family domain women in fact have a great deal of power, which has been overlooked. Women's power is pervasive when power is defined as the ability to bear, educate, and impact the personality, values, and beliefs of each new human being in society. Contemporary mothers are usually more intimately involved in children's lives than fathers, and so have more intergenerational influence in families. This situation has not changed, even with the increased participation of women in the workforce. However, gender-related differences in use of specific power resources and the nature of the decision-making process may vary with other factors, as reported by Godwin and Scanzoni (1989). Study results indicated that (marital) partners' emotional dependency (the love and caring for their spouse that each spouse reports) and the degree of commitment to their marital relationship influenced the decision-making processes that are used in the family. Data were collected via observation and self-reports from 188 married couples. In this sample, the more wives report loving their husbands, the less coercive tactics were used and the more consensus in decision making was likely. And the more committed husbands were to the marriage, the more control the wife had.

Clearly, most research about the effects of gender on power in relationships focuses on cross-sex [heterosexual] partnerships. The effect of gender on power may vary when the intimate parnters are gay or lesbian couples. Steen and Schwartz (1995) questioned whether the "pattern of dominance and support identified in heterosexual couples (and reflected in their communication patterns) carries over into homosexual couples" (p. 309). They concluded that gay male couples are much more likely to compete for dominant conversational position than are women, consistent with the general patterns described in the literature regarding differences in men's and women's power bases and related communication patterns. However, the authors caution the reader that ". . . homosexual couples are often critical of the role power can play in shaping a relationship" (p. 339), and so gay and lesbian couples may deliberately employ conversational techniques as a way of balancing power within their relationships.

AGE AND FAMILY LIFE CYCLE FACTORS

Family decisions and power among family members vary with the family's life cycle stage, as well. In childbearing families, there is an evolution from concentration of power in the hands of the adults when the children are young, to a more shared power arrangement as children move into adolescence. Before they have children, couples tend to be syncratic—discussing and mutually deciding on most major decisions between themselves (Blood, 1969). Later in the family's life cycle, when children are being raised and the system is more complex, each spouse usually has clearly defined areas of power and decision making, although major decisions are still jointly made. Corrales (1975) explains that when the dyad changes to a triad with the addition of a baby, some loss in the woman's power is often seen. Typically, adult partners discuss most areas less and less as time goes on, a sign that some estrangement from each other may also be occurring. During adolescence older children assume more power in the family than when they were younger. The shifts in power during the time when adolescents are in the home may be accompa-

nied by conflict revolving around the power distribution. In the later years of a childbearing family, the adult couple may return to a dyadic relationship, sharing in decision making and power. And, elderly persons in families often experience a decline in power, as they lose resources (Klein & White, 1996).

CULTURAL AND INTERPERSONAL FACTORS

Ethnic and religious differences among families also dictate different power arrangements. For instance, male dominance is commonly seen in unacculturated immigrant families from Europe, Asia, Latin America, Africa, and the Middle East. In traditional immigrant Asian families in which strong Confucian values are present, the male is ascribed the ultimate authority in the family. It is believed that men, having more important responsibilities, should be relieved of the mundane concerns of everyday life. "Thus, the wife is usually in charge of the budget and makes most of the economic decisions for the family. Although the husband is the head of the family, the wife is in charge of domestic life . . . the husband has orchestration power and the wife, implementation power" (Balswick & Balswick, 1995, p. 301).

Literature on Hispanic and African-American families describe the typical family to be male and female dominant, respectively. However, the stereotypes about male dominance in Hispanic families and female dominance in African-American families are questionable and have come under close scrutiny in recent years (see Chapters 19 and 20 for elaboration).

One important person variable is the resource of interpersonal skills. This includes the ability to argue convincingly and negotiate or bargain successfully, as well as manipulate, lie, and cajole. It is not uncommon to find a family member who has few of the objective resources that ordinarily facilitate dominance, but who actually controls much of family life through his or her masterful use of a broad repertoire of interpersonal skills (Turner, 1970).

SOCIAL CLASS

The term *social class* refers to a large group of people with relatively similar incomes, amount of wealth, life conditions, life chances, and lifestyles (Ropers, 1991). The terms *socioeconomic status* and *social status* are often used synonomously with the term *social class.* Wright and Leahey (2000) point out that "much of the sociological and psychological research has been confounded by social class differences among ethnic groups" (p. 83). Wright and Leahey point out the difficulties in discerning the effects of income and ethnicity on family functioning, and in light of our racist and classist history in America caution against misinterpreting findings related to social class. They, nevertheless, acknowledge that "Each class . . . has its own clustering of values, lifestyles, and behavior that influences family interaction and healthcare practices" (p. 83). Examples of classic differences in family power across social classes are presented below.

LOWER CLASS FAMILIES. Besmer (1967) summarizes the frequently seen power characteristics of poor families in the United States. The husband is more likely to proclaim authority because he is a male, although actually having to concede more authority to the wife due to the paucity of his resources. The father most generally loses influence in the family at lower socioeconomic levels as a consequence of his social and occupational inadequacy. An authoritarian theme is a strong underlying factor in the interpersonal relationships of the poor. There is a strong belief in the validity of strength as the source of power and on the rightness of existing patterns. An individual's dominance, rather than expertise and the merit of his or her suggestions, is relied on as the common source of decisions.

The lower-class wife often has more responsibilities than either the middle- or upper-class wife or the lower-class husband, and frequently has more influence in the family decision making than women in the other classes. This is especially true in the financial area, where the lower-class wife may feel that earning money is the man's responsibility and spending it wisely is the woman's.

WORKING-CLASS FAMILIES. In an early influential study by Komarovsky (1964), education was found to be the important determinant as to how authoritarian a family power structure was among working-class families; the higher the education, the more flexible and

"middle class" certain ideals and protocols in marriage became. The incidence of dominance by the husband declined with better education of the husband, and in contrast, patriarchal attributes were more prevalent among the less educated.

MIDDLE-CLASS FAMILIES. According to Kanter (1978), the most egalitarian or companion-based marriages seem to be found among the lower-middle-class, white-collar workers, perhaps as a result of the greater availability of the husband's time to share chores and act as a companion to his wife. Resource and expert power are more often used as bases for power in upper-middle-class families (Szinovacz, 1987). There is less research regarding families in upper social classes than about lower, working, and middle classes.

CLASSIFYING OVERALL FAMILY POWER STRUCTURE

Classifications systems are often used to state whether a family is dominated by one member (usually one spouse), has an egalitarian power structure, or has no effective leadership (is chaotic). Some authors point out that most of the classifications used to describe families are too simplistic and do not adequately reflect the dynamic qualities of family power or its complexity. Although an overall labeling of family power might neither be possible nor entirely accurate, we cannot overlook the parsimony of classification. If a family displays an overall dysfunctional power structure, a statement of this conclusion may serve as a family nursing diagnosis.

Two types of families have most often been described in the literature over the years: (1) the *patriarchal, traditional family* and (2) the *democratic, egalitarian, or modern family.* In the patriarchal, traditional [heterosexual] family, the father is the head of the family, with family power vested in his hands; and his wife, his sons, and their wives and children, and his unmarried daughters, are subordinated to his power. In contrast, the democratic modern, egalitarian family is based on the equality of husband and wife, with consensus in making decisions and increasing participation by children as they grow older (Burgess, Locke, & Thomas, 1963; Scanzoni & Szinovacz, 1980).

There has been a gradual shift from the traditional, patriarchal family structure toward a more democratic, egalitarian family structure. Nevertheless, men's and women's roles in the family are socioculturally defined and mediated, and family structure is not easily or quickly changed (Ellman & Taggart, 1993). As egalitarianism in the family becomes more prominent, changes in women's base for power are occurring, albeit slowly. Men are more likely to use expert power or direct informational power as a base for influence in the family rather than primary authority. Women, however, still use referent power, "helpless" power, and indirect informational power much more prominently. These bases for power are selected by women because of their greater acceptability to their mates. When women use expert power and direct informational power, they are sometimes seen as being "masculine" and "aggressive." While the common use of helpless power by women, however, is more acceptable to their spouses, it is not to their own self-esteem. As noted, women also have implementation power, but often not orchestration power. Research findings agree that workforce participation and achievement of higher education have given women more power in the family (Balswick & Balswick, 1995; Leslie & Korman, 1989).

Another frequently used typology for classifying power in the marital subsystem or family was developed by Herbst (1954). It divides marital power into *autocratic, syncratic,* and *autonomic* patterns. Autocratic power patterns exist when a single family member dominates the family. In these families, one individual makes decisions on family activities. Syncratic power patterns exist when both members of the marital dyad make decisions involving the family members. An autonomic power structure is present when the two partners share power but do this by functioning independently of one another in both decision making and their activities. Other authors refer to this pattern as the pattern found in an "atomistic" family.

One problem with Herbst's (1954) original typology is that he assumed that the power always rested with one or the other parent (or was shared). This is a constricting approach because the dominant individual may be a child, grandparent, or another family member in many family forms. Most research into family power has, in fact, dealt with conjugal power rather than family power, focusing on only husband–wife interactions to the exclusion of the child's role in the decision-making processes. The relative power of children in families has been found to be substantial and increasing with more egalitarian family power structures. In a recent article in *Time* magazine titled "Shifting the Balance of Power," Gibbs (2001) wrote that "Baby boomers are accused of raising the most spoiled generation ever, and everyone has a tale of out-of-control behavior . . ." (p. 3). She added that parents are "launching an urgent debate about how to treat them [children] with respect without sacrificing authority" (p. 3).

In contrast with the analysis and classification of marital power relationships, the categorization of the parent–child subsystem has usually been quite simple, for example, on a continuum from high to low parental control. In family process literature, derived mainly from family therapy, the categories most widely used are *symmetrical (balanced)* and *complementary (submissive–dominant)* relationships. Symmetrical and complementary role relationships are discussed in Chapter 12.

Lewis and associates (1976) developed a comprehensive model for summarizing a family's power structure that includes the chaotic or leaderless family not identified in the former models. Figure 11–1 modifies the model by Lewis and associates, incorporating the various types of power commonly observed in families. This continuum is suggested for use in assessing overall family power dimensions as well as subsystem power dimensions.

🦟 FAMILY POWER IN HEALTHY FAMILIES

Lewis and associates (1976) conducted in-depth interviews with a group of middle-class families to determine their psychosocial health status and the family structural characteristics with which health status was correlated. From their analysis of interviews and observations, they grouped families into three categories of health, from the severely dysfunctional to optimally healthy. It was generally found that the

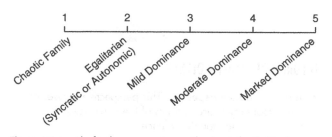

Figure 11-1. The family power continuum. The chaotic family (1) refers to a leaderless family, wherein no member has adequate power to make decisions effectively. In egalitarian syncratic and autonomic families (2), decisions and power are shared. In the syncratic form the decisions are made together; in the autonomic form the decisions are made independently. Dominance or power (3–5) ranges from marked, where there is practically absolute control by an individual and no negotiation, to mild, where there is a tendency for dominance and submissiveness, but most decisions are reached through respectful, mutual negotiation.

most severely dysfunctional families presented chaotic family structures (see Figure 11–1), and the most competent families presented flexible structures. These researchers emphasized that "the most direct measure of structure concerned the distribution of power or influence within the family" (Lewis et al., p. 209).

The power attributes of healthy families were seen to reflect the following:

> . . . the parental coalition played a crucial role in the determination of overall family competence. . . . Leadership was provided by the parental coalition as was a model of relating which appeared to be of great learning value to the children. Leadership was shared by the parents. . . . This trend toward an egalitarian marriage was in striking contrast to both the more distant marriages of the adequate families and the marital pattern of dominance and submission that so often was seen in the dysfunctional families. (p. 210)

In the healthy families, the parents, acting as a coalition, did not exercise their power in an authoritarian or rigid way but, within their style of leadership, left room for options and negotiation. Nevertheless, power and boundaries were clear; there was no confusion as to the position and power of family members. Generally, the father held the most power, the mother somewhat less, and the child distinctly the least power (Lewis et al., 1976). In contrast, all the severely disturbed families showed that

none of the family members had much power. The most inept families, the authors reported, had a powerless father and a strong coalition between mother and child. In families labeled as midrange, a strong, healthy parental–marital coalition did not exist. These families characteristically maintained rigid, authoritarian structures via dominance by one mate. Family control processes, such as rigid authoritarian structures, affect children in the family. Through modeling, children learn power-relevant behaviors such as coercive, Machiavellian, and/or violent behaviors (Straus, Gelles, & Steinmetz, 1980).

Minuchin (1974) agrees with Lewis and associates' findings when he asserts that the most important aspect of power within a family is the presence of a clear and functioning hierarchy in which the parents function as the executive subsystem and children have different levels of authority. For a family to function effectively there must also be complementary of functions, with the husband and wife accepting interdependency and working as a team.

POWER DYNAMICS AND FAMILY VIOLENCE

Family violence is recognized as one of our major public health problems today (Horner, 1998; Straus & Gelles, 1990; Wallace, 1996). The nature of the violence can include a range of violent, abusive, and neglectful actions and has "reached epidemic proportions" (Horner, p. 1). Although the basic mechanism of violence (use of physical force by one family member against another) is the same, there are at least five types of family violence, depending on who the abuser and victim are: spouse/intimate partner abuse (inclusive of gay and lesbian relationships), child abuse (physical and sexual), sibling abuse, elder abuse, and parent abuse. The first two types are more numerous and widely acknowledged than the others. One of the surprising findings of family violence researchers is that family violence may actually be increasing as women become more educated, obtain better jobs, and make a better income. Because these advances provide many women with more power and control than in the past, men may react more aggressively and violently in an effort to maintain or regain their declining power and control (Steinmetz, 1995).

The professional literature about family violence has mushroomed. Concomitantly, there has been rapid growth of research in this area. One of the main problems in examining family violence data and studies is that the terms *abuse* and *violence* are not conceptually equivalent terms; nor are they consistently defined in the literature. Straus and associates' (1980) definition of wife and child abuse refers to only those acts of violence that have a high probability of causing injury to the victim. Wallace (1996) defines family violence as "any act or omission by persons who are cohabiting that results in serious injury (physical or emotional harm) to other members of the family" (p. 3).

Family or domestic violence is not confined to any one social class or ethnic group. Most domestic violence is directly related to social stress in families (Wallace, 1996). The violent family is often one that is socially isolated (Gelles & Maynard, 1987). Those individuals who experienced a violent and abusive childhood are more likely to become abusers. The National Center on Child Abuse and Neglect estimates that 30 percent of individuals who were physically or sexually abused or extremely neglected as children become abusive parents themselves. The following sections describe three theoretical perspectives of family violence, followed by sections describing intimate partner abuse, child abuse, sibling abuse, parent abuse, and elder abuse.

THEORETICAL PERSPECTIVES OF FAMILY VIOLENCE

Three major theoretical perspectives used to explain the dynamics of family violence (the intraindividual, the sociocultural, and the social–psychological perspective) address unhealthy power characteristics in violent families (Table 11–3). In the intraindividual (within the individual) perspective, personality attributes of the abusive person and the victim are believed to "cause" abuse to occur and continue.

Sociocultural theories of violence focus on the macrolevel conditions of society that create a tendency for family violence (Steinmetz, 1995). Sexism, racism, ageism, poverty, inadequate housing, unemployment or underemployment, and opportunity disparities are societal conditions that create frustrations that are brought home to the family. They set up significant preconditions for violence to occur. Some

TABLE 11–3

THEORIES OF FAMILY VIOLENCE

- **Intraindividual Perspective:** This perspective focuses on the personality characteristics of the perpetrator and victim as "causing" family violence.
- **Sociocultural Perspective:** Sociocultural factors, related to societal or cultural differences in viewing violence as a way to resolve family problems, are described and analyzed.
- **Social–Psychological Perspective:** This perspective explains family violence as a function of the interface between the individual and society with respect to issues of power, control, social class (poverty), employment opportunities, and transfer of property.

Adapted from Steinmetz (1995).

family violence theorists believe that a society's general attitudes toward the use of physical aggression to resolve social problems are reflected in families' use of physical aggression. In any case, the impact of society's attitudes and norms on the family is always considerable. For example, the concept of the children being the property of parents—who are free to discipline as they see fit—is an ancient concept that has only recently been constrained (Steinmetz). Even today, the introduction of parental rights legislation in some states is evidence that some conservative parents still believe that they should have practically absolute power over how their children are cared for, educated, and disciplined.

Social–psychological perspectives about family violence examine the interface between the individual and society. Issues of power, control, social class, employment opportunities, and transfer of property are central to the analysis of family violence using this theoretical perspective. Steinmetz (1995) and others believe that power is a critical component of violence because (a) it characterizes and legitimates intrafamilial interactions between domestic partners or spouses and between parents and children; (b) it provides an indication of the value society places on each family member (e.g., the value of men over women); and (c) the power that is available to a specific family is based on the value that family is seen to have in the family's community (e.g., a prominent family has more value to the community than a poor family). Control, the outcome of having greater power, is also a crucial aspect of family violence, according to this theoretical perspective. Control includes direct control over another person, as well as control of resources, with poor and working-class families having fewer resources and, hence, less power and control.

INTIMATE PARTNER ABUSE

Although the use of physical force by one mate against the other (largely husbands against wives) has recently been recognized by the mass media and professionals as a significant social problem (Gelles, 1980; Straus & Gelles, 1990), it has been a commonly used tactic for the handling of frustration and stressors throughout our country's history and, as such, has been societally sanctioned in the past. Even though women are generally victims of spousal abuse, they can also be the perpetrators. Some studies have found that men as victims of spousal abuse are more common than people thought (Wallace, 1996). However, the abuse that women suffer is more common and more severe than the abuse men experience in spousal relationships (Wallace). Spousal abuse is defined by Wallace as "any intentional act or series of acts (physical, emotional, or sexual) that cause injury to the spouse" (p. 164). Horner (1998) notes that, according to the Bureau of Justice Statistics cited in Health Resources and Services Administration (HRSA) documents, there were more than 960,000 violent victimizations of women age 12 and older by an intimate partner between 1992 and 1996. In a subsample of the National Survey of Family and Households (n = 4088), the results indicated considerable underreporting of marital violence (Szinovacz & Egley, 1995).

Bolton and Bolton (1987) summarize research findings relative to the personality characteristics of the conjugal violence perpetrator:

> The need to control pervades the conjugal violence perpetrator's behavioral style. Although capable of controlling very little outside the home, his control in the home is absolute, extending through financial decisions, child care, sexual relationships, leisure time activities, and even menu. Domineering and hostile, this perpetrator acts out his dislike for authority figures through those who cannot exert authority over him: the weaker members of the family. (p. 126)

Abusive spouses can offer occasional warmth and protectiveness on their best days. It is this intermittent positive reinforcement that "locks" the victim(s) into the relationship. In other words, family relationships in abusive families are maintained through the abuse of power by the perpetrator and the dynamics of love, connectedness, and loyalty (Miller, 1989).

Abusive men/husbands may abuse, threaten, and intimidate women in such a way that the women feel powerless to change the relationship or to leave. The women may believe that they are to blame for the man's violent outbursts (Murray & Leigh, 1995). Women are more likely to be victims of domestic violence when they appear weak, vulnerable, and isolated—a person who is overcome by anxiety, guilt, and shame (Steinmetz, 1995).

Wallace (1996) believes that spousal abuse has multiple sources in society. For example, social stress, power differences in the marriage, women's dependency on their husband, alcohol abuse among husbands, pregnancy, and the marriage license (license being viewed as ownership and rights of control by any means) have all been found to be factors indicating a higher probability of spousal abuse (Wallace, 1996). Further, many studies have found that abusers have low self-esteem, abuse alcohol, and have experienced violence in the family of origin. Nevertheless, Lackey and Williams (1995) found married men (n = 424) who had developed strong attachments to their partner, friends, or relatives to be less likely to be violent to their female partner even though they had experienced violence in their family of origin.

Women who are beaten by their husbands often stay in the marriage with the hope that the husband will change, although statistics indicate this almost never happens. Also, many battered women lack alternatives (alternate places to live, financial resources). Many of these women remain very passive and are unwilling to run away because they often have come from families in which violence was customary, and thus see their predicament as part of "normal" married life. Moreover, some women say that they want to keep the family together and have very traditional values about family life. In fact, many wives are unaware that it is illegal for their husband to beat them up. Moreover, many batterers are "supermacho" types who will not let their wives go out alone, and follow and harass them if they try to run away, leaving the wives with the idea that they will never be able to become free (Benedek, 1978; Wallace, 1996).

Some wives do stay in the abusive relationships for many years, so that there may be many older women who are unrecognized, long-standing victims of abuse (Phillips, 2000). Other instances of partner abuse among older couples may occur following a remarriage in later years. The circumstances of abuse for older women may differ somewhat from younger couples, in part due to the time in history when the union was formed: Phillips wrote that

> For the most part, older women in this country are a breed apart from younger women. They are much more likely to have a death-do-us-part philosophy about marriage and . . . more likely to accept behaviors in their spouses as "normal" that younger women might term abuse. (p. 190)

Despite the vast numbers of wives who remain in marriages in which spousal violence is present, increasing numbers of wives and their children are leaving their home. The importance of leaving abusive relationships is truly a matter of life and death, as nearly a third of homicides of women are perpetrated by their husbands or boyfriends (Horner, 1998). In response to the trend of women leaving abusive relationships, shelters for battered women are now found in many communities across the nation. Woods and Isenberg (2001) cited evidence from multiple studies indicating that women may suffer from posttraumatic stress syndrome due to the violence they have experienced, and that there is a strong correlation between the severity of the abuse and the occurrence and severity of posttraumatic stress disorder (PTSD) among women who have left abusive relationships. Results of their own study indicated that the PTSD may be mediated by the women's adaptive capacity and their ability to redefine intimate relationships and learning to value themselves.

The effects of intimate partner violence is not limited to the abusive adults and the victim of the violence but extend to other family members. Parker (2000) estimated that between 3.3 million and 10 million children are exposed to spousal domestic violence each year, though they are not physically harmed. This exposure can result in multiple negative effects on their emotional, social, and cognitive development, including depression, aggressive behavior, and impaired school performance.

There has been increasing attention on the effects of parents' conflicts on children (Tschann, Flores, Pasch, & Marin, 1999) and the interactions between parental conflict and parenting behaviors (Lindahl & Malik, 1999) in diverse cultures (Rohner & Britner, 2000). Results indicate that the antecedents, power dynamics, and the nature of the violence are not easily accounted for, but rather are the result of complex relationships between intraindividual and societal factors. However, researchers agree that family members who engage in any one form of violence are likely to engage in other forms of violence (Horner, 1998).

Hall and Cummings (1997) found that the effects of partner and parent–child conflicts extended to grandmothers and grown children, though the nature of the negative effects and dysfunction varied depending on the role of the family member. Humphreys (2001) collected life history interviews from adult daughters of battered women and found that the effects of their parents' violence affected them well into adulthood. They described their suffering and their resilience. Results illuminated the adaptations the women made to family violence at different points, such as using vigilance in early childhood and involvement in activities outside the home when they were older.

Gay and lesbian family violence is believed by some researchers to be at the same rate as among heterosexual couples, or around 25 to 35 percent (Wallace, 1996). However, this form of violence has not been widely studied. Gay and lesbian families share emotions and financial responsibility in their relationship that can lead to conflict situations. Generally, both lesbian and gay abusers use similar types of violence on their victims as heterosexual couples, such as rape, threats, economic control, psychological or emotional abuse (e.g., humiliation, mind manipulation, isolation, and lying), homophobic control, breaking household items, assaults with weapons, biting, and scratching (Wallace, 1996).

CHILD ABUSE

Public awareness of child abuse did not come about until the 1960s when the diagnosis "battered child syndrome" was coined. Family violence as an academic topic of research remained virtually hidden until the early 1970s. Hence, the whole area of family violence and the important underlying family dynamics are relatively new for family health professionals.

The number of cases of child abuse appears to be rising rapidly; however, some of this rise is due to improved record keeping. Some family violence researchers believe that the incidence of child abuse has probably not changed dramatically from previous eras, but that the increase is due to greater public and professional awareness of child abuse and less public tolerance for it, as well as a better recording system (Straus et al., 1980; Straus & Gelles, 1990). However, according to the National Center on Child Abuse and Neglect (NCCAN), the number of children suffering abuse or neglect increased from 1.4 million in 1986 to 2.8 million in 1993.

Child abuse can be physical, emotional, or sexual, or a combination of any two or all three. Physical abuse in children has been defined as "any act that results in a nonaccidental physical injury by a person who has care, custody, or control of a child" (Wallace, 1996, p. 29). Child abuse has been found to occur in all social classes, races, and family forms and among both men and women (Vandewater & Lansford, 1998). Generally, children who are 5 years old or younger and older teenagers are at greater risk for experiencing abuse by their caretakers. Parental behaviors that are associated with physical abuse in children include life stress, loneliness, depression, anxiety, negative parenting attitudes and practices, poor conflict resolution in the marital relationship, and excessive alcohol use (Milner & Murphy, 1995; Straus & Gelles, 1990). The geographic characteristics of the family may put families at risk for child abuse. For example, Sachs, Hall, Lutenbacher, and Rayens (1999) found that geographic isolation in conjunction with daily stressors put rural mothers of low-birth-weight children at risk for depression and child abuse.

In child abuse, parents (both fathers and mothers) misuse their parental power to sexually or physically abuse their children (Murray & Leigh, 1995). Abusive parents have been found to be socially and psychologically troubled individuals who are less nurturant and have excessive authority and power needs (Steinmetz, 1995) as compared to parents who are not abusive. Even though all children are at risk for being physically abused, children who are difficult to manage or control may be at higher risk (Straus & Gelles, 1990; Wallace, 1996).

Children who have been sexually abused often react to abuse by changing their behavior. Feelings of guilt, shame, fear, and anger are often shown. These changed behaviors often manifest themselves in school; abused children may also experience sleep disturbances, have eating disorders, or show regressive or depressed behavior (Wallace, 1996). Briggs, Hubbs-Tait, Culp, and Blankemeyer (1995) studied 134 college students (67 males and 67 females) who had either been sexually abused, had a mother who was dying from cancer, or had a history of abuse. Students who had been sexually abused experienced more psychosocial problems than the other two groups.

An explanation of child abuse as the result of the interaction between the characteristics of the abuser and the social context are supported by the findings of a U.S. House Ways and Means Committee report (Harris, 1991). In this report, adult drug use has been implicated as a predominant contributor to child abuse. In child-protective service agencies in 22 states and the District of Columbia the most salient characteristic of the adult abuser was his or her use of drugs.

SIBLING ABUSE

Most of the discussion about the nature of family violence and physical child abuse can be applied to the discussion of sibling abuse. Sibling abuse has been defined as "any form of physical, mental, or sexual abuse inflicted by one child in a family unit on another" (Wallace, 1996, p. 101). Often, sibling abuse occurs when the older or more powerful sibling has control over another sibling (the victim). In addition, sibling abuse has been found to be higher in families in which child abuse and/or spousal abuse occurs (Straus & Gelles, 1990). The types of sibling abuse that have been reported are physical abuse (e.g., striking, kicking, punching); emotional abuse (e.g., name-calling, ridicule, degradation, exacerbating a fear, and destroying personal possessions); and sexual abuse (Wallace, 1996).

PARENT ABUSE

Another form of abuse is that in which children are old enough to now perpetrate violence against their parents. The children at one point were recipients of violence, and through role modeling learned that the use of violence was a feasible and an acceptable mode of expressing anger. In studies that examined this phenomenon, the children were adolescents. In the first national study published (Straus et al., 1980) of 2,143 intact families with adolescent children (10 to 17 years old), 9 percent of the parents reported experiencing at least one attack by one of their children, and 3 percent said they had experienced severe violence. In both single- and two-parent families, mothers were more likely to be the victims and sons the perpetrators (Steinmetz, 1987).

In data from another nationwide study of parent abuse (Agnew & Huguley, 1989), abusing adolescents were more likely to have friends who also assaulted their parents and approved of delinquency, including violence. These white adolescents who were weakly attached to their parents believed that the probability of official sanction for parental assault was low.

ELDER ABUSE

Elder abuse and neglect, according to a watershed 1985 report by a congressional subcommittee (Larsen, 1989) is a problem that is increasing nationally. In an extensive review of family violence literature, Wallace (1996) defines elder abuse as "conduct that results in the physical, psychological, or material neglect, harm, or injury to an elder" (p. 221). Phillips (1996) discusses controversies surrounding definitions of elder abuse, and argues for definitions (particularly legal definitions), which include intentionality, documentable harm, assignable responsibilty and vulnerability. Most of the early published articles represent personal observations and/or expert opinion. The research about elder abuse and neglect has increased markedly since the 1980s. One of the first surveys of elder abuse (Pillemer & Finkelhor, 1988) found that spouses were the most likely abusers of elders, with about equal numbers of men and women as victims. Other research indicates that older women are more likely to be victims of physical abuse and the abusers are most often men (Phillips, 2000).

One study of elder abuse, conducted by Steinmetz (1987), described circumstances under which elderly abuse occurred. Ninety-one percent of her sample was 70 years or older, and 85 percent had experienced diminished physical functioning. All elders shared a home with one of their children. The abusive techniques used by the caregiving children "ranged from screaming and yelling (30%); threatening to send elders to nursing home (8.5%); withholding food or medication (17%); . . . to physically restraining elder (7.5%) and slapping, hitting and shaking (2.5%). Overall, 12% of the caregivers had used physically abusive acts or the threat of physical violence in an attempt to maintain control" (p. 738). Families caring for an elderly parent that are experiencing high levels of stress are much more likely to be involved in elder abuse. Also, caregivers who perceive caregiving tasks to be stressful are more apt to engage in elder abuse (Pagelow, 1984; Steinmetz, 1987).

❧ ASSESSMENT OF FAMILY POWER

How does the family nurse measure or assess power in a family? This is the key question, and one for which there is no consensus concerning the appropriate methodology and focus. Studies of family power have been under criticism because of disagreement over how to measure family power, as well as other methodological limitations. Researchers in the past have relied heavily on the survey and structured interview schedule, with little direct observation to validate self-reported data. What has been consistently found, however, is that people are notoriously inaccurate in describing their own behavior. Hence, a combination of observation of family interaction with self-reporting by family members may provide more valid data about family power (Szinovacz, 1987).

Blood and Wolfe (1960) were among the earliest researchers to investigate the relationships between family task allocation and power in the area of that task. Later investigations indicated that such division of responsibility seldom reflected the dominant authority pattern. Reiss (1976) explained that division of labor may not indicate the family power structure, especially if the tasks were assigned based on family beliefs about gender roles rather than negotiated for other reasons. Johnson (1975) verified this difference between family power and task and responsibility allocation. She interviewed 104 Japanese-American wives in Honolulu. Part of the interview included specific questions about who was responsible for and made decisions in the major areas of family life. She then asked questions to determine the wives' overall freedom to pursue individual interests, counter to wishes of their husbands. When wives were queried about specific responsibilities and task allocation, they appeared more influential than the husbands. But when asked broadly stated questions pertaining to the wives' evaluation of their overall power as compared to her husbands' power, most of these wives placed themselves in a subordinate position, largely attributing this fact to their Japanese heritage and its norms regarding male–female roles. Legitimate power or tradition-derived power appeared to be operating here. Thus, while Japanese-American wives played active roles in decision making, they did so by virtue of a delegation of power from their husbands. In this instance, the husband assigned responsibilities while retaining final authority.

Safilios-Rothschild (1976b) wrote that one spouse may have the "orchestration" power while the other has "implementation power." She explains:

> Spouses who have "orchestration power" have, in fact, the power to make only the important and infrequent decisions that do not infringe upon their time but that determine the family life style and major characteristics and features of their family. They also have the power to relegate unimportant and time-consuming decisions to their spouse who can then derive a "feeling of power" by implementing those decisions within the limitations set by crucial and pervasive decisions made by the powerful spouse. (p. 359)

Hence, in this type of spousal power arrangement the wife is said to have "implementation power." In spite of the fact that implementation power is, in the last analysis, an inferior type of power, having control over implementation still confers power to the implementor.

Thus, family power is complex with many factors influencing family power structure, outcomes and decision-making processes. The overall family power can be difficult to assess, particularly during relatively brief encounters with a family or without all family members present. In spite of these difficulties, the following summary can be used to assist with applying the nursing process to family power.

POWER OUTCOMES

Who has the "last say" or "who wins"? Who makes what decisions? And how important are these decisions or issues to the family? More specific questions may be asked to elicit this information (validating when possible with observations). General questions followed by more specific questions in these areas may be helpful:

1. *Financial:* Who budgets, pays bills, and decides on how money is spent?
2. *Social:* Who decides on how to spend an evening or which friends or relatives to see?
3. *Major decisions:* Who decides on changes in jobs or residence?
4. *Child rearing:* Who disciplines and decides on children's activities?

A limitation is that overall power in the family often does not correlate well with specific task responsibilities (the issue of orchestration power versus implementation power).

DECISION-MAKING PROCESSES

What specific techniques are utilized for making decisions in the family and to what extent are these utilized?

1. Consensus decision making
2. Accommodation decision making
   a. Bargaining
   b. Compromising
   c. Coercion
3. De facto decision making

Specific questions eliciting decision-making techniques used focuses on how the family makes decisions.

POWER BASES

This area deals with the source from which the power of various family members is derived. To enumerate again, these sources are:

1. Legitimate power/authority
2. Helpless or powerless power

3. Referent power

4. Resource and expert power

5. Reward power

6. Coercive power

7. Informational power—direct and indirect

8. Affective power

9. Tension management power

Questions asked to elicit information on the source or bases of power might be either specific questions about who makes certain decisions and how (sometimes how also reveals the bases for power).

VARIABLES AFFECTING FAMILY POWER

Multiple variables affect family power. These are:

1. The family power hierarchy

2. Type of family form

3. Formation of coalitions

4. The family communication network

5. Gender differences

6. Age and family life cycle factors

7. Cultural and interpersonal factors

8. Social class

Recognizing the influence of these assessment areas will assist the family nurse in more fully appraising and interpreting family power attributes.

OVERALL FAMILY SYSTEM AND SUBSYSTEM POWER

From your assessment of all the above broad areas, are you able to deduce whether the overall family power can be characterized as dominated by an adult family member, child, or grandparent; as egalitarian, syncratic, or autonomic; as leaderless or chaotic? The family power continuum presented in this chapter can be used for a visual representation of the analysis. Power arrangements on this continuum in the 2 to 4 range have been found to be

healthy and satisfying patterns (if mild dominance is by husband).

To determine the overall power pattern, asking a broad, open-ended question is often illuminating. For example, the family nurse could ask both spouses and children if feasible: "Who usually has the last say about important issues? Who makes the important decisions involving the family? Who runs the family? Who wins the important arguments on issues? Who usually wins out if there is a disagreement? Who gets their way when adults disagree?" An important follow-up question is "Are you satisfied with how decisions are made and with who makes the decisions (i.e., the present power structure).

Subsystem power also needs to be assessed. Observation of adults' interactions, adult/parent–child interactions and sibling interactions and interview data are used to assess subsystem power characteristics (Olson & Cromwell, 1975).

✎ FAMILY NURSING DIAGNOSES

Understanding the power structure in the family is essential in formulating nursing diagnoses and effective nursing interventions. Several prime examples illustrate the importance of including this facet of the family assessment. When health care actions/decisions need to be made by the family, knowing who holds the power for this type of decision and for overall decisions, coupled with knowledge of how decisions are made, will guide the family nurse to speak to the appropriate persons with sensitivity as to how decisions take place.

Where families have a clear, intact power hierarchy that functions well for them, the nurse may want to support or reinforce this healthy structure (this is important in fostering confidence in parents). In this case, a family strength relative to family power could serve as a health promotional family nursing diagnosis, such as "family consistently uses consensual decision making." Where the parental executive subsystem is weak, the nurse may want to identify this as a family nursing diagnosis and plan ways to assist spouses/parents to strengthen this subsystem.

⁂FAMILY NURSING INTERVENTIONS

Nurses can be instrumental in addressing decisional conflicts and other power conflicts (McFarland & McFarlane, 1993). If family members are interested in addressing conflicts, the nurse may offer assistance in helping the family resolve their conflict(s) (McFarland & McFarlane, 1993). McFarland and McFarlane (1993), in describing the NANDA diagnosis "Decisional Conflict," present cogent guidelines for assisting nurses to help family members resolve this problem. Chapter 10 also has suggestions for helping families resolve conflictual communication.

If potential or actual family violence is identified, the nurse can assist in protecting family members. This goal may be accomplished by (a) recognizing and reporting child abuse; (b) supporting and referring abused spouses/intimate partners, elders, siblings, parents, the abuser, and the family unit; and (c) coordinating care to families and family members, working collaboratively with other health and welfare workers (Gilliss, Rose, Hallburg, & Martinson, 1989).

Another nursing intervention, derived from the empowerment model, is often appropriate in families in which one adult is more powerful than the other and the less powerful adult would like to increase her or his resources and power. The model was originally used with married couples, but could apply to other family subsystems. The empowerment model advocates that each family member (adult) use his or her resources to move the other from a position of weakness to greater strength. Balswick and Balswick (1995) elaborate on this notion, referring to a spousal subsystem as follows. Empowering is not merely one spouse yielding to the wishes of the other. It does not involve giving up one's power to empower others. Rather, empowering is the active and intentional process of each spouse developing and affirming power in the other. Each spouse is encouraged to reach full personal potential (p. 311). Hence, empowerment in this context means that each family member desires and assists the other to become all that he or she can be. Focusing on one another's autonomy rather than "control over" someone is a key thrust in the empowerment model. Working toward empowering one another can result in stronger but healthier interdependency in family relationships, as well as a greater sense of autonomy and mutual respect (Balswick & Balswick).

⁂SUMMARY

- Power, as viewed in this text, is one of the four interdependent structural dimensions of the family, and as such is a reflection of the family's unwritten family rules and underlying value system. Power structures vary greatly from family to family, and may be positive or dysfunctional.

- Power is the ability—potential or actual—of an individual(s) to control, influence, or change another person's behavior. Power always involves asymmetrical interpersonal relationships—one interactant exerts greater influence/control in the relationship.

- Power is manifested through decision-making processes in families. Decision making and family power are generally more shared in families now than in earlier decades.

- Because people are notoriously inaccurate in describing their own behavior, a combination of observation of family interaction with self-reporting by family members may provide more valid data about family power than self-reports alone.

- Examples of the source of power in families include legitimate authority, the power of the powerless, helpless power, referent power, resource power, expert power, reward power, coercive power, informational power, affective power, and tension management power.

- Three types of decision-making processes in families are consensus, accommodation, and de facto decision making.

- Men often develop or maintain power over women, often as a result of economic inequities. Parents almost always have more power than children do. In the egalitarian family, however, a clear gender and age-based power hierarchy may be absent.

- Ethnic and religious differences among families may dictate specific power structures in the family.

- Family power structure may also vary because of formation of coalitions, family communication networks, gender differences, family developmental stages, social class, and different family forms.

- Family power structure can be classified several ways (see Figure 11–1), to indicate whether a family is dominated by one member, has an egal-itarian power structure, or has no effective leadership.

- Three theoretical perspectives on family and intimate partner violence are the intraindividual, the sociocultural, and the social–psychological perspective. All present different explanations for the unhealthy power characteristics in violent families.

- Although the basic mechanism of violence (use of physical force by one family member against another) is the same, there are subtypes of family violence, depending on who the abuser and victim are: spouse/intimate partner abuse (includes violence in gay and lesbian relationships), child abuse (physical and sexual), violence between siblings, elder abuse, and parent abuse.

- Family assessment areas in the dimension of family power are described.

- Understanding the power structure in the family is essential in formulating nursing diagnoses and effective nursing interventions.

✿ FAMILY VIGNETTE: THE SIMPSON FAMILY

The Simpsons are a middle-class, white, stepparent family living in a suburban area. John Simpson, age 37, recently (8 months ago) married Sylvia, who had been divorced for 4 years. Sylvia (age 42) has three children, ages 13 (Joe), 10 (Mary), and 8 (Jimmie) from her former marriage. Mr. Simpson had no children from his former marriage. Mr. Simpson is a businessman; he owns and manages a hardware store. Mrs. Simpson is a registered nurse and works at a local hospital. Both have baccalaureate degrees from local colleges and their income level, due to their double income, is "quite comfortable." They live in a lovely, well-kept residential neighborhood. Their home is large and well furnished, containing four bedrooms, a living and family room, and a large, spacious kitchen. They moved to this particular community from the nearby city when they married and formed their new family. The Simpsons are bringing their 8-year-old child, Jimmie, to the family health center because of bedwetting (enuresis), hyperactivity, and inattention at school. He is being examined and interviewed by a pediatric nurse practitioner who is in the process of completing a family assessment and comprehensive history of Jimmie.

Sylvia, the mother, relates that things in the family have been difficult since John "moved in." "First we had to move and the children lost all their friends. And even though John used to come and take me out for the evening and visit with us—so that the children were able to get to know him—they now resent him terribly and I feel I'm in between the devil and the deep blue sea!"

When asked what seems to be the major area of family conflict and concerns, she mentions disciplining of the children. "John doesn't discipline them, which I wish he did, and when he does set some limits, due to my nagging, the children don't listen to him. Then, I have to come in and settle things myself. I married John because I felt the children needed a father to relate to. Their own father lives far away now and seldom keeps in contact with them. The children don't seem to respect John, and the only way he is able to manage them is by promising them something or threatening to punish them."

She says that she never fights or disagrees with her husband in front of the children (believing children should not hear such unpleasant things). But after the children go to bed, she finds herself berating John for not following through with his family obligations—paying bills, repairing the house, yard work, and so on. Sylvia sees herself as in charge of the children (primarily), housework, social affairs, cooking, and shopping, and feels that the rest is up to her husband. She does her work, in addition to a full-time job, and expects him to do his.

According to Mrs. Simpson, Joe, the 13-year-old, likes caring for his younger siblings, and Mary and Jimmie turn to him for help and advice if she is not home. She also comments that Joe is the child who really seems to resent John, and he speaks to her husband only when necessary, with most messages pertaining to the stepfather going through the mother.

When the nurse asks Sylvia about how the family arrives at the major decisions they have made since she and John became involved with each other—such as marriage, moving, and buying the house—Sylvia says that she initiated all three of these conversations. "I'm a practical person. I could see that marriage would be good for all of us, and so suggested it to John!" The nurse then asks, "And what was his answer?" Sylvia replies, "I don't remember exactly. I think he kind of hemmed and hawed around, and then, anyway, agreed, and I started making plans. He didn't want to move from the city or into such a big house, but I convinced him that it would be better economically and that the commuting time was reasonable for him. And I agreed to let him buy a more comfortable car to commute in, in return."

The pediatric nurse practitioner met with the whole family twice more to discuss their "identified" problem (Jimmie) and the family dynamics and family problems. At these meetings she notices that twice when she speaks to the parents and the children become noisy or disruptive, the older son, Joe, takes over, scolding them. In their discussion she observes that this is a family in which there is a proliferation of "do's" and "don'ts" about everything—from the time they get up in the morning until the time they go to bed at night. Feelings are not openly expressed, and the two youngest children directly answered the nurse's questions in a short, incomplete manner, looking to the mother for approval. The mother appears quite committed to a particular home schedule. John mentions that it is hard to fit into someone else's schedule and way of doing things. Joe confirms this point with the nurse in his statement, "We all know the rules better than he does, so why do we need him to tell us what to do?" (Mr. Simpson just sits quietly, and neither parent responds to Joe's hostile statement.) In discussing his own feelings and thoughts about the family, Mr. Simpson perceives that Jimmie may feel confused and insecure because of moving, their marriage, and the new school. He alludes to the difficulty he has faced in parenting his wife's children and to their negative reactions toward him. He also finds disciplining very hard because he never had children before and when he was growing up, was treated very permissively ("anything at all seemed to be okay with my parents"). He comments that "he tries to stay out of child rearing as much as possible."

Mr. Simpson appears to be passive and easygoing with his wife. In contrast, Mrs. Simpson initiates topics, leads discussions, and is quite "definite" and opinionated in her statements.

▪ STUDY QUESTIONS

Review the Family Vignette and answer the related questions.

1. Assess the family power patterns described in the above case.
   a. Who makes what decisions?
   b. What decision-making techniques are utilized?
   c. On what basis is family power derived?
   d. What variables affect family power?
   e. Using the family power continuum (see Figure 11–1), where would you place this family?
   f. If dominance, indicate dominant family member.

2. State a family nursing diagnosis for this family that focuses on the power dimension.

3. Propose two general family nursing interventions to assist the family with a family nursing problem in the power dimension area.

Answer the following questions.

4. Power is an important dimension in human relationships and groups because (select all appropriate answers):
   a. It is critical in understanding role relationships.
   b. It greatly influences the establishment and the maintenance of communication channels.
   c. It is the sole determinant on which an intimate relationship is formed and maintained.

5. Demonstrate your knowledge of several basic power concepts by matching the correct synonyms or definitions with the concepts in the left-hand column.

Concepts

___ a. Power
___ b. Authority
___ c. Family power
___ d. Decision making

Synonym/Definition

1. Influence
2. Legitimate power
3. Primary authority
4. Dominance
5. The outcome is control
6. Family group dominance patterns
7. One facet is decision making
8. Process whereby things get accomplished
9. Assessed within context of family interaction

6. Identify three limitations cited relative to studies of family power.

7. Match up the appropriate definition with the specific bases for power.

Bases for Power

___ a. Authority
___ b. Referent power
___ c. Reward power
___ d. Coercive power
___ e. Helpless power
___ f. Expert or resource power
___ g. Informational power (direct)
___ h. Informational power (indirect)
___ i. Affective power
___ j. Tension management power

Definition

1. Dominant person's obligation to assist the needy
2. Dominant person's greater knowledge regarding issue
3. Legitimate power
4. Tradition-based power
5. Based on positive identification with influencing individual
6. Belief in ability to inflict punishment
7. Based on belief in the ability to grant privileges
8. Way of controlling by managing present stress level in family
9. Based on having greater competency in a matter
10. Hinting or "putting suggestions into another's mouth"
11. The giving or withholding of care warmth, love (affection), and sex

Are the following statements in questions 8 through 10 true or false?

8. In cases in which the husband maintains power because of his control over money, this type of power is called expert authority.

9. Among traditional patriarchal families, reliance on direct informational power is quite common.

10. Primary authority is based on tradition and family members' acceptance of culturally based roles.

11. Identify and describe the three techniques used in making decisions.

12. Describe how each of the following variables affects family power.

    a. Family communication network
    b. Situational changes
    c. Ethnic influences
    d. Coalition formation
    e. Social class
    f. Developmental or life cycle changes

Choose the correct answers to the following questions.

13. The most commonly used and well-accepted typology of family power is:

    a. Democratic–patriarchal
    b. Companionship–authoritarian
    c. Husband dominated, egalitarian, wife dominated
    d. Autocratic, syncratic, autonomic
    e. Familistic–atomistic

14. Which type of overall power structure seems to be the least satisfying to both spouses?

    a. Husband dominated
    b. Wife dominated
    c. Syncratic
    d. Autonomic

15. What is the most outstanding contemporary trend relative to family power?

    a. The upsurge in traditionalism and conservatism
    b. The atomistic trend in the family
    c. The rise of the egalitarian, democratic family
    d. The rise of the matrifocal, matriarchal family

16. The healthy family, as described by Lewis and associates and Minuchin, is characterized by:

    a. A strong parent–child coalition
    b. A clear power hierarchy
    c. Husband having more power than wife
    d. A strong parental coalition

17. The following family roles and power relationships are frequently observed in poor families:

    a. Division of marital responsibilities is informal.
    b. Joint planning predominates.
    c. Father is bestowed titular authority.
    d. Father often plays a more passive, minimal role in the home.

18. Komarovsky found that the following factor played a significant role in the type of power structure present in working-class families:

    a. Occupational status
    b. Residence (city or rural)
    c. Education
    d. Ethnicity

From the following example, answer questions 19 and 20 below.

Mr. Gordon walked in the door while Mrs. Gordon was discussing child rearing with the community health nurse. Mr. Gordon immediately "took over" the conversation, voicing his opinion about every parenting comment made by the nurse or Mrs. Gordon. The children were heard to giggle about a couple of their father's assertions. Toward the end of the visit he shouted to the children to get up and clean the kitchen. The children did not respond but looked at their mother. She paused and then said, "Children, please go clean the dishes." With this request the children left for the kitchen.

19. In this situation, which one of the following most clearly describes the power and role relationships of the father and mother?
    a. Male dominance
    b. Children actually manipulate parents, playing one against the other
    c. Insufficient data to clearly define roles
    d. Mother acts as final arbiter and is dominant in parenting area

20. Data substantiating the above interpretation include:
    a. Father asserting role in an exaggerated manner
    b. His assertions being responded to by giggles from the children
    c. Need to show he is "leader"
    d. Children looking toward mother and responding to her request
    e. No response to father's requests

12

FAMILY ROLE STRUCTURE

CONTENT OUTLINE

LEARNING OBJECTIVES

1. Define and describe key terms relative to the family role structure.
2. Describe the roles of men, women, and grandparents and how family roles have changed in recent decades in the United States.
3. Define and give examples of informal roles that often exist in families.

4. Describe variations in family role behaviors related to family socioeconomic status, family form, family culture or ethnicity, family developmental stage and past role models of family members.
5. Discuss changes in family role structure when a family member experiences health alterations.
6. Apply the nursing process to a hypothetical family vignette in terms of family role structure.

In all known societies individuals live their lives enmeshed in a network of family rights and obligations called role relations (Goode, 1964). Family sociologists have often described the family as an interacting, interdependent set of roles that are in a state of dynamic equilibrium (Turner, 1970). Because of the critical nature that family roles play in the organization of the family, it is imperative for the family nurse to understand role relationships and, from this, be able to promote healthy role behaviors and identify role problems. Successful enactment of family roles is crucial for individual family members and for overall family functioning.

ROLE THEORY: DEFINITIONS AND KEY CONCEPTS

A *role* is defined as relatively homogeneous sets of behaviors that are normatively defined and expected of an occupant of a given social position. Roles are based on role expectations or prescriptions defining what individuals in a particular situation should do in order to meet their own or another's expectations of them (Nye, 1976, p. 7). *Position* or *status* is defined as a person's location in a social system. Role is subsumed under the concept of position (Merton, 1957). While roles are the behaviors associated with one who holds a particular position, position identifies a person's status or place in a social system. Every individual occupies multiple positions—adult, male, husband, farmer, Elks member, and so on (Biddle & Thomas, 1966; Hardy & Hardy, 1988). Associated with each of these positions are a number of roles. In the case of the mother position, the associated roles may include child caretaker and family health leader. Merton explains:

> A particular social status involves not a single associated role, but an array of associated roles. This is a basic characteristic of social structure. This fact of structure can be registered by a distinctive term, role-set, by which I mean that complement of role relationships which persons have by virtue of occupying a particular social status. (p. 3)

Thus, for each position a number of roles exist, each of which is composed of related sets of behaviors culturally defined as expected of persons in that position or status. The roles might, however, be shared with other members of a group. For example, the child care role is usually a shared responsibility of both parents in contemporary society.

ROLE BEHAVIOR, PERFORMANCE, AND ENACTMENT

Role behavior, role performance, and role enactment are all interchangeable terms that denote what a person actually does within a position in response to role expectations. Expectations and/or prescriptions for the sets of behavior appropriate for the basic social positions and their associated roles (family roles, occupational roles, etc.) evolve and are developed within a societal context.

Many of the roles associated with our basic social positions are learned within the family context. Societal role expectations are modified or refined as a result of an individual's exposure to role models and his or her individual personality—that is, his or her capacities, temperament, attitudes, and interests. In other words, an individual enacts particular roles based on societal expectations but modified by his or her identification with role models and individual personality characteristics. The outcome of an individual's role modification is the person's actual role behavior or performance. Figure 12–1 illustrates the process by which role behavior actually develops.

Roles are normatively or culturally defined; that is, the culture in which one participates and/or with which one identifies, prescribes, and proscribes the behavior of the occupants of various positions. However, "not all the family roles are equally normative" (Nye, 1976, p. 15). Jackson (1966) notes that some family roles are more "crystallized"—more clearly spelled out in terms of expected behavior—than others. For instance, in the past within the middle-class white American family, the affective (or therapeutic) role of the spouses was not crystallized; that is, it was not expected of mates to listen to each other's problems. Today, however, spouses see therapeutic support not as optional behavior but as an obligation, because it is a duty to help one's spouse. Thus, the therapeutic role for middle-class white American spouses has been "crystallized."

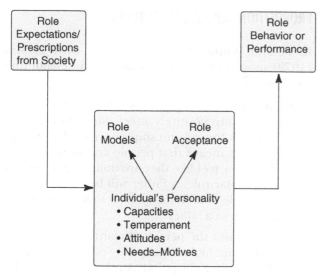

Figure 12–1. Development of role behavior.

One can infer the strength of a role (whether it is a strong norm or not) in a specific position by assessing the sanction(s) applied when the role is not performed. Certainly, social ostracism or criticism as a sanction against lack of role fulfillment, as in a mother's failure to attend open house at a child's school, is a lesser sanction than might result from failure to carry out the child care role adequately (e.g., when there is child neglect). Sanctions provide evidence that the society or parts of the society perceive a particular role to be sufficiently important that conformity to the norm be enforced.

ROLE SHARING, ROLE TAKING, AND RECIPROCAL/COMPLEMENTARY ROLES

Role sharing refers to participation of two or more people in the same roles even though they hold different positions. There is extensive role sharing in most families today. Sharply segregated role structures are unusual. An example of normative role sharing in the family is the case of the child socialization role where both mother and father usually jointly participate, in addition to school teachers, youth leaders, clergy, and so on. Another example is in the older family, where the retired couple often shares the housekeeper and shopping roles.

Another essential concept within role theory is that of *role taking*. In order for family members to

enact roles, they must be able to imagine themselves in the role of a counterpart, or role partner; in this way they are able to assign a role to the other and also better understand how they should behave in their own roles (Turner, 1970). Through socialization family members acquire a repertoire of roles through which they can act and interact with others. "Roles are never learned singly, but always as pairs or sets of interacting roles. Because the individual learns the role of alter [his role partner] while playing his own role, he is able to play the role of the alter when others in the situation are playing his usual role" (Turner, 1970, p. 215). Over a period of time, however, the self-conception incorporates certain roles and denies others, so that the individual no longer plays past roles.

Parsons and associates (1953) coined the concept of "the principle of *complementarity*," referring to the functional adequacy of roles in social situations that are based on the match between the performances and the expectations of partners in a relationship. The principle of complementarity is of great significance because it is chiefly responsible for that degree of harmony and stability that occurs in interpersonal relations (Spiegel, 1957). Whenever there is dissimilarity in expectations and performances of family roles, the potential for lack of role complementarity and possible conflict and stress exists. A role is interdependent with and patterned to mesh with that of a role partner. In other words, a role is always paired with a reciprocal role of another person. One can never look at a role in isolation. For example, one must look at the teacher's role together with the student's role, because both are necessary for either to function. Society specifies behaviors for each person in these reciprocal arrangements so that each will know what is expected of the role partner. Role partners are constantly influencing one another's role behavior through their many interactions with one another.

ROLE STRESS/STRAIN AND ROLE CONFLICT

Role stress occurs when a social structure, such as the family, creates very difficult, conflicting, or impossible demands for occupants of positions within that social structure (Hardy & Hardy, 1988). It is a characteristic of the social system, rather than of the person in the system. Role stress results in *role strain*—subjective feelings of frustration and tension. Role strain is also perceived and felt by the associated role partners (Hardy & Hardy).

Role conflict occurs when the occupant of a position perceives that he or she is confronted with incompatible expectations (Hardy & Hardy, 1988). The source of the incompatibility may be due to changes in expectations within the actor, others, or the environment. Several types of role conflict are discussed in the literature. *Interrole conflict* is when the norms or behavioral patterns of one role are incongruent with another role that the same individual simultaneously plays. Interrole conflict occurs when an individual's role complex—that is, the group of roles he or she enacts—involves several roles that are incompatible (Hardy & Hardy). This type of conflict is due either to the incompatibility of the behaviors associated with the various roles or the excessive amount of energy these roles demand, such as performing the student, employee, son, and child care roles simultaneously.

The second type of role conflict, *intersender role conflict* (LaRocca, 1978), occurs when two or more people hold conflicting expectations concerning the enactment of a role. An illustration of this second type of role conflict is the presence of conflicting expectations on how one's role, as a professional nurse should be performed. For example, the nurse manager may expect the nurse to delegate selected nursing tasks and to attend to the cost and efficiency; the patient may expect the nurse to personally provide sympathetic, nurturing care; and the nurse may expect to provide professional, competent care as defined by her or his profession.

A third type of role conflict is called *person–role conflict.* This type involves a conflict between the person's internalized values and the external values communicated to this person by others, throwing him or her into a state of role stress. This type of role conflict is similar to the second type, except in this case there is not a disparity in role expectations between people in the outer environment, but a role disparity with one's "inner" environment. One can think of the person–role conflict that results in families with young teenagers—when the teenager has one internalized notion of his or her role as a teenager and peers prescribe a very different role.

PROPOSITIONS ABOUT FAMILY ROLES

Klein and White (1996) summarize Burr et al.'s (1979) most useful propositions for understanding family roles:

- The quality of a person's role enactment in a relationship positively affects his or her satisfaction with the relationship (Burr et al., 1979, p. 70). This means that people are more satisfied when they feel like they are doing a good job in a particular role. A father will be more satisfied in his role as father if he feels that he is doing a good job as a father.

- The greater the perceived clarity of role expectations, the higher the quality of role enactment (Burr et al., 1979, p. 74). A role is defined as the normative expectations attached to a specific role in a social structure, and the more clearly defined the expectations are the easier it will be to enact the role (Klein & White, 1996). For example, the role of mother is defined by social norms about what is expected in the mother role. Mothers are expected to nurture and protect their young, but how this is achieved may change over time. In today's society, few mothers are expected to carry guns to protect their young from hostile others, yet in early pioneer days, mothers routinely used guns to protect their young from bandits, or other hostile forces.

- The more individuals perceive consensus in the expectations about a role they occupy, the less their role strain (Burr et al., 1979, p. 79). Rossi and Berk (1985) suggest that one critical aspect to a role is that expectations are shared or consensual. If a family member perceives that he is acting as expected in the role (e.g., the expectation of male partner as breadwinner), then he or she will experience little role strain. On the other hand, if role expectations for partner are not shared by other family members, role strain often develops.

- The greater the diversification of a person's roles, the less consensus the person will perceive in the expectations about those roles (Burr et al., 1979, p. 80). Family members often occupy multiple roles simultaneously (e.g., mother, wife, worker, sister, and friend), and there are multiple expectations for the multiple roles. When individuals are unable to fulfill role expectations or there is lack of consensus about the role, role strain develops.

- The greater the perceived role strain that results from performing a role, the less the ease in making the transition into the role and the greater the ease in making a transition out of the role (Burr et al., 1979, p. 86). The greater the role strain, the more difficult the adjustment or transition to a new role. For example, if a newly married person is unable to meet the expectations of the role of spouse, high levels of stress may result. The stress related to the role strain may lead to dissolving the relationship through divorce or by adopting unhealthy behaviors such as substance abuse to cope with the role strain.

FORMAL FAMILY ROLES

Family roles can be classified into two categories: formal or overt roles and informal or covert roles. Whereas formal roles are explicit roles that the family role structure contains (father–husband, etc.), informal roles are implicit, often not apparent on the surface, and are expected to meet the emotional needs of family members (Satir, 1967) and/or to maintain the family's equilibrium.

There are a limited number of positions defined as normative within the classic two-parent nuclear family. These positions are referred to as formal and paired, and consist of father–husband; wife–mother; son–brother; and daughter–sister. In the extended family (three-generation) more paired positions exist, and in the single-parent family fewer paired positions. Each of the normative positions of the family group is associated with related roles. Husband–fathers are expected to be wage earners and wife–mothers are often expected to take leadership roles in home management. In the single-parent family the mother often takes on the normative role responsibilities of both mother and father. In the stepparent family, the husband will often play husband–father, but because the children are biologically not his own, the father role is a quasi-father role (the role lacks crystallization).

Associated with each formal family position are related roles or clusters of more or less homogeneous behaviors. The family apportions roles to its family members in a manner similar to the way society apportions its roles: according to how critical the role performance is to the system's functioning. Some roles require special skills and abilities; others are less complex and can be assigned to the less skilled or to those with the least amount of power. When there are fewer persons in a family the number of persons to fulfill the formal roles is limited; there will be more demands and opportunities for family members to play several roles at different times. If a member leaves home or becomes unable to fulfill a role, someone else fulfills the role to keep the family functioning (Murray & Zentner, 1985, 1993).

MARITAL ROLES AND MARITAL RELATIONSHIPS

Nye and Gecas (1976) have identified eight basic roles making up the husband–father and the wife–mother social positions: provider, housekeeper, childcare, recreational, kinship role (maintaining relationships with paternal and maternal families), therapeutic (meeting the affective needs of spouse [or intimate adult partner]), sexual role. In this scheme the companionship role has been subsumed under the recreational and therapeutic roles.

Many people fail to separate parental roles from marital roles, but in reality the two roles are quite distinct, and marital roles should not be shortchanged due to overinvolvement in the parental roles. Marital roles are focused on the husband–wife interactions, while parental roles are focused upon the parent–child interactions and the parental responsibilities. In spite of their separateness, performance of marital roles will certainly have an impact on parental roles and vice versa.

Minuchin (1974) stresses the importance of couples maintaining a strong marital relationship. Children especially can interfere with the marital relationship, creating a situation in which a husband or wife may form a coalition with one of their children, which diminishes the close relationship between the parents. Maintaining a satisfying marital relationship is identified as one of the crucial family developmental tasks of the family as it progresses through its life cycle. In the previous discussion of

326 PART III FAMILY NURSING PRACTICE

family development in Chapter 5, the stress that children put on the marital relationship was made quite evident.

In addition to studies demonstrating the wide diversity of marriages, efforts have also been made to classify the types of dyadic (two-person) relationships. Described first by Bateson (1958) and later by Watzlawick and co-workers (1967), two types of basic relationships are found in dyadic relationships. These are termed complementary and symmetrical, with parallel relationships being a combination of the two. Dyads in *complementary relationships* exhibit contrasting behavior. One person is the leading, dominant personality and decision maker, whereas the other partner is the subservient follower (a typical "one-up and one-down" position). A strong element of dependency exists between adult partners who have a complementary relationship. The positive element in this type of relationship is that it allows one to give and the other to receive. The inherent danger lies in its tendency to become increasingly rigid, stifling the growth of both people. It is necessary that both partners of a complementary relationship play their "proper" role. If either partner does not continue to perform his or her respective functions, the relationship will come to an end, with each feeling disconfirmed by the other.

Symmetrical relationships are based on the equality of the partners. The partners demand equality through the character of their mutually exchanged messages and behavior, and each mate has the right to initiate action, to criticize the other's behavior, and to have a voice in family decisions. The positive aspect of this type of relationship is that it allows for mutual respect, trust, and spontaneity, with the optimal effect being that each partner is free to be himself or herself, knowing that each will be accepted and respected by the other. The danger inherent in this type of relationship is that the competitive aspect of the relationship may become overemphasized. When this happens there is increasing frustration and a decrease in cooperative behaviors (mutual assistance and support). Egocentricity by one or both partners may preclude the mutual accommodation and giving that is needed to enhance and nurture the intimate, affectional part of a marital relationship.

Parallel relationships are a third type of marital relationship introduced by Lederer and Jackson (1968). In parallel relationships, the dyad alternates comfortably between symmetrical and complementary relationships as they adapt to changing situations. Depending on the situation and the partner's areas of competence, there is an interchange and flexibility in relationship patterns. This switching from one pattern to the other restores the stabilizing properties when either pattern threatens to break down. Because of the greater flexibility and individual growth-enhancing properties (each partner being able to contribute according to his or her competencies and the situational needs), this type of relationship is seen as the most mature, healthy, and stable form of the three types. Developmentally, if maturation is allowed to occur, relationships should evolve in a person's lifetime from being complementary to being symmetrical and then to being parallel. If one visualizes this in terms of the dependency factor, relationships undergo a change from dependency (complementary) to independence (symmetry) to interdependence (parallelism). One qualification needs to be made here, however. The value judgment placed on these types of relationships and their perceived degree of maturity does not take into account the cultural background of the individuals involved. Parallel types of relationships may not be acceptable in some ethnic groups.

WOMEN'S AND MEN'S ROLES IN THE FAMILY

As women have moved from the home into the workplace in recent decades, their roles have changed, and correspondingly, their role partners' behavior has changed. Research shows changes in men's roles in the family are occurring, but at a slower pace than changes in women's employment and changes in family roles. Research on women's roles in the family has focused primarily on the effects of women's employment on the family and in allocation of roles (Elias, 1987; Goldenberg & Goldenberg, 2002; Spitze, 1988). The extent to which women retain the traditional sex-role obligations (child rearing, housekeeping, etc.) and simultaneously perform their work role has been analyzed. Role overload, role conflict, and role strain are documented in study after study as women move into the labor force and create careers for themselves. With the widespread advent of dual-earner families, there are three full-time jobs: the two adults' paid work and the family work.

When women work, their husbands typically share the roles of child rearing and housekeeping (Shaw, 1988). Research has consistently confirmed that the role behavior of husbands with respect to assuming more household activities appears to be changing (Spitze, 1988). For example, Coltrane (1997) wrote that men have doubled their contributions to many household chores while wives have decreased the amount of time spent on household chores. Nevertheless, Coltrane and others (John, Shelton, & Luschen, 1995) noted that men still do about a third as much housework as their wives. In one large study, wives spent 37 hours per week working at home while husbands only spent 20 hours per week (Hawkins, Marshall, & Meiners, 1995).

The increased involvement of husbands who have working wives appears to be mainly through increased involvement in childcare (Pleck, 1985). Coltrane (1997) noted there are still major barriers to father's full participation in family work, including job demands, the structure of their workplace, and limited social acceptance of the "daddy tracks" with work–family programs like flextime and parental leave.

However, congruence between beliefs about and enactment of provider and homemaker roles tends to foster marital satisfaction (McHale & Crouter, 1992; Perry-Jenkins & Crouter, 1990; Vannoy-Hiller & Philliber, 1992). In one study, gender-role identities and expectations were more important than socio-economic, life cycle, educational, or occupational status in determining marital quality (Vannoy-Hiller & Philliber, 1992). In another study, both husbands and wives reported that the division of family labor was the issue most likely to cause marital conflict (Cowan, Cowan, Heming, & Miller, 1991).

There is a rather extensive body of literature that shows that women are the kinkeepers in the family. Kinkeeping, or the kinship role, involves maintaining communication, facilitating contact and the exchange of goods and services, and monitoring family relationships (Hagestad, 1988). Women function as kinkeepers for both sides of the family. With this added family responsibility "the superwoman squeeze"—the overload experienced by middle-aged women who provide assistance to both children and two sets of parents in addition to working—is a real possibility.

Being the "sandwiched" generation and the "sandwiched" sex, middle-aged women are caught between the needs of parents with increasing life expectancies and children who remain dependent for a longer period of time and may need extra help during periods of marital and other personal disruption (Spitze, 1988). Just as many middle-aged women think they are getting off the "mommy track," they are finding themselves, due to the aging of their parents, getting back on "the daughter track." A U.S. House of Representatives report of 1988 (Beck et al., 1990) estimated that the average American woman spends 17 years raising children and 18 years helping aged parents.

Two other factors that have created concern, and thus research efforts, are the increased numbers of single-parent families created by mothers and fathers not marrying and by divorce, with many children being separated from their fathers. How these fathers maintain their fatherhood role with their biological children when separated from them is a major concern. Data by Furstenberg and Nord (1985) show that almost one-half of children had not seen their nonresidential parent in the past year. In 40 percent of all families in the United States, children are not living in the same home with their biological fathers (Stolberg, 1996a). How the father role is enacted when men remarry a woman with children is often problematic.

Kennedy (1989), in his review of the fatherhood literature, reports that the fatherhood role is described as the moral overseer, the distance breadwinner, and the sex role model. The moral overseer role predominated during colonial times. The prime role of moral overseer fathers is to exert moral leadership in the family. In contrast, the distant breadwinner is a provider who is uninvolved with child care. The father is a good provider, but does not have a direct influence on the life of the child. After World War II a new theory of gender identity began to emphasize the crucial role that fathers play in molding children's identity, particularly the son's identity. The "new father" began to be advocated in the 1980s and is viewed as an extension of the gender identity theory, modified by changes in the woman's role in the family. Kennedy describes "the new father's" role as:

> He is present at the birth; he is involved with his children as infants, not just when they are older; he participates in the actual day-to-day work of child care, and not just play; he is involved with his daughters as much as his sons. (p. 364)

In early research, the father's role was believed to be secondary to, or supportive of, the mother's role (Pedersen & Robson, 1969). Although the father was recognized as contributing to the family in unique ways, most early studies gathered data about the fathers role from the mother and children in the family. Newer research on the new father role has focused on fatherhood in the family life stages, satisfaction with the new father role, and rural/urban, cultural differences (Bronstein & Cowan, 1988; Kennedy, 1989; Lamb, 1987), and child consequences with and without father involvement (Snarey, 1993). Contemporary research has assessed fathers directly, with newer interpretations of how fathers enact their roles with children of varied ages. Based on several literature reviews (Bronstein & Cowan; Hanson & Bozett, 1987; Kennedy; Lamb; Snarey; Tiedje & Darling-Fisher, 1996), some interesting research findings in this area emerge (Table 12–1).

However, factors such as the father's own parenting, marital relationship, perception of the fathering role, feelings of insecurity, ability to express feelings, cultural expectations, and employment demands all influence fathering behaviors (Heath, 1976; Radin, 1981; Tiedje & Darling-Fisher, 1996; Wieser & Castiglia, 1984).

GRANDPARENTS' ROLES IN THE FAMILY

The roles of grandparents and even great grandparents are gaining attention, as the number of individuals who are grandparents and great grandparents grows larger each year. Grandparenthood is a heterogeneous experience, with there being wide variation on how the grandparent role is enacted. The historical context, age, ethnicity, social class, and gender of the grandparent and gender of the grandchild tend to produce significant differences in terms of how the role is enacted. For example, Cherlin and Furstenberg (1985, 1986) identified three styles of grandparenting in a sample of 510 grandparents: "the detached" (26 percent), who were low in both exchange and influence and saw their grandchild(ren) less than once a month; "the passive" (29 percent), who also scored low on both the above criteria but had seen their grandchild(ren) at least once or twice a month; and "the active" (45 percent), who scored high on exchange and influence regardless of their frequency of visiting. Many grandparents developed companionship relationships with their grandchildren—relationships that were easygoing and lighthearted.

TABLE 12–1

FATHER'S AND MOTHER'S FAMILY ROLE ENACTMENT

1. Findings from multiple studies agree that attitudes toward family roles are moving in the direction of egalitarianism and that child care and socialization roles are becoming the shared responsibility of both spouses (Hanson & Bozett, 1987; Lamb, 1987; Teachman, Tedrow, & Crowder, 2001).

2. Today's fathers are expected to be more actively involved in child rearing with children of all ages than in the past, and to a modest extent this is evidenced in study findings (McBride & Mills, 1993).

3. There is no evidence that maternal employment status affects levels of paternal involvement in child care.

4. Fathers spend more time on child care when children are younger (preschool and school age); they are more involved and interested in child care with their sons than with their daughters.

5. There are variations in the type of interaction fathers versus mothers have with their children. Mothers' interactions are dominated by caretaking activities, while fathers' interactions are more play oriented (McBride & Mills; Bridges & Connell, 1991).

6. If both parents are equally involved in infant care, there are no differences in parenting skills between mothers and fathers during the newborn period (Rustia & Abbott, 1993).

7. In a 40-year longitudinal study examining father involvement practices (Snarey, 1993), father involvement was positively linked to positive marital outcomes and children's educational and occupational mobility.

More recently, Baydar and Brooks-Gunn (1998) created a typology of grandmothers in the United States using data from a nationally representative sample of 2,095 grandmothers. The four types were (1) homemaker grandmothers (19 percent of the sample) who were not employed outside the home and provided care for their grandchildren on a regular basis; (2) young-and-connected grandmothers (23 percent of the sample) who were under 55 years old, employed, and cared for their grandchildren on a regular basis; (3) remote grandmothers (6 percent) varied in their employment status, lived with husbands, and did not provide care for their grandchildren; and (4) frail grandmothers (26 percent) who were older, lived alone, were in relatively poor health, and did not provide care for their grandchildren. The researchers found that the personal circumstances of the grandmothers correlated with the role they assumed with their children and grandchildren (e.g., the more adult children, the more likely that the grandmother would take a role in caring for some of her grandchildren). Bowers and Myers (1999) found that the experiences of caring for grandchildren may not be completely positive, and may in fact be quite stressful, depending on the degree of involvement and whether the grandchildren exhibit behavior problems. Difficult circumstances related to caring for grandchildren may negatively affect the grandparents' overall life satisfaction.

There is no consensus on whether grandparental involvement has direct positive effects on grandchildren's behavior. In most instances, indirect effects (through helping the child's parents) and symbolic influences play a greater role. And, in a study of 91 grandparents with 396 grandchildren, Fingerman (1998) found that the grandparent's relationship with grandchildren varied considerably depending on factors such as the personality of the individual grandchild.

The symbolic expressions of the grandparent role—the functions the role fulfills—are equally diverse and varied. Bengtson (1985) divides these symbolic functions of grandparenthood into (1) simply "being there" (simple presence); (2) acting as the national guard or family watchdog (being there to protect and give care if needed); (3) being an arbitrator (negotiator between parents and children); and (4) being an active participant in the family's social construction of its history (making connections between the families' past, present, and future).

Most of the research has been on grandmothers. Relatively little research has focused on grandfathers and virtually none on the growing number of great grandfathers (Hanson & Bozett, 1987). One of the crucial elements of the grandchild–grandparent relationship is the relationship between the grandparents and their children. The child's parents are found to determine the frequency of visits and encourage or discourage the development of a positive grandparent–grandchild relationship. Several researchers have observed that grandparents are more involved with grandchildren when parents are divorced or never married, especially when the grandparents are younger (Burton & de Vries, 1995). Moreover, African-American children have been observed to profit when grandparents play a more active role in their upbringing (Cherlin & Furstenberg, 1986). The grandparent role is also discussed in Chapter 5 in the section on the aging family.

FAMILY ROLE CHANGES

The roles of family members in the United States have become more variable, flexible, and complex. In the past, there was "women's work" and "men's work," and little role sharing existed except under special conditions. The family lived according to relatively rigid, traditionally established rules, which were maintained by the social and moral pressures of the entire society. Today, great variation in the roles of both genders is feasible. Expectations and practices differ tremendously. In one family, both adult members may be expected to work and jointly share in all family affairs and responsibilities; in another family, traditional roles are expected and performed; and in yet another situation, the single-parent family, the adult assumes the roles of both parents. Because the normative limits of family roles are so broad, a wide range of behaviors are accepted as appropriate depending on the situation. The requirements of the situation and the individuals in it often determine specific behaviors found in a role. Thus, individuals tentatively construct their roles in response to the cues given by other(s) in the situation (their role partners). Aldous (1996) notes that role performance in families today is increasingly the result of rolemaking due to the lack of prepared scripts in performing family roles. Instead, general norms serve as guides to role performance, but situational demands and interactions with others determine specific behaviors. Although role making allows more flexibility in roles, it may make roles more challenging and may lead to more conflict than if prescribed family roles existed.

The status and associated family roles of individuals change in many ways throughout a person's life cycle. The change in role relationships, expectations, and abilities is referred to as role transition (Meleis, 1975). Role transitions occur at clear demarcations of the family life, such as at marriage, divorce, and the death of a parent or spouse, as well as more subtly as an ongoing response to life experiences. A role change experienced by one family member necessitates complementary role changes by other family members.

The advent of role changes in families does not come without a cost to the individuals involved. Families often experience significant stress during role transitions. It is well recognized that when individuals deviate from normative role expectations and/or take on new roles, they may lack the role preparation or previous socialization needed to perform these new roles comfortably and adequately. In addition to lacking the necessary training, a family member may not feel that the new roles meet his or her interests or needs. Role changes such as those brought on by having a new baby, becoming a caretaker for an adult family member, or because of a father's new job, a mother's unemployment, divorce, or family relocation, may create role confusion, anxiety, and unhappiness in the family and may heighten familial conflict (Aldous, 1974, 1996).

The role change necessitated because of having a new baby illustrates the difficulty in making role transitions. Ventura (1987), in a qualitative study of middle-class couples, found that 35 percent of first-time mothers and 65 percent of fathers reported feeling stressed because of multiple role demands. At the third month postpartum, mothers described juggling parenting roles with home and work schedules and having very little time for themselves. Fathers portrayed stresses too, but these were linked to career and work responsibilities.

✎ INFORMAL FAMILY ROLES

An individual family member will play many roles in a family, both informal and formal, with some of these roles being shared. The existence of informal roles is necessary to fulfill the integrative and adaptive requirements of the family group. Kievit (1968) explains that:

> Informal roles have different requirements, less likely based on age or sex and more likely based upon the personality attributes of individual members. Thus, one member may be the mediator, seeking possible compromises when the other family members are engaged in conflict. Another may be the family jester, who provides gaiety and mirth on happy occasions, and a much-needed sense of humor in times of crisis and distress. Other informal roles may exist and emerge, as the needs of the family unit shift and change. In working with families, awareness of the informal roles may facilitate insight into the specific nature of problems faced and in turn possible solutions. Effective performance of informal roles can facilitate the adequate performance of the formal roles. (p. 7)

The following are some examples of other informal or covert roles described in the literature (Benne & Sheats, 1948; Hartman & Laird, 1983; Kantor & Lehr, 1975; Satir, 1972; Vogel & Bell, 1960). These informal roles may or may not contribute to the stability of the family—some of them are adaptive and others detrimental to the ultimate well-being of the family.

- *Encourager.* The encourager praises, agrees with, and accepts the contribution of others. In effect he or she is able to draw out other people and make them feel that their ideas are important and worth listening to.

- *Harmonizer.* The harmonizer mediates the differences that exist between other members by jesting or smoothing over disagreements.

- *Initiator–contributor.* The initiator–contributor suggests or proposes to the group new ideas or changed ways of regarding group problems or goals. Kantor and Lehr (1975) refer to this type of role as a "mover" role characterized by the initiation of action.

- *Compromiser.* The compromiser is one of the parties to the conflict or disagreement. The compromiser yields his or her position, admits error, or offers to come "halfway."

- *Blocker.* The blocker tends to be negative to all ideas, rejecting without and beyond reason. Kantor and Lehr (1975) label this role the opposer.

- *Dominator.* The dominator tries to assert authority or superiority by manipulating the group or certain members, flaunting his or her power and acting as if he or she knows everything and is the paragon of virtue.

- *The Blamer.* This role is similar to the blocker and the dominator. The blamer is a fault finder, a dictator, a bossy "know it all."

- *Follower.* The follower goes along with the movement of the group, more or less passively accepting the ideas of others, serving as an audience in group discussion and decision.

- *Recognition Seeker.* The recognition seeker attempts in whatever way possible to call attention to self and his or her deeds, accomplishments, and/or problems.

- *Martyr.* The martyr wants nothing for self but sacrifices everything for the sake of other family members.

- *The Great Stone Face.* The person playing this role lectures incessantly and impassively on all the "right" things to do, just like a computer. Satir (1975) calls this informal role the superreasonable.

- *Pal.* The pal is a family playmate who indulges self and excuses family members' behavior or his or her own regardless of the consequences. He or she usually seems irrelevant when family issues are discussed.

- *The Family Scapegoat.* The family scapegoat is the identified problem member in the family. As a victim or receptacle for the overt and covert family tensions and hostilities, the scapegoat serves as a safety valve.

- *The Placator.* The placator is ingratiating, always trying to please, never disagreeing, talking out of both sides of his or her mouth—in short, a "yes person."

- *The Family Caretaker.* The family caretaker is the member who is called upon to nurture and care for other members in need.

- *The Family Pioneer.* The family pioneer moves the family into unknown territory, into new experiences.

- *The Irrelevant One or Distractor.* The distractor is irrelevant; by exhibiting attention-getting behavior he or she helps the family avoid or ignore painful or difficult matters.

- *The Family Coordinator.* The family coordinator organizes and plans family activities, thereby fostering cohesiveness and combating family separateness.

- *The Family Go-Between.* The family go-between is the family "switchboard"—he or she (often the mother) transmits and monitors communication throughout the family.

- *The Bystander.* The bystander role is similar to "the follower" except in some cases more passive. The bystander observes but does not involve himself or herself; he or she acts like an outsider.

Two informal roles that warrant further discussion are the scapegoat and the go-between roles. The first of these is the scapegoat role, a role adopted by a member to preserve the family and maintain homeostasis. The family member who is constantly scapegoated (often a child) usually serves to divert attention from a disturbance between the spouses [adults].

The second informal role that is common in families is that of the go-between (Zuk, 1966). The mother usually takes the go-between or intermediary role. In this role the person acts as a "switchboard" between family members, relaying communication from one member to another. In so doing, the direct communication between other family members is blocked. As the switchboard through which all communication must go, the go-between assumes a covert position of power, and by passing along only those messages considered suitable, the go-between acts as a censor. She or he thus becomes a central figure in the family, acting as a confidant to its members. And as the center of the family communication network, the go-between is typically in charge of settling disputes and ensuring fairness to all sides. However, when disputes or conflicts do not become resolved, the go-between often gets blamed. Consistently having one person act as an intermediary is dysfunctional in that it is an emotional distancing mechanism and promotes estrangement between the other members of the family, because they are discouraged from communicating directly with each other.

Satir (1972) discusses the consequences of communicating via a third person. If the family habitually transacts business without all the members present, and also has little spare time, then family members get to know each other through a third person. "I call it acquaintance by rumor. The problem is that most people forget about the rumor part and treat whatever it is as fact" (p. 266).

The presence of a go-between role is revealed in the family's communication patterns. In interviews, it will be observed that the go-between answers for the children or other spouse when not directly questioned. In addition to talking for other family members, he or she usually gets in the way of messages sent or received by family members.

Family members learn about their informal roles through (1) role modeling; (2) filling in "vacuums" where they exist in the family (if there is no leader or decision maker playing the instrumental role, a member of the group will naturally emerge to fill this role); and (3) selective reinforcement that a child receives to behaviors he or she exhibits in the family. The child experiments with various roles in play, receives selective reinforcement for certain roles, and eventually finds informal roles that are comfortable.

Through selective reinforcement of certain behaviors by parents and significant others, children are molded to play specific informal, covert roles. This selective parental reinforcement may occur because of early labeling of the child; this labeling leads to a self-fulfilling prophecy. Parents label children for a variety of reasons: projection, comparison with siblings, past unresolved personal needs, and so on. A classic study of large families (Bossard & Boll, 1956) found that there were a number of specialized roles and labels given to the children. Eight informal roles, which result in or from labels, existed: (1) the responsible one, (2) the popular one, (3) the socially ambitious one, (4) the studious one, (5) the family isolate, (6) the irresponsible one, (7) the sickly one, and (8) the spoiled one. These labels are likely to exist in complementary pairs in a family. Thus, if a "sickly" child is identified in a family, the family usually labels another as the "healthy one"; if a "dumb one" is present, there is usually a "smart one."

Labeling limits the way an individual may act or develop. True negative labeling—in which adverse adjectives are consistently used—occurs when parents and/or significant others label a child according to an attribute or a behavior that indicates the child is inferior or unlovable. Because the parents see these labels as bad, the child sees himself or herself in the same light. Initially, parents condemn the child; later the child, through identification with parental labels, internalizes the parental label and condemns himself or herself. Negative labeling has been identified as an antecedent to both depression and lowered self-esteem (Mishel, 1974). As a result of early negative labeling and the internalization of these labels, individuals often develop certain limited ways of perceiving themselves and of reacting to others called "life games" or "scripts"; these restrict and limit a person's adaptability and repertoire of interpersonal skills (Lange, 1970). In other words, a script is written in early childhood based on messages and labels (both verbal and nonverbal) that a child receives from parents, such as parental perceptions of the child related to his or her worth, lovableness, sexual status, work, responsibility, and dependency. "Life patterns," which include suicide, obesity, and recurrent physical illness—especially when treatable and preventable—are all examples of tragic scripts (Lange, 1970).

VARIABLES AFFECTING ROLE STRUCTURE

As with the family power structure, there are major factors that influence both formal and informal roles. These factors include (1) social class, (2) family forms, (3) cultural/ethnic background, (4) family developmental stage, (5) role models, and (6) situational events—in particular health/illness problems (to be discussed under family roles during health alterations).

SOCIAL CLASS DIFFERENCES

Family roles are greatly influenced by the demands and necessities put on the family by the larger social structure. Thus, in response to our society's "benign neglect" of poor families, a variety of family role adaptations have evolved as a means of solving the recurrent problems and issues arising from being poor. Single-parent families comprise a significant portion of families living in poverty, and the proportion of working poor families is at a 30-year high (Leeds, 1996).

LOW-INCOME FAMILIES. Marital stability is more precarious among low-income families than in other social classes, with divorces being two to six times greater among families headed by unskilled laborers than among families headed by adults who are part of the professional middle class. The high rate of unemployment among groups who are very poor is a major stressor in the marital relationship and a significant cause of its dissolution.

Low-income families often have a relatively loose-knit structure, although the roles of the marital partners and their division of responsibilities are usually formal. In many poor families there is a sharp demarcation of family roles based on whether the jobs are located inside or outside the home. These firm lines of authority serve to reinforce the emotional distance of the mates. The husband generally plays a minimal role in the low-income family, often conceiving of his role as being simply the provider of money to meet material needs.

The parenting role has been of central importance to women from low-income families, and the mother is often more traditional in her outlook toward child rearing (e.g., a greater emphasis on respectability, obedience, cleanliness, and discipline of young children). In other words, the focus of parenting in the poor family is on fulfillment of maintenance functions—providing food for the children; making sure they eat, have adequate rest, bathe, get to school on time—and on the maintenance of order and discipline in the home. In comparison, middle- or upper-income families tend to place greater emphasis on developing self-reliance and independence in children and take more cognizance of developmental and psychological principles in the parent–child relationship (Kohn, 1977).

The older siblings in low-income families often participate in socializing with younger siblings—far more than is common in middle- or upper-class families. Childrens' peer groups in poor families are also very important, especially for boys who seek masculine models, given the central role of the mother and the more passive or "missing" role of the father in child rearing.

WORKING AND MIDDLE CLASS FAMILIES. Rubin (1976) studied blue-collar workers and their families and found that the more educated the husband, the greater the degree of companionship in marriage. This was confirmed by later studies. In contrast to working-class marriages in which a high degree of "gender segregation" exists within the family, companionship is a strong reason for the initiation and continuance of a marriage in middle-class families.

Working-class families generally tend to have more traditionally based family roles than middle-class families—the husband being more authoritarian in his role as head of the household (Dickinson & Leming, 1995). "The husband's world revolves around the provider role, while the wife has primary responsibility for the home and children in addition to working outside the home" (Dickinson & Leming, p. 185).

Child rearing is now generally a shared role of middle-class parents, and their role behavior toward their children differs qualitatively from the lower-class family. It has been pointed out that one major reason for this may be the unconscious molding of a child to survive in the world as experienced by the parents. For instance, if a family is poor, parents expect that their boys will probably have to work in positions in which obedience, respect for authority, and conformity are stressed. Hence, training that promotes creativity, questioning, and independence would be counterproductive to what the child needs in future adult work roles. In contrast, middle-class parents are more concerned with psychological growth, individual differences, independence, and self-reliance in their children. These traits, encouraged by middle-class parents, are functional to success in the middle-class occupational life (Kohn, 1969, 1977).

FAMILY FORMS

The majority of the families in the United States today are not the typical "idealized" two-parent traditional nuclear families, as detailed in Chapter 1. The family's role structure will vary along with variance in the family form. Because single-parent and stepparent families are probably the two most common nonnuclear family forms, these two types of family forms will be described in terms of their unique role arrangements and role stresses.

ROLES IN SINGLE-PARENT FAMILIES. The number of single-parent families has swelled rapidly in the last 15 to 20 years. Most single-parent families are headed by mothers, although fathers are increasingly heading single-parent families. About 17 percent of single-parent families are headed by men (U.S. Bureau of the Census, 1998). Men who are single fathers are typically better situated economically than women who are single mothers, due, in part, to the continuing disparities in education and income between men and women (Nortan & Glick, 1986; Teachman, Tedrow, & Crowder, 2001).

Two prominent role features of these families are (1) role overload and role conflicts, and (2) role changes of the single parent. The parent must fulfill both mother and father roles, without the support of a marital relationship. Single parents tend to be either overloaded with roles or in conflict over their various role commitments, because they have double tasks to assume. With a spouse to depend on, there is some role flexibility (if the child care and housekeeping roles are shared). And even though the single parent is freed from the responsibilities of marital roles, other adult relationships often enter in and create demands on the single parent's limited time. Because most single parents also work, high job/family role strain and reduced levels of wellness were found in a study conducted by Burden (1986).

Significant research has been generated by behavioral scientists who have studied the single-parent family relative to its long-term impact on children. Accumulated evidence from multiple studies consistently shows that children in single-parent families have greater problems (emotionally and behaviorally, than children from two-parent nuclear families (income level was controlled for in these studies). They are also twice as likely to drop out of high school and become teenage mothers (Popenoe, 1995).

ROLES IN STEPPARENT FAMILIES. With the tremendous increase in the number of divorces and remarriages (80 percent of the divorced remarry, one half within 3 years), there has been a tremendous increase in stepparent families (Glick, 1994). In 75 percent of these cases, this type of family form denotes the entry of a new husband and surrogate father (stepfather), rather than stepmother, into a previously established female-headed single-parent family. Stepparent families are at higher risk of serious problems than families of "first marrieds" or "second marrieds" with no children: 60

percent of all second marriages end in divorce (Kantrowitz & Wingert, 1990). One of the primary reasons for this is the greater complexity involved with integrating the stepfather into an already established family, coupled with the mixed allegiance the wife–mother experiences—to her new husband on the one hand and to her children on the other.

Role confusion, or role ambiguity, is a major source of stress for both stepparents and stepchildren (Coleman, Ganong, & Fine, 2000; Crosbie-Burnett, 1994). Perhaps the underlying issues creating role confusion for the stepfather and the resultant family disequilibrium are the issues of child rearing and disciplining of children (Hetherington & Stanley-Hagen, 2000). As discussed in Chapter 15, the diversity in child-rearing practices and values is great. Each parent draws on his or her own family background when defining child-rearing beliefs, practices, and discipline. And it is difficult to compromise in these values and beliefs because many of them are not objectively based. When parents enter into a relationship in which the stepfather heads the household but is not really the parent, synthesis of these values and rules is problematic. Furthermore, the children, through exposure to their natural parents' child-rearing practices, have developed their own behaviors and expectations of what is acceptable or unacceptable behavior, for both themselves and their parents. In the stepparent family the stepfather has no biological rights over the children—his wife must grant these to him. This places the stepfather in a rather untenable position.

When conflict arises over the disciplining of a child, the mother feels a natural right to decide the issue. If the stepfather disciplines the child, the mother will often become angry, or more often, indirectly strike back by undermining him. This latter course is particularly devastating to the entire family and often exacerbates the conflict, with the mother being torn between the loyalty to her children and to her husband. In addition, integrating the noncustodial biological parent, the kinship system of the stepparent, and the stepparent's children from a previous marriage may require further alterations in family roles (Bray, Berger, & Boethel, 1994). Children in stepparent families also have difficulties in adjusting to their new households. They are unsure of how to relate to both the stepparent and the biological parent of the same sex and experience loyalty conflicts (Crosbie-Burnett, 1994).

CULTURAL/ETHNIC INFLUENCES

Culturally or ethnically derived norms and values strongly influence how roles are carried out within a given family system. Knowledge of the core values, customs, and traditions of a particular ethnic group are important for interpreting whether family roles are functional. In some cultures, formal family roles are performed by extended family members who hold other family positions. A common example of this situation is when an uncle acts as a father surrogate in a single-parent family. Members of the extended family (such as a grandfather, uncle, or older brother) may, in some cultures, act as surrogate fathers even when the father is present, without causing any conflict or strained relationships. The maternal grandmother may also perform formal family roles, especially in African-American single-parent families (Burton & deVries, 1995).

Married couples who come from different ethnic backgrounds may experience differences in family role expectations. Because of the couple's dissimilar cultural backgrounds, the expectations that the spouses have of their roles and their spouse's roles often differ. Each marital partner may criticize the other for failure to carry out the marital or parental role as expected, while at the same time feeling guilty for not meeting the other's expectations (Hartman & Laird, 1983; Walsh, 1998).

FAMILY DEVELOPMENTAL STAGE

It is quite clear that the way in which family roles are enacted substantially differs from one life cycle stage of the family to another. For example, the role of parents changes as their role partners (their children), grow and change. The parenting behaviors and skills required to care for a dependent infant are quite different than the role behaviors demanded of the parent with an adolescent who is seeking maximum independence and differentiation from the family. Changes in family role patterns occur in many diverse family situations. For example, Haveman, van Berkum, Reijinders, and Heller (1997) studied families with a person with mental retardation to learn how their need for services, time demands, and caregiving burden changed over the family's life cycle. Analysis of data from 2,573 parents with children with mental retardation indi-

cated that ". . . although caregiving demands decreased from childhood, families perceived their tasks as less normative in adulthood, when most other families without a child with disabilities no longer cared for their offspring at home" (p. 422). The researchers noted that each life stage had unique challenges for the parents of the family member with mental retardation, some similar to families with nondisabled members and some situation-specific challenges.

And, the developmental stage of the parent at different points in the child's life will influence the fit in their respective developmental needs and tasks. For example, the developmental tasks for teen mothers for greater independence may be asynchronous with the infant's dependency needs.

ROLE MODELS

Our role behavior as parent or marital partner often imitates the roles we observed our parents playing. For example, it is not uncommon to find people tending to treat their children as their parents treated them in the past. With this observation in mind, family therapists have placed great importance on looking at the intergenerational aspects of clients' marital and parental roles.

When a family member is exhibiting or experiencing role problems (role transitions or role conflicts), assessing the role models of the troubled family member is helpful. This analysis is aimed at finding out about the early life of the family, when the individual was learning both his or her role and the counterpart's role (such as learning the role of a daughter, as well as a mother), and how those early experiences might have affected his or her present role behaviors and difficulties.

❧ HEALTHY FAMILY ROLE FUNCTIONING

Family homeostasis refers to the family's use of regulatory mechanisms to maintain stability or equilibrium in the family. Roles, both formal and informal, serve a homeostatic purpose in families. The family achieves homeostasis through adaptation—by altering the family structure such as family roles, and/or by bringing in outside resources. Turner (1970) remarks that once a system of formal and informal roles is established within the family, family processes proceed laboriously unless the members play their expected roles. This is because families become dependent on the existence of certain informal roles to be enacted so as to maintain family homeostasis. For example, if the family is used to having the middle daughter act as a mediator in disputes, this enables other family members to be less restrained in their sentiments and assures family members that she will step in to help resolve disagreements. When the mediating daughter is not present, conflicts are handled in a much less effective manner due to her absence, until family members learn new roles.

Family scholars and clinicians underscore the importance of role complementarity; compatibility of family roles and norms with societal and cultural norms; the presence of roles in families that meet the psychological needs of its members; and the ability of the family to respond to change via role flexibility (Ackerman, 1966; Glasser & Glasser, 1970; Messer, 1970; Olson, 1993). In addition, in a healthy family role allocation is reasonable and does not overburden one or more members. This results in all the necessary family functions being fulfilled.

🌿 FAMILY ROLES DURING HEALTH ALTERATIONS

Major situational life events confronting families unavoidably affect their role functioning. These situations are usually stressful events such as natural disasters, unemployment, or health alterations of family members. Chapter 16 elaborates on the entire area of the family's involvement in health care and health practices. This section focuses on family role structure during health alterations of family members, such as when someone develops a chronic illness or has a physical or mental disability. In most instances, when one person has health alterations, one or more family members assume caregiving role(s).

ROLE OF MOTHER IN HEALTH AND ILLNESS

An important role for women in most families is that of health leader and caregiver. Whatever criteria have been used in studies to measure health decision making and roles—including such measures as illnesses incurred and treated, medical and health services used, and primary source of family assistance—the pervasive and central role of the mother as prime health decision maker, educator, counselor, and caregiver within the family matrix has remained a constant finding (Finley, 1989; Litman, 1974). In this role, the mother defines symptoms and decides the "proper" disposition of resources. She also exerts substantial control over whether the children will receive preventive and curative services (Aday & Eichhorn, 1972; Rayner, 1970), and acts as the main source of comfort and assistance in times of illness (Litman).

One of the ways one can surmise the importance of the mother's health leader role is by observing what happens to her and the family when she is ill and unable to carry on her roles. Mothers usually assume the sick role only when it is absolutely mandatory, and then only reluctantly. Because her role performance is considered essential to family functioning, her illness tends to be quite disruptive and disorganizing (Mechanic, 1964). Usually, severe illness or prolonged incapacitation of the mother–wife is seen as a more serious blow to the family's functioning than is the incapacitation of the husband–father (although if his illness is prolonged, adverse economic reverberations are felt) (Litman, 1974; Giovannetti de Jesus & Bergamasco, 1998). If the mother becomes ill, often the oldest female child is expected to help the family carry on (Kahana, Kahana, Johnson, Hammand, & Kercher, 1994). Families need to understand the course of a health problem to facilitate flexibility of roles that involve children in caregiving and child-rearing responsibilities when a parent is ill (Rolland, 1994).

THE FAMILY CAREGIVER ROLE

Family members, and women in particular, play a vital role as primary caregivers not only for the frail elderly, but for many family members of all ages who are dependent, often due to chronic physical and/or mental disabilities. Their ability and willingness to provide care is often a critical factor in determining whether or not a disabled or ill member can avoid institutionalization.

Trends in family caregiving include increases in the numbers of caregivers with multiple caregiving responsibilities; grandchildren responsible for helping one or two older generations; and aging women without caregiver husbands due to high divorce rates (Brody, 1995). The consequences of caregiving may be negative or may include potential benefits. Previously caregiver research has focused on the negative outcomes—caregiver stress or burden—but more recently has shifted to examining physical and mental outcomes (Biegel, Sales, & Schulz, 1991). Biegel, Sales, and Schulz summarize caregiver problems: coping with the increased needs of the dependent family member caused by physical and/or mental illnesses. These include

> . . . coping with disruptive behaviors, restrictions on social and leisure activities, infringement of privacy, disruption of household and work routines, conflicting multiple role demands, lack of support and assistance from other family members, disruption of family relationships, and lack of sufficient assistance from human service agencies and agency professionals. (p. 7)

Different types of caregiving demands are associated with different types of role strain. Objective stressors, or patient characteristics, that are consistently associated with family caregiver strain include greater illness severity, suddenness of onset, and greater changes in preexisting patient behaviors (Biegel et al., 1991). In addition, the nature of the stress and role demands may change over the life of the caregiver and the dependent family member.

Robinson (1998) discovered a four-stage theory of women's experience in caring for a family member with a chronic illness. It begins with the diagnosis of a chronic illness for the family member and moves into an unbalanced second stage labeled "Women falling down and falling apart." The third stage involved therapeutic change through nursing intervention and moving beyond and overcoming problems. The fourth stage of Robinson's theory, labeled "taking charge of one's life," was characterized by the women achieving "life-enhancing balance between self and all other family members" (p. 285). These findings are consistent with other work emphasizing the importance of balancing caregiving demands with self-care. Carmack (1997) interviewed 14 caregivers

who were functioning well, and found that they balanced engagement and detachment, were pragmatic, and made conscious choices based on their own emotional needs. Carmack reported that these lay and professional caregivers, both men and women, set and maintained limits and boundaries with caregiving, and paid close attention to self-care as well as enacting their caregiving roles.

In a study of caregivers of older persons, the management of behavior problems was found to be a more powerful predictor of caregiver role strain than the management of physical problems (Harvath, Stewart, & Archibold, 1994). Reinhard and Horwitz's (1995) findings substantiate the burden that disruptive behaviors create. Caregivers of mentally ill relatives experience substantial role strain as the consequence of dealing with disruptive behaviors and having to provide instrumental and emotional assistance.

In a large study of primary caregivers who provide care to a spouse or parent with Alzheimer's disease or a related dementia (Aneshensel, Pearlin, Mullan, Zarit, & Whitlatch, 1995), one stressor experienced by caregivers was role overload (i.e., feeling overwhelmed by tasks and responsibilities). Caregivers report having role captivity, or a feeling of being involuntarily trapped in the role of caregiver as well as loss of intimate exchange in the caregiver–patient relationship because one of the role partners had "become someone else." Relationships of the caregiver to other family members, as well as work and other social roles, were often adversely affected.

Rolland (1994) presents a psychosocial categorization of illness that identifies onset, course, outcome, and degree of incapacitation as four major variables of illness and disability that have an impact on both ill family member and family performance. These characteristics can be used to anticipate the demands placed on caregivers.

Biegel and co-workers (1991) diagrammed variables that predict caregiver strain (see Figure 12–2). In their diagram, contextual variables that mediate the caregiver's reaction include caregiver demographic factors (gender, type of role relationship with patient, age, and socioeconomic status); preexisting psychological factors, relationship quality, family life stage, and social support. Some of these factors such as gender (female) and role relationship (spouses and parents) are consistently associated with greater caregiving burden whereas other variables show contradictory or more complex patterns. Although most caregivers are women who are socialized to the caregiving role, they exhibit greater adverse effects of caregiving than male caregivers (Pruchno & Resch, 1989).

The contributions of men to caregiving should not be overlooked. Men frequently provide support and affection to the primary caregiver. Many elderly husbands assume the role of caregiver if their wives become ill or disabled (Richards, 1996). In a study comparing the parent care experiences of women in different marital statuses (Brody, Litvin, Kleben, & Hoffman, 1990), married women were noted to have

Figure 12-2. Summary of variables predicting caregiver strain. *(From Biegel, D. E., Sales, E., & Schulz, R. (1991.) Family caregiving in chronic illness (p. 211). Newbury Park, CA: Sage. Reprinted by permission of Sage Publications.*

several advantages over women who did not have husbands. The husbands provided financial and socioemotional support and helped with instrumental tasks. Women who did not have husbands reported loneliness, lack of support, and lack of instrumental help in parental caregiving.

The caregiver's role varies according to his or her position or relationship to the care recipient; that is, the role is significantly altered when the caregiver is a spouse, parent, child, sibling, or friend. Mothers are the primary caregivers of chronically ill children (Shepard & Mahon, 1996). Spouses or adult children are most often the caregivers of the elderly. Parents care for their disabled adult children until they are no longer able to do so. Then a sibling usually becomes the primary caregiver (Roberto, 1993).

Another factor that increases the burden of the caregiving situation is a violation of social norms regarding roles. This often occurs in the following four situations: when children care for parents, when men or women perform household tasks that are typically performed by the other gender, when parents care for adult disabled children (Litwak, Jessop, & Moulton, 1994), and when siblings care for siblings (Avioli, 1989; Horwitz, 1993).

Although there are numerous caregiving stressors, many positive experiences in caregiving are reported. Some care recipients reciprocate through their expression of affection or appreciation, which may explain why some caregivers do not experience negative consequences despite providing physically demanding care (Carruth, 1996). In studying reciprocity in family caregiving, Walker, Pratt, and Oppy (1992) found that the majority of caregiving daughters perceived that they received valuable aid from their care-receiving mothers in return for their help. The contributions that the daughters received included love, information, advice, and money. Bulger, Wandersman, and Goldman (1993) noted that older parents caring for dependent adult children benefited from companionship and help with physical household work. While the assumption has been that occupying multiple roles, such as employee and caregiver, leads to negative effects such as role conflict and role overload, the emotional impact of combining multiple roles on employed caregivers has more often been found to be positive rather than negative (Neal, Chapman, Ingersoll-Dayton, & Emlen, 1993).

ROLE CHANGES DURING ILLNESS AND HOSPITALIZATION

In a period of crisis, such as that caused by the serious illness of a family member, the family structure is modified, the extent of modification depending on what degree the sick member is able to carry out his or her usual family roles and the centrality of the family roles or tasks that are vacated. The roles taken on by the mother are, as discussed previously, a good example of the centrality of a member's roles. When illness results in the vacancy of critical roles, the family often enters a state of disequilibrium in which role and power relationships are altered until new homeostasis is achieved (Fife, 1985; Hill, 1958).

Shared, balanced role functions often become impossible to maintain in couples when one partner becomes disabled. Negotiation of revised roles is often needed to prevent role strain and confusion (Rolland, 1994). In a study of the effects of a critical care illness on family members (Johnson et al., 1995), most family members reported changes in family roles and increased responsibilities as the result of critical care hospitalization.

There are two basic types of role changes that occur due to the loss or incapacitation of a family member. First, the remaining family members have enough inner and outer resources that they are able to take on the basic and necessary role obligations and tasks that the sick family member is unable to assume—this is the functional way the situation is managed. Second, they lack the needed inner and outer resources, and as a consequence, certain basic and necessary roles in the family are not performed or are performed unsatisfactorily. In other words, the adequately functioning family can either flexibly modify family roles to meet the demands of the situation or may call in resources and assistance from the outside to fill the vacuum. In dysfunctional families, however, this does not happen.

Because of the role changes necessitated due to the loss or incapacitation of a family member, role conflicts and role strain are often present, especially during the stage of family disequilibrium immediately following the loss or incapacitation, when family structure is in the transitional period. Either interrole or intrarole conflict may exist, as the family members are "forced" to accept new roles and have had little opportunity to learn these roles or to rearrange all their other role responsibilities. Role strain/stress is

often the outcome. The family members burdened with the acquisition of new roles may often feel worried, anxious, and guilty because of feelings that they are not doing a competent job in their new roles or that with these added responsibilities, their role complex is excessively demanding and unmanageable.

In a recent review of family nursing research regarding the impact of illness on families with a member experiencing ischemic heart disease, spouses frequently reported stress that was related to the need to assume additional household roles and health monitoring responsibilities (Artinian, 1989; Gillis, 1984; Gilliss, Sparacino, Gortner, & Kenneth, 1985; Hilgenberg, Liddy, Standerfer, & Schraeder, 1992; McRae, 1991; Nyamathi, 1987b; Stanley & Frantz, 1988; Tapp, 1995). Marital conflict related to role reversal and attempts of the healthy spouse to monitor noncompliance were also consistently reported (Caplin & Sexton, 1988; Hilgenberg et al.; McRae; Mishel & Murdaugh, 1987; Nyamathi, 1987a).

Once a family has achieved a new equilibrium in response to a sick member's inability to perform his or her roles adequately, a similar reintegration must take place when that member resumes his or her old place in the family unit. Understandably, having once gone through the process of adapting, the other members may well be reluctant to again "reshuffle" family roles and tasks, despite the recovery or reentry of the "lost" member. This reluctance is seen even in the most well-functioning families, because the process of reintegrating a family member entails the difficulties and problems that are part of any disorganization before a new (in this case, renewed) balance is achieved.

❧ ASSESSMENT OF FAMILY ROLE STRUCTURE

Families must respond to changes throughout their life cycle—sometimes due to normal developmental transitions and sometimes due to situational stressors they experience. Health stressors are one prime example of demands families face. Stressors/demands require family role changes. If family members do not have the requisite knowledge, skills, or emotional readiness for adjusting to the needed role changes, then numerous types of role problems may result. One important role of the family nurse in this regard is to assist families to identify role transitions so that information about the new role (anticipatory guidance) is provided to prevent or ameliorate role problems.

An assessment of family roles primarily focuses on the characteristics of the formal and informal role structure, coupled with a consideration of how sociocultural, situational, and historical factors affect family role structure. There are four broad areas for the assessment of the family role structure: the formal role structure, the informal role structure and types of relationships, role models, and variables affecting role structure. Each family member's position and roles are described by addressing the following questions:

Formal Role Structure

1. What formal positions and roles do each of the family members fulfill? Describe how each family member carries out his or her formal roles.

2. Are these roles acceptable and consistent with the family members' and family's expectations? In other words, are there any role conflicts present?

3. How competently do members perceive they perform their respective roles?

4. Is there flexibility in roles when needed?

Informal Role Structure

1. What informal or covert roles exist in the family, who plays them, and how frequently or consistently are they enacted? Are members of the family covertly playing roles different from those that their position in the family demands that they play?

2. What purposes do the identified covert or informal roles serve?

3. Are any of these informal roles dysfunctional to the family or family members in the long run?

4. What is the impact on the person(s) who play this (these) role(s)?

Role Models

1. Who were (or are) the models that influenced family members in their early life, who gave feelings and values about, for example, growth, new experiences, roles, and communication techniques?

2. Who specifically acted as role model for the mates in their roles as parents, and as marital partners, and what were they like?

3. If the informal roles are dysfunctional in the family, who enacted these roles in previous generations?

Variables Affecting Role Structure

1. *Social class influences.* How does social class background influence the formal and informal role structure in the family?

2. *Ethnic/cultural influences.* How is the family's role structure influenced by the family's ethnic and religious background?

3. *Developmental or life cycle influences.* Are the present role behaviors of family members developmentally appropriate?

4. *Situational events, including health and illness changes.* How have health problems affected family roles? What reallocation of roles and tasks have occurred? How have the family members who have had to assume new roles adjusted? Is there evidence of role stress and/or role conflict as a result of these role shifts? How has the family member with the health problem reacted to her or his change or loss of a role(s)?

✹ FAMILY NURSING DIAGNOSES

Family nurses frequently observe role problems. They may not, however, be identified as role problems, because there are so many interrelationships and overlaps between problems. Role problems may be stated as a family nursing diagnosis, remembering that role problems involve at least two people: the role occupant and his or her role partner(s).

Because role problems are usually very general, it is also useful to state defining characteristics and related factors.

In reviewing the list of nursing diagnoses approved by the North American Nursing Diagnosis Association (NANDA), the diagnoses given in Table 12–2 relate to role problems. It should be noted here that most of these diagnoses do not mention "role" in the diagnostic title, but actual and potential role problems could be a related nursing diagnosis. In NANDA, included under altered role performance are four more specific role problems: role transition, role distance, role conflict, and role failure. Defining characteristics of each of these types of role problems are seen in Table 12–3, as well as associated relevant nursing diagnoses.

In *A Pocket Guide to Nursing Diagnoses*, Kim, McFarland, and McFarlane (1995) list nursing diagnoses associated with medical diagnostic categories. For instance, for Alzheimer's type dementia many nursing diagnoses are listed, but five in particular dealing with role problems are identified. They are alteration in family processes, impaired social interaction, altered role performance, caregiver role strain, and risk for caregiver role strain. These diagnoses have been incorporated into the NANDA listing in Table 12–2.

FAMILY NURSING INTERVENTIONS

The Nursing Interventions Classification (NIC) Project at the University of Iowa has identified numerous nursing intervention approaches that may be used with families and are associated with actual or potential role problems (Table 12–3). These interventions are research based and are described in detail well in McCloskey and Bulechek's (1996) text, *Nursing Interventions Classification* (NIC). Johnson et al. (2001) have also written a text, *Nursing Diagnoses, Outcomes and Interventions,* which discusses the NANDA nursing diagnoses, nursing outcomes (NOC) and interventions (NIC).

ROLE SUPPLEMENTATION OR ROLE ENHANCEMENT STRATEGIES FOR ROLE TRANSITIONS

Johnson (1986) summarizes general nursing interventions appropriate for role transitions and role

---

TABLE 12–2

NANDA NURSING DIAGNOSES RELATED TO ROLE TRANSITIONS/ROLE PROBLEMS

Anticipatory Grieving	Role loss
Social Isolation	Role strain
Social Interaction, Impaired	Role change
Family Process, Altered	Role loss and strain
Parenting, Altered	Role conflict, role overload
Violence, Risk For, Directed at Others	Role change
Role Performance, Altered	Role conflict
Caregiver Role Strain	Role loss and role strain
Caregiver Role Strain, High Risk For	Role strain
Home Maintenance Management, Impaired	Role strain
Body Image Disturbance	Role strain
Ineffective Family Coping	Role loss, role insufficiency, or role ambiguity

Partially adapted from McFarland and MacFarlane (1993).

---

problems. Role transitions involve adding new roles and dropping others. Role transitions are created because of developmental changes and situational changes including health-related stressors. She refers to these interventions as "role theory strategies." Johnson's role theory strategies include helping family members identify significant cues of the other family members, clarifying expectations about the needed roles (family members identify their expectations for new roles) and strengthening the family members' abilities to enact a new role. Teaching strategies are used here.

Role supplementation or *role enhancement* is also suggested for role transitions. It consists of a set of interventions to assist family members to improve their role relationships and facilitate their role changes by clarifying and supplementing role behaviors

TABLE 12–3

ALTERED ROLE PERFORMANCE NURSING DIAGNOSES (NANDA) WITH DEFINING CHARACTERISTICS AND RELEVANT NURSING INTERVENTIONS (NIC)

ROLE TRANSITION

- Feelings of anger and depression
- Change in usual pattern of responsibility
- Change in capacity to perform role
- Inability to achieve desired role
- Refusal to participate in role

ROLE DISTANCE

- Uncertainty about role requirements
- Lack of knowledge of role
- Different role perceptions

ROLE CONFLICT

- Confusion
- Frustration in role (intrarole or interrole conflict)
- Ambivalence about role
- Inadequate problem-solving skills
- Incongruent or incompatible role expectations

ROLE FAILURE

- Withdrawal
- Loss of role skills
- Inability to achieve desired role
- Refusal to participate in role
- Difficulty learning new roles

MAJOR INTERVENTIONS

- Coping Enhancement
- Role Enhancement

SUGGESTED INTERVENTIONS

- Anticipatory Guidance
- Caregiver Support
- Counseling
- Decision-Making Support
- Emotional Support
- Family Support
- Health System Guidance
- Mutual Goal Setting
- Spiritual Support
- Support Group
- Support System Enhancement
- Values Clarification

OPTIONAL INTERVENTIONS

- Family Involvement Promotion
- Insurance Authorization
- Body Image Enhancement
- Cognitive Restructuring
- Family Therapy
- Mood Management
- Normalization Promotion
- Socialization Enhancement
- Substance Use Prevention

Sources: McFarland & McFarlane (1993); Johnson, Bulecheck, McCloskey, Dochterman, Maas, & Moorhead, (2001).

(McCloskey & Bulechek, 1996; Meleis & Swendsen, 1978). Role supplementation strategies can also be preventive, in this case used to clarify role insufficiency (Morehead, 1985). They consist of components, strategies, and process. The two components are (1) role clarification, understanding the specific information and cues needed to enact the role; and (2) role taking, being able to imagine yourself in a particular role and assuming the perspective of the other person. Roles are paired and learned in pairs. Hence, if an individual learns the expectations of a parenting role, theoretically he or she should also know the role of the role partner, in this case the child.

The strategies used to accomplish role clarification and role taking are role modeling, role rehearsal, and reference group interactions. Through role modeling, the desired behavior is performed by the health professional for the family member to imitate; the imitation eventually becomes part of the family member's own behavioral repertoire (Goldenberg & Goldenberg, 2000). For example, a family nurse may serve as a role model for a caregiver by showing how to assist an elder who has had a stroke how to walk safely.

Role rehearsal is a second role supplementation strategy suggested by Meleis (1975). Here, the role behavior and reactions of significant others are mentally enacted. This strategy is very helpful when a new role can be anticipated. This mental practice prepares the individual for a future role change. The nurse can effectively use role reversal with parents, marital partners, and in parent–child and sibling relationships. Helping family members to rehearse their interactions is good anticipatory guidance.

The third role supplementation strategy is initiation of *referrals to reference groups*. Reference groups are groups with which an individual or family identifies. Self-help groups can become powerful reference groups for individuals and families. Self-help groups assist their members to adapt to their new roles by sharing feelings and perceptions in the group and offering practical solutions to vexing issues related to the new role. Nurses often initiate referrals of family members struggling to learn a new role to self-help groups and, in some cases, lead a self-help group or act as a consultant to the group.

The process used in role supplementation is communication. Through communication, new information needed to enact the new role or role options can be shared. Feelings can be ventilated—such as feelings of anger, depression, and frustration over difficulties in learning the new role. Exploration of family members' perception of what has changed and how the role change has affected them is a vital area to discuss. And lastly, through communication, clients should be encouraged to seek out new information and explore role options themselves.

INTERVENTIONS FOR ROLE STRAIN

There are several ways to address *role strain*. Family nurses can explore the following options with family members who are experiencing role strain:

1. Redefining the role in terms of what behaviors are considered adequate role performance, for instance, educating caregivers about ways to enhance functioning among their disabled family members (Jacob, 1999).

2. Examining an individual's role complex (the various roles the role occupant plays) and setting priorities within a role and among roles.

3. Role bargaining or role negotiation with role partners so that role occupants achieve a set of roles that collectively are relatively equitable and rewarding. Role negotiation involves influencing the members of one's role set so that they agree to changes in the role and the allocation of resources.

4. Reduced interaction with role partners. If, however, role partners have a high interdependency on each other, this tactic usually leads to unsuccessful role bargaining and role distancing. Partial withdrawal from interaction may relieve role strain when the interdependency is not so great and when diminished interaction is possible (Hardy & Hardy, 1988). This suggestion is often not possible in family relationships.

For primary caregivers who are strained in their caregiver role, respite care and participation in self-care groups are recommended (Dell Orto, 1988; Jacob, 1999). Studies of caregiving role strain and reports from family support groups indicate that regularly scheduled periods of respite are essential to counter role fatigue and stress (Pallett, 1990). Respite care refers to temporary care of disabled individuals for the purpose of providing relief to the primary caregiver (Dell Orto). Friends and family sometimes serve as surrogate caregivers.

Nurses can assist families in locating community resources for respite care, such as adult day care, temporary nursing home placement, and/or intermittent home care. Unfortunately, there is a scarcity of funding for respite services. Pioneering efforts have been made by groups and organizations to implement respite care programs for the caregivers with family members who are developmentally, physically, or mentally disabled or who have chronic mental illness. Some family caregiving situations are very intense, and without respite or home care, family stress may increase with accelerated deterioration in family functioning. Still, some caregivers may hesitate to accept respite care and may need encouragement to work through their concerns so that they may benefit from available respite services (Strang & Haughey, 1998).

Participation in a formal self-help support group for caregivers has proved to be important in boosting morale and preventing social isolation for the caregiver (Jacob, 1999; Pallett, 1990). Feelings and frustrations, as well as practical solutions, are shared in groups. Additional interventions to reduce caregiver burden include caregiver education and skill training (Schmall, 1994).

INTERVENTIONS FOR ROLE INADEQUACY

Role inadequacy refers to a role occupant not fulfilling the role behaviors that are a part of that role. In this type of role problem, role expectations are set by society and they are in conflict with the role occupant's behavior. Support and counseling strategies, as well as teaching strategies, should be used here. Family members need to understand role requirements; they very much need information, because knowledge deficits are usually present. Focusing on clarifying perceptions and fostering awareness of prevailing expectations is recommended. In addition, in working with immigrant families, showing respect for role behaviors that are culturally derived and comparing the role occupant's customs with expected practices in their new country is suggested.

Many fathers in our society are not undertaking the father role that is expected of them today. Hanson and Bozett (1987) and Kunst-Wilson and Cronenwett (1981) recommend several tactics for nurses to use to promote greater active participation by fathers in family health care. These suggestions include:

1. Encourage fathers to attend clinics with their children and to attend prenatal clinics and family planning clinics with their partners/wives.

2. Encourage fathers to participate in men's support groups and resource centers if they need support to undertake new father roles.

3. Encourage father's participation in birthing and parenting classes.

4. Encourage fathers and mothers to negotiate infant and child care roles. Role sharing and

role negotiation involves an agreement among involved persons regarding the behaviors that are expected in an associated role.

5. Support fathers' active involvement in labor, delivery, and newborn care in the hospital or birthing center.

INTERVENTIONS FOR ROLE CONFLICT

Interventions for role conflict cover both intrarole and interrole conflicts. Guidelines for this problem include the following:

1. Before intervening, plan strategies to reduce or resolve role conflict. To do this, determine the sources of stress and the type of role conflict present.

2. Actively listen, encouraging expression of frustration with role conflict.

3. Encourage role partners who are in conflict to discuss their perceptions and feelings about the roles in question.

4. Encourage family members to discuss their feelings and perceptions together and assist them in problem solving.

5. Assist family to set priorities.

6. Family members should meet together to discuss role incompatibilities. The nurse, acting as a facilitator, encourages family members to explore role incompatibilities and to come up with a different allocation of roles or perhaps different role expectations.

INTERVENTIONS FOR ROLE FAILURE

Role failure implies that the client has tried to carry out the role, but has failed. Role failure addresses the lack of knowledge and skills for a particular role and perhaps the needed emotional or developmental readiness. Strategies are aimed at resolving role failure problems and assisting family members to achieve satisfactory role competence. Teaching about role requirements is paramount. Supportive counseling involves encouraging family members to voice their concerns and questions about their new role(s). Because clients are often disappointed and frustrated about the new role, recognizing and praising each successful behavior is important. Strengths and resources that the client possesses should also be recognized and supported.

In conclusion, family nurses are able to effectively assess and intervene to assist families with role transi-tions and role problems. In assessing formal and informal family roles, our understanding of family strengths and resources is also enhanced. This sup-plies us with important data for planning interven-tions to resolve health problems.

❧ SUMMARY

- Individuals live their lives enmeshed in a net-work of family rights and obligations called role relations. Adequate role functioning is crucial for the individual and for the family as it is through the performance of family roles that family functions are fulfilled.

- Role behavior, role performance, and role enactment are all interchangeable terms that denote what a person actually does within a posi-tion in response to role expectations.

- Role sharing refers to participation of two or more people in the same roles even though they hold different positions.

- Role taking refers to family members' ability to imagine themselves in the role of a counterpart, or role partner, and thereby better understand how they should behave in their own roles

- Role complementarity refers to the functional adequacy of roles based on the match between the performances and the expectations of part-ners in a relationship. A role is always paired with a reciprocal role of another person. One can never look at a role in isolation.

- Role stress occurs when a social structure creates very difficult, conflicting, or impossible demands for occupants of positions within that social structure.

- Role conflict occurs when the occupant of a position perceives that he or she is confronted with incompatible expectations. The source of the incompatibility may be due to changes in expectations within the actor, others, or the environment.

- Formal roles are explicit roles and informal roles are implicit roles within families. Informal roles are played to meet the emo-tional needs of individuals and/or to maintain the family's equilibrium. An individual family member plays many roles in a family, both informal and formal, with some of these roles being shared.

- Major factors influencing the formal and infor-mal family role structure include social class, family form, cultural/ethnic background, family developmental (life cycle) stage, role models, and situational events such as health alterations of family members.

- Eight basic roles making up the husband–father and the wife–mother social positions are the provider role, the housekeeper role, the child care role, the recreational role, the kinship role (maintaining relationships with paternal and maternal families), the therapeutic role (meet-ing the affective needs of spouse [or intimate adult partner]), and the sexual role.

- As women have moved from the home into the workplace in recent decades, their roles have changed, and correspondingly, their role part-ners' behavior has changed. There is much more flexibility and variation in men's and women's roles in families now than in decades past.

- Grandparenthood is a heterogeneous experi-ence, with wide variation in how the grandpar-ent role is enacted. The historical context, age, ethnicity, social class, and gender tend to pro-duce significant differences in grandparents' role enactment.

- In healthy families, role allocation is reasonable and does not overburden one or more members and results in family functions being fulfilled in healthy families. In dysfunctional families, role allocation is problematic.

- In most instances, when one person has health alterations, one or more family members assume caregiving role(s). Family members, and women in particular, play a vital role as primary caregivers for family members of all ages who are dependent, often due to chronic physical and/or mental disabilities. The consequences of caregiving may be negative or may be seen in a positive light by caregivers.

- In a period of crisis, such as that caused by the serious illness of a family member, the family structure is modified, the extent of modification depending on what degree the sick member is able to carry out his or her usual family roles and the centrality of the family roles or tasks that are vacated.

- There are four broad areas for the assessment of the family role structure: the formal role structure, the informal role structure, types of role models, and variables affecting role structure.

- Role problems may be stated as a family nursing diagnosis, remembering that role problems involve at least two people: the role occupant and his or her role partner(s). Because role problems are usually very general, it is also useful to state defining characteristics and related factors. NANDA diagnoses related to roles are identified.

- There are numerous nursing interventions related to family roles, including interventions for role supplementation, role strain, role inadequacy, role conflict, and role failure.

⚘ FAMILY VIGNETTE: THE GREEN FAMILY*

Mr. and Mrs. Green are a young couple, married for 3 years, with a 2-year-old son. The 23-year-old husband is a garbage collector, earning $28,000 a year. He completed two years of high school; his 22-year-old wife is a high school graduate. (But the family nurse commented: "It is hard to believe in view of her poor vocabulary and illiterate handwriting that she had completed high school." The husband said: "She was sort of a dumbbell at school, but people liked her and she got through.")

Mr. Green is a slim, tall man, slow moving and soft-spoken. When asked what he liked about himself, he replied, "People tell me I'm easygoing but not a chump." The assessor observed his deceptively lazy attitude as the manner of a man who thinks that most people, particularly women, become too excited about things and foolishly so. He reports that he quit school at 14 because he did not like it. Since then he has held a number of unskilled jobs. Concerning his present occupation as garbage collector, he stated: "People laugh at you for being in this line of work. I don't know what's so funny about it. It's got to be done. There is no future in it, though, and the pay is terrible. I'm going to make a break for it as soon as I can. Everybody's looking out for me now, and something is bound to turn up pretty soon."

Both Mr. Green and his wife express satisfaction with their sexual relations and with the marriage in general. Mr. Green is in charge of the outside of the house and repairs to their home, and Mrs. Green is in charge of the interior of the home and the child.

A good deal of the communication between them is nonverbal. This type of communication pattern began during their courtship. When asked whether her husband had said he loved her when he proposed, Mrs. Green answered, "He just got softer and softer on me and I could tell that he did and we got to necking more and more and he wanted to go all the way and I didn't want to unless we were going to get married." The nurse asked whether he had ever said out and out that he could go for her or wanted her or anything like that. Mrs. Green said, "No, we don't go in for that kind of stuff." When she told him she was pregnant, "He looked a little funny when I told him, but he didn't say much. You know that's what's going to happen. After a while, when I began to show a lot, he asked me sometimes how I felt."

Mrs. Green was asked to describe their quarrels. She said they quarrel little, but when they do, it is about such things as his failure to help move the furniture or her failure to do something he demands. "We just get over it." He might "crab around and then he would know that he had been mean to me and makes it up." There is no conversation about such quarrels, but Mr. Green helps to dry the dishes or asks her if she likes a television program or wants something else. Mrs. Green felt that talking does no good, since it might worsen things.

When asked whether they like to talk about what makes people tick or to discuss the rights and wrongs of things, each said in separate interviews, "No, we don't hash things over." Mr. Green added, "It's either right or wrong—what is there to discuss?"

This "conversation of gestures" between Mrs. Green and her husband contrasts sharply with the communication characterizing her relationships with female relatives and friends. On many counts Mrs. Green reveals her emotional life to the latter. And this extends to spheres of experience beyond the "feminine world" of babies, housework, or gossip.

Mrs. Green sees her sister and her mother daily. "Oh yes," she said about her sister, "we tell each other everything, anything we have on our minds. We don't hold nothing back. We discuss the children, the house, cooking, and 'female things.'" But when asked whether she can talk to her husband, she answered, "Sure, I can talk to him about anything that has to be said." Her view is that "men and women do different things; he don't want to be bothered with my job of cleaning and children and I don't want to be bothered with his. He makes the big decisions and I don't have to bother with it. Sometimes we got to do the same things, something around the house and we have to tell each other."

When asked what helped her when she was in the "dumps," Mrs. Green replied, "Talking to my sister or my mother helps sometimes." When asked directly whether conversations with her husband ever have a similar effect, she replied, "No."

Mr. Green enjoys an active social life with his male friends and relatives. Mr. Green revealed to his father and his brother his fears that Mrs. Green is making a "sissy" out of their son, and he regularly consults with them about his occupational plans. He does not discuss the latter topics with his wife because "there is no need of exciting her for nothing. Wait until it's sure. Women get all excited and talk too much."

Mr. Green thinks the world of the fellows in his own clique whom he sees after supper several times a week and on Saturday afternoons. Mrs. Green does not always know where he meets his "friends" when he leaves in the evenings. Mr. and Mrs. Green testified independently that having a beer with the fellows is the best cure for his depressions.

*Adapted by permission of Random House, Inc., from Blue-Collar Marriage, by Mirra Komarovsky with the collaboration of Jane H. Phillips. Copyright 1962, 1964, 1967 by Random House, Inc.

■ STUDY QUESTIONS

Review the Family Vignette and answer the related questions.

1. Both marital partners characterized this marriage as "happy." This was because:
   a. Both come from same social class.
   b. Both shared the same marital role expectations.
   c. Both were denying how really alienated they were from each other and how unsatisfactory their marriage was.
   d. Their sex life was adequate.

2. This marriage illustrates:
   a. The mates' lack of understanding of one another.
   b. An insufficient amount of communication in meaningful areas of family life.
   c. That marital companionship is not essential to make a satisfactory marriage.
   d. That both mates did not communicate openly with anyone.

3. This type of marriage is frequently seen in:
   a. Low-income families
   b. White, skilled, working-class families
   c. Disorganized families
   d. Middle-class white families

4. Through the couple's communication we can gather that:
   a. Both mates carry out traditional male–female roles.
   b. Mrs. Green would rather move out and be with her sister and friends.
   c. Mr. Green's occupational role is of central concern to him.
   d. Mr. Green desires to raise his son to be "a man."

5. Which type of relationship does this marriage most closely fit?
   a. Symmetrical
   b. Parallel
   c. Complementary

6. Complete a brief description of the couple's formal roles from what can be inferred from the narrative.

7. If the wife was going to vocational school and began to question her husband's traditional sex roles in the family, what kind of role problems might result? (Name at least one.)

8. Suggest two strategies to ameliorate or resolve the role problem identified in question 7.

Answer the following questions.

9. Match the correct definition or description with the appropriate term.

Terms	Definitions
a. Role	1. Status
b. Position	2. Incompatibility of the role(s) (intrarole or interrole)
c. Role enactment	3. A set of behaviors of an occupant of a particular social position
d. Socialization	4. The process of learning family and adult roles in preparation for societal responsibilities
e. Role conflict	
f. Reciprocal role	
g. Role strain	5. Balancing in family structure to maintain stability
h. Family homeostasis	6. Joint participation in fulfilling same role
i. Role sharing	7. Complementary role
	8. The worry or guilt felt as a result of difficulty with role enactment or presence of role conflict
	9. The actual behavior exhibited in a role

Questions 10–12: Are the following statements true or false?

10. A most functional way of maintaining equilibrium in a family in the face of change is by use of role flexibility.

11. The principle of complementarity states that there must be a match in expectations and performance of roles by role partners in order for stability and harmony to be present in the relationship.

12. Paired relationships in the family refer to father–son and mother–daughter relationships.

13. Identify three commonly seen differences in role structure between low- and middle-income families.

14. List five examples of informal roles seen in the family, indicating which of them could be functional.

15. The maintenance of informal roles is vital to the family because (select the best answer):

a. It relieves the role overload of some members.
b. Without covert roles the family could not exist.
c. Each formal role has an associated informal role.
d. Through the assumption of informal roles, family homeostasis is maintained and individual socioemotional needs are met.

16. Why are both formal and informal roles important to assess?

17. Give reasons why labeling is restrictive to an individual's growth and development.

18. Identify two role characteristics of single-parent families that act as stressors to the family and its members.

19. What are two prominent role problems within the stepparent family?

Questions 20–22: Are the following statements true or false?

20. When a family member is ill, the functional way of handling the situation is to leave the roles unfulfilled until he or she returns.

21. Role flexibility suggests that family members have the motivation and capacity to shift and reenact new roles when needed.

22. Middle-class parents are generally more concerned with promoting self-reliance and independence in their child-rearing practices, while lower-class parents stress respect and obedience.

23. Male caregivers experience greater adverse effects of caregiving than female caregivers.

FAMILY VALUES

❧ CONTENT OUTLINE

❧ LEARNING OBJECTIVES

1. Define the terms *values, family values, beliefs, norms,* and *family rules,* and explain their significance relative to family assessment.

2. Describe common outcome of a disparity in values between the health worker and the client.

3. Identify and briefly explain four recent important changes that have taken place in society related to family values.

4. Discuss the core value orientations of American society in terms of their significance today and their interrelationships with each other.

5. Identify variables that influence the family's value system and that create value conflicts.
6. Discuss an aspect of family life that should be included in the nursing assessment of family values.

7. State the nursing diagnosis that reflects potential or actual problems that may arise when the family faces value conflicts.
8. Describe the meaning and purposes of the value clarification process.

Because the value system is one of the four highly interdependent structural dimensions of a family, family health assessment is not complete without an analysis of a family's central values. Understanding what is important to a particular family is vital in terms of assessment, diagnosis, and health care intervention, for the health care practitioner knows that what a family believes and values affects both the family's and its members' behavior. Moreover, when family values and beliefs are identified, nurses may better understand family dynamics and behavior.

As health care professionals, nurses have the tendency to diagnose or label a family as pathological when they deviate from the dominant cultural values and norms. Most research on families is based on the mainstream or dominant culture (described later), and we must be particularly cautious about extrapolating these findings to all social classes and cultural groups, whose life conditions and traditions differ greatly from those of mainstream American culture.

An accurate assessment of a family's value system should help to tailor nursing interventions to a particular family or groups of similar families. Nurses need to work within the family's value system and to relate services to goals that are important to the family being assisted. For instance, it is well accepted that "ideas and methods which least affect the patient's habits, beliefs, and values meet less resistance than those that attempt to alter existing behavior patterns and values" (Dougherty, 1975, p. 441).

In assessing a family's value system, it is also imperative for health care providers to recognize their own priorities and values and to examine carefully how their values and attitudes subtly—and sometimes not so subtly—affect family-centered care. One ultimate goal in assessing family values is to demonstrate to families an appreciation of, and respect for, different value systems (Clemen, 1977).

❧ BASIC DEFINITIONS

VALUES

One of the most developed definitions of value is by Rokeach (1973): "A value is an enduring belief that a specific mode of conduct or end-state of existence [such as freedom] is . . . preferable to the opposite or converse mode of conduct or end-state of existence" (p. 5). Values are central features of an individual's belief system due to their enduring quality; they are not short-lived attitudes. Values serve as guides to action (Rokeach).

Values serve as general guides to behavior. Within families, values guide the development of family beliefs, norms, or rules. For instance, if a person values health and feels it is a desirable state, he or she is much more likely to engage in preventive health care and salubrious health habits. In addition, there will be a moral injunction (a norm or family rule) against "bad" health habits.

Values are not static. As an individual's or a family's development evolves over time, and as particular situations in society, within a person's or family's life, demand a shift of priorities, the potency or primacy of certain values changes. Furthermore, families and individuals rarely behave according to consistent value patterns. Certain values compete with other values, which are held simultaneously, such as the competition between valuing individualism and freedom versus valuing familism (meeting of the family's needs before personal needs). Also, certain values are not amenable to conscious identification, whereas others are consciously held.

There is a hierarchical nature to values. Some values are more central, molding or influencing most aspects of family lives, while other values are more peripheral and have less influence, involving only certain aspects of family lifestyle and daily functioning.

FAMILY VALUES

Family values are defined as a system of ideas, attitudes, and beliefs about the worth of an entity or concept that consciously and unconsciously bind together the members of a family in a common culture (Parad & Caplan, 1965). The family's cultural heritage is a prime source of a family's value system and norms. In turn, the family group is a prime source of family members' belief systems, value systems, and norms regarding the nature and meaning of the world, their place in it, and how to reach personal goals and aspirations.

A family's configuration of values ascribes meaning to certain critical events and at the same time suggests ways to respond to these situations. This configuration of values provides definitions of the time dimension; contains concepts concerning the responsibility and worth of the individual members of the family; ranks certain commonly held life goals; imposes a framework within which the pursuit of risks connected with the pleasure impulse takes place; defines what messages, thoughts, and feelings should and should not be shared and with whom; and finally, involves a system of sanctions.

Values are learned from the family of origin, which is the basic transmitter of societal or cultural values from one generation to the next. The family of origin assimilates societal and cultural values and modifies them somewhat to match with its own values. Societal values change, with some values becoming more important than others. These value changes and swings have a great influence on the family, profoundly affecting its own values, norms, and ultimately its behavior.

Family values are not only a reflection of the society in which an individual or family resides, but also of the subculture(s) with which the individual or family identifies. Most persons belong to a number of subcultures based on social class, ethnic background, occupation, gender, peer group, religious affiliation, and so forth. Subcultures exist within the larger, dominant culture, and so aspects of that value system also pervade the subculture. Members of a particular subculture respond to both subcultural and dominant value systems, although at different moments the values of one or the other may be more relevant to the individual or family. Obviously, the greater the degree of congruence between a family's subcultural values and the community's values, the easier the individual's and family's adjustment, and the greater degree of success the family will have in relating to the community.

Families will often have values that they cannot realize. Sheer practical necessity can often distort a family's values in everyday life so that they become unrecognizable (Graedon, 1985). In assisting families, both their values and actual behaviors need to be understood—for what families say is important may be at striking variance with their actual behavior. In anthropology, this is referred to as the real or manifest (family's actual behavior) versus the ideal (the family values espoused) (Leininger, 1978). The variance between the ideal and real is typically due to the family making a pragmatic adaptation to a particular social and historical context. Poor ethnic minority families have often had to compromise their values or ideals due to the harsh realities of their world.

BELIEFS

Wright, Watson, and Bell (1996) state that "beliefs are the lenses through which we view the world. Beliefs are the bedrock of our behavior and are the essence of our affect. Beliefs are the blueprints from which we construct our lives and intermingle them with the lives of others" (p. 3). The term *belief* has been used synonymously with attitude, explanation, premise, construct, assumption, preference, and values. Beliefs guide the individual's and family's actions (Wright & Leahey, 2000). Thus, beliefs and behaviors are intertwined with and connected to each other. The choices a family makes evolve from their beliefs, which in turn are evolved from their value system. A family's belief system is learned, is shared, and persists over time. Beliefs have deep social and cultural roots. A discussion of family beliefs about health and illness is presented in Chapter 16.

NORMS

Norms are patterns of behavior considered to be right in a given society and, as such, are based on the family's value system. They are also modal behaviors. In other words, norms prescribe the appropriate role behavior for each of the positions in the family and society and specify how reciprocal relations are to be maintained, as well as how role behavior may change with the changing ages of occupants of these positions (see Chapter 12).

FAMILY RULES

Family rules are a more specific reflection of the family values than are family norms. Rules refer to the specific regulations the family maintains as to what is acceptable behavior and what is not. The family rules, guided by more abstract values, provide the stability, commonality, and guidance family members need. Holman (1979) suggests that family rules form the family miniculture, the shared meanings that define the individual character of each family as different from all other families.

An example of how family rules express the value system by which the family operates is seen in some Latino families. The high value of familism among Latino families translates to the norm and family rule that members of the extended family are all part of the *"familia,"* and are to be treated as such. Values are also determinants of family rules about communication—perhaps what is discussed and not discussed and with whom. Recall the high value that respect for elders, especially fathers, has in some families, with a resultant family rule being to not openly challenge the father's decisions or actions.

Family rules are reflective of the family's level of functioning. Whall (1986b) corroborates this association by stating that in general "it is fair to say that dysfunctional families have dysfunctional rules since one begets the other" (p. 100).

DISPARITY IN VALUE SYSTEMS

DIVERSE SOCIAL VALUES

Conflicts inevitably exist between families and society because there are so many factors and experiences that serve to alter an individual's or a family's values and norms. Issues or unresolved conflicts are often present because traditional and emerging sets of norms exist simultaneously, both within and outside of the family. Within communities, certain groups and individuals resist emerging norms and cling vehemently to more traditional patterns, whereas other individuals and groups find traditional patterns unacceptable and adhere to a new set of norms and values. The result of this social change is that areas of major conflict arise. Although our society values its pluralism, where both traditional and emerging value systems and patterns can exist side by side, this social diversity played out in the family results in conflict and confusion. A very common family value issue concerns the meaning of marriage itself for the individuals involved. Traditionally, marriage has been viewed as sacred and binding; today, among those persons espousing emerging social values, marriage is increasingly viewed as merely a contract that can easily be voided when either or both parties have legitimate grievances.

CLASH OF VALUES BETWEEN DOMINANT CULTURE AND SUBCULTURE

Another common source of value conflict is the clash between the values of the dominant culture and a family's cultural reference group. When we consider the family as the mediating agent between the culture (or the wider society) and the individual, it follows that a basic incompatibility in values between the family's reference group and wider society generates certain value conflicts, which increase stress within the family as a system and also negatively affect family members. Larrabee (1973), a Cheyenne Indian, describes this clash of values and one of its effects:

> In trying to teach our young about themselves, we must tell them about the Indian values of compassion, respect for elders, sharing, and wisdom. We want our children to have these values and to know about them. When our children go to school and are told by the teacher that they must learn to be saving instead of sharing, the child becomes confused. This terrible conflict of values contributes to the high suicide rate among our youth.

The same observations about a clash in values is found in the literature about Asian-American parents who retain their traditional values and their children (particularly adolescents) who take on the American values of independence, individualism, and assertiveness. This is a commonly cited value conflict problem brought to counseling and discussed more in depth in Chapter 20 (Hong, 1996; Pedersen, Draguns, Lonner, & Trimble, 1996).

The findings of Cleveland and Longaker (1972) confirm the disruptive effects value conflicts have on the ethnic family. Based on extensive data collected from interviews, home visits, testing, and therapeutic sessions, they concluded that the emotional problems in the family members who were studied were a function of two processes: (1) a value conflict between the society the family resided in and the family itself, and (2) a culturally recurrent mode of self-disparagement linked to the failure of individuals to adjust to incompatible value orientations.

CLASH OF VALUES BETWEEN GENERATIONS

As mentioned previously, a third source of value conflict within families lies in generational differences in values. A family may be composed of several generations of individuals, each bringing to the family group his or her generationally based values. Value conflicts are inevitable when grandparents hold traditional values, when parents operate by a combination of traditional and emerging (progressive) values, and the children are influenced by emerging values. This conflict between generations is especially prevalent if the family household is an extended family or a family with adolescents. This generational clash of values is also magnified among first-generation immigrant families from non-Western countries (Hong & Ham, 1992).

DIFFERENCES BETWEEN THE FAMILY MEMBERS AND THE HEALTH CARE PROFESSIONAL

One of the primary stressors in relationships between health care workers and family clients is the social distancing created because of social class and/or cultural value differences. When the professional and the family do not possess the same basic beliefs and values, the results are often divergent goals, unclear communication, and interactional problems. As professionals working within the mainstream health care systems, nurses generally uphold the values of the dominant culture of which the health care system is a part. These are generally white, Anglo-Saxon, Protestant (WASP) values. Brink (1976) described the American nurses' value system thusly:

> The American nurse, educated in the United States, falls within the "Old Yankee" classification of value systems. American nurses are future-oriented, belong to a doing-oriented profession, are individualistic in decision-making, but lineally-oriented in the health institution, believe that disease is controllable, and view the human being as neither good nor evil, but ill. (pp. 63–64)

Additionally the average age of the traditional nurse is about 44. Value conflicts may arise when new nurses of the younger generation (generation x) interact with their peers (baby boomers) and with a rising client population of elderly patients.

This picture of health providers' having one common value orientation does not negate the reality that many nurses and nursing students come from diverse cultural and social class backgrounds and possess their own configuration of more particular values and goals, while also conforming to the central values of the health care system of which they are a part. Families, on the other hand, come from all walks of life and, more often than not, hold different values than the health care worker does. Because the class and cultural backgrounds of many clients differ from those of the health care professional, the possibility of value conflicts is present (Lauver, 1980).

VALUE CHANGES IN AMERICAN SOCIETY

Since the 1960s, the United States, as well as the world at large, has witnessed a profound revolution in ideas, values, and norms. Most of the literature suggests that the Civil Rights Movement marked the beginning of America's cultural revolution. Because of turbulent events in society and the family, a widening social stratification, a rise in poverty, a growth in consumerism and materialism (Lebey, 2001; Samuelson, 1986), globalization of our economy, and most recently the threats of terrorism, American cultural values are continually being shaped and modified. Although the family has been widely perceived as threatened by multiple societal events and concomitant value shifts, turning the tide back to "the good old traditional days" appears futile, in spite of fervent efforts by some fundamentalist and reactionary groups to do so.

Profound physical, social, and technological changes have also taken place. For example, in the last 200 years, the United States quadrupled in physical size and its population grew 52 times greater. We have gone from an overwhelmingly rural society to a highly urbanized nation. Whereas only 1 percent of Americans were high school graduates in 1800, 76 percent of Americans now graduate from high school. And more recently, the country changed from an overwhelmingly white, Anglo-American country to one with increasingly significant Asian, African-American, and Hispanic populations.

A number of authors (Aldous, 1996; Koten, 1987; Glick, 1989; Schwartz, 1987; Yankelovich & Gurin, 1989) have suggested that the vitality of the traditional values (the Protestant ethic, essentially) has declined. Surveys of Americans and their values and lifestyles indicate that Americans, particularly middle-class Americans, are a very heterogeneous group today. There is no one overarching core value orientation today like there was in the 1960s and 1970s. Koten of the *Wall Street Journal* agrees that there is no longer one set of values to which the middle class subscribes. "There are fewer things that everybody wants and fewer things that everyone feels compelled to do" (p. 25).

Shifting values have fueled institutional changes throughout society. Both Family Service America (1984) and Scanzoni (1987) describe surveys in which Americans, according to the values they reported, were divided into three groups. At one end of the continuum were the "traditionalists," those who espoused traditional values, such as preserving the good old days, duty, obligation, and hard work. At the other end of the continuum were the "new wave," the "progressives," those espousing emerging values of self-fulfillment, freedom, and individualism over authority. The middle-of-the-continuum group was composed of the vast majority of Americans. They val-

ued some of the old and some of the new values and goals. Scanzoni reports that in one national survey 20 percent were traditionalists and another 20 percent new wavers or progressives, while 60 percent were middle-of-the-roaders. Most sociologists explain that our values are in a state of flux or transition. The increasing proportion of families that are either single-parent, blended, or cohabiting families, coupled with the widespread acceptance of divorce, lends evidence to the shifting from traditional, conventional values to individualistic, utilitarian values (Glick, 1989; Teachman, Tedrow, & Crowder, 2001).

Despite the continual clash between the new and traditional values and the resultant modification in values and priorities, a substantial amount of continuity in the American value system has, however, prevailed. A discussion of American society's core value orientation, coupled with the recent value shifts, provides the foundations for understanding our primary family values today. Some of these values are of lesser importance today and others are of greater importance. A discussion of this shift in priorities follows.

MAJOR VALUE ORIENTATIONS

In spite of the declining state of the secularized Protestant ethic and the existence of other strongly conflicting values, a cluster of core values still molds and shapes, to a varying degree, American society, and thus also shapes family life and the behavior of health care professionals. (See Table 13–1 for a listing of America's core values.)

PRODUCTIVITY/INDIVIDUAL ACHIEVEMENT

Individual achievement and productivity have been consistently identified as key traditional values in this society (D'Antonio, 1983; McKinley, 1964; Williams, 1960). Success and achievement, the reputed outcomes of being productive, are corollary social values (Stewart & Bennett, 1991). In the middle class, extensive emphasis is placed on personal achievement, especially occupational achievement. This focus can cause interpersonal and familial conflict when work achievement must compete against a concurrent

TABLE 13–1

AMERICA'S CORE VALUES

- Productivity/Individual achievement
- Individualism
- Materialism/The consumption ethic
- The work ethic
- Education
- Equality
- Progress and mastery over the environment
- Future time orientation
- Efficiency, orderliness, and practicality
- Rationality
- Quality of life and maintaining health
- Tolerance of diversity

value that the individual holds regarding the role he or she must fulfill within the family (Kaufman & Uhlenberg, 2000). Carlson and Kacmark (2000) found that individuals who valued work over family experienced greater family interference with their work and less family satisfaction.

Because so much apprehension surrounds the individual's choice of occupational goals, there is often a postponement in selecting one's career. Many Americans also have not learned how to relax and enjoy life, as seen by their anxious preoccupation with activity and productiveness and the enormous numbers of people suffering from stress-related illnesses. Another behavioral consequence of our achievement value is its effects on individuals who do not have the required position and role adequacy for productiveness. For those people, the emphasis on achievement often leads to a lack of goals and/or to alienation.

In order for a value to continue to mold a person's goals and behavior, a powerful system of social sanctions and rewards must be present. According to McKinley (1964), there are four major rewards available to the "successful," which are referred to as the

"American Dream": material possessions, interpersonal approval and status, control over others, and control over self (autonomy).

Kluckholm (1976) refers to the normative interpersonal behavior valued in American society, or its national character, as being exemplified in the "doing orientation." Its most distinctive feature is its demand for action in terms of accomplishment and in accord with external (societal) standards. The person who "gets things done" is seen as productive. The person who finds ways to do something and is the rational problem solver is much esteemed. Along with "doing" is a dominant value of keeping busy; "Idle hands are the devil's workshop" (Stewart & Bennett, 1991).

Various types of interpersonal sanctions are employed against those individuals who are "unproductive," including the unemployed, those on welfare, or those who choose values markedly different from society's values. These responses range from gossip, laughter, and ridicule to social ostracism, isolation, or rejection. Members of society will vary their reactions depending on the society's evaluations of where the responsibility for unproductiveness lies and how important the deviation is. As a result of society's disapproval, many times the individual adopts those same attitudes toward himself or herself (i.e., low self-esteem, lack of self-worth), a phenomenon referred to as "the self-fulfilling prophecy."

In middle-class and affluent families, the focus on productivity and individual achievement has extended from the adults in the family to their children. Tofler and DiGeronimo (2000) state "this generation of parents wants not only to encourage and protect but also to push, push, and shove their children to the front of the line" (p. xvii). Parents are consumed with raising high-achieving children and are taking the fun out of childhood. Children are removed from neighborhood playgrounds to be placed in music classes, organized sports, SAT preparation classes, and modeling competitions. Tofler and DiGeronimo (2000) assert that "pushing children to be the very best has great potential for detriment to the healthy person inside the child" (p. 9). As parents encourage high achievement in their children, the difficulty becomes identifying and defining the difference between encouragement and exploitation, and between support and the pursuits of a distorted parenting model. When the external benefits of the child's achievement (fame, financial gain, social recognition, respect) become primary goals for the adult, then the stage is set for toxic and detrimental outcomes to the child and to his or her development over time. Table 13–2 summarizes guidelines that can be used to keep parental involvement with high-achieving children within the normal and supportive boundaries.

TABLE 13–2

GUIDELINES FOR PARENTAL SUPPORT OF HIGH-ACHIEVING CHILDREN

- Parents should acknowledge the child as a unique individual with his or her own separate physical and psychological attributes.

- Parents should be able to recognize the child's psychological and physical needs and then make and prioritize decisions based on these requirements rather than on their own wishes, ambitions, and fantasies.

- Parents should be able to acknowledge and distinguish between their own feelings of anger and disappointment (as well as their pride and pleasure) and the child's feelings; they should not project their own feelings onto the child.

- Children should never feel that parental love is contingent on winning or excelling in any one educational, sporting, career, or social endeavor.

- Parents must retain the power to make parental decisions. It is crucial that parents make tough—even courageous and unpopular—but developmentally appropriate, responsible judgments for the child.

- Parents should encourage developmentally appropriate independence, autonomy, and decision-making skills in their children. They should not, however, hide behind that independence when important, even critical, decisions are made.

- Social and financial benefits of the child's achievements should be a dividend rather than a primary (or even a disguised primary) goal for the adult.

Source: Adapted from Tofler & DiGeronimo (2000).

INDIVIDUALISM

In the numerous writings about value changes in American society and the family, there is agreement about the rising importance of individualism today (Bellah, Madsen, Sullivan, Swidler, & Tipton, 1986; Glick, 1989; Orthner, 1995; Schwartz, 1987). According to Lesthaeghe (1983), individual freedom of choice is one of our central social values in Western societies. The trend toward more individualism and independence and away from familism and collectivism has weakened but not killed the ideal of permanence in marriage. This value trend has also caused a shift from a child-centered to a self-centered culture (Elkind, 1994). This transformation means that people are becoming less firmly rooted in the traditional institutions of family, community, and organized religion and more committed to individual goal attainment—unfettered by traditional obligations (Orthner; Rossi, 1986). Based on demographic trends, other authors also emphasize that people in Western societies are becoming "averse to long-term commitments and increasingly focused on individual autonomy and detachment." (Rossi, p. 123). Some authors (Elkind; Popenoe, 1995) believe that the individualistic trend has gone too far for the good of society, the family, and the individual. They state that until recently, there has been a balance between helping community and family (collectivism) and helping oneself. This balance has become lopsided as individuals become more focused on their own pursuits.

Individualism is the reverse of the traditional Christian doctrine of the ethic of reciprocity in which "you are your brother's keeper," or of familism, where family needs take precedence over family members' needs. Individualism suggests that every person has to make it on his or her own merits. A large survey conducted by Bellah and associates (1986) confirmed the centrality of personal autonomy and individualism in the United States.

Individualism also involves the associated values of self-reliance and self-responsibility. The prevalent belief remains that "strong" persons can control their own lives and, by that reasoning, it must follow that lack of such control is evidence of the person's own weakness. Self-fulfillment is another value closely associated with individualism.

Many families who belong to other ethnic groups do not share this same value of individualism (Sillars,

1995). Many of these families have a familistic orientation, whereby there is much sharing and interdependency between extended family members. In highly familistic cultures, an individual's identity and place in society may be defined more by family than by individual achievement (Sillars).

MATERIALISM/THE CONSUMPTION ETHIC

The possession of money and goods is not only an essential reward for being productive, but is also a central value of society in and of itself. This value is referred to as materialism (Stewart & Bennett, 1991). Samuelson (1986) writes about "the discovery of money" and society's increasing preoccupation with wealth as a measure of achievement. Money and wealth are both the foundation for power and prestige and the primary symbol of success and achievement. Money has been consecrated as a value over and above its use in procuring goods and services or for its enhancement of power. Society, through its major institutions, reinforces this cultural emphasis except perhaps among the lower class. These institutions join to provide the disciplining and training required for an individual to retain this elusive goal and to be properly motivated by the promise of gratification.

Along with materialism has come a relaxation of prohibitions against expressiveness and hedonism (Orthner, 1995). In a society in which the consumption of goods has become a fundamental value, people are enjoined to cease being ascetic and self-denying and to abandon guilt about spending and expressing their pleasure impulses. Political leaders encourage Americans to spend, spend, spend and thus keep the economy healthy.

The moral values of thriftiness and saving were parts of the Protestant ethic. As with other traditional values, their importance arose partly from the short supply of material goods and money that existed in the past. In fact, often the ability to save and conserve was critical to survival.

In more recent times, Americans seem to have entirely disregarded these values (except perhaps by members of the older generation) as evidenced by our habits of acquiring vast goods and constantly replacing material items. Toffler (1970) calls this "planned obsolescence." We have acted as if there

were a limitless supply of goods and resources. This consumption ethic has now largely replaced the thrift ethic, and the "put-away" society has become the "throw-away" society (Inkeles, 1977). In our current technocratic society, many goods are so inexpensive that replacement is viewed as cheaper than repair.

We may now be seeing a modest swing back to "conservation" goals, however. There is a noticeable attitudinal change among some Americans that our habits of waste and enormous consumption of the world's resources must be altered. More concern is voiced about ecology, dwindling resources, environmental impact, and the impact of globilization on people and the environment. In spite of these encouraging signs, however, Americans continue to consume goods and resources at increasingly high levels.

THE WORK ETHIC

The rule of "He who does not work should not eat" expressed the deadly struggle of the early settlement and frontier days in our country and explains the primacy of this ethic due to the objective conditions of want that existed historically. As part of Puritanism and the Protestant ethic, however, work literally became an end in itself, not the means to an end. Americans were obsessive about work, and even today we meet individuals who are "workaholics." Although the work ethic has lost much of its potency today, it is still part of our dominant culture and is still upheld by our societal institutions (Stewart & Bennett, 1991). The success of modern industrial states remains dependent on "mean and lean" businesses and work-oriented individuals.

According to Inkeles (1977) and Glick (1989), in the 1960s and 1970s, the ethic of hard work was eroding quickly. Increasing numbers of Americans during that period considered the most important attributes of a job to be high pay and short hours, instead of the intrinsic importance of the work itself, or of a promise of advancement. Yankelovich and Gurin (1989), surveyors of American values, noted a change in this trend in the 1980s. They observed many Americans returning to a view of the workplace as a site for self-expression of competence, creativity, and satisfaction. A resurgence in entrepreneurship in the 1990s accompanies the renaissance of the work ethic.

The scarcity of work and jobs has certainly augmented the return of the work ethic. Even if the work ethic is not the central overriding value today that it was in the past, it remains strong, primarily because of its basic tie to the value of materialism and the consumer ethic. People value work because of the financial gains associated with that work.

Recent times are characterized by an almost constant sense of insecurity in relation to work. Ryan (1999) states that nearly half the population worries that someone in their household will be out of work. Parents no longer expect their children to have a higher standard of living than themselves, despite the fact that those children are drawing in more income and working more hours than they did. Many families have experienced a work layoff, or expect large scale layoffs to be a permanent part of the modern economy (Ryan). Despite U.S. governmental interventions to maintain a steady economy, external factors such as terrorist attacks on American soil and a weakening global economy threaten citizens' ability to find gainful employment. Besides fear of losing a job, changes in the American work culture have contibuted to several other stressors which impact the family system. These include:

- Lowering of worker compensation (decline in health benefits and retirement options) families

- Conversion of full time positions to part time and temporary positions that have no benefits

- Increased use of overtime, rotating shifts, and longer shifts

These stressors create conditions in which family members are fearful of missing work to care for children, reluctant to change jobs (even if they dislike the work) for fear of losing benefits, and sacrificing time with the family in order to manage the extra hours they are being required to put in on their job (Ryan, 1999).

EDUCATION

Education is seen by the middle class as the means to achieve productivity and to "get ahead." The value placed on education is closely aligned with the work ethic, materialism, individualism, and progress. Although education is much more emphasized among the middle and upper classes, its value has also become more prominent within the working class (Inkeles, 1977) and many immigrant families.

Unfortunately, while Americans may hold dear the idea that every child deserves the opportunity to receive a good education, many educators believe that where academic achievement is concerned, we are a second-rate nation (Bempechat, 2000). Demographic, societal, and economic changes that took place from the 1960s through the 1990s have led to an increased number of children who are at risk for school failure and behavior problems (e.g., drug and alcohol abuse, promiscuity). Factors that contribute to this decline in academic performance include poverty, single parenthood, parents with low levels of education, limited English proficiency, and a fear of making children feel negative about themselves if we do not academically promote them (despite their actual academic abilities). Children are constantly entertained from birth by television, videos, computer games, and the Internet. They are not socialized to seek information or to learn on their own, despite the fact that there is a trend toward self-directed learners and Web-based education. Bempechat believes that we are a nation that does not value academic excellence. Winning basketball players are given more acclaim (and financial rewards) than are exemplary students, writers, or mathematicians. Children are disciplined by their coaches for missing a practice, while parents are complaining that children should not be required to do homework. Today's challenge is to rethink education while at the same time accommodate the growing desire to create children who are "well-rounded." We need to acknowledge that children need opportunities to grow and express themselves in a variety of ways, while still putting these activities in a context that places academic achievement firmly at the top of every family's list of priorities (Bempechat).

EQUALITY

The value of equality has become more important in American society than it was in the past (Stewart & Bennett, 1991), although it is only a partially realized value. The dominant culture of the United States values equality in personal relationships much more than many other cultures do. Antiauthoritarianism is still a very important characteristic of present-day American society. Children express dissatisfaction when their parents use arbitrary or coercive power, feelings that are derived from the family values favoring egalitarianism, as well as expectations resulting from parents fostering participation, independence, and autonomy.

On the other hand, a hierarchical and authoritarian emphasis exists in large-scale organizations. Individual achievement and status hold greater value than equality does. Running through the whole of our society is the thread of nonegalitarian beliefs and practices concerning interpersonal relations with people of different ethnic groupings and women. Recurring manifestations of prejudice and bigotry are still ongoing problems for much of our population.

Smelzer and Halpern (1978) clearly point out the clash between individualism/individual achievement and equality. If the priority in the society is on individual achievement, this produces greater inequality in the society, which then leads to a call for equality. Prioritizing equality generates a counterreaction as well. The fact that these values are inherently "at odds with each other" is not so surprising—what is surprising, however, are the oscillations that have occurred in recent times concerning the saliency of these two competing values or cultural themes (Smelzer & Halpern). During the 1960s and early 1970s, equality was prioritized, as seen in the liberal ideas and programs of the "Great Society," the Peace Corps, and affirmative action and civil rights programs. Beginning in the late 1970s, the pendulum swung back again—with a dismantlement of programs that fostered the value of equality, and a return to the more conservative values of achievement and individualism. A return to more conservative values of achievement and individualism can be seen in the recent legislative fights over affirmative action and welfare reform.

In spite of the resurgence of conservativism, individualism, and achievement values, equality still is recognized as a central cultural value. The importance of equality is closely linked with an increasing tolerance of diversity and the growing tendency to pursue individualistic personal goals, where freedom, independence, and autonomy, as well as greater expression of feelings, are paramount. There is renewed interest in social justice and community

action as reflected in texts of social action research and participatory research paradigm.

The rise of egalitarianism is reflected in American family life. According to the noted historian Toynbee (1955), the most vital revolution of our time has been the emancipation of women, because women's emancipation affects family life by moving marital relationships closer to equality. A men's movement has followed suit, encouraging men to go beyond their occupations in defining their male identity. This male emancipation encourages reinvestment in families, homes, and communities, and has led to an increasing number of men taking on the homemaker role as their wives particpate full time in the labor force (Zimmerman, Northen, & Seng, 1999). In addition to the women's movement and the affirmative action programs, there has been considerable progress in protecting the rights of the mentally ill and of children. These legislative trends demonstrate the continued potency of equality as a value (Stein, 1997).

In the health care field, the value of, and commitment to, equality is seen in the recurring concerns about equal access to health care for all persons (universal coverage). This value, though, runs into competition with the value of individual freedom of choice. As health care reforms occur, the fight between these two often opposing values becomes evident.

PROGRESS AND MASTERY OVER THE ENVIRONMENT

Kluckholm (1976) refers to this value orientation as involving the "man–nature relationship issue"—for example, whether human beings are viewed as (1) subjugated to nature, (2) as part of nature, or (3) as dominant over nature. Traditional Spanish-American culture in the American Southwest illustrates the first relationship. To the rural, traditional rancher in the Southwest in the past, there was little or nothing that could be done if a storm damaged range lands or disease destroyed flocks. He or she simply accepted these events as inevitable. This fatalistic attitude may also be found in dealing with illness and death in a statement such as, "if it is the Lord's will that I die, I shall die" (p. 69).

The second relationship, in which humans and nature are viewed as aspects of a harmonious whole, is found in many of the North American Indian tribes and traditional Chinese cultures.

The dominant American culture, however, conceptualizes the man–nature relationship as being that of humans against, or over, nature (Stewart & Bennett, 1991). Natural forces are seen as things to be overcome, mastered, and utilized by people. Americans build bridges, blast through mountains, create lakes and massive dams, and exploit all of nature's resources—all to serve humankind. The conflict between this "lord of nature" value as opposed to the value of harmony plays out in conflicts between environmentalists, who seek to protect endangered species and to preserve natural resources, and developers interested in economic growth.

It is this general attitude of being able to solve any problem and to overcome seemingly impossible obstacles that is referred to as progressiveness. Change is seen as progress or going forward (Stewart & Bennett, 1991), even though it sometimes seems that the pendulum swings backward. Innovativeness and openness to new experiences is highly valued, as is optimism or confidence that striving and change are positive (Inkeles, 1977).

FUTURE TIME ORIENTATION

All societies must deal with three time dimensions—past, present, and future. All cultures have some conception of the past, all have a present, and all give attention to the future time dimension. They vary, however, in the emphasis they place on each dimension. The time orientation in the United States is toward the discernible future (Daly, 1996; Stewart & Bennett, 1991). For example, Kluckholm (1976) and Murillo (1976) report that in contrast to Americans, unacculturated Mexican-Americans are more present oriented. Historically, China and Japan, on the other hand, were societies that put their main emphasis on the past. Ancestor worship and strong family traditions were both expressions of this time orientation. Many modern European countries, such as England, have also tended to stress the past more than America does.

Most middle-class Americans, regardless of ethnic heritage, place their emphasis on the future (Tripp-Reimer & Lively, 1988), which we anticipate optimistically will be "bigger and better." Past ways are considered "old fashioned." The value put on the future correlates closely with the value on change and progress. A Frenchman, Servan-Schreiber, wrote, "We Europeans continue to suffer progress while Americans pursue it, welcome it and adapt to it" (Inkeles, 1977, p. 1). A more recent text, "Who Moved My Cheese?" stresses that if you do not change, you may become extinct (Johnson, 1998).

EFFICIENCY, ORDERLINESS, AND PRACTICALITY

In frontier society, being practical—learning to improvise and make the best out of one's resources—was tied to survival. Individuals and families concentrated on obtainable goals in the immediate situation—"If it works, it must be good." Today, this same kind of pragmatism views technical advances with great appreciation, especially those resulting in savings of time and manpower—after all, "time is money."

Science is highly valued as an endeavor through which efficiency, practicality, and progress can be achieved. The way we treat food and the manner in which we consume it are expressions of values we hold. Seventy percent of households today have microwave ovens and 40 percent have personal computers (Weiss, 2000). These figures suggest that we have a strong faith in the efficacy of technology, and that we appreciate the speed at which these machines work and, therefore, save us time.

RATIONALITY

Rationality and reason are highly valued in our society (Herberg, 1995). In order to be efficient, orderly, progressive, productive, and practical, one must be rational and be able to react by problem solving and by logically thinking through one's situation and goals. Foresight, deliberate planning, allocation of resources in the most efficient way, and long-term gratification are necessary. Rationality became a prime value during the Enlightenment in the late 1700s and early 1800s. Science was a natural outgrowth of this rational philosophy, because it depends on the same logical cognitive approach to the world and its problems. Applied science is highly esteemed in the dominant culture as a tool for controlling nature and the environment. This value has led to the "rational scientific man" becoming the exemplar of our society.

By contrast, women have historically been stereotyped with the opposite of these desirable attributes; women have been deemed irrational, illogical, emotional, and intuitive. This stereotype is diminishing as women move into cognitively challenging fields and succeed admirably. In addition, there is growing attention to the validity of a variety of "ways of knowing" that are more reflective of women's understanding. These different viewpoints provide a wider repertoire for solutions to life issues, and are also reflected in greater respect for qualitative methods in research, counterbalancing scientific methods grounded in rational traditions.

QUALITY OF LIFE AND MAINTAINING HEALTH

People today are becoming increasingly interested in making qualitative changes in their lives. These include such lifestyle improvements among adults as curtailing smoking, making dietary changes, and partaking in self-help stress reduction and other mental health programs. People are also making environmental alterations in their lives, such as moving from city and suburbia to small towns and rural environments, and participating in creative and leisure endeavors. All these activities signify a basic modification of values to a more introspective orientation where personal and familial happiness and personal independence in decision making have greater priority. While it is difficult to measure how highly health is valued and how widespread this shift is, available evidence suggests that maintaining health is becoming a major value within the American hierarchy of values (Harris, 1984; Institute of Medicine, 2000; Yankelovich & Gurin, 1989). This is especially true when it comes to valuing public health measures, such as immunizations and clean, safe water supplies (Stewart & Bennett, 1991). The importance of this value is probably influenced not only by social class, but also by age and ethnicity.

Additionally, most families value being an active and equal participant in their health care decisions as opposed to being a passive recipient of health care interventions. Patients' rights and advocacy for all family members (including children) to have a voice in their health care decision making are tenets being supported by politicians, by institutional policy makers, and by professional organizations (McAiley, Hudson-Barr, Gunning, & Rowbottom, 2000). The advent of a revised Patient's Bill of Rights and the use of advance directives are two examples of the united efforts to ensure that families have a voice in the decision-making process that affect the health of their members. Despite these activities, the health care community continues to struggle with an image of being uncaring and uncommunicative with the families they serve (Levine & Zuckerman, 2000). The perception is that as long as the family agrees with the medical advice, harmony prevails. When the family disagrees or raises concerns of their own, conflict can occur. Levine and Zuckerman recommend that to support the values of both the health care provider and the family we move toward an ethic of accommodation. That is, health care providers continue to work toward family-sensitive policies and practices. This can be achieved by ensuring that health care providers have an understanding of family dynamics and illness and that the participants agree to establish a partnership that respects and values open communication and mutual decision making as the foundation of their relationship.

TOLERANCE OF DIVERSITY

A notable change toward greater tolerance for diversity continues to emerge as a core value of American citizens. Diversity within families means that there are different types of families who use a multitude of ways to meet their needs for reproduction, cohabitation, nurturance, economic cooperation, affection, protection and meaning (Allen, Fine, & Demo, 2000). Diversity also extends to different cultures, religious beliefs and views of male/female rights in society. Perhaps due to the civil rights and antiwar movements of the 1960s and/or because of the increasing number of minorities in the United States, a greater tolerance of diversity has been noted (Boulding, 1976; Koten, 1987; Rubin, 1999).

Weaver (1976) states that the major and most significant result of the civil rights movement, the women's movement, and growing ethnic consciousness has been the growth of questioning of cultural assumptions held by Americans for generations, such as the myth of the melting pot. "Rather than having values of a subcultural group dissipated and absorbed by the dominant culture, these groups have undermined the values and assumptions of the dominant culture" (p. 123).

Another myth or assumption that is being challenged is the notion that the white middle-class family ideal popularized by the sitcoms in the 1950s was the historical norm for most families, and that diversity in our family forms and structures is a recent phenomenon. The reality is that there has never been a single family model in the United States and change has been a constant feature of every kind of family (Coontz, Parson, & Raley, 1999). For instance, Native American family arrangements of the past ranged from simple monogomy (usually with divorce rights) to various forms of multiple marriages. The African-American cultural legacy is one of extended-kin networks. The distinct *barrio* culture among Hispanic families has been present since Mexicans began migrating to America. These examples remind us that change in family life and diversity in family life have been constants in American history (Coontz, Parson, & Raley).

FAMILY VALUES

The family's value system is thought to be heavily influenced by the society's core values, as well as by the values of the family's subcultural and other reference groups. Family changes in values and norms are very much connected to, and rooted in, fundamental shifts in the values and norms in North American society (Orthner, 1995).

Basic family values embedded in our culture have not changed dramatically, according to Orthner (1995), but our family norms and rules guiding family behavior have. Norms are guidelines for behavior and both norms and family rules, particularly those associated with family roles, have been relaxed or lost over the past several decades. Norms related to sexual behavior and marriage, as well as those linking marriage and pregnancy have also changed. Today, with traditional family roles changing, most men and women are uncertain of what is expected of them in their family roles (Orthner).

David Elkind (1994), a renowned child psychologist, holds a more gloomy view about the shift in values and norms in the American family than does

Orthner (1995), a sociologist. In Elkind's analysis of how the family has been impacted by societal changes, he sees that an imbalance in family values has taken place—as society emphasizes the importance of individualism and individual achievement (as seen in descriptions of recent generations being the "me generation").

Elkind calls the postmodern family the "permeable family," a family that is more open, more fluid, more flexible, more vulnerable to outside pressures, and not as protective of children. In this permeable family, each family member (as soon is he or she is able) is supposed to be "independent, competent, achievement-oriented, and able to go it alone" (Elkind, 1994, p. 75). Although parents in permeable families have more personal freedom and lifestyle choices to pursue their own individual interests, their children suffer. Hence, there is an imbalance in values, favoring individualism over family togetherness and familism. The postmodern family is individual centered, not child centered. Elkind points to the change in family forms as evidence of the widespread permeable family. Single-parent families were the fastest growing family structure in America in the 1990s, with more couples choosing divorce or opting not to marry when pregnancy occurs. We have also seen a growth in blended families due to the increasing divorce rate and subsequent remarriage.

Nevertheless, because families have special functions within the larger societal context, they subscribe to a combination of certain values that guide family life. Families create their own family miniculture or family paradigm—an enduring structure of shared beliefs, convictions, and assumptions about the social world (Reiss, 1981; Fitzpatrick & Ritchie, 1993). These shared beliefs are largely based on the family's past experiences. Families develop their own paradigm as an extension of how they deal with hardships and crisis. Family belief systems can have a more internal locus of control (mastery over nature) or external locus of control (situations are governed by external factors beyond the family's control) (Rolland, 1988, 1993).

A family's value and belief system shapes its patterns of behavior toward the health problems that they face. Family values and beliefs shape the views families have of stressful situations and of how they should respond to them. In other words, family beliefs and values determine how a family will cope with health and other stressors. "A family's beliefs about mastery strongly affect the nature of its relationship to an illness and to the health care system" (Rolland, 1993, p. 464). A family with a mastery orientation may believe it can control and solve almost every problem it faces. In this case, the family would use more active, assertive coping strategies, such as seeking out new information or community resources to resolve or control the problem. Conversely, a family less oriented toward mastery and control and more oriented toward passive acceptance may believe in accepting whatever happens. They may cope by resigning themselves to God's will, or to fate. Often, such families view disease progression and outcomes as a matter of chance and tend to establish marginal relationships with health professionals (Rolland, 1988). These families are often called "fatalistic" (Boss, 1988). Fatalism needs to be distinguished from acceptance, according to Boss. Fatalism is the belief that everything is predetermined by a higher power or "powerful others." The family feels powerless to change what is preordained to happen. Families that are fatalistic are those that because of their cultural, socioeconomic, and environmental conditioning, feel a sense of powerlessness to change the course of events.

In situations that are hopeless, with loss inevitable and control impossible, the mastery-oriented and fatalistically oriented families typically behave quite differently. The mastery-oriented family will be less likely to give up hope, even with terminal illness, but will experience much more stress than the fatalistically oriented family, which will accept the situation using strength they receive from "passive forbearance," seeking peace and serenity and perhaps seeking strength from prayer and meditation.

❧MAJOR VARIABLES AFFECTING FAMILY VALUES

There are several important variables or factors that greatly influence whether a family assimilates the "major value orientation" of American society, or whether differences in priorities and values or divergent norms operate. Three important variables are the family's social class and ethnicity (both of which are discussed in Chapter 8) and the family living arrangement or structure (e.g., divorced families, gay and lesbian families) (Creed, 2000; Lebey, 2001). Other important variables include a family's degree of acculturation to the dominant culture, generational differences, geographical location, and familial and personal idiosyncrasies.

FAMILY'S SOCIOECONOMIC STATUS

Because a family's socioeconomic status shapes the family lifestyle, it also is a powerful factor in family values. The dominant American core values are in large part middle-class values. Poor families may share American dominant values such as productivity and work, but will be unable to achieve what they value because of their limited resources (the difference between the ideal and the real as previously mentioned). Relative to the time dimension, poor families are likely to be more present-time oriented than the middle class. Among some poor families, for example, time and appointments are perceived as "flexible"; that is, events will start when everyone involved arrives. Middle-class families, in comparison, hold the dominant time value and expect punctuality and good time-management skills. These families are typically future oriented and are therefore likely to save and plan for the future (Giger & Davidhizar, 1999).

FAMILY'S ETHNICITY AND ACCULTURATION

Ethnic background makes a major difference in how important each of the core American values are to a family. For instance, Irish-American families place a high value on independence. Irish culture is replete with many sayings that illustrate the importance of this value. "You've made your bed, now lie in it" tells a married family member not to bring his or her problems home to the parent. In contrast, the Italian-American family could hardly imagine this being uttered (Foley, 1986). In the Chinese culture, group cohesiveness, social deference, obedience, and social order are valued. Chinese-American parents have been traditionally concerned that their children's behavior be culturally appropriate and desirable. Children are taught to listen to parents and elders and to follow the parents' guidelines without any objection (Xiao, 1999). Table 13–3 provides a description of core values of several ethnic groups.

A family's degree of acculturation to dominant cultural values also varies widely. The more acculturated the family members, the more they subscribe to modern American core values.

GEOGRAPHICAL LOCATION (URBAN, SUBURBAN, OR RURAL)

Whether a family resides (or has resided for a long period of time) in a rural, urban, or suburban community also plays a significant role in shaping their values. In terms of country versus city residence, rural dwellers tend to be more traditional and conservative than their urban or suburban counterparts. Suburban communities are primarily residential and

---

TABLE 13–3

CORE VALUES OF SELECTED CULTURALLY DIVERSE, TRADITIONALLY ORIENTED FAMILIES

- Irish-American: Independence, strong religious orientation, highly verbal, humor, sociability

- American Indian: Living in harmony with nature, spiritual inspiration, folk healing, respect for elders, authority, and children, collectivism (family and tribe), ethnic pride

- Italian-American: Familism, traditional male–female roles, loyalty through personal relationships

- Jewish Americans: Value education, success, family, and community connections; encouragement of children; commitment to democratic principles

- African-Americans: Strong bonds and support from kin and friendship, flexibility in family roles, strong religious commitment and participation

- Asian-Americans: Respect for elders, familism, harmony and interdependence in relationships, filial piety, saving face, ancestor worship, respect for authority, education and achievement orientation

- Asian Indians: Purity, sacrifice, passivity, spirituality

- Latinos: Familism, respect for authority and elders, strong religious orientation, people valued for their character rather than their success, greater present-orientation

---

Sources: Billingsley (1992), Harrison et al. (1994), Herberg (1995), Ho (1992), McGoldrick (1993, 1996), Stauffer (1995). (Also see Chapters 18–20 of this text.)

---

middle class, and usually espouse more middle-class urban cultural values. In contrast, urban, inner-city populations are diverse, generally containing families from the whole social class spectrum, as well as families from various ethnic and racial groups; thus, urban families usually show a greater diversity of values, although generally tending to hold more liberal social and political views.

Marketers have used the concept of "clusters" to define and identify the shared lifestyles of American families in order to target consumers of their products and services. Weiss (1988, 2000) describes neighborhood clusters, which are used by corporations, political parties, and religious groups (Table 13–4). These clusters, or neighborhood types, are based on a target marketing system developed by the Claritas Corporation. Data from the U.S. Census Bureau and a host of consumer surveys and public opinion polls were all analyzed to identify the values shared by groups of families who come from similar demographic segments of the United States. Americans cluster themselves by income, age, education, values, and political ideology in neighborhoods that repeat themselves around the country. The premise underlying this clustering strategy is that where you live determines how you live. Finances, education, and a host of other socioeconomic factors can have a deep impact upon how the family members express their values, and upon how they are catagorized by advertisers, politicians, and religious groups in relation to their presumed values.

GENERATIONAL DIFFERENCES

Another variable influencing the values and norms of a family is which generation(s) its members belong to. There are "generational" value systems in the United States. Most core values are instilled at an early age by parents (Lustig, 1988). Yet, core values are also altered by society's value shifts. For instance, certain values were predominant when persons were in their early adulthood years in the 1950s. These individuals are now most likely in the phase of retirement/aging or the contracting family phase, and they retain many of their traditional work-oriented Protestant ethic values (values that have more potency in their lives than for younger adults today). McLeod and Cooper (1996) and Slater (1970) illustrate the drastic differences in

TABLE 13—4

AMERICA'S NEIGHBORHOOD TYPES

CLUSTER	DEMOGRAPHIC SNAPSHOT	PRIMARY AGE GROUP	MEDIAN HOUSE-HOLD INCOME (2000)	% OF U.S. HOUSE-HOLDS
Blue Blood Estates	Elite super-rich families	35–54	$113,000	.8
Winner's Circle	Executive suburban families	35–64	80,600	1.9
Country Squires	Elite exurban families	35–54	75,600	1.0
Kids & Cul-de-Sacs	Upscale urban families	35–54	61,600	3.0
Money & Brains	Sophisticated townhouse couples	45–64	59,000	1.1
Second City Elite	Upscale executive families	35–64	58,800	1.7
Urban Gold Coast	Elite urban singles and couples	Mixed	58,300	.5
Executive Suites	Upscale white-collar couples	25–44	58,000	1.2
Pools & Patios	Established empty-nesters	45–64, 65+	58,000	1.9
God's Country	Executive exurban families	35–54	57,500	2.7
Upward Bound	Young upscale white-collar families	25–44	54,500	2.0
Young Literati	Upscale urban singles and couples	25–44	52,100	1.0
American Dreams	Established urban immigrant families	35–54	51,700	1.4
Greenbelt Families	Young middle-class town families	24–44	46,700	.9
Big Fish, Small Pond	Small-town executive families	35–54	46,000	1.9
Boomers & Babies	Young white-collar suburban families	25–44	46,000	1.3
Big Sky Families	Midscale couples, kids, and farmland	35–54	45,200	1.5
New Empty Nests	Upscale suburban fringe couples	45–64, 65+	45,100	1.8
Young Influentials	Upwardly mobile singles and couples	Under 24	44,100	1.1
Blue-Chip Blues	Upscale blue-collar families	35–64	41,700	2.2
Suburban Sprawl	Young suburban townhouse couples	Under 24, 25–34	41,000	1.8
New Homesteaders	Young middle-class families	35–44, 45–54	38,800	2.0
Middleburg Managers	Midlevel white-collar couples	55+	37,800	1.5
Middle America	Midscale families in midsize towns	25–44	37,300	1.3
Gray Power	Affluent retirees in suburban cities	55–64, 65+	36,300	2.0
River City, USA	Middle-class rural families	35–54	35,700	2.0
Urban Achievers	Midlevel white-collar urban couples	25–34, 65+	35,600	1.6
Big City Blend	Middle-income immigrant families	25–54	35,500	1.0
New Eco-topia	Rural white- or blue-collar and farm families	35–64, 65+	35,300	1.0

(continued)

TABLE 13–4 *(CONTINUED)*

AMERICA'S NEIGHBORHOOD TYPES

CLUSTER	DEMOGRAPHIC SNAPSHOT	PRIMARY AGE GROUP	MEDIAN HOUSE- HOLD INCOME (2000)	% OF U.S. HOUSE- HOLDS
Red, White, & Blues	Small town blue-collar families	35–64	34,800	2.0
Bohemian Mix	Bohemian singles and couples	Under 24, 25–34	33,700	1.7
Shotguns & Pickups	Rural blue-collar workers and families	35–54	33,300	1.7
Agri-Business	Rural farm town and ranch families	45–54, 55–64, 65+	32,300	1.7
Starter Families	Young middle-class families	Under 24, 25–34	32,200	1.6
Boomtown Singles	Middle-income young singles	Under 24, 25–34	32,000	1.2
Upstarts & Seniors	Middle-income empty-nesters	Under 34, 55+	31,800	1.2
Old Yankee Rows	Empty-nest middle-class families	25–34, 65+	31,500	1.4
New Beginnings	Young mobile city singles	Under 24, 25–34	31,400	1.4
Gray Collars	Aging couples in inner suburbs	55–64, 65+	31,400	2.1
Mid-City Mix	African-American singles and families	Under 24, 25–44	31,400	1.3
Sunset City Blues	Empty-nesters in aging industrial cities	55–64, 65+	31,400	1.8
Mobility Blues	Young blue-collar/service families	Under 24, 25–34	30,900	1.6
Latino America	Hispanic middle-class families	Under 24, 25–34	30,100	1.3
Military Quarters	GIs & surrounding off-base families	Under 24, 25–34	29,200	0.5
Blue Highways	Moderate blue-collar/farm families	35–54	27,000	2.2
Golden Ponds	Retirement town seniors	55–64, 65+	26,000	2.0
Rural Industria	Low-income blue-collar families	Under 24, 24–34	26,000	1.6
Back Country Folks	Remote rural, town families	45–64, 65+	25,600	1.8
Rustic Elders	Low-income, older, rural couples	45–64, 65+	25,200	1.9
Grain Belt	Farm owners and tenants	45–54, 55–64, 65+	22,600	2.0
Scrub Pine Flats	Older African-American farm families	55–64, 65+	21,600	1.5
Smalltown Downtown	Older renters and young families	Under 24, 25–35, 65+	21,500	1.9
Single City Blues	Ethnically mixed urban singles	Under 24, 25–34. 65+	19,600	1.7
Mines & Mills	Older families, mines and mill towns	55–64, 65+	19,600	2.0
Family Scramble	Low-income Hispanic families	Under 24, 25–34	19,400	2.0
Norma Rae-ville	Young families, biracial mill towns	Under 24, 65+	19,400	1.4
Hometown Retired	Low-income, older singles and couples	55–64, 65+	18,800	1.3

TABLE 13–4 (CONTINUED)

AMERICA'S NEIGHBORHOOD TYPES

CLUSTER	DEMOGRAPHIC SNAPSHOT	PRIMARY AGE GROUP	MEDIAN HOUSE-HOLD INCOME (2000)	% OF U.S. HOUSE-HOLDS
Towns & Gowns	College town singles	Under 24	18,600	1.4
Hispanic Mix	Urban Hispanic singles and families	Under 24, 24–34	17,600	1.4
Hard Scrabble	Older families in poor, isolated areas	55–64, 65+	17,400	2.0
Southside City	African-American service workers	Mixed	15,800	2.0
Inner Cities	Inner-city solo-parent families	Under 24, 25–44	15,000	2.1

Source: From The Clustered World by M. Weiss. Copyright © 2000 by Michael J. Weiss. By permission of Little, Brown and Company, (Inc.)

values when they compare the value of the "youth generation," the "me generation," and "generation X" with the old values of the dominant (adult) culture.

FAMILY ASSESSMENT

An understanding of the prevailing value system of American society and how societal values affect the family, as well as an understanding of some of the variables influencing family values, provide the foundation for assessing family values. Nurses and health care professionals should use this foundational information discretely, however. Studies and descriptions address group tendencies not particular families and individuals. Therefore, assessments must be individualized, recognizing the unique family values and norms of families. Assessing specific values to which a family adheres and the generational, cultural, and developmental value differences among family members will lead to detection of value conflicts within the family, between the family and its macrosystem, and between the family and health care providers.

Assessment of a family's values is very helpful in motivating a family to take preventive or restorative health action or to make health decisions. Elkins (1984) reminds us that the basis for motivation is derived from a family's value system—what is important and unimportant to it and how important different values are. Although health for its own sake may not be a high value in a family's list of priorities, helping the family see that other very important values will be adversely affected if health actions are not taken (such as a parent not being able to work) may be a way of motivating a family. Elkins (1984) explains this motivational strategy:

> A client's value system can serve as a guide in choosing positive reinforcers for client progress toward goals. The client must believe that the behavior change will result in something of greater value to him—a good return on his investment. The nurse can help the client see the results. Any behavior change requires an investment of self, time, and possibly money, all of which are high on the value scales of most people. In reinforcing newly acquired behavior, the community health nurse, by understanding the client's values, can direct the intrinsic and extrinsic rewards so that the client perceives them as being more valuable than the old behavior patterns. (p. 279)

Given that values cannot be observed directly, they must be inferred from assessment of family structure, functions, and coping styles. This is because these dimensions are strongly influenced by the underlying values held by family members. When family values and beliefs are identified, this information will help the family nurse to better understand the reasons for family behavioral patterns.

One way of simplifying the assessment of family values is for the health care provider to make use of a "contrast and compare" method. This involves comparing and contrasting a specific family's values with those of the dominant American culture. This enables the assessor to identify various areas that need assessment and to appraise how much conformity or disparity in values exists between the dominant culture and the family. The family nurse can then hypothesize as to the impact of this disparity on the family. If an assessor is familiar with the values and norms of a specific ethnic group, then this same comparison process could be applied, using the family's cultural reference group as a basis for comparison (see the assessment areas listed in Table 13–5). To illustrate the "compare-and-contrast" process more concretely, a list of central values can be utilized as a guide for this assessment. Using a list of central values of the dominant culture or of the family's subcultural reference group on one side of the assessment form identify the family's values on the other side. The assessor can then discuss a family's particular values in each of these areas. This listing should help in identifying the specific values to which the family adheres. Table 13–5 summarizes the assessment questions to evaluate family values and beliefs.

FAMILY NURSING DIAGNOSES

Family nursing diagnoses in the area of values are not common. This is because family value problems are generally considered to be underlying causes (related factors) of other problem areas that are more behaviorally oriented. One family nursing diagnosis about family values is "Value Conflicts." If a Value Conflict diagnosis is made, then the system in which the problem resides (between "whom") must be specified—such as "Value Conflict between grandparents and grandson"—and defining characteristics and related factors included. Value Conflicts are often seen as a contributory factor to family problems in the other structural dimensions (communication, power, and roles) or in the functional areas (affective, socialization, and health care) or in coping.

FAMILY NURSING INTERVENTIONS

Knowledge of family values is important data for the nurse to have in order to establish realistic goals and intervention strategies with the family (Elkins, 1984). In addition, understanding the relationship of the family's values to the values of community agencies will help the nurse suggest more value-appropriate community resources when making a referral.

In the nursing literature, only one intervention strategy is specifically discussed in the area of values—that is, value clarification. The family nursing interventions described under role conflict (see Chapter 12) and communication conflicts (Chapter 10), should be appropriate for value conflict problems with only slight modification.

VALUE CLARIFICATION

Value clarification is a technique or process used to increase a family's awareness of value priorities as well as the degree of congruency between the family members' values, attitudes, and behavior. Because values are a basis for decision making and coping, helping families reaffirm their existing values, clarify their values, or reprioritize their values will help them become more autonomous and responsible for their own health (Wilberding, 1985).

In addition to moralizing (telling a person, usually a child, what is right and wrong) and role modeling, the value clarification process assists both children and adults to think critically about their values and to undertake the process of valuing (Raths, Harmin, & Simon, 1978). Value clarification, Kirschenbaum (1977) explains, is an approach that uses questions and activities designed to teach the valuing process. These exercises help people to apply the valuing process to value-rich areas of their lives. Once values become clearer, it is easier to see dissonance between

TABLE 13–5

FAMILY ASSESSMENT: FAMILY VALUES

1. **BEGIN BY COMPARING AND CONTRASTING THE FAMILY'S VALUES TO THE VALUES OF THE CULTURE**

AMERICAN CORE VALUES	THE FAMILY'S VALUES
1. Productivity/Individual achievement	1.
2. Individualism	2.
3. Materialism/The consumption ethic	3.
4. The work ethic	4.
5. Education	5.
6. Equality	6.
7. Progress and mastery over the environment	7.
8. Future time orientation	8.
9. Efficiency, orderliness, and practicality	9.
10. Rationality	10.
11. Quality of life and maintaining health	11.
12. Tolerance of diversity	12.

2. **DISPARITY IN VALUE SYSTEM**

- To what extent is there congruence between the family's values and the family's reference group and/or interacting systems like the educational and the health care systems and the wider community?
- To what extent is there congruence between the family's values and each family member's values?

3. **FAMILY VALUES**

- How important are the identified values to the family? (Rank order the family values.)
- Are the values consciously or unconsciously held?
- Are there any value conflicts evident within the family?
- How do the family's social class, cultural background and degree of acculturation, generational differences, and geographic setting (rural, urban, suburban) influence the family's values?
- How do the family's values affect the health status of the family?

values and behavior; if an individual values health, the dissonance should be reduced by changing his or her health-related behaviors.

A perplexing issue occurs when value clarification is used during the consultation and it becomes evident that the client's values differ greatly from the nurse's values. Is the nurse able to accept differing values without resorting to moralizing? This is an ethical question that must be addressed before undertaking value clarification. According to Wilberding (1985), the ultimate issue is whether the family nurse can accept the client as being an autonomous self-care agent.

There are numerous value clarification tools mentioned in the literature. Pender (2001) has developed and adapted tools and exercises to help individuals and families clarify their values. Pender believes that the nurse interested in health promotion should assist clients with value clarification and value changes. She explains that:

- Value clarification involves increasing personal or group awareness of value priorities and the degree of consistency among values, attitudes, and behavior.

- Value change addresses the reprioritization of values, abandonment of existing values, or acquisition of new values and subsequent attitudes and behavior change.

Assisting family members with value changes is an intervention discussed in rehabilitation nursing. Persons with disabilities and their families need to reprioritize when certain values are no longer possible to operationalize. This process is a crucial one for the client with a disability and his or her family to accomplish in adapting to the disability in a functional manner. Pender (2001) adds one caveat about the use of value clarification. She states that value clarification should be used cautiously with individuals who have emotional problems or with families who are markedly dysfunctional.

CROSS-CULTURAL COUNSELING APPROACHES

In working with families of various ethnic backgrounds, approaches to counseling need to be adapted to make the counseling interventions more culturally relevant and, thus, more effective. An understanding of the family's values is essential in order to select the correct counseling approach. For instance, in the traditionally oriented family from a culture that is familistic, counseling should be directed more toward relationships of the collective (the extended) family. In collectivistic environments, the paramount concern is the promotion and maintenance of intrafamily and interpersonal harmony and being able to fit into the group (Gudykunst, 1991). For families who are individualistic in their value orientation, counseling could be concentrated more on the individual family members. A basic goal in this case might be to assist family members with their own issues and concerns in order to raise their self-esteem or self-growth (Draguns, 1996). When dealing with family issues, expression of the individual family members' perceptions and feelings should be sought. This approach may not be appropriate in families with a hierarchical family structure where the father is the head of the family.

Another example where counseling may need to be adapted in order to be more culturally appropriate is in the area of the time dimension. Anglo-Americans value punctuality or "being on time," and have the attitude that "time is money" and hence, should not be wasted. In traditional families from present-oriented cultures, time does not have the same meaning or significance. "Things happen when I get there" may be the attitude, causing clients to show up for appointments on the right day, but not at the right time. Use of time may also be of concern because of the increase in time stress (not enough time, too much to do in too little time) that is perceived by various members of the family that may lead to generational and gender conflicts within the family (Daly, 1996, 2000). Counseling may assist the family to recognize their varying perceptions of time, as well as determine ways to preserve family time.

❧SUMMARY

- The value system is one of the four highly interdependent structural dimensions of a family.

- A value is an enduring belief that a specific mode of conduct is preferable to the converse mode of conduct.

- Family values are defined as a system of ideas, attitudes, and beliefs about the worth of an entity or concept that consciously and unconsciously bind together the members of a family in a common culture.

- Values serve as general guides to behavior. Within families, values guide the development of family beliefs, norms, or rules.

- Values are learned from the family of origin, which is the basic transmitter of societal or cultural values from one generation to the next. Family values are not only a reflection of the society in which the individual or family resides, but also of the subculture(s) with which the family identifies.

- The term belief has been used synonymously with attitude, explanation, premise, construct, assumption, preference, and values. Beliefs guide the individual's and families' actions.

- Norms prescribe the appropriate role behavior for each of the positions in the family and society and specify how reciprocal relations are to be maintained, as well as how role behavior may change with the changing ages of occupants of these positions.

- Family rules are the specific regulations the family maintains as to what is acceptable and what is not.

- Conflicts and disparity exist in value systems because of diverse social values, clashes of values between the dominant culture and various subcultures and clashes of values between generations.

- Value differences are often noted in the relationship between consumers and health care providers. When these differences occur the results are often divergent goals, unclear communication, and interactional problems.

- Value changes in America have occurred as the population has increased and become more diverse, as society has changed from an overwhelmingly rural society to a highly urbanized society, and as technology and the global economy have altered our understanding of our daily lives.

- The major value orientations that continue to mold and shape the American way of life include:

- Productivity/Individual achievement
- Individualism
- Materialism/The consumption ethic
- The work ethic
- Education
- Equality
- Progress and mastery over the environment
- Future time orientation
- Efficiency, orderliness, and practicality
- Rationality
- Quality of life and maintaining health
- Tolerance of diversity

- A family's value and belief system shapes its patterns of behavior toward health problems. Family values and beliefs shape the views families have of stressors and how they should respond. In other words, family beliefs and values determine how a family will cope with health and other stressors.

- A family's socioeconomic status shapes the family lifestyle; it also is a powerful shaper of family values. The dominant American core values are in large part middle-class values.

- Ethnic background makes a major difference in how important each of the core American values are to a family.

- Whether a family resides (or has resided for a long period of time) in a rural, urban, or suburban community also influences family values.

- There are "generational" value systems in the United States. Although most core values are instilled at an early age by parents, they are altered by society's value shifts that occur over time and in response to various sociopolitical events.

- Assessment of family values must be individualized, recognizing the unique family values and norms. Assessing specific values to which a family adheres and the generational, cultural, and developmental value differences among family members leads to a detection of value conflicts.

- A helpful assessment method to evaluate family values involves comparing and contrasting a specific family's values with those of the dominant American culture. This enables the health care professional to identify various areas that need assessment and to appraise how much conformity or disparity in values exists between the dominant culture and the family and the impact of the disparity on the family.

• Family nursing diagnoses in the area of values are not common. This is because family value problems are generally considered to be underlying causes (related factors) of other problem areas that are more behaviorally oriented.

• Value clarification is a technique or process used to increase a family's awareness of value priorities as well as the degree of congruency between family member values, attitudes, and behavior. Because values are a basis for decision making and coping, helping families reaffirm their existing values, clarify their values, or reprioritize their values will help them become more autonomous and responsible for their own health.

• In working with families of various ethnic backgrounds, counseling approaches need to be adapted to make the counseling interventions more culturally relevant.

❧ FAMILY VIGNETTE: THE GARDINER FAMILY*

The Gardiner family members are Harry, age 37; May, 28; Len, 11; Joanie, 7; and Ann, 3. This African-American family came to the attention of the public health nurse working in a pediatric outpatient clinic when the family missed several appointments arranged for Len at the diabetes and urology clinics. Although appointments to the diabetes clinic were kept occasionally, no urology visit was made, and the chart showed that the mother had reported continual bedwetting at one time.

Len was originally diagnosed as having juvenile diabetes when he was hospitalized at age 6. After the child was diagnosed and stabilized, the family was counseled as to treatment regimen. Subsequently, four hospitalizations occurred because of diabetic crises.

During the nurse's first visit, Mrs. Gardiner appeared very anxious, explaining that she always anticipates "bad news" about Len. In response to inquiries about Len's missed clinic appointments, Mrs. Gardiner seemed indifferent, stating that they have been too busy and that arranging child care for Ann was a problem. On a later visit other factors, more covert, which contribute to the family's reluctance to keep Len's appointments were noted. The mother's statements clarify these factors: "When they told me what was wrong with Len I worried day and night and wouldn't let anyone play with him or take him any place. I was constantly with him. Then I decided I couldn't worry like that anymore. I know he really isn't sick. No one could play as hard as he does and still be sick!" Mrs. Gardiner seemed unwilling to discuss Len's fainting episodes except to say they were Len's way of getting attention. She also declined to discuss his four diabetic crisis hospitalizations.

Data concerning the health status of other family members were also noted. Mrs. Gardiner was of average weight and neatly dressed. She was quite gregarious as long as she could control the conversation. Her knowledge about nutrition and other aspects of family welfare important to her—shelter, cleanliness, adequate child care arrangements, regular school attendance—were satisfactory. Mrs. Gardiner claims good health, although she has not received any preventive care from a physician, with the exception of prenatal care late in the pregnancy.

Mr. Gardiner had been in the Army many years ago and since this time has been under the care of a Veterans Administration Hospital for bouts of depression. He regularly receives tranquilizers and occasional counseling. His wife reported that his physical health is average, stating: "He doesn't get sick or go to the doctor, but he sure is tired all the time."

Joanie, the 7-year-old, was reported to be in good health, attended school regularly, and was doing all right there. Her mother termed her "a good girl." Ann, the preschooler, was active, friendly, and appeared healthy. Mrs. Gardiner complained of her "overactivity." She explained that Ann was constantly "into things" and interfered with her efforts to keep the house clean and picked up. Ann's health supervision is irregular and her immunizations incomplete. After well-baby care was completed at 1 year, health care has been sought only for acute illnesses.

The family's economic situation has been unstable. Mr. Gardiner works irregularly in a factory, while Mrs. Gardiner works off and on at a car-washing business. To supplement their insufficient earnings, they receive welfare.

Mrs. Gardiner's primary expressed concerns had to do with her husband's lack of responsibility for helping with the household and child care tasks, as well as his overall neglectfulness and his irregular employment. She openly berated her husband in front of the nurse and their children, complaining that he did not bring home enough money for the family to live on and lacks interest in the home, the children, and money matters. Mr. Gardiner sat silently as his wife verbally complained about him.

There was an impression of little communication or companionship among family members, except in those areas related to the daily activities of living and taking care of the apartment. The children's play was kept at a minimum due to the noise they created. Most communication was in the form of commands from the mother to the husband and children. Mrs. Gardiner states that she is constantly working to keep the home clean, meals ready, and the children cared for. The home was viewed as a place to be kept clean and organized, so that everything was put away. The children were expected to be "seen but not heard," to be home exactly on time, to attend school regularly, to keep themselves and their surroundings clean, and to obey and respect their mother. There were no toys or reading materials visible. The only discernible source of recreation for the entire family was the television set, which was on constantly. Family recreational pursuits were practically unheard of. Life was virtually task oriented, and no enjoyable and fun activities were included.

The family lives in a low-income housing project, for which they are charged a minimum rent. Kitchen equipment, food, and clothing storage facilities are adequate, as are their furnishings. Although the outside appearance of the housing project is dirty and visually in a state of disrepair, the inside of their apartment is orderly and well maintained.

Mr. and Mrs. Gardiner dropped out of high school in the ninth and tenth grades, respectively, in order to start working to help out their parents. No further education or skill training has been received since that time. Relatives do not reside near them, nor are they affiliated with any religious or other community groups.

The community in which the family lives is part of a large inner-city area that is deteriorating rapidly. Transportation and social, health, and welfare facilities are easily accessible. Shopping for food and other necessities is limited to small neighborhood shops since they do not own a car. The schools and churches are nearby. The mother feels the neighborhood is crime-ridden (which the nurse confirmed), and hence she has kept the children indoors most of the time.

* Family case study adapted from Sobol and Robischon (1975).

▮ STUDY QUESTIONS

Review the Family Vignette and answer the related questions.

1. From the limited information contained in the family case study, what are the salient values operating in this family? (Use the assessment process that was suggested in this chapter.)

2. How important are these identified values to the family?

3. Are these values consciously or unconsciously held?

4. Are there any value conflicts evident within the family itself?

5. Given that value conflict between husband and wife is the family nursing diagnosis in this case, discuss briefly one intervention strategy that could be used here (given spouses are interested in discussing this area).

Choose all correct answers to the following questions.

6. It is true that:
   a. Values are defined as a system of ideas and beliefs that bind families together.
   b. Values serve as general guides to behavior.
   c. The family is the basic transmitter of values.
   d. Values are relatively fixed and change very little over time.
   e. All values have the same or similar weight as far as their influence and centrality in a person's life are concerned.

7. The best definition of norms is:
   a. Patterns of personal behaviors.
   b. Patterns of behavior considered "right" in a given society.
   c. Role behaviors or expectations associated with family positions.
   d. Clustering of attitudes and beliefs.

8. Family rules are related to family values in which of the following ways?
   a. Family rules generate family values.
   b. Family rules are specific manifestations of family values.
   c. Family rules and family values are distinct concepts and have no overlapping meaning.

9. List and briefly explain four major, recent value changes that have occurred in society and within families.

10. Individualism is criticized for "going too far." Identify which of the following choice(s) reflect(s) critics' concerns regarding the impact of this trend on the family:

   a. Individualism encourages excessive concern with achievement.
   b. Familism is impacted negatively.
   c. An imbalance is created between individualism and family togetherness.
   d. Child-centeredness has decreased with growth in individualism.

11. Value clarification is a process that helps people to (choose the one correct answer):

   a. Identify their values.
   b. Change their values.
   c. See the difference between their values and family rules.
   d. Question the rights and wrongs about their values.

12. Many ethnic families do not share the same value of individualism that mainstream Americans do (answer true or false).

13. Several values cluster together, comprising the central configuration of values in the dominant culture. List six values.

14. Four variables that influence the family's value system are described. List these.

Choose the correct answers to the following questions.

15. Which of the following are sources of value conflicts?

   a. Generational differences
   b. Social class differences
   c. Acculturation differences
   d. Idiosyncratic (personal) differences

16. One of the concepts germane to social class is that when a family and its reference group do not subscribe to the central core values of a society (select all correct answers):

   a. The adjustment to wider society is relatively easy.
   b. The family is able to gain compliance from society.
   c. The more difficult the family adjustment to community life becomes.
   d. The family experiences social stigma.

14

THE FAMILY AFFECTIVE FUNCTION

LEARNING OBJECTIVES

1. State three reasons why the affective function is a vital family function.

2. Describe seven components of the affective function in healthy families.

3. Name two underlying values and/or priorities present in energized families related to affective function.

4. Describe the impact that individual and family stressors can have on family affective function.

5. Using a family vignette, complete an assessment of the affective function. Propose a family nursing diagnosis in the area of the affective function. Suggest two family nursing interventions to ameliorate and/or resolve the above affective problem.

It is generally recognized that the family exists to fulfill basic functions necessary for the survival of the species (societal needs)—procreation and child rearing. Additionally, the family acts as the mediator between society and the individual. The family forms the matrix in which personal needs are met. Social organizations and institutions such as schools and social service agencies now share in fulfilling many of the traditional functions of the family. A number of extremely vital functions, however, remain. Perhaps the most important of these functions are socialization (see Chapter 15) and the affective function. Major functions of the millennium family include nurturing, partnering, communicating, adapting, respite (Janosik & Green, 1992), and emotional support of family members. The affective function is a means to achieve family tasks of physical care, reproduction, teaching, personal growth and development, bonding, and providing purpose and meaning (Friedemann, 1993a). Another significant family function is the health care function, covered in Chapter 16.

IMPORTANCE OF THE AFFECTIVE FUNCTION

The affective function deals with the internal functions of the family—the psychosocial protection and support of its members. A substantial amount of research exists confirming the positive influence of healthy personal and familial ties on individual health and well-being (Singer & Ryff, 2001). Positive social relationships correlate with better health outcomes, longevity, and decreasing levels of stress. Conversely, family life can also contribute to stress and dysfunctional coping with consequences that can be detrimental to physical health (e.g., difficulty sleeping, high blood pressure, lowered immune response) (Singer & Ryff, 2001).

The family accomplishes the task of supporting the healthy development and growth of its members by meeting the socioemotional needs of its members, starting with the early years of an individual's life and continuing throughout his or her lifetime. Fulfillment of the affective function is the central basis for both the formation and continuation of the family unit (Satir, 1972). An individual's self-image and his or her sense of belonging is derived through primary group (family) interactions. Moreover, the family serves as a primary source of love, approval, reward, and support.

Loveland-Cherry (1996) points out that affection among family members produces a nurturing emotional climate that positively influences growth and development and a sense of personal competence. Family nurturance is essential for health promotion behaviors and healthy outcomes.

The family assumes a heavy responsibility in attempting to fulfill the role of meeting its members' socioemotional needs, especially as many families move frequently and often do not have the social support systems they need. Moreover, today's families are generally smaller, and there are fewer members to share the tasks of meeting each other's needs for companionship, love, and support.

Because the affective function is vital for both survival and the functioning of the family as a whole and for its individual members, assessment and intervention in this area are crucial. Both supportive counseling and education are critical strategies employed by professionals in helping families strengthen their relationships and to meet each other's needs more satisfactorily. Consideration of the affective function is particularly vital in working with young families with newborns and infants, in which parent–infant relationships are significant in terms of their long-term impact on the child's and family's future.

COMPONENTS OF THE AFFECTIVE FUNCTION

The affective function involves the family's perception of respect for and care of the psychosocial needs of its members. Through fulfillment of the affective function, the family enhances the qualities of humanness, the stabilization of personality and behavior, relatability (ability to relate intimately), and self-esteem of family members (Table 14–1).

MAINTAINING MUTUAL NURTURANCE

First and foremost, fulfilling the affective function involves creating and maintaining within the family a system for mutual nurturance. Recall that in Chapter 13 on family values, one important family value was that the family should serve as a haven for warmth,

TABLE 14–1

SOCIOEMOTIONAL ATTRIBUTES OF HEALTHY FAMILIES

- A social milieu for the generation and maintenance of affectional bonds within family relationships, where one is first loved and given to, and in turn learns to love and give in return.

- An opportunity to develop a personal and social identity tied to family identity.

- An opportunity for individuals to be themselves. The family provides a home base or haven where its members are permitted to be themselves—to express their true feelings and thoughts (e.g., hostility with less fear of consequences) and to experience security and love without fear of rejection.

support, love, and acceptance. A prerequisite to achieving mutual nurturance is the basic commitment of an adult couple both to each other and to a nurturing, emotionally satisfying initimate/marital relationship. This becomes the emotional foundation on which the parents build their supportive structure. The nurturing attitudes and behavior flowing from parents and siblings to younger children will result in a return flow from children to parents as well. Brown (1978) views this flow as a spiral phenomenon. As each member receives affection and care from others in the family, his or her capacity to give to other members increases, with the result being mutual support and emotional warmth among family members.

Mutuality and reciprocity are the key concepts. Parents give emotionally to children; in turn, this emotion is received by the child and is reciprocated to both parents and siblings. The opposite also occurs: Rejecting and angry parents breed angry and rejecting responses in their children. By maintaining the kind of family emotional environment in which family members respond adequately to one another, the family provides the opportunity for individuals to form and to maintain meaningful relationships not only with family members, but with other individuals also.

Within a marriage or domestic partnership, the need to maintain mutual nurturance can be achieved by determining the most important emotional needs of the domestic partners/spouses and how effectively they are in meeting those needs for one another. Harley

(1994), a psychologist and marriage counselor, utilizes an Emotional Needs Questionnaire to assist the thousands of families he has worked with to determine their needs within their marriage. From the families he has counseled, five basic needs of men and five basic needs of women have consistently emerged as sources of marital problems when these needs are not met (Table 14–2). Though the categories may not apply equally to everyone, they do provide some insight into the unique emotional needs of marital partners. Harley points out that most often failure to meet these needs is not due to selfish unwillingness to be considerate, but rather is due to the ignorance that these needs even exist.

DEVELOPMENT OF CLOSE RELATIONSHIPS

By fulfilling of the family's affective function, individual members develop the ability to relate intimately or closely with others. Intimacy is vital in human relationships, because it fulfills the psychological need for emotional closeness with another human being and allows individuals in the relationship to know the full range of each other's uniqueness.

An infant usually first experiences an intimate relationship with his or her parents, beginning with early mother–infant bonding. The relationship continues

TABLE 14–2

BASIC NEEDS OF MEN AND WOMEN IN A MARITAL RELATIONSHIP

HIS FIVE MOST BASIC NEEDS	HER FIVE MOST BASIC NEEDS
1. Sexual fulfillment	1. Affection
2. Recreational companionship	2. Conversation
3. An attractive spouse (in their eyes)	3. Honesty and openness
4. Domestic support	4. Financial support
5. Admiration	5. Family commitment

Source: Adapted from Harley (1994).

to grow and develop during the years that follow in the family of origin. When achieved, this sense of closeness and trusting gives the person the confidence to reach outside the family confines and establish close and emotionally satisfying relationships with others. As young adults then form their own families, this sense of intimacy and closeness is continued and may be passed on to the next generation (in childbearing families). Conversely, if early bonding and a sense of trust and intimacy does not occur in the family of origin, the individual will not have the confidence and ability to relate intimately with others. Unfortunately, this inability to trust others is usually passed on to the next generation unless some intervening factor such as personal experiences and growth at a later stage in life occurs (Bowen, 1978; Byng-Hall, 1995).

Closeness of relationships within the family are not equal among all family members. It is well established in the literature that children feel differently toward mothers and fathers and toward stepfathers and biological fathers (Thornton, Orburch, & Axinn, 1995). There is strong evidence that the father's relationship with the children is often mediated by the mother, while a mother's relationship with her children is more independent of the father. A study by Barber and Thomas (1986) found that emotional ties varied depending on the gender of the child and the parent. The researchers surveyed 527 largely Mormon college students about their relationships with their parents. Fathers were found to be more physically affectionate to daughters, while mothers showed the same amount of physical affection to children of both sexes. Mothers typically had more companionship with daughters, and fathers with sons. Physical affection was found to be positively associated with self-esteem in both sexes. Another study (Wenk, Hardesty, Morgan, & Blair, 1994) using longitudinal data from 762 children, ages 7 to 11, showed that children's perceptions of emotional and physical parental involvement were equally important to the well-being of both boys and girls. Feeling loved and respected by parents and having time with parents fosters self-esteem and mental health in children.

There is also strong support that a healthy, functional marital/domestic partner relationship does, indeed, strengthen many dimensions of the parent–child relationship. If marital/partnership problems exist in a family, the father is the family member who most often becomes isolated or who most often withdraws from close family ties (Volling, Notaro, & Larsen, 1998; White, 1999).

Family members gain a great deal of social support from the close relationships they have developed within the nuclear and extended family system. A myth prevalent in the American culture is that American families have shifted away from the structure of an extended, multigenerational family, to one that is nuclear. In truth, however, nuclear families have always been the predominant family form. The change that has occurred over the last decade has been in the size of the nuclear family. Whereas once the nuclear family consisted of 8 to 10 children, today's family size has been reduced dramatically. With the decline in family size, a concurrent decline has occurred in the number of secondary kin (aunts, uncles, and cousins) in most families. On the other hand, life expectancy has increased. Many children today are able to experience close family ties with four living grandparents, and often with one or two great-grandparents. In previous generations, children did not have these elder family members present to offer emotional, material, or informational support. Many grandparents provide day care services to their grandchildren. Additionally, technology and the ease of travel have erased the negative impact of distance in creating close bonds between older family members and their children's families (Castiglia, 1999).

MUTUAL RESPECT BALANCE

The literature of parent–child guidance presents a well-respected approach to parenting termed the mutual respect balance (Colley, 1978). When operationalized, it helps family members to fulfill their affective function. The primary thrust of this approach is that families should maintain an atmosphere in which positive self-regard and the rights of both parents and child are highly valued. It is accepted by all family members that each person in the family has his or her own rights as individuals, as well as developmental needs specific to his or her age group. A mutual respect balance can be achieved when each family member respects the rights, needs, and responsibilities of other members (Colley, 1978).

Positive communication patterns (showing empathy, reflective listening, and supportive comments) between children and their parents is a key factor in the development and maintenance of moral-judgment agreement between family members and subsequent respect for varying moral views. Children who experience negative communication patterns (e.g., hostility and criticism) within their family system are less likely to accept parental moral views and parental moral authority (Olson et al., 1983; White, 2000). Maintaining a balance between the rights of individuals in the family means creating an atmosphere in which neither parents nor children are expected to cater to the whims of the other. Parents need to provide sufficient structure and consistent guidelines so that limits are set and understood. At the same time, enough flexibility must also be built into the family system to allow for freedom and for room to grow and develop individual identities. Mutual nurturance is also made possible when a mutual respect balance exists.

BONDING AND IDENTIFICATION

The sustaining force behind the perception and satisfaction of the needs of individuals in the family is called *bonding* or *attachment,* terms that are used interchangeably by theorists. Attachment, according to Wright and Leahey (2000, p. 100) refers to "a relatively enduring unique emotional tie between two specific persons." Bonding is first initiated in a new family within the marital/domestic partner relationship. This is when a couple discovers common interests, goals, and values and finds that the relationship validates each of them, carries with it certain tangible benefits (prestige, peer relationships, community privileges, etc.), makes possible the meeting of certain goals that could not be accomplished alone (e.g., having children), and provides mutual enjoyment and comfort due to their sustained contact with each other (Perry, 1983; Turner, 1970). Bowlby (1977) called the development of this emotional tie "falling in love." This same kind of bonding or attachment develops later between parents and children and between siblings as they continually and positively relate to each other.

The attachment between a mother and her newborn infant is crucial because early parent–infant interactions affect the nature and quality of later attachment relationships, and in turn these relationships influence the child's psychosocial and cognitive development (Ainsworth, 1966). Identification is the critical element in bonding, and it is at the heart of family relationships. Turner (1970) explains that in its most uncomplicated definition, identification refers to "an attitude in which a person experiences what happens to another person as if it had happened to himself" (p. 66). In other words, when a family member identifies with another member, he or she experiences the joys and sorrows of the other as if these experiences were his or her own.

In order for bonding or attachment to occur in family relationships, positive identification must first be present. As the most pervasive aspect of attachment, identification may be based on sympathy or on libidinal mechanisms or may be solely derived from the internalization of the attitudes of the other person whom the family member cares for and depends on. Once established, the long-term consequence of identification and bonding is a change in the individual's self-image toward the characteristics of the other person with whom he or she has identified. Through identification, children attempt to imitate the behavior of their parents (the parents with whom they identify become their role models). As the child's identity is enhanced by the learning of behaviors, attitudes, and values of parents, a bond is formed. Through identification and bonding, parents gain referent power (see Chapter 11) over their children.

The identification or identity bond depends on positive, giving responses from people in the relationships. Even an infant rewards the mother early in their relationship by feeding, snuggling up, letting the mother comfort him or her, and so forth. For bonding to be effective, there must be support and enhancement of a person's identity through his or her association with another. "Whenever a child shows admiration towards his parent or spontaneously gives affection, the gratification that the parent feels activates a response bond" (Turner, 1970, p. 72).

One facet of the response bond is the general sensitivity, caring for, and responsiveness of the other member(s) in the relationship. A sense of closeness and a desire to continue sharing together occur when one's communication is accepted and appreciated, and feelings are supported. Bonding may also exist because of special needs that one person meets for the other person. For instance, a dominant, controlling person may bond with a submissive type—with both having their special needs satisfied in the relationship.

The duration of close relationships is also a factor to be considered. Even though the bonding between newlyweds is intense, and the relationship between mother and a newborn child profound, loss of the newly married mate or newborn may not be felt as severely when compared to a loss that occurs after the relationship had persisted for a long period of time. As family members closely involved with each other continue their relationship, old bonds become intensified and new, stronger bonds emerge; these stronger bonds unite these individuals together in a unique, sustaining relationship. These attachments are not transferable—that is, no other person(s) can replace a particular member. Because these enduring bonds are not initially present, and grow through a close, sustained involvement, Turner (1970) terms these bonds *crescive bonds*.

Although crescive bonding sounds like a natural phenomenon, it is not inevitable, and in some situations crescive bonds do not develop. Turner (1970) discusses two factors that inhibit their growth. First, bonds that are situationally based (based on the existence of certain specific needs or circumstances), such as those bonds that meet certain developmental needs that an individual will possibly outgrow, or task-oriented bonds, are far more vulnerable to weakening and eventual breakage. Second, bonding relationships based on contractual agreements, rather than sacred linkages, are also more vulnerable to dissolution, because contracts involve mutual obligations. In this case, if one partner fails to live up to his or her part of the contract, the contract can become invalid. Marriages are seen by many in this light. In sacred linkages, the basis for staying together is felt to be religious beliefs, family, tradition, and/or ethical–moral obligations/one's duty. The parent–child bond is still seen as sacred and immutable. (A case in point: States do not legally permit a parent the right to disown their minor children.)

Assessing the nature of the attachment and quality of the affectional ties between each set of relationships in the family has been suggested by several family therapists and nurses (Minuchin, 1974; Wright & Leahey, 2000). The bonds between family members can be illustrated using an attachment diagram (Figure 14–1A). The diagram visibly portrays the level of attachment between various members of the fam-

ily. Wright and Leahey point out that there is no "right" level of attachment or "best" attachment configuration. Rather, families should demonstrate a variety of attachment relationships in which all family members of whatever age and position in the family feel they have a reliable network of attachments to form a secure family base (Byng-Hall, 1995; Wright & Leahey. Attachment networks will change among family members as they progress through various stages of the family life cycle. For instance, the attachment diagram for a newly married couple should demonstrate close emotional ties between the spouses while at the same time they negotiate a different relationship with their families of origin. This configuration usually changes as the adults become caretakers to young children (see Figure 14–1B).

SEPARATENESS AND CONNECTEDNESS

One of the central, overriding psychological issues involving family life is the way in which families meet their members' psychological needs, and how this affects the individual's identity and self-esteem. During the early years of socialization, families mold and program a child's behavior, thus forming his or her sense of identity. Minuchin (1974) further explains: "Human experiences of identity have two elements—a sense of belonging and a sense of being separate. The laboratory in which these ingredients are mixed and dispensed with is the family, the matrix of identity" (p. 47).

Children's sense of belonging comes from being a part of, or connected to, a family—playing the roles of child and sibling. The development of a sense of separateness and individuation occurs as children participate in roles within the family and in different family events and situations, as well as through involvement in activities outside of the family. As children grow, the parents progressively allow them more autonomy to meet their own unique needs and interests (Minuchin, 1974).

In order to perceive and to meet the psychological needs of family members, the family must achieve a satisfactory balance of separateness or autonomy and connectedness (Peterson, 1995). Family members are both connected to and separate from one another. Each family handles the issues of separateness and connectedness in a unique fashion, some families

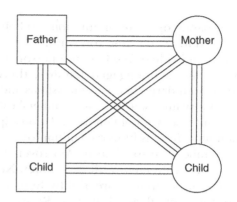

Figure 14–1. **(A)** An example of an attachment diagram. Shows how the newly married couple adjusts ties with their family of origin and builds strong ties with each other. **(B)** The second diagram illustrates how attachment between the spouses may change with the introduction of children. *(Adapted from Wright & Leahey, 2000).*

placing much more emphasis on one facet than on the other. The balance between autonomy and connectedness is often shaped by a family's cultural background and its life cycle stages.

Both conditions are basic and are constitutive of family life. The young infant begins the separation process at about 6 months. Through the formative years, he or she forms an identity, while individuation and growth continue throughout his or her lifetime. Nonetheless, connectedness is equally basic, taking a variety of forms from physical proximity to intense involvement that excludes other interests (Handel, 1972).

The family needs to provide opportunities for the mastery of this duality. An important role for family members is that they must help other family members want to be together and to develop and maintain cohesiveness or connectedness. On the other hand, the family must gradually provide appropriate amounts of freedom and avenues of expression for members to individuate and to become separate individuals.

It is important to note how much of family life is regulated by power considerations. Parental authority—its scope and the manner of its exercise—is one of the forces shaping the patterns encouraging individuality (separateness) and cohesion (connectedness). Parents differ in how extensively they impose their image on their children. When parents expect children to do all the adapting, there is little room for negotiating, and the chances of promoting individuality are hampered.

Also, families vary in how quickly they push their children toward separateness and how intensively they encourage connectedness—that is, how soon they expect their children to grow up and to separate from parents. Some parents encourage babyish, dependent behaviors in their children, while others pressure their children to act more adult at an early age. The pace set for their children's growing up is often based on the parents' aims for themselves and their children. For example, if both parents are working and see dependency as a burden that is frustrating to their goals, they will push their children at a faster pace to become self-sufficient and independent. As in other dimensions of family life, parental ideas about child growth and development and the acceptability of various behaviors are also influenced by the family's culture and social class background (Handel, 1972; Peterson, 1995).

In assessing separateness and connectedness within a family, Hartman and Laird (1983) look at the characteristics of the family in terms of enmeshment–disengagement (a continuum). Minuchin (1974) originally generated the concepts of enmeshment and disengagement in families. He refers to an enmeshed family as one in which individual and subsystem boundaries (like spousal subsystem boundaries) are continually violated by members outside those boundaries. In enmeshed families, family members interpret or speak for each other and are super-sensitive to family members' signals for help. Enmeshed families are families that do not allow room for separate opinions or autonomous behavior. Members tend to be too close (overinvolved) and too restrictive of individual freedom and personal identity. Conversely, in disengaged families, there are closed, rigid boundaries between subsystems and individuals, and very little sensitivity to members' calls for assistance. In these types of families, relationships are too distant and there is little recognition or meeting of family members' personal needs. Moreover, there is an absence of involvement with each other. Neither extremes on the continuum are healthy. In their studies of troubled families, Minuchin, Rosman, and Baker (1978) found that certain types of families are generally enmeshed, including psychosomatic families and families with school phobic and schizophrenic children.

Similar work evaluating family cohesion (connectedness–separateness continuum) and adaptability has been carried out by Olson and McCubbin (1982). The theorists have developed a model that has been used extensively to assess the above two dimensions of marital and family behavior. In FACES (Family Adaptation and Cohesion Model), family cohesion is defined as the emotional bonding that family members have toward one another and the degree of individual autonomy they experience. Family adaptability is the ability of the marital or family system to change its power structure, role relationships, and relationship rules in response to situational and developmental stress. The model hypothesizes the following:

- Couples/families with balanced cohesion and adaptability will generally function more adequately than those at extreme dimensions.

- Couples/families will change their cohesion and adaptability to deal with situational stress and life changes in their family life cycle.

- Positive communication skills will facilitate couples and families to balance cohesion and adaptability.

The model describes four levels of each dimension (cohesion and adaptability) and identifies 16 distinct types of marital and family systems. Table 14–3 describes the clinical and research indicators of variables that can be used to diagnose and to measure the family cohesion dimension. Families that are in the separated or connected levels allow family members to experience being both independent from and connected to their family. Conversely, disengaged or enmeshed families tend to function only at these extremes and are not expected to change their behaviors (Olson & McCubbin, 1982).

NEED–RESPONSE PATTERNS

The affective component of family relationships needs to be evaluated in terms of the extent to which family members seem to care for and about each other (Hartman & Laird, 1983). Parad and Caplan (1965) address this concern in their discussion of the assessment of the need–response patterns in families. This concept is essentially synonymous with that of the family affective function. Mutual nurturance, respect, bonding, and separateness–connectedness aspects emerge as vital prerequisites or necessary corequisites to satisfactory need–response patterns in families (Table 14–4).

Three separate and interlocking phases are inherent in a family's affective response to these needs. First, family members must perceive the needs of the other members within the constraints of the family's culture. Next, these needs must be viewed with respect and seen to be worthy of attention (as discussed under mutual respect balance). Finally, these recognized and respected needs must be satisfied to the extent possible in light of family resources. It is especially propitious if family members each have confidants within the family with whom they can unburden themselves.

This triad of perception, respect, and satisfaction of family members' needs is very much influenced by American sociocultural perspectives—viewing individuals as separate persons who are deserving of recognition and respect as well as a fair share in the family's resources. This tendency to view family members as unique, evolving individuals corresponds with the high value this society places on individualism.

A family's sensitivity to, and perception of, the individual member's actions and needs varies greatly. Most families fall somewhere between extreme sensitivity (a sign of enmeshment), high responsiveness to individual member's input, and extreme insensitivity and unresponsiveness to individual members' inputs (sign of disengagement).

The extent to which basic psychological or socioemotional needs are met also varies depending on

TABLE 14–3

FAMILY COHESION DIMENSION

	DISENGAGED (VERY LOW COHESION)	SEPARATED (LOW TO MODERATE COHESION)	CONNECTED MODERATE TO HIGH COHESION)	ENMESHED (VERY HIGH COHESION)
Emotional Bonding	Very low	Low to moderate	Moderate to high	Very high
Independence	High independence of family members	Moderate independence of family members	Moderate dependence of family members	High dependence of family members
Family Boundaries	Open external boundaries. Closed internal boundaries. Rigid generational boundaries.	Semi-open external and internal boundaries. Clear generational boundaries.	Semi-open external and internal boundaries. Open internal boundaries. Clear generational boundaries.	Closed external boundaries. Blurred internal boundaries. Blurred generational boundaries.
Coalitions	Weak coalitions, usually a family scapegoat.	Marital coalition clear.	Marital coalition strong.	Parent–child coalitions.
Time	Time apart from family maximized (physically and/or emotionally).	Time alone and together is important.	Time together is important. Time alone permitted for approved reasons.	Time together maximized. Little time alone permitted.
Space	Separate space both physically and emotionally is maximized.	Private space maintained; some family space.	Family space maximized. Private space minimized.	Little or no private space at home.
Friends	Mainly individual friends and seen alone. Few family friends.	Some individual friends. Some family friends.	Some individual friends. Scheduled activities with couple and family friends.	Limited individual friends. Mainly couple or family friends seen together.
Decision Making	Primarily individual decisions.	Most decisions are individually based, able to make joint decisions on family issues.	Individual decisions are shared. Most decisions made with family in mind.	All decisions both personal and relationship must be made by family.
Interests and Recreation	Primarily individual activities done without family. Family not involved.	Some spontaneous family activities. Individual activities supported.	Some scheduled family activities. Family involved in individual interests.	Most or all activities and interests must be shared with family.

Source: Olson, D., & McCubbin, H. (1982). Family stress, coping, and social support (pp. 48–68). Courtesy of Charles C Thomas, Publisher, Ltd., Springfield, Illinois.

TABLE 14–4

THE SOCIOEMOTIONAL NEEDS OF FAMILY MEMBERS

1. Love for one's own sake
2. A balance between support and independence with respect to tasks
3. A balance between freedom and control
4. The availability of suitable role models

Adapted from Parad & Caplan (1965).

the family's own social support system. Some families have a greater, more involved social network, such as an extended family, from which to draw support. In these families, meeting family members' psychosocial needs can be accomplished by individuals who are both inside and outside of the nuclear family or household. In contrast, families that are truly isolated from social support systems—closed families—have limited outside resources and hence depend primarily or solely on nuclear family members to meet all their psychological needs. Naturally, this latter state imposes a great burden on family relationships, because probably no one person can meet all of another person's needs.

THE THERAPEUTIC ROLE

The therapeutic role of spouses is discussed in Chapter 12 as one of the emergent roles increasingly expected of mates entering into marital and family life from all social classes, but particularly in the middle class. This role is quite similar to the adults' domestic partner role in meeting the affective needs of their mates. While the affective function describes the broad mental health function of the family—as a group designed to meet the psychological needs of its members—the therapeutic role describes an important socioemotional role within the marital/adult partner subsystem. Primarily, the therapeutic role that spouses/domestic partners play is problem oriented. It involves listening to each other's problem, sympathizing, giving reassurance and affection, and offering help in solving the problem. In Nye's (1976) study of spousal roles, he reported that both husbands and wives indicated that mates have the duty to enact this role. This finding has been confirmed by Harvey (1994) who found that the needs of men and women are similar in marriage, with both needing their spouse to listen and assist in problem solving and guidance when asked.

This role has been explained by Nye (1976): "The behavior . . . is therapeutic in assisting the spouse to cope with and, hopefully, dispose of a problem with which he is confronted" (p. 111). When this role is extended to include the rest of the family, children and adults alike, some very important elements of family behavior come to light. Nye continues: "Listening and giving the family member an opportunity to verbalize, acting as a 'sounding board' for the ideas or reactions of the other, supplying additional information, concepts, or insights, and taking concrete actions in sharing the solution of the problem are all involved" (p. 115). Some of these behaviors, of course, would not be appropriate (therapeutic) in relating to a young child or infant, but with older children, much of the same therapeutic, assistive relating can occur.

THE AFFECTIVE FUNCTION IN ENERGIZED FAMILIES

Pratt (1976) conducted a large survey in the mid-1970s and from this classic study described how healthy, functional, or, as Pratt calls them, *"energized"* families achieve their affective function. She states:

A feature of energized family structure . . . is the tendency to provide autonomy and to be responsive to the particular interests and needs of individual family members. . . . This includes the tendency not only to accept, but to prize individuality and uniqueness, and to tolerate disagreement and deviance. Respect and acceptance are given unconditionally, without continuous comparison of the person to others or to prescribed standards. . . . The family members are encouraged in their various endeavors, especially in seeking new areas of growth and in developing their creativity, imagination, and independent thinking. (pp. 84–85)

This description provides a basis for comparison. One important caveat, however, is that this study was completed with largely middle-class white families. A family's social class and cultural variability must be considered in evaluating what is healthy and less healthy behaviors in a family in regard to the manifestations of optimal affective functioning.

THE FAMILY UNDER STRESS: THE AFFECTIVE FUNCTION

Maintaining a nurturing familial environment is often a formidable task, as many stressors tend to disrupt family homeostasis and make family members less sensitive and loving toward each other. Threats to affective functioning include health-related stressors.

When the affective needs of family members are not being adequately perceived and addressed due to the stress in a family member, health alterations and distress signals from one or more family members become apparent. These symptoms of family dysfunction may include emotional responses such as anger, anxiety, and depression; delinquent or acting-out behaviors; and somatic complaints and illness of family members. This dysfunction may inhibit affective functions within family relationships, resulting in a downward-spiraling process until some positive step is taken to curtail further disorganization and to reverse the tailspin.

Parad and Caplan (1965) do not believe that the temporary periods of low response to members' needs are necessarily harmful to their emotional health. However, persistent, long-standing need frustration is deleterious. Even a temporary inattentiveness to a family member's needs may be harmful if the loss occurs when that individual is particularly vulnerable, such as during a critical phase of a child's development.

Family health professionals note that family problems and dysfunctions generally become worse or more apparent during the terminal phase of an illness or during bereavement (Rolland, 1994). When the family is grieving, conflicts in the family often become overt and the affective needs of family members are usually not recognized and/or acknowledged. The death of a family member is probably the most catastrophic event for families (Arnette, 1996). With

death comes profound loss. People who are closest to the person who has died are immediately affected by the loss. Eventually, as in an earthquake, the whole system of relationships is shaken (Gelcer, 1986).

The seriousness of this event is demonstrated in the higher mortality rates of spouses up to two years after the death of a mate. Bereaved persons are at higher risk for multiple diseases. These are primarily the chronic diseases of middle and late age. The excess risk of mortality due to bereavement is higher among widowed men than women (Kosten, Jacobs, & Kasl, 1985). Some studies found increased risk of death in the first six months of bereavement (Bowling & Windsor, 1995). A recent study found that middle-aged people who lost spouses, siblings, and siblings-in-law generally adjusted more poorly than did either younger or older individuals and were more prone to health problems in the bereavement period (Perkins & Harris, 1990). Chapter 17 provides a more thorough discussion of the impact of stress and grief on the individual and family system.

Concerning childhood bereavement, it has been well documented that bereaved siblings show a higher level of behavior problems compared to standardized norms for age and sex. Studies report that between one fourth and one third of bereaved siblings have serious problems. These problems include behaviors such as sleep problems, poor school performance, and attention seeking. Grief behaviors in children tend to be internalizing behaviors (Birenbaum, Robinson, Phillips, Stewart, & McCown, 1990; Davies, 1995; Mahon & Page, 1995; McCown & Davies, 1995). Some additional research (Worden, Davies, & McCown, 1996) compares the adjustment of children following a parent's death as compared to a sibling's death. Approximately one fourth of the children in each group had behavior problems. However, boys scored higher in the parent loss group and girls scored higher in the sibling loss group. Reasons for these gender differences were unclear.

Family members' psychological needs for support are much greater during the period when a family member is dying and after the death. If the family member's death is unexpected, stress and grief will be more extreme. When death is prolonged over a period of months or even years, stress is continuous and circumstances are ambiguous. Family members are often left emotionally depleted in terms of helping themselves or supporting others in the family. Other stressors occur after a death in the family (numerous arrangements that must be made, settling of the estate, medical bills, and family role transitions); it is easy to see how the adult member(s) would have difficulty supporting child members of the family. This is often a time when the family's social support system (both formal and informal) can play an important role in supporting grieving families. Functional families also pull together during this period and try to share their grief and to support each other. Elements of this process have been described by McCubbin and McCubbin (1993) in the Resiliency Model of Family Stress, Adjustment, and Adaptation (see Chapter 17).

A salient affective need of family members during the time of a major loss is to be able to grieve for the loss. Constructive grief work depends on the ability of the social support network (family and the family's social network) to be permissive of feelings, positively accepting them and supportive of those who grieve. Family members' energies should be directed to the actual loss as experienced both collectively and individually. When feelings are shared there needs to be an open stage for discussing, recalling, memory associating, and reliving of past events. Moreover, certain beliefs may need to be confronted, especially when guilt is expressed based on irrational assumptions of a person's responsibility for events that were beyond the control of that person.

Children also need to be able to grieve. Sharing feelings and thoughts with children and communicating with them at their cognitive and emotional levels of maturity are most important. The parents' handling of death when comforting children and adolescents is most significant in terms of helping them with their psychological needs (Shapiro, 1994). Those families who are open to expressing their emotions are more successful in adjusting to the loss of a family member (McClowry, Gilliss, & Martinson, 1989). For long-term adjustment, it is also important for children to review the death event at each new developmental phase in order to reintegrate the experience with a more mature level of understanding.

Several articles have been written about the similarity between divorce and death in a family in terms of adjustment to the loss. Increased risk of illness and distress has been found among both recently divorced and widowed adults. The impact of certain factors on adjustment to widowhood and divorce (economic, social support, cause of divorce/death,

timing of event, and attachment) makes a difference as to how difficult both divorce and widowhood are (Kitson, Babri, Roach, & Placidi, 1989).

FAMILY ASSESSMENT

The evidence gathered to illustrate the bonds between family members is largely subjective. Both observational and interview data can be used. Observations about relationships include expression of feelings toward a family member as well as signs of closeness or distancing (kissing, hugging, eye contact, smiling, comforting, cuddling, sitting close or far away). Verbal (interview) data include responses to questions about how close member A is to member B. For example, how do A and B get along? What's their relationship like? Which of the siblings is closer to parent A? Also historical information often gives clues as to how close a relationship is. An example is the case of the mother who has constantly cared for the chronically ill child in hospital and home, while the father and older child have rarely been involved in caregiving. Table 14–5 provides questions that can be utilized to appraise the family affective function. To assist in summarizing the answers to some of the questions an attachment diagram is recommended. Attachment diagrams depict both the strength and quality of the affective relationship or emotional ties between members of the family. The focus is on the relationship and the reciprocal nature of the affectional tie. Figure 14–2 illustrates an attachment bond and the symbols used in these diagrams. Present relationships are diagrammed rather than past relationships. Bonds that are very close or very negative (conflictual) are typically maladaptive, although situational crisis sometimes forces very close relationships on a short-term basis and these very close relationships serve a necessary supportive purpose.

FAMILY NURSING DIAGNOSES

A myriad of family problems may be manifested in families where the psychological or affective needs of family members are not being adequately fulfilled. A number of North American Nursing Diagnosis

TABLE 14–5

AFFECTIVE FUNCTION ASSESSMENT QUESTIONS

1. **Mutual Nurturance, Closeness, and Identification**
   - To what extent do family members provide mutual nurturance to each other?
   - How supportive of each other are they?
   - Is a sense of closeness and intimacy present among the sets of relationships within the family?
   - How well do family members get along with each other?
   - Do they show affection toward each other?
   - Does mutual identification and bonding or attachment appear to be present? (Empathetic statements, concerns about others' feelings, experiences, and hardships are all indications of this being present.)

2. **Separateness and Connectedness**
   - How does the family deal with the issues of separateness and connectedness?
   - How does the family help its members want to be together and maintain cohesiveness (connectedness)?
   - Are opportunities for developing separateness stressed adequately, and are they appropriate for the age and needs of each of the family members?

3. **Family Need–Response Patterns**
   - To what extent do family members perceive the needs of the other individuals in the family?
   - Are the parents and spouses able to describe their children's and mate's needs and concerns?
   - How sensitive are family members in picking up cues regarding others' feelings and needs?
   - Are each member's needs, interests, and differentness respected by the other family members?
   - Do they show mutual respect toward each other?
   - How sensitive is the family to each individual's actions and concerns?
   - Are the recognized needs of family members being met by the family and, if so, to what extent?
   - What is the process for emotional release (unburdening) in the family?

Note: For the above questions it is suggested that a list of the family members be included with their needs identified (as perceived by family members) and the extent to which these needs are being met.

Association (NANDA) diagnoses may be appropriate when there is ineffective family affective functioning (Table 14–6). In these cases, an inability to meet the affective needs of all family members would be a defining characteristic.

FAMILY NURSING INTERVENTIONS

For interventions related to the NANDA diagnoses mentioned previously, the reader is referred to Carpenito (2000) and McCloskey and Bulechek (2000). General suggestions for assisting families to better meet the psychosocial needs of their members are briefly explained in the present section.

INTERVENTIONS PROMOTING HEALTHY NEED–RESPONSE PATTERNS

The assessment of this area (asking members to tell the nurse about each family member, what his or her psychological needs are, and if family members are responding to these needs) functions as an intervention in and of itself. Therefore, some preparation should precede the assessment, such as explaining to the family that each person has his or her own individual emotional needs, that many of these needs are based on the person's developmental stage, and that family members must recognize these needs and respond to them as much as possible—without interfering with one another's needs. In large families or families that are not psychologically oriented, this may be new information. In fact, there is a misperception by some parents that children should be treated exactly the same, so that no favoritism is involved. With this belief, parents often don't recognize each child's unique qualities. Teaching the family members about individual and family growth and developmental characteristics may be very helpful for sensitizing parents to their children's affective needs.

Another strategy for helping family members, especially the parents, become more sensitive to individual family members' affective needs is by asking, "What is Johnnie like?" When parents respond to this question, and the nurse asks further questions about the child's unique qualities, comments

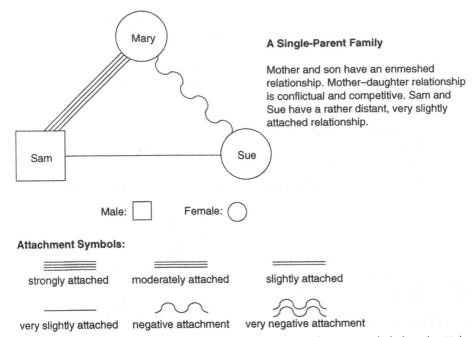

A Single-Parent Family

Mother and son have an enmeshed relationship. Mother–daughter relationship is conflictual and competitive. Sam and Sue have a rather distant, very slightly attached relationship.

Male: ☐   Female: ◯

Attachment Symbols:

strongly attached   moderately attached   slightly attached

very slightly attached   negative attachment   very negative attachment

Figure 14–2. An example of an attachment diagram. Shows a single-parent family. Mother and son have an enmeshed relationship. Mother–daughter relationship is conflictual and competitive. Sam and Sue have rather distant, very slightly attached relationship. *(Adapted from Wright & Leahey, 2000.)*

can then be made that interpret a child's behavior so that parents better reframe their perceptions of the child. For example, a mother says her son's incessant talking means that he is a spoiled brat. The family nurse relabels the behavior, helping the family see the son as feeling anxious and wanting his parents' attention.

PROMOTING MUTUAL NURTURANCE

To help families maintain or initiate mutual nurturance, communication patterns in the family need to be analyzed (Chapter 10). Parents need to feel that they are the ones who must stop circular patterns of angry, rejecting, or dysfunctional communication that sabotages affective function. For instance, they can ignore messages that start the dysfunctional pattern going, or they can learn not to initiate these kinds of interactions and instead communicate with the child so that mutual respect is shown. If parents understand the dynamics of problematic interactional patterns and are aware of what is happening,

they can take definitive steps to change dysfunctional communications. (See Chapter 10 for more elaborate discussion.) Nurses can act as communication role models to families and help them see that a more healthy mutual respect balance can be achieved in family interactions.

ASSISTING FAMILIES WITH CLOSENESS–SEPARATENESS ISSUES

Closeness–separateness problems may be due to a lack of knowledge and inhibition by family members as ways in which they can positively demonstrate aspects of the affective function toward one another. Parents may be modeling their own parents' behavior patterns with each other and to their children and there may be unresolved intergenerational problems. In health settings, overcloseness or enmeshment is a much more common problem than disengagement. In some families, the adult member(s) may become oversolicitous and overprotective of a family member who has a serious or disabling illness. In some cases,

TABLE 14–6

NANDA DIAGNOSES FOR INEFFECTIVE FAMILY AFFECTIVE FUNCTIONING

DIAGNOSIS	EXAMPLE
1. Interrupted Family Processes	The family is under stress and all the family members' energies are being diverted to handle the stressor, thereby neglecting or overlooking family members' psychosocial needs.
2. Impaired Parenting	A family with marked dominance by the mother (mother is very controlling) and marked passivity by father does not allow oldest adolescent son to individuate or separate from the family, thereby not meeting his psychosocial needs.
3. Risk for Impaired Parenting	The same as the above family example, except the oldest son is in fifth grade and has not entered puberty. Because of the mother's controlling, overbearing mothering, the potential for a problem occurring when the son reaches adolescence is very great.
4. Dysfunctional Grieving	Dysfunctional grieving is being extended to include the grieving family—which is grieving dysfunctionally. The usual family dysfunction is the denial of the death in the family. (Ineffective denial could also be stated.) A family rule is established that it's not all right to talk about the loss, to express feelings about the loss, or to recall memories of the loved one or events where the loved one was present. The memories, feelings, and thoughts are not shared, leading to other problems: psychosomatic illness, depression, pseudomutuality, emotional cutoff, and emotional distancing of family members from each other.
5. Compromised Family Coping	Mother has been hospitalized for one week due to having surgery. She is the primary nurturer in the family—to both the husband and children. The husband–father has attempted to give the children attention and love, but they (ages 2 and 3) are upset and resentful that their mother abandoned them.
6. Disabled Family Coping	Within this family the wife and husband (both are remarried) have two children—a son, age 10, from the husband's previous marriage, and a daughter, age 5, from the mother's previous marriage. The son has been labeled the troublemaker in the family, and is outwardly called this. The daughter is labeled the "sweet one," and comparisons of the children's personality differences are made when the parents get angry at the son.
7. Risk for Other-Directed Violence	These problems could also be present given the situation in which family members' psychosocial needs are not being adequately met.

the whole family may be highly resonant (or hypersensitive) to the "identified patient's" needs.

If enmeshment is a long-standing problem in a family and is of the intensity that family members' growth and development is being significantly impeded, family therapy may be needed, and a referral should be initiated if the family concurs with this diagnosis. Minuchin (1974), a noted family therapist, would work to restructure the enmeshed family, while Bowen (1978), another noted family therapist, would work on helping a fused family member(s) become more differentiated (more separated from the family).

ASSISTING FAMILIES WITH GRIEVING

Several authors have presented guidelines to facilitate grief resolution following a loss or death in the family (Corless, Germino, & Pittman, 1995;

McClowry et al., 1989; Kahn, 1990; Shapiro, 1994). In order to help family members who are in anticipatory grief (a family member is dying) or have experienced a loss and are now processing through their grief, family nurses need to understand tasks of family members during this difficult time. Tables 14–7 and 14–8 highlight information that can be useful in helping families engage in a healthy grieving process. A central thrust of the family nurse should be to help family members achieve patient–family member affective functioning. Rando (1986) suggests that to achieve this end family nurses can assist by helping to "maintain the relationship between the dying person and family by encouraging open communication to the extent the family style allows" (p. 75). Another intervention family-focused nurses make is assisting the family to assume new roles. One way to assist family members to adjust and to take on additional duties and make practical plans is having family conferences. A third exceptionally important intervention is to facilitate the expression of emotions and support the family members in their grief. Family members need to know that their feelings are normal and part of the grief process that needs to occur. Fourth, assisting the family to understand and absorb pertinent medical communication about the course of illness and treatment is a central role of the family nurse. Holding family conferences to explain illness, treatment concerns, and the dying process are very helpful. Last, family nurses need to assist family members, family friends, and even other health professionals in better understanding of the large variability in how grief is experienced. The nurse should not compel the family to subscribe to a belief that there is a normal experience of grief and also a pathological reaction (Moules & Amundson, 1997). Grief is a powerful emotion that cannot be bound by time restrictions, cultural traditions, gender or age-based assumptions, nor does it fit into the parameters of some discrete theoretical model. Each family situation is unique, and each family member is unique in their expression and management of personal loss.

TABLE 14–7

STRATEGIES TO HELP THE FAMILY FACING THE LOSS OF A FAMILY MEMBER THROUGH DEATH

- Family members should keep the dying person involved in family decisions as long as possible, so that he or she feels some sense of control and that his or her opinions still matter.

- The well family members need to individuate from the dying family member. They must come to grips with reality that the loved one will die, and to start contemplating the future without the loved one.

- Family members need to begin dealing with the reallocation or shifting of roles in the family to establish a new family homeostasis. This shifting of roles is often very difficult and family system functioning is precarious.

- Family members need to learn to manage the feelings aroused by the terminal illness and death. Sadness, guilt, anger, memories, and reactions to past losses are common emotions that need to be shared and managed.

- Family members need to face reality in terms of discussion of what needs to be done when death occurs (medical requirements, funeral arrangements, finances, etc.).

- Family members need to "say goodbye." This should be done by each family member—verbally or nonverbally. This critical area requires support and role modeling from caregivers. Family members need to know when death is imminent.

Adapted from Rando (1986).

TABLE 14-8

STRATEGIES TO ASSIST THE FAMILY AFTER THEY HAVE EXPERIENCED A LOSS

- Remind families that grief exerts tremendous stress on even the most loving relationships.

- Explain how family members may mourn individually and differently, depending on their ages and gender.

- Encourage bereaved parents to show their emotions to youngsters to help them understand what constitutes appropriate grieving behavior.

- Alert parents to the special needs of young children, who may feel guilty about the death of a family member because of unresolved disputes or rivalries.

- Recommend that parents be watchful of their teenagers' responses to death through withdrawal, the use of alcohol or drugs, or sexual activity.

- Encourage the lines of communication between all family members (parents to grandparents, grandparents to granchildren, parents to children, etc.) remain open at all times.

- Explain that our society has grown uneasy with death and grief, which can prevent loved ones from knowing what to say or do to help.

- Caution families to expect especially difficult times during major holidays.

- Encourage family members to use events such as the person's birthday or date of death as ways to remember and celebrate the life they shared with the deceased family member.

Sources: Bowden, Dickey, & Greenberg, 1998; Moffitt, 2001.

SUMMARY

- Fulfillment of the affective function is the central basis for both formation and continuation of the family unit.

- The affective function involves the family's perception of respect for, and care of, the psychological needs of its members.

- Fulfilling the affective function involves creating and maintaining a system within the family for mutual nurturance. This requires a basic commitment of a couple to each other and a nurturing, emotionally satisfying marital/intimate relationship.

- Through the affective function, individuals develop the ability to relate intimately or closely with one another. This process begins at birth as the infant bonds to his or her parents, and continues as family members are added.

- Families should maintain an atmosphere in which positive self-regard and the rights of both parents and children are highly valued.

- Bonding and identification occur when a couple discovers common interests, goals, and values and finds that the relationship validates each of them, carries with it certain tangible benefits, makes possible the meeting of certain goals that could not be accomplished alone, and provides mutual enjoyment and comfort due to their sustained contact with each other.

- Crescive bonds refer to enduring bonds that develop over time between family members, characterized by shared values and goals that are intensified by shared experiences and memories.

- Families must strive to achieve a balance between separateness and connectedness among family members. When separateness and connectedness are well balanced, families are better able to deal with situational stress and life changes.

- The enmeshed family is one in which individual and subsytem boundaries are continually violated by members outside those boundaries. Members tend to be too close and too restrictive of individual freedom and personal identity.

- Disengaged families are characterized by closed rigid boundaries between subsystems and individuals and evidence very little sensitivity to members' calls for assistance. Relationships are too distant and there is little recognition or meeting of family members' personal affective needs.

- Family members must perceive the needs of one another within the constraints of the family's cultural heritage. These needs must be viewed with respect and must be seen to be worthy of attention (as discussed under mutual respect balance) and must be satisfied to the extent possible in light of family resources.

- The therapeutic role that spouses or domestic partners play is problem oriented. It involves listening to each other's problems, sympathizing, giving reassurance and affection, and offering help in solving problems.

- Energized families are characterized by mutual acceptance of the uniqueness of family members, respect and acceptance of each other, and the capacity to encourage and to applaud the growth and achievements of family members.

- Maintaining a nurturing familial environment can be threatened when a member faces a severe illness or the family experiences the loss of a member. Family dysfunction can occur when these stressors arise. The emotional responses to this dysfunction can include anger, anxiety, depression, delinquent behaviors, acting-out behaviors, and somatic complaints and illness.

- To assess the affective function of the family, several questions can be asked in order to evaluate the family's perceived and actual ability to meet the emotional needs of its members. An attachment diagram can be used to illustrate the nature of the emotional ties that connect family members to one another.

- Ineffective family affective functioning may be seen in families struggling with illness, the loss of a family member, or the addition of a family member, as well as in families where perceived individual needs are no longer being met.

- Effective interventions to help families better meet their affective function include:
  - Teaching family members about basic family (and human) affective needs.
  - Teaching family members about family growth and developmental characteristics.
  - Asking members to share their interpretation of the behavior and actions of other members, and assisting families to reframe their understanding of these behaviors.
  - Assisting families to improve their communication patterns.
  - Helping families analyze the amount of closeness or individual freedom they afford one another, and providing suggestions on how to balance separateness and connectedness.
  - Assisting families to gain support from each other and from their communal support system in times of grief or loss.
  - Counsel and support families facing the loss of a family member through death.

❧ FAMILY VIGNETTE: THE NICHOLS FAMILY*

Mrs. Ruby Nichols, a 34-year-old obese woman, came to the mental health clinic because, she said, "I just don't know what to do." She was crying hysterically and unable to respond to further questioning. After remaining with her for an hour, the nurse was able to elicit that her 5-year-old foster daughter was being removed from her home per court order. Welfare funds, her only support for herself, her unemployed husband, and their five children, were being terminated in a week, leaving her unable to pay the bills or buy enough food for her family.

Although Mrs. Nichols was still tearful and depressed, she was able to be driven home by a community worker.

The following day the nurse made a visit to the Nichols' home. Mrs. Nichols related the following history: Ruby and John Nichols had been married 15 years. Four children were born of the marriage: Priscilla, 13; Cindy, 10; John Jr., 6; and Lisa, 4. They also had a foster daughter, Ann, age 5. The couple had known each other a year before their marriage in their hometown of Smithfield, Louisiana. John was an unskilled laborer, but had always managed to be employed. Ruby had attended business school prior to the marriage and was employed as a bookkeeper until the first child was born. She described her early marriage as fine except for moving so many times, caused by John's meddling mother. The family would move to get away from his mother, but she would always manage to locate them and appear on the scene. "We were a healthy, happy family and everything was fine as long as John's mother stayed away." Ruby related that this source of conflict between herself and John was resolved each time by a move on their part. However, according to Ruby, she and John never really discussed their mother-in-law problems. Following each new move, Ruby would join clubs and organizations to make new friends and John's work provided a similar opportunity for him. John also spent several evenings a week in the local bar, "shooting the bull" with the boys from work.

The family's last move was six months ago. After two months, John lost his job and was unable to find another. This resulted in the family's going on welfare, which Ruby and John felt ashamed of, as they had always prided themselves on paying their own bills. Shortly after this, John's mother found the family and moved into town. When she came to visit, a bitter argument ensued regarding John's mother and since then John had been staying away from home and drinking a lot. Moreover, three months ago Ruby had abdominal surgery, which was followed by complications and a prolonged hospitalization period. During her absence from home, the role of mother was assumed by Priscilla, who managed well with the help from the next door neighbor, Mrs. Law.

Ruby was released from the hospital three weeks ago as sufficiently recovered to stay at home. When she got home she perceived that the children had functioned very well in her absence; in fact, she felt that they did not need her and even seemed to resent her. John remained away most of the time and was minimally involved in family life both during her hospitalization and after her return home.

A week ago, Ruby learned of the court's decision to remove Ann from the home and the termination of welfare funds. Ruby felt herself becoming less and less able to manage and admitted to depression and suicidal thoughts. However, her concern for her children prevented her from doing anything self-destructive. The next-door neighbor, Mrs. Law, realizing the gravity of the family's situation, told Ruby to go to the mental health clinic for help.

Subsequent visits to the family revealed that the children were having problems and that Ruby had difficulties relating to their problematic behaviors. It was observed that the children and parents did not discuss these problems or their concerns with each other, and that there was no movement toward sharing their feelings about Ann's leaving, the mother-in-law's disruptive influence, or Ruby's health problems.

Priscilla, age 13, seemed to resent Ruby's return, because it meant the loss of her mothering role. She and her mother have engaged in frequent arguments over the discipline of the younger children, what they should wear, and how they should act. The arguments usually ended with Priscilla leaving the house for long periods of time without telling Ruby where she was. This caused Ruby to worry. Priscilla was not interested in school, her main interest being to grow up as quickly as possible and emulate her mother. She also wanted desperately to be independent and make her own decisions in life. Ruby had weaned Priscilla early in terms of her being self-sufficient at home; from age 6 on, Priscilla was caring for her younger siblings and helping her mother out in the home.

Cindy, age 10, seemed unaffected by the situation. She was quite involved with her school activities and Campfire Girls and spent much time in these activities and at her friends' homes. Priscilla and Cindy evidently have a closer sibling relationship than the other siblings do. Cindy tells all her secrets to Priscilla when she is upset, worried, or needs someone to talk to.

John Jr., a first grader, was refusing to go to school. Every morning it was now a struggle to get him off to school. He would cry and hang on to his mother. His teacher reported poor school work and lack of attentiveness when he was present.

Lisa, age 4, displayed similar clinging behaviors to those of John Jr. She seemed frightened when her mother left the home and was wetting the bed again after having no problems in this area for two years. Both John Jr. and Lisa frequently questioned their mother about the recent absence of Ann. They asked if Ann went away because she was bad.

On the third contact between the family (the parents) and the nurse at the mental health clinic, the nurse asked the parents to describe each child, what he or she was like, and what personal needs or problems they were trying to assist their children with at that time. It was noted that specific information on each child was difficult to obtain. For instance, these general statements were made: "Oh, he (she) is just the average 6-year-old" (or whatever age applied), or "Priscilla's just like all other teenagers, wanting her way all the time," or "I treat all my children the same, regardless." They were able to recognize, though, Priscilla's need to care for her younger siblings and to be independent, but were not open to her staying away from the family very much, or developing a set of friends outside the family with whom she might have frequent social contact.

The mother also recognized that Lisa was very attached to and dependent on her, and needed reassurance that her mother would be back when she left home. Additionally, both parents thought Ann's leaving was threatening to the younger children, who might think this might happen to them if they misbehaved. Ruby was trying to spend more time with Lisa to help her with her fears over the mother's separation and Ann's leaving. John showed interest in comforting and being involved with Lisa also, since Lisa always responded in "such a cute, loving way to her daddy," according to the mother.

Both parents are able to show affection and warmth to the younger children (John Jr. and Lisa), but do not feel that it is appropriate to be so physical when they get older. It was noted that the parents were not physically affectionate to each other and seemed emotionally distant during the interviews. Ruby says that they have never shared their personal concerns with each other much. She said, "It takes another woman to understand my feelings. I used to confide in Priscilla a lot, but since she is upset with me, I haven't been able to talk with her."

*Vignette used in Chapter 17 and adapted from Black (1974).

■ STUDY QUESTIONS

Review the Family Vignette and answer the related questions.

1. To what extent do family members perceive and meet the affective needs of other family members?

2. Does a mutual respect balance exist, where each member shows respect for the other's feelings and needs?

3. To what extent do family members provide mutual nurturance to each other? How supportive of each other are they?

4. Is a sense of closeness and intimacy present among the sets of relationships within the family? How compatible and affectionate are family members toward each other?

5. Does mutual identification and bonding appear to be present?

6. How does the family deal with the issues of separateness and connectedness?

7. Propose one family nursing diagnosis in the area of family affective function.

8. Recommend two family nursing interventions to resolve or ameliorate the above problem.

Answer the following questions.

9. Discuss three reasons why the affective function is so important.

10. The need–response pattern includes not only the perception of family members' needs and the meeting of these needs in the family. What other component is part of this pattern, the component that makes meeting the needs possible?

11. The results and goals of achieving a balance in familial mutual respect are (select appropriate answers):

    a. Members of the family do not encroach on the rights of the other individuals in the family.

    b. No family members are expected to cater to the whims of other family members.

    c. Parents treat children as people, not "inferiors" (objects to be manipulated and dominated).

    d. Children do not develop "brat" syndrome, in which they seek and receive gratification for their needs, but fail to consider the needs, rights, and responsibilities of parents.

12. Match the four terms and/or concepts in the right-hand column with definitions and descriptions in the left-hand column.

Definitions/Descriptions	Terms/Concepts
a. Responsiveness of other member(s) to a family's positive feelings toward them.	1. Bonding or attachment
	2. Identification
b. Empathy or role making.	3. Crescive bonds
	4. A response bond

  c. Sustaining force behind perception and satisfaction of family members' needs.

  d. Develops in familial relationships where there is continuity and positive interaction.

  e. Grows in intensity with time.

  f. Identification precedes it.

  g. Parents obtain referent power when this is present.

  h. Receiver's reaction to sender's affection and warmth.

13. What is the parental task relative to dealing with connectedness and separateness?

14. The spousal/partner therapeutic role differs from the family affective function in that (select all appropriate answers):

  a. They do not differ; both are synonymous terms.

  b. The spousal/partner therapeutic role deals with a subsystem rather than with an entire family system.

  c. The therapeutic role is largely problem focused, whereas the affective function covers therapeutic aspects and other supportive and nurturing elements.

  d. The family affective function deals only with being sensitive to family members' feelings, while the therapeutic role suggests more skilled assistance.

15. Pratt describes energized families and how they can achieve their affective function. From her description, list two salient values or priorities that energized families display relative to this area.

16. What are ways the nurse can interview to support the family experiencing grief due to a loss of a family member?

THE FAMILY SOCIALIZATION FUNCTION

LEARNING OBJECTIVES

1. Define socialization in relation to child-rearing families.
2. Describe shifts in societal attitudes toward children and child rearing over recent decades.
3. Describe how changes in gender roles of men and women have influenced child rearing.
4. Summarize contradictory reports about the effects of day care on children's well-being.
5. Describe changes in expectations for children and adolescents.
6. Give examples of how legislative action affects child care and children.

7. Explain the relationships between selected theories and family socialization function.
8. Discuss the role that culture plays in socialization patterns, particularly child-rearing practices.
9. Explain the role that social class plays in socialization and identify some broad differences in socialization of children of working-class and middle-class families.
10. Provide examples of socialization patterns unique to selected, nontraditional family forms (families of single-parents, stepparents, and lesbian/gay parents).
11. Apply the nursing process to a hypothetical family vignette in terms of family socialization patterns.

The family is more specialized in its function today than it has ever been. Nevertheless, one vital responsibility has remained a primary focus of the family: the socialization or the rearing of children. The nurse is frequently in a position to influence, support, and assist the socialization process in families. This chapter defines and discusses socialization processes, the social context for child-rearing families, contemporary socialization patterns, theories related to children's socialization, and the influence of culture, social class, and family form on parenting patterns. The chapter concludes with nursing practice guidelines (assessment areas, family nursing diagnoses, and intervention).

SOCIALIZATION: DEFINITIONS AND INFLUENCES

Socialization begins at birth and ends only at death. It is a lifelong process by which individuals continually modify their behavior in response to the socially patterned circumstances they experience. It includes internalizing the appropriate sets of norms and values for the teenager of 14, the young professional of 25, the parent of 29, the grandparent of 55, and the retired person of 65.

Socialization embraces all those processes in a specific community or group whereby humans, through their significant lifetime experiences, acquire socially patterned characteristics (Honigman, 1967). Translated into role terminology, the concept of socialization refers to "the process of development or change that a person undergoes as a result of social interaction and the learning of social roles" (Gecas, 1979, p. 365). Child-rearing practices are subsumed under the rubric of socialization and are the primary focus of this chapter. The terms "socialization," "socialization process," "child rearing," "parental behavior," and "parent–child interaction" are used interchangeably in both this chapter and in the child socialization literature in general (Gecas).

Most often, socialization proceeds informally and inexplicitly, so that changes made in response to altering cultural and environmental conditions go quite unnoticed. Through socialization, people learn to live with others in groups and come to play gender and age-linked roles considered appropriate for their social context.

In the family, socialization refers to the myriad of learning experiences provided within the family. These experiences are aimed at teaching children how to function and assume adult roles in society. The child is taught language, the roles he or she is expected to assume at various stages of life, sociocultural norms and expectations of what is right and wrong, and relevant cognitive structures. Reiss (1965) points out that the nurturant socialization of children is found universally within the family structure. It is the family, particularly the parents, who transmit their cultural knowledge to the next generation. Parents are responsible for ferrying children from birth through the various developmental challenges and life events to adulthood.

Children's socialization also occurs through their experiences outside of the family, such as interactions with adults at their schools. Hillary Rodham Clinton (1996) points out the importance of people outside the immediate family for children:

> "Children exist in the world as well as in the family. From the moment they are born, they depend on a host of other "grown-ups"—grandparents, neighbors, teachers, ministers, employers, political leaders, and untold others who touch their lives directly and indirectly. Adults police their streets, monitor the quality of their food, air, and water, produce the programs that appear on their televisions, run the businesses that employ their parents, and write the laws that protect them. Each of us plays a part in every child's life: It takes a village to raise a child." (pp. 11–12)

Clinton also noted the indirect influences of other people on children through "radio, television, newspapers, books, movies, computers, compact discs, cellular phones, and fax machines" (p. 13), and wrote about how extrafamily influences may be invaluable or destructive to children's well-being. The values or lessons learned outside the home may support or conflict with the family's own lifeways and socialization patterns. A case in point is the recent immigrant family, where the school system teaches children values and norms that contradict the non-Western values and norms the immigrant parents have and are trying to transmit to their children.

One aspect of the socialization process of particular relevance for nurses is the child's acquisition of health concepts, attitudes, and behaviors. Typically, the mother is the family's primary health educator and leader. She has the responsibility for deciding whether a family member is sick, whether or not to initiate treatment, and what kind it should be. She is usually responsible for teaching her children basic health habits and attitudes and, as they grow older, how to care for themselves.

Another important and integral task of socialization is the inculcation of controls and values—giving the growing child (and adult) a sense of what is right and wrong and the internal controls needed for self-discipline. The development of morality has been described by Kohlberg (1970) and Gilligan (1982) as a developmental process evolving over childhood and adolescence. By identifying with parental figures and experiencing consistent responses to their behavior, children develop a personal value system and a set of morals that is greatly influenced by the family (Baumrind, 1996).

It is clear and notable that many variables affect child outcomes. As noted earlier, parents share the socialization function with other important institutions and the wider community. Children themselves vary greatly in their temperament and behavioral traits (Dadds, 1995; Kileen, 1995) and influence the way parents relate to them. In fact, there is a recent school of thought that the general family environment may be less significant than genetic influences on children's behavior and child outcomes (Bussell & Reiss, 1993). Regardless of whether environment or heredity is most influential, both factors are indisputably sources of variation in children's behavior.

Changes in traditional socialization patterns, responsibilities, and time-honored methods are now occurring at a greater rate than ever before. The dilemma of who will teach children important sociocultural traditions, how and where these are to be learned, and at what age and stage are the questions we have struggled with in the past and will continue to debate into the future.

SOCIETAL CONTEXT FOR CHILD-REARING FAMILIES

No matter which society we observe, the attitudes and approaches to the care and rearing of children are congruent with the social, moral, religious, and economic values of that society at a particular period of time. Over time, the place of children in our society has changed. Extraordinary gains have been made in the understanding and care of children. But along with such advances, new social and economic pressures and realities have introduced other attitudes and concerns.

Goodman's observations in 1978 of these events suggest that something had changed in the relationship between adults and their children over recent decades. Goodman commented on the reemergence of a hostile relationship between adults and children, and expressed a concern for the untoward effects of this generational conflict:

> Now, increasingly, parenthood is regarded as a personal, individual decision—a "lifestyle," whatever that may be—made apart from community interests. Kids are listed not as economic assets, but as financial liabilities. Each year, someone tallies up the cost of raising them as if they were sides of beef. And each year, someone else tallies up their cost to the local town or city and wonders if they are worth it. In many places, the voters are saying "no." (p. E1)

Elkind (1994), a noted child development educator, laments over the changes that have occurred in the postmodern, contemporary family. He notes: "In the modern nuclear family [the family of the 1950s and 1960s] binding sentiments were largely child-centered in the sense that they give preference to the well-being of children and required the self-sacrifice of parents. In the post modern permeable [contemporary] family, however, the sentimental ties have been transformed and are now more likely to be adult centered to the extent that they favor the well-being of parents and adults and require self-sacrifice from the young" (p. 38). Elkind states that the pendulum has swung in favor of fulfilling adult needs and has led to a "family need imbalance," where children and youth are under greater stress than adults. Elkind asserts, "Children are under substantially greater stress because the world is a more dangerous and complicated place to grow up in, and in part, because their need to be protected, nurtured, and guided has been neglected" (p. 201).

Child development experts mirror Goodman's concern about societal attitudes toward children. Elkind (1994) says that there are times in history when children fare better than others. But there is no question about it: Children are generally not well cared for in our society today. Child advocacy organizations cite statistics that show the declining lot of children (e.g., increased poverty, infant mortality, delinquency, teen pregnancy, and child abuse) (Children's Defense Fund, 1995).

Some authors such as Popenoe (1995) and Lasch (1977) suggest that institutional "overseeing" of the training needs of children has resulted from parents' disenchantment with traditional family roles, as well as their waning commitment to child rearing. It is also argued that part of this decline in enthusiasm for raising children stems from the difficulties parents feel in trying to fulfill their primary roles due to increased economic and employment pressures and increased personal needs for their own development and self-expression (Elkind, 1994; Popenoe).

The feminist movement of the 1970s increased the options in women's lives. However, many women experience role overload as they carry out all their old roles, in addition to new ones (Woodward, 1990). Experts tell parents to spend "quality time" and "meaningful" time with their children, but even this is difficult to squeeze in between a multiplicity of other priorities. In a recent national survey, 84 percent of parents said they are having a tough time balancing work and family responsibilities (Mehren, 1996).

In response to the increasing numbers of dual-earner families, Broom (1998) studied the effects of maternal employment on both the children and on the parents' marriage. She found that employed mothers showed significantly greater sensitivity interacting with their infants, compared to nonemployed mothers. However, marital satisfaction was less among the dual-earner parents than among single-earner couples. These findings are consistent with the family systems perspective, and consideration of the different patterns of child socialization, depending on the family circumstances.

Green (1994) and his co-authors in the influential book, *Bright Futures: Guidelines for Health Supervision of Infants, Children and Adolescents,* reiterate Elkind's (1994) concerns about children when they state that children face new and troubling issues today due to major economic, social, and demographic changes affecting families. As part of these pressures, parents spend less time with their children and children have less contact with extended family members. There is increased geographic mobility, a shortage of quality day care services, diminished neighborhood involvement, and widespread family restructuring of relationships.

The professional advice given to parents may be a reflection of the child's changing status in a particular time in society. When one examines the shifts in the advice given to parents over the past 60 years, the fluctuating philosophies and anxieties of a highly industrialized and technological society appear evident. Elkind (1994) and Osborne (1995) note these changes in child-rearing advice across the decades:

- 1910s and 1920s: Spank them, deprive them.
- 1930s and 1940s: Ignore them, reason with them.
- 1950s and 1960s: Love them and spank them lovingly.
- 1970s: Use firmness with love.
- 1980s and 1990s: Apply parenting "techniques" advocated by parenting experts.

Methods of child rearing have changed drastically over the decades (Table 15–1). In the 1920s, influenced by Watson, a behaviorist, firm, controlled child-rearing practices were in vogue. In the 1960s and 1970s, there was a return to a permissive, more relaxed way of child rearing. In the 1990s, more democratic strategies characterized by a combination of rational control, mutual communication, and high levels of affection were in vogue (Bodman & Peterson, 1995).

Elkind (1994) and Osborne (1995) also observed a shift from an emphasis on the nurturing aspects of parenting pervasive in the previous three decades to an emphasis on using scientifically based "parenting techniques," which are more democratic and encourage mutual communication, but are also more structured and rule oriented. Simultaneously, the controversy about the relative influence of "nature versus nurture" in children's behavior continues (Cowley, 1995). More sophisticated techniques for assessing

TABLE 15-1

CHANGING CHILD-REARING VIEWS AND PRACTICES

From one generation to the next, parents and pediatricians have altered the way they feed, teach, and discipline their children. Some examples across the decades:

	1900s–1910s	1920s–1930s	1940s–1950s	1960s–1970s	1980s	1990s
BREAST-FEEDING						
	Nursing popular although many well-to-do women used wetnurses.	Commercially prepared formulas popular as a convenient and progressive way of nourishing infants.		A return to nursing promoted by women's groups and pediatricians as healthier and providing more nurturance.	Nursing overwhelmingly preferred by middle-class white women, less popular with African-Americans and Latinos.	Nursing preferred by middle-class white women, while less popular among Latinos and African-Americans.
THUMB-SUCKING						
	Attitudes not uniform, although often discouraged.	Prohibited by most parents and physicians.	Allowed along with pacifiers.	Encouraged, along with pacifiers.	Offered, along with pacifiers but neither discouraged nor encouraged.	Offered to children until a certain age and then are taken away to prevent orthodontic, overbite problems.
POTTY TRAINING						
	Enemas and bowel irrigation popular methods of "cleaning" babies.	Begun as early as 2 months of age.	Delayed until 6–18 months.		Child determines time to begin, usually between ages 2 and 3.	May be "hurried" because of need for mother to place child in child care center where children need to be potty trained.
DISCIPLINE						
	Children expected to act like small adults.	Strict and early discipline advocated.	Common sense and nurturance urged.	Permissive era of child rearing.	Moderate discipline that is age appropriate.	
LEARNING						
	Moral training began early.	Nursery schools proliferated as early education became popular.		Early reading advocated along with early training for disadvantaged children.	"Super babies" urged to be treated normally; day care increasingly becomes a national issue.	Providing many avenues for learning and stimulation. Older children are seen as competent and less in need of guidance and protection.

Partially adapted from Elkind (1994),, Roack (1988).

405

physiological variables have led to renewed arguments about whether most human development and behavior is biologically based rather than being strongly influenced by environmental or parenting variables. Cowley comments that "Asking whether nature or nurture is more important is like asking whether length or width is a better gauge of size" (p. 52).

Review of the various historic and contemporary attitudes and approaches to children illuminates the obvious; children have always generated an "air of ambivalence" that permeates society and influences its values and beliefs in the care and rearing of its young. Certainly, the ambivalence that exists regarding children extends throughout society. The increased use of drugs and alcohol among school-aged children and adolescents, along with their myriad of other health and social problems, only increases this feeling of ambivalence. Still, in the middle of conflicting values and beliefs about children and their place in society, an attempt is also being made to adapt to such ambivalence, change, and conflict by emphasizing the importance of the family in child rearing and "revaluing" the parent–child dyad relationships.

In contrast to some researchers who emphasize the biological basis of child behavior, many continue to focus on the impact of the home environment. For example, Blum (2000) collected data from 90,000 adolescents across the country to learn about health-related experiences. He found that "Across all of the health outcomes examined, the results point to the importance of family and the home environment for protecting adolescents from harm" (p. F9). Blum specifically urged parents to restrict adolescents' access to tobacco, alcohol, and firearms in the home in order to minimize the opportunities for dangerous or unhealthy practices.

❧ CONTEMPORARY SOCIALIZATION PATTERNS

A real need exists to assess the changes that have occurred in family socialization patterns and the impact on child rearing and the long-term effects of these new social relationships and arrangements on children. We cannot say with certainty what the impact will be of increased equity in parenting roles, reassignment of traditional male–female parenting practices, varied family forms, or realignment of traditional cultural values with those of new host cultures. These changes suggest issues that nurses will inevitably face in caring for emerging families of the future.

Parents may be overwhelmed with parenting issues and with conflicting advice from many sources. Pediatricians and other child care specialists have become the grandmothers of the 1990s. The tendency for parents to rely on the judgment of others may have been carried to the extreme. One example of this trend is from an article in the *Los Angeles Times* by Dr. Joyce Brothers (1990), a psychologist, on "Testing Parenting Philosophies." Dr. Brothers asks her readers eight questions about "What does being a good parent mean?" Scientific answers are then supplied to correct any faulty information the reader might have; from this short article it is clear that scientific knowledge has become the acceptable basis for parenting decisions in mainstream America.

Child care experts report that parents are worried, confused, and uncertain. Parents dash to work and hand their children to a variety of relatives, nannies, sitters, nursery and elementary schools, day care centers, neighbors, and recreational, social, and religious organizations for after-school and weekend activities (Elmer-Dewitt, 1990). They are not raising children the way they were raised and they have little idea of how their children will turn out (Elmer-Dewitt).

CHANGES IN GENDER ROLE SOCIALIZATION

Masculine and feminine adult roles are changing in families, and as they change, so do the socialization experiences of children. Research on gender roles in child rearing demonstrates modest changes in child care roles of parents, although there has been more father involvement in child care activities, particularly when children are older. Mothers remain the primary caregivers through the preschool years of children's lives (Thompson & Walker, 1991). Regardless of children's ages, mothers are typically more involved in the daily lives of their children than fathers, who tend to take a "helping" or "assistive" role in child care. Relative to father involvement, there seems to be two divergent trends. On the one hand, more and more fathers are involved in child care either by choice or by necessity (both working parents, job loss, single fatherhood, etc.). On the other hand, the absence of fathers is reaching epidemic proportions (Stolberg, 1996b). Father participation (or a father substitute) is critically needed for positive child outcomes (Snarey, 1993).

In working-class families, gender roles in child care usually follow the more traditional pattern. Men and women tend to have segregated roles in which mothers are responsible for home and family, including child care, and fathers are the primary wage earners (Hughes & Perry-Jenkins, 1996). According to Hughes and Perry-Jenkins, working-class wives place very little responsibility on their husbands for the child care and emotional support of their children. Child rearing is more gender based than in middle-class parents.

Discontinuity with prior practices is evident in many aspects of child rearing including sex-role behavior and expectations. Motherhood has come to occupy a less significant aspect of many women's adult lives who are from acculturated families. Many mothers are wage earners, and so socialization practices are changing. There are fewer sex-based differences in socialization patterns (Hoffman, 1977; Scanzoni & Szinovacz, 1980). Most parents today are being encouraged to socialize their children in a more androgynous fashion, that is, not as identified with a specific gender. Moreover, there are emerging concerns that the feminist emphasis on eliminating gender-based roles and creating more life options for girls has led to role confusion for many boys. Levine (1995) wrote that

> ". . . many experts now say we've been driving our little boys crazy. We send them out in the world each day with outdated, confusing messages about how they should act and what it means to be a man. They must be stoic but empathetic, strong yet vulnerable, tough but never too forceful. They must be masculine while embracing their feminine side." (p. E1)

A number of new books about raising boys speak to the gender role angst of many boys (Pollack, 1999; Gurian, 2000). Pollack argues that many parents are still enforcing outdated gender guidelines for boys and he encourages more flexibility in the "boy code" in parenting. Others, such as Gurian, emphasize the biological bases for gender differences in behavior and call for acknowledging and channeling the behavior differences into moral and ethical development to counter the societal messages, which encourages violence and chaos in boys' lives.

DAY CARE AND SOCIALIZATION OF YOUNG CHILDREN

Day care is the top-priority issue for working parents. The proportion of working women who have children continues to rise. Rapid growth in women's participation in the workforce means a concomitant growth in child care for preschool through school-aged children (after-school programs for those in school). A major worry for many parents is deciding who can assist them with child care while they are at work (Kelleher, 1996). Child care is usually expensive, and even when parents can afford day care, accessibility and quality are often inadequate (Dickinson & Leming, 1995). Parents and some social scientists share the concern that day care is ultimately not as good for the child as the parent's care. For instance, Levine (1988) argues that there is compelling evidence that "day care" children suffer more from diseases and emotional problems (separation anxiety) than children who remain at home with mother. These children are poorly socialized when they are sent to day care too soon or for too long.

Hofferth and Phillips (1987) reported their own evaluation of the research on the effect of mothers' employment and found no consistent positive or negative impact on the child. A growing body of research indicates that children of satisfied working mothers tend to do well. The children demonstrate positive adaptation, self-esteem, and self-aspirations (*Los Angeles Times* Editorial, 1996). A large number of school-aged children—almost 15 percent according to one national survey—go home alone after school (Kelleher, 1996). For a great majority of school-aged children their "self-care" works out satisfactorily. But for some, it does not. For these latch-key children, supervision or after-school programs are needed. After-school hours are a very important and formative part of a child's day.

CHANGES IN EXPECTATIONS FOR CHILDREN AND ADOLESCENTS

Child development experts believe that today's child is being pushed to act like an adult long before he or she is developmentally ready to do so. Many middle-class and affluent parents have the tendency to push their children to overachieve, to become "super babies" or "super kids" (Roack, 1988; Tofler & DiGeronimo, 2000). Many children are being pressured to read before kindergarten and are left unsupervised after school. Some hurried children develop into "harried teens," expected not only to achieve in school but to shop, cook, and care for the family as well (Libman, 1988). Part-time employment at minimum wage during high school has also risen sharply, but only about 11 percent of adolescents in school save rather than spend their earnings from part-time employment.

Increasing numbers of young adults are taking longer to finish college, longer to establish a career, longer to leave home, and longer to become independent with families of their own. Many more young adults are living at home after they graduate from school or are cohabiting. With the unprecedented rise in cohabitation, over 50 percent of all men and women live together before marriage (Popenoe and Whitehead, 1999). These changes reflect a change in some of our values—consumerism, narcissism, individualism, and instant gratification (Orthner, 1995; Woodward, 1990). These values are learned through role modeling and other socialization experiences in and outside of the home.

LEGISLATION AFFECTING CHILD CARE AND CHILDREN

There have been dramatic changes in this century in the laws concerning child care and protection, as well as numerous changes in the concepts of children's rights, parental rights, duties, and responsibilities. The legal system presents a sometimes contradictory picture of expectations of parents. In the past, the father was regarded as the "natural guardian" of the child and was free to punish his child within reasonable boundaries. Some of the most frequently used disciplinary practices of the past are being redefined as unacceptable, ill advised, or even detrimental. Physical punishment, from spanking to more severe punitiveness, is being redefined as child abuse by some researchers of child abuse (Gelles, 1990; Steinmetz, 1995).

In the past, loss of parents' rights over the care and discipline of their children could occur only in extreme cases when a "fit person" order was made by the court. The Children's Act of 1975 evidenced a disenchantment with the natural family as inevitably providing the best care for the child. This change was brought about following the death of a child after being returned to her natural mother. This situation served to strengthen the rights of foster parents, as well as direct the appointment, in appropriate circumstances, of a person to act as guardian of the child or young person in order to safeguard his or her interests.

Legally, children's rights are now widely recognized by the American courts. For instance, in many states, children are entitled to the protection of a lawyer if they are accused of committing a delinquent act and have to appear in court. Greater civil rights for children make clear to parents that children are no longer considered their property and that outside authorities and agencies have the legal right to question parental actions.

In spite of this recent legislation, children are still inadequately protected in our society. The rise in child abuse is evidence of this. Since 1985, there has been a 40 percent increase in the number of reported cases of child maltreatment (Green, 1994). Baumrind (1994) believes that escalating child maltreatment is symptomatic of societal neglect of the "forgotten half" of our populace. (See Chapter 13 for discussion of family values.)

Another area where children are not adequately protected is in the area of day care (Belsky, 1995). There are no minimum federal standards to protect the safety and well-being of children in day care centers (Dickinson & Leming, 1995). And widespread noncompliance with state regulations means that the quality of child care in the United States is frequently poor to minimally adequate (Scarr, 1995).

Child advocacy groups have voiced grave concern about the 1996 welfare reform legislation whereby deep cuts are being made in aid to families with dependent children. Welfare recipients with young children are being forced into the workplace; immigrant families who are not citizens are being denied welfare benefits. The rights of the children in these two types of families are not being protected (Kelleher, 1996).

⚘THEORIES RELATED TO SOCIALIZATION

Theoretical perspectives from psychology and sociology form the foundation for the socialization literature. This section reviews relevant concepts from developmental theories and theoretical perspectives about the processes of socialization, and how variations in parental support and control affect children.

DEVELOPMENTAL THEORIES

The most important socialization task for parents is in establishing and guiding the next generation (Erikson, 1963). Erikson's concept of generativity demonstrates an understanding of the importance of socialization for continuity. In Erikson's discussion of generativity versus stagnation, he describes the mature person's need for and dependence on the younger generation. Erikson asserts that when this stage is not fulfilled, regression to an obsessive need for pseudo-intimacy takes place, often with a pervading sense of stagnation and personal impoverishment. Bronfenbrenner (1974) embellishes on the importance of this developmental stage in his com-

ment that we must bring adults back into the lives of children and children back into the lives of adults.

Achieving the motivation for continuity between the generations has become something of a dilemma, because it is difficult to foster the concept of continuity in a time of discontinuity and change. Past traditions, values, and social norms to many parents seem emptied of their utility for the day-to-day functioning of their families. The lack of traditions in families may have subtle, yet important, disruptive effects on the ability of parents to socialize children for continuity. In light of the array of available information on child rearing, the nurse frequently is one of the health care professionals assisting parents to sort out and understand their children's needs and their own responsibilities. In this regard, Friedman (1957), five decades ago, suggested five definitive stages through which parents progress and the appropriate child-rearing task for each period. Each stage reflects the major problems in the child's development with which the parent is grappling. These stages have been observed in a wide variety of sociocultural settings and ethnic groups, as well as in single-parent families, and the basic concepts appear to be universal. The five stages of parent development are outlined in Table 15–2.

TABLE 15–2

STAGES OF PARENT DEVELOPMENT

STAGE OF CHILD DEVELOPMENT	STAGE OF PARENT DEVELOPMENT	PARENTAL TASK
I. Infant	Learning the cues	To interpret infant needs
II. Toddler	Learning to accept growth and development	To accept some control while maintaining necessary limits
III. Preschooler	Learning to separate	To allow independent development while modeling necessary standards
IV. School-ager	Learning to accept rejection without deserting	To be there when needed without intruding unnecessarily
V. Teenager	Learning to build a new life—having been thoroughly discredited by one's teenager	To adjust to changing family roles and relationships during and after the teenager's struggle to establish his/her identity

Adapted from Friedman (1957).

SOCIALIZATION PROCESSES

The biggest theoretical breakthrough in the area of child socialization has been the recognition that parent–child relationships are dynamic and interactive (Bodman & Peterson, 1995; Broderick, 1993; Brody, 1994; Rollins & Thomas, 1979). Most research and theoretical discussion up until recently presented a static unidirectional model of parent causation; that is, parents have certain child-rearing techniques, and with these they mold the behavior and attitudes of the child. This one-sided lineal perspective ignored the prior history of interaction between parent and child, as well as the specific immediate antecedent responses of the child to the parents. This "social mold" theory blamed the mother for the child's later problems. Chess (1983), a well-known child development researcher, explains:

> Although the mother's role in child development is significant, development proceeds through a series of interactions with many others, including the father, siblings, teachers, and peers. Other factors that influence child development include individual neuro-chemical, genetic, and temperamental characteristics of the child. The point, then, that no one factor is overriding makes linear unidimensional models of child development obsolete. (p. 6)

It is crucial that family nurses are cognizant of the influence that the children's characteristics can have on families and vice versa (Dadds, 1995). Today, using a systems circular causation model in which feedback loops exist, children are viewed as active organisms who contribute significantly to the nature and course of the evolving parent–child relationship. Children are viewed as shaping parents' behavior and parents as shaping children's behavior. For successful parenting to occur, there needs to be a "goodness of fit" between the child and his or her environment (the expectations and demands of caregivers are consonant with the child's skills and potentials) (Chess, 1983).

Although there has been an extensive amount of research in the area of parent–child socialization, the cultural variable has been largely ignored in the past and the social class variable not disentangled from the cultural variable. However, there is evidence to suggest that family size affects children's socialization

as well. Growing up in a small family constitutes a qualitatively different developmental and child-rearing experience than growing up in a large family. Children from small families tend to receive more attention than children from large families. Research has linked these differences to intellectual development and school performance (Feiring & Lewis, 1984).

In summary, earlier research studies based their investigations on social mold conceptualizations, while later research emphasized bidirectional systemic models (Peterson & Rollins, 1987).

PARENTAL SUPPORT AND CONTROL

The most powerful models explaining effective parenting are those combining parental support and control. Parents have been most effective when they combine a high level of support with authoritative control (Gecas & Seff, 1991). Parental support is one of the most robust factors associated with positive child outcomes (Gecas & Seff). Rollins and Thomas (1979), in an in-depth review and analysis of child-rearing research, which has primarily studied white parents and children, state that there is sufficient empirical evidence to support the following propositions about the effects of parental support.

1. Especially for boys, the greater the supportive behavior of parents toward children, the greater such culturally valued child behaviors as self-esteem, academic achievement, creativity, and conformity.

2. In most instances, a positive relationship is found between parental support and cognitive development in children.

3. The greater the parental support, the greater the moral behavior of children and conformity to adult standards.

4. The greater the parental support, the greater the self-esteem, internal locus of control, and instrumental competence in children.

In summary, parental support was consistently found to have a positive association with all aspects of social competence in children, with the exception of creativity. Here a curvilinear relationship was revealed. Creativity increases in conditions of low to moderate parental support and decreases in moderate to high parental supportive conditions. Creativity also decreases as parental coercion increases.

Different styles of parental control have been found to have opposite socialization consequences (Gecas & Seff, 1991). Baumrind (1978) classifies parental styles of discipline and control into indulgent permissive, authoritative, and authoritarian. The permissive parental style is characterized by being accepting and nonpunitive in dealing with the child's behaviors. In contrast, the authoritarian style of discipline and control stresses obedience to rules and parents' authority. Control is based on force, threat, or physical punishment. Finally, the authoritative style of discipline and control stresses a rational, issue-oriented, "give-and-take" way of dealing with the child. Control is based on reason and explanation. Authoritarian and indulgent permissive styles are associated with negative or unfavorable socialization outcomes, while authoritative control has positive socialization outcomes. Hence, of the three styles, Baumrind advocates the third, asserting that it can produce reasonable conformity without loss of autonomy or self-assertiveness.

Epstein and associates (1982, 1993) studied behavioral control in normal and troubled families over the last 30 years. They discovered that a flexible behavior control style, in which there were reasonable standards and an opportunity for negotiation and change, was the most effective control style. This style is more likely to be present in normally functioning families. In contrast, a chaotic, unpredictable behavior control style was the least effective and found most frequently in dysfunctional families.

CULTURAL VARIATIONS IN SOCIALIZATION PATTERNS

The context in which child rearing and socialization patterns occur was identified by Kardiner (1945), a cultural anthropologist. He stated that:

- Techniques that members of any society employ in the care and rearing of children are culturally patterned and will tend to be similar, although never identical, for various families within the society.

- Culturally patterned techniques for the care and rearing of children differ from one society to another. (p. vi)

Parents from different ethnic backgrounds use child-rearing techniques that are derived from their unique set of cultural values and role expectations. They draw their parenting practices from the culture(s) with which they identify. Because the process of child rearing is cross-culturally so intricate, social scientists have specialized in studying different age groups and different cultures, with some researchers conducting longitudinal studies. Work in this area has revealed that despite individual variation, children demonstrate patterned behavior that is linked to the culturally patterned behavior of their caretakers.

Cultural factors in socialization are exceedingly difficult to disentangle from environmental, social, and psychological considerations (Julian, McKenry, & McKelvey, 1994). In fact, the relative influence of each is often a matter of conjecture and speculation. Over the years, however, specific cultural responses have been studied and have increased our understanding of the variety of socialization patterns among various ethnic and culturally divergent groups. Nevertheless, one serious limitation of this research is that the samples are primarily mothers. Research has focused on maternal parenting, not paternal parenting. Research about paternal involvement in child rearing is sparse (Julian et al.).

One example of cultural differences comes from Caudill's comparative research (1975) of infant caregiving in middle-class families in Japan and the United States. Caudill found that mothers in the two cultures engage in subtly different styles of caretaking that have, however, strikingly different effects. Generally, the American mother seems to encourage her baby to be active and respond vocally, whereas the Japanese mother acts in ways that she believes soothes and quiets her child. By the age of 3 to 4 months, the infants of both cultures seem to have already learned responses appropriate to these different patterns. The striking discovery is that the responses of the infants are in line with certain broad expectations for behavior in the two cultures: in America the expectation that individuals should be physically and verbally assertive, and in Japan that individuals should be physically and verbally restrained.

In middle-class America, the mothers perceive their babies as separate and autonomous beings who are expected to learn to do and think for themselves. The baby is seen as a distinct personality with his or her own needs and desires, which the mother must learn to recognize and care for. She does this by helping her infant learn to express these needs through her emphasis on vocal communication; the baby can thus "tell" her what he or she wants so that the mother can respond appropriately. In contrast, the Japanese mother views her baby much more as an extension of herself; psychologically, the boundaries between mother and infant are blurred. As a result of this emphasis on close attachment, the mother is likely to feel that she knows what is best for the baby. There is then no perceived need for the infant to tell the mother what he or she wants. Because of this orientation, the Japanese mother does not place much importance on vocal communication and instead stresses physical contact (Caudill).

It is not clear in this study what social class the Japanese mothers are from, which is another variable to consider when looking at differences. In cross-class studies of infants in the United States, researchers have often found that middle-class mothers talk more to their infants than mothers in lower socioeconomic groups. Therefore, differences found in this and other cross-cultural studies may possibly be due to differences in social class or to the interaction of social class and culture.

In looking at the influence of ethnicity in African-American compared to white, non-Hispanic parents, parental socialization practices of African-American parents mirror those of the wider community. Nevertheless, there is one added dimension to child rearing that is present in African-American families. Because of a history of persistent racial prejudice and discrimination, explicit racial socialization (i.e., teaching of coping skills for survival in a prejudiced society) is clearly a distinctive feature of child rearing (Taylor, 2000). A stricter parenting style is believed to be necessary to develop the coping abilities to deal with racism and discrimination. This is buttressed with extensive parental support and open communication.

Lin and Fu (1990) in comparing Euro-Americans' to Chinese-Americans' parenting patterns, discovered that Chinese-Americans exert more parental control and discipline. Chinese-American parents tend to be more achievement oriented and demand more self-control and self-discipline in their children. Parents' demands and control are mixed with devoted sacrifice on the part of the mother, who remains supportive and physically close to the child. This authoritarian child-rearing pattern might seem undesirable from a Western perspective, but to the Chinese culture, this child-rearing pattern is felt to lead to high achievement in their children (Baumrind, 1996).

Many modern parents have never been taught as children how to care for infants and other small children. In contrast, Whiting (1974) notes that in traditional societies in which women have important roles in the subsistence economy, children are required to act as nurses to their younger siblings. In all the agricultural societies she studied, mothers designate a child, usually between 7 and 8 years of age, to be their assistant. Mothers in these same subsistence cultures need to be freed to return to work in the fields, and therefore believe that 7- or 8-year-old children can be trained to be capable caretakers for younger children. In Navajo society, children are required to assume child care responsibilities as soon as they are able, starting with "herding" other children as early as age 3 (Phillips & Lobar, 1990).

These examples indicate the need for a cross-cultural approach to our understanding of families and their child-rearing patterns. Ho (1987), a family therapist, believes that a cross-cultural perspective is crucial in working with families. Considerable intraethnic variation exists within cultural groups. For example, Martinez (1988) found that Mexican-American mothers' child-rearing patterns varied considerably, though most mothers used authoritarian or authoritative child-rearing techniques.

The role of the father varies widely in child rearing from culture to culture, even though these roles are socially and culturally defined (Lamb, 1987). In traditional Asian, Islamic, and Hispanic families, the father's role in child care and socialization is deemphasized. He disciplines and controls the children, while the mother provides nurturance and support, as well as takes care of children's day-to-day needs (Erickson & Gegas, 1991; Ho, 1987). In traditional Native American society, the father is responsible for teaching his children, particularly his sons when they are older, and for acting as a role model. The ultimate power and authority is vested, however, not in the mother or father, but in the community as a whole (Phillips & Lobar, 1990; Mirandé, 1991).

SOCIAL CLASS DIFFERENCES IN SOCIALIZATION

Although it is now well accepted that a child's socialization is influenced by the social class position of his or her family, there is little information about the distinctions that may exist between the social classes relative to child-rearing practices. Ethnocentric or stereotyped notions about the differences that exist between low-income, middle-income, and upper-income families abound. It is not uncommon to find that in dealing with families in a health care setting child-rearing patterns that differ from a white middle-class standard are often seen as deviant, dysfunctional, and/or unacceptable. Most practitioners continue to evaluate families in terms of their own middle-class standards. Nurses are often bothered, uncomfortable, or shocked by behavior they perceive as careless, overdependent, aggressive, pretentious, or uninhibited. Class differences in definitions of what is considered to be good or bad child rearing, normal or abnormal, acceptable or deplorable, present possible barriers to the therapeutic relationship between the nurse and the family. "When evaluating lower class behavior we need to keep in mind that behaviors and attitudes considered maladaptive by white, middle-class standards may be quite adaptive given the conditions of lower-class family life" (Erickson & Gegas, 1991, p. 116).

Stemming from several reviews of child-rearing studies that examined the social class differences in parenting (Gecas, 1979; Julian et al., 1994; Peterson & Rollins, 1987), there is a consensus about the relationship between social class and child-rearing behaviors. These major empirical generalizations can be made on the basis of a number of studies:

1. Middle-class parents tend to use an authoritative, democratic parental style, while lower-class parents tend to use a more authoritarian, autocratic parental style.

2. One of the most consistent results in the literature is that low-income families rely more heavily on physical punishment as a means of disciplining and controlling the child, while middle-class parents use more psychological techniques (e.g., use of guilt or shame). Inter-

estingly, earlier studies showed a greater difference between the lower and middle classes than later studies.

3. Middle-class families are more likely to encourage a democratic or egalitarian parent–child relationship, while low-income families are more likely to encourage a more authoritarian or autocratic parent–child relationship.

4. The higher the social class, the more likely that parental affection and involvement will be greater.

5. The higher the social class, the greater the parents' emphasis on independence (Bronfenbrenner, 1969).

6. Language (linguistic ability) is more highly developed in middle-class children. Low-income parents rely more on the use of commands and imperatives, whereas middle-class parents tend to explain the reasons for a rule or request. Middle-class parents tend to use reasoning and "psychological techniques" and tend to be more verbal in interactions with their children.

OTHER VARIABLES INFLUENCING CHILD REARING

Social class and culture are only two of the variables that influence child-rearing patterns (albeit sociocultural variables appear in studies to explain the most variance in child-rearing practices). Parental behavior and socialization techniques are also influenced by the amount of stress and strain parents experience, parents' idiosyncratic ways of coping and parenting, the resources available to them, and the issues related to varied family forms. For example, the ages of both parents and children influence child-rearing patterns: A teenage girl who becomes a mother may not be developmentally mature enough to meet the needs of her newborn, especially if the baby is fragile or premature (Holt & Johnson, 1991) and specific family forms are related to specific child-rearing issues.

FAMILY FORM AND SOCIALIZATION

Most of the research and literature on child-rearing patterns applies to the two-parent, dual- or single-earner nuclear family. Single-parent and stepparent families are two common family forms with unique patterns of socialization, and child outcomes. However, other family forms are gaining more attention as the stigma associated with varied family forms diminishes and the respect for individual and family diversity grows. As Allen (1997) points out, lesbian and gay parents exemplify the concept that "families are constructed by a variety of biological, adoptive, and chosen kin ties"(p. 196). This section discusses the socialization patterns in single-parent families, stepparent families, and families of lesbian and gay parents.

SINGLE-PARENT FAMILIES

Twenty-six percent of all family units in the United States were single-parent families in the last decade (Figure 15–1). Of these, 88 percent were mother headed and 12 percent were father headed. In 1991, 15.3 million American children (24.3 percent of all children under 18 years of age) lived with one parent only, an increase of 12.4 percent since 1970 (see Figure 15–1). The growth of single-parent families is due primarily to a high rate of divorce, the increase in births to never-married teenage mothers, and the growth of father-headed families (Bianchi, 1995; U.S. Bureau of the Census, 1993b). There is considerable difference in the proportion of single-parent families among the social classes and ethnic groups (see Chapter 1 for further detail).

Child rearing among single parents is difficult, especially if there are no other adult caregivers available to assist the parent. Single parents struggle against the dual demands of providing financial and emotional support for their children (Weiss, 1994). Poverty and employment of the single parent (usually the mother) add to the difficulty in child rearing (Bowen, Desimone, & McKay, 1995).

Extensive research has been conducted on the effects of the single-parent family on the children—their educational attainment, work, and income.

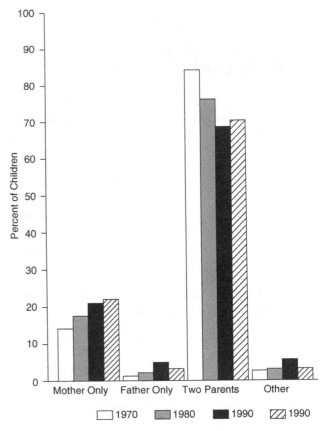

Figure 15–1. Living arrangements of American children under 18 years of age. (Source: U.S. Bureau of the Census, 1988, 1992, 1996.)

Abundant evidence now exists that children from single-parent families have less success in school, lower earnings, and lower occupational prestige than children reared in intact two-parent families. This has been found even when education and income level of the single parent are controlled (Mueller & Cooper, 1986; Nock, 1988; Popenoe, 1995). Moreover, the difficulties that mother-only families have are reflected in the finding that single mothers report less satisfaction in their parenting role (Fine, Donnelly, & Voydanoff, 1986).

STEPPARENT FAMILIES

In the stepparent family, the stepfather's role confusion and resultant family disequilibrium are related to difficult issues in child rearing (see Chapter 1). Each parent draws on his or her own family background when defining child-rearing beliefs, practices, and discipline. When adults enter into a stepfamily relationship, the stepfather becomes a husband but is not really the parent, and agreement about child-rearing rules is often problematic. Furthermore, the children have developed their own behaviors and expectations of what is acceptable or unacceptable for both themselves and their parents through exposure to their natural parents' child-rearing practices.

In the stepparent family, the stepfather has no legal rights over the children, as he has no biological relationship to them, and whatever parental rights he may have must be granted to him by his wife. This places the stepfather in a rather untenable position. When conflict arises over the disciplining of a child, the mother feels a natural right to decide the issue. If the stepfather disciplines the child, the mother may either directly become angry, or, more often, indirectly strikes back by undermining him. This latter course is particularly devastating to the entire family and often exacerbates the conflict, with the mother being torn between the loyalty to her children and to her husband (Furstenberg & Nord, 1985; Visher & Visher, 1993).

In a study of 232 remarried families, Hobart (1987) found that depending on whose children they are, children had different statuses in the family. For instance, first-class children were those born to the remarried couple, second-class children were those from the wife's previous marriage, and third-class children were those from the husband's previous marriage. Parents reported that the most positive relationships were with their shared children. Parent–child relationships varied considerably in the remarried families, and relationship problems were perceived as affecting the spousal relationship.

GAY/LESBIAN FAMILIES

A *Healthy People 2010* companion document for lesbian, gay, bisexual, and transgender (LGBT) health notes that the most cited estimate of the number of gay and lesbian adults is 10 percent in the male population and 5 to 6 percent in the female population. However, the authors of the companion document note that these estimates may be inaccurate as there is limited agreement about criteria for defining someone as LGBT and uncertainty about whether people who might consider themselves LGBT are identified in surveys.

Lesbian, gay, bisexual, and transgender adults are members of many families, often parenting children in a variety of circumstances. For example, Savin-Williams and Esterberg (2000) discuss current knowledge about lesbian–gay families, including (a) families in which parents are heterosexual but the children are lesbian, gay, or bisexual; (b) children of lesbian or gay parents; how these children have fared; and (c) lesbian and gay adults who are parenting children together.

Ahmann (1999) explained that gay and lesbian adults commonly bring children into their relationships from earlier heterosexual unions. She also noted that "In other families, children are in foster care with or are adopted by gay or lesbian adults" (p. 531). Ahmann cited other authors (Gold et al., 1994; Harrison & Silenzio, 1996), who wrote that "Increasingly, gay men may father children through arrangements with friends or surrogates and lesbians may conceive by alternative (artificial) insemination with known or unknown donors" (p. 531). This section focuses primarily on families with gay and lesbian parents in contemporary America. However, many of the issues presented may apply to families with bisexual or transgendered parents as well.

The source of many of the unique issues in the families of lesbian or gay parents are rooted in heterosexism and/or homophobia. Heterosexism refers to assumptions that heterosexuality is the only acceptable life option and hence is superior, more natural and dominant than other sexual orientations (Dunn, 2001). These assumptions continue despite evidence that homosexuality has occurred in societies throughout history. Heinrich (1996) noted that discrimination against homosexual individuals has diminished in recent years, as evident in use of the term *domestic partnerships* for committed homosexual couples and other changes in public policies.

Dunn (2001) points out that heterosexism and homophobia impact lesbian parents in three key areas:

1. Heterosexism and homophobia contribute to the oppression of lesbians and are responsible for the lack of social and legal recognition of lesbian [and gay] parents and their partners.

2. They create a barrier to accessing services, as lesbian [and gay] parents may feel they should conceal their sexual identity from health providers.

3. They inhibit the "coming out" process, and may contribute to the feeling that lesbian mothers [and gay fathers] should conceal their lesbian identity for the sake of their children.

A number of authors (Heinrich, 1996; Savin-Williams & Esterberg, 2000) have written about the effect of public policies that neglect or reject the needs of gay and lesbian families. Heinrich noted that

> "American society has traditionally discriminated against homosexual individuals by declaring sexual acts between same-gendered partners illegal, not recognizing gay marriages as legal, and denying custody or adoption of children to same-sex partners. Homosexual partners have no legal rights during illness, cannot cover one another with health insurance benefits, and cannot be listed as next of kin on records." (p. 295)

Even as many of these policies are changing to be more equitable, such as ability to add domestic partners to health insurance policies, other public policies reflect an ongoing belief among the heterosexual majority that lesbian (or gay) adults are not fit as parents (Heinrich, 1996; Mitchell, 1996). Allen and Demo (1995) note that most of the research about lesbian and gay families tends to problematize the families and fails to recognize the diversity among LGBT families. Understandably, lesbian mothers may believe it is not prudent to be candid with health providers about their own sexual identity or family form.

In truth, results of many studies contradict stereotypes and prejudices about parenting effectiveness of lesbian and gay adults. Fitzgerald (1999) reviewed 20 years of research about the development of children with gay and lesbian parents and concluded that

> Children with lesbian and gay parents are developing psychologically, intellectually, behaviorally, and emotionally in positive directions, and that the sexual orientation of parents is not an effective or important predictor of successful child development. (p. 57)

Strickland (1995) reviewed research about gay- and lesbian-parented families and wrote that "The overall emotional well-being of gay men and lesbians, as well as children raised in gay and lesbian families,

is as psychologically healthy as that of their heterosexual counterparts" (p. 137).

Nevertheless, there may be specific issues related to the residual negative societal attitudes about gay and lesbian families. For example, Gershon, Tschann, and Jemerin (1999) examined the perceived stigma, coping, disclosure, and self-esteem among adolescents with lesbian mothers. Their results supported the need for interventions to assist adolescents with social coping skills related to stigma and self-esteem, and urged educational efforts to eradicate stigmatizing attitudes in the wider community. Another example is the problem encountered by lesbian mothers, when one is the biological mother and the other is the "stepmother" with no recognized relationship to the child. Ahmann (1999) quoted a story told by a lesbian mother:

> As a lesbian family, we are faced with a dilemma. Often, especially in a medical emergency, we "come out" to others before we know what their reactions will be. It is frightening enough to turn your child's care and/or life over to medical practitioners you do not know. Not knowing if that practitioner has a strong prejudice toward your family is a very real added burden." (p. 533)

Barriers to providing sensitive care to families with lesbian or gay parents could be decreased through providing nurses and other providers with accurate information about lesbian and gay families—replacing their negative perceptions and stereotypes (Eliason, 1996). Another suggestion from the professional literature is to remove assumptions about implied heterosexual relationships and family form in family assessment forms; for example, asking clients who they consider to be "family" and using the terms *family member* or *parent* rather than husband and wife.

🌿 FAMILY ASSESSMENT AREAS

Before discussing the assessment of family socialization patterns, it is important for the nurse to be very clear about his or her own biases, attitudes, and expectations that might interfere with assessing family child rearing accurately. Because families have diverse sociocultural backgrounds and forms, some families will have child-rearing styles that the nurse believes are better or worse than others. Most health care specialists who work with families with children assume that the parents are somehow at fault when a child acts in a "socially unacceptable way" or is sick. This covert attitude functions as a barrier, making it difficult for the nurse to sustain a respectful and an effective role with the family. In the nursing assessment of families, the following questions will provide useful data from which to identify potential or actual problems and plan care accordingly.

1. What are the family's child-rearing practices in the following areas?
   a. Behavior control, including discipline, reward, and punishment
   b. Autonomy and dependency
   c. Giving and receiving of love
   d. Training for age-appropriate behavior (social, physical, emotional, language, and intellectual development).
2. How adaptive are the family's child-rearing practices for their particular family form and situation?
3. Who assumes responsibility for the child-care role or socialization function? Is it shared? If so, how is this managed?
4. How are children regarded in the family?
5. What cultural beliefs influence the family's child-rearing patterns?
6. How does social class influence child-rearing patterns?
7. Is this a family that is at high risk for child-rearing problems? If so, what factors place the family at risk?
8. Is the home environment adequate for children's needs to play (appropriate to children's developmental stage)? Is there age-appropriate play equipment/toys in the home?

FAMILY NURSING DIAGNOSES

Observing family strengths and problems within the area of family socialization are very common occurrences for family nurses working in schools, pediatrics,

community health, family primary care, and mental health. This makes actual and potential family nursing diagnoses within this area most germane. Family strengths may be covered under "potential" family nursing diagnoses or may be stated as strengths, eliminating the use of family nursing diagnoses. Recalling that the family socialization function covers child rearing, parent–child relationships, and parental behavior, the area is quite broad.

As with the other family dimensions, North American Nursing Diagnosis Association (NANDA) diagnoses were reviewed to identify which diagnoses appear to incorporate actual and potential family socialization problems. The following is a list of the NANDA diagnoses (2001) that may be relevant to family socialization patterns:

Nursing Diagnoses

- Interrupted Family Processes
- Health-Seeking Behaviors (health-promotion diagnosis)
- Deficient Knowledge
- Parental Role Conflict
- Impaired Parenting
- Risk for Impaired Parenting

Possible Outcomes of Socialization Problem (Possible Defining Characteristics)

- Delayed Growth and Development
- Self-Care Deficit
- Ineffective Health Maintenance
- Deficient Knowledge
- Situational (or chronic) Low Self-Esteem
- Social Isolation
- Impaired Social Interactions
- Risk for Violence: Directed at Others
- Noncompliance

Two significant NANDA nursing diagnoses that appear to be directly related to a family socialization problem are Interrupted Family Processes and Impaired Parenting. Interrupted Family Processes is a more general family nursing diagnosis, but can be used when specific defining characteristics are included. Defining characteristics which could be related to this diagnosis are (McFarland and McFarlane 1993):

- Parents do not demonstrate respect for each other's child-rearing practices.
- Rigidity in function and roles.
- Family does not demonstrate respect for individuality and autonomy of its members.
- Inappropriate or inconsistent family roles.

The other nursing diagnosis, which is more specific to child-rearing problems, is Impaired Parenting. The defining characteristics of this diagnosis directly apply to the areas subsumed under family socialization. Table 15–3 is included in this text because this diagnosis is so appropriate here. As previously mentioned, defining characteristics and related factors should accompany the diagnosis.

Identifying parents at risk for child-rearing problems—indicating Potential Altered Parenting—is critical. To name some high-risk groups, they include parents in crisis situations or under stress; teen parents; single parents with limited financial or personal resources or inadequate social support; parents with serious physical or psychological problems; and parents who have premature infants or infants or children with serious or chronic health problems.

🌿 FAMILY NURSING INTERVENTIONS

The Iowa Intervention Project (McCloskey & Bulechek, 1996) has developed listings and descriptions of a broad range of nursing interventions. In most cases, these interventions have been linked to NANDA nursing diagnoses. For instance, Altered Parenting, the NANDA diagnosis, is linked with 22 interventions (see Table 15–4). The interventions that follow are relevant to health promotional, preventive diagnoses, as well as health restorative types of diagnoses in the area of family socialization. The italicized nursing interventions are particularly germane to and/or focused on family socialization diagnoses.

- Child protection, child
- Active listening
- Animal-assisted therapy

- *Anticipatory guidance*
- *Attachment promotion*
- Behavior management (for overactivity/inattention, sexual)
- Behavior modification
- Behavior modification, social skills
- Coping enhancement
- Counseling
- Decision-making support
- *Developmental enhancement*
- Emotional support
- Family integrity promotion
- Family involvement
- Family mobilization
- Family process maintenance
- Family support
- Family therapy
- Infant and newborn care
- Learning facilitation
- Learning readiness enhancement
- *Normalization promotion*
- *Role enhancement*
- Socialization enhancement
- Support group
- *Support system enhancement*
- *Teaching (many areas)*

In addition to the broad listing of possible nursing interventions that are relevant in the family socialization area, five intervention areas are discussed more in-depth: supporting parents, making interventions socioculturally appropriate, making interventions appropriate for single-parent and stepparent families, teaching and anticipatory guidance, behavior modification, and initiating referrals to parenting programs and early intervention programs.

MAKING INTERVENTIONS SOCIOCULTURALLY APPROPRIATE

In all nursing care, assessments and interventions based on appropriate sociocultural data are impor-

TABLE 15–3

PARENTING, ALTERED (NANDA) NURSING DIAGNOSIS

Definition: The state in which one or more caregivers demonstrate a real or potential inability to provide a constructive environment that nurtures the growth and development of his/her/their child (children)

DEFINING CHARACTERISTICS

Major (must be present)

- Inappropriate and/or non-nurturing parenting behaviors
- Lack of parental attachment behavior

Minor (may be present)

- Frequent verbalization of dissatisfaction or disappointment with infant/child
- Verbalization of frustration of role
- Verbalization of perceived or actual inadequacy
- Diminished or inappropriate visual, tactile, or auditory stimulation of infant
- Evidence of abuse or neglect of child
- Growth and development lag in infant/child

RELATED FACTORS

Individuals or families who may be at risk for developing or experiencing parenting difficulties:

Parent(s): Single, addicted to drugs, adolescent, terminally ill, alcoholic, abusive, acutely disabled, emotionally disturbed, accident victim

Child: Of unwanted pregnancy, mentally handicapped, of undesired gender, hyperactive characteristics, with undesired characteristics, terminally ill, physically handicapped

SITUATIONAL (PERSONAL, ENVIRONMENTAL)

Related to interruption of bonding process secondary to illness (child, parent), relocation, incarceration

Related to separation from nuclear family

Related to lack of knowledge

Related to inconsistent caregivers or techniques

Related to relationship problems (specify): Marital discord, stepparents, divorce, live-in partner, separation, relocation

Related to little external support and/or socially isolated family

Related to lack of available role model

Related to ineffective adaptation to stressors associated with illness, economic problems, new baby, substance abuse, elder care

MATURATIONAL

Adolescent

Related to the conflict of meeting own needs over child's

Related to history of ineffective relationships with own parents

Related to parental history of abusive relationship with parents

Related to unrealistic expectations of child by parent

Related to unrealistic expectations of self by parent

Related to unrealistic expectations of parent by child

Related to unmet psychosocial needs of child by parent

Source: Carpenito, L. J. (2000). Nursing diagnosis: Application to clinical practice (8th ed). New York: Lippincott-Williams/Wilkins.

TABLE 15–4

NURSING INTERVENTIONS FOR NURSING DIAGNOSIS OF PARENTING, ALTERED

Parenting, Altered: *Definition:* Inability of the primary caretaker to create an environment that promotes the optimum growth and development of the child.

EXAMPLES FOR OUTCOME OF CHILD DEVELOPMENT FOR A CHILD AGED 2 MONTHS

Major Interventions

- Family integrity: Promotion
- Childbearing family parent education: Infant
- Parenting promotion

Suggested Interventions

- Anticipatory guidance
- Attachment promotion
- Bottle-feeding
- Breast-feeding assistance
- Family involvement promotion
- Family process maintenance
- Family support
- Infant care
- Lactation counseling
- Parent education: Infant
- Role enhancement
- Teaching: Infant nutrition
- Teaching: Infant safety

Optional Interventions

- Abuse protection
- Support: Child
- Behavior modification
- Caregiver support
- Environmental management
- Attachment process
- Health system guidance
- Newborn care
- Respite care
- Sibling support
- Support system enhancement
- Surveillance

EXAMPLES FOR OUTCOME OF CHILD DEVELOPMENT FOR A CHILD IN MIDDLE CHILDHOOD (6–11 YEARS)

Major Interventions

- Developmental enhancement: Child
- Parent education: Child-rearing family
- Parenting promotion

Suggested Interventions

- Anticipatory guidance
- Family integrity promotion
- Family involvement promotion
- Mutual goal setting
- Spiritual support
- Substance use prevention
- Teaching: Individual
- Value clarification

Optional Interventions

- Abuse protection support: Child
- Counseling
- Family process maintenance
- Family support
- Family therapy
- Health system guidance
- Sibling support
- Sports-injury prevention: Youth
- Sustenance support

Source: Johnson, M., Bulechek, G., McCloskey, J., Dochterman, J. M., Maas, M., & Moorhead, S. (2001). Nursing diagnoses, outcomes and interventions: NANDA, NOC, & NIC linkages (pp. 229 & 233). St. Louis: Mosby.

tant, whether counseling a mother, teaching a child, supervising a medical therapy, or coordinating community resources to resolve identified problems. In each case, the nurse should focus on the relevance to the family and not on his or her own values or child-rearing techniques. For example, some families can accept and respond to recommendations for improving the diet of their children if the parents are given an explanation that ties in with their own values (e.g., if the children are fed better, they will behave better and the family will be less stressed). In other families, however, having well-nourished children is valued in and of itself, and so a direct teaching approach is used.

TEACHING AND ANTICIPATORY GUIDANCE FOR VARIED FAMILY FORMS

Parents often want information about normal developmental behavior of children. They may need information about the importance of modeling the behavior they wish children to adopt, the importance of actively listening and communicating with their children, and the importance of respecting and supporting their children (Schor, 1995). Parents may be referred to some of the books about children and parenting concerns if this is a way they use to gain information. Goldenberg and Goldenberg, two family therapists, have written an excellent book entitled *Counseling Today's Families* (2002), with guidelines for counseling various family forms, including single-parent and remarried families, gay and lesbian couple families, dual-career families, cohabiting heterosexual couple families, and culturally diverse families. For both health professionals and parents, three American Academy of Pediatrics books are quite instructive: Shelov's *Caring for Your Baby and Young Child* (1991); Schor's *Caring for Your School Age Child* (1999); and Greydanus's *Caring for Your Adolescent* (1991).

INITIATING REFERRALS TO EARLY INTERVENTION PROGRAMS

Early intervention programs have been shown to reduce child abuse, improve behavior, and improve school performance (Smith, 1995). For families at

risk with children with special needs and young, high-risk mothers, early intervention has become one of the cornerstones of treatment (Kang, Barnard, & Oshio, 1994; Smith). Intervention that is interdisciplinary and comprehensive is incorporated in these programs. Regional developmental centers are examples of such services. Family nurses often serve as case managers (coordinating interdisciplinary services), as monitors of the developmental progress of children, as assessors of the home and family environment, and as health educators and counselors to families with respect to children's developmental and health care needs. Counseling is directed at providing family support; it can also involve helping families obtain food stamps and other community resources, and counseling parents about child rearing of children with special needs and disabilities (Healy, Keesee, & Smith, 1985; Kang et al.).

INITIATING REFERRALS TO PARENTING PROGRAMS

Family nurses also initiate referrals to parenting programs. Working closely with the schools and health and other social agencies, family nurses coordinate a variety of resources and a wealth of necessary information to assist families in coping with the complexities of raising children in a changing world of challenging expectations. Hammer and Turner (1985) and Osborne (1995) have identified different approaches and types of parenting programs popular in communities today. Five of the most popular are described here:

1. *Parent Effective Training (PET):* This first approach/program is based on humanistic psychology and stresses the importance of parent–child communication and parents' listening to and understanding the feelings of children. Gordon's book, *Parent Effectiveness Training* (1970), and the programs that use Gordon's principles help parents gain the skills needed to be supportive to children.

2. *Behavior Modification:* The second type of program/approach uses behavior modification techniques to help parents deal with specific child behavioral problems. Behavioral models of parent education focus on shaping desirable behavior in their children. Behavior modifica-

tion principles are also used in helping parents with child behavior control problems. Because behavior modification is based on the premise that all behavior is learned, this intervention is likewise based on behavioral learning principles. After gaining a baseline of a child's problematic behavior, so that the frequency of behavior and antecedents to the problem behavior are known, a structured program of reinforcements is implemented. Positive, negative, and neutral reinforcements may be used; although most behaviorists primarily recommend the use of positive reinforcement. This approach can be quite helpful if there are specific child behaviors that parents want to eliminate or modify, and parents can understand the program and have the resources to follow through with the planned, structured approach. Written contracts are developed that detail the planned intervention, so as to guide the parents and health professional (Johnson, 1986; Jones, 1980).

3. *Developmental Approach:* The third approach/program to parent education is a life-span, developmental psychology approach. The goal of this type of program is to teach parents about their children's development. Parents need to know what to expect of their children and what realistic expectations to have. Most of the very popular parenting books use this approach (i.e., Gesell, Spock, Ilg and Ames, Elkind).

4. *Family Systems Approach:* The fourth approach or type of parenting program is based on family systems theory. This approach is a family counseling approach, which focuses on unhealthy relationships/dynamics in the family. It assumes that once these unhealthy interactions/relationships are mended, parents can more successfully parent.

5. *Guidelines for Discipline:* Discipline is undoubtedly one of the prime areas about which parents seek help. Hammer and Turner (1985) and others have developed guidelines to help parents discipline more effectively (see Table 15–5).

By discussing parents' expectations of their role, the family nurse may identify sources of frustration, confusion, and gaps in information. By initiating referrals to parent education programs, conducting parent groups and client education sessions, and providing support and encouragement, parental role transition and confidence can be facilitated.

ＳUMMARY

- The family is more specialized in its function today than it has ever been. Nevertheless, one vital responsibility has remained a primary focus of the family: the socialization or the rearing of children. Socialization embraces all those processes in a specific community or group whereby humans, through their significant lifetime experiences, acquire socially patterned characteristics. In the family, socialization is a lifelong process and involves a myriad of learning experiences provided within the family. These experiences primarily are aimed at teaching children how to function and assume adult roles in society.

- There has been a shift from an emphasis on the nurturing aspects of parenting pervasive in the previous three decades to an emphasis on using scientifically based "parenting techniques," which are more democratic and encourage mutual communication, but are also more structured and rule oriented.

- Masculine and feminine adult roles are changing in families, and as they change, so do the socialization experiences of children. We cannot say with certainty what the impact will be of increased equity in parenting roles, reassignment of traditional male–female parenting practices, varied family forms, or realignment of traditional cultural values with those of new host cultures.

- A growing body of research indicates that children of satisfied working mothers tend to do

TABLE 15–5

GUIDELINES TO PARENTS ON DISCIPLINING CHILDREN

- Parents' goals in disciplining should not be punishment for wrongful actions, but rather punishment to assist children to control their behavior; develop self-discipline, optimal competence, and moral character; accept responsibility for their behavior; and consider the needs and feelings of others.

- Within a responsive and supportive parent–child relationship, prudent use of punishment is a necessary disciplinary strategy.

- Discipline works best when tailored to the individual child and the specific situation.

- Children need consistent discipline from loving parents.

- Failure to discipline can produce serious rebellion and "acting out" behavior during the adolescent period.

- Children want and need structure and limits.

- With young children, when parents decide to use punishment for a given act:

  1. The punishment should immediately follow the act.
  2. The punishment needs to be both deserved and understood.
  3. The punishment needs to be related to the act.

- Parents should remain calm and focus attention on the child's behavior (not the child himself or herself) when disciplining.

- Parents should refrain from venting their own anger at the child's expense.

- Although spanking is acceptable and normative in some cultures, its use should be carefully evaluated, as research has shown negative outcomes relative to children's later behavior. The effectiveness of spanking must be viewed within the cultural context.

Sources: Baumrind (1996); Dickinson & Leming (1995); Giles-Sims, Straus, & Sugarman (1995); Greydanus (1991); Hammer & Turner (1985); McCubbin & Dahl (1985).

well. However, child development experts believe that today's child is being pushed to act like an adult long before he or she is developmentally ready to do so.

- Legally, children's rights are now widely recognized by the American courts. In spite of this recent legislation, children are still inadequately protected in our society.

- Theoretical perspectives from psychology and sociology form the foundation for the socialization literature, with key concepts drawn from developmental theories, theories about the processes of socialization, and how variations in parental support and control affect children.

- It is now well accepted that a child's socialization is influenced by the social class position of his or her family. For example, child rearing is more gender based in lower-class families and there

are differences in usual methods of discipline across social classes.

- Parents from different ethnic backgrounds use child-rearing techniques that are derived from their unique set of cultural values and role expectations. They draw parenting practices from the culture(s) with which they identify. Cultural factors in socialization, however, are exceedingly difficult to disentangle from environmental, social class, and psychological considerations.

- Most of the research and literature on child-rearing patterns applies to the two-parent, dual- or single-earner nuclear family. Single-parent and stepparent families are two common family forms with unique patterns of socialization. However, other family forms are gaining more attention as the stigma associated with varied family forms diminishes and the respect for individual and family diversity grows. Lesbian and gay parents exemplify a broad conceptualization of family as inclusive of a variety of biological, adoptive, and chosen kin ties.

- It is important for the nurse to be very clear about any biases, attitudes, and expectations that might interfere with assessing family child rearing accurately.

- Areas of assessment of the family socialization patterns include identifying the family's child-rearing practices, determining whether the socialization practices are adaptive, and identifying factors influencing socialization patterns (such as sociocultural background and family form).

- Nursing diagnoses for family socialization may be quite broad, as this function relates to child rearing, parent–child relationships, and parental behaviors. Family strengths may be covered under "potential" family nursing diagnoses or may be stated as strengths. Examples of possible nursing diagnoses are impaired parenting and risk for impaired parent/infant/child attachment.

- Interventions related to family socialization patterns are relevant for health promotional, and preventive diagnoses, as well as health restorative types diagnoses. Examples of relevant interventions in this area include teaching and anticipatory guidance and referral to early intervention and to parenting programs.

✿ FAMILY VIGNETTE: THE CHIN FAMILY

Mr. and Mrs. Chin, ages 50 and 45, respectively, moved 10 years ago to San Francisco from Hong Kong. The Chins operate a small cleaners, and the family income has always been low despite the long, hard hours of work of both parents. They have four children: Harold, 23, who is at the California School of Technology studying engineering; Lee, 22, who is a registered nurse; John, 17, who is in high school and an excellent student; and Joe, 10, who is attending fifth grade. All the children (including the older ones) are always busy working. John and Joe work extremely hard on their studies, and with schoolwork and home chores there is little time left over for playing or getting into "mischief." The parents have greatly encouraged their children to pursue higher education and academic achievement. Through their accomplishments, the Chins feel the children have brought honor to them.

During the home visit, all the children were observed to be respectful of their parents' authority. In the presence of their parents, the two youngest were quiet and did not interject comments or express themselves until directly asked a question, at which time they answered quickly while looking to their mother for approval.

Mrs. Chin states that her husband is strict in child rearing and that if the two younger boys who are still living at home disobey, he administers immediate corporal punishment. Mrs. Chin relates that a misbehaving child in the Chinese community is considered "not trained," meaning that the parents are to blame; thus, a child's wrongdoing brings shame and dishonor to the whole family.

When Mrs. Chin was asked how she raised her children, she related that she cuddled and fondled them a lot while they were little, but as soon as they became preschoolers, she gradually withdrew her expressions of love and physical hugs and kisses. From school age on, she and her husband have pushed their children to become independent and responsible. Both parents said that they had emotionally removed themselves somewhat from their children, lest their children lose respect for them.

The parent–child relationships appear to be more restrained and formal than in most American families. However, though muted, one was still able to feel the obvious respect and caring they feel for each other.

■ STUDY QUESTIONS

Review the Family Vignette and answer the related questions.

1. Describe how the family dealt with the following areas of child rearing: discipline, rewards, punishment, moral training, autonomy, initiative, creativity, dependency, giving and receiving of love, and training for age-appropriate behavior (social, physical, emotional, language, and intellectual development).

2. How adaptive are the family's child-rearing practices for their particular situation (social class, culture, environment, etc.)?

3. Who assumes responsibility for the child care role or socialization function? Is it shared and, if so, how?

4. How are children regarded in the family?

5. What cultural beliefs are operating in their child-rearing practices?

6. Identify a family nursing diagnosis in the area of family socialization.

7. Identify an intervention appropriate to the diagnosis identified in question 6 above.

Answer the following questions.

8. Which of the following is the best definition of socialization?
   a. The act of learning to relate to people
   b. The training provided to function in a social environment
   c. The social and psychological development of a child
   d. Child-rearing practices

9. The central task involved in socialization of children revolves around teaching them how to function and assume adult roles in a society. Subsumed under this main task are several more specific tasks. Name three of these.

10. Culture plays a dominant role in socialization. Explain briefly.

11. Which of the following research findings are true about research in family socialization? (select all correct answers)
    a. The "social mold" theory continues to be the prominent theoretical perspective used.

b. Parental control and parental support are two major parenting variables found to influence child outcomes.

c. Androgynous socialization leads to later problems in child adjustment.

12. Social class is another vital variable influencing a family's socialization patterns. Social class makes a difference because (select the best answer):

a. By virtue of experiencing different life conditions, families from various social classes have varying conceptions of social reality and what is desirable, feasible, and most important.

b. Social class determines how parents deal with the world and their children.

c. Being in one social class or another gives a family a limited view of the world and consequently limits its child-rearing techniques to those with which the family is familiar.

13. Research concerning social class differences in child-rearing patterns found that (answer true or false):

a. The white-collar family stresses respect and obedience more than the blue-collar family does.

b. Conformity and individualism are both emphasized more by middle-class versus working-class families.

c. Middle-income families rely more on reasoning and talking things over with children, while low-income families tend to use punishment more as a way of disciplining children.

14. Identify several important changes and/or issues affecting child rearing in our society.

15. Addressing self-examination of child-rearing biases, what particular beliefs and attitudes do you hold that might limit your effectiveness in working with parents and children in the area of parenting or child rearing?

THE FAMILY HEALTH CARE FUNCTION

LEARNING OBJECTIVES

1. Recall the various ways in which the family carries out its health care function.

2. Identify three salient factors that influence a family's conceptualization or definition of health and illness, and whether they seek health care.

3. Explain the significance of the Health Belief Model and the Health Promotion Model for family nursing practice.

4. Summarize Pratt's findings and conclusions concerning how adequately the American family performs its health care function.

5. Discuss the basic aspects that need to be assessed when completing an appraisal of a family's (a) dietary practices, (b) sleep and rest practices, (c) exercise and recreational activities, (d) therapeutic and recreational drug, alcohol, and tobacco practices, and (e) self-care practices.

6. Identify potential environmental and hygiene practices that could negatively affect family members' health.

7. Describe the basic health promotion and preventive measures recommended for adults and children, including general medical care, vision and hearing examinations, immunizations, dental care, and use of alternative therapies.

8. Describe what should be included and recorded in a family health history.

9. Identify nursing diagnoses that are applicable to the family as they participate in health prevention, health promotion, and health maintenance activities.

10. List and define four intervention strategies that are used to assist families to modify their lifestyle.

For the family health professional, the health care function is a vital component of family assessment. To place this function in perspective, it is one of the five family functions that entail the provision of physical necessities: food, clothing, shelter, and health care. Shelter (housing and family's neighborhood and community) was discussed previously in Chapter 9 as part of environmental data.

From the perspective of society, the family is the basic system in which health behavior and care are organized, performed, and secured. Families provide health promotion and preventive health care, as well as the major share of sick care for their members. Furthermore, families have the prime responsibility for initiating and coordinating services rendered by health care professionals (Pratt, 1977, 1982).

There has been a pervasive assumption that as the family has become more specialized in its functions its health care function has been lost—being transferred to the doctor's office and hospital. And yet the tremendous role families play in the provision of health care to family members is clearly evident to health care professionals.(The reader is referred back to Chapter 1, which discusses in depth the role of the family in relation to the entire spectrum of health and illness concerns.) With the acknowledgment that major improvements and maintenance in health occur primarily through environmental and personal lifestyle modifications and commitments, the family's central role in assuming responsibility for its members' health is strengthened (Pratt, 1982). Therefore, it is our belief, supported by Pratt (1976) and Forrest (1981), that the provision of health care is indeed a vital and basic family function. We believe that education and counseling for family self-care should be a primary goal of family nursing practice.

FAMILY BEHAVIORS RELATED TO HEALTH AND ILLNESS

Health practices and the use of health care services vary tremendously from family to family. Two primary reasons for this diversity in health care practices are family differences in both conceptualizations of what constitutes health and illness and their health beliefs relative to seeking health care and following through with health care actions.

DIFFERENCES IN CONCEPTUALIZATIONS OF HEALTH AND ILLNESS

Conceptualizations of health and illness vary widely from culture to culture, region to region, and family to family. The prevalence of a disease in a community and gender, social class, and ethnic differences are additional factors that influence a family's conceptualizations of health and illness. How a family or family members define health and illness has important ramifications for family nursing practice. The family's definition of health needs to be clarified so that the nurse knows what goals and priorities are important to the family, as well as what possible areas of health education are present.

THE UBIQUITY OF HEALTH PROBLEMS. Some health problems endemic to whole communities or groups may be taken as a matter of course rather than defined as illness. Social customs and norms often determine whether particular behaviors are considered sick or healthy (Jahoda, 1958). A family, neighborhood, community, or society must label a condition or certain behaviors as an illness or disability before that illness or health condition can be considered a health problem to that group. The frequency of a condition often influences whether the condition is labeled an illness or not. For instance, if practically everyone in a community is suffering from malnutrition, the associated fatigue will probably be considered normal. A case in point: In America today, we accept colds and dental caries, which occur so frequently, as annoyances that are a part of normal living, and most sufferers of colds or toothaches do not consider themselves ill.

GENDER AND SOCIAL CLASS FACTORS.   Woods and associates (1988) uncovered some interesting gender and social class findings in their research, which addressed women's definitions of health. In an attempt to measure the concept of health from a woman's perspective, these researchers interviewed a sample of 528 women living in the Pacific Northwest on the meaning of health. The women, ranging in age from 18 to 45, representing diverse cultures, marital status, and educational and socioeconomic levels, reported a rich variety of health definitions. The health complaints most frequently reported by the sampled women were: defining health as a clinical notion (e.g., not being ill, having no aches, pains, or headaches), as a positive affect (e.g., sense of well-being, feeling good), as feeling fit (having stamina and strength, able to be active), as practicing healthy lifestyles (e.g., not smoking, eating a balanced diet), and as being in harmony (e.g., feeling spiritually whole, where life is in balance, feelings of contentment). Women who had more formal education and/or higher incomes reported images of health in which there was a positive sense of "exuberant" well-being. The women who were educationally and/or economically less advantaged tended to conceptualize health more pragmatically—as the absence of symptoms, the ability to perform their usual roles, and the ability to adapt to the demands of their environment. The study findings suggest that the women from higher social classes probably have more opportunity to develop images or conceptualizations of health that go beyond the limits of clinical symptomatology, role performance, and adaptive notions.

Recent reports confirm that men are more "out of touch" with their health and with the health care system. Three times as many men as women do not see their physician on an annual basis. A quarter of men surveyed said they would wait "as long as possible" before seeking health care. The barriers to health care seeking by men have been primarily noted to be psychological. That is, men are uncomfortable about discussing health issues with a doctor. Other contributing factors include the lack of health insurance (3 in 10 working men are uninsured) and culture (i.e., Latino men were twice as likely to avoid seeking medical care than Anglo men) (Marquis, 2000).

SOCIAL CLASS DIFFERENCES.   People from the same ethnic background and from a similar socioeconomic status often share comparable attitudes, myths, and values concerning their health (Spector, 2000). This has been particularly documented in poor communities (McLachlan, 1958; Lewis, 1961). Kane and associates (1976) point out that the interpretation given to "health" by the poor is a natural consequence of the living conditions in which they find themselves. Irelan further explains:

> Their entire orientation is colored by the fact that they live with other poor people; they take on the perspectives of those around them and reinforce each other's beliefs and values. The way they cope with health problems is traceable either to the material situation of poverty itself, to the social structure of poverty, or to the aspects of the life outlook of poverty—the ideals, values, and beliefs to which the poor man adheres. (Irelan, 1972, pp. 56–57)

People have different ways of defining whether they are sick or well. Some people feel they are sick only when they can no longer work or carry on their usual daily activities and roles; others are very attuned to their physiological functioning and recognize even minor symptoms or signs as an indication of disease and illness. A third orientation to illness is that people are sick simply when they are not feeling well.

Baumann (1961) demonstrated these differences in an early study she conducted of middle-aged and older chronically ill clinic patients from working-class and lower socioeconomic backgrounds and freshmen medical students in their first three years of medical school, who were generally from middle- and upper-middle-class backgrounds and in their early 20s. She compared the two groups according to their definitions of health and illness. Baumann found the three prevailing basic orientations to wellness and illness mentioned above existed in the two groups: (1) a subjective feeling of well-being or ill health (the feeling-state orientation), (2) an absence or presence of general or specific symptoms (symptom orientation), and (3) a state of being able or unable to perform usual activities (a performance orientation). Consistent with American society's productivity value orientation, both groups (representing both age and socioeconomic differences) mentioned an activity orientation in their conceptualization of health and illness. The clinic patients tended to identify subjective feelings as being a significant factor in their definition (supporting Koos's conclusions [1954] that people with less education are less articulate in their thoughts about illness), while the freshmen medical students identified the presence or absence of symptoms as the second criterion in their definition of health and illness.

Koos (1954), in a classic study, demonstrated that socioeconomic position greatly influenced an individual's interpretation of symptoms—that is, whether symptoms are perceived as symptoms of illness or not, and when present, whether they constitute indications that medical care should be sought. He found that as one descends the social class ladder, less symptom recognition and perceived need for medical services existed among the study population. Middle-class workers were found to be much more knowledgeable about disease symptoms, while the working-class and lower-class persons showed less recognition of symptoms as being signs of ill health and therefore did not view these symptoms as indicating a need for medical attention. Thus, Koos and Baumann (1961) were consistent in their findings that the more educated a family is, the better the family's knowledge of health usually is. With the increased use of home computers and access to the World Wide Web, many families who can afford these resources in their home are more informed about health care issues based on their data searches. Certainly, determining any family's level of knowledge about a condition cannot be automatically assumed by their socioeconomic level, rather this would have to be assessed with every client. Also, certain family members, generally the mother, may be better informed. Women have consistently been found to have acquired more health education information due to their health role in the family.

Social class differences are also quite pronounced relative to a family's overall priorities. In lower-class families, health is often a lower priority than jobs, food, and shelter, unless a health crisis presents itself.

ETHNIC DIFFERENCES.   The family's ethnic background is another major factor influencing family members' conceptualizations and beliefs of health and illness. Arthur Kleinman, an anthropologist and psychiatrist, developed an Explanatory Model of Health and Illness, which describes how cultural factors govern individuals' perception, labeling, explanation, valuation of symptoms, health and illness definitions, prognosis, treatment, and health promotion. Kleinman (1988) and his associates (Kleinman, Eisenberg, & Good, 1978) make an important distinction between disease and illness. Disease is the health care professionals' biomedical understanding of the health problem, while illness is the patient's personal and unique understanding and definition of what is happening to him or her.

According to Kleinman, cultural factors determine the importance of the various domains of influence. These domains shape people's explanations of health and illness and what they think they should do about health. The three domains of influence that Kleinman identifies are the professional, popular, and folk domains of influence. Within the professional domain, individuals learn about diseases and treatment from a health professional perspective. Within the popular domain, which is the most powerful of the domains of influence, family, relatives, and the lay community are sources of health and illness information and beliefs. According to Kleinman and associates (Kleinman, Eisenberg, & Good, 1978), in 70 to 90 percent of all health situations, the popular domain of influence is consulted first. The last domain of influence is called the folk domain, whereby nonprofessional healers such as curanderas/curanderos, Native American medicine men, or herbalists provide explanations about health events. In unacculturated families, both the popular and folk domains of culturally derived influences are transmitted by family and community across generations.

Western societies typically root their explanations of health and illness in natural phenomena (as opposed to supranatural phenomena) and scientific findings; that is, the causes of health problems are thought to be infection, mechanical injury, tumor growth, or stress induced. In non-Westernized ethnic groups and societies, families often hold explanatory belief systems in which health and illness are viewed as resulting from social or supranatural causes or from an imbalance (like hot and cold or yin and yang) in the body. These explanations are usually holistic explanations—recognizing the interrelationship between the mind and body and between the individual and his or her social environment. The view of treatment of an illness is generally congruent with the beliefs about the cause of the problem (Kleinman, 1980). For example, if the health problem is thought to be caused by disturbed social interactions, social interventions are preferred (Friedman & Ferguson-Marshalleck, 1996). In Native American cultures, "sings" and sand paintings may be the therapies used when social interaction and support are needed for problems emanating from interpersonal problems.

HEALTH BELIEFS ABOUT HEALTH CARE SEEKING AND HEALTH ACTION

Another major factor identified as influencing health practices is an individual's and a family's health beliefs about seeking care and taking health action. Two related issues are discussed here: (1) the factors that lead to the readiness and intention of an individual to seek health care services and improve his or her lifestyle (i.e., change personal health behaviors), and (2) the variables that influence health promotion and preventive actions themselves (personal health practices and use of health services).

HEALTH BELIEF MODEL. The most comprehensive scheme for looking at disease prevention and illness detection behavior is the Health Belief Model (Berkanovic, 1976), which has been subjected to testing in a wide variety of preventive and curative health areas. It has been modified several times since its inception and is a useful tool for systematically analyzing personal health behavior, predicting such diverse activities as preventive health actions, medical care utilization, delay in seeking help, and compliance with medical regimens.

The Health Belief Model utilizes Lewin's theories that stress that it is the world of the perceiver that determines what he or she will do, not the physical environment, except as this environment is viewed by the individual. Lewin identifies some aspects of life as having a negative valence (negatively valued), some as having a positive valence (positively valued), and some as having a neutral valence. Individuals seek to avoid the negatively valued aspects, whereas they try to incorporate the positive aspects into their lives.

The original model (Figure 16–1) deals with explaining preventive health actions—that is, strategies for avoiding the negatively valued regions of illness and disease. In order for an individual to take preventive action to avoid disease, he or she would need to believe that:

- He or she was personally susceptible or vulnerable to the disease.

- The illness was at least moderately severe, so that the consequences of acquiring the disease would significantly disrupt the person's life.

- Taking a particular action would be beneficial in that it would reduce susceptibility to, or severity of, the disease.

- The benefits are outweighed by the barriers, such as costs, pain, time, inconvenience, and embarrassment.

The susceptibility and seriousness of the disease are perceived factors that are not dependent on fact but on the person's personal beliefs. Both of these individual perceptions become the "readiness" factors leading to the perceived threat of a disease. In this model, there are modifying factors (demographic, sociopsychological, and structural) that are posited to modify perceived susceptibility, severity, perceived benefits versus costs, and cues to action. Cues to action refer to the immediate stimuli needed to trigger recognition in the person's mind of the susceptibility and seriousness of a disease (the threat), and the need for taking action to reduce the threat (Redding, Rossi, Rossi, Velicer, & Prochaska, 2000; Rosenstock, 1974).

In newer, modified health belief models, the readiness factors have been extended to include both the perceived feelings of the susceptibility and seriousness of the health problem (the threat) and positive motivation to maintain, regain, or attain wellness.

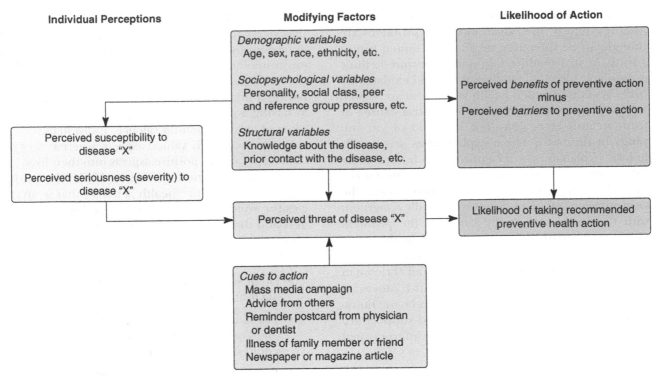

Figure 16–1. Diagram of the (original) Health Belief Model. *(From Rosenstock, 1974, p. 7.)*

This motivational factor includes concern about, and the salience of, health matters in general, willingness to seek and receive medical direction, plans to comply, and existence of positive health practices (Becker, 1974; Redding et al., 2000; Rosenstock, 1974).

The model has been used extensively to assist in determining why people engage in certain activities that will or will not promote their health and well-being. These studies have shown consistently that the benefits of certain health behaviors (e.g., physical activity) may not serve as enough impetus for action when the individual believes that the barriers or perceived risks are not fully understood or seem to be high (Clarke, Lovegrove, Williams, & MacPherson, 2000; Cousins, 2000; Grubbs & Tabano, 2000). For instance, Cousins found that women aged 70 and older often feel physically vulnerable and are unsure about their actual risks and/or the benefits of an exercise program. Thus, in the face of this uncertainty, these women report medical reasons why they should be excused from fitness-promoting exercise.

HEALTH PROMOTION MODEL. Pender, Murdaugh, and Parsons (2001) extended the Health Belief Model into the Pender Health Promotion Model, which is complementary to other models of health protection. Health promotion focuses on movement toward a positively valenced state of enhanced health and well-being. The negatively valenced states of illness and disease appear to have minimal motivational significance for health-promoting behavior. Pender suggests that a desire for growth, expression of human potential, and quality of life provides the motivation for health-promotive actions.

Pender's Health Promotion Model (Figure 16–2) builds on previous health belief models. The revised model (Pender, Murdaugh, & Parsons, 2001) theorizes about the relationships among individual characteristics and experiences, behavior-specific cognitions and affect, and behavioral outcomes. In Pender's model, individual characteristics and experiences include the effect of prior related behavior and personal biological, psychological, and sociocultural factors. Although personal factors are thought to

Figure 16–2. Revised Health Promotion Model. *(From Pender, 1996, p. 67.)*

influence the likelihood of engaging in health-promoting behavior, some personal characteristics cannot be changed and, thus, are seldom incorporated into nursing interventions.

The core of the revised Health Promotion Model emphasizes the importance of behavior-specific cognitions and affect as the primary motivators of behavior. These variables could be especially significant for nurses to consider, as they are subject to modification through nursing interventions. The six behavior-specific cognitions and affect considered to be of major motivational significance in encouraging an individual to engage in health-promoting behaviors have been identified within the model as: perceived benefits of action, perceived barriers to action, perceived self-efficacy, activity-related affect, interpersonal influences, and situational influences. Behavior-specific cognitions and affect that are hypothesized to be directly related to health-promoting actions include positive perceptions of the anticipated expected outcome, minimal barriers to action, feeling efficacious and skilled, positive feelings about the health behavior, presence of family and peer social support, positive role models, and availability of environmental contexts that are compatible, safe, and interesting (Pender, Murdaugh, & Parsons, 2001).

In Pender's model, behavioral outcomes are influenced by a person's sense of commitment to a plan of action with identified specific strategies, and the capacity of the person to repress competing demands and preferences. Health-promoting behavior is the action outcome in the model. Pender and associates emphasize that health-promoting behavior is ultimately directed toward attaining positive health outcomes for the client that should result in a positive health experience throughout that person's lifetime.

In summary, important aspects to remember about the health belief models is that they are rational decision-making models in which the occurrence of personal health behavior is thought to be influenced by factors identified in The Health Belief Model and Pender's Health Promotion Model.

In regard to implications for family health care, these models emphasize the significance of the family's and the family members' belief system. If a family perceives a threat and if avenues are then presented to the family for reducing the threat, such as accessible and effective screening, health services, lifestyle improvements, and education, the family will be more likely to act positively on its behalf. A health practitioner should not use the fear tactic to build up anxiety and readiness without offering an effective and accessible remedial action to handle and reduce the threat.

✺ HOW WELL FAMILIES PERFORM THE HEALTH CARE FUNCTION

The health care function is not only an essential and basic family function but one that assumes a central focus in healthy, well-functioning families. However, fulfilling the health care function for all family members may be difficult due to external and internal challenges. Pratt (1976, 1982) suggests that the reasons families have difficulties providing health care for their members lie with both (a) the structure of the family structure and (b) the health care system. Pratt found that when families had wide associations with organizations, engaged in common activities, and used community resources, they used health care services more appropriately. Also, personal health practices were enhanced when husbands were actively involved in internal family affairs, including matters concerning the health care system.

In order for families to become a primary and effective health resource, they must become more involved in the health care team and the total therapeutic process (Krozy, 1996; Levine & Zuckerman, 2000). This implies an egalitarian relationship with health care providers in which both parties can openly express their opinions and negotiate services that meet their particular needs and interests. Levine and Zuckerman ask:

> "Why do physicians and other health care professionals, including lawyers and bioethicists, so often view families as 'trouble'? And why do families so often see medical professionals as uncaring and uncommunicative? Presumably everyone wants the same goal—recovery or the best possible outcome for the patient. And yet trouble clearly exists." (p. 5)

Pratt (1976) acknowledges that it is not possible for families to become highly responsible about their health care function if health care professionals exclude them from participating in medical management. Such a partnership role is needed whether promotive, preventive, curative, or rehabilitative health needs are under consideration. People must be treated as responsible adults, not passive children, if professionals wish them to assume self-responsibility.

Not only must the family be in partnership with health care providers in directing and implementing its own health care, but clients should also be the ultimate decision makers and managers of those health issues affecting their welfare and lives. In order for clients to engage in effective self-care, they must have the knowledge and skills needed to provide good health care. This means that families need access to the primary sources of health information. Thus professionals must be willing to extend their role to include health education directed toward family self-care and family empowerment (Courtney, 1995; Institute of Medicine, 2000; Rafael, 1995).

Most families appear to recognize the need to assume strong management of their own health care (Levine & Zuckerman, 2000). However, both professionals and the health care industry—hospitals, pharmaceutical companies, supply companies, and the health insurance industry—discourage it. Data from

Pratt's study revealed that families who were most effective in obtaining appropriate medical services and who practiced a wellness lifestyle on their own were the families referred to as "energized" families. These families assertively sought and verified information, made discriminating decisions, and negotiated aggressively with the health care system, rather than passively accepting and complying (Pratt, 1976, 1982).

Another reason that families are having difficulties providing health care to their members is the lack of access to care. Race and level of income and education contribute to class differences in health care service access and utilization. Minority populations and those with lower levels of income and education utilize preventive health care services less frequently. Nonwhite populations spend fewer days in the hospital, see a physician less often, and are more likely to be treated in a hospital outpatient department than in a physician's office (United States Department of Health and Human Services [U.S. DHHS], 1989a). For such groups, poor experiences with the health care system are likely to lead to low rates of service utilization for health examinations and treatments.

One major factor explaining differences in access and utilization patterns of medical services is the lack of health care insurance coverage (Kozol, 2000). Approximately two thirds of the U.S. population is covered by employment-related coverage, either individually or through groups sponsored by those other than employers. A total of 74.5 percent of the insured population is privately insured. Ten percent of the population receives coverage from publicly funded programs such as Medicare and Medicaid, according to data obtained from survey findings conducted by the National Center for Health Services Research. Despite use of these public funds, elder Americans now pay about one fifth of their income on out-of-pocket health care costs such as premium and prescription drugs. An estimated 16.3 percent of the population, or 44.3 million Americans, remain without private insurance or public coverage to help pay medical needs (ACP-ASIM, 2001; Centers for Disease Control and Prevention [CDC], 1999; Himmelstein & Woolhandler, 1994; *Los Angeles Times*, 2001).

About two thirds of the uninsured are employed workers and their families. This group represents the largest number of uninsured persons. Uninsured workers are typically part-time or self-employed, work for small establishments, earn low hourly wages at or near the minimum wage, and work in industries characterized by seasonal or less technical employment such as agriculture, construction, manufacturing, and sales. Individuals who are poor and from minority backgrounds are at highest risk of being uninsured. More than one third of Hispanics had no health insurance in 1996, and blacks were more likely than either Hispanics or whites to have only public insurance (Agency for Health Care Policy and Research [AHCPR], 1996). In addition, workers from certain occupations have a high rate of being uninsured. Other population groups that are especially vulnerable for being uninsured and underinsured include children, unmarried young adults, older women, lower-middle-income groups, and families without a working adult who are living at or near the poverty line (Himmelstein & Woolhandler, 1994) (see Table 16–1).

Many families who do have insurance are underinsured, preventing them from getting comprehensive health care. Furthermore, many poor families who

TABLE 16–1

SELECTED SUMMARY OF PEOPLE WITHOUT HEALTH INSURANCE

White	12.9%
Hispanic	32.0%
Black	18.5%
Native American or Alaska Native	26.8%
Asian and Pacific Islander	18.0%
Males	14.9%
Females	13.1%
Under 18 years of age	11.6%
18–24 years of age	27.3%
65 years or older	0.7%
Household income less than $25,000	22.7%
Household income $75,000 or more	6.9%
No high school diploma	26.6%
Bachelor's degree or higher	7.1%

Source: http://www.census.gov.

TABLE 16–2

HARMFUL IMPACT EXPERIENCED BY AMERICAN FAMILIES WITHOUT INSURANCE

- Less likely to have a regular source of care
- Less likely to have had a recent physician visit
- More likely to delay seeking service
- More likely to report they have not received needed care
- Less likely to use preventive services
- Less likely to seek prenatal care
- More likely to have higher mortality and specifically higher in-hospital mortality
- Three times more likely than privately insured individuals to experience adverse health outcomes
- Four times as likely as insured patients to require both avoidable hospitalizations and emergency hospital care

Source: Data from ACP-ASIM. (2001).

are covered by Medicaid are treated in busy emergency departments and outpatient clinics of public hospitals where care may be fragmented and episodic (Center for Health Economics Research, 1993). There are deleterious outcomes associated with not having health insurance, including a higher mortality rate (Table 16–2) (ACP-ASIM, 2001).

❧HEALTH CARE PRACTICES

Promotion of health practices within the family is a basic goal of family nursing. It becomes critical to gain information regarding the family's health practices to assist the family in health promotion and maintenance. One indication of the family's level of health care functioning is the overall level of health of its family members. This is often inferred by gathering information as to the incidence of disease per member in a specific period of time, realizing, of course, that the ages of individuals and their environment play major roles in the genesis and incidence of disease. Large families and families with young children, for example, have a greater incidence of disease per family. Troubled, problematic families are

found to have less resistance to disease and thus have higher rates of disease than families that are functioning well.

Hundreds of thousands of Americans die prematurely each year of diseases caused primarily by unhealthy lifestyles. These unnecessary mortalities result from heart disease, cancer, accidents, hypertension, cirrhosis of the liver, and diabetes. Recognizing the significance of lifestyle in promoting the health of Americans, the U.S. Department of Health and Human Services published *Healthy People 2000,* a platform for action to help bring the American people toward their full health potential. The report identifies three broad goals: "increase the span of healthy life for Americans, reduce health disparities among Americans, and achieve access to preventive services for all Americans" (U.S. DHHS, 1991, p. 6). *Healthy People 2010* builds on the initiatives pursued over the past two decades. Measurable objectives have been established to serve as the basis for the development of state and community plans to improve the overall health of U.S. citizens. The leading health indicators that will be used to measure the health of the nation include:

- Physical activity
- Overweight and obesity
- Tobacco use
- Substance abuse
- Responsible sexual behavior
- Mental health
- Injury and violence
- Environmental quality
- Immunization
- Access to health care

The economic and cultural diversity of families speaks to the need to adapt health promotion activities to the needs of minorities, the impoverished, and special ethnic groups. Although the U.S. Bureau of the Census (2000a) reports a noticeable trend in delays and declines in childbearing, single-parent families are on the upsurge. The number of families headed by single mothers has increased 25 percent since 1990, to more than 7.5 million households in the United States (Kantrowitz & Wingert, 2001). This family structure often results in poverty with the children living outside of marriage 7 times more likely to experience poverty and 17 times more likely to be on welfare when they are adults (Kantrowitz & Wingert).

Teenage pregnancy and abortion rates have been declining in the 1990s, but are still very high. Abortion rates were down nearly a third between 1990 and 1997 among teenagers 15 to 19 years of age, with teenage birth rates falling 17 percent from 1990 through 1999 (Ventura, Mosher, Curtin, & Abma, 2001). Teenage pregnancy is not a new phenomenon; however, there is a change in the context within which it occurs (i.e., pregnancy outside of the context of marriage) (Brooks-Gunn & Chase-Landsdale, 1995). Thus, adolescent pregnancy is viewed as particularly problematic because of the vulnerability of and lack of resources of the mother. Not surprisingly, pregnancy is the chief cause of women leaving school. Within marriage, early pregnancy (within the first two years) detracts from marital adjustment.

The physical health of mother and child is a major issue, documented in obstetrical and perinatal studies. Birth intervals of between two and four years and a maternal age in the 20s are the most favorable factors for reducing maternal and infant mortality and morbidity. Optimal family size, spacing, and timing of births also reduces infant mortality (Cohn & Lieberman, 1974).

The rate of planned pregnancies is growing, as is the number of women or couples who are using contraceptives (Abma, Chandra, Mosher, Peterson, & Piccinino, 1997). Forty-five states, as well as the District of Columbia, have enacted legislation allowing teenage girls under the age of 18 to obtain contraceptives without parental consent. Yet a large proportion of sexually active adolescents and young adult women are not receiving family planning services (Chilman, 1988). Furthermore, contraceptive use is known to be less among black and Hispanic teenagers (72 percent and 53 percent, respectively) at first intercourse than among white teenagers (83 percent) (Abma et al.).

Inconsistent patterns of contraceptive use are attributed to inaccessibility of services, and the fractious debate about the role of government in providing such services (Brooks-Gunn & Paikoff, 1993). Religious and sociopolitical factors have interceded to reduce women's and couple's reproductive rights. As of the early 1990s, due to pro-life opposition, the struggle to keep present services available is of growing concern. Public funding for family planning initiatives, as well as abortion, has been cut and services gravely curtailed for women who are poor and young.

In addition to the need for more health care clinics and permissive legislation for teenagers to receive care, effective sex and family planning health education programs need to be devised and implemented in schools, religious institutions, and health agencies. Such services should be focused not on the general premise that family planning is an end in itself, but on the health benefits of family planning to the individual and to the growth and development of the family.

In addition to looking at the family's overall perceived health status, illness patterns of family members and the issues of birth control and conception, the family's health practices are fruitful assessment areas, providing relevant areas for client education. Eight primary areas of health practices will be explored in this section:

- Family dietary practices
- Family sleep and rest practices
- Family exercise and recreational practices
- Family therapeutic and recreational drug, alcohol, and tobacco practices
- Family self-care practices
- Environmental and hygiene practices
- Medically based preventive practices
- Alternative therapies

FAMILY DIETARY PRACTICES

Poor dietary practices leading to obesity is a primary example of the results of an unhealthy lifestyle. Many Americans are overweight and gain weight as they grow older. About 55 percent of American adults are overweight, with men more likely to be overweight than women (CDC, 1999). Being overweight is linked to high blood pressure, heart disease, certain types of cancer, arthritis, breathing problems, and other illnesses (Akande, Van Wyk, & Osagie, 2000; U.S. DHHS, 1995). Cardiovascular disease is now recognized as a disease of childhood, as obesity increases in young children. As individuals age, to stay at the same weight, they must balance the amount of energy taken in food (caloric intake) with the amount of energy the body uses (caloric output). Physical activity is an important way to use up food energy. Many Americans spend too much of their day in sedentary activities that require little energy. In addition, many Americans of all ages now spend a lot of leisure time each day engaging in passive activities, for example, watching television.

The kinds and amounts of food people eat affect their ability to maintain their weight. High-fat foods contain more calories per serving than other foods and increase the likelihood of weight gain. However, even when people consume less high-fat foods, they can still gain weight from eating too much of foods high in starch, sugar, or protein. In 1998, less than one fourth of adults reported eating recommended daily amounts of fruits and vegetables and less than 71 percent of high school students reported the same (CDC, 1999).

Foods from the base of the Food Guide Pyramid should serve as the foundation for meals. Foods from the grain group, along with vegetables and fruits, are the basis of healthful diets (U.S. DHHS, 1995). Diets high in fat, saturated fat, cholesterol, and salt contribute to Americans' risk for chronic disease. According to the American Cancer Society, approximately 30 percent of all cancer deaths are attributable to dietary factors (CDC, 1999). Obesity, high blood pressure, high blood cholesterol, and elevated serum glucose can be modified by a balance of a healthy diet and sufficient physical activity. Because obesity has been repeatedly demonstrated to be one of the key precursors to chronic illness and shortened longevity, assessing the family's caloric intake and comparing this to their actual caloric need becomes germane to practice. Additionally, children must learn to make healthy food choices to manage their weight so they do not have to struggle with weight issues later in life.

Encouraging all family members to keep a three-day food diary is very helpful in assessing both the quality of their family's diet and how it meets individual nutritional needs. Such a record, three sequential days' intake (two weekdays plus one weekend day), is a stronger indication of a family's eating patterns than is the record of only a single day's intake. A 24-hour food history may not truly represent the family's usual eating patterns (Lacey, 1989). Dietary variations that may occur among individual family members during the day should be included in the journal. Active participation by all family members in completing the food record will enhance the discovery of what family members eat, and where their dietary strengths and deficiencies lie. The three-day nutrition intake record is an excellent base for assisting families to assess their present nutritional status and begin to develop nutritional goals. The family food diary offered in Figure 16–3 may be used as a guide for data collection.

Assessment of the family's food choices should be a collaborative effort between the family and the nurse. Are a variety of foods consumed from the food guide pyramid each day? Specifically, does the diet contain 6 to 11 servings from foods in the grain group, 3 to 5 servings from the vegetable group, 2 to 4 servings from the fruit group, and 2 to 3 servings from the dairy group and the meat and beans group.

	Food Served	Quantity	Comments (Factors Such as Place, Activity, Money)
Breakfast			
Snacks (between meals)			
Lunch			
Snacks (between meals)			
Dinner			
Snacks (between meals)			

Figure 16–3. Family dietary diary (record of family dietary intake for three days).

Are adequate amounts of dark green or deep yellow fruits or vegetables consumed each day to meet vitamin A requirements? Are vitamin C–rich fresh fruits and dark green leafy vegetables part of the daily diet? Are low-fat dairy products consumed to meet calcium and vitamin D requirements? Other aspects of the family nutrition analysis should include evaluation for the amount and quality of dietary fat, intake of cholesterol and saturated fat, patterns of complex carbohydrate and fiber intake, consumption of sugar and artificial sweeteners, sodium use, processed food intake, alcohol consumption, coffee and tea intake, and the use of dietary supplements.

In analyzing a three-day food record, the family nurse should determine individual variances. Are any individual family members underweight or overweight for their height and age group? What does each person eat (types of food and quantity) in relation to the family's dietary practices? By learning about family food practices, preferences, and individual dietary habits, the nurse and family will gain a holistic picture of family dietary patterns. For instance, is Johnnie's state of obesity and extensive tooth decay due to his eating excessive amounts of sugars and carbohydrates? If so, is this part of the family's customary diet, along with sedentary activities and poor dental hygiene? Or does the family serve well-balanced meals and is Johnnie's sweet intake at school a reflection of other problems? Does the family require the child to eat at specific mealtimes, or do they allow some variance in scheduling in association with the child's internal hunger drives (Johnson, 2001)?

Food fads, reduction diets, special dietary beliefs, or culturally based food patterns—such as dietary practices based on a traditional Jewish, Mexican, or Italian pattern, or special food practices based on a philosophical or health commitment such as that held by many vegetarians—need to be appraised. Understanding the family's value system and beliefs underlying their food practices is also important and serves as a suitable foundation for later work with the family on any modification that might be needed.

Additional information relevant in assessing family dietary practices includes an awareness of the function of mealtimes for the family and the family's attitude toward food and mealtimes. Does the family eat together (all meals, only dinner, etc.)? Is mealtime (when they are together) a social, pleasurable experi-

ence? How are the meals handled when the family does not eat together? When families are more atomistic or individualistic (each family member doing his or her own "thing"), junk foods and a less adequate diet are often found. When family members do not congregate for at least dinner, it is difficult for the family to interact and share with each other, because mealtime is often the one opportunity families have to enjoy each other's company and share important and pleasurable experiences, thoughts, and feelings.

Do parents use the giving and withholding of food as reward and punishment? Where this occurs, the child learns to associate food with approval (love) and disapproval (rejection). Pairing food and social needs for love and acceptance is an unhealthy linkage, as counselors who treat the obese will attest.

SHOPPING, PLANNING, AND PREPARATION PRACTICES

What are the shopping arrangements? Where is food purchased? Does the family plan for the week or several days at a time, or do they operate on a meal-to-meal basis, shopping for each meal or one day at a time? (The latter is certainly an inefficient means in terms of time and money.) What kind of budgetary limitations exist in their food shopping? If the need is present, does the family use food stamps? Is food storage and refrigeration adequate? What are usual ways in which food is prepared (fried, boiled, microwaved, eaten cold, variety of means)? Who is responsible for the tasks of shopping, planning, and meal preparation? Although we generally assume that the mother–wife is responsible, it is sometimes a role shared with the spouse and/or older children.

FAMILY SLEEP AND REST PRACTICES

Sleep is a necessary function for quality living; it fulfills several physiological needs, such as energy conservation, restoration, and protection against exhaustion (Kick, 1996). A major factor in determining how much sleep family members require is age. Newborns need between 16 and 18 hours of sleep distributed over every 24-hour period. Infants in the first 6 months of life sleep progressively more in the night than in the day, with requirements for 10 to 12 hours of rest nightly and usually two to three daytime naps by the end of the first year. Toddlers will sleep 8 to 12 hours nightly and have one daytime nap. The preschool-aged child requires 10 to 12 hours of sleep. The average school-aged child requires 9 to 10 hours of rest each night. The need for sleep declines for adolescents to about 7.5 hours daily. Young and middle-aged adults require 6 to 8 hours of sleep. Elderly sleep requirements drop to an average of 6.5 hours. An increase in overall health status, improved mental status, and increased longevity has been positively correlated with regular, adequate rest and sleep habits (Baker, 1985; Bowden, Dickey, & Greenberg, 1998).

Every family has patterns for sleeping, even though in some families these patterns may be erratic due to crowding in the family's home, different work or school schedules, illness, or because of caregiving needs as in the family with a new baby. Assessment of the family's sleep should begin with a sleep history. The nurse should assess if any individual family member has trouble sleeping (insomnia) and if so, what specific type of trouble—falling asleep, or awakening early without being able to resume sleeping. Frequency and severity of the insomnia should be elicited. Often, sleeping difficulties are due to inadequate sleeping arrangements in the home. A simple sleep diary or log individually kept by each family member may provide additional insight into identifying sleep disturbances.

A deficiency in knowledge of family members' sleep requirements, and what makes a good sleep routine, may be found. New parents may be confused about their baby's irregular sleep schedule. Older adults may lack understanding regarding normal sleep requirements and changes that occur with aging. Many families lack a knowledge of the effects that sedatives and other prescribed drugs, over-the-counter drugs, and illicit drugs have on sleep. The nurse should elicit information from the family as to the possible etiologies of any identified sleep pattern disturbances.

FAMILY PHYSICAL ACTIVITIES AND RECREATIONAL ACTIVITIES

Regular physical activity promotes general health. Less sedentary or more vigorous activity may help reduce body fat and disease risk. Despite the proven benefits of physical exercise, 28 percent of adults are sedentary and 60 percent of adults do not engage in regular, sufficient activity (CDC, 1999). These patterns are learned all too early. In 1997, it was noted that 51 percent of high school students were not enrolled in a physical education class (CDC). Among the priorities for health promotion established by the U.S. Public Health Service's *Healthy People 2010* (U.S. DHHS, 2000), physical activity and fitness is listed first. The current public health recommendation regarding physical activity states that every adult should accumulate 30 minutes a day or more of moderate physical activity on most, preferably all, days of the week (Burns, 1996). Additional research indicates that those who meet these standards may derive additional health and fitness benefits by becoming more physically active or by including more vigorous activity in their daily life (Dinger, 1999; Pate et al., 1995). The recommendation emphasizes physical activity as opposed to exercise, which some people find difficult to fit into their daily schedules. Experts agree that intermittent episodes of physical activity are more beneficial than remaining sedentary. To meet the recommendation, an individual must accumulate the 30 minutes of moderate-intensity physical activity on at least five of the seven days of the week (Table 16–3). Studies show that adults who began physical activity after years of inactivity had reduced mortality rates when compared to those who remain sedentary (Paffenbarger et al., 1993). When exercise and physical activities are made family activities, everyone in the family benefits, and important lifelong habits are established.

RECREATIONAL ACTIVITIES. The importance of family recreation in maintaining healthy family life is consistently recognized in family literature and research (Zabriskie & McCormick, 2001). Although each family member has his or her own special leisure-time activities, families also need to have regular family-centered activities in which all members can share and enhance their life together. These activities may be religious, educational, recreational, civic, or cultural in nature. Family rituals and celebrations, most commonly held during holidays or birthdays, are also important times when families come together to

TABLE 16-3

PHYSICAL ACTIVITY RECOMMENDATIONS

Guideline: Accumulate at least 30 minutes of moderate-intensity physical activity on most, preferably all, days of the week.

- Accumulation of physical activity throughout the day is a reasonable alternative to setting aside an uninterrupted period of time for physical activity each day (e.g., 10 minutes in the morning, 10 minutes in the afternoon, 10 minutes in the evening).

- Examples of moderate-intensity physical activity include general cleaning of the house, using a push mower to mow the lawn, playing golf (walking or carrying the clubs), and walking briskly (3–4 mph).

- Physical activity should be completed on at least five of the seven days of the week.

- Increase in physical activity beyond the 30 minutes of moderate-intensity activity yields additional health benefits.

- Previously sendentary people who begin physical activity programs should start with short sessions (5–10 minutes) and gradually build up to the desired level of activity.

- Adults with chronic health problems (i.e., heart disease, diabetes) should consult a physician before beginning a new program of physical activity.

Source: Adapted from Pate et al. (1995).

renew their ties and sense of continuity as a family and to enjoy each others' company.

Recreational activities refers to those activities that are apart from the obligations of work, family, and society and to which individuals turn at will for relaxation, diversion, self-development, or social participation. Family recreation entails maintaining and strengthening of family bonds, having fun together, sharing feelings, reducing tension, and improving family members' feelings about their family (Geba, 1985; McCown, 1996; Zabriskie & McCormick, 2001). Families should be urged to incorporate more exercise, such as hiking, biking, swimming, and physically active games into their family recreational activities.

These activities also have the benefit of promoting physical fitness in families.

Changing values of society have made quality of life, high-level wellness, and self-fulfillment through work and leisure more prominent today. In the family today, family-centered recreation has in some ways declined in importance because of competing leisure-time opportunities for individuals and because of so many dual-worker families. Other factors, however, are responsible for making family recreation a continuing significant family activity: longer paid vacations, shorter working hours, more three-day weekends, and greater accessibility to recreational facilities, at least for more affluent families.

Researchers also report that family members believe that not enough time is spent in family leisure-time activity (Smith, 1985). It is from the family that individuals learn to value certain lifestyle patterns, including healthy recreational pursuits such as those involving exercise as well as leisure time and group/team work. The family is the context in which healthy recreational, leisure-time, and exercise patterns are established (McCown, 1996).

Research on family recreation has focused on its positive effect on marital and family satisfaction, family unity, and marital stability (Hill, 1988; Smith, 1985). For instance, Gerson (1960), in studying married college couples, found a positive relationship between a number of leisure-time factors and marital satisfaction. West and Merriam (1969) discovered a positive correlation between outdoor recreation and family solidarity. Hill, applying attachment theory to her study, found that spouses' shared recreational time was predictive of marital stability.

Kelly (1978) concluded that the family is a central social context of leisure. He observed that the home is the most common locale for leisure-time activity, and that family members are the usual companions for most kinds of weekday, weekend, and vacational leisure. Stinnett (1979), Otto (1973), and McCubbin and McCubbin (1988) validate the important role family leisure-time activity plays in family life by including indicators of family recreational activity in their lists of family strengths—such as spending time together, having common interests, having fun together, and having family traditions, celebrations, and rituals.

Keeping the family subsystems strong and functioning effectively is crucial to family health. Recreational activities involving the subsystems as well as the whole family are viewed as a major family strength. Based on a family assessment, when nurses find that a family is lacking in cohesiveness or bonding, the fun of being a family, social supports, or active recreational activity or is under stress, the promotion of regular, more frequent family recreation and leisure-time activities may be indicated. McCown (1996) identifies the nurse's role in promoting active family recreation as including modeling behaviors, providing education, and contracting for client self-care. Hence, family nurses are urged to be good role models of an active, healthy lifestyle that incorporates family recreation; to act as health educators and counselors for families in need of increasing their recreation and other leisure-time activities; and to use behavior modification and contracting as one mechanism to assist families to acquire additional healthy lifestyle patterns such as family recreation and exercise.

FAMILY'S THERAPEUTIC AND RECREATIONAL DRUG, TOBACCO, AND ALCOHOL PATTERNS

The consumption of medications is ubiquitous in America, with over-the-counter drugs most often used (60 to 70 percent of the time). In a society where pills are regarded as a panacea for everything from sexual problems to headaches, it is no wonder that major community health problems exist in Americans' substance-using practices. Use of such substances is viewed as "hip" and "cool" by many adolescents, college students, and mid-career and older-aged citizens. Such practices, in moderation, can have a relatively benign impact on individual health and overall family health practices. However, extensive use of these substances can impact family members' health as well as family finances, family relationships, and family stability. Health care professionals need to be most concerned with helping teenagers because smoking, drinking, and recreational use of drugs often begin during these years.

OVER-THE-COUNTER AND PRESCRIPTION MEDICATIONS. Families use a significant amount of over-the-counter medication as an alternative to professional care for health prob-

lems that are seen as being too trivial to seek medical care for, or that are conditions that the family can adequately handle. A national survey discovered that one half of those sampled undertook self-medication for sore throats, coughs, colds, and upset and acid stomachs. Home over-the-counter medication was found to not be limited to gastrointestinal and upper respiratory complaints, but also covered other body system problems, including the central nervous system, urogenital tract, and skin (Roney & Nall, 1966). Home medication is also frequently used as a supplement to professional treatment. Professional treatments are often altered or modified by patients, as seen in the extensive modifications made to diet and insulin regimen by diabetic patients. Prescribed medications, furthermore, are often not taken by patients as directed. One study reported a medication rejection rate of 50 percent (Linnett, 1970).

It is important to assess the family's use of over-the-counter and prescription drugs, particularly for nurses working in primary care and home health care. Nurses should ask about what drugs family members take and for what purpose. By identifying drugs commonly used by the family, the assessor can look for possible side effects or harmful interactive effects. Also, drug usage can tell the nurse something about how the family and/or the family members cope with life events and health problems, as well as how they define health and illness.

Some over-the-counter drugs commonly taken by Americans are potentially harmful, or at best unnecessary. The regular use of laxatives and painkillers is an example. Although most of the fatal medication poisonings are caused by prescribed medications, with barbiturates heading the list, 20 percent are caused by over-the-counter drugs. Of the nonfatal drug poisonings, aspirin is the leading offender, primarily because of its tendency to produce gastrointestinal bleeding. In homes where young children are present, storage of drugs and other hazardous substances in safe childproof containers and cupboards is imperative. This is vitally important given that the incidence of poisoning among young children is very high.

One important factor leading to medication poisonings is the tendency of older family members to save and reuse medicines years later. Many nurses who have cared for older patients in their homes will attest to the fact that families will hoard medicines prescribed many years ago. Many of these containers do not even contain the name and dosage of the drug. Such medications undergo change over time and, at best, become ineffective. Often families end up using their old medicines to treat a family member who they perceive to be experiencing the same or similar symptoms as the person for whom the drug was originally prescribed. The possible misdiagnosis by the family presents a further hazard.

In assessing the drug use of older family members, as part of a home health visit, the nurse must find a way to tactfully review the kinds and the age of the drugs stored in the house. By doing so, the nurse will be able to go over with the family both the new and old medications and their usage, which may influence the family to properly dispose of drugs that are old and/or unmarked.

RECREATIONAL DRUG USE.   Drug abuse involves the regular taking of a deleterious or noxious quantity of any drug, prescribed or illicit, over a period of time. The family exercises a profound influence on the onset and continuity of patterns of substance abuse by family members and provides a context for communication of knowledge, skills, and attitudes about substance abuse. Positive social reinforcement (modeling by parents or esteemed family members of substance abuse behavior patterns) may play a major social influence in contributing to youth drug use (Baumrind, 1985). At the other end of the continuum, families may highly discourage substance abuse and openly communicate that illicit drug use is contradictory to family values.

Those family members who do become severely drug dependent most often need specialized treatment in order to recover. A wide range of treatment is available through public and private entities. Recovery treatment centers that incorporate the family into their plan of care are more effective in their treatment of the substance abuser.

In 1999, an estimated 14.8 million Americans (6.7 percent of those 12 years and older) were current illicit drug users. This number is lower by approximately one quarter from the 1979 peak level of 20 million current users, yet also demonstrates a level that has remained virtually constant since 1992. Some downward trends have been noted over the past few years among youths 12 to 17, decreasing from 11.4

percent in 1997 to 9.0 percent in 1999 (CDC, 1999). The discussion that follows summarizes concerns related to the most common forms of illicit drug use assessed in the United States.

Marijuana is by far the most prevalent drug used by illicit drug users; approximately 77 percent of current illicit drug users were marijuana or hashish users in 1995. Between 1994 and 1995, the rate of marijuana use among youths aged 12 to 17 increased from 6 percent to 8.2 percent, continuing a trend that began during 1992–1993 (U.S. DHHS, 1996). In 1995, an estimated 9.8 million Americans were current marijuana or hashish users. This represents 4.7 percent of the population aged 12 and older.

A second illicit drug that is widely used is **cocaine.** In 1994 and 1995, an estimated 1.5 million Americans were current cocaine users. This represents 0.7 percent of the population aged 12 and older. Rate of cocaine use had declined from 5.7 million in 1985 to 1.4 million in 1992, but has since risen somewhat (U.S. DHHS, 1996). Most clinicians estimate that approximately 10 percent of those who initially use cocaine "recreationally" will go on to serious, heavy use. Cocaine is one of the most powerfully addictive of the abused drugs and is available in several forms. It is usually sniffed or "snorted" nasally as a white powder and is absorbed through the mucous membranes of the nose. It can also be injected in liquid form, or it can be smoked after chemical conversion to a purified form known as "freebase" or "crack." Compulsive cocaine use may develop even more rapidly if the substance is smoked rather than ingested intranasally.

Estimates of **heroin** use from the National Household Survey on Drug Abuse (U.S. DHHS, 1996) are considered very conservative due to probable undercoverage of the population of heroin users. Estimates of lifetime heroin prevalence have generally remained at around 2 million since 1979, and no significant changes in recent years have been detected. The estimated number of current heroin users was 117,000 in 1994 and 196,000 in 1995. A major concern associated with heroin intravenous drug users is the increased risk for acquired immune deficiency syndrome (AIDS). Since January 1, 1989, data from the National Institute on Drug Abuse indicates that 30 percent of all AIDS cases involve IV drug abuse. Minorities are overrepresented among IV drug users. Among heterosexual IV drug abusers, a disproportionate number (80 percent) of persons with AIDS are African-Americans and Latinos.

Methamphetamine, also known as "crank," "meth," or "speed," once associated with blue-collar workers and biker gangs, is now gaining increased popularity among college students and young professionals. The estimated number of persons who have tried methamphetamine in their lifetime was 4.7 million, 2.2 percent of the population in 1995. In 1994, the estimate had been 3.8 million (U.S. DHHS, 1996). A frightening form of methamphetamine is a new-comer called ice. Produced in rocklike form, ice is smoked. The drug enters the body faster and its effects are longer lasting when compared to cocaine. Also called crystal meth, it is often odorless, colorless, and tasteless.

Hallucinogens such as lysergic acid diethylamide (LSD), phencyclidine (PCP), mescaline, and peyote continue to be a significant problem in the United States. Chronic users of these drugs report memory loss, speech difficulties, depression, and weight loss. When given psychomotor tests, PCP users tend to have lost their fine motor skills and short-term memory. Mood disorders occur. The rate of current use of hallucinogens increased from 0.5 percent in 1994 to 0.7 percent in 1995. Among youth aged 12 to 17, the rate increased from 1.1 percent to 1.7 percent (U.S. DHHS, 1996).

During the 1988 to 1989 survey (Turner, 1990), it was found that the use of **inhalants,** and the **nonmedical use of psychotherapeutic drugs** such as sedatives, tranquilizers, stimulants, and analgesics, decreased to less than 2 percent of the population, being slightly higher for females than males.

TOBACCO USE. The American Cancer Society estimates that cigarette smoking is responsible for one in five deaths in the United States, or more than 430,000 deaths per year (CDC, 1999). Cigarette smoking is the leading cause of preventable death in the United States (Manley, 1996). An estimated 66.8 million Americans aged 12 and older used a tobacco product in 1999. This represents a smoking rate of 30.2 percent of the population. No significant differences in smoking rates have been found by race or ethnicity. Education level affects smoking rates as demonstrated by a consistent decrease in the smoking rate in groups with a higher level of education (U.S. DHHS, 2000). Every day, nearly 3,000 youths

aged 18 and younger become daily cigarette smokers. In 1997, 36 percent of high school students smoked, with a reported range in smoking from 16 percent in Utah to 47 percent in Kentucky (CDC). Significant reductions (approximately 3 percent) in cigarette use among youth have been noted in recent surveys (U.S. DHHS). Factors associated with young people using tobacco products include nicotine dependence, public attitudes about smoking, knowledge of health consequences, tobacco marketing, and peer and parental influences (CDC; Ragon & Mouzon, 1999).

Tobacco use increases the incidence of heart attacks and strokes, pneumonia and other lung diseases, and even deaths of low-birth-weight babies whose mothers' smoking habits played a significant role in the stunted development of their unborn infants. In 1997, the direct medical cost associated with smoking was more than $50 billion, or about 7 percent of the total cost of health care in the United States.

ALCOHOL USE. Alcohol, another lifestyle hazard, is used by more Americans than any other drug, including cigarette tobacco. According to national data, approximately 105 million Americans (47.3 percent) report current alcohol use. Approximately 14 million Americans (7.4 percent) meet the diagnostic criteria for alcohol abuse or alcoholism. About 45 million persons engaged in binge drinking, and about 12.4 million Americans were heavy drinkers. Alcohol usage rates have not significantly changed since 1994 among all age groups (U.S. DHHS, 2000). Euro-Americans continue to have the highest rate of alcohol use at 56 percent. Rates for African-Americans and Hispanic-Americans were 45 percent and 41 percent, respectively. Men were more likely than women to be binge and heavy drinkers. In contrast to the pattern for tobacco use, the higher the level of educational attainment, the more likely the use of alcohol (U.S. DHHS, 1996). Male youths are more likely to drink alcohol than female youths. Other factors associated with high use in adolescents include older age, father-absent homes, and not being in school (e.g., not participating in school activities and extracurricular activities) (Parker, Calhoun, & Weaver, 2000). More than one half of American adults have a close family member who has or had alcoholism, and one in four children younger than 18 are exposed to alcohol abuse or alcohol dependence in the family (U.S. DHHS, 2000).

Nearly one half of all deaths from motor vehicle crashes are alcohol related. There is considerable evidence that drinking is associated with violence, with almost one in four violent crimes reporting that the offender had been drinking prior to committing the crime (U.S. DHHS, 2000). The economic cost of alcohol abuse was estimated at $184.6 billion in 1998. The health care costs of alcohol abuse were estimated at $26.3 billion, and work productivity losses were estimated at $134.2 billion (U.S. DHHS).

Drinking excessive amounts of alcohol increases the risk of coronary heart disease, hypertension, stroke, chronic liver disease, some forms of cancer of the oral pharynx, neurological diseases, osteoporosis, nutritional deficiencies, and many other disorders. Even moderate drinking carries some risk in circumstances that require neuromotor coordination and judgment (e.g., driving vehicles, working around machinery, and piloting airplanes or boats). Alcohol consumption during pregnancy can damage the fetus, cause low infant birth weight, and lead to fetal alcohol syndrome.

In considering drug habits, the family nurse must assess the use of medications as well as the consumption of caffeine, alcohol intake, smoking, and recreational drugs. Smoking and alcohol intake should be assessed in terms of who uses either substance, how much, when, and under what situations or circumstances. Is the use of tobacco or alcohol by a family member(s) perceived as a problem by that person or other family members? Among drinking members, does the use of alcohol interfere with their capacity to carry out their usual activities? How long has the present use of alcohol continued? What was the pattern of drinking in the past?

FAMILY'S SELF-CARE PRACTICES

When assessing a family, especially one in which members are experiencing health problems, the nurse must assess the family's ability to provide self-care, the family's motivation, and its actual competence in handling health matters. A family needs to have an understanding of its own health status and/or health problems and of the specific steps needed to improve or maintain its health in order to be responsible for its own self-care (Johnson, 1984). Self-care practices involve preventive practices, as well as diagnosis, home treatment of common and minor ambulatory health problems, and all the procedures and treatments prescribed for the care of illness of a family member. For example, a family may be giving medications, using special appliances, changing dressings, and carrying out special exercises and diets.

Many studies have demonstrated the benefit of individuals participating in annual screening activities, such as those to detect cancer. However, the use of such preventive services remains relatively low. For instance, in 1997–1998, only 30 percent of Americans aged 50 or older had a sigmoidoscopy (detects precancerous polyps and colorectal cancer), and only 27 percent of American women reported having mammography screening (CDC, 1999).

How adequately is the family able to handle the responsibilities of these therapies? Estimates from the literature report that 75 to 85 percent of all health care is provided by self or family, with self-care being the predominant illness response in the older population (Hickey, 1988). These percentages hold whether or not people have access to professional health services (Levin, Katz, & Holst, 1976). There are no firm data demonstrating that lay-initiated self-care is less effective than professional care (which is about 35 percent effective), or less dangerous (professional care involves 20 percent iatrogenic ill effects and 4 to 11 percent complications from nosocomial infections) (Levin, 1977).

An assessment of the family's self-care abilities, focusing on the family's knowledge, motivation, and motor skill strength or coordination necessary to carry out the physical tasks of care, provides the foundation for evaluating the need for nursing intervention. In identifying the family's strengths, resources, and potentials, the nurse should not overlook the possible stressful effects of caregiving on the family unit. Families that assume the major health care responsibility for members who are frail or suffering severe health problems may experience high levels of physical and emotional strain. Financial burdens may also contribute to a family's level of strain. Studies have shown that women caregivers tend to exhibit higher levels of stress than males. Adult daughter caregivers especially have been found to experience greater familial conflict and household disruption, particularly when they are married with dependent children (Bass & Noelker, 1987; Cantor, 1983).

ENVIRONMENTAL AND HYGIENE PRACTICES

Environmental practices consist of habits or patterns that positively or negatively affect the family's or its members' health status. For instance, is the family regularly exposed to smoke, herbicides, asbestos, lead, or other harmful substances? Noise pollution may also be harmful, as well as water pollution and radiation exposure. More and more evidence demonstrates the adverse effects of long-term, low-level exposure to noise and to chemicals in our air, water, and food. A discussion of environmental concerns relative to the home, neighborhood, and community is presented in Chapter 9.

The family's hygiene and cleanliness practices may also be considered as forms of environmental practices. Although cleanliness is not "next to godliness," there are several general health habits that reduce the possibility of infection and its spread:

1. Washing hands before meals and after toileting.

2. Using separate towels for each family member. When an infectious skin condition such as scabies or impetigo is present, sharing towels can be an infection route.

3. Drinking from separate cups and glasses that are clean. In families with several children and an overworked and overwhelmed mother, sharing of baby bottles and cups is commonly seen.

4. Bathing and cleanliness. Although this is certainly needed, community-based nurses have been overly critical of the families they visit in terms of degree of family cleanliness. We need to carefully differentiate between family hygiene practices that are, in fact, deleterious to health and those that are contrary to our own habits and customs but are not harmful.

Safety practices could also be included here, but were included in Chapter 9 as part of environmental data.

MEDICALLY BASED PREVENTIVE MEASURES

ANNUAL PHYSICAL EXAMINATION. Although the annual physical examination can detect early-stage disease in the absence of symptoms, there is considerable controversy as to whether such examinations are effective when performed for routine screening of asymptomatic persons. Moreover, there is little scientific evidence that healthy persons experience better outcomes as a result of head-to-toe physical examinations. The U.S. Preventive Services Task Force concluded that health care clinicians should invest most of their time during annual appointments in talking with clients about health behaviors and a healthy lifestyle rather than performing physical examination procedures and tests (Woolf & Lawrence, 1996).

On the other hand, a selective health promotion/disease prevention–oriented physical examination on a regular and periodic basis, and tailored to the client's age, race, and sex, is vital and serves several purposes. It provides the necessary information to jointly establish with the client a health maintenance plan. The preventive health assessment identifies risk factors particular to an individual; for example, an adult who smokes and whose father died of heart disease should be counseled about heart risk factors. The rationale is that a person with that health profile has twice the risk of incurring heart disease as an individual who does not smoke and has no family history of disease.

Major genetic risk factors are related to heredity, sex, race, and age. For instance, individuals whose families have had a history of heart disease at early ages or diabetes have an increased likelihood of inheriting a predisposition toward those diseases. Thanks to their hormones, premenopausal women are less likely to have myocardial infarctions than men of the same age group. African-Americans have more than twice the chance of developing hypertension than whites. And generally, the older one gets, the greater the chance of developing a chronic illness.

This does not imply, however, that the above risk factors are inevitable harbingers of future events. In fact, susceptibility to certain diseases can actually be reduced if an attempt is made to attenuate risk factors by improving one's lifestyle and seeking routine, preventive health care.

What should be included in the annual health assessment of the well adult? Standards have been established for both general pediatric and adult populations. Figure 16–4 provides a sample of the age chart for periodic health examinations of the general adult population. A wide range of charts are available from the American Academy of Family Physicians (*www.aap.org*).

What are the family's feelings about having a "physical" when they are well? Past practices of the family may be a gauge to their feelings; nevertheless, a lack of periodic well-care may also be a function of inaccessibility to, ignorance about, and/or the costs of such services. In order to ascertain the reasons behind not receiving health examinations, more direct questions may be warranted.

VISION AND HEARING EXAMINATIONS. Health assessments should be supplemented by vision and hearing examinations. This is particularly important, because glaucoma and hearing loss can be detected and can usually be treated effectively or prevented. Children should have periodic vision and hearing examinations done as part of their well-baby and preschool care. During the school years, children are periodically given a Snellen test, a rough screen for common vision problems. Because hearing difficulties can lead to serious behavioral and learning problems in school, children should be routinely given an audiometric test during the early school years. Primary care practitioners should also complete rough screening for hearing during well-child care visits (Green, 1994).

Adults who wear glasses need an eye examination annually, unless visual changes are noted sooner. For others, every other year is adequate. The eye examination should include tonometry testing for detection of glaucoma, which is recommended on a yearly basis for all adults over 40 years of age. If families do not know of an eye specialist to call, it is helpful to review with the family the difference in training and focus of an optician, optometrist, and ophthalmologist. If, while eliciting a family medical history, the nurse finds a history of glaucoma in the family, he or she should stress an annual eye examination even more vigorously, as there is now overwhelming evidence of a higher incidence of glaucoma among siblings and offspring of patients with

the disease than among the rest of the population (Perkins, 1973).

Although asymptomatic adults may not need annual audiometric testing, if hearing difficulties are noted or an individual is at high risk, testing is indicated. Progressive hearing loss can occur from exposure to certain types of noise. If a client is exposed to a high level of noise at work or at home, the nurse should inquire into his or her use of ear protectors and past hearing examinations. Hearing loss can also occur with age, due to vascular insufficiency of the cochlea. Smokers have greater hearing loss than nonsmokers, as smoking reduces the blood supply by vasospasm induced by nicotine, by atherosclerotic narrowing of the vessels, and by formation of thrombi in the vessels (Diekelmann, 1977).

IMMUNIZATION STATUS. The most important and specific measure against preventive disease is that of immunization (Green, 1994). At least 75 to 80 percent of susceptible children must be immunized to effectively protect a community from preventable communicable diseases (Garner, 1978). Promotion of immunization services is a vital and integral part of family health care.

In 1985, through legislative regulation of immunization requirements for school attendance and provision of free immunizations for those who were in need, a 96 percent overall immunization level was achieved in the school-aged population (U.S. DHHS, 1985). Unfortunately, however, the level of immunized children has dropped. We must refocus our attention on immunizing preschool and infant populations, as the immunization levels in 1994 were reported to be as low as 58 percent (Wong, 1995).

For infants and children, the list of recommended immunizations has grown and continues to change as new vaccines are licensed and recommended (Table 16–4) (American Academy of Pediatrics, 2001). Smallpox vaccinations are no longer advised, as the risk of untoward reactions to the vaccine are now greater than the risk of contracting the disease. Flu vaccines and tuberculin skin tests are also recommended for certain age groups and under certain situations. (The condition and age of the person and the community incidence and exposure risk are important variables here.) Booster shots of diphtheria and tetanus are recommended for adults every 7

American Academy of Family Physicians

Family Practice | Clinical Info | CME | Practice Management
About the AAFP | Products & Services | Careers | Publications

ACADEMY my
Members: Log in to
customize this site
and create your own
web site!

AAFP Home   Search: [   ] GO   more options

Table 3 General Adult Population

Clinical preventive services for adults, based on the AAFP Summary of Policy Recommendations for Periodic Health Examinations

	18	25	30	35	40	45	50	55	60	65	70	75

SCREENINGS
- ➤ BLOOD PRESSURE — (SR) Periodically
- ➤ HEIGHT & WEIGHT — (R) Periodically
- ➤ LIPID DISORDERS (men) — (SR) Either a fasting lipid profile or a nonfasting total cholesterol and HDL cholesterol
- ➤ LIPID DISORDERS (women) — (SR) Either a fasting lipid profile or a nonfasting total cholesterol and HDL cholesterol
- ➤ COLORECTAL CANCER — (R) Order FOBT (annually), sigmoidoscopy, barium enema or colonoscopy
- ➤ VISION — (R) Perform Snellen acuity testing
- ➤ HEARING — (R) Question about hearing impairment

Women:
- ➤ BREAST CANCER — (SR) Mammography & clinical breast exam every 1-2 years
- ➤ CERVICAL CANCER — (SR) Pap smear at least every 3 years
- ➤ CHLAMYDIA — (SR) Age 25 or younger and sexually active

COUNSELING
- ➤ OBESITY — (R) Counsel to maintain caloric and nutrient balance
- ➤ CORONARY ARTERY DISEASE, HYPERTENSION, OBESITY, DIABETES — (R) Counsel to engage in regular physical activity as appropriate for age
- ➤ ACCIDENTAL INJURY — (R) As appropriate for age (child safety seats/seat belts/bicycle & motorcycle safety/smoke alarms/poison control center numbers/driving while intoxicated)
- ➤ AUTOMOBILE ACCIDENTS — (R) Counsel problem drinkers about dangers of driving while intoxicated
- ➤ STDs — (R) Counsel regarding risks of STDs and how to prevent them

Women:
- ➤ OSTEOPOROSIS — (R) Counsel to maintain adequate calcium intake from age 11 and older
- ➤ MOTHERS OF INFANTS — (SR) Breastfeed infants through at least 6 months of age
- ➤ WOMEN PLANNING TO BECOME PREGNANT [1] — (SR) Prescribe 0.4 - 0.8 mg/day folic acid supplementation (from at least 1 month prior to conception through the first trimester of pregnancy)
- ➤ WOMEN NOT PLANNING A PREGNANCY [2] — (R) Prescribe 0.4 mg/day folate supplementation
- ➤ BREAST CANCER — (R) Counsel regarding potential risks and benefits of mammography
- ➤ PERI-MENOPAUSAL WOMEN — (SR) Hormone replacement therapy counseling

Men:
- ➤ PROSTATE CANCER — (R) Discuss risks and uncertain benefits of screening

Tobacco Users:
- ➤ PARENTS WHO SMOKE — (SR) Discuss harmful effects of smoking on children's health
- ➤ TOBACCO USERS — (SR) Tobacco cessation counseling on a regular basis
- ➤ PATIENTS DESIRING TO QUIT — (SR) Discuss pharmacotherapy as an adjunct for smoking cessation
- ➤ RISK OF TOBACCO USE — (R)

(Right margin, vertical: UPPER AGE LIMITS SHOULD BE INDIVIDUALIZED FOR EACH PATIENT)

1 Women planning to become pregnant who have not had a previous pregnancy affected by a neural tube defect

2 Women not planning a pregnancy but of childbearing potential who have not previously had a baby with a neural tube defect

(SR) Strongly Recommend:
Good quality evidence exists which demonstrates substantial net benefit over harm; the intervention is perceived to be cost effective and acceptable to nearly all patients.

(R) Recommend:
Although evidence exists which demonstrates net benefit, either the benefit is only moderate in magnitude or the evidence supporting a substantial benefit is only fair. The intervention is perceived to be cost effective and acceptable to most patients.

(NR) No Recommendation Either For or Against:
Either good or fair evidence exists of at least a small net benefit. Cost-effectiveness may not be known or patients may be divided about acceptability of the intervention.

(RA) Recommend Against:
Good or fair evidence which demonstrates no net benefit over harm.

(I) Insufficient Evidence to Recommend Either For or Against:
No evidence of even fair quality exists or the existing evidence is conflicting.

Age Charts | Clinical and Research | AAFP Home | Search

Figure 16–4. Age chart for periodic health examination: General adult population. *(Source: American Academy of Family Physicians (2001). Age charts for periodic health examinations. Available at www.aafp.org/exam/table3.html.)*

TABLE 16—4

RECOMMENDED CHILDHOOD IMMUNIZATIONS

Hepatitis B

Diphtheria, tetanus, and pertussis

Haemophilus influenzae type B

Inactivated polio

Pneumococcal conjugate

Measles, mumps, and rubella

Varicella

Hepatitis A (in selected areas)

---

to 10 years, because both of these diseases are serious and are endemic in the United States today.

When completing an assessment of the immunization status of family members, the types of immunizations received, dates, and any adverse reactions to immunization should be recorded.

DENTAL HEALTH. Dental health practices are essential in maintaining good teeth throughout an individual's life span. The prevalence of dental ill health is widespread, especially among low-income families. Dental health care includes both preventive care and curative health practices. In order to maintain high-level dental health, a combination of personal habits or practices, as well as preventive care by a dentist and/or dental hygienist, should be carried out. The four basic elements for dental health maintenance are:

1. Regular preventive dental services, including dental examination, x-rays, cleaning, education, and, for children, topical fluoride treatments when indicated. The American Academy of Pediatrics (1995) recommends children have dental checkups, cleaning, and fluoride treatments twice a year.

2. Use of fluoridated water, or if unavailable, prescription for daily oral fluoride liquid or tablets for children.

3. Regular brushing and flossing of teeth after meals.

4. Reduced amounts of certain types of fermentable carbohydrates in the diet. All fermentable carbohydrates have the potential of contributing to the development of dental caries by supplying the raw materials necessary for bacteria in the mouth to produce tooth-decaying acid. Fermentable carbohydrates include sugars, such as found in fruits, honey, and sweets; and cooked starches such as found in bread and potatoes (Loe, 1988).

A survey conducted by the National Institute of Dental Research (NIDR) found that an estimated one half of the nation's school children aged 5 to 17 have no tooth decay at all. This represents a 36 percent reduction in caries from NIDR studies conducted at the beginning of the 1980s (Loe, 1988). According to dental experts factors that have contributed to the improvement in children's dental health include the widespread use of fluoride, the increased application of sealants, improvement in personal oral hygiene, the receipt of regular professional dental care, and the rise in awareness of the effects of eating habits on the teeth (Loe, 1988).

Fluoride, which can be found in the drinking water supply in some communities, or which is prescribed by dentists as an oral supplement, is recognized as the most effective agent available to protect teeth from decay. Less helpful but still effective are the various means of applying fluoride topically, including the application of fluoride solutions by many dentists, or the self-administration of fluoride rinses or gels by the patient (American Dental Association, 1988). With a combination of fluoride treatment and sealants, the incidence of dental caries can be reduced by 90 percent (American Academy of Pediatrics, 1995).

For adult Americans, periodontal disease continues to be a major dental problem and is the chief cause of tooth loss. Gum disease is thought to affect at least three out of four adults and may strike 95 percent of the population at some time (Kandzari & Howard, 1981; Loe, 1988). Gum disease can be slowed down or prevented by careful attention to brushing, flossing, and regular professional dental care.

The family nurse, in teaching families about dental health and hygiene, may wish to check the mouths of some of the children or adults for plaque buildup or bring some disclosing solution that they can use to detect plaque themselves. Dental health education should stress that teeth should be brushed at least twice a day after meals, and the sooner the better, to prevent sugars from remaining in the mouth. The object of brushing is to remove plaque and food particles from the teeth, which is done by effective friction of the toothbrush (a soft-bristled one) against the surface of the teeth. The importance of using dental floss once a day to supplement brushing should also be advised, because some surfaces of the teeth and teeth–gum junctions are inaccessible by brushing alone (American Academy of Pediatrics, 1995).

Families (both children and adults) need thorough demonstrations of an effective method for brushing teeth. Due to limited dexterity, children may need some help brushing their teeth until they are between ages 7 and 10. Newer methods of brushing teeth are much more effective than the older vertical (from gum line or down) method taught in the past. Regular, after-meal brushing and flossing teeth is considered essential in the prevention of dental caries, gum disease, and periodontal disease.

Treatment of dental problems has not been mentioned except in passing, but is also of vital importance. Although prevention has been stressed, early detection and treatment of dental and gum problems will certainly keep more serious problems from developing. Malposition problems—over- and underbites, causing unequal exertion of pressure on teeth—are targets for early detection in children. Orthodontia may be needed to correct these problems, which if untreated could later cause periodontal disease and speech problems, as well as result in cosmetic ill effects (American Academy of Pediatrics, 1995).

COMPLEMENTARY AND ALTERNATIVE THERAPIES

Over the past decade, there has been a growing interest in complementary and alternative therapies in managing health care promotion, prevention, and treatment practices. These practices range from use of supplemental vitamins and herbs to seeking the services of a chiropractor, acupuncturist, massage therapist, or folk practitioner (Table 16–5). While initially shunned by most medical practitioners, there is a growing acceptance and implementation of these therapies among health care providers and the gen-

TABLE 16–5

COMPLEMENTARY AND ALTERNATIVE MEDICINE THERAPIES

Acupuncture

Acupressure

Aromatherapy

Biofeedback

Folk remedies (e.g., cupping and moxibustion in Eastern religions)

Healing touch

Herbal supplements

Home remedies

Hypnotherapy

Lifestyle diets

Manipulation (chiropractic, osteopathy)

Massage

Meditation

Megavitamins

Nutritional supplements

Pastoral/spiritual counseling

Relaxation therapy

eral population (Boutin, Buchwald, Robinson, & Collier, 2000; Brolinson, Price, Ditmeyer, & Reis, 2001; Harvey-Walker, 1998). Older adults (aged 65 and older) appear less likely to seek alternatives to conventional medical doctors for their care (Foster, Phillips, Hamel, & Eisenberg, 2000; Wellman, Kelner, & Wigdor, 2001). Treatment of children with complementary therapies is more common and is frequently undertaken by parents without the knowledge or advice of their pediatrician (Ottolini et al., 2001). Many patients are selecting complementary and alternative medicine (CAM) therapies to adjunct their medically based therapies for diseases and conditions such as rheumatic disease, attention deficit disorder, asthma, Alzheimer's disease, cancer, sleep problems, and symptoms associated with menopause. Concerns among medical practitioners remain focused on the safety and efficacy of these treatments (Parascandola, 2000). For instance, older adults most commonly choose to use chiropractic and herbs, both of which may be problematic in the elderly, compounded by the fact that their medical practitioner may be unaware of these practices (Foster et al.). Additionally, medical practitioners place themselves at risk by using or prescribing therapies without appropriate preparation in their use and without a substantial research base to ensure the safe use of such practices.

The family health history must include direct and specific questions related to the use of complementary and alternative therapies. The family nurse should determine the specific practices being used by each family member, the frequency of these practices, and the individual's perception of their health benefits. Additionally, the nurse should explore with the family whether or not they have shared their use of these practices with their medical care provider. If this has not been done, the family should be highly encouraged to do so to ensure that the care modalities indeed remain "complementary" to each other. As with all health care practices, use of alternative therapies should not be discouraged if indeed the family is able to associate a perceived benefit from the program of care and the actions are not harmful to them.

🌿FAMILY HEALTH ASSESSMENT

HEALTH CARE FUNCTION

As discussed in this chapter, an assessment of the family's health care function includes aspects of health beliefs, health perceptions, and specific health practices. Table 16–6 summarizes the pertinent assessment questions that can be used to determine more about the family and their health practices.

FAMILY HEALTH HISTORY

This area is significant for several reasons. First, family histories will often identify familial risk factors. Second, the family's experience with certain diseases

might possibly have resulted in fears, myths, or misconceptions about these illnesses. Family nurses should be sensitive to these possibilities and may want to explore family members' beliefs in this area further. Third, through eliciting a family medical history, the family nurse will learn more about both families of orientation and the current family group and thus gain a better understanding of the family's past and present.

The family medical history includes an identification of past and present environmentally and genetically related diseases of the family of orientation—going back to maternal and paternal grandparents and including aunts and uncles and their children. Besides ascertaining the general health status of all these individuals, family-centered nurses should specifically inquire about the presence of the following diseases, because individuals often forget to mention important familial diseases:

1. Environmentally related diseases (to which family members might be or have been exposed).
   a. Psychosocial problems (e.g., depression, schizophrenia).
   b. Infectious diseases: typhoid fever, tuberculosis, sexually transmitted diseases, hepatitis, diarrheas (dysenteries), and skin diseases (scabies, lice, impetigo).
2. Genetically linked diseases: epilepsy, diabetes, cystic fibrosis, developmental disabilities, sickle cell anemia, kidney disease, hypertension, heart disease, cancer, leukemia, vision and hearing impairments, hemophilia, allergies, and asthma.

Including family history information on the family genogram (see Figure 8–1) is a useful way of recording this information. The family genogram should include the age of members, whether the individual is living or deceased, the cause of death, level of general health, and presence of acute or chronic disease/disability.

FAMILY HEALTH RECORDS

Families change health practitioners often and are seen at several agencies or by different specialists for

TABLE 16–6

HEALTH CARE FUNCTION

ASSESSMENT QUESTIONS

1. **Family's health beliefs, values, and behaviors**
   - ✓ What value does the family assign to health? Health promotion? Prevention?
   - ✓ Is there consistency between family health values as stated and their health actions?
   - ✓ What health-promoting activities does the family engage in regularly? Are these behaviors characteristic of all family members, or are patterns of health-promoting behavior highly variable among family members?
   - ✓ What are the family's health goals?

2. **Family's definition of health–illness and its level of knowledge**
   - ✓ How does the family define health and illness for each family member? What clues provide this impression, and who decides?
   - ✓ Can the family observe and report significant symptoms and changes?
   - ✓ What are the family members' source of health information and advice?
   - ✓ How is health information and advice transmitted to family members?

3. **Family's perceived health status and illness susceptibility**
   - ✓ How does the family assess its present health status?
   - ✓ What present health problems are identified by the family?
   - ✓ To what serious health problems do family members perceive themselves vulnerable?
   - ✓ What are the family's perceptions of how much control over health they have by taking appropriate health actions?

4. **Family dietary practices**
   - ✓ Does the family know food sources from the Food Guide Pyramid?
   - ✓ Is the family diet adequate? (A three-day food history record of family eating patterns is recommended.)
   - ✓ Who is responsible for the planning, shopping, and preparation of meals?
   - ✓ How are the foods prepared?
   - ✓ How many meals are consumed per day?
   - ✓ Are there budgeting limitations? Food stamps usage?
   - ✓ What is the adequacy of storage and refrigeration?
   - ✓ Does mealtime serve a particular function for the family?
   - ✓ What is the family's attitude toward food and mealtimes?
   - ✓ What are the family's snack habits?

5. **Sleep and rest habits**
   - ✓ What are the usual sleeping habits of family members?
   - ✓ Are family members meeting sleep requirements that are appropriate for their age and health status?
   - ✓ Are regular hours established for sleeping?

TABLE 16–6 (CONTINUED)

ASSESSMENT QUESTIONS

- ✓ Do family members take regular naps or have other means of resting during the day?
- ✓ Who decides when children go to sleep?
- ✓ Where do family members sleep?

6. Physical activity and recreation

- ✓ Are family members aware that active recreation and regular aerobic exercise are necessary for good health?
- ✓ Do usual daily work activities allow for physical activity?
- ✓ What types of family recreational pursuits and physical activities (i.e., jogging, bicycling, swimming, dancing, tennis) are family members engaged in? How often? Who participates?
- ✓ Do common daily activities performed by family members require a moderate level of energy expenditure? Do family members spend at least 30 minutes nearly every day participating in moderate or heavier physical activity?
- ✓ What are the recreational/leisure-time activities of the family subsystems (spouse subsystem, parent–child subsystems, and sibling subsystems)? How often do these activities occur? Who participates in them?
- ✓ What are the family's beliefs about the relationship of physical activity to health?
- ✓ Exploring the family members' feelings about the family's leisure-time/recreational activities (satisfaction with time spent and types of activities).

7. Family therapeutic and recreational drug, alcohol, and tobacco practices

- ✓ What is the family's use of alcohol, tobacco, coffee, cola, or tea? (Caffeine and theobromine are stimulants.)
- ✓ Do family members take drugs for recreational purposes?
- ✓ How long has (have) family member(s) been using alcohol or other recreational drugs?
- ✓ Is the use of tobacco, alcohol, or prescribed/illicit drugs by family members perceived as a problem?
- ✓ Does the use of alcohol or other drugs interfere with the capacity to carry out usual activities?
- ✓ Do family members regularly use over-the-counter or prescription drugs?
- ✓ Does the family save drugs over a long period of time and reuse?
- ✓ Are drugs properly labeled and in a safe place away from young children?

8. Family's role in self-care practices

- ✓ What does the family do to improve its health status?
- ✓ What does the family do to prevent illness/disease?
- ✓ Who is (are) the health leader(s) in the family?
- ✓ Who makes the health decisions in the family?
- ✓ What does the family do to care for health problems and illnesses in the home?
- ✓ How competent is the family in self-care relative to recognition of signs and symptoms, diagnosis, and home treatment of common, simple health problems?
- ✓ What are the family's values, attitudes, and beliefs regarding home care?

(continued)

TABLE 16–6 (CONTINUED)

HEALTH CARE FUNCTION

ASSESSMENT QUESTIONS

9. **Environmental and hygiene practices**

These questions are already covered under family environmental data.

10. **Medically based preventive measures**

   ✓ What are the family's history and feelings about having physicals when well?

   ✓ When were the last eye and hearing examinations?

   ✓ What is the immunization status of family members?

   ✓ Do family members use fluoridated water, or is a daily fluoride supplement prescribed for the children?

   ✓ What are the family's oral hygiene habits in regard to brushing and flossing after meals?

   ✓ What are the family's patterns of simple sugar and starch intake?

   ✓ Do family members receive regular preventive professional dental care including education, periodic x-rays, cleaning, repair, and, for children, topical or oral fluoride?

11. **Complementary and alternative therapies**

   ✓ What alternative health care practices do family members use?

   ✓ How often do they participate in these practices and for what reasons do they initiate these practices?

   ✓ How does the family member feel these practices will benefit his or her health?

   ✓ Have these practices been undertaken in coordination with other medically based services?

12. **Family health history**

   ✓ What is the overall health of family members of origin and marriage (grandparents, parents, aunts, uncles, siblings, and offspring) over three generations?

   ✓ Is there in the past or present a history of genetic or familial diseases—diabetes, heart disease, high blood pressure, stroke, cancer, gout, kidney disease, thyroid disease, asthma and other allergic states, blood diseases, or any other familial diseases.

   ✓ Is there a family history of emotional problems or suicide? Are there any present or past environmentally related family diseases?

13. **Health care services received**

   ✓ From what health care practitioner(s) and/or health care agency(ies) do the family members receive care?

   ✓ Does this provider(s) or agency(ies) see all members of the family and take care of all their health needs?

14. **Feelings and perceptions regarding health services**

   ✓ What are the family's feelings about the kinds of health services available to it in the community?

   ✓ What are the family's feelings and perceptions regarding the health services it receives?

   ✓ Is the family comfortable, satisfied, and confident with the care received from its health care providers?

   ✓ Does the family have any past experience with family health nursing services?

   ✓ What are the family's attitudes and expectations of the role of the nurse?

TABLE 16–6 (CONTINUED)

ASSESSMENT QUESTIONS

15. **Emergency health services**

   ✓ Does the agency or physician the family receives care from have an emergency service?

   ✓ Are medical services by current health care providers available if an emergency occurs?

   ✓ If emergency services are not available, does the family know where the closest available (according to their eligibility) emergency services are for both the children and adults in the family?

   ✓ Does the family know how to call for an ambulance and for paramedic services?

   ✓ Does the family have an emergency health plan?

16. **Source of payment**

   ✓ How does the family pay for services it receives?

   ✓ Does the family have a private health insurance plan, Medicare, or Medicaid, or must the family pay for services fully or partially?

   ✓ Does the family receive any free services (or know about those for which it is eligible)?

   ✓ What effect does the cost of health care have on the family's utilization of health services?

   ✓ If the family has health insurance (private, Medicare, and/or Medicaid), is the family informed about what services are covered, such as preventive services, special medical equipment, home visits, and so forth?

17. **Logistics of receiving care**

   ✓ How far away are health care facilities from the family's home?

   ✓ What modes of transportation does the family use to get to them?

   ✓ If the family must depend on public transportation, what problems exist in regard to hours of service and travel time to health care facilities?

different health problems. With passing years, memories fade as to what happened when, underscoring the need for families to keep records of the year-by-year medical events of each family member.

Educating families about the importance of maintaining family medical records is a way to assist families to become responsible for their health care. The data the family maintains will aid new practitioners and may also obviate the need for redundant, expensive, and time-consuming laboratory and diagnostic tests. Moreover, the information in the family medical record may result in faster and more accurate diagnoses.

When family members have multiple health alterations and are seeing more than one practitioner concurrently, it is especially critical to have medical record information. It is very important to maintain immunization records for children; for adults, diagnostic and laboratory tests, diagnoses, medications taken, and any adverse reactions to them should be carefully recorded.

The following broad areas of health information need to be included in the family health history:

- Maternity record

- Children's heights and weights

- Adults' weight records
- Childhood diseases
- Diseases or conditions afflicting members of older generations
- Accident records
- Major surgeries, illnesses, and hospitalizations
- Immunization records
- Allergies
- Corrective devices (e.g., glasses, hearing aids, dental plates, special shoes)
- Blood groups and Rh factors
- Blood pressure; other laboratory tests performed

🐝 FAMILY NURSING DIAGNOSES

There are many family nursing diagnoses related to the family health care function. Certainly, family nursing diagnoses that lead to health-promotional or educational strategies are appropriate, because knowledge deficits of family members are commonly observed. These knowledge deficits about health care are common. Knowledge deficits are seen in the various areas discussed in this chapter, such as dietary practices, rest and sleep patterns, physical activity and recreational practices, drug and alcohol use, lifestyle practices, and use of health care services. The North American Nursing Diagnosis Association (Carpenito, 2000; McFarland & McFarlane, 1997; North American Nursing Diagnosis Association [NANDA], 2001) individual and family nursing diagnoses that are behaviorally oriented and deal with the family health care function include:

- Altered Health Maintenance
- Caregiver Role Strain
- Deficient Knowledge (specify)
- Health-Seeking Behaviors (specify)
- Ineffective Health Maintenance
- Ineffective Therapeutic Regimen Management

- Ineffective Family Therapeutic Regimen Management
- Noncompliance (specify)
- Risk for Caregiver Role Strain
- Self-Care Deficits

Nursing diagnoses related to family health promotion may be subsumed under health-seeking behaviors. Carpenito (2000) explains that health-seeking behaviors in the family context pertains to a state in which a family or family members who are in stable health actively seek ways to alter personal health habits and/or the environment in order to move toward a higher level of wellness.

The family nursing diagnosis of "Altered Health Maintenance" identifies health care practice areas where the family or family members demonstrate actual or potential inadequate health practices. Carpenito (2000) extended this diagnosis to the family and said that the diagnosis pertains to a state in which a family or family members are at risk of experiencing a disruption in health because of an unhealthy lifestyle or lack of knowledge to manage a condition. Specific examples of problems under this broad diagnosis are ineffective or inadequate dental care practices, dietary practices, preventive health care practices, and family planning.

Family nurses are challenged to assist the family unit in identifying areas of health risk, in establishing relevant health goals, and in planning for lifestyle changes that will continue as an ongoing family commitment. For health-promotion planning to be effective, it must be compatible with the family's cultural beliefs and practices. Awareness of the family's cultural interpretation of health, illness, and health care is essential prior to embarking on specific goal-oriented interventions. In addition, family goals should be recorded and then prioritized by the nurse and family together. Major sources of stress, along with any recent or current family developmental or situational transitions, also require consideration prior to intervention. Collaboration of the entire family in expressing concerns, setting health goals, and planning for lifestyle modifications should increase the effectiveness of the nursing interventions.

FAMILY NURSING INTERVENTIONS: GUIDELINES FOR LIFESTYLE MODIFICATIONS

An important role for the family nurse is working with families to plan lifestyle modifications so that health goals can be met. Pender and associates (2001) describe useful approaches that may be considered in initiating and supporting family behavior alterations. Specific strategies that nurses may apply in initiating family lifestyle changes include self-confrontation, cognitive reframing, modeling, operant conditioning, and stimulus control.

SELF-CONFRONTATION

The first technique, self-confrontation, is based on the assumption that clients make changes when they recognize incompatibilities within their own beliefs, values, and behaviors, or between their own behaviors and those of individuals they hold in esteem and wish to emulate. Once this comparison occurs and contradiction is experienced, the client is more likely to change values, attitudes, and behaviors to achieve greater consistency with the self-concept. The nurse, in reviewing family lifestyle, can provide feedback to families by suggesting areas of inconsistencies between family beliefs or values and current behavior patterns. Contradictions that are of most concern to the family should be the focus for intervention. An example of using this strategy can be found in a family that highly values good nutrition as an essential ingredient in maintaining health and believes its diet is well balanced. Yet family members admit to regularly consuming "fast foods" for lunch during the week. A family that is confronted with this inconsistency between its beliefs and actual dietary patterns hopefully will be more motivated to change its behavior.

COGNITIVE REFRAMING

Cognitive reframing consists of assisting families to understand and resolve past issues by helping them to view the situation from a different perspective. The nurse utilizing this approach should counsel family members on recognizing the irrationality or the constraining nature of certain beliefs and helping them to view the issue from a new, different facilitative perspective (Wright, Watson, & Bell, 1997). An example of this would be where all of a family's members are overweight and firmly convinced that "none of us will ever be thin; we have always been heavy." Cognitive reframing as an intervention promotes the acquisition of rational positive self-statements and contributes to clients feeling an increased sense of personal control that is present oriented, rather than based on past beliefs.

MODELING

Modeling is a common strategy used in behavior therapy. It is based on the premise that some learning will occur through observation of role models, beginning with early childhood and continuing through to adulthood (Bandura, 1977). Modeling is especially helpful when clients are uncertain as to what behavior is necessary in order to achieve a specific goal. Clients should identify with their role models in order for this technique to be effective, with family members and nurse working together to select suitable models. The family nurse is in a position to positively influence family health behaviors by being a role model of healthful living. He or she does this by demonstrating skills that the family seeks to learn, by providing needed health education, and by expressing encouragement to promote desired family behavior. Modeling may also be used in community organized health promotion classes, and in self-help groups such as Weight Watchers or Alcoholics Anonymous. Self-help groups function by offering a setting for role modeling and mutual support (Roth, 1996b).

OPERANT CONDITIONING

Operant conditioning, based on the principle that behavior is determined by its consequences, can be an effective behavior modification strategy. Desirable behavior is reinforced to increase the probability that the behavioral will be repeated. Positive reinforcers, or rewards, are more effective motivators of behavioral change than negative reinforcers or punishments. Nurses applying this intervention strategy should work with families to choose behavior to be changed. Schedules should be developed of how to gradually move toward selected targeted health-generating behavior, and reinforcement contingencies should be set up. In order to attain family goals, a nurse–family contract with planned rewards for desired behavior and incremental successes may be implemented in order to promote responsibility for all family members. Contracting can be enjoyable for the entire family, with family members serving as an important source of motivation for each other. Pender and associates (2001) suggest that operant conditioning works best if the behavior to be reinforced is countable, so that reinforcement may be used correctly.

STIMULUS CONTROL

In stimulus control, attention is directed toward changing the antecedents rather than the consequences of behavior as addressed in operant conditioning (Pender et al., 2001). This method of behavior control suggests that by changing events that precede undesirable behavior, it is possible to decrease or eliminate such action and increase successful behavior. Stimulus control concentrates on arranging environmental cues to promote only the desired behavior. The original Health Belief Model and Pender's Health Promotion Model agree that cues are important factors in promoting health behavioral change. Nurses should work with families to accomplish stimulus control by accurately identifying under what conditions desirable behavior occurs more frequently, and under what circumstances undesirable behavior is prompted. Nurses should offer instruction on how to develop sensitivity to appropriate cues and counsel families on ways to facilitate opportunities for encountering those that are appropriate. Behavioral cues may be taken from a variety of sources. Examples of possible sources include contact with health care professionals, significant others, and the communication media, or visual stimuli from the environment such as viewing others participating in the target activity. In addition to environmental cues, nurses can further influence desired action by encouraging families to develop a positive set of internal cues such as "feeling good," or an increased sense of self-esteem. External cues, such as having a family member or friend invite you to an aerobic exercise class, can be combined with internal cues, such as remembering feeling more energetic after exercise sessions. Multiple cues potentiate each other.

✺ SUMMARY

- Conceptualizations of health and illness vary widely from culture to culture, region to region, and family to family.

- A family, neighborhood, community, or society must label a condition or certain behaviors as an illness or disability before that illness or health condition can be considered a health problem to that group.

- Three times as many men as women do not see their physician on an annual basis. A quarter of men surveyed said they would wait "as long as possible" before seeking health care. The barriers to health care seeking activity by men are primarily psychological.

- The three basic orientations to wellness and illness are: (1) a subjective feeling of well-being or ill health (the feeling-state orientation), (2) an absence or presence of general or specific symptoms (symptom orientation), and (3) a state of being able or unable to perform usual activities (a performance orientation).

- The anthropologist Kleinman makes a distinction between disease and illness. Disease is the health care professionals' biomedical understanding of the health problem, while illness is the patient's personal and unique understanding and definition of what is happening to him or her. The authors state that cultural factors determine the importance of the various domains of influence.

- The Health Belief Model posits that: in order for an individual to take preventive action to avoid disease, he or she would need to believe that he or she was personally susceptible or vulnerable to the disease; the illness was at least moderately severe, so that the consequences of acquiring the disease would significantly disrupt the person's life; taking a particular action would be beneficial in that it would reduce susceptibility to or severity of the disease and the benefits are outweighed by the barriers, such as costs, pain, time, inconvenience, and embarrassment.

- The revised Health Promotion Model emphasizes the importance of behavior-specific cognitions and affect as the primary motivators of behavior. These variables could be especially significant for nurses to consider, as they are subject to modification through nursing interventions. The six behavior-specific cognitions and affect considered to be of major motivational significance in encouraging an individual to engage in health-promoting behaviors have been identified within the model as: perceived benefits of action, perceived barriers to action, perceived self-efficacy, activity-related affect, interpersonal influences, and situational influences.

- Pratt suggested that the reasons why families are having difficulty providing health care for their members lies with both (1) the structure of the health care system and (2) the family structure.

- Major factors explaining differences in utilization patterns of medical services include the lack of health care insurance coverage, lack of services for special populations (i.e., teenage males), the perception by families of the health care system and the health care provider, and the lack of partnership between the health care provider and the family in mutually addressing health care issues.

- Assessment of dietary practices should include the amount and types of food the family eats, the social behaviors associated with dietary practices, and the meal planning, shopping, and preparation practices of the family.

- Sleep and rest patterns are assessed to determine if individual members are getting the required number of hours of rest and if not, what factors may impact the ability to sleep.

- Individuals are recommended to participate in 30 minutes a day or more of moderate physical activity on most, preferably all, days of the week. This activity can and should include recreational activities shared with other family members.

- When assessing drug, alcohol, and tobacco practices among family members, a thorough investigation of prescribed, over-the-counter, and illegal substance use practices should be made.

- For a family to be responsible for its own self-care, it needs to have an understanding of its own health status and/or health problems and the steps needed to improve or maintain its health. Self-care practices involve not only preventive practices, diagnosis, and home treatment of common and minor ambulatory health problems, but also all the procedures and treatments prescribed for the care of illness of a family member, such as giving medications, using special appliances, changing dressings, and carrying out special exercises and diets.

- The family's hygiene and cleanliness practices should include good handwashing, good personal hygiene, and discouraging the sharing of food and utensils.

- Medically based preventive measures employed by the family include completing an annual physical examination, seeking vision and hearing screening, seeking regular dental care, and ensuring that all family members are immunized.

- The use of complementary and alternative therapies to address health issues is expanding. The health care provider must thoroughly assess for these practices and, where appropriate, introduce, encourage, or discourage their ongoing use.

- The family medical history includes an identification of past and present environmentally and genetically related diseases of the family of orientation—going back to maternal and paternal grandparents and including aunts and uncles and their children.

- Types of family nursing diagnoses that are often found in the area of the family's health care function include those that lead to health-promotional or educational strategies, because knowledge deficits of family members are commonly observed.

- Nurses and other health care professionals can assist families to attain a healthier lifestyle by modeling such behaviors themselves.

- Specific lifestyle modification strategies have been suggested as possible nursing interventions to support families to increase their health-promoting activities and attain their family health goals.

- Specific strategies that nurses may apply in initiating family lifestyle changes include self-confrontation, cognitive restructuring, modeling, operant conditioning, and stimulus control.

❧ FAMILY VIGNETTE: THE DIAZ FAMILY

The Diaz family immigrated to the United States from Guatemala 10 years ago. The family is composed of Mr. and Mrs. Diaz, both aged 53, and three children ranging in ages from 15 to 25. Mrs. Diaz has been brought to a free clinic by her husband because of complaints of chronic diarrhea that include severe cramping. Mrs. Diaz has curtailed her activities due to her fear of having a bowel "accident." She primarily stays within her home watching television and cooking for the family. Their daughter is getting married in one month, and their eldest son, a U.S. Marine, has recently been deployed to a confidential location in the Middle East. When introduced to Mr. and Mrs. Diaz the family nurse notes that they are both obese. The daughter, who has driven them to the clinic, is also overweight for her age and height.

■ STUDY QUESTIONS

Review the Family Vignette and answer the related questions.

1. Identify specific areas of health care function that you would want to assess.

2. State the potential lifestyle issues that may contribute to Mrs. Diaz's current health problem.

3. Select a nursing diagnosis that focuses on the need for lifestyle change by the Diaz family.

4. List health care practices you would encourage the Diaz family to employ at this time.

Answer the following questions.

5. Which of the following are major ways that the family carries out its health care functions? (Select all appropriate answers.)

   a. Family provides preventive health care to its members at home.
   b. Family provides the major share of sick care to its members.
   c. Family pays for most health services received (directly or indirectly).
   d. Family has prime responsibility for initiating and coordinating health services.
   e. Family decides when and where to hospitalize its members.

6. List three primary factors that influence a family's conceptualizations of health and illness and whether they seek health care services.

7. Name the three basic orientations used to define health and illness (according to Baumann). Keeping in mind the two groups studied, correlate those two groups with their health orientation.

8. Describe what Koos's central research findings were.

9. Recall in The Health Promotion Model the behavior-specific cognition and affect variables suggested as influencing the likelihood of engaging in health-promoting behaviors. What other modifying factors are thought to contribute in activating health-promotion behaviors?

10. Pratt found that most American families were not adequately performing their vital health care function. On what basis did she draw this conclusion? What are three basic reasons for this inadequacy?

11. Kleinman's Explanatory Model of Health and Illness is significant because (select best answer):

   a. It explains what kind of health beliefs a family is likely to have
   b. It brings out the importance of culture in forming health explanations
   c. It discusses the important role that popular and folk domains of influence have

12. List four assessment areas to cover when appraising a family's dietary practices.

13. The following is a list of several areas that should be assessed under family's sleep and rest practices: number of hours usually slept each night by family members, who takes regular naps during day or what other rest techniques family members use, and where family members sleep. What important area(s) has (have) been omitted?

14. Formulate three basic questions to ask a family in relation to its physical activity practices.

15. Which of the following substances constitute drugs that need to be assessed by the family completing a family health assessment? (Select all appropriate answers.)

   a. Coffee, tea, cola, and cocoa (caffeine intake)
   b. Alcohol use
   c. Over-the-counter medicines
   d. Tobacco use
   e. Recreational drugs such as marijuana and cocaine

16. List five examples of complementary or alternative care practices.

17. An appraisal of self-care practices involves an assessment of:

   a. Preventive and diagnostic practices
   b. Home treatment practices, including home care of family members who are sick or disabled
   c. Determination of the family's ability to provide self-care
   d. (Fill in) _____

18. Which of the following family nursing intervention strategies would be appropriate in assisting a family with school-aged children to change the children's dental health practices in the area of brushing and flossing teeth? (Select all correct answers.)

    a. Cognitive restructuring
    b. Modeling
    c. Operant conditioning
    d. Stimulus control
    e. Self-confrontation

19. Safety was a major area covered under environmental practices. Identify two general areas of health advice related to family safety.

20. Name four salient general health education areas for families to learn about concerning dental health.

21. Which of the following measures are generally recommended for plaque control? (Select all appropriate answers.)

    a. After-meal toothbrushing
    b. Reduction in dietary sucrose
    c. Daily flossing of teeth
    d. Use of an antiseptic mouthwash twice a day

22. A family medical history consists basically of two parts. First, information would be elicited about each family member (going back to maternal and paternal grandparents and aunts and uncles) and his or her present and past health status. What would be the second area of assessment?

FAMILY STRESS, COPING, AND ADAPTATION

LEARNING OBJECTIVES

1. Describe the importance of family coping strategies and processes.
2. Present evidence of changes in family life that indicate how well families are coping.
3. Define and differentiate the meanings of these terms and concepts: stressor, stress, crisis, individual coping, family coping, and adaptation.

4. Explain what coping tasks are appropriate for each of the three time phases of stress.
5. Identify three major variables involved in the development of crisis or successful resolution of the problem (noncrisis), according to Hill's family stress theory.
6. Discuss the way in which the Resiliency Model is an extension of Hill's family stress theory.

7. Explain the purpose of the Family Inventory of Life Events scale and what life events are most stressful to families.

8. Briefly describe four functional coping strategies used by families and four dysfunctional adaptive strategies used by families.

9. Differentiate whether specific coping strategies are functional, dysfunctional, or both (could be either healthy or unhealthy).

10. Describe two nursing interventions designed to maintain or promote family social support.

11. Give an example of how family coping differs according to gender, culture, and the health status of the family.

12. Utilizing a family case example:
    a. Assess the family in terms of family stressors, strengths, perceptions, coping strategies, and adaptation.
    b. Identify one family nursing diagnosis in the area of family coping.
    c. Propose two family nursing interventions appropriate for resolving or ameliorating the problem.

Families constantly face the need to modify their perceptions and lives. The stimulus for this change comes from within and without. The normal, continually evolving developmental needs of all the family members, in addition to the presence of unexpected situations involving family members, make up the inner demands for change. The external stimuli for change come from the changing society as it interacts with the family during the family's life cycle. In this regard, "We live in turbulent times, on the edge of uncertainty" (Walsh 1998, p. 3).

This chapter begins by discussing the importance of family coping and how well families are adapting to the continual challenges they face. Basic concepts related to family stress and coping literature are briefly defined and later elaborated upon. Two family stress theories are explained and the concepts within these theories defined. The process of family coping, as well as the various internal and external family coping strategies, are detailed. Finally, dysfunctional family adaptive strategies are presented as well as guidelines for family nursing assessment, diagnosis, and intervention.

❧HOW WELL FAMILIES ARE COPING

Continual demands force the family to adapt in order for it to survive, continue, and grow. Family coping processes and strategies are essential for making this possible. A family's perceptions and handling of its problems through use of various resources and coping strategies are crucial to the family's success in dealing with the demands placed on it.

Most important, moreover, family coping processes and strategies serve as vital processes or mechanisms through which the family functions are made possible. Without effective family coping, the affective, socialization, economic, and health care functions cannot be adequately achieved. Hence family coping processes and strategies constitute the underlying processes that enable the family to enact its necessary family functions.

Assessing family resources, coping strategies, and processes provides the foundation for assisting families in their adaptation and in their attainment of a higher level of wellness. Achieving a higher level of wellness is the goal or the raison d'être of family nursing practice. Strengthening and encouraging adequate adaptive responses and capacities, as well as reducing the actual and potential stressors from within and outside the family, are part of this broad and encompassing goal. Whether the family is essentially healthy or dysfunctional or somewhere in between (in their location on the health–illness continuum), the family health nurse is still dealing with the same issue: assisting families to help themselves achieve a higher level of functioning or wellness within the context of their particular aims, aspirations, and abilities.

Families in the United States have great strengths but face considerable challenges today (see Chapter 1). One of the main strengths of U.S. families is their **durability** (Fine, 1992). Despite all the technological changes that have occurred in society, families are still the basic institution where individuals are socialized and nurtured. Other strengths of American families are their ethnic and structural diversity (i.e., the array of family forms such as nuclear, intergenerational, single-parent, stepparent, cohabiting, and gay and lesbian). Non-nuclear family structures have reached a greater level of acceptance today than before, although many of these families and their members still face discrimination in school, workplace, and community settings. U.S. families also can be characterized by their **resilience** (Fine, 1992; Walsh, 1998). Despite all the economic, social, and political pressures, most families can be considered to be functioning quite satisfactorily. The majority of adults in the United States are employed, are in relatively good health, have meaningful social relationships, and have at least a high school education (Fine).

The continual challenges families are confronted with typically are associated with changes in American family life. Structural and situational changes in American family life—increased cohabiting, more single-parent and stepfamilies, higher divorce rates—as well as downsizing of both small businesses and major corporations (resulting in decreased employment opportunities, need for dual earners for financial survival), and a growing elderly population—all create both new opportunities for growth and increased stress and demands for coping to fulfill family functions (Leeds, 1996).

Families cope with and adapt to stressful life situations on a daily basis. In addition, over the life course, families also need to cope with situational (unexpected) stressors such as acute or chronic illness in child, adult, or elderly members; abusive behavior; alcohol or drug abuse; adolescent pregnancy; and/or accidental death or injury. Today there is a growing realization that these unexpected acute and chronic health problems produce "family diseases" (Foreman, 2001).

From early research and theoretical efforts the picture of how well families were adapting to stress and change was that the family was merely a reactor to stress, a "defensive" manager of resources, with much tendency towards dysfunction. Fortunately, this trend is changing. Many subsequent investigations have shifted away from the dysfunctional emphasis to a more positive and broadened interest in the wide array of resources and coping strategies families utilize. Thus, the healing resilient properties of families and their ability to "bounce back" and grow after adversity has received greater emphasis. With this focus, families tend to be seen as resilient social change agents, innovative and surprisingly effective under stressful conditions (Burr, Day, & Bahr, 1993;

Burr et al., 1994; McCubbin & McCubbin, 1993; Walsh, 1998).

BASIC STRESS AND COPING CONCEPTS

The following concepts are foundational to the literature on family stress, coping, and adaptation.

Stress is the response or state of tension produced by the stressor(s) or by the actual/perceived demand(s) that remains unmanaged (Antonovsky, 1979; Burr, 1973). It is the tension or strain within a person or social system (e.g., family) and is a reaction to a pressure-producing situation (Burgess, 1978). Because stress or tension in a family is so difficult to measure, researchers and practitioners alike often assess stressors.

Stressors refer to the initiating or the precipitating agents that activate the stress process (Burr et al., 1993; Chrisman & Fowler, 1980). The precipitating agents that activate stress in the family are life events or occurrences of sufficient magnitude to bring about change in the family system (Hill, 1949). Family stressors can be interpersonal (inside or outside of the family), environmental, economic, or sociocultural events or experiences.

Those stressors that occur "off-time" or out of sync with chronological or social expectations, such as early widowhood, are much more difficult for families (Walsh, 1998). Moreover, stressors that are perceived as losses and are ambiguous (unclear) have greater negative effects on families; diminished family morale and greater family conflict are mentioned in this regard. Ambiguous losses include physical absence of family member—"leaving without saying goodbye," unexpected catastrophic loss created by war, natural disaster, relocation, imprisonment, desertion, bioterrorism, or health problems (dementia, chronic mental illness, addictions), affairs, adoption, and divorce (Boss, 1999).

The accumulation (pile-up) and magnitude of stressors in a family's life gives an estimate of the amount of stress the family is experiencing (Olson et al., 1983). McCubbin and Patterson (1983a). The concept of pile-up of family life stressors is defined as the sum of developmental (expected) and situational (unexpected) events as well as intrafamily strains (tensions in relationships among family members).

Family member/family perceptions refer to the interpretations family members singularly or collectively make of their experiences. Perceptions color the nature and gravity of possible family stressors, because families react not only to the presence of actual stressors, but also to events as they perceive or interpret them. A family's perceptions are of paramount importance. It is significant to note that families that are crisis prone consistently tend to perceive events in a distorted, subjective manner. Events that healthy families would look at objectively and/or positively as a challenge are viewed by crisis-prone families as threatening and overwhelming. In these cases extensive stress is experienced, which in turn taxes family adaptive capacities.

Coping consists of problem-solving efforts by an individual faced with demands highly relevant to his or her welfare, but taxing the person's resources (Lazarus, Averill, & Opton, 1974). Pearlin and Schooler (1978) add the notion of presumed effectiveness of coping responses when they define coping as any response (behavioral or perceptual–cognitive) to external life strains that serves to prevent, avoid, or control emotional distress. Simply stated, coping efforts or behaviors are positive or negative, problem-specific, active strategies geared toward addressing a problem. Coping is a term that is limited to actual behaviors or cognitions people employ, not to resources they potentially could use.

Family coping denotes a family group level of analysis (or an interactional level of analysis). Family coping is defined as an active process where the family utilizes existing family resources and develops new behaviors and resources that will strengthen the family unit and reduce the impact of stressful life events (McCubbin, 1979). By shifting from the individual level to a family level of coping, coping becomes much more complex. Because of the difficulty in assessing family coping efforts, most family coping studies describe a combination of individual and family coping responses made by family members and the family. Family coping responses or behaviors are the specific actions or cognitions that family members employ when adapting to stress (McCubbin, McCubbin, Nevin, & Cauble, 1981), while coping patterns and strategies are similar responses that cluster into homogeneous sets. Family and individual coping strategies develop and change over time, in response to the demands or stressors being experienced (Menaghan, 1983).

A **family crisis** has been defined as a continuous condition of disruptiveness, disorganization, or incapacitation in the family system (Burr, 1973; McCubbin & McCubbin, 1993). A crisis results when a family's current resources and adaptive strategies are not effective in handling the stressor(s) (see Figure 17–1). Hence, a family crisis refers to a disruptive state or period in a family's life when an extremely stressful event or series of events significantly taxes the family's resources and coping abilities, with no resolution of the problem in sight. The family's usually effective problem-solving skills become useless or diminished during this psychosocial emergency (Kus, 1992).

There are two types of situations that can put families into a crisis: developmental and situational events. Developmental or maturational events are those stemming from a family's experience in the process of the psychosocial growth of members (e.g., becoming a parent; child maturing as adolescent; retirement). They are inherent within the stages of the normal life cycle of both the family and its members. Situational events are not common or normally expected, such as the death of a child or serious illness of one of the family members. Depending on a family's resources, coping abilities, and perceptions of these events, developmental and situational events can become crises for the family. In contrast to this negative view of family crisis, crisis has also been seen as a "wake-up" call, heightening family members' attention to what really matters in life (Walsh, 1998).

Adaptation is a process of managing the demands of the stressors through the use of resources, coping, and problem-solving strategies. The outcome is an altered state of functioning that may be positive or

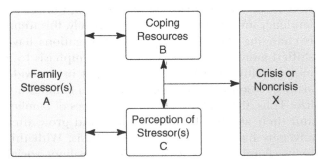

Figure 17–1. Hill's Family Stress Theory (1949). *(Adapted from McCubbin & Patterson, 1983b.)*

negative, resulting in the increase or decrease of a family's state of wellness (Burgess, 1978). For example, seeking help from community agencies may be a very positive move when outside assistance is needed to help a child with learning problems, but the same adaptive strategy may be negative if it becomes the predominant way a family solves its problems. This is because the family does not learn to utilize its own inner resources.

Family adaptation is functionally defined by McCubbin and McCubbin (1993), as a "process in which families engage in direct responses to the extensive demands of a stressor, and realize that systemic changes are needed within the family unit, to restore functional stability and improve family satisfaction and well-being" (p. 57). According to McCubbin and McCubbin, adaptation involves the process of restructuring family patterns of functioning. In a concept analysis by Clawson (1996) that focused on family adaptation to chronic illness of a child family member, family adaptation was defined as an ongoing family system process used to achieve adaptive tasks in a chronic illness situation. Both of these definitions emphasize that family adaptation is a process that takes place over time when family members are adapting to stressful life situations such as caring for a child with chronic illness. When the family is successful in its response to stressors, it moves through the situation with relative ease and a positive outcome results. This is called bonadaptation (Rungreangkulkij & Gilliss, 2000). Family adaptation is also defined as an outcome (the family's level of family functioning) in family stress and coping theories.

Family coherence refers to a key natural resistance resource in individuals and families. This dispositional quality serves to promote health and well-being. In Antonovsky's writings (1979, 1998) about a sense of coherence (SOC) it is clear that the sense of coherence is seen as more of an individual attribute rather than a family attribute. Later, however, family theorists have maintained that families can also possess a strong sense of coherence as one of the family meanings that influence demands and resources of families (Patterson, 1988b). Antonovsky defines SOC as follows:

> a global orientation that expresses the extent to which one has a pervasive, enduring, though dynamic, feeling of confidence that 1) the stimuli deriving from one's internal and external environ-

ments in the course of living are structured, predictable, and explicable; 2) the resources are available to meet the demands posed by these stimuli; and 3) these demands are challenges worthy of investment and engagement (Antonovsky, 1998, p. 22).

Family coherence is a dispositional world view. Families who have a strong sense of coherence have the confidence that the world is comprehensive (internal and external stimuli are predictable and structured), manageable (available resources are present to address demands), and meaningful (demands are seen as challenges worth investing in (McCubbin et al., 1998).

Family resilience is defined as the adaptational processes in family systems. A family resilience approach to working with families builds on the competencies and strengths of family members and families, enabling health care providers to shift from a pathogenic model to a strength-based model—one in which we see families as being challenged, not "broken," by adversity (Walsh, 1998).

🐾 TIME PHASES OF STRESS AND COPING STRATEGIES

Nurses need to be aware of the time phases of stress, as well as the coping strategies family members and the family unit might use during each of the three time periods.

ANTESTRESS PERIOD

In the period before actually confronting the stressor (such as the hospitalization of a child), anticipation is sometimes possible; there can be an awareness of impending danger or the perceived threat of the situation. If families or helping persons can identify a future stressor, anticipatory guidance as well as preventive coping strategies may be sought or provided to weaken or reduce the impact of the stressor.

ACTUAL STRESS PERIOD

Coping strategies during the period of stress usually differ in intensity and kind from those utilized prior to the onset of the stressor and stress. There may be very basic survival, defensive strategies used during this period if the stress in the family is extreme. With tremendous energy expended in dealing with a stressor(s) and stress, many family functions (some that may be crucial to family health) are often temporarily set aside or are inadequately performed until the family has the resources to deal with them again. An example of the latter situation is when families totally organize their family life around the care of a member with a chronic illness. In these situations they may become very dysfunctional over time as the developmental needs of the healthy members go unmet and the developmental course of family life is distorted (Reiss, Steinglass, & Howe, 1993). The most helpful coping responses during stressful periods are often intrafamilial (to be discussed later), and the seeking of spiritual support (Friedman, 1985; Pravikoff, 1985).

POSTSTRESS PERIOD

The coping strategies employed following the initial acute stress period, termed the posttrauma phase, consist of strategies to return the family to a homeostatic, balanced state. To promote family wellness during this phase, the family needs to pull together, mutually express feelings, and solve its problems (Burgess, 1978) or seek out and utilize familial supports for resolving the stressful situation. Four possible poststress outcomes have been cited: (1) family functioning at a higher level than before; (2) family functioning at the same prestress level; (3) family functioning at a lower level than before; or (4) family dissolution (i.e., separation, divorce, abandonment) (Mederer & Hill, 1983). When a family ends up functioning at a lower level of wellness or in a state of family dissolution, family members often need professional assistance to help them increase their repertoire of effective coping strategies (Reiss, Steinglass, & Howe, 1993).

✺ FAMILY STRESS THEORIES

Family stress theory has evolved over the last 50 years, as evidenced by the array of models cited in the literature. This evolution is depicted in Table 17–1. Here

the major theories/models are identified and compared with earlier model(s).

Two family stress theories, one emphasizing the precrisis stage (the ABCX Model) and one emphasizing postcrisis (the Resiliency Model) are discussed in this text as useful guides for nurses working with families managing stressful situations. One of the differences between these two models is that in the ABCX Model (Hill, 1949) a crisis situation is viewed as a negative outcome for the family, but in the Resiliency Model (McCubbin & McCubbin, 1993), crisis is viewed as a challenge—as an indication that the family must make some fundamental changes in how it usually functions in order to adapt to stressor events (McCubbin & McCubbin, 1993). Each of these models are now discussed.

HILL'S FAMILY STRESS THEORY

Hill's (1949) classic landmark, family stress theory is the most eloquent, parsimonious model for describing the factors producing crisis or noncrisis in families. Based on research Hill conducted on war-induced separation and reunion, he developed a family stress theory called the ABCX Model in which he identified a major set of variables (factors A, B, C, and X) and their relationships that led to family crisis/noncrisis. He also theoretically described a postcrisis "roller coaster" adjustment process that families went through. These two parts of his theoretical framework have remained virtually unchanged for the last 50 years. Moreover, this theory has been the basis for many research studies in the family stress and coping area, and has been foundational to the work of Caplan (1964) and other clinicians in generating practice theory and principles in crisis intervention.

The ABCX framework has two parts. The first is a proposition dealing with the determinants of family crisis: "A (the event and related hardships) interacting with B (the family's crisis meeting resources) interacting with C (the definition that the family makes of the event) produces X (the crisis)" (Hill, 1965, p. 36). The second part is a more process-oriented statement regarding the course of adjustment following a crisis. Hill (1965) explains that the course of family adjustment following a crisis involves (1) a period of disorganization, (2) an angle of recovery, and (3) reorganization and a new level of family functioning.

Figure 17–1 presents a visual representation of an adaptation of Hill's model. To elaborate further on Hill's model, this model explains what precipitates a crisis in one family and not in another. As seen in Figure 17–1, there are three basic factors involved.

The first is the actual presence of stressors or stressor-events (factor A). The second basic factor influencing the outcome—crisis or noncrisis in dealing with a stressor is the family's resources and use of coping mechanisms (factor B). Major stressors initially force stereotypic defenses. Later, coping efforts emerge. If the family does not make use of its resources and coping mechanisms from its repertoire of possible responses, the result is the same as if the family did not possess the coping resources. However, the intervention is easier in this case because it is less difficult to assist families to utilize past coping patterns than to help families learn new ways of responding.

Third and most important of the three contributing factors is the family's perception and interpretation of the stressors or stressor-events (factor C).

TABLE 17–1

THE EVOLUTION OF FAMILY STRESS THEORY

THEORY/MODEL	THEORIST AND YEAR	DESCRIPTION OF THEORY
ABCX Model	Hill (1949)	Factors A (stressor), B (family's crisis-meeting resources), and C (family's definition of the stressor event) interact to produce X (crisis or noncrisis). Theory was developed after World War II to explain families' responses to war separation and reunion.
Double ABCX Model	McCubbin & Patterson (1982)	Hill's model was modified, whereby the A factor was expanded to include original stressor and pileup of stressors. The concept of coping was also added and seen as a key explanatory variable, leading to different levels of family adaptation. The model first described postcrisis adaptation in families who had husbands/fathers missing in action in the Vietnam war and later in families adjusting to childhood chronic illness (Faux, 1998)
Family Adjustment and Adaptation Response (FAAR) Model	Patterson (1988)	This model, built on the Double ABCX model, emphasizes potential positive outcomes. The model is consistent with many studies that focused on family and individual coherence and resilience (Antonovsky, 1979). Situational and global meanings (such as family coherence) are viewed as influencing both the demands/stressors (strains and hassles) and capabilities (resources and coping behaviors). The demands versus the capabilities leads to different levels of family adjustment (precrisis) and family adaptation (postcrisis).
The Resiliency Model	McCubbin & McCubbin (1993)	This model builds on the previous three models and emphasizes the strengths and resiliencies of families (see text for detailed discussion). New explanatory concepts were added: newly established patterns of functioning (family types) and the family's schema or world view. The coping variable was broadened to include problem solving.

Lazarus and co-workers (1974) emphasize that it is the person's or group's cognitive appraisal of the stressor that influences what coping efforts are made as well as the final outcome. Recall that families that consistently perceive and define events and their situation as threatening and dangerous rather than challenging will most likely be crisis prone. Functional families are able to see events as understandable and manageable.

Factor X deals with crisis or noncrisis. Hill (1965) discusses this factor in terms of crisis-proneness in families. Crisis-proneness describes how families handle the B and C factors of the theory. When families are crisis-prone, they tend to experience stressor events (A) with greater frequency and greater severity and define these (C) more frequently as crises. These types of families are more vulnerable to stressor events also because of the meager resources and coping abilities (B) they possess. In addition, they typically fail to learn from past crises, leading them to see new stressor events as threatening and crisis provoking.

The X factor tends to be seen by Hill as an "either/or" outcome, although gradations of crisis or noncrisis certainly exist. The disorganizing effects of crisis in the family are seen in family relations and role performance of family members. Hill (1965) observed that sexual behavior of the marital couple was a most sensitive index of the presence of crisis (Hill, 1965).

Subsequent to Hill's seminal theory building, other family stress models have been built on Hill's original work. The most recent family stress model emphasizes the factors that influence the family's postcrisis response.

THE RESILIENCY MODEL OF FAMILY STRESS, ADJUSTMENT, AND ADAPTATION

The Resiliency Model of Family Stress, Adjustment, and Adaptation (McCubbin & McCubbin, 1993, 1996) is a theoretical framework that also emphasizes family adjustment and adaptation when families experience stressful life situations (McCubbin, McCubbin, Thompson, & Thompson, 1998). The Resiliency Model builds on the earlier work of Hill's ABCX stress model (Hill, 1949, 1958) as well as later family stress models (McCubbin & McCubbin, 1987, 1989; McCubbin & Patterson, 1983a). The main emphases

of this model is on the **resiliency** of families or their ability to recover from adverse events. It is a strengths-based model, which highlights what strengths and capabilities influence the process of resiliency.

The Resiliency Model is based on four fundamental assumptions about family life:

> (a) Families face hardships and changes as a natural and predictable aspect of family life over the life cycle; (b) families develop basic strengths and capabilities designed to foster the growth and development of family members and the family unit and to protect the family from major disruptions in the face of family transitions and changes; (c) families develop basic and unique strengths and capabilities designed to protect the family from unexpected or normative stressors and strains and to foster the family's adaptation following a family crisis or major transition and change; and (d) families benefit from and contribute to the network of relationships and resources in the community, particularly during periods of family stress and crises. (McCubbin & McCubbin, 1991, p. 3)

In the Resiliency Model (Figure 17–2), families' responses to stressful life events and transitions occur in two phases: (1) the adjustment phase, and (2) the adaptation phase.

THE ADJUSTMENT PHASE OF THE RESILIENCY MODEL. The adjustment phase of the model depicts family response to events that do not present major hardships and require only minor changes in how the family unit is currently functioning *or* the *initial* response of the family to a more major event. Situations that may require only adjustment by the family could be family vacations, a family member's brief acute illness with complete recovery, or a family member receiving a ticket for a minor traffic violation. Families who experience such stressors will adjust to the stressor by calling on the families' established ways of functioning with only minor changes being made: the family's definition of the stressor (family appraisal), the family's existing resources and family problem-solving and coping abilities. However, if minor changes in family functioning are not adequate to manage these events, then the family moves into a crisis situation and the adaptation phase of the model.

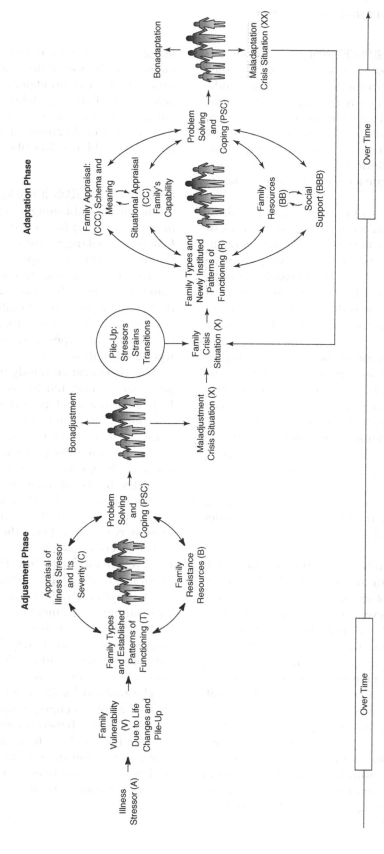

Figure 17–2. The Resiliency Model of Family Stress, Adjustment, and Adaptation. *(From: McCubbin, M. A., & McCubbin, H. I. (1993). Families coping with illness: The resiliency model of family stress, adjustment and adaptation. In C. Danielson, B. Hamel-Bissel, & P. Winstead-Fry (Eds.), Families, health, and illness: Perspectives on coping and intervention (pp. 21–63). St. Louis: Harcourt Health Services.*

THE ADAPTATION PHASE OF THE RESILIENCY MODEL. In this model, the crisis situation is not necessarily viewed as pathological or detrimental to the family, but rather indicates that the family needs to make fundamental structural or systemic changes in functioning in order to adapt to the situation. In other words, old ways of functioning are no longer adequate and new solutions must be found. Both developmental and situational stressors can create a crisis and require adaptation by the family.

Crises in the family call upon the family unit to make some systemic family changes to adapt to stressful life situations and restore stability to family member and family unit functioning (McCubbin & McCubbin, 1993). Therefore, family crisis is viewed as a necessary precondition in order for the family to adapt to stressors or demands that family members are experiencing (see Figure 17–3) (McCubbin & McCubbin, 1993).

In the adaptation phase of the model (see Figure 17–2), response to a crisis situation is determined by the pile-up of demands, stressors, transitions, and strains, as well as the strengths and capabilities of the family unit. These include newly established patterns of functioning; the family's appraisal of how the demands are being met and the family's world view; resources within individual family members, the family unit, and the community; and the family's existing and newly developed problem-solving and coping responses. Each of the major variables in the model are subsequently described.

PILEUP OF DEMANDS. Families are often dealing with more than one stressor at a time. In the Resiliency Model, six categories of stresses and strains are identified: (1) The stressor event and associated hardships (e.g., when families of children with chronic asthma need to stabilize the family environment in the home by keeping the air clean and dust free, not having pets, and asking family members to give up smoking); (2) normative transitions (e.g., birth of children, children entering school, adolescent stage, retirement); (3) preexisting family strains (e.g., difficulty getting along with an ex-spouse); (4) situational demands (e.g., work hours increase or extensive requirements for work-related travel with frequent absences from family); (5) consequences of the family efforts to cope (e.g., one member quiting his or her job to care for a member with chronic illness, which decreases family income; or the use of drugs and alcohol as a coping strategy); and (6) intra-family strains and social ambiguity—lack of clear guidelines from both within and outside the family as to how to manage this situation, such as what to do about infertility or having miscarriages (McCubbin & McCubbin, 1993).

NEWLY INSTITUTED PATTERNS OF FUNCTIONING. The importance of the family establishing new patterns of functioning in a crisis is emphasized in the Resiliency Model. Instead of looking at just one aspect of family functioning at a time, two aspects of functioning are considered simultaneously to construct a "family type." Family types are defined as the set of family attributes that explain how the family functions as a unit (McCubbin & McCubbin, 1993). Although there may be many family types or combinations, three family types are briefly described.

The **regenerative family** type is characterized as possessing family hardiness and family coherence. Family hardiness refers to the internal strengths and durability of the family unit and is comprised of the family members' ability to work together and have a commitment to solve problems; an ability to see stressors and change as challenges rather than enormous obstacles that family members cannot surmount; and the feeling that the family has some influence in how things turn out and that it can achieve some degree of mastery or control over the situation.

Family coherence is the second major characteristic of regenerative families. This concept was defined previously in the section defining basic concepts.

The **rhythmic family** type focuses on family time and routines (e.g., mealtime and bedtime routines); and the valuing of these times and routines as an integral part of daily family life. These routines provide predictability and comfort for the family during times of stress and crisis.

The **resilient family** type highlights family flexibility (the ability to change) and family bonding (emotional closeness between family members). Families who are high on both hardiness and coherence, time and routines and the valuing of these, and flexibility and bonding have been found to be better able to adapt to stressful situations (McCubbin, Thompson et al., 1988).

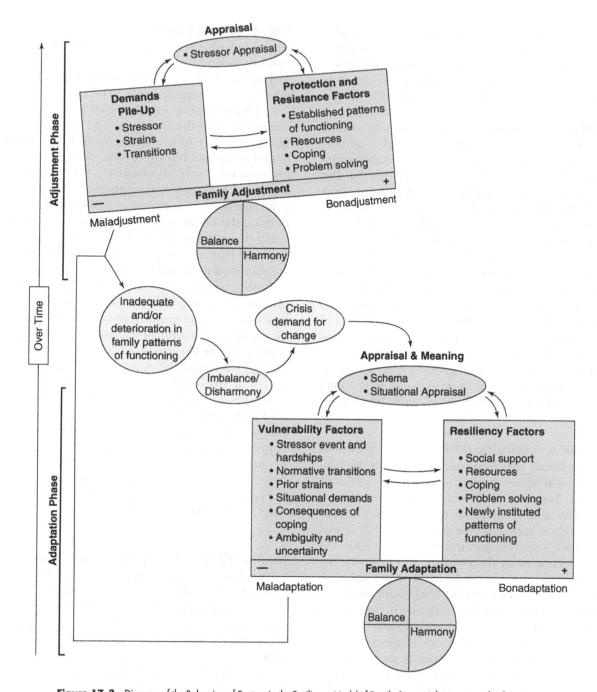

Figure 17–3. Diagram of the Balancing of Factors in the Resiliency Model of Family Stress, Adjustment, and Adaptation.

RESOURCES. Resources are those attributes and supports that are available for use by the family in crisis situations. McCubbin and McCubbin (1993, 1996) emphasize three different sources and levels of resources: the individual, the family unit, and the community. Resources of individual family members may include: (1) intelligence, (2) knowledge and skills, (3) personality traits (e.g., optimism), (4) physical health, and (5) emotional health such as self-esteem or sense of mastery. Family unit resources may include organization, decision-making skills, and conflict-resolution abilities. Community resources include both personal support (e.g., relatives, friends) and institutional support (e.g., health care services) that are available outside the family.

SOCIAL SUPPORT. Social support can be a vital help to families in crisis. Social support will be described more fully later in this chapter but in the Resiliency Model, social support is defined as "information exchanged at the interpersonal level that provides: (a) emotional support (individuals in the family believe that they are loved and cared for); (b) esteem support (family members believe that they are respected and valued); and (c) network support (family members believe that they belong to a network of communication where mutual support and understanding is emphasized)" (Cobb, 1976, cited in McCubbin & McCubbin, 1993, p. 48). In addition, McCubbin and McCubbin also emphasize (d) appraisal support (information that allows family members to assess how well they are doing), and (e) altruistic support (information received as goodwill from others for giving of oneself). Community resources can be a valuable source of social support if the family is willing to access and use this source of support.

FAMILY APPRAISAL IN ADAPTATION PHASE. In the adjustment phase, the family appraisal encompasses only the family's definition of the stressor (the first level of family appraisal). Two additional levels of appraisal are introduced in the adaptation phase of the model. The family's situational appraisal (the second level) is viewed as the family's shared assessment of the stressor, the hardships created by the stressor, and how well the family is managing these demands (McCubbin & McCubbin, 1993). This second level of appraisal may bring about changes in how a family is coping and functioning. *Family schema* or *world view* is the third level of family appraisal. This level of appraisal refers to the families' view of shared values, goals, and expectations that is constructed over time. This level of appraisal is influenced by the family of origin of the adult family members, the cultural and religious background of the family, and societal norms and values. The family world view is usually quite stable, but can be altered by the occurrence of catastrophic events such as the premature death of a young father in an accident or the birth of a child with Down syndrome.

PROBLEM SOLVING AND COPING. In the Resiliency Model, coping behavior is defined as the effort and resources families use to manage a stressor (McCubbin & McCubbin, 1993). Thus, resources are what the family possesses and coping is what the family does. Four strategies of coping are identified in the model: (1) action to reduce the demands (e.g., putting a disabled family member in a nursing home), (2) action to obtain additional resources (e.g., finding home nursing care for disabled member), (3) managing tensions and relieving stress (physical exercise, doing enjoyable activities together as a family), and (4) reappraising the situation using reframing strategies (e.g., being thankful for the good things, believing you are doing all that is possible). Reappraisal and reframing are discussed more fully later in the chapter.

Problem-solving communication also influences how families adapt. In the Resiliency Model, two types of family communication are identified: (1) incendiary or a conflict-escalating type of communication, which increases stress and tension (e.g., yelling, screaming, blaming tactics); and (2) affirming or a stress-reducing type of communication, which has a calming, supportive, and soothing effect on family members' interaction. Telling members they are doing a good job, conveying warmth and appreciation, and listening to concerns are examples of this type of communication. Families that have lower levels of incendiary and higher levels of affirming communication have been found to adapt better (McCubbin & McCubbin, 1991).

FAMILY ADAPTATION. In the Resiliency Model, family adaptation, is the outcome. It describes the outcome of the family's efforts to manage their stressful situation (Rungreangkulkij & Gilliss, 2000). Family adaptation is depicted as occurring at two levels: individual to family and family to community (McCubbin & McCubbin, 1993). At the first level, family adaptation occurs after the family has accepted changes in its functioning in order for the family to work together as a unit. At this level, families are able to carry out their functions—affective, socialization, health care—effectively without compromising the physical health and emotional well-being of family members. At the second level, family adaptation occurs through daily transactions and interactions between the family and community. Families adapting to stress need to adapt at both the individual-to-family and the family-to-community levels of functioning because change at one level influences family functioning at the other level (McCubbin & McCubbin, 1993, 1996). If the family is not able to make these changes or a new stressor challenges the family's existing level of adaptation, the family can move back into a crisis situation (see Figure 17–2).

STRESSORS AND THEIR IMPACT

Families are daily bombarded with tension-producing stimuli, some of which are only mildly irritating and hardly noticed, such as traffic noise and poor housing, and some of which are potentially or actually devastating to families, such as marital disruption or the loss of a child (McCubbin & Patterson, 1991; Pearlin & Turner, 1987). As depicted in the Resiliency Model (McCubbin & McCubbin, 1993), families are seldom dealing with a single stressor at a time but are often exposed to both normative and situational stressors stimultaneously.

For over 50 years researchers have realized the great quantitative and qualitative differences that stressors have on individuals. As early as 1949, researchers systematically studied the quality and quantity of life changes and their impact on the health of individuals (Holmes & Rahe, 1967). From these studies, weights were assigned to a variety of life events (both positive and negative life changes) that were associated with poor health outcomes (Nickolls, 1975). From these early studies, researchers developed family-based tools that assessed life changes in families. The most widely used tool is the Family Inventory of Life Events and Changes (FILE) (McCubbin, Patterson, & Wilson, 1983) (see Table 17–2). The FILE (McCubbin, Patterson, & Wilson) is an instrument that can be used to assess the pile-up or accumulation of family stressors in a family.

On the FILE each of the 71 life events is weighted as to how stressful it is. The seven most stressful life events in the *total* FILE scale are: (1) a child member died; (2) a parent or spouse died; (3) spouse or parent was separated or divorced; (4) the presence of physical or sexual abuse or violence in the home; (5) a member became physically disabled or chronically

TABLE 17–2

THE MOST STRESSFUL LIFE EVENTS (WEIGHTED SCORES) BY SUBSCALE IN THE FAMILY INVENTORY OF LIFE EVENTS AND CHANGES SCALE (FILE)

FAMILY LIFE CHANGES	VALUE
LOSSES	
A child member died	99
A parent/spouse died	98
Married son or daughter was separated or divorced	58
MARITAL STRAINS	
Spouse/parent was separated or divorced	79
Spouse/parent has an "affair"	68
Increased difficulty with sexual relationship between husband and wife	58
FAMILY LEGAL VIOLATIONS	
Physical or sexual abuse or violence in the home	75
A member went to jail or juvenile detention	68
A member ran away from home	61
ILLNESS AND FAMILY "CARE" STRAINS	
A member became physically disabled or chronically ill	73
Increased difficulty in managing a chronically ill or disabled member	58
Increased responsibility to provide direct care/financial help to husband's/wife's parents	47
INTRAFAMILY STRAINS	
A member appears to depend on alcohol or drugs	66
A member appears to have emotional problems	58
Increased difficulty in managing teenage child(ren)	55

(continued)

TABLE 17–2 (CONTINUED)

THE MOST STRESSFUL LIFE EVENTS (WEIGHTED SCORES) BY SUBSCALE IN THE FAMILY INVENTORY OF LIFE EVENTS AND CHANGES SCALE (FILE)

FAMILY LIFE CHANGES	VALUE
PREGNANCY AND CHILDBEARING STRAINS	
An unmarried member became pregnant	65
A member gave birth to or adopted a child	50
A member had an abortion	50
WORK–FAMILY TRANSITIONS AND STRAINS	
A member lost or quit a job	55
A member stopped working for an extended period	51
A member retired from work	48
FINANCE AND BUSINESS STRAINS	
Went on welfare	55
A member started a new business	50
Change in agriculture or stock markets, which hurt family income	43
TRANSITIONS "IN AND OUT"	
Young adult member left home	43
A member was married	42
A member moved back home or a new person moved into the household	42

Source: Adapted from McCubbin, Patterson, & Wilson (1983).

ill; (6) spouse or parent has an affair; and (7) a member went to jail or juvenile detention. Table 17–1 illustrates the three most stressful items under each of the nine subscales of the FILE. Families with a higher accumulation of life events (i.e., higher scores on the FILE) have been found to have lower family function-ing and poorer health of family members (McCubbin & Patterson, 1991).

Family life strains and stressors stem from multiple factors, suggesting how difficult it is to assess families. We have tended to think that in order to eliminate a problem one would need to find a way to eliminate or treat a particular causative factor, rather than view the situation more broadly. By assessing the balance between the stressors (their duration and strength) and the nature and strength of supportive or protective elements, both intrafamilial and extrafamilial, one can either attempt to eliminate or reduce the potency of stressors or to build up and strengthen the family's resources.

FAMILY COPING STRATEGIES

Family and individual behavioral, cognitive, and emotional coping strategies are conceptualized as being problem or situation specific. Different circumstances and different problems demand different solutions; that is, different coping responses need to be employed. Burr and associates' study (1994) confirmed that coping strategies were stressor specific. For example, the cognitive strategy of "accepting the situation" was helpful for 90 percent of displaced homemakers, but perceived as more harmful by 39 percent of couples managing infertility problems. These researchers concluded that if displaced homemakers accepted their situation, they could then go on to seek more education, find employment, and build new relationships. In contrast, accepting the situation for infertile couples meant they were giving up on having a biological child and this was not helpful for them (Burr et al.).

Hence, family stress scholars have suggested that using a variety of coping strategies to cope with stress is more important than using one or two particular coping strategies all the time (Burr, Day, & Bahr, 1993; Burr et al., 1994; McCubbin, Olson, & Larsen, 1991). Burr and associates found the most harmful coping behaviors to be: keeping feelings inside (suppressing emotions), taking out feelings on others (in relationships), keeping others from knowing how bad the situation was (lack of communication), and denying, avoiding, or running away from the problem. Without being specific as to the particular situational and family context, the real functionality of any behavioral pattern cannot with certainty be determined. However, families do have certain coping styles or propensities, which also influence the particular types of coping efforts the family brings to bear on a problem.

Another way to view family coping is to look at whether the coping strategies come from within the family or rely on supports and resources outside the family. In this text family coping strategies are classified here as internal or external to the family system (see Table 17–3). It is assumed that the following coping strategies are usually functional—although perhaps the exclusive/predominant or inappropriate use of a particular coping strategy could produce dysfunctional family outcomes.

INTERNAL FAMILY COPING STRATEGIES

Under internal family coping strategies, three general types of intrafamilial coping strategies are discussed: family relationship strategies, cognitive strategies, and communication strategies.

RELATIONSHIP STRATEGIES

Family Group Reliance. Certain families when under stress cope by becoming more reliant on their own resources. Pulling together is one of the most important processes in weathering storms in families' lives. Families accomplish this by creating greater structure and organization in the home and family. Established family time and routines such as those involving mealtime, bedtime, household chores, visits with extended family, and the valuing of these routines can be a source of strength and predictability when the family is under stress (McCubbin & McCubbin, 1991). When families establish greater structure, it is an attempt to have greater control over their lives. This usually involves tighter scheduling of members' time, more tasks per family member, a more close-knit organization, and a more rigid, prescribed routine. With the closing of family boundaries comes a call for greater family organization and control of members, coupled with the expectation that members will be more self-disciplined and conforming. Families utilizing greater control, if successful, also achieve greater integration and cohesiveness.

TABLE 17–3

FAMILY COPING STRATEGIES

INTERNAL FAMILY COPING STRATEGIES

Relationship strategies
  Family group reliance
  Greater sharing together
  Role flexibility

Cognitive strategies
  Normalizing
  Controlling the meaning of the problem by reframing and passive appraisal
  Joint problem solving
  Gaining of information and knowledge

Communication strategies
  Being open and honest
  Use of humor and laughter

EXTERNAL FAMILY COPING STRATEGIES

Community strategy: Maintaining active linkages with the community

Social support strategies
  Extended family
  Friends
  Neighbors
  Self-help groups
  Formal social supports

Spiritual strategies
  Seeking advice of clergy
  Becoming more involved in religious activities
  Having faith in God
  Prayer
  Seeking renewal and connectedness in communion with nature

Source: Partially adapted from Burr, 1994; McCubbin, Olson, & Larsen, 1991; Walsh, 1998.

This type of family coping usually stems from the influence of the traditional Protestant ethic, which values and sees self-control and self-sufficiency as particularly necessary during hardship periods. Concomitant with structuring is a need for some families to be "strong" and to learn to conceal feelings and master tension within themselves. However, "strong" families sometimes have weak bonds. A case in point is a study by Reiss and associates (1986). The researchers observed that members with a chronic illness in "strong" families who rigidly adhered to the medical regimen for their end-stage renal disease died sooner than family members with a chronic illness who took a day off from their strict treatment regimen to spend time with the family, have a meal together, and socialize (Reiss et al., 1986). Thus, rigidity and control can be helpful in managing stress, but if carried to extreme, appear to be detrimental to both individual and family functioning.

Burgess (1978) points out that this particular coping strategy, involving self-discipline among family members, may be very necessary *initially* in stressful situations such as when parents are confronted with a serious accident at home. They must maintain composure and the capacity to problem solve, because they then are responsible for their own lives and those of their children. And, in fact, Pearlin and Schooler (1978) found that self-reliance was an efficacious coping response in the area of enacting one's marital and parental roles. Time management is one particular coping response that follows within this broader coping strategy.

Walsh (1998) notes that some self-reliant families who are dealing with chronic or serious health problems may look pathologically enmeshed. The high cohesion they display, however, may be functional and even necessary in the context of their health situation. It must also be mentioned that this strategy can be dysfunctional if the need for control is not tempered by the need to accept that which cannot be controlled and in situations in which outside help is needed but not sought. For example, a family caregiver for a member with Alzheimer's who does not seek outside help when the member's condition deteriorates to needing total physical care may seriously impair his or her own physical and mental wellbeing. Also if family group reliance becomes a habitual, pervasive mode of adaptation, the needed flexibility is lost.

Greater Sharing Together (Strengthening of Family Cohesion). One way of bringing the family closer together and maintaining and managing stress levels and the necessary family morale is by sharing of feelings and thoughts, and engaging in joint family experiences or activities. Greater sharing together produces higher family cohesion, a family attribute that has received wide attention for being a central family attribute (Olson, 1993). Olson views family cohesion as "the emotional bonding that family members have toward one another" (p. 105). Extreme families are either very high or very low on cohesion. When families are very high on cohesion, the family is said to be enmeshed and there is little individual independence or autonomy. In these types of families, members seek satisfaction and connection primarily within the family and children are slower to leave home (Walsh, 1998). When the family is disengaged or is very low on cohesion, family members are not close to one another and have little commitment to the family unit. Families that have moderate levels of cohesion tend to be more functional and better able to adapt to stress (Olson). The level of cohesion that is functional for the family also is influenced by cultural background; higher levels of cohesion in certain cultural groups are both desirable and functional.

The most crucial relationship requiring cohesiveness or sharing together in the family system may be between the spouses or adult partners, particularly in middle-class families. A confiding relationship, especially between mates, in which individuals can talk intimately about themselves and their concerns has been shown to be critical for good psychological health in times of stress.

Greater cohesion and sharing of concerns and feelings are also very advantageous in reducing the family tension level due to acute or serious illness or other major stressor. High family cohesiveness is especially helpful when a family has been traumatized, because family members are in much greater need of support (Figley, 1989). In these times of crisis family members can be highly connected and rally together as well as respect the differences among family members (Walsh, 1998).

A family's involvement in family rituals that have meaning and value to the family is another way in which the family shares together. Rituals in families are repeated social processes or patterns of interaction that preserve the family identity and give family members a shared definition of the world (Hartman

& Laird, 1983). An excellent cultural example of a family ritual is the traditional Jewish custom of sitting shivah for a 7-day period after a funeral in which relatives and close friends visit with the bereaved family and share their thoughts and feelings, providing mutual emotional support and nurturance.

Leisure-time family activities are especially important coping resources to rejuvenate a family's cohesiveness, morale, and satisfaction (McCubbin & McCubbin, 1991; Olson, 1993). Like so many sayings, the adage "A family that plays together, stays together" contains much truth. This coping strategy is ultimately aimed at building greater integration, cohesiveness, and resiliency in the family.

Role Flexibility. Because of the rapid and pervasive changes in our society and hence in family life, role flexibility, especially among mates, constitutes a powerful type of coping strategy. Olson (1993) and Walsh (1998) have emphasized that role flexibility is one of the major dimensions of family adaptation. A family must be capable of adapting to changing developmental and environmental changes. When the family copes successfully it is able to maintain a dynamic balance between change and stability. Role flexibility allows for this balance to continue.

The spouse or adult partner subsystem's ability to role share and change roles when needed is very important. In research on levels of functioning of grieving families, Davies and colleagues (1986) corroborated the importance of role flexibility of mates as a functional coping strategy. They found that the degree to which family roles were flexible or rigid differentiated levels of functioning in their sample of grieving families, with flexible roles associated with better functioning. In research on the long-term success of couple relationships, flexibility in roles was crucial in helping couples evolve and cope with the multitude of challenges in their lives (Walsh, 1998).

COGNITIVE STRATEGIES

Normalizing. Another functional family coping strategy is the tendency for families to normalize things as much as possible when they are coping with a long-term stressor that tends to disrupt family life and household activities. Multiple authors have used the term "normalizing" to conceptualize how families manage a member's disability (Faux, 1998; Knafl, Deatrick, & Kirby, 2001).

Davis (1963) was the first researcher to use the term "normalization" to describe a family's response to illness or disability. He found that families with children who had polio normalized their situation by minimizing the abnormalities in the child's appearance, participating in usual activities, and maintaining ongoing social ties. Normalization is a family management process that is often preferred in families with chronic health problems. It is an ongoing process that involves acknowledging the chronic condition but defining family life as normal, defining the social effects of having a member with a chronic condition as minimal, and engaging in behaviors that show others that the family is normal (Deatrick, Knafl, & Murphy-Moore, 1999; Knafl & Deatrick, 1986; Shepard & Mahon, 1996). Families "normalize" by maintaining rituals and routines. This helps families cope with stress and promotes a sense of continuity over time, so important for normalizing a family's situation (Fiese, 2000).

Research from George Washington University of families dealing with end-stage kidney disease demonstrated that the families coping by normalizing actually fared better in terms of the sick member's course of illness than families where all activities of the family were scheduled around the health needs of the sick member (Cornille, 2001).

Controlling the Meaning of the Problem by Reframing and Passive Appraisal. In a large study of American adults, one of the primary means Pearlin and Schooler (1978) found to be effective in coping was by use of the mental mechanism—controlling the meaning of the problem. This cognitive coping strategy ameliorates or cognitively neutralizes threatening stimuli that are experienced in life. Numerous research studies have shown that individuals and families who possess "an optimistic bias" tend to do better than those with a "hard take" on reality (Walsh, 1998). As mentioned earlier, the interpretation given to events can make the difference between overresponding to a situation (wherein the family experiences great stress), reacting in a realistic way (wherein the situation is seen objectively, appraised accurately), and underreacting (wherein an element of denial may be present and less stress is elicited). Two ways to control the meaning of the problem are presented here; reframing and passive appraisal.

In the family mental health literature, *cognitive reframing* is encouraged most often as a way for controlling the meaning of a stressor. The terms "optimistic beliefs" and "positive appraisal" (Burr, Day, & Bahr, 1993; Folkman, Lazarus, Dunkel-Schetter, De Longis, & Gruen, 1986) are also used synonymously. Families that use this coping strategy tend to see the positive facets of life's stress-producing events, as exemplified by the making of positive comparisons ("count your blessings"; "it could have been worse"); selectively ignoring the negative aspects ("I've learned a lot from this negative experience"); and making the stressful events or experiences less important in terms of the family's hierarchy of values (Chesler & Barbarin, 1987; Pearlin & Schooler, 1978). Walsh (1998) emphasizes that having a positive outlook is a key process in family resilience. It is characterized by family members' having confidence in overcoming "the odds," holding an optimistic view of events, having sustained hope, and focusing on strengths and potential. Miller (2000) concurs with Walsh and other authors—that holding positive views and maintaining hope are crucial coping mechanisms, particularly when confronted with cancer and other life-threatening illnesses.

Reframing is an individual or family perceptual way of coping and is often influenced by family beliefs. Families have shared perceptions or shared subjective realities, and the reframing process will be influenced by these perceptions. Rolland emphasizes that individual and family beliefs function as a cognitive map that guide family actions and decisions. Beliefs can, in that way, be in harmony with the families' world view, family paradigms, and family values. According to Rolland families develop paradigms or belief systems about how the world operates. These beliefs shape how families experience and interpret their environment and are an important factor in the family's process of reframing and redefining its situation. The role of religion and spirituality also plays an important role in forming beliefs. Families will note in stressful situations that they believe that "God would not give us anything we couldn't manage" or that "God will help us through this situation." The importance of beliefs is highlighted in the clinical practice of Lorraine Wright and associates (Wright, Watson, & Bell, 1996). These clinicians/researchers have found that examining family members' beliefs and intervening where constraining beliefs prevail are powerful ways to help families with the alleviation of their suffering.

A second way families control the meaning of a stressor(s) is by *passive appraisal*, sometimes referred to as a passive acceptance. Here families use a collective cognitive coping strategy of viewing the stressor or stressful demand as something that will take care of itself over time and about which there is nothing or little that can be done. As Boss (1988) points out, passive appraisal can be an effective stress-reducing strategy in the short run, especially in cases where nothing can be done. By passively accepting the situation, a family may more easily tolerate the inevitable or immutable. However, if this strategy is used consistently and over time, its use inhibits active problem solving and change in families and can be detrimental to family adaptation.

Joint Problem Solving. Joint problem solving among family members is a family cognitive and communication coping strategy that has been extensively studied via laboratory research methods by a group of family researchers (Klein, 1983; Reiss, 1981; Strauss, 1968) and in the natural setting (Chesler & Barbarin, 1987; Epstein et al., 1993; Figley, 1989). Focusing on the routine and expectable disruptions in family life, researchers have looked at the differences in families' use of joint problem solving. Joint problem solving can be described as a situation where a family jointly is able to discuss a problem at hand, search for a solution governed by logic, and reach a consensus on what to do based upon a fully shared set of cues, perceptions, and suggestions from the various family members. Effective family problem solving involves seven specific steps: (1) identifying the problem, (2) communicating about the problem, (3) coming up with possible solutions, (4) deciding on one of the solutions, (5) carrying out the action, (6) monitoring or making sure that the action was carried out, and (7) evaluating the entire problem-solving process. By incorporating these problem-solving strategies into family life, families are believed to function more effectively (Epstein, Bishop, Ryan, Miller, & Keitner, 1993). Reiss calls families that use effective problem-solving processes environment-sensitive families. These types of families see the nature of a problem as being "out there" and do not try to make the problem an internal one.

Figley (1989) and Walsh (1998) identified solution-oriented or collaborative problem solving as being a type of functional coping leading to family resilience. Confidence in family problem-solving is necessary for this strategy to be effective. McCubbin,

Olson, and Larsen (1991) point out that families need to "know" they have the strength and power within themselves to solve their own problems and face their problems "head-on."

Gaining Information and Knowledge. Families that are more cognitively based respond to stress by seeking knowledge and information concerning the stressor or potential stressor. This is particularly true in the case of serious or life-threatening health problems. By gaining useful information, this increases the family's feelings of having some control over the situation and reduces their fear of the unknown; it also helps the family to appraise the stressor (its meaning) more accurately and to take the needed action.

Parents who actively cope with parenting by seeking out new information and other resources demonstrate positive results and feelings of coping well with parenting responsibilities (Pearlin & Schooler, 1978). Provision of information is often one of the major ways nurses and other health care professionals intervene with families. Many studies have borne this out. For example, providing information related to self-care and early recognition of children's asthma symptoms resulted in significant reduction in emergency room visits for intervention groups (Alexander, Younger, Cohen, & Crawford, 1988; Fitzpatrick, Coughlin, & Chamberline, 1992); and programs focusing on informing families about asthma medication observed improvement in the child's asthma management after the intervention (Barnett, Fatis, Sonnek, & Torvinen, 1992; Hunter & Bryant, 1994). Assisting families to use the Internet effectively to gain accurate and current information is an increasingly important role for family nurses to play in helping families cope (Stone, 2001).

COMMUNICATION STRATEGIES

Being Open and Honest. As Chapter 10 notes, good communication is vital to family functioning (see this chapter for greater detail). However, it becomes even more crucial during periods of family stress and crisis. Family members who demonstrate greater openness, honesty, clear messages, and feelings and affection are needed at these times (Oliver, 1998; Walsh, 1998). Satir (1998) observed that communication in functional families is direct, open, honest, and clear. Openness refers to being communicative in sharing of ideas and feelings.

Collaborative problem solving, discussed as a cognitive coping strategy, is also a communication coping strategy, which facilitates family coping and adaptation.

Use of Humor and Laughter. Studies of resilience emphasize that humor is invaluable in coping with adversity (Walsh, 1998). Humor not only can bolster spirits, it can also bolster a person's immune system to encourage healing. For families as well, a sense of humor is an important asset. It can contribute to improving the family's attitude toward its problems and health care and to relieving their anxiety and tension. Wooten (1996) asserts that humor and laughter can be viewed as self-care tools to cope with stress whereby the ability to laugh can give one the feeling of power over the situation. Humor and laughter can support a positive and hopeful attitude instead of feelings of helplessness or depression in a stressful situation. "Encouraging care humor—members' laughing with one another—can revitalize families in distress" (Walsh, p. 116). Recent studies have shown that stronger families (those with more strengths and resources) used humor more often than more vulnerable families. Moreover, humor is associated with a positive outlook on family life and social situations (Hickman & Starr, 2001). It should be noted, however, that even though humor is identified here as functional, if it is used repeatedly to mask direct emotional expression and cover up and shun problems, its use is obviously dysfunctional.

EXTERNAL FAMILY COPING STRATEGIES

Although internal coping strategies are crucial, most authors writing in this area today also emphasize the necessity for families under stress to bring in or receive greater external information, tangible goods, services, and support. External family coping strategies of maintaining active community linkages and using social support systems and spiritual strategies are addressed in this section.

COMMUNITY STRATEGY: MAINTAINING ACTIVE LINKAGES WITH THE COMMUNITY. This category refers to a continuing, long-term, and general family coping effort, not one geared to alleviate any one specific stressor. In this case, family members are active participants (as active members or in leadership positions) in clubs, organizations, and

community groups. Recall that one of the assumptions in the Resiliency Model (McCubbin & McCubbin, 1993) is that families contribute to and benefit from an active network of community supports and services. The rationale for the importance of this linkage as a coping effort is grounded in systems theory, which states that any social system must have a movement of information and activity across its boundaries if it is to perform its functions (Whitchurch & Constantine, 1993). Because the family alone cannot serve all its member and group needs without enrichment from other sources, the initiation and promotion of growth-producing relationships within the neighborhood, town, and wider society is essential (Pratt, 1976). Creative community connections can be made to meet family members' needs—such as having elderly family members who lack family contact provide assistance in understaffed child care centers (Walsh, 1998).

USING SOCIAL SUPPORT SYSTEMS. Using social support systems within the family's social network is a very major and crucial external family coping strategy. "Personal ties are a ubiquitous part of life, serving important social, psychological and behavioral functions across the life span" (Singer & Ryff, 2001, p. 73). Linkages with the social world are especially vital to families with health problems (Singer & Ryff; Walsh, 1998). In addition to extended families and the whole network of professional services, experts, and organizations, there exists a great reservoir of potential help: kin, friends, neighbors, employers, fellow employees, class-mates, teachers, and groups with which a family shares common interests, goals, lifestyles, recreational involvements or social identity. Subcultural and refer-ence groups are examples of these types of groups. The family's social networks serve as a third "set of players" for the family wrestling with making suitable arrangements or in need of support, guidance, and advice (see Table 17–4 for coping strategies used by family members in the area of social support).

Definition of Concepts. In this discussion two closely related key terms are social support and social network. **Social network** (Hall & Wellman, 1985) refers to a weblike structure comprising one's relationships. "Families are profoundly influenced by this web of ties and they are active agents in modifying and adapting these communities of personal relationships to meet ever-changing circumstances" (Milardo, 1988, p. 14).

TABLE 17–4

SOCIAL SUPPORT COPING STRATEGIES IDENTIFIED ON F-COPES QUESTIONNAIRE

The following statements from the F-COPES questionnaire were identified by respondents as effective ways they coped as a family in the area of social support.

INFORMAL SOCIAL SUPPORT NETWORKS

Social Support of Extended Family

- Sharing our difficulties with relatives
- Asking relatives how they feel about problems we face
- Seeking advice from relatives

Social Support of Friends

- Seeking encouragement and support from friends
- Sharing concerns with close friends
- Seeking information and advice from persons in other families who have faced the same or similar problems

Social Support of Neighbors

- Asking neighbors for favors and assistance
- Sharing problems with neighbors

Social Support of Self-Help Groups

- Seeking help and support from others with the same con-cerns and problems

FORMAL SOCIAL SUPPORT NETWORKS

Seeking professional counseling

Seeking information from health care providers and other professionals

Source: Partially adapted from McCubbin, Olson, & Larsen (1991).

Within a family's social network are friends and work associates, neighbors, and community networks (church and community groups and agencies); pro-fessional networks (including health care providers and other professionals); self-help groups; and extended and immediate kin (Pilisuk & Parks, 1983).

In contrast, **social support** "focuses on the nature of the interactions taking place within social relation-ships as these are evaluated by the individual" (Roth, 1989, p. 91) and their supportive value, as evaluated by the individual or family (Roth, 1996b). Cohen and Syme (1985) further clarify the difference between social support and social networks: "While social network may be defined as the structure of the relationship, social support is the function of the relationship" (p. 11).

Most researchers see social support as including both tangible instrumental support (transactions in which direct aid or assistance is given) and emotional/informational support (House & Kahn, 1985; Thoits, 1982). House and Kahn (1985) include these two components of social support in their four types of support: instrumental, informational, appraisal, and emotional.

In the social support/social network literature these terms refer to individuals, not family groups. To focus on the aggregate level of analysis—the family—these terms need to be modified.

Family social support refers to the social supports that are perceived by family members to be available/accessible to the family (the social support may or may not be used, but family members perceive that supportive persons are ready to provide aid and assistance if needed). Family social support can either be internal family social support, such as spousal support or sibling support; or external family support—the social supports external to the nuclear family (within the family's social network). A family's social network is simply that social network of the nuclear family itself.

Although there are voluminous descriptions of social support, only a few articles discuss family social support (Friedman, 1985; Kane, C. E., 1988; Roth, 1996b). Kane defines family social support as a process of relationship between the family and its social environment. The three interactional dimensions of family social support are reciprocity (the nature and frequency of reciprocal relations); advice/feedback (the quality/quantity of communication); and emotional involvement (the extent of intimacy and trust) in the social relationships.

Family social support is a process that occurs over the life span, with the nature and type of social support varying in each of the family life cycle stages. For instance, the types and quantity of social support during the stage of marriage (before a young couple have children) is drastically different than the social support types and amount needed when the family is in the last stage of the life cycle. Nevertheless, in all life cycle stages, family social support enables the family to function with versatility and resourcefulness. As such, it promotes family adaptation and health.

Sources of Social Support. According to Caplan (1974) there are three general sources of social support. These consist of spontaneous, informal networks; organized supports not directed by professional health care workers; and organized efforts by health care professionals. Of these, the informal social network (defined above as the family's social network) is viewed as the group providing the greatest amount of help in times of need.

The duration and permanency of support systems vary. Some family support systems are long-term, composed of continuous sets of individuals and groups that assist the family in more general life issues such as developmental tasks and situational crisis (e.g., a loss of family member). Other support systems may be crisis oriented, dealing with specific issues and are short-term in duration (Hupcey & Morse, 1995) such as a group of families who all have a member in the intensive care unit at the same time.

Purpose of Social Support Systems. It is widely accepted that people who are in supportive social environments are generally in better condition than their counterparts without this advantage. More specifically, because social supports are thought to attenuate or buffer the effects of stress as well as enhance an individual's or family's mental health directly, social support is a crucial coping strategy for families to have available in times of stress. Social support also may serve as a preventive strategy to reduce stress and its negative consequences (Roth, 1996b). A case in point is a study of families with young disabled children. In these families, the use of social supports was highly associated with family strengths (Judge, 1998).

Caplan (1976) explains that the family has eight supportive functions including informational support (the family serves as a collector and disseminator of information about the world); appraisal support (the family acts as a feedback guidance system, guides and mediates problem solving, and is a source and validator of member identity); instrumental support (the family is a source of practical and concrete aid); and emotional support (the family serves as a haven for rest and recuperation and contributes to emotional mastery) and boosting the morale of the family.

Emotional support and task-oriented support are the primary coping purposes. Extended family and close friends fulfill the first of these key purposes. They encourage members to communicate freely about their personal difficulties. When the family shares its problems with this support system, it is offered individualized advice and guidance in keeping with the family's traditions and values. The superiority of extended family and close friends over professionals who do not know the family, in terms of giving help and advice, is often expressed by clients (Friedman, 1985). After all, who knows the family better than these supportive individuals? Can health care professionals have the same keen sense of uniqueness of a particular family that close friends and family have? And who has the greater and more lasting interest in the family's welfare and happiness? The answers to these questions speak of the vital nature of informal social networks. The family's informal social network also can provide feedback to the family about its expectations, perceptions, and priorities; this, in turn, can improve the family's communication with outside community supports (Wade, Howell, & Wells, 1994).

The second primary purpose support systems achieve is that of task-oriented assistance that extended family, friends, and neighbors often provide. An important element of this assistance is not only telling family members how to find sources of care and assistance in the community, but also giving direct assistance. In our society, usually only close relatives will provide extensive long-term help. Assistance from extended family also takes on the form of direct help, including continuing and intermittent financial aid, shopping, care of children, physical care of elders, performing household tasks, and practical assistance in times of crisis (Caplan, 1974).

Hence, extended families provide critical social support to nuclear families today. Most adults live in communities in which they maintain one or more contacts with a living parent or other close relative. In the Latino community, extended family ties have remained particularly strong; extended family ties are also stronger in Asian-American and African-American families than with Anglo-American families. In Anglo-American families typically the strongest supportive tie within the extended family network is between mother and daughter. Litwak (1972) referred to the common American form of

family as "the modified extended family," emphasizing that it consists of two or more nuclear families, linked to one another by a web of economic interdependence, mutual aid, and social interaction.

The absence of assistive relationships can generate a sense of vulnerability, especially where use of these assistive relationships (e.g., the extended family) is an important culturally derived way of coping. For instance, Friedman (1985) found that the absence of extended family support was much more disruptive in Latino versus Anglo families that had a child with cancer. Another case in point, where absence of social support made a difference, was in a study by Murata (1995). Murata studied family stress, social support, and sons' behavior problems in 21 low-income inner-city African-American mother-headed families. In her sample, higher family stress, greater behavioral problems of sons, and higher levels of depression were all positively associated with the mothers' perceptions of having lower levels of social support.

The management of chronic illness is an example of a situation in which the type of family form often makes a difference in terms of the availability of adequate social support. Chronic illness often necessitates substantial economic, social, and psychological resources and having an extended family to call upon is often vital to the family management of the chronic illness. Single parent, blended, and dual-worker families may not have the same ability to access needed support during these high demand periods.

Extended kin are reported in research studies to be the preferred source of assistance for long-term crises and more extensive problems such as chronic illness, yet some families do not have these family ties to fall back on (Pilisuk & Parks, 1983). A good example of the lack of the extended family resources are recent immigrant families, many of whom settle here without extended family members being able to join them. If women in the extended family (the caregivers in our society) work, outside assistance typically has to be brought in, in areas where support for the dependent relative is not possible (Brody & Schoonover, 1986).

Inadequate Use of Social Networks. There is both concern and evidence that many people do not seek needed external help (Pearlin & Schooler, 1978). Several factors inhibit families, especially those families with an Anglo-Saxon heritage, from fully utilizing these resources. First, the belief exists that professional services are often best, but because they are very costly and often beyond the family's means, no outside help is sought. Second, while the family is thought of as a place where individuals can let down their defenses and receive and give support and care, some believe that in facing the outside world the family should exhibit independence and self-sufficiency (Walsh, 1998). Despite the fact that family members often yearn to be interdependent, to be supportive of others outside of the family, and to receive support in return, a feeling persists that asking for help or support is a sign of weakness and fallibility. Thus, when a family "fails" to handle its own problems, it should be prepared to turn to paid professionals to resolve the problem.

In the case of family "failure"—that is, where the family is unable to succeed solely through its own means—professional services hopefully are available. The services available to the lower-income family or to those who cannot pay full fees, however, are often inadequate or inaccessible (Wilson et al., 1995). Unfortunately, professionals, rather than encourage self-care and self-control, sometimes rob families of their control over their own problems and, ironically because of their lack of real understanding and knowledge of the family, may very well provide unsatisfactory solutions (Hogue, 1977).

In contrast to closed families who inadequately utilize informal social support, it has been suggested that open families are able to define their boundaries more loosely and flexibly. Because such boundaries allow for a greater exchange of resources, these families are better able to use the family's informal social network.

A family's use of its own informal social network as a resource for assistance will alter the use of professional services in a more appropriate direction, namely, for those specialized or complex needs that cannot be met by the family's social support system or self-care resources.

Mutual Aid or Self-Help Groups.   Self-help or mutual support groups (the terms are used interchangeably) are defined as small groups of peers who come together to share a common problem and through mutual assistance to resolve or ameliorate the problem (Steiger & Lipson, 1985; Trainor, 1983). Even though the extended family and other informal social networks usually serve as primary sources of support for many individuals and families, self-help groups are another very important source of social support

(Pender, 1996). Many family members find that they need to share and seek help from others who have the same concerns. Moreover, their usual support system does not adequately provide for these needs, some of which are more specialized in nature. Hence, participating in a self-help group provides a supportive and/or assistive system to share experiences and coping strategies, to exchange information and access new resources, to seek companionship and make personal experiences more bearable (Maffeo, 1997; Miller & Katz, 1992).

Individuals and families join mutual aid groups as a coping strategy to meet a wide variety of special needs and almost every conceivable problem. Self-help groups include a broad gamut of organizations, established with varied purposes and processes. Increasingly, self-help groups are being formed to assist families (particularly the caregivers) of those afflicted with a particular illness or disability. Examples of these types of groups are Candlelighters for families with childhood cancer, Al-Anon for families of alcoholics, and Adult Children of Alcoholics. Many groups welcome both the person with the identified problem and family members, such as Make Today Count for clients and family members of persons with life-threatening illness, and Mended Hearts for clients and families of people who have had heart surgery.

There is a tremendous growth in urban areas of recovery-oriented self-help groups for family members with addictions (the addicted person and his or her "codependents"). This rapid growth is evidence of the extent to which addictions (alcohol, drugs, eating, gambling) are problems today, as well as the tendency for families to use self-help groups for coping with these growing problems. More recently, support/education groups also have been formed for prevention of such problems. The DARE (drug awareness resistance education) program to prevent drug use in children and adolescents is one example.

Some self-care groups, such as PFLAG (parents and friends of lesbians and gays) provide education, support, and understanding for this often marginalized group; parents of murdered children band together to share their grief and rage; Vietnam veterans' groups are alternative caregiving systems; some groups are an expression of democratic, political ideals, such as the National Organization for Women (NOW); and some are vehicles for promoting individual change, such as

Parents Anonymous and Alcoholics Anonymous. Self-help groups maintain face-to-face, telephone, newsletter, and/or computer support networks among members. Computer support networks, due to the growing and widespread use of the Internet, have become a major type of self-help group.

Research on the outcomes of self-help group participation has indicated that self-help group participation is useful cognitively, through providing beneficial information, attributing meaning to the problem (Shapiro, 1989) and assisting with problem-solving skills; and emotionally, through providing a network of support for expressing feelings and encouraging grief work. Groups enable its members to pool their experiential knowledge and profit from others' experiences. They provide role models of successful adaptation and reinforcement for successful coping. And lastly, by helping other group members, it is found that those individuals help themselves (Trainor, 1983).

SPIRITUAL SUPPORTS. Although most people think of seeking and relying on spiritual support as being an individual coping response, several studies have reported that family members find it a family way of coping too (Burr, Day, & Bahr, 1993; Chesler & Barbarin, 1987; Friedman, 1985; McCubbin, Olson, & Larsen, 1991; Olson et al., 1983). Spiritual and religious beliefs, often the most fundamentally held beliefs of individuals and families, are at the core of all family coping and adaptation (Walsh, 1998; Wright et al., 1996). These beliefs are powerful forces in enhancing family resilience. Core secular and sacred beliefs anchor us in the dizzying vastness of the great unknown we call reality, and thus our beliefs define reality (Taggart, 1994). Spirituality refers to an overarching belief, involving an

> active investment in internal values that bring a sense of meaning, inner wholeness and connection with others. It may involve belief in an ultimate human condition or set of values toward which we strive; a belief in a supreme power; or belief in a holistic oneness with the human community, nature, and the universe (Walsh, 1998, p. 70).

Transcendence and connectedness are typically embedded in definitions of spirituality (O'Neil & Kenny, 1998). These fundamental spiritual beliefs can be embedded in a formal religious structure or outside of formal religion (O'Neil & Kenny).

Numerous studies have shown the clear linkage between spiritual well-being and an individual's or a family's enhanced ability to cope with stress and illness (Humphreys, 2000; O'Neil & Kenny, 1998). Religion is a powerful and pervasive force in shaping families (Miller, 2000). Research on family and individual coping and resilience consistently finds that spiritual supports are critical for supporting a family's belief that they can overcome adversity (Wright et al., 1996). Belief and faith in God and prayer were identified as a very important way families coped with life-threatening stressors in three studies of families (Friedman, 1985; Pravikoff, 1985; Rehm, 1999), while in another large survey of 1,200 white middle- and upper-middle-class Lutherans, use of religious supports were ranked as very helpful in dealing with everyday life problems (Olson and associates, 1983). Burr and associates (1994) also noted that seeking advice/comfort from members of the clergy, as well as becoming more involved in religious activities were very positive spiritual coping ways. And finally, Walsh (1998) notes that some people obtain spiritual connectedness and renewal by being in communion with nature—in walking through the mountains, viewing a sunset, watching the waves hitting the shore.

Spiritually based ways of coping vary significantly cross-culturally. A case in point was a study by Friedman (1985). In this study of 55 families with a child with cancer, half the families were Anglo and half Latino. Latinos, in comparison to Anglos, relied much more heavily on religion as their most important way of handling their child's cancer. Ethnic differences in family coping with respect to the helpfulness of spiritual supports were quite evident.

The use of spiritually based coping may also vary depending on the life cycle of the family (Olson and associates, 1983). For instance, families in the Olson et al. study reported that they used spiritual supports less during the early stages of family life, but used spiritual supports more thereafter.

It is widely agreed that spiritual beliefs offer comfort and meaning to family members and families experiencing suffering and adversity (McLeod & Wright, 2001). These sustaining beliefs help families to endure acute life-threatening experiences, tolerate chronic, long-term strains, and ultimately to maintain the family unit.

🕷DYSFUNCTIONAL FAMILY COPING STRATEGIES

Whereas functional families experiencing stress tend to act in a direction that reduces stress, dysfunctional families tend to use habitual defensive strategies that tend not to dissipate the stress or eliminate or attenuate the stressor (Epstein et al., 1993; White, 1974). Dysfunctional coping strategies temporarily reduce stress, but the stress returns because the underlying stressors are not dealt with. Stress-reduction strategies can be functional or dysfunctional. The difference here is that dysfunctional strategies have long-term deleterious effects on family members and the family.

Families use various specific dysfunctional strategies in attempting to cope with their problems. In most cases these strategies are selected unconsciously, often as responses that their families of origin used in attempting to adapt.

As might be expected, the literature dealing with dysfunctional coping patterns is much more voluminous than the literature dealing with healthy ways of solving familial problems. This literature has been generated primarily by family and other psychotherapists interested in family interaction and process among their troubled clients.

Because no all-encompassing typology or classification of family dysfunctional coping strategies exist in the literature, the classification in Table 17–5 was devised to identify the major types of family dysfunctional coping strategies. It should be noted that each of these dysfunctional family coping strategies is used to reduce family stress or tension.

DENIAL OF FAMILY PROBLEMS

Denial is a defense mechanism used by family members and the family as a whole. On a short-term basis, family denial is often functional, as it allows the family to "buy time" to protect itself while gradually accepting painful events. But in the long run, denial is dysfunctional for a family.

DENIAL AND EMOTIONAL EXPLOITATION OF FAMILY MEMBERS.
There are several overt exploitive ways that families can reduce tension for the family as a group at the emotional expense of one or more family members.

TABLE 17–5

TYPOLOGY OF DYSFUNCTIONAL FAMILY COPING STRATEGIES

DENIAL OF FAMILY PROBLEMS

- Denial with emotional exploitation of family members: Scapegoating, use of threat
- Denial seen through family belief system: Family myth
- Denial seen through communication patterns: Triangling
- Denial maintained through emotional distancing: Pseudomutuality
- Extreme dominance/submission patterns: Authoritarianism

FAMILY DISSOLUTION AND ADDICTIONS

- Loss or abandonment by family member
- Drug and/or alcohol addiction

FAMILY VIOLENCE

- Spouse abuse
- Child abuse
- Sibling abuse
- Elder abuse
- Parent abuse
- Gay/lesbian abuse

Under this broad category of denial and emotional exploitation, two family dysfunctional patterns are briefly discussed: scapegoating and the use of threat.

Scapegoating. Scapegoating is a dysfunctional coping mechanism because although it reduces the tension level of the family system and makes the continuance of family homeostasis possible, it does this at the expense of the emotional health of one of its members—the scapegoat or "the identified patient" (Fischer & Wampler, 1994; McCreery, 1981). The scapegoat's function is to effect a total clearance of the emotional ills that beset the family. This pattern is fairly common in troubled families and can be recognized when a family has achieved unity and cohesiveness while at the same time negatively labeling and stigmatizing one of its members. The identified patient or scapegoat is "selected" to be the focus of the family's difficulties, thus hiding the real problems within the family (e.g., the marital relationship).

How is the scapegoat selected? First, the person must not be someone who has great significance for family survival; thus, children are by far the most common choices for being scapegoats. Children are in a relatively powerless position, cannot separate from family, are pliant to behavioral changes, and can adopt the roles parents assign to them. Usually, the first child is more vulnerable, because in a faulty marriage further strained by the advent of a child, the stressful marital difficulties are quickly displaced onto the first available and "appropriate" object—the first child. A particular child may also be selected because of his or her age or sex, intelligence, health status, developmental stage, resemblance to another family member with negative attributes, or simple availability. Also, a family member who has already been negatively labeled is particularly vulnerable to scapegoating (Klose, 1995; Roberts, 1975).

How does the scapegoating process start and continue? The scapegoating process often starts when families are faced with some unresolved tension that hinders their natural development. For example, when couples are experiencing marital stress they may be having deep-seated fears about the marital relationship but at the same time need to deny that the problem exists (Bell & Vogel, 1968; Hardwick, 1991). The family's problem is perceived to be insoluble and beyond its resources and coping abilities. Because of this, the situation is felt to be a threat or danger to the family's survival and the life goals of its members. Concomitantly, the tension and stress levels rise and throw the family into a state of disequilibrium.

As a result of increased stress level and precarious family stability, the family attempts to reduce tension through the exploitation of one or more of its members. Scapegoating reduces family tensions, because tensions, hostilities, and guilt can be directed toward (or displaced onto) the identified problem member. Furthermore, the scapegoat begins taking on the assigned roles, which started as negative labeling and later became internalized (i.e., into the role of being the scapegoat).

When scapegoating has become an established family adaptive mechanism, family homeostasis is achieved. There is open acknowledgment and labeling of the identified patient or scapegoat. Psychic economy results as group tensions are attenuated by the displacement of anxieties, guilt, and hostility onto an object acceptable to the value system of the family.

Later, when the problem has been further walled off, the individual is reclassified in the family structure as a "problem member" different from all other family members. Although the scapegoat is the victim of hostile projections, because the family is an interactive system, the scapegoat concomitantly works to maintain his or her position as a scapegoat. The parents, to avoid criticism of their treatment of their scapegoated child, define themselves as being victimized by the "problem child" (Hajal, 1990; Vogel & Bell, 1960). Eventually the outside world verifies this differentness by also labeling and stigmatizing the scapegoat. Such labeling maintains the family system's dysfunctionality.

Why would the scapegoat maintain his or her unpleasant role? The answer lies in the self-fulfilling prophecy: a person does what is expected and responds to the reinforcement he or she receives to maintain a certain role. Reinforcement consists of secondary rewards of extra attention, even if negative, and exemption from responsibility.

If the scapegoat leaves the family, is removed by the community, or does not enact the proper role (because of psychiatric treatment), the family will face another homeostatic crisis. At that time the scapegoat may step back into the former role or a new scapegoat may be selected.

In summary, the scapegoating mechanism can be viewed as functional for the family on a short-term basis, in that the scapegoat produces family equilibrium, but it is dysfunctional in the long run for the emotional health of the exploited member and, for that matter, the health of all family members and the family unit.

Use of Threat. Threat is a dysfunctional coping strategy used to keep the family together at the expense of the emotional health of its members. Threat can be viewed as a recurrent family dynamic in some troubled families (Gagne, 1992; Smoyak, 1969). This technique is employed by an extremely enmeshed family to produce and maintain connectedness and discourage members' efforts to individuate and achieve separateness (Walsh, 1998). The purpose of doing so is to ensure the survival of the family.

Gagne (1992) and Smoyak (1969) describe the control technique involved in using threat. The initial basis for needing this means of ensuring family survival is that the family system views its surrounding environment as hostile and threatening. The family feels that the only way it can survive is to stick together as a closed family system. Family preservation then becomes emphasized over the individual needs of its members, and the family value of connectedness becomes elevated to a place of high importance to maintain the family. Minuchin (1974) and Olson (1993) refer to these families as "enmeshed;" Bowen calls them "undifferentiated" families (Miller & Winstead-Fry, 1982).

When one or more family members acts in an autonomous, individualistic fashion, the other family members become threatened by the separating individual's impending breach with the family, and thus take action to bring him or her back into the fold. They may do this by themselves threatening to leave the family system, including threats of suicide or self-destructive acts; by threatening social ostracism, and forbidding reentry into the family; by threatening an aggressive act against the separating individual; or by threatening emotional rejection—withdrawal of affection and support. These maneuvers, if successful, result in the "deviant" family member's retreating from his or her separatist efforts and again conforming to the value of connectedness. Furthermore, once reintegrated, this individual may then take part in sanctioning another member who attempts to individuate.

Forcing deviating members back into the family so that all members espouse connectedness restores the family's equilibrium. However, individuals from such families have severe adjustment problems when they leave the family environment, because they have not learned autonomy, self-directedness, and how to relate effectively with the outside world.

DENIAL SEEN THROUGH FAMILY BELIEF SYSTEM: THE FAMILY MYTH. Through the family's belief system, myths can be created about the family that obscure reality and deny some of the real issues and problems within the group. These problems are perceived as either too painful to be brought out in the open or as unnecessary to discuss because doing so will only make things worse (Byng-Hall, 1988). A family myth refers to beliefs that are generated in response to the unfulfilled wishes and expectations of the family, instead of being based on a rational and objective appraisal of the situation (Battiste, 1975). Family myths are made

up of "a series of fairly well integrated beliefs shared by all family members, concerning each other and their mutual position in the family life, beliefs that go unchallenged by everyone involved, in spite of the reality distortions they may conspicuously imply" (Ferreira, 1963, p. 457).

As wish-fulfillment fantasies, family myths are established early in the family life cycle to serve as a defense against the limitations that the reality of family life imposes. Family myths thus tend to suspend reality. The more myths a family has, the less realistically that family can judge a situation and the fewer the alternatives it has to draw from. For instance, if a myth exists that the mother is "frail" and needs to be protected and helped, then during times of the father's absence, the family's role flexibility is diminished because the mother's ability to function in an instrumental role is stifled by the family myth.

Myths are inner images of the family group, not only the facade that the family holds out to outsiders. Examples of these family myths are: "We all like to do things together"; "We stay married only because of the children"; "Father is the strong one"; "We're a happy family" (Battiste, 1975). Battiste further explains when to suspect that family myths are operating: "When these inner images a family has of itself seem to not ring true to the outside observer, but when the family clings tenaciously to them, one is probably on the track of a family myth" (p. 101).

As previously mentioned, most family myths begin in the early days of the family, when relationships are being formed and cemented. Family myth formulas for togetherness are sought to promote closeness and set limits on possible untoward interpersonal reactions. Circular, repetitive communication patterns, as well as roles, power, and value characteristics develop based on a myth, which in turn, preserves the family unit (Pillari, 1992).

Occasionally, during a time of family crisis, a family myth will be used as a balancing mechanism. As a means of achieving homeostasis, the myth is called into play when a family experiences stress that threatens to disrupt family functioning. Thus, the family myth functions as a defensive mechanism in that it prevents the family from destroying itself by maintaining, and sometimes even increasing, the level of family organization through the establishment of patterns set up as part of the family myth—a myth such as, "When in times of distress, we all help each other" (Peters, 1974).

On the surface, one might say that this "coping" strategy is functional—after all, it provides satisfaction for the family, automatic agreement, a common frame of reference, and stabilizing reassuring rituals. However, it is a dysfunctional adaptive mechanism because it narrows the vision of reality and the choices or alternatives available. Members react to family issues in a stereotypical, nonindividualized way and become limited in their repertoire of responses used to deal with significant issues and life problems. Thus the growth of the family and its members is stifled because, in the presence of family myths, they will not acquire the feelings of confidence and growth that come from meeting life's problems head-on and confronting life's disappointments with a broad range of possible solutions (Battiste, 1975; Price, 1990).

DENIAL SEEN THROUGH COMMUNICATION PATTERNS: TRIANGLING. Another way of reducing stress either on a short-term or long-term basis within the family is through the use of triangling. This concept was developed by Bowen (1976), a noted family therapist, and applies to the reduction of tension in a dyadic relationship by adding a third member, who then absorbs and diffuses the ongoing tension in the dyadic relationship (Goldenberg & Goldenberg, 2000). In other words, bringing in a third member relieves the emotionality between the original two by shifting the tension to the new dyadic member and making one of the initial partners into an "outsider." The balance of forces within triangles is fluid and may shift either frequently or over long periods of time. In periods of very high stress, a system will triangle in more outsiders, again reducing the stress within the family (Goldenberg & Goldenberg; Miller & Winstead-Fry, 1982).

For instance, a husband and wife may be involved in an unsatisfactory, argument-laden relationship that results in neither of their needs being met. Triangling in a third person, one of the couple's children, reduces the marital relationship strain. Both mates begin to focus on the child, although one mate usually develops a dyadic relationship with the child and the other mate becomes the third person—the outsider. This process forces the child to take sides: for one parent and against the other. The parent who forms the close relationship with the child tries to fulfill his or her emotional needs through the parent–child relationship, putting new unrealistic demands on this relationship, so that often the newly formed dyad also becomes strained. As a result, the outside parent may again be triangled in, resulting in a shift back to the marital dyad. "If a triangled person remains in this position for a period of time, it is quite possible he/she will develop some physical or emotional problem as an outlet for his/her anxiety" (Francis & Munjas, 1976, p. 38).

Triangling is included here as a dysfunctional coping strategy because it is a commonly used way in which to reduce interpersonal tension within the family without treating the underlying ills of the situation (Juni, 1995). Although triangling can be looked on as a phenomenon occurring to some extent in all emotionally laden interactions, and especially in dyadic ones under stress, the pervasive use of this stress-reducing mechanism over a long period of time may be considered to be dysfunctional because it does nothing to alleviate the stressor and is injurious to long-term emotional needs of family members.

DENIAL MAINTAINED THROUGH EMOTIONAL DISTANCING: PSEUDOMUTUALITY. Pseudomutuality may be classified as a long-term dysfunctional coping strategy because it maintains family homeostasis at the expense of meeting the family's affective function—that is, recognizing and responding to the socioemotional needs of its members (Schreiber, 1992). The real problem, the inability to foster and maintain intimate, close, affective relationships, is covered up by a facade of solidarity and cohesiveness among family members.

Pseudomutuality has been defined as "a type of relatedness in which there is a preoccupation of family members with a fitting together into formal roles at the expense of individual identity" (Wynne et al., 1958, p. 205). As with the use of threat, individual separateness or individuality is forbidden. Individual differentness or divergence is perceived as leading to disruption of the relationship and must therefore be avoided. The use of threat is sometimes used in families displaying pseudomutuality.

These families may desire closeness and intimacy but are afraid of it and are unable to reach one another on a feeling level. Affective communications are almost nil. Each family member strives for relatedness, but feels that other members block his or her efforts at closeness.

To the outside world these families usually present a picture of family solidarity, because their face-saving needs are great. However, they are able to approach this desire only through much formalized or ritualized action, such as giving gifts, celebrating birthdays, holidays, and so forth.

Pseudomutuality is a long-term coping strategy used by families. It presents a stifling structure that constricts autonomy and diminishes self-esteem of family members.

EXTREME DOMINANCE/SUBMISSION PATTERNS: AUTHORITARIANISM.
Submission to marked domination is included in this section as a long-term dysfunctional coping strategy, because through the submission of family members to a dominant, ruling figure, usually the husband/father, family equilibrium is achieved. This again, is at the emotional expense of the subordinates and less obviously, the dominator. Peace and balance may be accomplished on either a short- or long-term basis, but when these outcomes are forced, anger rages beneath the surface—to be either repressed, with conformity and dependence on the outcome, or expressed as depression, somatization, or acting-out behaviors of defiance, antisocial acts, and destructiveness.

Authoritarianism refers to the tendency to give up one's independence due to feelings of powerlessness and dependency and to fuse self with somebody or something outside one's self in order to acquire the power or strength felt lacking. In an authoritarian family, people renounce their own personal integrity and become part of an unhealthy, submissive-dominance symbiosis. The submissive family members are very dependent on the dominant individual. Life as a whole is felt by the submissive members to be something overwhelming, all-powerful, and uncontrollable. There may also be defiant family members in these types of families who react to the domination with resistance. Interestingly enough, the dominating family member is also dependent on his or her subordinates, because the need for power and control is paramount. Along with having absolute power over the other family members and making them into instruments to be used and exploited, the dominator holds the feeling, "I rule you because I know what's best for you" and "I have done so much for you, now I expect something in return."

As with all the other dysfunctional coping strategies, all members in these families suffer. This authoritarian symbiosis curtails efforts of family members to individuate, grow, and become self-directed and independently proficient in life. Moreover, they learn only two ways of relating to people—either as the ruler or the ruled. With this background they perpetuate these roles in all their other relationships and transmit these interpersonal patterns to the next generation. The types of families that fit into this category are those families that do not negotiate on issues, and where the dominant one seeks no input from others before decisions are made.

Many families are mildly husband-dominated and function very effectively. It is only when this dominance pattern becomes exaggerated that it becomes a dysfunctional way to adapt to life's stressors.

Cultural patterns must be taken into account when examining whether authoritarianism is an adaptive strategy the family is using. For instance, both Hispanic and Asian families are traditionally patriarchal. However, even in these families marked domination is not salubrious and does not follow the social mores of these cultures.

These dysfunctional coping strategies—scapegoating, use of threat, perpetuation of family myths, triangulating, pseudomutuality, and authoritarianism can lead to dysfunctional family adaptation. The family may dissolve through abandonment, separation, or divorce or exhibit psychosomatic illness or patterns of family violence or addiction. Nurses in family health care settings often encounter families in these situations.

FAMILY DISSOLUTION AND ADDICTION

To reduce tension or stress in the family, the family members may physically or psychosocially separate from each other. This includes loss of a family member through abandonment, separation, or divorce, and psychosocial loss of family member through the member's involvement in an addiction (e.g., alcohol, drugs, gambling). Only the addicted family is discussed here.

THE ADDICTED FAMILY.
While most persons recognize that alcohol and drug addictions are diseases, too few recognize them as "family diseases" (Al-Anon Family

Groups, 2000). Addictions of family members are being understood today as family system problems rather than as individual problems. Alcohol and drug use have been found to have an intergenerational pattern. Abusive drinking in young adults has been found to be influenced by dysfunction in the family of origin (Fischer & Wampler, 1994). Steinglass and associates (1987) explained how alcoholism is a family systems problem when they examined the family system of the alcoholic. In *The Alcoholic Family*, they clearly demonstrated the role that alcohol plays in reducing tension in the family and maintaining homeostasis (albeit, short-lived). Their research charts the developmental course of alcohol abuse in the family and explains the role that other family members play as co-dependents or enablers of the problem drinker. The 10-year study upon which *The Alcoholic Family* was based challenges many of the commonly held notions about alcoholism and proposes a family systems approach for treating alcoholism.

The role of drugs in families is similar to that of alcohol—only the substance is changed (it should be noted that many individuals are addicted to more than one drug or to drugs and alcohol). Certainly, the recent growth in drug use, particularly among teenagers aged 12 to 17 years (Savage, 1996), and addictions has had a tremendous influence on the health care system and treatment modes. In addition to professionally led recovery programs, self-help groups following the 12-step program, originally developed to assist alcoholics, are mushrooming nationwide. Many theories have been applied to explain and treat addictions: family systems theory, chemical dependency therapy, child abuse theories, and group therapy theories.

Concerns for family members is evidenced in the literature and in the growth of self-help groups for the adult and teenage children of the alcoholic persons. Adult children of alcoholics have been profoundly affected by growing up in an alcoholic family, as growing up in these types of families places specific and constant strains on all the family members (Al-Anon Family Groups, 2000). Easley and Epstein (1991) often found that adult children of alcoholic parents who used passive appraisal of the problem, attempted to avoid the problem or blame themselves and are more likely to have poorer adult functioning. Steinglass and co-workers (1987) described the tension stress level in alcoholic families as being like the ocean tides—always changing, with continual ups and downs and maneuvers to keep the system afloat.

Researchers have found that binge drinking by the member with alcohol dependency is more stressful for the family than when a member has steady drinking habits. In the case of binge drinking, the family never knows exactly when the member will decide to engage in heavy drinking (i.e., go on a "binge"). Family members are in a constant state of tension, worrying about whether the member's behavior will disrupt family plans, embarrass them in public places, or require intervention (i.e., taking away car keys). Families of steady drinkers, on the other hand, know that the alcoholic member is a continuous abuser of alcohol. Hence, there is less uncertainty and unpredictability in that person's behavior and they grow accustomed to the addicted member not performing family roles and responsibilities (Jacob, 1992).

A third type of family addiction is problem gambling—where one or more family members are addicted to gambling. This is largely a hidden and unrecognized addiction (Pavalko, 1999).

FAMILY VIOLENCE

Extreme uses of threat, scapegoating, and authoritarianism can result in family violence. Family violence is recognized as one of our major public health problems today (Gelles, 2000; Wallace, 1996). The professional literature about child abuse, child neglect, and spouse abuse has mushroomed, and there is concomitant rapid growth of research in this area.

Chapter 11 contains a much more in-depth discussion of family violence, since family violence is viewed as a control and power issue. Please refer to this chapter for a more comprehensive coverage of this important area.

Wallace (1996) defines family violence as "any act or omission by persons who are cohabitating that results in serious injury (physical or emotional harm) to other members of the family" (p. 3). Family or domestic violence is not confined to any one social class. Most domestic violence is directly related to social stress in families (Wallace). The violent family is often one that is socially isolated (Gelles & Maynard, 1987).

There are six types of family violence, depending on who the abuser and victim are. These are: partner abuse, child maltreatment (child abuse and neglect), sibling abuse, elder abuse, parent abuse, and gay and lesbian abuse. The first two types are more numerous and widely acknowledged than the latter four.

Partner Abuse.   Although the use of physical force by one mate against the other (largely husbands against wives) has recently been recognized by the mass media and professionals as a significant social problem (Gelles, 2000; Straus & Gelles, 1990), it has been a commonly used tactic for the handling of frustration and stressors throughout our country's history and, as such, has been societally sanctioned in the past. Even though women are generally victims of spousal abuse, they can also be the perpetrators. Some studies have found that men as victims of spousal abuse are more common than people thought (Wallace, 1996). However, the abuse that women suffer is more common and more severe than the abuse men experience in spousal relationships (Wallace).

Child Maltreatment (Child Abuse and Neglect).   Public awareness of child abuse and neglect did not come about until the 1960s when the diagnosis "battered child syndrome" was coined.

Child abuse can be physical, emotional, or sexual, or a combination of any two or all three. Whereas child abuse includes physical injury, child neglect involves the inadequate giving of essential emotional and physical care to a child. Physical abuse in children has been defined as "any act that results in a nonaccidental physical injury by a person who has care, custody, or control of a child." (Wallace, 1996, p. 29)

Child abuse has been found among both men and women. In fact, research on child abuse often finds that mothers are slightly more likely than fathers to abuse or kill their children (Gelles, 2000). Generally, children who are 5 years old or younger and older teenagers are at greater risk for experiencing abuse by their caretakers. Parental behaviors that are associated with physical abuse in children include life stress, loneliness, depression, anxiety, negative parenting attitudes and practices, poor conflict resolution in the marital relationship, and excessive alcohol use (Milner & Murphy, 1995; Gelles). Even though all children are at risk for being physically abused, children who are difficult to manage or control may be at higher risk (Straus & Gelles, 1990; Wallace, 1996).

Sibling Abuse.   Sibling abuse has been defined as "any form of physical, mental, or sexual abuse inflicted by

one child in a family unit on another" (Wallace, 1996, p. 101). Often, sibling abuse occurs when the older or more powerful sibling has control over another sibling (the victim). In addition, sibling abuse has been found to be higher in families where the child abuse and or spousal abuse occurs (Straus & Gelles, 1990). The types of sibling abuse that have been reported are: physical abuse (e.g., striking, kicking, punching); emotional abuse (e.g., name-calling, ridicule, degradation, exacerbating a fear, and destroying personal possessions); and sexual abuse (Wallace).

Elder Abuse.   Elder abuse and neglect is a problem that has increased nationally (Larsen, 1989) and only recently been studied (Gelles, 2000; Steinmetz, 1987). It is estimated that over two million elderly people are abused each year in the United States (Lynch, 1997).

Wallace (1996) defines elder abuse as "conduct that results in the physical, psychological, or material neglect, harm, or injury to an elder" (p. 221). One study of elder abuse, conducted by Steinmetz (1987), described circumstances under which elderly abuse occurred. Ninety-one percent of her sample were 70 years or older and 85 percent had experienced diminished physical functioning. All elders shared a home with one of their children. Family members' (children and spouses) who are caring for an elderly sick/disabled member and experiencing high levels of stress are much more likely to be involved in elder abuse. Also, caregivers who perceive caregiving tasks to be stressful are more apt to engage in elder abuse (Pagelow, 1984; Steinmetz, 1987).

Parent Abuse.   Another hidden form of abuse is that in which children are old enough to now perpetrate violence against their parents. The children at one point were recipients of violence, and through role modeling learned that the use of violence was a feasible and acceptable mode of expressing anger. In studies that examined this phenomenon, the children were adolescents and usually teenage boys (Gelles, 2000).

Gay and Lesbian Abuse.   Gay and lesbian family violence is believed by some researchers to be at the same rate as among heterosexual couples or around 25 to 35 percent (Wallace, 1996). However, this form of violence has not been widely studied. Gay and lesbian families share emotions and financial responsibility in their relationship that can lead to conflict situations. Generally, both lesbian and gay abusers use similar types of violence on their victims as heterosexual couples.

FACTORS INFLUENCING COPING

GENDER DIFFERENCES IN COPING

Men and women use different coping strategies. Out of the 80 coping strategies examined by Burr and associates (1994), men and women differed significantly in the use of ten coping strategies. Women found it more useful to reach out to others, share their concerns or difficulties with friends and relatives, openly express positive and negative feelings and emotions, and spend time on self-development and hobbies. On the other hand, men tended to use more withdrawal strategies such as trying to keep feelings inside, trying to keep others from knowing how bad things were, and using alcohol more. Other gender research confirms Burr and associates' findings. For instance, Jordan et al. (1991) found that women place greater value on closeness, sharing, and intimacy in their relationships. Research on coping among dual-career men and women across the family life cycle (Schnittger & Bird, 1990) also revealed gender differences in coping. In Schnittger and Bird's study, women, when compared to men, coped significantly more often by delegating, using social support, using cognitive reframing, and limiting their avocational activities such as recreation and hobbies.

SOCIOCULTURAL VARIATIONS IN FAMILY COPING

It is clear that family coping patterns vary across culture and social class. An example of family coping differences in Latino versus Anglo families was previously described under Spiritual Supports. Recall that Latino families relied more heavily on religion (faith in God and prayer) than Anglo families. Another example of family coping differences was found in a recent newspaper article describing how families from non-Western cultures do not have the same need to control and manage their own family members' serious end-of-life decisions (Carey, 2001). Carey, a journalist, asserts that not everyone wants straightforward information (as do Anglo middle-class generally). In many cultures paternalism has a role and some families want health care providers, not the family or the ill family member, to make health care decisions (Carey). This, then, is an example of how the family coping strategy "gaining of information and knowledge" would not be a preferred way of coping with these families.

Social class variations in family coping also exist. For example, more affluent, educated families typically have a greater need to manage and control their own health care and therefore utilize more the family coping strategies of "gaining information and knowledge." Poor families may also feel less confident in their ability to control their own destiny, and in these cases may use "controlling the meaning of the problem by passive appraisal."

IMPACT OF HEALTH ALTERATIONS

As mentioned earlier, the type of coping individuals and families employ is situation specific. With lesser demands placed on a family (e.g., everything is going well and family members are healthy), certain types of long-standing coping patterns may typically prevail, such as "maintaining active linkages with the community." But with the advent of adversity (whether from health stressors or other types of stressors—economic, environmental, etc.), the usual ways of coping are typically not sufficient, and a wider array of family coping strategies are brought forth to address the challenges. These could involve all the different family coping strategies previously described, although certain family coping ways are more widely identified in the literature. These are: greater use of family reliance, use of spiritual supports, gaining of information and knowledge, normalization, and employment of cognitive strategies such as reframing and passive appraisal.

FAMILY ASSESSMENT AREAS

There are both structured, tested family coping scales, which are used for research and clinical practice (see Table 17–6 for a summary of the three most

TABLE 17–6

FAMILY COPING ASSESSMENT TOOLS

Tools	Supporting Theories or Models	Concepts Measured	Administration & Scoring	Advantages	Limitation
CHIP Coping Health Inventory for Parents (McCubbin, McCubbin, Nevin, & Cauble, 1981)	• Social Support Theory • Family Stress Theory • Coping Theory	• Family coping • Parents' coping • Health care communication coping	• 45 Self-report coping behaviors • Hand scored	• Each parent can complete the tool to get a picture of how helpful family's coping strategies are • Can be used as pre- and posttest with intervention program aimed at improving coping	• Not designed to evaluate children's perceptions of helpfulness of family coping.
CICI: PQ Chronicity Impact and Coping Instrument: Parent Questionnaire (Hymovich, 1983)	• Crisis Theory • Coping Theory	• Impact of child's chronic illness • Perceptions of stressors • Coping strategies	• 48 items • Scoring unknown	• Identifies areas relevant for nursing interventions • Can be used to measure outcome of intervention strategies	• Only for family with chronically ill child
F-Copes Family Crisis Oriented Personal Evaluation Scales (McCubbin, Olson, & Larsen, 1987)	• Double ABCX Model	• Available family resources within and external to family in coping with family crisis	• 30-item Likert scale • Easily administered • 3 scales evaluate internal family coping patterns • 5 scales evaluate external family coping patterns	• Identifies family's repertoire of coping behaviors (internal and external)	• Applicable to use with families in crisis.

Sources: Partially adapted from Bowden, Dickey, & Greenberg, (1998) and Touliatos, Perlmutter, & Straus (1990).

widely used tools), as well as the following assessment questions, where information is gathered from family members via interviewing, observation, and reports/data from other sources.

The following questions are relevant to consider when appraising family stressors, strengths, perceptions, coping strategies, and adaptation.

FAMILY STRESSORS, STRENGTHS, AND PERCEPTIONS

1. What stressors (both long and short term) are being experienced by the family? Refer to the Family Inventory of Life Events Scale for examples of significant stressors. Consider environmental and socioeconomic stressors. What is the strength and duration of these stressors?

2. What strengths counterbalance the stressor? Is the family able to handle the usual stresses and strains of daily family life? What resources does the family possess to address the stressors?

3. What is the family's definition of its situation? Is it realistic, hopeful, seen as a challenge? Is the family able to act based on a realistic and objective appraisal of the stressful situation or event? Or is the prime stressor(s) seen as overwhelming, insurmountable, or in some way distorted?

FAMILY COPING STRATEGIES

4. How is the family reacting to the stressors it is experiencing? What coping strategies are being used? What coping strategies has the family employed to deal with what types of problems? Do family members differ in their ways of coping with their present problem? If so, how?

5. To what extent does the family use the following internal coping strategies (see Table 17–3)?
   - Family group reliance
   - Sharing of feelings, thoughts, and activities (strengthening cohesiveness)
   - Role flexibility
   - Normalizing
   - Controlling the meaning of the problem by reframing and passive appraisal

- Joint problem solving
- Gaining of information and knowledge
- Being open and honest in family communication
- Use of humor and laughter

6. To what extent does the family use the following external coping strategies (see Table 17–3)?
   - Maintaining active linkages with the community
   - Using spiritual supports
   - Using social support systems

Informal support systems:
- Does the family have meaningful ties with friends, relatives, neighbors, social groups, and community organizations that provide support and assistance when needed?
- If so, who are they and what is the nature of their relationship?
- Or does the family have little or no contacts with friends, neighbors, relatives, social groups, or community organizations? If so, why? Does the family harbor dissatisfaction or hostility to possible sources of social support?

Hogue (1977) suggests that these types of questions be asked to elicit information on the family's support system. She says that it is more acceptable with clients to move from life events already identified and ask:

"Who helps you with . . . ? If you have any problems about . . . who would you talk to, get help from?" Asking general, then more specific questions is helpful. For example, "Who helped you through retiring from your job?" (general), "Who or what kind of help have you had with the financial concerns most people have when they retire?" (specific). Another useful question is, "Who has helped you through tough situations in the past?" (p. 77).

Formal support systems:
- What health and health-related services and persons assist the family?
- What is the significance and strength of these relationships?

To obtain further social support network information, both the genogram and the ecomap are suggested. Figure 8–1 depicts the family genogram. The

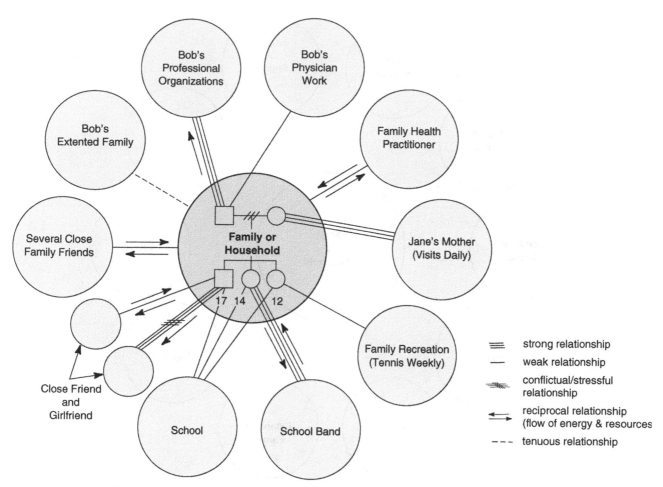

Figure 17–4. Example of family ecomap.

genogram identifies primary kin within the extended family (these are the parents' siblings and parents).

The ecomap graphically depicts the family's relationships and interactions with its immediate external environment. This tool assists the family and family health provider to visualize the family social network and, to some extent, how family members are perceiving and/or receiving social support. Figure 17–5 is a blank ecomap that family members and the nurse may jointly complete.

To complete the ecomap, place the family in the middle circle, and significant people, organizations, and agencies in the outer circles. The nature of the relationships between the family and its various contacts are indicated by lines. Straight lines show strong relationships, dotted lines tenuous relationships, and

slashed lines conflictual/stressful relationships. The wider the straight lines, the stronger the relationship. Arrows may be used to show the direction of energy and resources within a particular relationship (Hartman, 1978; Wright & Leahey, 1994). Figure 17–4 shows an example of an ecomap. By using both the family genogram and family ecomap in assessment, the family nurse is able to get a fuller view of the family and its social network and supports.

7. What dysfunctional coping strategies has the family used or is the family using? Are there signs of any of the dysfunctionalities listed below? If so, record their presence and how extensively they are used.

- Scapegoating.
- Use of threat.

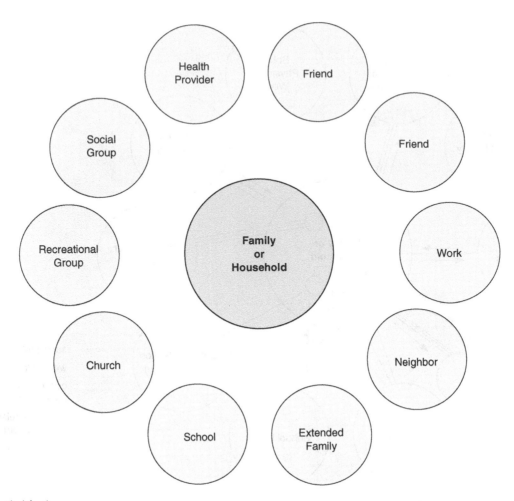

Figure 17-5. Blank family ecomap.

- Family myth.
- Triangling.
- Pseudomutuality.
- Authoritarianism.
- Family dissolution.
- Alcohol and/or drug abuse.
- Family violence (spouse, child, sibling, elder, or gay and lesbian).
- Child neglect.

ADAPTATION

8. How is the family managing or functioning? Are the family stressors/problems being adequately managed by the family? What has the impact of the stressor(s) been on family functioning?

9. Is the family in crisis? (One of the primary tasks of a family nurse is detecting when a family is in crisis.) Is the existing problem(s) part of a chronic inability to solve problems (i.e., is the family crisis-prone)?

TRACKING STRESSORS, COPING, ADAPTATION OVER TIME

When family nurses work with families over time, it is useful to track or monitor how the family is doing relative to stressors, perceptions, coping, and adaptation. Is the family starting to recover, bringing forth helpful coping processes, or is it staying at the same level of adaptation, or showing evidence of diminished adaptation?

✿FAMILY NURSING DIAGNOSES

Many family nurses find the North American Nursing Diagnosis Association (NANDA) nursing diagnoses useful in identifying family problems in the areas of family stress and coping. According to the NANDA classification (NANDA, 2000), there are 12 nursing diagnoses that are germane for family stress, coping, and adaptation problems:

1. Ineffective Family Management of Therapeutic Regimen
2. Readiness for Enhanced Family Coping
3. Compromised Family Coping
4. Disabled Family Coping
5. Risk for Other-Directed Violence
6. Interrupted Family Processes
7. Dysfunctional Family Processes: Alcoholism
8. Dysfunctional Grieving
9. Impaired Home Maintenance
10. Spiritual Distress
11. Risk for Spiritual Distress
12. Readiness for Enhanced Spiritual Well-Being

Each of these family nursing diagnoses have been linked to interventions and outcomes via the work of the Center of Nursing Classification at the University of Iowa. The text *Nursing Diagnoses, Outcomes, and Interventions* (Johnson, Bulechek, Dochterman, Maas, & Moorhead, 2001) describes these linkages. See Table 17–7 for an example of linkages for family coping diagnoses. The coping diagnoses are also summarized in this section.

The diagnosis of *Readiness for Enhanced Family Coping* is family-systems based and is appropriate for situations where the family nurse's goals are to assist families in coping effectively with the family demands/stressors. Families may be successfully adapting at this time, but are anticipating certain future health stressors and in need of information to promote health and prevent problems in the future.

TABLE 17–7

SAMPLE OF LINKAGES BETWEEN FAMILY NURSING DIAGNOSIS, INTERVENTIONS, AND OUTCOMES

NURSING DIAGNOSIS: FAMILY COPING: COMPROMISED, INEFFECTIVE

OUTCOMES	MAJOR INTERVENTIONS
Caregiver—Emotional health	Emotional support
Caregiver—Patient relationship	Respite care
Caregiver stressors	Caregiver support
Family coping	Caregiver support
Family normalization	Coping enhancement
	Family involvement promotion
	Family mobilization
	Family process maintenance
	Family support
	Normalization promotion

Abbreviated and adapted from Johnson et al. (2001). Suggested and optional interventions (in greater detail) are identified on pp. 115–117 of this text.

The diagnosis of *Compromised Family Coping* is appropriate to use when the family assessment data show that the family is employing coping strategies that are ineffective for resolving present stressors and when family member(s) are providing insufficient, ineffective, or compromised support to the sick member. Because of the use of ineffective coping strategies, its functioning or adaptation is compromised.

The diagnosis of *Disabled Family Coping* is used "when the behavior of one or more family members incapacitates the family or its members to therapeutically adapt to the existing health challenge" (McFarland & McFarlane, 1993, p. 943). Although the generation and description of this diagnosis was guided by family systems theory, the above definition is ambiguous in terms of how family coping is used. Family coping in this text refers to the coping behaviors or responses made by a subsystem, such as parent–child or spousal subsystem, or the family as a whole—indicating an interactional level. Hence, the use of this diagnosis for family coping diagnoses should not include individual coping or adaptive responses; the outcome "disabling" would then refer to the family outcome(s).

Although *Disabled Family Coping* can be long or short term, the family is having greater difficulties adapting when this diagnosis is used than when the previous diagnosis is used (NANDA, 2000). Family health and growth are adversely affected here.

In reviewing the diagnosis of *Risk for Other-Directed Violence*, the diagnosis, defining characteristics, and suggested interventions are focused on the potentially violent individual. Using a family-centered approach, each of these areas needs to be broadened to incorporate the family system and the family members at risk.

🐝 FAMILY NURSING INTERVENTIONS

Because of the breadth of coverage in this chapter, family nursing interventions are outlined here. See Chapter 7 for a more detailed description of family nursing interventions. Interventions are based on family assessment data pertaining to family stressors, perceptions of stressors, family strengths, coping, and adaptation, as outlined in the assessment section, as well as on the identified family nursing diagnoses.

ASSISTING FAMILY TO DECREASE RISK FACTORS

Family nurses can, using a preventive perspective, counsel families about the need to reduce exposure to or overload of stress. In addition, it is important to provide anticipatory teaching. In this regard, family nurses can assist families by helping them to anticipate and prepare for threatening situations. One way of helping them anticipate what may happen is by giving them information about anticipated events (Walsh, 1998).

ASSISTING FAMILIES AT RISK TO COPE

These guidelines are recommended:

- **Encourage all family members to be involved,** especially fathers, and help them form a working alliance when needed. Ways to involve family members include: (1) encouraging care by family members during hospitalization; (2) including family members, along with the patient, to be involved in health care decisions, (3) encouraging family members to maintain close family relationships; (4) teaching caregivers; (5) encouraging respite for primary caregivers by having other family members pitch in; and (6) encouraging family members to share their life stories with each other; this helps family members gain a greater compassion and empathy for each other.

- **Mobilize families** by helping families to recognize, identify, and utilize family strengths and resources to positively influence sick family member's health (Johnson et al., 2001).

- **Praise family efforts and accomplishments.** Support adaptive coping strategies that families and family members are using to reduce family tension, control the meaning of the stressor(s), and eliminate stressor(s). Provide positive feedback and commendations to family members regarding their coping and shared efforts to problem solve.

- **Based on a recognition and respect for a family's values, interests, and goals, support families.** Johnson et al., (2001) lists many general ways family-oriented nurses can do this. Some of the most relevant of their suggestions are:

- Fostering realistic hope
- Listening to family members relative to their perceptions, feelings, concerns, and interests
- Facilitating communication between family members so that they are more open, honest, and sharing of their thoughts and feelings with each other
- Orienting family members to health care settings and systems
- Providing necessary information to assist families to make informed health care decisions
- Advocating for families
- Introducing family members to other families undergoing similar problems/experiences
- Arranging/referring families to self-care, support groups
- Provide families with literature and Internet resources/references

- **Teach families effective ways of coping** to promote and maintain family health (see Table 17–7). Psychoeducational programs may be very useful programs to educate families. These are programs focused on both the illness and family coping. These programs recognize not only the need for families to gain the health knowledge needed for care, but also the psychosocial aspects of care and family concerns (Campbell, 2000).

- **Encourage families to normalize their family life and family distress** as much as possible. Normalization promotion activities include encouraging family members to maintain family habits, rituals, and routines, assisting them to alter a prescribed treatment regimen to fit the family's normal schedule (Knafl, Deatrick, & Kirby, 2001) and helping them see that their distress and reactions to adversity are "normal," common, and predictable and that they are not deficient for not solving their problems themselves (Walsh, 1998).

- **Help families receive the spiritual support they need.** "Nurses now recognize spiritual needs and value spiritual care" (O'Neal & Kenny, 1998, p. 277) as a way of helping family members cope with adversity and their daily life challenges. The ways this is done varies; these suggestions are mentioned in studies addressing nursing interventions to help clients meet their spiritual needs: listening, "presence," having therapeutic

conversations, support of individual and family religious practices, fostering integrity within people, fostering holistic care, promoting interpersonal bonding, respecting and enhancing personal and familial searches for meaning, and providing spiritual resources for families (Clark & Heidenreich, 1995; Johnson et al., 2001; McLeod & Wright, 2001; O'Neal & Kenny).

- **Help families reframe and relabel their problem situation** in order to cast a more positive light and to attenuate families' constraining views and responses (Wright, Watson, & Bell, 1996; Walsh, 1998). Reframing can alter destructive, blaming processes, can overcome impediments to change, and can generate hope. Problems can be depathologized and seen as normative, expected, and transitional stressors (Walsh). This intervention has become a very significant and effective one in helping families cope and grow through their experiences. Wright, Watson, and Bell, leaders in family nursing, have written an entire book on how health professionals can assist families by challenging their constraining beliefs and thus helping them to alter and replace those beliefs with beliefs that facilitate positive change and alleviate family suffering.

- **Refer crisis-prone families.** For families that are employing ineffective family coping strategies, the family nurse should differentiate between whether the family is chronically dysfunctional (in that case referral for more long-term therapy is indicated) or in acute crisis but functioning within normal limits until the onset of the stressor(s). In this case, family crisis intervention principles and an empowerment perspective are suggested as guides to family interventions.

- **Help families enhance and utilize their social support systems.** Social support system interventions are designed to extend or enhance functioning of clients' informal and formal social networks (Stewart, 1993). Of course, interventions should be matched to meet the assessed need. In formulating interventions, Stewart advises nurses to consider the desired intensity and type of support needed and desired, the client's other personal resources, the timing of the intervention, the potential drain of resources in support networks, and the appropriate target or level of intervention (i.e., the client, the informal social system, particular key support persons, and groups or community organizations).

Social support can be mobilized by: (a) reinforcing families' positive patterns of help seeking; (b) helping family members improve the quality of support received by the family's social network. This can be done by helping family members to reanchor themselves into a network that is more responsive to their present emotional needs or reorient themselves to sectors of their network containing more appropriate psychosocial resources; (c) helping them explore and access untapped social support systems: and (d) fostering affiliation among families who face similar stressful circumstances (use of self-help groups).

USE OF SELF-HELP GROUPS. Nurses are increasingly aware of the value of self-help groups for family members who need support to overcome or cope with a stress-

ful life experience. The following interventions in this particular area can be most facilitative to families:

- Seeking information about groups offering assistance to individuals and families.
- Collaborating with such groups.
- Understanding how these groups enhance and complement professional services.
- Referring family members and families to appropriate groups.
- Creating new groups or encouraging others to do so when there is a lack of a needed self-help group (Trainor, 1983).
- Counseling groups of family members who have formed support groups to help them with particular problems they are facing.

SOCIAL NETWORK FAMILY THERAPY. In family therapy, the social network family therapy approach is an innova-

TABLE 17–8

INTERVENTIONS FOCUSED ON ENHANCING FAMILY'S SOCIAL SUPPORT SYSTEM

TARGET	INTERVENTION STRATEGIES
Particular significant support persons (e.g., daughter, spouse)	Contacting person(s) and encouraging them to assist if possible. Informing significant support person(s) of need. Providing resources or information on how to seek resources. Correcting inaccurate/inhibiting beliefs about client's need.
Informal social support system (e.g., extended family, neighbors, friends, social groups/ organizations)	Informing persons/groups of need. Bringing informal social system members together to provide support collectively. Fostering social network's communication with each other. Referring client/family to self-help group or community organization.
Formal social support system (e.g., health, transportation, welfare, educational, recreational)	Initiating referral to community agency to provide outside assistance and services, e.g., transportation, home health care. Communicating with agency regarding client's need to share information about client with agency and about agency with client; also to coordinate services.
Client(s): family or family members	Targeting negative attitudes and beliefs regarding seeking assistance from others. Helping families identify their strengths and vulnerabilities. Helping families establish new supportive relationships and maintain old relationships. Enhancing support appraisal for families prone to devalue ties. Reinforcing positive efforts family make to reach out for support.

Source: Pearson (1990); Roth (1996); Stewart (1993); Voux (1990).

tive strategy aimed at mobilizing family social support for family in distress. Here the family's social network is mobilized—that network of people with whom the family in crises has a social relationship (extended family, friends, neighbors, and other associates). Healing is believed to come from within this social unit as it is brought together to support the distressed family (Jones, 1980). Social network family therapy takes place in the home setting with the family and its large social network, which is assembled to create a nurturing and healthy social matrix.

See Table 17–8 for a listing of social support interventions.

FAMILY CRISIS INTERVENTION PRINCIPLES.
Family crisis intervention extends crisis intervention theory by incorporating a family focus. Very briefly, family crisis intervention is a short-term practice model for families experiencing crisis or stress to help them cope with present stressor(s) and future stressor(s). It involves many of the ideas already espoused but emphasizes the following practice guidelines. The crisis intervenor: (a) defines the precipitating stressor event and hazardous life events, (b) assesses the family's interpretation of the event(s), (c) assesses the family's resources and methods for coping with stressors, and (d) assesses the family's state of functioning. Based on this model, a supportive yet focused problem-solving approach is used to assist the family to mobilize resources (its own and community resources) to resolve the present crisis, and to learn how to prevent and cope with future stressful experiences (Kus, 1992). Families are coached to help them make sense of the crisis and its meaning and to help them feel confident that they will receive needed help. Another intervention deals with helping families reframe their situation and to look back at how they have coped with previous crises for lessons on how to cope with the present crisis. In addition, families are provided with referrals and help obtaining resources.

EMPOWERING FAMILIES.
Boss (1988) and Figley (1989, 1995), family researchers and clinicians, describe an approach involved with empowering families. Their suggestions extend and enrich the family crisis intervention model. Boss points out that for families that

have been traumatized or victimized, learned helplessness is a common family reaction. If helplessness can be learned, she reasons, then helplessness can be unlearned. Empowerment comes when family members regain their self-esteem and self-confidence and take pride in the family as a team, regaining control over what happens to the family collectively and individually, making sense out of what happened by finding some meaning to the problem(s), and sharing with other family members while actively attempting to prevent the problem or event from reoccurring. Reassuring families that their reactions to traumatic situations are common and predictable, thereby "normalizing" their situation, is an effective supportive technique (Figley, 1989).

Figley implies that empowering families is as much a philosophical attitude toward working with traumatized families as it is engaging in certain specified activities. When he views and treats troubled families, his approach is tempered by his genuine respect for the natural resourcefulness and strengths of families. In the following passage, he explains this perspective:

> I try to empower the family by creating the kind of intervention context that results in the resolution of the traumatizing experience but, just as importantly, that results in the family's giving themselves most of the credit for the accomplishment. Moreover, this approach makes the family feel more confident to face any future traumatic experience equipped with the necessary information, skills, and problem-solving methods. (p. 42)

PROTECTING FAMILY MEMBERS WHO ARE AT RISK FOR VIOLENCE

This goal may be accomplished by:

1. Recognizing and reporting child abuse.

2. Supporting and referring abused spouses, elders, siblings, parents, gays and lesbians, the abuser, and the family unit.

3. Coordinating care to families and family members, working collaboratively with other health and welfare workers (Gilliss et al., 1989).

REFERRING FAMILIES THAT EXHIBIT MORE COMPLEX FAMILY COPING PROBLEMS AND DYSFUNCTION

When family stress and coping problems of families are beyond the services the family nurse can provide, referral and follow-up of ongoing family counseling or therapy is often indicated. Referral to a counselor who uses a family systems approach is often quite helpful.

❧SUMMARY

- Many evolutionary and revolutionary changes continue to take place in society and correspondingly in families over time. How families cope with stressful changes differs, although it is believed that generally American families are resourceful and resilient in their adaptation to change. Nevertheless, a wide range of responses occur when adversity strikes.

- Some families adapt very well to stressors and strains by changing patterns of functioning, using resources and helpful coping strategies to manage the stress. These families successfully fulfill their family functions and have satisfactory relationships with the community.

- Other families utilize harmful or dysfunctional coping strategies that may only temporarily reduce stress. Outcomes for these families may include family violence, family dissolution, and addictions.

- Family nurses and other health care professionals who are in contact with families in both institutional and community settings are in key positions to assess family stressors, perceptions, strengths, coping, and adaptation, and intervene with these families to bring about more optimal family adaptation.

- The basic stress and coping concepts are defined in this chapter and consist of definitions of stressors, family member/family perceptions, stress, coping, family coping, family crisis, adaptation, family adaptation, family coherence, and family resilience.

- There are three phases of a family's experience with a stressful situation: the antestress period, the actual stress period, and the poststress period. Assessment and intervention strategies may differ depending on the phase of stress the family is in.

- Two family stress theories are described: the ABCX Model, which emphasizes the precrisis stage, and the Resiliency Model, which emphasizes the postcrisis period and is strength based. Both of these models are useful guides for nurses working with families managing stressful situations.

- Families experiencing adversity are dealing with not one stressor, but a pileup of stressors stemming from multiple factors, which accumulate over time. One instrument assessing the pileup of family stressors is discussed: the Family Inventory of Life Events (FILE).

- Families and family members use a wide array of family coping strategies to address stressful situations. Behavioral, cognitive, and emotional coping strategies are identified and discussed relative to their impact on family functioning. Functional family coping strategies are divided into internal and external family coping strategies, depending on whether the strategies are intrafamilial or extrafamilial.

- Internal family coping strategies consist of (a) relationship strategies: family group reliance, greater sharing together—strengthening of family cohesion, and role flexibility; (b) cognitive strategies: normalizing, controlling the meaning of the problem by reframing and passive appraisal, joint problem-solving, and gaining information and knowledge; and (c) communication strategies: being honest and open and use of humor and laughter.

- External family coping strategies consist of maintaining active community linkages, using social support systems and seeking spiritual supports.

- Using social systems is particularly vital when families lack the necessary internal resources and coping abilities. Sources of social support, the purposes of social support systems, the issue of inadequate use of social support by families, and the importance of mutual aid or self-help groups are discussed.

- In addition to the internal and external family coping strategies, the mental health literature identifies dysfunctional family coping strategies. The following strategies families use to deal with stress and adversity are injurious to either or both family members and the family on a long-term, consistent basis: (a) denial of family problems—scapegoating, use of threat, family myth, triangling, pseudomutuality, and authoritarianism; (b) family dissolution and addiction; and (c) family violence—partner abuse, child maltreatment, sibling abuse, elder abuse, and gay and lesbian abuse.

- Men and women use different coping strategies. One important difference is that women tend to reach out to others, while men use more withdrawal strategies.

- Sociocultural variations in family coping also exist. Social class differences affect families in terms of the availability of coping resources. Cross-cultural coping variation is pervasive among families and often is manifested as a difference in the extent to which families and family members rely on certain types of coping to help them with crises.

- Family coping strategies are situation-specific. Health alterations, viewed as "family diseases," bring forth demands for coping that may not be used in everyday life. Certain coping strategies are widely cited as very helpful here (e.g., social support, spiritual support, and gaining information and knowledge regarding the "family disease").

- To complete an assessment of family stress and coping, specific questions are posed relative to each of the major concepts in this area. These questions focus on family stressors, strengths, and perceptions, family coping (internal, external, and dysfunctional coping strategies), and family adaptation.

- Six NANDA family nursing diagnoses are applicable to the family stress, coping, and adaptation areas.

- Family nursing interventions in this area are many and diverse. They involve preventive approaches (risk reduction), as well as how to help high-risk families to cope. The interventions cover increasing family involvement, mobilizing the family, supporting adaptive coping strategies, teaching families ways of coping effectively, normalization promotion, helping families reframe and relabel their problems, helping families receive spiritual support, helping families use and mobilize their social support systems, and intervening using family crisis intervention and empowerment principles. Family nursing interventions also include protecting family members at risk for family violence, referring families who have complex, long-standing problems, and educating families.

✎ FAMILY VIGNETTE: THE NICHOLS FAMILY

Mrs. Ruby Nichols, a 34-year-old white obese woman, came to the mental health clinic because, she said, "I just don't know what to do." She was crying hysterically and unable to respond to further questioning. After remaining with her for an hour, the nurse was able to elicit that her 5-year-old foster daughter was being removed from her home by protective services. Welfare funds, her only support for herself, her unemployed husband, and their five children, were being terminated in a week, leaving her unable to pay the bills or buy enough food for her family. Although Mrs. Nichols was still tearful and depressed, she was able to be driven home by a community worker.

(continued)

The following day the nurse made a visit to the Nichols's home. Mrs. Nichols related the following history.

Ruby and John Nichols had been married 15 years. Four children were born of the marriage: Priscilla, 13; Cindy, 10; John Jr., 6; and Lisa, 4. They also had a foster daughter, Ann, age 5. The couple had known each other a year before their marriage in their home town of Smithfield, Louisiana. John was an unskilled laborer, but had always managed to be employed. Ruby had attended business school prior to the marriage and was employed as a bookkeeper until the first child was born. She described her early marriage as fine except for moving so many times, caused by John's "meddling mother." The family would move to get away from his mother, but she would always manage to locate them and appear on the scene. "We were a healthy, happy family and everything was fine as long as John's mother stayed away." Ruby related that this source of conflict between herself and John was resolved each time by a move on their part. However, she and John never really discussed her mother-in-law problems according to Ruby. Following each new move, Ruby would join clubs and organizations to make new friends and John's work provided a similar opportunity for him. John also spent several evenings a week in the local bar, "shooting the bull" with the boys from work.

The last move was six months ago. After two months John lost his job and was unable to find another. This resulted in the family going on welfare, which Ruby and John felt ashamed of, as they had always prided themselves on paying their own bills. Shortly after this, John's mother found the family and moved into town. When she came to visit, a bitter argument ensued regarding John's mother and since then John had been staying away from home and drinking a lot. Moreover, three months ago Ruby had abdominal surgery, which was followed by complications and a prolonged hospitalization period. During her absence from home, the role of mother was assumed by Priscilla, who managed well with the help from the next door neighbor, Mrs. Law.

Ruby was released from the hospital three weeks ago as sufficiently recovered to stay at home. When she got home she perceived that the children had functioned "very well" in her absence; in fact, she felt that they did not need her and even seemed to resent her. John remained away most of the time and was minimally involved in family life during her hospitalization, as well as presently.

A week ago she learned of the court's decision to remove Ann from the home and the termination of welfare funds. Ruby felt herself becoming less and less able to manage and admitted to depression and suicidal thoughts. However, her concern for her children prevented her from doing anything self-destructive. The next-door neighbor, Mrs. Law, realizing the gravity of the family's situation, told Ruby to go to the mental health clinic for help.

Subsequent visits to the family revealed that the children were having problems and that Ruby had difficulties relating to their problematic behaviors. It was observed that the children and parents did not discuss these problems or their concerns with each other, and that there was no movement toward sharing their feelings about Ann's leaving, the mother-in-law's disruptive influence, or Ruby's health problems.

Priscilla, age 13, seemed to resent Ruby's return, because it meant the loss of her mothering role. She and her mother have engaged in frequent arguments over the discipline of the younger children, what they should wear, and how they should act. The arguments usually ended with Priscilla leaving the house for long periods of time without telling Ruby where she was. This caused Ruby to worry. Priscilla was not interested in school, her main interest being to grow up as quickly as possible and emulate her mother. She also wanted desperately to be independent and make her own decisions in life. Ruby had "weaned" Priscilla early in terms of her being self-sufficient at home: from age 6 on, Priscilla was caring for her younger siblings and helping her mother out in the home.

Cindy, age 10, seemed unaffected by the situation. She was quite involved with her school activities and Campfire Girls and spent much time in these activities and at her friends' homes. Priscilla and Cindy evidently have a closer sibling relationship than the other siblings do. Cindy tells "all her secrets" to Priscilla when she is upset, worried, or needs someone to talk to.

John Jr., a first grader, was refusing to go to school. Every morning it was now a struggle to get him off to school. He would cry and hang on to his mother. His teacher reported poor school work and lack of attentiveness when he was present.

Lisa, age 4, displayed similar clinging behaviors to those of John Jr. She seemed frightened when mother left the home and was wetting the bed again after having no problems in this area for two years. Both John Jr. and Lisa frequently questioned their mother about the recent absence of Ann. They asked if Ann went away because she was "bad."

On the third contact between the family (the parents) and the nurse at the mental health clinic, the nurse asked the parents to describe each child, what he or she was like, and what personal needs or problems they were trying to assist their children with at that time. It was noted that specific information on each child was difficult to obtain. For instance, these general statements were made: "Oh, he (she) is just the average 6-year-old (or whatever age applied)," or "Priscilla's just like all other teenagers, wanting her way all the time," or "I treat all my children the same, regardless." They were able to recognize, though, Priscilla's need to care for her younger siblings and to be independent, but were not open to her staying away from the family very much, or developing a set of friends outside the family with whom she might have frequent social contact.

The mother also recognized that Lisa was very attached to and dependent on her, and needed reassurance that mother would be back when she left home. Additionally, both parents thought Ann's leaving was threatening to the younger children, who might think this might happen to them if they misbehaved. Ruby was trying to spend more time with Lisa to help her with her fears over the mother's separation and Ann's leaving. John showed interest in "comforting" and being involved with Lisa also, since Lisa always responded "in such a cute, loving way to her daddy," according to the mother.

Both parents are able to show affection and warmth to the younger children (John Jr. and Lisa), but do not feel that it is appropriate to be so "physical" when they get older. It was noted that the parents were not physically affectionate to each other and seemed emotionally distant during the interviews. Ruby says that they have never shared their personal concerns with each other much. "It takes another woman to understand my feelings. I used to confide in Priscilla a lot, but since she is upset with me, I haven't been able to talk with her."

■ STUDY QUESTIONS

Read the Family Vignette and answer the related questions.

1. What short- and long-term stressors are impinging on the family? What strengths counterbalance these stressors?

2. Is the family able to act based on a realistic and objective appraisal or perception of the situation?

3. How is the family reacting to stressful situations? Both functional and dysfunctional coping strategies should be described.

4. Estimate the family's level of adaptation. How well do you think the family is functioning?

5. Based on your assessment of this family, state one family nursing diagnosis in the area of family stress and coping.

6. Propose two family nursing interventions that address the identified family nursing diagnosis.

Answer the following questions.

7. Family coping is vitally important because (select the best answer):
   a. It is the mechanism through which family functions are made possible.
   b. It provides opportunities for family members to learn.
   c. It leads to problem solving and mastery over family issues and stresses.
   d. It either eliminates stressors or leads to stress-reduction activities.

8. Changes in family life in North America come from within and outside the family. Major recent changes in families include (select all correct answers):
   a. Families are becoming more isolated from kin.
   b. There is greater diversity of family forms.
   c. Marriage rates have declined, especially in early 20s age group.
   d. Divorce rates are dropping dramatically.
   e. Poverty has increased significantly among working poor families.

9. Match the definitions in the right-hand column with the concepts and terms in the left-hand column.

Concepts/Terms	**Definitions**
a. Crisis	1. A family's dispositional worldview.
b. Family coherence	2. Active, effective adaptive efforts.
c. Family resilience	3. The precipitating or initiating events or agents that generate stress.
d. Stressors	4. A process of restructuring to adjust to change.
e. Stress	5. The strain, disequilibrium produced by threat or actual existence of stressors.
f. Adaptation	6. Positive adaptational processes in families.
g. Coping	7. In the presence of the stress and stressors, the family's failure in use of effective coping strategies.

Are the following statements true or false?

10. In the antestress period, anticipatory guidance would be contraindicated.

11. Defensive tactics are often necessary adaptive responses during the actual stress period.

12. During the poststress period, coping tactics consist of strategies to return the family to a homeostatic state.

Answer the following questions.

13. McCubbin, Patterson, and Wilson (1983) developed the Family Inventory of Life Events and Changes Scale (FILE) to (select the best answer):

    a. Identify positive correlation between stressors and stress.
    b. Assess pile-up of life events and strains experienced by families.
    c. Identify cause-and-effect relationships between number of life change events and presence of illness.
    d. Assess correlation between stress and wellness.

14. In the Resiliency Model an indicator of family adaptation is (select the best answer):

    a. Family is experiencing no stress.
    b. Family has not gone into crisis.
    c. There is a "fit" between the family and the community.
    d. Family members do not have a chronic illness.

15. When families experience adversity, there is no single stressor involved. A pileup of stressors results. In the Family Inventory of Life Events (FILE) scale, which of these events generally generate stress?

    a. Change in father's employment
    b. Marriage of one of the children in family
    c. Birth of baby
    d. Death of child
    e. Divorce of parents

16. Select four functional family coping strategies (two internal coping resources and two external coping strategies) and describe each of these briefly.

17. Select four dysfunctional family coping strategies and describe each of these briefly.

18. Identify two social support system interventions family nurses employ to help families cope:

    a. Provide direct assistance.
    b. Foster social network's communication with each other.
    c. Replace professional services.
    d. Refer family to self-help group.

19. Indicate which of the following family coping strategies are functional (F) or dysfunctional (D) or which could be either (E), depending on the situation.

    a. Family group reliance
    b. Scapegoating

    c. Pseudomutuality

    d. Sense of humor

    e. Increased linkage with community

    f. Spouse violence

    g. Child neglect

    h. Triangling

    i. Social support systems

    j. Seeking of information

    k. Role flexibility

    l. Controlling the meaning of the problem by reframing

20. The purpose(s) for families utilizing threat as a control mechanism is (are) to:

    a. Maintain authoritarian structure within the family.

    b. Maintain or reinstate connectedness within the family.

    c. Ensure the survival of the family group.

    d. Decrease family members' attempts to behave in an autonomous, individualistic manner.

21. Frank Stanton, 89, has advanced Alzheimer's disease and is living with his son, 62, and his son's girlfriend, age 50. Both his son and son's girlfriend work full time. Frank hasn't left the house in months, but just recently was seen wandering the neighborhood. A neighbor reported her observations to the police. What family coping problem may be present?

CULTURAL DIVERSITY AMONG FAMILIES

In the last section of this book, a description of families from America's three largest minorities or ethnic groups is presented, in order to show the significance of cultural variation in family life. After a brief overview of each of the ethnic groups, the Friedman Family Assessment Model (discussed in Chapters 7–17 and Appendices A and B) is used as a framework for describing the family groups. Chapter 8 provides the foundational sociocultural content for these chapters.

THE LATINO FAMILY

❧ LEARNING OBJECTIVES

1. Identify what peoples constitute Latinos and their respective percentages of all Latinos.

2. Discuss why the Latino family has not integrated into the mainstream of American society to the extent that other ethnic groups have.

3. Explain why the rate and nature of acculturation of Latinos is both complex and multifaceted.

4. Describe how the Latino population differs socioeconomically from the general U.S. population.

5. Compare American core values with traditional Latino values.

6. Describe briefly how the traditional role and power structure of the Latino family is changing.

7. Describe two general socialization patterns among Latino families.

8. Identify the most important structural change occurring in Latino families today.

9. Recognize the functions and primary role of these folk healers: yerbero, curandero, santeria, espiritualisto, and brujo.
10. Recall several common Latino folk illnesses.

11. Identify two central culturally derived family coping patterns of Latinos.
12. From the family vignette, explain three health care practice implications based on Latino culturally patterned beliefs and practices.

Family nurses are increasingly aware of the need for a transcultural and pluralistic perspective in working with diverse ethnic, religious, and cultural groups in American society (Friedman, 1990). There is both a demographic imperative and a practice imperative for having a good understanding of the Latino family.* The sheer numerical growth of this group in the United States and the fact that Latino family members tend to have more frequent and serious health problems provide additional rationale for becoming knowledgeable about the Latino family and its family life patterns.

✎ LATINO DEMOGRAPHIC PATTERNS

Latinos are persons residing in the United States whose ancestries are from the 22 Latin American countries in the Western Hemisphere, most notably Mexico, Cuba, Puerto Rico, and Central and South America (Suarez & Ramirez, 1999). Eleven percent of the U.S. population is now Latino (U.S. Bureau of the Census, 2000b). Recent census projections report that the Hispanic-American population is rising sharply and will after the turn of the century become the largest ethnic minority group in the United States (Larmer, 1999), and with more than one third of the Latino population being under 18 and a high birth rate, the population boom is just beginning. Mexican-Americans are the largest ethnic group within the larger Latino population in the United States (58.5 percent). Puerto Ricans constitute 9.6 percent of Hispanic-Americans, while Cubans make up 3.5 percent and South and Central Americans constitute 8.6 percent of Hispanic-Americans. According to the 2000 census, almost 18 percent of Latinos are classified as "other," many of whom have a mixed Latino ethnic heritage (McDonnell, 2001; U.S. Bureau of the Census).

According to data from the Immigration and Naturalization Service, more than at any time since World War I the U.S. population increase is driven by immigration, both legal and illegal. Immigrants—7 to 9 million over the 1990–2000 decade—are largely from Mexico and Asia (Alonso-Zaldiver & Fields, 2001).

The rapid and large growth in the Hispanic-American population is confirmed by historical trends (U.S. Bureau of the Census, 1990, 2000). In 1960, there were 3.1 million Latinos; in 1970, 9.1 million; in 1980, 14.6 million; in 1990, 26.5 million; and in 2000, 35.5 million. Whereas the white non-Hispanic population in the United States increased 9 percent from 1990 to 2000, the Latino population increased 24.4 percent during the same period.

Latinos are more concentrated in some regions of the United States—primarily in the Southwest. California is now one third Latino, while Texas is about one fourth Latino (McDonnell, 2001). The 2000 census also reported that Latinos have moved briskly into the midwest, southern, and eastern regions of the United States. Many Latinos are recent immigrants (Larmer, 1999; Ortiz, 1995).

What specific factors are involved in the tremendous increase in the Latino population? The rate of natural increase (births over deaths) among Hispanics is 1.8 percent, one third higher than for African-Americans. The fertility rate of Latinos is over 50 percent greater than that of whites (Hayes-Battista, 1990; Larmer, 1999). Hispanic immigration (legal and illegal) is running at the astonishing rate of an estimated 1 million people per yer. The booming economy of the 1990s and job opportunities throughout the United States have attracted more illegal immigrants than in previous decades (McDonnell, 2001). Extrapolating from these figures, Hispanics will outnumber African-Americans shortly after the turn of the century (see Figure 18–1).

Whereas African-Americans are united by race and a common historic experience of slavery, Hispanic-

---

* The terms Latino and Hispanic-American are used interchangeably in the literature and throughout this chapter. Today, Latino appears to be the preferred term because of its greater geographical coverage, as well as economic and political accuracy (Falicov, 1998; Hayes-Battista & Chapa, 1987).

Figure 18–1. Dramatic changes expected in ethnic portrait in United States, 2005–2050. *(Source: Larmer, 1999.)*

Americans are united by three powerful forces: their language (Spanish, except for Brazilians who speak Portuguese), their strong adherence to Roman Catholicism, and their common values and beliefs rooted in a history of conquest and colonization (Garcia-Preto, 1996). Nevertheless, there are also many factors that divide them into diverse groups.

The focus of research on the Hispanic-American family has been overwhelmingly on the Mexican-American family, which is more homogeneous than the larger Hispanic-American grouping. In spite of Mexican-Americans being more homogeneous, this subgroup of Latinos evidences great intraethnic variation also. People of Mexican heritage vary by country of origin (United States or Mexico) and self-identification. In addition, socioeconomic, generational, regional, and idiosyncratic factors account for further intragroup diversity (Falicov, 1982).

Mexican-Americans are a blend of both Indian and Spanish cultures and races. Most Mexican-Americans are *mestizos,* of mixed Caucasian and Indian blood lines (Kuipers, 1995). Generally speaking, first-generation individuals speak Spanish and

identify themselves as "Mexicano," whereas second- and third-generation people of Mexican descent speak English and Spanish and usually identify themselves as Mexican, Chicano, or Mexican-American.

THE LATINO INTERFACE WITH AMERICAN SOCIETY

The major waves of Latino immigrants came to the United States after World War II. The pattern and timing of the migration usually has corresponded with economic depression and/or political turmoil in the immigrants' native land (Garcia-Preto, 1996). The Latino historical interface with the United States has varied by subgroups. The Mexican experience is described first.

THE MEXICAN-AMERICAN EXPERIENCE

The pattern of labor utilization of Mexicans and Mexican-Americans provides a significant path for understanding the growth and obstacles to the Mexican-American subculture's assimilation into the American cultural mainstream. Historically, Mexican immigration has been closely tied to southwestern labor needs (Gonzalez, 1991). For decades, job-starved Mexican nationals worked competitively and at lower wage scales than Mexican-Americans either by crossing the border daily or coming over as *braceros.* The bracero program, now defunct, permitted Mexican workers in the 1940s and 1950s to work under contract to the United States when the supply of field workers in this country was evaluated as insufficient (McLemore & Romo, 1985; Suarez & Ramirez, 1999).

Mexican-Americans, because of their proximity to Mexico, the fluidity of the border, and the exploitation of the Anglo-dominated agricultural system, have never been able to participate in the usual social processes used by European immigrants to become integrated into and socially mobile within the mainstream of American society (Hayes-Battista & Chapa, 1987; Queen & Haberstein, 1974).

A vast majority of Mexican-Americans have been, and continue to be, isolated from wider society by religion, language, culture, and social class. In the major population centers of Mexican-Americans, there is, however, a growing, influential, emergent middle-class community. Language has served a vital role in maintaining the culture: The Mexican-American family, more than other immigrant families, has continued to speak its native language—Spanish—in the home and community. Social class has also served to isolate Mexican-Americans who are poor from the mainstream of the American middle-class society.

Furthermore, Anglos' discriminatory practices and stereotypical view of the Latino culture have created further problems of social integration. Adding to this situation is the view that some Mexican-Americans hold, that the *gringo* is someone from a world alien and hostile to their own way of life (Castro, 1978; Garcia-Preto, 1996).

Compounding the problem of incompatibility between the larger society and the Mexican-American culture is the social and political ferment being generated by the drastic increases in the population of Spanish-speaking immigrants, mostly Mexican and Central American, in many of the areas in the Southwest. The passage of two anti-immigration propositions in California (Proposition 187 and Proposition 209) in the 1990s are evidence of the politicization of the immigration influx (Falicov, 1996). The vast influx of Latinos, particularly illegal immigrants, has been a prime source of conflict, dissension, and lack of acceptance in communities.

Mexican-Americans, the largest Latino group, collectively have low family incomes, high labor force participation for men and increasing labor force participation for women, and the lowest educational attainment and largest average household size of all Latino groups (Zinn & Wells, 2000). For Mexican families who live in the border states, there is typically a traveling back and forth between the bordering countries. Recurrent separations and reunions among family members add stress to families already struggling with economic and migratory challenges.

THE CENTRAL AMERICAN EXPERIENCE

Immigration from Central America (Guatemala, El Salvador, and Nicaragua primarily) has been recent and dramatic. With civil war, poor socioeconomic conditions, and violation of human rights rampant in the three above-mentioned countries from the 1970s on, record numbers of refugees and illegal immigrants have come to the United States. Political refugees from these countries have not been recognized by the U.S. government; hence, until recently, when amnesty regulations took place, many Central Americans were forced to remain hidden (Conover, 1993).

THE PUERTO RICAN EXPERIENCE

Puerto Rican families began migrating to the United States in great numbers after World War II. Most came for economic reasons and settled in the Northeast, particularly in New York City. Their pattern of immigration has been a back-and-forth one—going back to the island and then returning for jobs and economic stability. However, migrating here has not been easy for them; one third of all Puerto Ricans on the mainland are unemployed and poor (Garcia-Preto, 1996). They are the most economically disadvantaged of all major Latino groups (Zinn & Wells, 2000).

THE CUBAN EXPERIENCE

Cubans arrived in the United States in large numbers in the 1960s, after Fidel Castro won the revolution of 1959 and established a harsh communistic society. The United States at that time opened its doors to Cubans fleeing Castro's government. A second wave of Cubans came in the 1980s, escaping Cuba in boats. Most Cubans live in four states: Florida (concentrated in Miami or "Little Havana"), New Jersey, New York, and California (Garcia-Preto, 1996). Cuban families have higher incomes and substantially lower poverty rates than do other major Latino groups (Zinn & Wells, 2000).

FAMILY–SOCIETY INTERFACE: EFFECT ON FAMILY LIFE

The type and quality of the interchanges between the family and the external social system significantly affects internal family activities and integration. A major way this occurs is through children's school participation and the parents' employment experiences. For instance, the lower- or working-class Latino male has often been unemployed or employed in menial minimally paying positions that constantly erode his self-esteem. He often has had very little access to resources that could change his situation, and has had few effective means of making institutions in society respond to his needs. This damaging, limiting process invariably diminishes the internal functioning and role relationships within his family. It has an adverse effect on family leadership and the integration and solidarity of families and their members.

❧ENVIRONMENTAL ISSUES

Most Latino families are immigrants. Their migration transports them to a new, foreign, social, and physical terrain. Bombarded by these differences, they attempt to recreate aspects of the culture they left behind. Cubans, Puerto Ricans, Central Americans, and Mexicans tend to live in urban ethnic, segregated neighborhoods that serve as buffers against culture shock, giving them some sense of continuity with their native culture (Falicov, 1998). In spite of this community buffer, immigrant families are faced with the threat of discrimination and intrusion by the Immigration and Naturalization Service.

Many new immigrants are preoccupied with the tasks of basic survival—adjusting to a new social environment, new jobs, new neighborhoods, new friends, and new social networks. For some, this process can take years, or even a lifetime.

Immigrants may have witnessed the terror and violence that recently has dominated the Central American region. Hence, when working with refugee Hispanic families, assessing the degree to which family members' past trauma is affecting their current health and adjustment is a primary assessment consideration (Hernandez, 1996).

❧THE ACCULTURATION ISSUE

Sociologists have assumed in the past that Hispanic-Americans would become acculturated (make the transition from traditional values and behaviors to modern, Western values and modes of behavior) and that length of time living in the United States was positively associated with modernization, implying that the longer an individual or family is exposed to a dominant culture, the more adoption of the host culture occurs. Although such a formulation has some

explanatory value, it fails to delineate which aspects of ethnicity and culture persist over time or the demographic and sociopsychological factors that are likely to affect the acculturation process.

Because of the above shortcomings and the implication inherent within the acculturation notion that the "American" family is the ideal and the "un-American" family less desirable, there is a tendency to move away from acculturation as the sole and central framework for explaining the changes in Latino families. Also, in spite of intergenerational differences, Latino families exhibit a wide range of differences in the extent to which they are acculturated to Anglo society.

Increasing attention is now being devoted to the study of ethnic identity among Latinos by more objective empirical methods. There is growing recognition that families can be both "modern and ethnic" at the same time (Baca-Zinn, 1981) or bicultural or bifocal—possessing the capacity to see the world through two different value lenses (Falicov, 1966). Latinos retain a strong sense of ethnic identity, regardless of the number of generations in the United States (Vega, 1995).

There has been tremendous criticism of published Hispanic-American family literature in the early social science literature. Much of the criticized literature is based on opinion and personal observation (Jaramillo & Zapata, 1987). Researchers in their writings failed to recognize and account for the many societal processes (work situation, educational institutions, socioeconomic constraints) affecting the Latino family. Oversimplifications and inaccuracies were inherent in the broad generalizations made about Latino families (Vega, 1995). In addition, most studies were limited to the lower-class Mexican-American family, and social scientists tended to paint pictures of "black and white" stereotypes of family life and family roles—many times in a pejorative, ethnocentric manner. Current family science literature on the Hispanic-American family fortunately is "more concerned with understanding the accommodations, vulnerabilities and resilience of the Latino family . . ." (Vega, p. 5).

Although acculturation has been the primary process used to describe differences between Mexican-American families, this is an uneven process and some cultural patterns seem to be retained regardless of length of residency in the United States. The pace of acculturation is more rapid among children than parents. The acculturation process unfortunately may also involve adjusting to minority status, diminished life opportunity, and dangerous environments (Vega & Amaro, 1994).

Cultural adaptation varies by socioeconomic status, number of generations in the United States, and ability to speak English (Sorofman, 1986; Vega, 1995). Also, families in urban California areas tend to be more acculturated than are families living in more rural areas, such as in Texas (Dickinson & Leming, 1995).

Even though Mexican-Americans undergo acculturation as evidenced by a decrease in cultural awareness and/or ethnic loyalty, some things do not change. In particular, the importance of the extended family does not wane. In fact, the extended family appears to grow in structure and function when studied across several generations (Velez-Ibanez, 1996). Latinos also tend to maintain strong ties to their language (Parra & Guarnaccia, 1998).

✷ SOCIOECONOMIC STATUS OF LATINOS

Although most Latinos have come across the border in search of jobs, higher wages, and better working conditions, many experience discrimination in employment, housing, and education. Skin color, language difficulties, and Spanish surnames have all contributed to the continued isolation, discrimination, and exploitation Latinos have experienced (Falicov, 1996; Kuipers, 1995).

The impact of social class stratification has received sparse attention in the literature about the Hispanic-American family, and yet must be taken into account. Social class stratification of Hispanic-Americans reflects their disadvantaged social class status. The proportion of Mexican families in the various social classes does not conform to the American social class distribution of families. Instead, social class distribution is more restricted, reflecting limited social mobility. According to Vega and co-workers (1983), there are basically four classes in Mexican-American society: the underclass, the low income, the working class, and the middle class.

The underclass is composed of new immigrants who are still in the transition process, while the low-income families are still poor, but have stable unskilled, low-paying employment and residential stability. This is probably the largest group of Hispanic-American families today (Fulwood, 1996).

The other large Latino social class group in most urban areas is the urban working class. Working-class parents have achieved stable employment in skilled or semi-skilled occupations and are not economically marginal like the under- and lower-class Latinos.

The middle class is similar to the Anglo-American middle class in that it is a nuclear unit and predominantly English speaking and young. Education is highly stressed and a significant proportion of men are in the skilled trades or in business. In Southern California, recent research reveals a substantial, steadily growing Latino middle class. Data here show that the longer immigrant families reside in the United States, the more likely they are to become middle class.

Two indicators of Hispanic-American families' precarious status are income and education. In 1995, it was estimated that the median Hispanic family income was about 50 to 63 percent of the median U.S. income (Fulwood, 1996; Ortiz, 1995). Educationally, Latinos are at a disadvantage compared to Anglos. For example, 66 percent of Latino adults reported in a recent survey that they never attended college, whereas 41 percent of Anglos reported not going to college (Larmer, 1995). Their median family income is less than two thirds the median family income of all U.S. families, although there is a considerable income range among Latinos (U.S. Census Bureau, 1996).

A significant factor that lowers Latinos economic status is family size. Latinos tend to have larger families and more children than non-Latinos. Hence the ratio of dependence, or the number of persons who rely on the income of the family head, is considerably larger for Latinos than for non-Latinos. With larger families and a reduced salary, 27 percent of all Latino families have incomes below the poverty level (Figure 18–2). Latinos are over twice as likely to be poor, when compared to the white U.S. population (see Figure 18–2). Cuban families are the exception when discussing the socioeconomic status of Hispanic-American families. They currently earn 17 percent more in income than other Latino subgroups. Their success is explained by their migration pattern. The large Cuban migration of the 1960s primarily

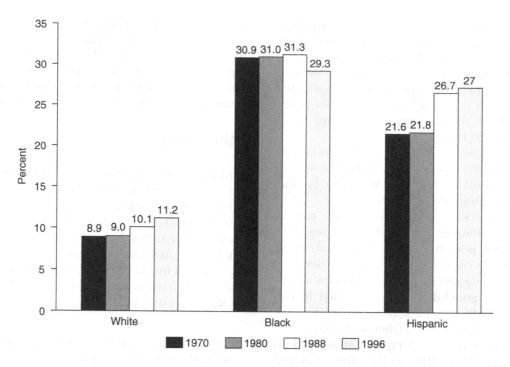

Figure 18–2. Percentage of U.S. population below the poverty line, 1970, 1980, 1988, and 1996 by ethnicity. There were 36.4 million or 13 percent of persons in the United States below the poverty level in 1996. *(Sources: U.S. Bureau of the Census, 1980, 1990, and 1996, cited in Fulwood, 1996; and Zinn & Wells, 2000).*

included white, educated professionals who had the resources to improve their status here. In addition, being white, they faced no color barrier (Bernal & Shapiro, 1996).

THE NORMATIVE FAMILY FORM

Due to the deep commitment to family, more Latinos live in traditional nuclear families (two parents with children) than white or African-American persons. According to 1990 Los Angeles County, California, data, 47.1 percent of Latinos lived in nuclear families, while 24.6 percent of whites and 21.8 percent of African-Americans lived in nuclear two-parent families (Hayes-Battista, 1990). The idealized Latino family is the extended family, although the extended family living under one roof is not common. Nevertheless, relatives often live nearby and other than nuclear family members often live in the same household (Miller, 1986). In addition to living in traditional nuclear and

extended families, a variety of household arrangements are found among Latinos. Immigration contributes to this variety of family forms, such as binational families, single-parent families, and multiple-family households (Zinn & Wells, 2000).

Children traditionally do not separate from their families of origin psychologically or socially. As children grow up and marry, their families become extensions of the original unit, even though they probably do not live within the same household. The mother's and father's kin are generally of equal importance, with special recognition given to the mother's sisters. Both sets of grandparents are revered. First cousins are especially important secondary kin and are somewhat like sisters and brothers (Keefe, 1984; Queen & Haberstein, 1974).

The Latino family is typically described as a large and cohesive kin group including both lineal and collateral relatives. Strong and extensive linkages beyond the nuclear family are present, with all relatives having reciprocal rights and duties. In other words, the extended family system, as a concrete manifestation of a familistic orientation, refers to that network of relatives including primary kin (siblings, children, and parents) and secondary kin (aunts, uncles, cousins, nieces, nephews, grandparents).

New immigrants, especially those who are undocumented, tend to live in multiple family arrangements. Single immigrant men tend to live together in the same household to conserve money and other resources (Chavez, 1986).

Godparents (compadrazgo) may hold an important place in the family, although the presence and/or role of godparents in Mexican-American families today is more limited (Ramirez & Arce, 1981). Compadrazgo refers to the ritual kinship pattern whereby a special linkage is established between two families or two persons by the baptismal ritual. Compadres provide co-parenthood in time of need but also generate social and interpersonal cohesion, and godparents and godchildren are expected to visit each other and cultivate a close relationship (Kuipers, 1995; Falicor, 1998; Queen & Haberstein, 1974).

Recently, the number of teenage Latino mothers has risen sharply. From 1983 to 1993 there was a 45 percent increase in the number of Latino teenage pregnancies. Some of these girls remain home with their parents, some marry, and some establish female-headed families of their own. Reasons given for the sharp rise are: a taboo against discussing sex in the family; a religious prohibition against abortions; inaccessibility of family planning services; and girls' perceptions of the women's role as being to stay home and have and raise children (Roan, 1995).

Puerto Rican families have a much greater proportion of families headed by women than other Latino groups. Thirty-nine percent of all Puerto Rican families in 1990 were identified as female headed, versus less than 20 percent of Mexican and Cuban families being female headed (Ortiz, 1995).

❦FAMILY STRUCTURAL CHARACTERISTICS

The descriptions of the Latino family that follow are culled primarily from the last two decades. Even then, the nurse should particularly keep in mind the possible bias of social class. The nurse also needs to keep in mind that cultural norms tend to refer to what ought to be, and that these cultural perscriptions sometimes do not coincide with how things "really" are in families. Because recent research has clarified the wide variation of behavior in Hispanic-American families and has dispelled some of our stereotypes of these families, many of the traditional classic descriptions of family life and roles are now viewed as inaccurate.

FAMILY VALUES

Cultures "hang together" on the basis of commonly shared value orientations. For traditional Hispanic-Americans, orienting values are present and pervasive, although their actual adherence to these values in family life varies. Nevertheless, "an appreciation of their existence and potential impact on family life provides an invaluable perspective for understanding cultural behaviors and expectations" (Vega, Hough, & Romero, 1983, p. 199).

FAMILISM. The major theme dominating both the classic and modern portrayal of the Latino family is the deep importance of the family to all its members. The set of norms or values related to the importance of the family is referred to as familism. Here "the needs of the family collectivity supercede the needs of each individual family member" (Grebler, Moore, & Guzman, 1970, p. 369). Familism, the opposite of individualism, denotes a set of rights and obligations pertaining to members of a kin network. Family membership and belonging are a source of great pride. Interdependencies are seen as both healthy and necessary. When strong familistic attitudes prevail, role obligations are seen as mandatory (Casas & Vasquez, 1996; Diaz-Guerrero, 1975; Goldenberg & Goldenberg, 2002; Heller, 1976).

Mexican-American family values reinforce the system of mutual obligations, support, and reciprocity. Vega and associates (1983) explain that other values must also be mutually acknowledged in order for mutual support and reciprocity to occur.

> These [values] are mediated by certain values which have received broad attention in the literature: *orgullo* (pride and self-reliance), *dignidad* (dignity), *confianza* (trust and intimacy), and *respecto* (respect). (p. 199)

Table 18–1 compares American and traditional Latino values in some of the major areas of family

TABLE 18–1

AMERICAN AND TRADITIONAL LATINO VALUE DIFFERENCES

AREA/ISSUE	AMERICAN CENTRAL VALUE ORIENTATION AND PATTERN	TRADITIONAL HISPANIC-AMERICAN VALUE ORIENTATION AND PATTERN
Family	Americans see themselves as individuals first and as members of families second.	Latinos see themselves as members of families first and as individuals second.
Self versus kin obligations	American culture stresses individuality and independence from family after a certain age. Self-reliance, autonomy, and achievement are emphasized.	Latinos believe in ethic of reciprocity within family and kinship group and interdependency.
Respect and authority structures	Americans value democratic ideals and egalitarianism (to a much greater extent). The elderly do not receive great respect. The authority of the masculine role is gradually diminishing as a result of the societal trend toward egalitarianism.	Greater value on male leadership and respect toward the elderly and toward authority figures.
Progress versus tradition	Americans value progress and change.	Hispanic-Americans show more reverence and respect for tradition.
Work	Work and productivity are central, often prominent values of the Anglo culture. Work often becomes a value in itself (more true in the past than today).	Work is seen as a necessity in order to live. Other life experiences—social and emotional experiences—are valued more than work.
Materialism	Materialism is a central American value. Possession of material goods is seen as a sign of success and becomes an end in itself. Cynosures of society are the businessman and financier.	Material objects are viewed as necessities and not as ends in themselves. Social status and prestige are more likely to be derived from an ability to experience things directly and/or through social and family relationships rather than through past successes and accumulation of wealth. Hispanic-Americans generally have great reverence for philosophers, poets, musicians, and artists.
Time	"Time is money." Punctuality is equated with goodness and being responsible.	Time is a gift to be enjoyed. More flexible attitude toward time. "Wasting time" is not understood. Punctuality is not an important moral value.
Present versus future time orientation	Making plans for the future is highly valued as a means of getting ahead. Future oriented.	Enjoyment of the present. Less concern for always living for the future. More present oriented.
Interpersonal relationships	Americans value openness and directness in communications. (Americans are viewed as being blunt and succinct by Hispanic-Americans.) Use of kidding to get messages across more indirectly is	Latinos value diplomacy, smooth and pleasant social relationships, and tactfulness, and show concern and respect for others' feelings and dignity. Their manner of expression is more elaborate and indirect. They value

(continued)

TABLE 18–1 (CONTINUED)

AMERICAN AND TRADITIONAL LATINO VALUE DIFFERENCES

AREA/ISSUE	AMERICAN CENTRAL VALUE ORIENTATION AND PATTERN	TRADITIONAL HISPANIC-AMERICAN VALUE ORIENTATION AND PATTERN
Interpersonal relationships (continued)	acceptable. In interpersonal conflict situations, Americans value "leveling," open dissent, and criticizing each other. Value rational expression of thoughts and not emotional expression as much.	agreement, respect, and courtesy, and are very sensitive to criticism regardless of manner presented. They value being expressive and showing feelings toward other persons.
Environmental responses	Americans are less sensitive to the environment and its various forms of stimulation.	Hispanic-Americans value greater sensory stimulation within their environments, using a fuller range of senses to experience their environment (vivid colors, expressive music and art, spicy foods).
Relationship to environment	Americans see themselves as mastering the environment.	Latinos place more value on living in harmony with the environment.
Education	Education is highly valued as means to success and way to be productive. Education is correlated with work and productivity values.	Education is valued but has often been inaccessible, with schools being culturally incongruent with traditional Hispanic-American values. Also, many Latinos are not in tune with success and scientific, individualistic values associated with American education.
Religion	Most Americans are more secular today.	Religion is more highly valued. Over 95% of Hispanics are Roman Catholic. Acceptance of God's will is widespread way of coping.

Adapted from Andrews (1995), Falicov (1996), Garcia-Preto (1996), Marin & Marin (1991), Murillo (1976).

and personal life. Although clear differences are identified here, again it needs to be stressed that in both American and traditional Hispanic-American families heterogeneity abounds and intraethnic variation is, indeed, great.

Traditional Latino values, with the exception of familism and a religious orientation, are more prominently found among the unacculturated and the poor. Moreover, social class status is a prime determinant of the viability of traditionalism (Falicov, 1998; Goldenberg & Goldenberg, 2002; Moore, 1970).

VALUE CONFLICTS. One of the serious problems that occurs as the Latino family interfaces with the larger society is that value conflicts arise. Hispanic-American children's socialization experiences (in school and in the *barrio*) often provoke value conflicts between the generations. Many of the primary values of the Latino family are incongruent with American core values. For example, American core values stress individualism, pragmatism, and efficiency, whereas in Latino homes, familism, a more personal, rather pragmatic, efficient manner is valued. This naturally poses significant adaptation problems for Latino families and individuals (Goldenberg & Goldenberg, 2002; Hernandez, 1996). For instance, when Latino children start school, they soon learn that they and their families are "out of synch" with the wider society.

Vega and co-workers (1983) point out that in low-income areas where Mexican-American families live in *barrios;* the *barrio* also is a powerful socializer.

> The *barrio* has an independent culture and tradition that is neither Mexican alone nor middle class Anglo-American. (p. 205)

Expectations and sanctions for not conforming to values and social roles within the family are probably more rigidly defined and controlled among Latinos than Anglos, but nonconformity outside the home is typically not rigidly controlled, as parents perceive limitations on their ability to control the external environment.

FAMILY ROLES AND POWER

The early classic literature about Latino cultures takes cognizance of male dominance in the home. Here, the father is described as unquestionably the head of the family, as well as being "hard, unyielding, and strong," exemplifying the traits of *machismo* (Castro, 1978). Paz (1973), a noted Mexican author, and Ingoldsby (1995b) have described the *macho* or masculine role as incorporating the following elements of arbitrary power: superiority, fearlessness, aggressiveness, insensitivity, hypersexuality, and invulnerability. Along with the Latino male's authoritarian role, he is characterized as providing for his family in the best possible manner he can, priding himself on being the sole provider and being economically self-sufficient. As a father, he is expected to protect mother by demanding that the children obey and assist her. Latino fathers in the past were less involved with parenting. Today, they may be involved in child care only peripherally or do quite a bit of child care, along with being playful and affectionate with their children (Falicov, 1998).

In this same literature, the ideal mother is seen as a soft, nurturing, and self-sacrificing woman, with her traditional and positive role of being in the home, with responsibility to her husband and to her children (Falicov, 1998). In fact, her status and roles are usually defined solely by her marriage and her children.

There has been much criticism over this stereotyping of Hispanic-American family roles, both of the conclusions reached and of the theoretical models underlying these past studies (Mirandé, 1991). The focus of recent studies is toward understanding gender roles as flexible and responsive to environmental conditions (Vega, 1995). Empirical studies show that patterns of absolute male dominance in conjugal decision making have never been the behavioral norm among Mexicans either in the United States or Mexico (Cromwell & Ruiz, 1979; Grebler et al., 1970; Hawkes & Taylor, 1975). Although the family structure is described as male dominant, the evidence generally suggests the presence of a more egalitarian structure and process, especially when the wife works or when the family is not poor (Hernandez, 1996; Ybarra, 1982). Moreover, the influence and predominance of *machismo* and the presence of female submissiveness and lack of power are equally controversial generalizations being challenged in Latino family literature as studies refute the existence of these stereotypes (Falicov, 1998). Latino scholars on the family argue that there is much diversity within the Latino family and that many of its present adaptations are due to discrimination and socioeconomic barriers.

Several authors have noted the influence that immigration, urbanization, social mobility, and acculturation have on the Hispanic-American family. The Latino family is being subjected to many of the same societal changes that the Anglo family is facing.

Given the increasing occupational opportunities for women and the wish for a higher standard of living, more and more Latino women are working. Latino women's participation in the workforce has increased rapidly and almost equals that of American women generally (Falicov, 1996). As with Anglo families, when women take advantage of educational opportunities and find employment outside the home, their self-image and role expectations change considerably. Working, educated Latino women are espousing new aspirations for independence and finding greater flexibility and choice of options.

Thus, education and labor force participation of Latino women are causing revolutionary changes in the Latino family. Traditional male–female roles are changing, particularly among younger and middle-class couples. Many women, especially the younger ones, are challenging women's traditional roles (Baxter, 1996). In the urban areas, the *chicanitas* (adolescent girls) are joining social clubs and gangs. Young Latino women express a need for greater equality in the family and society. The husband/father's pervasive power has given rise to the wife/daughter's sense of injustice, particularly as they are exposed to American mores and values.

Moreover, large families and the difficulties of the husband–father in finding employment with good wages compromises his ability to provide adequately for the family, which tends to diminish the base for his authority. Thus, the more noteworthy and profound change, as noted in recent studies, revolves around the declining primary authority of the male and the greater egalitarianism of spousal roles. Given women's emancipation, generational conflicts, and the decline of the male's patriarchal authority, the Latino family is facing substantial transition and occasion for stress.

FAMILY COMMUNICATION PATTERNS

Strong affective communication patterns are characteristic of many Latino families. There is much warmth and affection shown between mother and children when children are young. In traditional families, respect is shown by children to parents and elders, and females to males of the family. Affiliation, cooperation, and smooth, pleasant relationships that avoid conflict are stressed (Falicov, 1996).

The Spanish language, being more emotionally expressive and elaborate than English, shapes the cognitive structure of its speakers. Interpersonal relationships are noted for their tones of respect and hierarchical relationships. As seen in the summary of values in Table 18–1, Hispanic-Americans value courtesy, respect, maintaining one's dignity, diplomacy, tactfulness, expressiveness of feelings (emotionality), and agreement (Falicov, 1996). Kidding and open confrontation are not generally sanctioned, because the need to show respect and to "save face" are important.

FAMILY FUNCTIONAL CHARACTERISTICS

THE FAMILY SOCIALIZATION FUNCTION

Children are at the center of family life (Wilkinson, 1987). Also, sex role distinctions through child-rearing

practices appear to be reinforced in most Latino families. A male is taught how to think and behave like a man, and a female like a woman (Mirandé, 1985). The authority of the parents is unquestioned throughout life. In addition to being the authority in families, parents demand *respecto* (respect) from their children (Falicov, 1998).

Traditionally, the raising of children has been the mother's job, while the father's role has been to work and to form associations with his *compadres* (godparents). However, as with American families generally, this rigid demarcation of roles is rapidly declining. Much more sharing of the child care role is occurring among Chicano couples (Mirandé, 1979).

Hispanic-American babies are wanted, cherished, and pampered. They are regarded as *angelitos*, untouched by evil and sin. Parents and older siblings respond to young children in very indulgent, affectionate ways (Queen & Haberstein, 1974). There is a longer state of interdependence between mother and child than in Anglo families (Falicov, 1996).

Differences in child rearing and disciplining are notable among Latino families of diverse social classes. Although parental desires for their children may not vary, the ability to realize aspirations does, and hence socialization experiences are clearly varied between social classes (Vega et al., 1983). In more recent studies of child-rearing patterns among Latinos, some researchers have discovered substantial diversity, ranging from permissive, to authoritarian, to authoritative parenting styles. More acculturated mothers tend to use authoritative parenting (Martinez, 1993).

Socialization strains are common among immigrant Hispanic families. Researchers have found that children acculturate at a faster rate than adults in the family—a difference that leads to profound intergenerational conflicts (Goldenberg & Goldenberg, 2002). These conflicts are then aggravated by parental attempts to gain control over their children and children rejecting parental efforts (Hernandez, 1996; Vega, 1990).

THE FAMILY HEALTH CARE FUNCTION

Among Latinos, the structure and values of the family are important influencing factors relative to understanding an individual's health attitudes and practices. The importance of familism is seen in how family members define family health. In one recent qualitative study, young Mexican-American parents talked about what family health meant to them. They spoke of family health in terms of family unity and being together. One parent explained, "Well, we have to be together, no? We have to do everything in order to be together" (Niska, Snyder, & Lia-Hoagberg, 1999, pp. 224–225). One can also better understand the shorter longevity and the higher mortality and morbidity rates of Latinos versus the general American population when the high percentage of this group living at or below the poverty level is taken into account (Angel, 1985). The health of family members is affected by their living conditions, the community resources, and the social environment.

Health care needs are diverse and depend largely on the specific vulnerabilities and risks associated with social class, environmental, occupational, and lifestyle patterns. Major health problems and poor access to health care are concentrated among the poor, the least assimilated, the illegal migrant, and the migrant worker (Angel, 1985; Zambrana, Dorrington, & Hayes-Battista, 1995).

HEALTH CARE BELIEFS AND PRACTICES. Early studies of health care behavior of Hispanic-Americans emphasized the widespread use of folk medicine (Madsen, 1964; Saunders, 1954). Saunders asserted that Mexican-Americans considered health care as encompassing both scientific and folk cures. Research on Mexican-Americans in the Southwest shows that folk medicine and beliefs still persist in rural and urban areas among the lower class (Farge, 1975; Keefe, 1981).

Use of folk healing in the urban areas appears to have declined considerably, except among recent, immigrant and poor families. In Keefe's (1981) large study of Mexican-Americans in three southern California communities, there was little indication that *curanderismo* (Mexican traditional folk medical care system) was used. Only 7 percent of the respondents in Keefe's second survey consulted a *curandero* in the last year and one half of those did so only for a minor medical problem. *Curanderismo* was adhered to most frequently among recent Mexican immigrants who came to the United States after the age of 15, were Spanish-speaking, identified themselves as "Mexicano," and were in the lowest socioeconomic stratum. The respondents who had used

curanderos believed that folk healers were superior for curing folk illnesses, for curing minor ailments not serious enough to require a doctor's care, and for treating illnesses that physicians could not cure (Keefe).

Recent studies of Hispanic folk health practices demonstrate that Hispanic-Americans who use folk medicine do not rely entirely on folk prescriptions for cure, but consider them an important adjunct in expediting solutions to various health problems (Herrera & Wagner, 1974; Mikhail, 1994) or as appropriate for certain folk illnesses (Mikhail).

Regardless of the degree to which folk medicine is relied upon, there is no empirical evidence indicating that folk medicine and scientific medicine are mutually exclusive systems (Farge, 1975; Kay, 1978; Keefe, 1981; Nall & Speilberg, 1978). Urban Mexican-Americans appear to readily accept modern health care, sometimes supplementing folk medicine with modern medical care or vice versa. Usually, there is little incompatibility perceived between the indigenous and the scientific forms of health care.

When both systems of health care are used in health settings (folk medicine and Western medicine), this is called "complementary health care." Some clinics in California are now delivering this type of care. Physicians and nurse practitioners work cooperatively with indigenous (folk) health practitioners (herbists, *curanderos*), or in some cases use herbs for certain symptoms or illnesses.

TRADITIONAL HEALTH BELIEFS. Latinos typically maintain a dual system of beliefs and practices concerning health problems and health care—mainstream medical approaches and traditional folk beliefs and remedies (Felicov, 1998; Trevino, Weber, Reza, & Reyes, 1999). Most of the Latino health beliefs are based on assumptions and traditional practices that have evolved over centuries. In the blending of older European, Spanish-Catholic, and Indian traditions, three basic aspects of Mexican and Latin American traditional folk health concepts and practices emerge. One aspect is concerned with the specific health beliefs and practices. A second aspect consists of a set of ritualistic acts that are believed to improve health. And lastly, the use of folk practitioners or *curanderos* has evolved (Gonzales, 1976; Harwood, 1981).

Folk medicine does not treat symptoms of disease conditions alone. Folk medicine views the sick person as a whole psychobiocultural and spiritual being in relationship to the natural and supernatural environments. Whereas Western medicine focuses on epidemiology and pathophysiology, Latino folk medicine focuses on holistically treating the person.

Mexican-American. Basic to Chicano health beliefs and practices are the health philosophies and ideologies of the culture that circumscribes these beliefs and practices. The basis for many health beliefs derives from notions about the importance of maintaining equilibrium (a balance between "hot" and "cold" or between "wet" and "dry"). Human beings are viewed holistically, as being in harmony and unity with the natural and supernatural environments. Health is a result of maintenance of this natural state of balance between humans and the natural and supernatural worlds. Illness and disease stem from a loss of homeostasis or balance (Dorsey & Jackson, 1976; Spector, 2000).

Preventive beliefs and rituals are exercised to promote this balance. Prayers, relics, faith, herbs, and spices are all used to ward off disease or to prevent complications of long-term illness. Two examples of the Chicano's concern with maintaining balance are in the consumption of hot and cold foods and in prenatal health practices. To achieve the necessary balance in the body, foods thought of as "hot" (heavy foods, meats, fatty or spicy foods) are eaten with "cold" foods (vegetables, ice cream), which are considered soothing and fresh to the body (Spector, 2000). Because pregnancy is seen as a delicate time when imbalances occur easily that can cause great harm to the fetus, the practice of the mother's wearing keys on the night of the lunar eclipse is thought to be protective. Mothers are also urged to maintain good diets, exercise, and take herbs and teas recommended by the *yerbero* (herbalist) or health leader in the family, thus maintaining the delicate balance during the months of pregnancy (Dorsey & Jackson, 1976).

In addition to disease being caused by "imbalances," disease also may be inflicted on an individual as a form of supernatural punishment for wrongdoing (Clark, 1970). Folk illnesses can be caused by a variety of circumstances, although most folk illnesses are believed to be intimately related to faulty social relationships (Herrera & Wagner, 1974; Prattes, 1973).

Some of the specific folk health beliefs, as expressed in form of folk illnesses, are the following:

Mal de ojo (bad or evil eye) is believed to be a result of excessive admiration or desire on the part of another. *Mal de susto* (illness from fright) is a syndrome believed to be the result of an emotionally traumatic experience. *Empacho* (indigestion) is believed to be caused by food clinging to the wall of the stomach in the form of a ball. *Caida de la mollera* (fallen fontanel) is the one illness that is felt to affect children only and is attributed to a child's being dropped and as the result of a fall. *Mal puesto* (sorcery) is considered to arise as a consequence of one of three kinds of social relationships: (1) a lover's quarrel, (2) unrequited love, or (3) as a reflection of individiousness between individuals or nuclear families (Falicov, 1996; Giger & Davidhizar, 1999; Herrera & Wagner, 1974; Spector, 2000).

In recent studies of Mexican-American families, mental illness is not the "dreaded affliction" and stigma of "enduring madness" to the person and family that it once was. The majority of Latinos in one study described serious mental illness as being a problem of the emotions and of *nervios* (a noun that describes physical distress, emotional disturbance, and social dislocation) (Parra & Guarnaccia, 1998). Mental illness, in other studies, was described by Latinos as being on a continuum that ranged from "being nervous" and "suffering from nerves" to having a "mental failure and being crazy" (Parra & Guarnaccia). For the treatment of mental illness, Latinos will use either or both folk healing practices and mainstream psychotherapy. They tend to underutilize mental health services. This is partially due to their health beliefs about mental illness, but also due to their lack of health insurance coverage and the lack of trained bilingual and bicultural counselors (Goldenberg & Goldenberg, 2002).

THE PROCESS OF SEEKING HEALTH CARE. Typically, in the traditional lower-class Latino family when an individual becomes ill, he or she usually consults the health expert in the family and tries to cure the illness with home remedies (prayers, diet, herbal remedies). If this does not relieve the symptoms depending on the type of health problem, he or she may consult a physician, folk practitioner, or sometimes both. Of the folk practitioners, the *yerbero* and then the *curandero* are often consulted. The types of healing or remedies prescribed are reflective of the healer's perceptions of etiology. In folk medicine, much of the healing is geared toward restoring the necessary equilibrium or preventing disequilibrium. There are specific household remedies, such as those for being wet and chilled and those for menstruation. Spiritualistic practices are also appropriate for helping with illness considered supernatural in origin. Prayers and ritualistic activities are performed by *espiritualistas,* family, and patient. Herbs are extensively used for treating a multitude of illnesses, some of which have been found scientifically to have great benefit (Dorsey & Jackson, 1976; Giger & Davidhizar, 1999).

FOLK HEALERS.   Clark (1970), an anthropologist, explains why traditionally oriented Mexican-American people may consider folk healers to be vital for meeting their health needs.

> Folk healers are not professionals in the sense that they have formal training in the art of medicine or earn their living by their practice; they are members of the community who are regarded as specialists because they have learned more of the popular medicinal lore of culture than have other barrio people; use language which patients understand and vocabulary familiar to patients; never dictate what must be done, advise the patient what she or he considers appropriate. (p. 207)

There are several levels and types of folk practitioners in most Latino communities, as described below.

Yerbero(a).   The herbalist is an expert in the source, purposes, and derivatives of herbs and spices useful for cure and prevention of disease. As a grower and distributor of herbs, as well as a teacher about their uses, the *yerbero(a)*'s position in the community is one of respect and esteem. Patients will often try family remedies first, herbs from the *yerbero* second, and a visit to the *curandero* and/or physician third (Dorsey & Jackson, 1976; Giger & Davidhizar, 1999).

Curandero(a).   The *curandero(a)* is the most respected and specialized of folk healers in the Mexican-American

community (Kuipers, 1995). The following characteristics of *curanderismo* have been noted: (a) *curanderos* are chosen through divine calling and live in the community; (b) they usually have their practice in their home and their reputation is established by their successes; (c) if respectable, they will not try to cure someone who is incurable, critically ill, or "hexed" (under the influence of a witch or magic); (d) most prescribe prayers, teas, poultices, and herbs; and (e) they do not charge fees, but do accept donations from families (Dorsey & Jackson, 1976; Prattes, 1973; Spector, 2000).

Espiritualisto(a).   This person is a spiritualist who has the ability to analyze dreams and fears, foretell the future, and treat some supernatural and magical diseases (those caused by *brujos*).

Brujo(a).   The *brujo(a)* is skilled in the use of magic and witchcraft and can cast spells or hexes on individuals, as well as remove those cast by other magicians. They are honored out of fear rather than admiration (Dorsey & Jackson, 1976; Giger & Davidhizar, 1999).

Most of these above descriptions of health care practices and beliefs are those of Mexican-Americans. Central Americans tend to have similar practices and beliefs. Puerto Ricans, however, have some differences in their health beliefs and practices. Folk diseases are somewhat different. In addition, treatments for hot and cold diseases (food, medicines) are categorized as "hot," "cold," and "cool." Some Puerto Ricans believe in spirits and spiritualism. *Santerias,* similar to *espiritualistos,* are folk healers who use spiritual means for healing. The origins of the *santerias* were in Nigeria, and health practices were brought to the Americas in the 1500s during the slavery period (Spector, 1991).

ACCESS TO AND ATTITUDES ABOUT WESTERN HEALTH CARE

There is increased reliance on physicians and "scientific health care" among second- and third-generation Latinos. Significant barriers to utilization of health care still exist, especially among the poor and recent immigrant groups. Many Latinos work in the secondary job market, characterized by low wages, poor working conditions, and limited or no health care insurance. A lack of job-based health insurance (59 percent of working

Latinos in California have no job-based health insurance) translates into serious health risks (Levan, Brown, Hayes, & Wyn, 1999). Access to Western health care has also been problematic for many Latinos due to the problems associated with language barriers and cultural differences between Anglos and Latinos. Lack of access fuels underuse of health services, misuse of emergency rooms, and delayed treatment, that is, waiting until the illness is more serious (Zambrana et al., 1995). The widespread lack of health insurance benefits and the cultural tradition that "suggests that bad health, though unpleasant, is something that one endures" (Bullough & Bullough, 1982, p. 79) are barriers to seeking health care. Moreover, when a Hispanic-American is in need of medical assistance, he or she is expected to turn to the family first in order to have these needs met. Only when familial resources have been exhausted or circumstances are unusual, is it acceptable for the traditional Latino to seek outside help (Bullough & Bullough).

Mexican-Americans generally tend to dread illness and hospitalization more than Anglos do. Perhaps this is due to higher mortality rates or the poorer health that Chicanos experience. Certainly, the family cannot afford the huge medical expenses. The estrangement Latinos often feel when dealing with the health care system also contributes to their apprehension of being sick, injured, or hospitalized (Trevino et al., 1999).

Many authors have mentioned that Latino feelings about health providers and the "scientific" or Western health care systems are usually negative. There are several reasons for this:

1. Health providers use their own medical jargon, which is incomprehensible to poor Latino clients.

2. Linguistic barriers exist. Less than 5 percent of physicians in California are Latino and relatively few speak Spanish.

3. The provider's ignorance and arrogance regarding Latino's traditional beliefs and practices make families feel alienated and uncertain.

4. Latinos generally object to clinical, cold, objective attitudes of physicians and nurses and to their concept of efficiency, which involves a time orientation that values speed and results rather than getting to know the patient.

5. For fear of jeopardizing their families' immigration status, many Latino immigrants will not apply for government assistance (Farge, 1975; Herrera & Wagner, 1974; Trevino et al., 1999).

In contrast to the above literature that portrays Hispanic-Americans as being negative about Anglo health care, Friedman (1985), in a study of 27 Latino families who had a child with cancer, found the parents to be overwhelmingly positive about their Western health care providers. Not only were parents satisfied with the ongoing care they and their children were receiving, but they also expressed confidence in their doctors and nurse practitioners. They saw these providers as "healers" who were very helpful in assisting them to cope with their child's illnesses.

FAMILY STRESSORS AND COPING STRATEGIES

Latino families collectively are likely to experience a greater number of major stressors when compared to Anglo families. Certainly poverty, discrimination, cultural conflicts, the immigration experience, social and geographic mobility, and language barriers are primary sources of stress. Substandard housing, inadequate health care and education, and poor employment opportunities are widespread. Immigrant families are identified as a very high-risk group in terms of being candidates for family instability and individual health problems (Zambrana et al., 1995).

Based on the Hispanic-American family literature, seeking of social support from the extended family and of spiritual support appear to be two central culturally derived family coping strategies.

FAMILY SUPPORT

Previous studies have empirically demonstrated that the Latino extended family is stronger and more active in providing both instrumental and emotionally supportive assistance than the Anglo family, and thus serves as an important family coping strategy (Falicov, 1998; Sotomayor, 1991). This was empirically confirmed in a study by Friedman (1985). Friedman predicted that there would be differences in family coping between Anglo and Latino families. To examine this hypothesis, she sampled 28 Anglo and 27 Latino families that had a child with childhood cancer. Friedman's findings demonstrate that the extended family, especially secondary kin, and religion are significantly more important family coping strategies of Latino families than of Anglo families.

A well-articulated system of linked nuclear family households exist through which Latino families meet their various life needs. Clearly established patterns of reciprocal help and mutual aid are found between and among extended family members (Falicov, 1998; Mirandé, 1977; Vega et al., 1983). This system offers assistance and feelings of security. An example of reciprocity is seen when a poor family becomes too large to support all of its members and, as a result, a child or some of the children are raised by grandparents, uncles, or aunts. Godparents may also be vitally supportive persons in Latino families (Falicov).

SPIRITUAL SUPPORT

The church, religion, prayer, and reliance on God and saints appear to be more important to Latinos than to Anglos (Rehm, 1999; San Miguel, Morrison, & Weissglass, 1999). In Friedman's (1985) study, Latino parents reported that "God, prayers, and faith" were the most important way Latino families coped with their child's cancer. In terms of the predominant religion among Hispanic-American families, 90 percent are Catholic. Mexican Catholicism, it should be noted, varies from American Roman Catholicism. Mexican Catholicism is described as a blend of both Catholicism and pre-Cortesian Indian beliefs and ideology (Kruszewski, Anthony, Hough, & Ornstein-Galicia, 1982). The basic Catholic premise that God governs one's life and ultimately takes it from us permeates the traditional Hispanic attitude toward illness.

FATALISM/PASSIVE APPRAISAL

The extent to which Latino families employ fatalism as a passive appraisal type of coping strategy is not entirely clear in the literature, and certainly has been controversial, due to the early anthropological studies that stereotyped all Mexican-Americans as being fatalistic. Yet, Mirowsky and Ross (1984) and Neff and Hoppe (1993) did find a greater tendency for Latinos

to be fatalistic than Anglos, especially among those Latinos with a stronger ethnic heritage. Fatalism can be looked at as implying a sense of vulnerability and lack of control in the presence of adversity, or as an adaptive response to uncontrollable life situations (Neff & Hoppe). Poor families' realistic assessment of their possibilities has been called fatalism, "contentment with their lot," and lack of concern. All imply pathology, differentness, and wrongness. Martinez (1976) warns that it is this sort of stereotyping that leads people in positions of dominance and control to expect stereotyped behavior and to act accordingly.

CONTRASTS WITH ANGLO FAMILIES

In addition to spiritual and family supports being more important in Latino families, in Friedman's (1985) study, Anglo in comparison to Latino families reported that spousal support, helpfulness of friends and neighbors, and obtaining medical information were more important family coping strategies. Besides these apparent ethnic differences, social class of parents also made a difference in family coping patterns. For example, spousal support was reported as a more helpful way of coping by both the middle-class Latinos and Anglos—who generally have more of a companionship type of marriage than lower- or working-class individuals have.

Vega and associates (1986) also studied ethnic differences (Anglo and Latino) in family coping—in the areas of family cohesion and family adaptability. When comparing families with respect to these two patterns, they found no significant ethnic differences. Both the Latino and Anglo families appeared to be functioning within healthy boundaries in terms of cohesion and adaptability.

One of the major considerations pertaining to culturally derived family coping strategies is the concern about what happens to a family when culturally derived coping strategies are not available. Researchers speculate that the consequences of the Latino family being heavily reliant on family support (and usually not on support from friends or neighbors) may have adverse effects when the extended family is not present (Keefe, Padilla, & Carlos, 1978; Vega et al., 1983). When these families do not have a local extended family network, they will sometimes be without other social supports, leaving them less able to cope with stress. Friedman (1985) confirmed the increased vulnerability to stress that Latino nuclear families, who were unsupported by extended families, experienced under the prolonged stress of childhood cancer. These families showed much greater familial strains (greater family conflict) and expressions of parental distress.

FAMILY NURSING ASSESSMENT

The family nurse needs to consider to what extent the characteristics of Latino families described in this chapter are applicable to the family they are caring for. Also, to what extent does a family member, or the family as a whole, identify with their culture of origin or with mainstream American culture? Different families, as well as different members within a family, may differ in their cultural identification. Rather than there being a discrete dichotomy between Latino and mainstream American culture, a continuum exists with an infinite number of positions present that individuals and families may take.

Recall the cultural assessment guidelines in Chapter 8 relative to the key questions to ask or observations to make. In addition, the following several assessment areas are particularly germane when working with Latino families.

- With immigrant families, asking the question "What is your country of origin?" and listening to the family members' stories of immigration help to build an understanding about the country and culture the family left behind and their reasons for leaving (Garcia-Preto, 1996).

- Assessment of the Hispanic-American family's environment is often crucial. This includes the physical as well as the social environment. If the family is an immigrant family, are they suffering from the loss of their traditional social support network, which was left behind in their country of origin?

- Are language and lack of familiarity with U.S. institutions interfering with their access to health and other community services?

- Evaluating the extent to which a family subscribes to traditional folk or indigenous health

practices and to Western health care should be part of a cultural assessment. As mentioned earlier, it is common for families to subscribe to both forms of health care, depending on the health problem and access to Western health care. The family nurse in community-based settings must be sensitive to the use of dual systems of health care. In fact, it is often necessary to ask a family whether they are trying any traditional Latino medical remedies. The family nurse should approach this issue in a respectful and understanding manner, rather than unwittingly hinting that Latino medical practices are inferior or unacceptable. If done properly, such a discussion will convey the nurse's cultural competence to the family, and will contribute to the therapeutic alliance between family and nurse (Hong, 1993; Hong, Lee, & Lorenzo, 1995). The family nurse should not interfere with non-Western health care practices as long as they are not detrimental to the client. In fact, when folk remedies are not harmful, support and encouragement of these in combination with Western health treatments (called complementary health care) show respect for the clients' values, beliefs, and practices (Sheppard, 1990).

FAMILY NURSING INTERVENTIONS

Chapter 8 discusses culturally based family nursing interventions appropriate for working with culturally diverse families. Based on Latino culturally patterned beliefs and practices, as well as family characteristics, family nursing interventions specific to the Latino family are discussed in this concluding section.

Interactions with Latino families need to be respectful, friendly, and warm, with sensitivity shown toward clients' feelings and their need to maintain their dignity (Goldenberg & Goldenberg, 2002). Avoiding direct confrontation with a traditional Hispanic-American family member and being alert to subtle, indirect messages are also important. A polite and mild disagreement from a client may actually mean a strong disagreement and hence should be clarified with the client in a nonthreatening manner.

In addition, because the Latino tends to respect authority figures and look at health care professionals in this light, attempting to form an egalitarian partnership type of nurse–client relationship may not be most effective. The Hispanic client may feel more comfortable with a hierarchical relationship and a structured instructive approach.

Family nurses, particularly those in community health and primary care, need to be alert to and understanding of the social environmental problems and institutional discriminatory barriers faced by less acculturated, poor Hispanic-American families (Gallegos, 1991). When referring families who have experienced these barriers to different service agencies, coordinating and streamlining referrals and intake procedures as much as possible will minimize confusion and ensure better outcomes. It is well to remember that other family problems may supersede the resolution of health problems. Helping a family tackle their other health-related problems, often by making well-coordinated referrals, may leave the way open for the family to engage in solving their primary health concerns.

Applying knowledge about the traditional Hispanic-American family structure and lifestyle patterns, the family nurse should be sensitive to the role and expectations of different family members, such as the authority of the parents, especially the father, and the grandparents, especially the grandmother, in the area of health care and child rearing. She or he should also be respectful of the special strengths of Latino families (Goldenberg & Goldenberg, 2002). Family nurses should not expect a Latino client to make a significant health decision until he or she has a chance to consult with family members. For client compliance, the family needs to feel positive about the health decision and feel that the recommended treatment will work. The importance of the family members' mutual responsibility should be recognized. Family health professionals should make an effort to consult with those family members who have authority in the family. Meeting with the extended family members to discuss a seriously or chronically ill family member's diagnosis and treatment plan is often an excellent way to bring the family into the health care planning and decision-making process.

Recognizing that belief in folk illnesses maintains a strong cultural pattern among traditional Latino families, family nurses who work with these families should become familiar with traditional health beliefs and practices, including folk illnesses, healing practices, and indigenous health care systems (e.g., *curanderismo*). Those family members who hold folk beliefs and/or use folk medicine or folk practitioners generally will not discuss these ideas and practices with Western health care practitioners unless asked about directly (Huff & Kline, 1999).

It is best to emphasize to the adult ill family members their responsibility for the family (Rankin & Stallings, 2001) and to encourage the whole family or the extended family to adopt a new health program—such as dietary regimens or obtaining immunizations—rather than encouraging a sole individual to go it alone. People may be more influenced by what other significant family members say and do than by what the health care practitioner recommends. Monroe (1990) explains why many Latinos have not been getting the message about health-promotive behavior.

> Health messages need to use traditional Latino family values. . . . In effect, telling a Latino to exercise more and to eat a low-fat diet generally does not work if the implied short-term payoff is that a person will be thinner or feel better. Latinos, like American Indians, tend to see things more in a social context. . . . It's not all me, me, me. It's more of "How will that affect my family? I will live longer; therefore, my family will be better off." It is easy to see the effect of this lack of culturally appropriate health messages in the Latino community. (p. E1)

Planning programs to fit Latino cultural patterns and values is an extension of this latter suggestion. Because family involvement and participation work best, planning of family-oriented programs is recommended. Fostering of family-oriented rather than individually oriented self-care is another way of stating the above suggestion. Our own cultural bias may be for self-care and individual effort, but for the Latino who values familism, assisting the family to become competent makes more sense.

Family members, including the extended family, may want to take an active role in the treatment/rehabilitation of the ill member. It is important to allow all members of the extended family to ask questions and participate in the treatment/rehabilitation as much as possible.

❧SUMMARY

- There is both a demographic and practice imperative for family nurses to have a good understanding of Latino families. This understanding is essential for providing culturally appropriate and competent care.

- Latinos are persons residing in the United States whose ancestries are from the Latin American countries in the Western Hemisphere—Mexico, Puerto Rico, Cuba, and South and Central America, 22 countries in all.

- Demographically, there has been a massive surge in Latino immigration to the United States in the last decade. By 2005, Latinos will be the largest minority group in the United States. They are relatively young and have a high birth rate, meaning the population boom is just beginning.

- The largest Latino group is from Mexico (59 percent), followed by Puerto Rico (10 percent), South and Central America (9 percent), and Cuba (4 percent). Other Latinos account for 18 percent, according to the 2000 census data.

- The major waves of Latino immigrants came to the United States after World War II. The historical interface with the United States has varied by Latino group.

- The Latino family–U.S. society interface usually comes via children's school participation and parents' employment. Children's school participation has resulted in value clashes between school (exemplifying American values) and traditionally held family values. The occupational interface has often been problematic also in that lower- and working-class Latinos have often experienced job discrimination, unemployment, and employment in menial, minimally paying jobs.

- Educationally, occupationally, and economically, Latinos, with the exception of Cuban-Americans, are substantially disadvantaged when compared with Anglo-Americans.

- Although acculturation of Latino families has been a primary process used to explain Latinos adaptation to American culture, research has found that the process is complex, uneven, and incomplete. Latinos typically acculturate in many areas, but retain culturally derived patterns in other areas, such as the centrality of the extended family and their love for their own native language. Latinos can be both "modern and ethnic" at the same time.

- To understand Latino families today, one must understand their immigration experience (since many Latinos are immigrants) and the environmental challenges they face.

- Due to a deep commitment to family, more Latinos live in traditional nuclear families today than white or black families. Nevertheless, there are a growing number of varied family forms among Latinos today—such as single-parent families, binational families, and multiple-family households.

- Past descriptions of Latino families in the literature have often been erroneous. Many of these descriptions did not consider social class variation and perpetuated negative stereotypes.

- Several Latino values were discussed. These are the primacy of *familism* and with this, the concomitant family values of familial mutual obligations, support, and reciprocity.

- Value conflicts between the generations are commonplace in Latino families. Exposure to American values comes through school, work, and living in the barrio.

- Although family roles are changing in many Latino families, the father still holds a place of primary authority and respect in the family. The traditional role of wife is being a nurturing, self-sacrificing woman and mother. The role of women in the family is changing as they become educated and join the workforce.

- Communication and socialization patterns in Latino families are heavily influenced by culture. Table 18–1 discusses these differences, as well as other major differences between Anglos and Latinos.

- Many Latino families, especially those who have recently migrated to the United States and/or who are poor, hold traditional folk health beliefs and use folk health practices and practitioners, especially for folk illnesses, as well as Western health care.

- For Latinos, significant barriers to utilizing Western health care still exist. These barriers are largely due to lack of job-based health insurance, Latino health beliefs, linguistic barriers, the way Western health care is delivered (seen as clinical, cold, and confusing), and reticence applying for governmental assistance because of the fear that one's immigration status might be jeopardized.

- Culturally derived family coping includes seeking and using extended family support and spiritual support, as well as fatalism/passive appraisal.

- Certain family assessment areas and interventions are recommended as being particularly germane, given the Latino family structure, lifestyle, beliefs, and practices.

✎ FAMILY VIGNETTE: THE LOPEZ FAMILY

The Jorge Lopez family came to the hospital to visit the father's mother, Mrs. Lupe Lopez, age 65, who was hospitalized with newly diagnosed diabetes and is quite distraught. The younger Lopez family consisted of Jorge, the father, age 42; Marie, the mother, age 40; Luciana, the older daughter, age 13; and Lupita, the younger daughter, age 12. Mrs. Lopez lives with one of her daughters and her daughter's three teenage children. The Jorge Lopez family came from Puerto Rico one year ago and now live in New York City. Family members speak little English, although the girls are picking it up rapidly in school. During the visit the father was observed as being outspoken in his communication with his own family. He was respectful and kind to his mother. He works double shifts as a janitor, while his wife works part time cleaning houses. Jorge and Marie, when asked their ethnic background, stated they were Puerto Rican and preferred to speak Spanish whenever possible.

The younger Lopez family's main concern was for the health of Jorge's mother. Reluctantly, the father conveyed to the nurse that the whole family believed that Mrs. Lopez did not have diabetes, but became ill because of "nervios" and "sugar," created by bad family conflicts in the home. The family also believed that giving the mother certain herbs and restoring harmony in the Lopez family (the mother and her daughter and her children) would heal the mother. They wanted to take their mother home and, after consulting the rest of the extended family, take her to an herbalist (yerbero) and a spiritualist (an espiritualisto or a santero) before any decision could be made about the mother's treatment.

▪ STUDY QUESTIONS

Review the Family Vignette and answer the related questions.

1. As the primary family nurse caring for Mrs. Lopez, what is your cultural assessment of the family?

2. What information would you like to have about the family (as part of your assessment)?

3. What family nursing interventions would be appropriate in working with this family?

Answer the following questions.

4. What peoples constitute Latinos? Which of these subgroups are most numerous in the United States?

5. Several important factors have adversely influenced the Latino family's integration into American society, even though some of these same factors may be "positive" for the family. Give three of these factors.

Are the following statements true or false?

6. Familism refers to the Mexican-American's propensity to marry early and have a family.

7. In the Latino family, the male and older person have both traditionally held positions of respect.

8. Male dominance in the Latino family is widespread, the evidence indicating that the father–husband holds absolute power.

9. The institution of having *compadres* among Mexican-American families refers to the custom of having godparents. This custom is, however, declining as a result of acculturation.

10. Which of the following are criticisms that Latino family scholars and researchers have made about the early writings by social scientists?

   a. They are pejorative.
   b. They tend to describe the Latino family as homogeneous.
   c. The literature discusses only the middle-class family.
   d. They assume that acculturation will occur uniformly across all facets of family life.
   e. They view the family from a systems, ecological perspective.

11. For each of the following American central values, explain what the corresponding traditional Latino value is:

Area	American Core Value	Traditional Latino Value
Family	Americans see themselves as an individual first, a family member second.	
Work	Productivity and work are central and prominent values. Work often becomes an end rather than a means to an end.	
Materialism	Possession of material goods is a symbol of success. The greater the accumulation of goods, the greater the prestige.	
Time and punctuality	"Time is money." Punctuality is a moral value equated with being responsible.	
Interpersonal relationships	Americans value openness and directness in communication, as well as rationality versus emotional expressiveness.	

Are the following statements true or false?

12. The most profound structural change occurring in the Latino family today is the resurgence of the value of familism.

13. Democratic ideals and verbal facility in negotiation are taught at a young age in the Latino family.

14. The ethic of reciprocity in the Latino family has to do with the exchange that takes place between spouses when they role share.

15. Match the description of the folk healer with the type of folk healer.

    1. *Yerbero*   a. Herbalist
    2. *Santeria*   b. Deals with supernatural illnesses
    3. *Respecto*   c. Practices witchcraft or magic
    4. *Espiritualisto(a)* d. Puerto Rican folk healer
    5. *Brujo(a)*   e. Healer of folk illnesses in the Mexican-American
    6. *Curandero(a)*   community
                          f. None of the above

16. Fill in the name of each of the following common Mexican folk illnesses from this list of possibilities (mental illness, *empacho, susto, mal de ojo, mal puesto, caida de la mollera*).

    a. "Bad eye," resulting from excessive admiration or desire on the part of another
    b. Disease given by God or a *brujo* as a hex or punishment on the patient
    c. Affliction caused by food adhering to the stomach wall in the form of a ball
    d. Fallen fontanels (in infants)
    e. Sorcery
    f. Illness caused by fright or emotionally traumatizing experience

17. Based on what is known of Latino families, and of families in general, identify which of the following practice suggestions would be most appropriate for which group (Latino family, A; all families, B).

    a. Separation of hospitalized patient from family member(s) should be considered very carefully.
    b. Client should not be expected to make a significant health care decision until he or she has had a chance to consult with the family.
    c. It is best to attempt to have the whole family adopt a health-promotion or maintenance program.
    d. Other family problems may take precedence over health problems, and thus the health worker may have to help the family with its other problems in order for it to be able to resolve health needs.
    e. Families need to be spoken to in terms and concepts they understand and suggestions need to appeal to their basic values.
    f. An authoritative approach, whereby the health professional conveys expertise and confidence in his or her ability to "heal," is expected.

18. Identify two primary culturally derived family coping strategies of Mexican-Americans. Based on knowledge about culturally derived family coping strategies and an assessment of a Latino family's coping responses, state one practice implication.

THE AFRICAN-AMERICAN FAMILY

✎ LEARNING OBJECTIVES

1. Identify what populations constitute African-Americans.
2. Name one demographic trend among African-Americans and explain the factors associated with that trend.

3. Briefly discuss the status of the African-American family today, relative to the growing middle class and the underclass.
4. State an opinion on what the most important limitation of past black family literature is and why.

5. Discuss the most prevalent black family forms and why they are different from white family forms.
6. Identify three important coping strategies of African-American families.
7. Broadly describe differences in socialization among middle-class, working-class, and lower-class African-American families.
8. Identify two traditional folk practitioners and folk remedies that existed in black American communities in the past.

9. Compare the family roles and power structure of black middle-class, working-class, and lower-class families.
10. Explain two family nursing assessment considerations based on African-American cultural patterns.
11. Explain three family nursing interventions based on African-American cultural patterns.

According to Census 2000, African-Americans are the largest racial/ethnic minority group in the United States. African-Americans are geographically and socioeconomically very diverse. Nevertheless, they share both cultural origins (coming from Africa centuries ago and enduring the legacy of slavery) and the necessity to manage the stress produced by discrimination and other social and institutional barriers. Most African-Americans' ancestors came directly from Africa. Some, however, came from Africa originally, but more recently from the West Indies or Central or South America.

In this chapter, both African-American and black are used to describe this racial/ethnic group. The current literature addressing the black/African-American family also uses both terms interchangeably.

"The family is one of the strongest and most important traditions in the black community" (Franklin, 1988, p. 23). It is unclear as to how much of this tradition is part of the African legacy and how much was developed in the New World.

The development of the contemporary African-American family is overshadowed by the disastrous legacy of slavery. During the era of slavery, the black family existed only by the consent of the slave owner for the purposes of perpetuating the system and improving the slave owner's economic status. The black family was not autonomous or self-sufficient. Slaves were able to construct family units when it suited the needs of the slave owners. These units often were mother centered, with the mother–child relationship primary and the husband–wife and father–child relationships tenuous (Rainwater, 1971).

❧ AFRICAN-AMERICAN DEMOGRAPHIC PATTERNS

African-Americans comprise approximately 12 percent of the American population. It is projected that by 2005 they will be the second largest minority group—Latinos will be more numerous then. Over 81 percent now live in urban areas (U.S. Bureau of the Census, 2000a). The percentage of African-Americans in the population will rise slowly and in the year 2050 is projected to constitute 14 percent of the U.S. population (Rosenblatt, 1996) (see Table 8–1). Two striking developments have occurred within the black population in the United States since the civil rights movement of the 1960s. One is the emergence of an authentic, large, and economically strong middle class—better educated, better paid, better housed than for any group of African-Americans in the past (Cose, 1999; Gelman et al., 1988; Hutchinson, 1988). The other development is the emergence and growth of the black underclass (Cose; Taylor, Chatters, Tucker, & Lewis, 1990). In 1997, 27 percent of all black Americans were poor as compared to 11 percent of all white Americans (Fulwood, 1996; Cose) (see Figure 18–2).

The black middle class grew in the 1990s, while the black underclass increased to approximately three times larger than it was in the 1970s and 1980s (Cose, 1999). This group, as discussed in Chapter 8, generates a disproportionate share of the social pathology associated with living in a ghetto—poverty, unemployment, high welfare rates, high rates of homelessness, high crime rates, gang warfare, drugs, dropouts, and teenage pregnancies. Poverty has hit black children particularly hard. For example, in 65 percent of African-American mother-headed families, children are poor. Black children are three times more likely to be poor than white children (see Table 8–5).

The opportunities of the last three decades resulted in the underclass becoming isolated from the more educated and ambitious blacks who took advantage of opportunities to move to more middle-class neighborhoods and away from the ghettos. For the underclass left behind, the statistics in Table 19–1 bespeak their disadvantaged condition.

With a large proportion of African-Americans in poverty and the simultaneously rising proportion of African-Americans at the higher income levels (Cose, 1999; Malveaux, 1988), a polarity of economic extremes exists within the black community (Levy, 1988; Taylor, 2000). It is important to emphasize this diverse complexion of black families in America. Despite the large number and worsening status of the black underclass, the majority of African-Americans have experienced substantial economic improvements, although certainly more improvement is needed (for instance, the median black income is still only 62 percent of the median white income) (Cose).

TEENAGE PREGNANCIES AND SINGLE-PARENT FAMILIES

The very high number of black teenage pregnancies and resulting single-parent families, which then live in poverty, is a major societal and family health concern. The majority (two thirds) of out-of-wedlock births, however, are not to teenagers, but to adult women over the age of 20 (McAdoo, 1995). The proportion of single-parent families is much higher among African-Americans when compared to Anglo-Americans—45 percent versus 13 percent of all households, respectively (U.S. Census Bureau, 2000a). According to some sociologists (Meisler & Fulwood, 1989; Staples, 1985, 1989), the cause of the large number of black single-parent families is the shortage of marriageable black males in the underclass.

MARRIAGES: DELAYED AND DECLINING

The marital status of black parents is changing. "Marriage is becoming a minority lifestyle for black parents" (McAdoo, 1995, p. 23). Marriages are being delayed until the late 20s (a trend in the

TABLE 19–1

AFRICAN-AMERICAN FAMILIES: EVIDENCE OF THE SERIOUS PROBLEMS AFRICAN-AMERICAN FAMILIES FACE

- Twenty-nine percent of all African-American families live in poverty.
- African-Americans continue to make on the average about 60% of what white Americans make.
- A black man over 24 is twice as likely as a white man to be unemployed.
- The rate of unemployment for black youth is more than double that of white youth.
- Black children are three times as likely to live in poverty and in female-headed families than white children.
- Sixty percent of African-American children live in poverty.
- More than one in six black households live in dilapidated homes.
- Twenty percent of all African-American families live in public housing.
- The divorce rate among African-Americans is twice as high as Anglo-Americans.
- A black baby is three times more likely than a white baby to have a mother who dies in childbirth or a mother who received no prenatal care.
- Black Americans are disproportionately represented among the homeless (e.g., in New York City, 73% of the city's homeless are black even though only 25% of the city's population is black).
- Black teenagers and young adults are nearly five times as likely as their white counterparts to die of AIDS.

Sources: Clinton (1995), Edelman (1997), Fulwood (1996), Schulte (1995), and the U.S. Bureau of the Census (2000b).

United States generally, but more pronounced among blacks). Moreover, marriage rates are declining considerably. Only 44 percent of black adults were married in 1991, compared to 64 percent in 1970. Most of those who are not married are not divorced. They are persons who have never been married. The level of marriage is important both for economic reasons (two parents make a higher household income—often enough to take them out of poverty) and for marital stability. The literature discusses several reasons for delayed marriages and a decline in marriages. The sex-ratio imbalance (more available, marriageable women than men) is identified as the primary factor. There are approximately 32 men for every 100 women in the African-American marriage pool. The imbalance is caused by a high death rate of black teenagers and young adults; a high rate of male incarceration; men's high unemployment rate; women's higher educational attainment; men's poorer health status; and a growing incidence of suicides among black men. Women's increasing economic independence and labor force participation has also made marriage less attractive for some African-American women (McAdoo; Taylor, 2000).

RISING NUMBER OF TROUBLED AFRICAN-AMERICAN MEN

There is widespread concern about the declining status of black adult men in both the African-American and general community (Heady, 1996). Black males place at the bottom of nearly every social indicator—highest unemployment, highest infant mortality rate, lowest life expectancy, and poorest educated (Harris, 1990; Savage, 1990). Poverty is three times higher among black adult males than among their white male counterparts. In 1995, according to a national survey report (the "Sentencing Project"), 30 percent of young black men (20 to 29 years) were under the supervision of the criminal justice system, and to add to this tragedy, young black men are murdered—almost always by other black men—at 10 times the rate of white men in the same age group (Brownstein, 1995). So bad is the black males' situation that the National Association for the Advancement of Colored People (NAACP) calls the black male an "endangered species."

THE AFRICAN-AMERICAN FAMILY: A LEGACY OF VULNERABILITY AND RESILIENCE

Accounts of the African-American family portray two opposing pictures—one of incredible resilience (the family displaying resilience, adaptive coping strategies, and a mood of optimism [African-American Monitor, 1999] in the context of a harsh past and present environment) and the other of an endangered family with major problems in race relations, living with racism and poverty (Cose, 1999; Greene, 1995; Ingrasia, 1993; Johnson, 1997).

The good news about black families is that the black middle class is doing very well, relative to their past. All indicators of success (e.g., employment, home ownership, reading and math proficiency, infant mortality rate) are up, while indicators of dysfunction (crime, births to single women, poverty) are down. In the past few decades, black families' fortunes and prospects have soared. The discouraging news, however, is that not all black Americans have enjoyed this prosperity. Despite all the progress made, there is still a considerably large number of black families who are working but poor or are part of the underclass. Moreover, America is still intensely segregated across all socioeconomic levels relative to residential living patterns (Cose, 1999; Craig & Clymer, 2000).

Staples (1989), a noted family sociologist, brings into perspective the present and future status of African-American families. He summarizes the problems of the black family as being the same as in the past century. Problems are primarily poverty and racism. A major stressor in black family life is the psychological and social pressures of racism in the everyday environment. This is termed *mundane extreme environmental stress* in some of the literature (Peters & Massey, 1983; Peters, 1997).

Race relations continues to be a major barrier to integration of African-Americans; white and black Americans often see the same world in drastically different ways, and in spite of remarkable progress made in black and white relations, a considerable rift still exists. President Clinton, in addressing the University of Texas (1995), spoke of the responsibility of all Americans to acknowledge injustices and to help heal the division between the two races. He stated:

White America must understand and acknowledge the roots of black pain. It began with unequal treatment first in law and later in fact. African Americans indeed have lived too long with a justice system that in too many cases has been and continues to be less than just. The record of abuses extends from lynchings and trumped-up charges to false arrests and police brutality. The tragedies of Emmett Till and Rodney King are bloody markers on the very same road. (p. A12)

Although the future of black middle-class families looks positive, the future of black families in the underclass looks dim. Black men continue to experience widespread problems, as noted in Table 19–1, while black women and their roles are in a state of transition—paralleling some changes in American women generally (decreased fertility and greater liberation) (Staples, 1989).

STATUS OF AFRICAN-AMERICAN FAMILIES: CRITICISM OF THE LITERATURE

There has been extensive criticism in the past of both governmental reports and of the writings of social scientists about black families (Taylor, 2000). The most controversy over governmental reporting was directed toward a report of Daniel P. Moynihan, then Assistant Secretary of Labor, who wrote a report that identified the black family with a "tangle of pathology" and with a deterioration of black society. He concluded that black families were falling apart, basing his conclusions on a myriad of statistical data showing such phenomena as numbers of absent fathers, children on welfare, and juvenile delinquency. This well-known, highly controversial report marked the beginning of the continuing debate and dialogue about the status of the black family, and more importantly, what/who was the victim and the cause. The real debate often centered around who was "to blame" for the multitude of problems besieging black lower-class families. Is it the family itself, the societal treatment of African-Americans, or a combination of both external and

internal factors? (As we know from other studies, the most potent force for family behavior is external factors, particularly economic constraints.)

Although Moynihan pointed out that the societal treatment of blacks was ultimately to blame, this statement was hidden among the extensive evidence of the black family in trouble. His report also suggested that the black family itself, as a result of its weakening, possessed characteristics inimical to its welfare. Moynihan identified the black family's matriarchal structure as a key contributor to the deterioration of the black family.

Billingsley (1968) and other scholars of the black family disagreed. They see the black family as a resilient and adaptive system and maintain that black families survived their long journey from Africa to urban America by developing characteristic strength—chiefly a sense of extended family that provides support and nurture during crisis or parental absence (Billingsley, 1992; Greene, 1995; Hill, 1971; Taylor, 2000).

One of the significant points of clarification to come from the debate about the status of the black family is that the issues concerning the black family concern the black lower-class family (Taylor, 2000). Notwithstanding the recognition that racism exists against all black Americans, the black middle-class family varies greatly from the lower-class and underclass family. It is similar to its white counterpart in family lifestyle and does not manifest the extensive strains of the poor black family.

The African-American family, regardless of social class status, has been repeatedly termed a matrifocal structure, forced into this family form because of the separation of husband and wife during slavery and more recently because of economic realities, welfare restrictions, and a lack of available, marriageable black men (Clinton, 1995). But according to Billingsley (1992) and Willie (1976), this assertion about the black families' matrifocal structure does not properly account for the total range of black families in our society. First, a majority of adult black men and women work to support their families. Although still well below the proportion of two-parent white families with children, about one third of black families are two-parent families (Cose, 1999; Glick, 1997).

The black family has adapted to the larger society in various ways, with the common experience of racial discrimination, oppression, and economic adversity playing very significant roles. Economic stressors include the stressors of poverty, under- and unemployment, housing, and health care (McAdoo, 1995). Billingsley (1992), a black sociologist, believes that the various structures and functions of black families have resulted largely as adaptive reactions to varying socioeconomic conditions and stressors that threaten black families' survival.

STUDIES OF AFRICAN-AMERICAN FAMILIES BY SOCIAL SCIENTISTS

As with the Mexican-American family literature, there has also been extensive criticism of the writings of social scientists about the black family (Johnson, 1997). Dodson (1988) criticized black family literature as inconsistent, poorly conceptualized, and flawed in terms of research designs. Hill and co-workers (1993) cited the ubiquity of inadequate research perspectives that have guided African-American family research and social policy.

The early black family literature of the 1960s and 1970s generally saw black families that deviated from mainstream white family lifestyles as deviant or pathological. Using the deficit theory (Peters, 1981), the root problem was often believed to reside within black families themselves. Social scientists and the media alike tended to view black families as homogeneous: poor and in trouble. A case in point is an analysis of black family articles published in the *Journal of Marriage and the Family* from 1939 to 1987 (Demos, 1990). In these articles sources of distortion were identified. A culture-of-poverty thesis was a prominent focus throughout the surveyed years and was an obvious source of distortion about the African-American family. This focus, encouragingly, has diminished considerably in recent years (Taylor, 2000).

In the last two decades a number of researchers (McAdoo, 1983; Peters, 1981; Staples, 1985) have looked at black families with a more positive theoretical perspective and also by social class (Billingsley, 1992; Coner-Edwards & Spurlock, 1988; McAdoo, 1982). Having this more positive view, black family life is viewed from a cultural variant perspective (Johnson, 1997). This is also an ecological, systems perspective, one that views black families as viable, functional, and interacting within mainstream soci-

ety. "This approach assumes that most Black families have developed patterns of behavior and child-rearing attitudes and practices which are appropriate to the values and constraints within their own lives" (Peters, pp. 73–74). Unique aspects of black life are not necessarily taken as reflections of pathology (Johnson; Taylor, 2000).

One important deficiency among black American family literature is the paucity of research about blacks who come from diverse countries and cultures. Greater attention must be given to black American immigrant families who come from the West Indies, Central and South America, and Africa (Johnson, 1997).

AFRICAN-AMERICAN FAMILY FORMS AND KINSHIP SYSTEM

Thirty-five percent of all black families with children under 18 were nuclear two-parent families in 1997 (Cose, 1999). Although the female-headed single-parent family is commonly seen (45 percent of all black families were single parent in 2000 according to the U.S. Bureau of the Census [2000a]), the modal and ideal black family is still considered the traditional nuclear two-parent family.

EXTENDED FAMILIES

One of the distinctive characteristics of black families is the fact that a much higher proportion of black than white family households have extended family members living with them (Glick, 1997; Taylor, 2000). Many of the black families that are not nuclear in form consist of groups of relatives such as grandparents and their grandchildren, brothers, sisters, and other relatives. Sometimes non–blood relatives (fictive kin) are also part of the extended family (Glick). Approximately 1 in 5 African-American families is extended, compared to 1 in 10 white families (Taylor). Working-class and middle-class black families may have an older relative living in the home providing child care while both spouses work. In the poorer family, the more common pattern is of an older female relative bringing under her wing a younger woman and her children.

Three-generation households typically exist when there is no husband present. Most married couples have their own apartment or home.

One of the primary cultural patterns noted in the black family literature is the strong reliance on the extended family (McAdoo, 1995). The concept of the extended family among African-Americans can mean that family members live in the same household or in separate households. Parent–child bonds across the life course are very close (Taylor et al., 1988). Young black couples prefer to live near their families of origin. Strong kinship bonds are also evidenced by the high frequency with which African-American families take relatives (especially children under 18) into their households. Black families have developed their own network for the informal adoption of children (Hill & Shackleford, 1986). Babies born to unmarried girls and women are frequently kept in the home; in 1978 fully 90 percent of such black children were reared by parents or relatives, whereas in white families only 33 percent of children born to unmarried girls and women were kept in the home.

Historically, the tradition of living together as an extended family may have come from West African cultures (Hines & Boyd-Franklin, 1996). In any case, the extended family has served as a means of pooling resources (Taylor, 2000; Thornton, 1995). Extended families, regardless of social class, provide reciprocity and a collective network, helping one another and sharing goods and services (Hines & Boyd-Franklin). Today, especially among the poor, financial resources, food, emergency care, and child care are extensively shared among the extended family (Peters & Massey, 1983; Taylor et al., 1988). Child care is often provided by relatives. This is called "multiple mothering," meaning that grandmothers, aunts, cousins, close friends, or people considered as kin to the child's mother carry out parental roles. They provide emotional support, tangible child care assistance, and alternative parent role models (Greene, 1995). The grandmother, especially the maternal grandmother, has been the most prominent provider of child care.

Today, many of the grandmothers are very young themselves (between 27 and 39). A considerable number of these young grandmothers are feeling resistant to taking on another role—that of grandparenthood—because they still are involved in young adult roles themselves (Burton & Bengtson, 1985; Burton & de Vries, 1995). Parenting "a second time

around" can be very stressful, especially when the grandparenting is due to a parent's drug or child abuse problems (Haglund, 2000).

SINGLE-PARENT FAMILIES

Single-parent families are more numerous among African-Americans than other ethnic groups (see Figure 1–6). A delay in marrying, never marrying, and a high rate of divorce (twice as high as whites) are reasons for the high number of single-parent black families (McAdoo, 1995). In 2000, according to the U.S. Bureau of the Census, 43 percent of all African-American families are mother-headed families. Another 2.4 percent are father-headed families. Of these single-parent families, two thirds of births were to unmarried mothers in 1992 (U.S. Bureau of the Census, 1993). Never-married mother-headed families are likely to be poor and often young. Fatherless families are generally more troubled economically and socially. Children who grow up without fathers are disadvantaged educationally, interpersonally, and psychologically. In many single-parent families, an extensive network of other family members, family friends, and neighbors participates in the rearing of and caring for the children (Greene, 1995).

FAMILY VALUES AND COPING STRATEGIES

The black family's culturally derived values or ideology is basically conservative; that is, adult members believe in the traditional family structure, church, hard work, and strong kinship bonds. However, for the poor some of these traditional values have not been realizable, particularly the value of the traditional family structure. It is important to recall here that values are the ideals or "what should be," and the real culture is "what actually is." There sometimes is a dissonance between culturally derived family values and the structural conditions in society, particularly for lower-class and underclass black families. Staples (1985) describes this dissonance as being created because the black male is prevented from fulfilling his normative familial roles, primarily that of being the provider for the family. The adaptation of family life that has occurred is seen in the large numbers of households headed by women and out-of-wedlock births. The majority of adult women are not married and living with spouses. Moreover, two out of every three marriages end in divorce (the divorce rate for whites is also high, about 50 percent).

This analysis is presented to emphasize the point that sheer practical necessity often distorts one's values in everyday life and makes family values—what family members say is important—very different from actual behavior. Hence, some coping strategies—that is, how families respond to the demands placed on them—are more prominently found in the working- and middle-class families, and are discussed in those sections. These coping strategies that are characteristic of African-Americans regardless of social class are addressed here.

The several core coping patterns common to African-Americans as identified in the black family literature are:

1. Strong religious commitment and participation.
2. Strong bond with and support from kin and friends.
3. Flexibility in family roles.

These are crucial strengths of the black family (see Figure 19–1). Elaborations on the above coping strategies follow.

STRONG RELIGIOUS COMMITMENT AND PARTICIPATION

A strong commitment to and participation in religion has served as a primary means of coping and decision making for both the black individual and family (Paniagua, 1994; Smerglia, Deimling, & Baresi, 1988). A religious orientation was a major aspect of the lives of Africans transported here as slaves. During the era of slavery, the church played a vital role in helping black Americans cope with the oppression of slavery. It was through the church that blacks learned to use religion as a means to survive (Hill, 1971). Black churches today are descendants of the black church during slavery, where old-time religion and preaching were the mainstay of black family life (Pipes, 1997). Pipes (1988), in studying the old-time religion and preaching, explains that its purpose was to "stir up, to excite the emotions of the audience as a means for their escape from an impossible world" (pp. 55–56).

The black church is a central institution in African-American communities. In times of crisis, religion and the church-sponsored social services have been significant supportive elements in revitalizing hope for African-Americans (Goldenberg & Goldenberg, 2002; Ho, 1987). The church provides emotional, spiritual, intellectual, and social satisfaction (Hines & Boyd-Franklin, 1996). It is also an important avenue for gaining musical expression and leadership opportunities. Many black families identify elaborate church networks in which their minister and other church "sisters and brothers" are an important informal social network for the family and particularly for the older women members (Boyd, 1982). Hence, religion often plays a central role in family life, providing a powerful spiritual, social, and emotional resource (Bagley & Carroll, 1995; McGoldrick, 1993).

STRONG BONDS AND SUPPORT FROM KIN AND FRIENDS

Black families generally have a strong support system composed of kin and friends. As such, this social network represents crucial ways for families to cope. The kin and friendship help–exchange system supplements black families by sharing material, emotional, and social resources (Goldenberg & Goldenberg, 2002) as well as emergency assistance (Taylor et al., 1988) and care for sick members, children, aging parents, and grandparents (Benin & Keith, 1995).

The genesis for strong kinship has been traced back to the traditional African culture (Nobles, 1974). The tradition survived the splitting up of fami-

Figure 19–1. Strengths of the African-American family (common cultural patterns). *(Source: Adapted from McAdoo, 1995, 2000.)*

lies during slavery and has served to assist the family to deal with the harsh environment in such a way as to ensure survival, security, and self-esteem of its members. Black Americans need support and family involvement, conclude Taylor (1990) and Ellison (1990), who found in research on social support patterns of black Americans that higher levels of familial involvement and subjective family closeness were positively associated with greater family life satisfaction and personal happiness, respectively.

Black "extended families" are not necessarily drawn along "bloodlines" (Greene, 1995; Hill, 1971). There may be a number of nonkin people (fictive kin) who function in important roles in families. It is common practice for long-time friends and neighbors to be brought into the family circle (Carrington, 1978). White (1972), in his study, observed that a number of "uncles, aunts, big mamas, boyfriends, older brothers and sisters, deacons, preachers, and others operate in and out of the African-American home" (p. 45). Nonrelatives were often found to be as influential as relatives, according to one study of black social supports (Manns, 1988). African-Americans from lower-class backgrounds have been found to have a greater number of kin and nonkin in their social network than those from working- and middle-class backgrounds; the larger network serves to offset more adverse life experiences (Manns; McGoldrick, 1993).

FAMILY ROLE FLEXIBILITY

Probably the most efficacious family coping strategy in terms of assisting the family to function effectively is the black family's role flexibility, complementarity, and shared decision making (McAdoo, 1988; Peters, 1981; Taylor, 2000). The fluid interchanging of family roles emerged out of economic imperatives of black life (Ho, 1987). In most black families both parents have always had to work outside the home to make ends meet; hence, both parents shared the task of provider, as well as the domestic and child care responsibilities. African-American women have worked outside the home for decades and still are more likely to combine child rearing and work (Benin & Keith, 1995). Thus, African-American men are not threatened by their wives' employment; having a working mate has fostered more egalitarian spousal relationships (Hines & Boyd-Franklin, 1996).

Although roles vary considerably between families, sharing of household and child care tasks between spouses is more common than in white families (McAdoo, 1983). Older children in large families become responsible helpers, participating in caring for younger siblings and sometimes working part time to augment the family income. Family teamwork and cooperation are stressed.

Role flexibility within the nuclear and extended family is mobilized in times of crisis. For families experiencing problems such as separation, illness, hospitalization, death, substance abuse, or unemployment of a family member, being flexible in who does what in the family can make a difference between successful adaptation and maladaptation.

✸THE FAMILY SOCIALIZATION FUNCTION

In African-American families, children are extremely important and valued. If the mother cannot handle them, extended kin will generally take a more active role in rearing and caring for the children (McGoldrick, 1993). While men have well-defined, significant family roles, women-centered child care has been the norm (Thornton, 1995). African-American women are described in the literature as "all sacrificing mothers" and "the strength of the family" (Hines & Boyd-Franklin, 1996).

Research findings from ecologically oriented and comparative studies represent the most informative and enlightened types of child-rearing studies involving black Americans. In the ecologically oriented studies, it is assumed that black families encourage the development of skills, abilities, and behaviors necessary to survive in their environment (Peters, 1997). In the comparative studies, relevant differences between Anglo and ethnically diverse families are examined using a relativistic perspective. In general, according to Peters, black families are reported to be strong, functional, and flexible in their socialization practices. The values of sharing, reciprocity, collective actions, and cooperation are emphasized (McBridge, 1995).

Black Americans provide a home setting that is culturally different from that of white Americans.

Children are raised to adjust to the special stress of poverty (in the case of lower-class families) and discrimination, as well as the "ambiguity and marginality of living simultaneously in two worlds—the world of the Black community and the world of mainstream society" (Peters, 1981, p. 233). Greene (1995) explains that black parents must prepare their children to function adequately within the dominant culture without internalizing the dominant culture's negative messages about African-Americans. Parents must teach their children to "make psychological sense out of their disparaged condition, deflect hostility from the dominant group and negotiate racial barriers under a wide range of circumstances" (Greene, p. 30). Explicit racial socialization is a distinctive child-rearing technique black parents use to prepare their children for life in America (Thornton, 1995).

Discipline techniques of black parents are reported in some child-rearing research studies to be more direct and strict, emphasizing obedience rather than being psychologically oriented. This stricter parenting style across social class lines is seen as a pragmatic and realistic adaptive practice necessary for survival in an inimical, harsh environment. Open communications and high levels of family support buffer parental strictness (Bartz & Levine, 1978). Also, a high value is placed on getting along with others (Julian, McKenry, & McKelvey, 1994; Peters, 1997).

A blurring of gender roles was found by some researchers (the stress was on getting the job done rather than matching the job to the child's sex). Parents generally socialize children of both sexes the same until early adolescence. At that time sex-based differences in socialization emerge.

In large families, there are clear differences in the responsibilities children are given depending on their birth order, with, for example, the oldest child having authority over the younger children and the firstborn receiving special preparation for a leadership role in the family (Lewis, 1975).

The oldest or an older child may be "parentified." This is especially so when both parents work, there are many children, or the family is mother headed. The child who assumes parental responsibilities may be developmentally unprepared, and hence the role becomes a stressor, or the parental child may successfully engage in that role and develop responsibility and maturity beyond his or her years (Hines & Boyd-Franklin, 1996; Minuchin, 1974).

Although child-rearing literature describes mothers' roles in terms of being child centered in their child rearing, less is known about the role of the black father. What has primarily been written has focused on the negative impact of the absent black father (McAdoo, 1997). Research recently has shown that although fathers were often not living with their children, they often participated meaningfully in the child's care and socialization (Hines & Boyd-Franklin, 1996; Hunter, Pearson, Ialongo, & Kellam, 1998). Where fathers are in the home, researchers have reported a greater sharing of housekeeping and nurturing of children than white fathers (McGoldrick, 1993). The most common interactional pattern of fathers and their children appears to be warm, nurturant, and loving (McAdoo). In several studies, African-American fathers evidenced greater interest and involvement in their children's socialization when compared to white, Asian, and Hispanic fathers (Julian et al., 1994; McAdoo). Father involvement, especially with adolescents, has been found to be most relevant in helping sons avoid problem behaviors and in helping daughters prevent psychological distress (Salem, Zimmerman, & Notaro, 1998).

Significant caretaking others (kin and nonkin) play an important role in encouraging educational and occupational achievement, according to a study of black achievers (Manns, 1997). These findings confirm that the child-rearing role is often a shared one—involving "multiple mothers" and fathers.

Maternal interactive behavior with children and other child-rearing practices are found to differ by social class. As discussed in Chapter 15, socialization practices of parents are molded by what they envision their children needing to adapt to the world as they see it. Because the worlds of the middle, working, and lower classes are so varied in terms of the skills and behaviors that are adaptive, it stands to reason then that child-rearing patterns would also differ. These differences are addressed later.

✾THE FAMILY HEALTH CARE FUNCTION

HISTORIC REVIEW

A brief review of historic African-American health practices is instructive for a comprehension of the present-day situation. After slavery and during the reconstruction period in the South, a rise in the use of folk remedies and the midwife or "granny" occurred (Kroska, 1985). As late as 1962, the black midwife was still delivering 42 percent of black babies in the state of Mississippi (Harrison & Harrison, 1971). Their use in the South has been discontinued as a result of legal prohibitions. The use of the conjure doctor, voodoo or hoodoo man, or witch doctor—a practice brought from West Africa—also continued throughout the postemancipation period. Certain diseases were thought to be caused by God or the supernatural; one effect was a belief in fatalism among rural black Americans.

African-American traditional folk illnesses are divided into two main categories: (1) natural illnesses that occur when a person fails to maintain harmony in the physical or spiritual world; and (2) unnatural illnesses that occur when a person has fallen victim to a hex, curse, or spell (Huff & Kline, 1999; Matthews, 1987). The most common modality to treat illness is prayer. Laying on of the hands and rooting are also mentioned as folk remedies. Rooting is a voodoo practice wherein a person (typically a woman) is consulted as to the etiology of the illness. She then prescribes an appropriate treatment, often a magical ritual (Spector, 2000).

The use of conjure doctors, magical thought patterns, folk practices, and feelings of fatalism are all health attitudes that migrated north with poor black families. Immigrants from Haiti and Jamaica bring traditions of spiritualists, herbalists, and voodoo with them also. In some black ghettos today, some lower-class black families continue to use herb doctors, spiritualists, and faith healers.

USE OF FOLK MEDICINE AND HOME REMEDIES TODAY

As medical care has become more accessible to black Americans, the use of folk medicine and practitioners has declined considerably. Particularly among the working and the middle classes, only isolated home remedies remain as reminders of the days of "grannies," conjure doctors, and folk health practices. Nevertheless, folk medicine for a limited number of health problems has remained important in the urban ghettos and in the rural South. Low-income black families commonly make use of patent medicines and home remedies, secure medical

advice from friends, and are reluctant to seek professional health care. Often, the poor black person will endure blatant symptoms of ill health such as unexplained weight loss, abdominal pain, and frequent breathlessness without seeking care. For families of low socioeconomic status and/or families that feel socially and culturally alienated from available health care, the period of delay is generally longer. These families will usually exhaust all the home remedies known to kin and friends before feeling forced to turn to health care facilities for help.

Older women are the common repository of folk remedies in today's black families. Bullough and Bullough (1982) explain that home remedies may have their origins in magical beliefs or have a logical, empirical basis. Two of the more common purely magical actions are putting a knife under the bed of a woman in labor to cut the pain and wearing amulets or charms to ward off disease. Empirical modalities include massage, heat, and tub baths for rheumatoid arthritis, and the application of poultices and the use of herb teas for colds.

HEALTH CARE ACCESS BARRIERS

A considerable proportion of black Americans have serious problems obtaining health care. This is in large part due to the fact that many poor black Americans do not have health insurance or Medicaid.

One in five (22 percent) of nonelderly African-Americans are uninsured, well above the percentage for whites (15 percent) (Cunningham, Levan, Brown, & Wyn, 1999). Although Medicare and Medicaid access leads to increased usage, often poor families cannot pay the supplemental costs (Thornton, 1995).

U.S. health statistics provide evidence of the inaccessibility of health care for many black Americans. The differences in the health status of blacks and whites have been well documented in the United States for decades. Health disparities exist relative to all the major chronic diseases (Hayward, Crimmins, Miles, & Yang, 2000). Poor families avoid the expenses of preventive health care, and receive poorer and later prenatal care.

Because many African-Americans live in urban, crime-ridden, overcrowded ghettos with dilapidated housing (Edelman, 1997), the health of these individuals is adversely affected. Racism, poverty, and unhealthy lifestyle patterns are contributory factors to the widening health disparity between the health status of white and black Americans (U.S. Department of Health and Human Services, 1993). The positive correlation between poor general health status and poverty and unsanitary, overcrowded, poor environments provides evidence of the negative impact of the environment on health (Stokes, 1974). Violence in these neighborhoods claims more young lives than any other health problem (Griffin, 1994).

Another reason why African-American clients may delay care is their feelings of discomfort and mistrust in going to a white health facility (Spector, 2000). New African-American patients sometimes feel strange, unwelcome, uncomfortable, or mistrustful of white health facilities. There may have been so much difficulty working through the system to be cared for that a patient will come in assuming he or she is not going to be treated well (Monroe, 1989). These apprehensions and negative feelings lead some black clients to delay seeking health care.

SOCIAL CLASS DIFFERENCES

To cope with the sociocultural stresses of daily living—racism, discrimination, and economic distress—the African-American family has adapted by developing a variety of family structures, including the patriarchal, egalitarian, and matriarchal forms. The differences in family structure and function can be understood better when one looks at the social class differences. Sociologists Eshleman (1974) and Billingsley (1992) state that the most important variable in understanding the lifestyle of black families is social class. The impact of socioeconomic status on family structure is seen in the statistics with respect to one- and two-parent families. In black families with incomes below the poverty line, only 20 percent of children live with both parents, while in black families where incomes are above the poverty line, three times more children live with both parents (U.S. Bureau of the Census, 1993).

A sense of peoplehood (common ethnic identity) is present among African-Americans regardless of socioeconomic status. Even though lower-class and upper-class black families exhibit dramatic differences in lifestyles and family life, they still share a common experience and strong ethnic/racial identity that makes them feel as "one people," distinct from non-black families, regardless of their social class similarity.

Billingsley (1992), a black family sociologist, has done the most work on black family social class characteristics. He has identified distinct social class strata in the African-American community. The social class strata are based primarily on family income and source of income, supplemented by educational, occupational, and lifestyle data. These strata include: (a) a small black *upper class* with high incomes and substantial wealth; (b) a *middle class,* primarily composed of skilled and professional white-collar workers; (c) a *nonpoor working class,* composed of unskilled and semiskilled workers above the poverty line; (d) the *working poor,* composed of workers with unskilled, low-paying jobs who are living below the poverty line; and (e) the *nonworking poor* made up of families in which no members are working—described in the literature as the "underclass."

AFRICAN-AMERICAN UPPER- AND MIDDLE-CLASS FAMILIES

In 1990 black middle-class and more affluent upper-class families comprised about 42 percent of all black families in the United States (Billingsley, 1992). Billingsley reported that the more affluent black upper class increased from 6 to 14 percent from 1983 to 1990, a reflection of the growing number of well-educated black professionals. The black middle-class group is still growing also—from 25 percent in 1986 to 29 percent in 1990.

The black middle class is a diverse group, represented by a broad spectrum of income, occupational, and educational levels. They are usually skilled and professional white-collar workers and small business owners, whose education ranges from completion of high school through postdoctoral education.

Most families are nuclear in form, generally consisting of husband, wife, and two or three children. Because of their dual employment, cooperative work and team effort of husband and wife are needed. Thus, many family tasks such as cooking, cleaning, and shopping are shared, and there is extensive adaptability or flexibility of roles. Spouses are partners out of economic necessity and have an egalitarian pattern of interaction (Taylor, 2000; Willie, 1976). Egalitarian patterns include the sharing of decision making by spouses and more democratic communication patterns than white middle-class families (Willie & Greenblatt, 1978).

The middle-class black family's value system and, consequently, its socialization patterns are largely congruent with those of the dominant culture (Coner-Edwards & Edwards, 1988). Value conflicts emerge as a continual problem, however, because black and white cultures have different value orientations (Benjamin, 1991). For the middle-class African-American, there typically is extensive involvement in the nonblack world. This demands that middle-class blacks have the ability to live in two worlds simultaneously (termed being bicultural), managing dual sets of values, expectations, roles, ways of communicating, and behaviors (Woodward, 1994).

Racist attitudes and practices are still commonly experienced by African-Americans within our institutions (e.g., work, education, the media, housing) (Woodward, 1994). Because middle-class black parents may not expect, because of discrimination, to get the full benefits for their efforts, they tend to be more protective of their children and act as a buffer between the outer world and the family, to help their children develop their potential while maintaining their self-esteem (Greene, 1995; McAdoo, 1995).

Social class variability in how black parents rear their children is seen. For instance, middle-class mothers are more vocal with their infants than are lower-class mothers. During later periods of development, middle-class parents arc less coercive, restrictive, and arbitrary in their disciplining than lower-class parents. Middle-class parents use more reasoning, support, and communication of democratic approaches and less physical punishment with their children than do lower-class parents (Peterson & Rollins, 1987).

Recent research on the role of black fathers in socialization indicates that middle-income and affluent black fathers look much like their white counterparts in terms of their relationships with their children. John McAdoo (1997, 1988b) has noted that when economic status rises within the black family there is an increase in the active participation of black fathers in the socialization of their children. Most middle-class fathers are observed to be warm, nurturant, and loving in their interactions with their children. Some studies also report that black middle-class fathers are more restrictive and controlling toward their children than white middle-class fathers (McAdoo, 1997, 1988a).

Parents tend to be active participants in church affairs, the church serving not only important emotional and spiritual needs but also as a central institution for black social life (Willie, 1976; McGoldrick, 1993).

Additionally, grandparents, older siblings, or extended family members usually play a more active role in the socialization process than in middle-class white families (Greene, 1995; Peters, 1997). It is interesting to note, however, that for upwardly mobile black families, the connection with extended family members who have not moved up can be stressful or guilt producing. A sense of responsibility and an obligation is felt toward those who assisted individuals in moving up or who have not moved up as they have (Coner-Edwards, 1988).

AFRICAN-AMERICAN NONPOOR WORKING-CLASS FAMILIES

The nonpoor working class have been numerically declining beginning in the 1980s. The primary cause of this erosion in the nonpoor working class is found in the larger society. The shift from a manufacturing economy to a service economy has reduced the number of factory and manufacturing jobs and created low-paying service jobs (Billingsley, 1992; Taylor, 2000).

These families tend to be nuclear households, but usually have more children than do black middle-class families. There is also a greater likelihood that a relative or boarder may be part of the household. Both parents generally hold jobs. Men tend to work in semiskilled factory, restaurant, or janitorial positions and women are frequently employed at a similar level in community institutions. The parents have often not completed high school, but desire more education for their own children, and encourage the more motivated children to go to college. Couples usually marry early and begin a family very soon after marriage.

The relationship between husband and wife usually takes on an egalitarian character, because cooperation for getting by and survival is a necessity. Because husbands carry out traditional provider roles, women generally have more economic control in matters pertaining to the home and children (Greene, 1995).

Additionally, there is a tendency toward some flexibility concerning child care tasks based on the sex of the child. Finally, the mother also takes on the social liaison role, primarily with the school and the church.

Respectability is important among black working-class families, with the ownership of one's own home and the good character of one's children being important symbols of the attainment of this value. Of great significance is one's family. The size of the family may be a source of pride for the parents, as the bearing and rearing of children is considered to be an important responsibility. Working-class parents often make great personal sacrifices for their families and kinship relationships are strong (Willie, 1976; McGoldrick, 1993).

Again, religion and the church play a central role in the lives of these families. And the church is often second only to the home as the emotional center of black life (Fellows, 1972; Hines & Boyd-Franklin, 1996).

In regard to child rearing, parents raise their children to assure that they receive the skills and attitudes necessary to survive in the world as the parents perceive it. Thus respectfulness, obedience, conformity to rules, and being "good" are stressed. A strong work ethic exists. During childhood, children are assigned household chores as part of their family responsibility and are encouraged to seek away-from-home jobs for pay when old enough.

Fulfilling the affective functions in the family poses difficulties because of the long hours both parents usually work to provide the necessities of life. Most black working-class families have to give up doing things together as a whole family. Many husbands hold down two jobs, and it is not uncommon for spouses to work different shifts to cover child-care responsibilities (Billingsley, 1992; Willie, 1976).

AFRICAN-AMERICAN LOWER-CLASS FAMILIES: THE WORKING POOR AND THE NONWORKING POOR

In 1993, the black American poor family comprised about 29 percent of all black families (Fulwood, 1996), while in 1999 the black American poor family had declined to 23.6 percent of all black families (see Figure 1–3) (U.S. Bureau of the Census, 2000b).

Still the proportion of African-American poor is over three times higher than in the white lower class. Poor black families largely live in the urban inner-city poverty areas (Levy, 1988), where social isolation and all the consequences of poverty exist.

Black lower-class families can be divided up into those that represent the working poor and those in the nonworking poor, the underclass—a group remaining at the bottom of the social ladder and increasingly estranged from mainstream patterns and norms of behavior (Wilson, 1987). The black underclass increased considerably in size in the 1970s and 1980s due to economic changes and declining governmental programs. It decreased in size in the 1990s, although welfare reform, instituted in 1999, might create more underclass families in the future. The underclass is described more fully in Chapter 8.

Most poor married couples have their own households, although poorer black households are much more likely to be single-parent families (Glick, 1997). It is common to find extended families also, consisting of the grandmother and the mother and her children, and perhaps other relatives and/or fictive kin. Moreover, lower-class black families generally have more children than either the poor white family or the working- or middle-class black family.

In the lower class, desertion and divorce are chief causes for family disruption, although single-parent families are usually not entirely devoid of a male presence. Often, the mother will have a boyfriend who visits frequently and acts as companion to the family. Boyfriends and biological fathers often play supportive roles, assisting mothers financially and emotionally (Staples, 1989). If a husband–father is present, he is often unemployed, with the mother on welfare or working in an unskilled job. Even when either spouse is working, the possibility of unemployment or underemployment is a continual threat.

The primary feature of lower-class African-American families is their low-income status. Due to the families' impoverished state, they are coerced into making various adaptations, some of which are heavily criticized by the wider society. These adaptations include multigenerational living arrangements and taking in boarders or foster children for pay. Adult heterosexual relationships may involve both marital and parental responsibilities in the absence of marriage. Poor households sometimes forgo conventional morality in order to provide an expedient arrangement for earning sufficient money to live on. Movement and instability are great in areas of jobs, residence, and relationships.

Adolescent girls and boys from poor black families tend to have sexual experiences at an early age and have children earlier than their counterparts in the working and middle classes. Premarital pregnancy, though not condoned, is accepted by the family after the fact, as is the belief that, although it may be desirable, it is not necessary to have a man around the house in order to have and raise a family. Many teenage mothers are not marrying today, but raising their children alone, usually with the help of their mother, extended family, and friends. Via the process of informal adoption, some young mothers arrange for their children to be raised by kinfolk (Staples, 1989; McAdoo, 1995).

Marriage is looked upon ambivalently and in many cases negatively by both sexes, because of the stresses and strains associated with family life (Goldenberg & Goldenberg, 2002; Rainwater, 1971). This ambivalence and negativity has a reality base. Much greater marital instability exists, generally due to economics (unemployment) and affectional problems (extramarital relationships).

One of the prevailing myths or stereotypes about the black lower-class family is that it is matriarchal (female dominated) in structure. There is much convincing evidence that among married couples in the black lower class this is not the case (Cromwell & Cromwell, 1978; Dietrich, 1975; Scanzoni, 1971; Staples, 1976). Dietrich asserts that matriarchy is not normative in the poor black family. "The study, relying on self-report data from eight samples of black wives in intact nuclear families, reported a predominance of egalitarian decision-making structures in every study population" (Cromwell & Cromwell, p. 750). Cromwell and Cromwell's study of lower-class black married couples in Kansas City also suggests that egalitarian decision making predominates.

Because a majority of lower-class African-American families are female-headed, single-parent families, by definition these families are matrifocal. The mother makes most of the necessary decisions and has the greatest sense of responsibility for the family. There is intense loyalty between mothers and grandmothers and their children or grandchildren. Mothers extend every effort to assist their children, even into adulthood, and the grandparents often take on the child care role and act as prime socializers. Strong loyalty and reciprocity also exists among siblings. The problem here is that when one person is in need, all of the siblings are probably struggling too. Nevertheless, they share their already overcrowded living quarters and often give whatever assistance they can.

The family's values are distinct and different from the wider society's values, thus helping to create the malintegration of this group within and the stigmatization by society of the black lower class. A few selected values will be explained. Fatalism is a common value and one associated with poverty. African-American lower-class families learn to hope for little and expect even less. Men and women get sexually involved, but are afraid to trust and commit themselves to each other due to their experience of repeated disappointments. Dependency, rather than self-sufficiency, is an orientation—not really valued, but accepted as a reality and a way to "get by" (e.g., it is all right to lean on extended family and on society by receiving welfare). A lack of valuing the achievement and work ethic is apparent, as is the lack of valuing education and future planning. In this regard, it must be remembered that family values are modified by family experiences and become a reflection of what families can aspire to and expect in life.

Irrespective of social class, kinspeople (grandmothers, aunts, cousins, older siblings) play a more active role in the socialization of African-American children than is true of white families (Hines & Boyd-Franklin, 1996). In lower-class, three-generation, maternal households, it is the grandmother who is expected to stay at home with the young children (infants and preschoolers), because the mother has the right to continue outside activities (Burton & Bengtson, 1985; Burton & de Vries, 1995).

Rainwater (1971) described the African-American lower-class family as having little sense of the awesome responsibility of caring for children that the middle-class parent experiences. Although the confinement of being home with infants and preschoolers is also difficult for black mothers and grandmothers, there is not the constant solicitousness that is seen when observing working- and middle-class mothers from various ethnic backgrounds care for their infants. "Multiple mothers" help defray the responsibility of 24-hour child rearing (Greene, 1995).

In single-parent poor homes, the maternal household is generally run with a loose organization. Children learn at an early age to fend for themselves, especially if the family is large, with school-aged children beginning to shop, cook, go to bed and school on their own, and watch after themselves when mother is gone. Lower-class, three-generation, maternal homes are busy with kin and friends coming and going at all times of the day and evening on an unplanned basis. This openness of the home, in part, may be a reflection of the mother's sense of impotence in facing the street system. Although the mother often tries to keep children away from the street when they are young, as they grow older it becomes increasingly futile, and she may finally give up, disengage, and let the children have their freedom. Black ghetto street life increasingly involves gangs, drugs, criminal activity, and lack of good role models (Billingsley, 1992; Griffin, 1994). Poor parents often disengage themselves from their school-aged or adolescent sons when they feel they are powerless to change the direction of their lives.

FAMILY NURSING ASSESSMENT

The family nurse needs to consider to what extent the characteristics of African-American families described in this chapter are applicable to the family they are caring for. Also, to what extent does a family member, or the family as a whole, identify with their cultural heritage or with mainstream American culture? Different families, as well as different members within a family, may differ in their cultural identification. Rather than there being a discrete dichotomy between African-American and mainstream American culture, a continuum exists with an infinite number of positions present that individuals and families may take.

Recall the cultural assessment guidelines in Chapter 8 relative to the key questions to ask or observations to make. In addition, the following several assessment areas are particularly germane when working with African-American families.

REPLACING STEREOTYPES WITH INFORMED KNOWLEDGE

Stereotypes about the African-American family must be replaced with informed knowledge about cultural similarities and differences. This includes traditional folk beliefs and practices. In this regard, family nurses "working with African Americans must be willing to expand the 'definition of family' to more extended kinship systems" (Hines & Boyd-Franklin, 1996, p. 70). Behavior that is not congruent with white middle-class standards should not be prejudged and negatively labeled as deviant or dysfunctional, but evaluated and viewed within the family's cultural and situational context (Billingsley, 1992; Mitchell, 1982). Understanding the broader social and political context in which poor black families live is also essential in working with this group.

ASSESSING FAMILY STRESS AND COPING PATTERNS

Gathering information on the nature and perception of stressors a family is confronting and how a family is coping are crucial assessment areas, especially when there is a crisis. Because social support from extended family and friends is generally so vitally important, asking about available support and the roles family members play can be very helpful. Asking about the role religion and church play or could play in helping the family cope is also suggested.

DEALING WITH CLIENT DISCOMFORT AND MISTRUST

Health care professionals must be aware of the discomfort and alienation poor black families frequently feel toward white health care facilities. An African-American family's inactive or nonverbal participation during a first interaction with a health care provider may simply represent the family's initial discomfort or mistrust of the health care provider (Ho, 1987). Interactions need to be warm, sensitive, and respectful of clients' needs, beliefs, and feelings. Communicating respect is key to successfully engaging families and making them feel comfortable.

With regard to dealing with the black client's initial discomfort and mistrust, some of the ethnic family literature suggests that it is helpful, but not necessary, to have a health care professional be of the same cultural or racial background as the client. However, this is many times not possible or practical. Successful assessments and educational and counseling interventions are still accomplished with black families when the family nurse is of another cultural background and he or she is informed, empathetic, sensitive, and concerned. Hines and Boyd-Franklin (1982) caution counselors to proceed slowly with family assessments, since many black families are suspicious of white counselors, whom they may view as prying into their family secrets.

✿FAMILY NURSING INTERVENTIONS

Chapter 8 discusses culturally based family nursing interventions appropriate for working with culturally diverse families. Based on African-American family structural and functional characteristics, family nursing interventions specific to the African-American family are discussed in this concluding section. The key notion here is that family nurses and other health professionals need to design intervention strategies, methods, and materials to the specific cultural characteristics of African-Americans.

ENCOURAGING THE USE OF EXTENDED FAMILIES, SOCIAL NETWORKS, AND SELF-HELP GROUPS

In intervention, family nurses should incorporate important people who the family identifies as part of its extended family and social network into the plan of care.

In this regard, because the extended family often provides a substantial amount of direct assistance as well as emotional support, this family resource should be considered when working with families. For the older or disabled person, help from extended family is often an invaluable asset that makes the difference between the client having to be placed in a nursing home or cared for in the home. For the family with young children, the assistance of the extended family support system is a central family strength and should be capitalized on in counseling families.

The importance of the role of the older adult woman or grandmother in the family should be especially recognized in working with African-American families. Parent–child bonds usually exist across the life span and are of critical importance for the provision of assistance (Taylor et al., 1988). Grandmothers are often the repository of both child care expertise and health remedies. They can serve as both a crucial asset and also as a stumbling block if their central role in health matters is not appreciated and they are not brought into important family health decision making.

In addition to recognizing the importance of extended families, in particular grandmothers and older adult women, it is also important to recognize the role of fathers and encourage them to get involved with their children's care when possible (Hines & Boyd-Franklin, 1996).

Community-based family nurses can facilitate the formation of self-help groups. Murata (1995) recommends that family nurses take this approach in helping single parents with parenting. She suggests locating organizations such as churches within the African-American community to sponsor parenting groups. "Providing single mothers with the opportunity to meet to discuss family and childrearing concerns and to form friendships that provide social support can be important" (Murata, p. 59).

ENCOURAGING THE USE OF SPIRITUAL AND CHURCH SUPPORT

African-Americans are grounded in religion and spirituality and these beliefs contribute to their survival skills (Bagley & Carroll, 1995). Because the church plays a vital role in the life of most African-Americans, a family's church may be an important resource to utilize in assisting families with serious or long-term health problems. This resource may be especially useful in helping women because they tend to show more involvement with church activities than African-American men. If tangible and emotional supports and counseling from a particular church are available, it may be advisable to include church members in family interviews or in health decision making and planning (Paniagua, 1994).

ASSISTING WITH HEALTH-RELATED FAMILY PROBLEMS

Poor families, from any cultural group, have survival needs that often supercede the resolution of health problems. Family nurses should recognize that their role needs to be enlarged in order to assist families with their problems of greater priority. Only after these more pressing problems are resolved can any real energy be given to health needs (Boyd-Franklin, 1989). Improvement in educational, environmental, social service, and employment opportunities for poor black families is crucial in elevating their health status.

PROMOTING FAMILY-CENTERED HEALTH REGIMES

In recognition of the powerful influence the family exerts on personal behavior, the whole family should be encouraged to adopt a new health-promotion program, if appropriate, rather than involving only the identified client.

EMPHASIZING STRENGTHS AND EMPOWERMENT

In working with African-American families, it is much more effective to emphasize the family's and family members' strengths than its deficits. Exploring the resources black families have (e.g., the church, the extended family, "multiple mothers," role flexibility, etc.) invites families to feel a greater sense of control, optimism, efficacy, and empowerment. Teaching families how to use power appropriately within the family system and when dealing with external systems is an important counseling role (Goldenberg & Goldenberg, 2002). This positive approach is especially crucial in working with black families because of their experiences with racism and discrimination (Paniagua, 1994).

❧ SUMMARY

- African-Americans are the largest ethnic/racial minority group in the United States (12 percent of the U.S. population). Although geographically and socioeconomically diverse, they share common cultural origins and stress produced by long-standing societal discrimination.

- Demographically, a polarity of economic extremes exist within the black community. There is the emergence of a large, economically strong middle class, and concurrently, there is the emergence and growth of a black underclass. The black underclass is desperately poor, with high rates of unemployment, welfare, crime, gang participation, drug and alcohol abuse, homelessness, and teenage pregnancies.

- Five other major demographic trends among black Americans are a very high rate of teenage pregnancies and single-parent, mother-headed families; the delay of marriage until the late 20s; the decline in marriage rates; and the rising number of troubled black men.

- The African-American family, as described in the social science literature, has a legacy of vulnerability (past writings stressed this aspect) and resiliency (present writings recognize the strengths of black families).

- A major stressor in black family life is the psychological and social pressure of racism in the everyday environment. For the lower class, poverty is the other major stressor.

- There has been extensive criticism of both governmental reports and social science writings about black families. Past governmental reports tended to blame the victim, rather than looking at the social and economic constraints in society that have shaped black Americans' family behaviors.

- In the last two decades, black family literature and research has become less biased. A number of researchers have described and analyzed black families with more positive theoretical perspectives and by social class.

- To adapt to environmental challenges, black American families live in a variety of family forms. Single-parent families are most numerous, followed by nuclear families and then extended families.

- The extended family, consisting of grandparents and their grandchildren, brothers, sisters, other relatives, and/or fictive kin, is much more common among black families than among white families. These three-generation families provide a vital collective network for sharing of scarce resources and services.

- Black single-parent families are more numerous than white single-parent families. The primary problem of this family form, especially when the mother heading the family is young, is poverty.

- Several core coping patterns or strengths of black families include: (a) a strong religious commitment and participation, (b) a strong bond with and support from kin and friends, and (c) family role flexibility.

- Socialization of children varies by social class. In all classes, children are extremely important and valued. If the mother cannot care for them, extended kin will generally step in and help.

- As medical care has become more accessible to black Americans, the use of folk medicine and practitioners, as well as home remedies, has declined considerably. Nevertheless, for a limited number of health problems home remedies may be used, especially among black families living in urban ghettos and the rural south.

- A significant number of African-Americans have serious problems obtaining health care. Often the problem is the lack of health insurance.

- The differences in African-American families can best be understood by looking at social class differences in family structure and function. Social class differences are discussed in upper- and middle-class families, nonpoor working-class families, and lower-class families (the working poor and the nonworking poor or underclass). Values and lifestyles differ considerably across these social classes.

- Several family assessment areas are discussed: (a) replacing stereotypes with informed knowledge; (b) assessing family stress and coping patterns; and (c) dealing with client discomfort and mistrust.

- Five family nursing interventions are discussed: (1) encouraging the use of extended families, social networks, and self-help; (2) encouraging the use of spiritual and church support; (3) assisting with health-related family problems; (4) promoting family-centered health regimes; and (5) emphasizing strengths and empowerment.

❧ FAMILY VIGNETTE: THE WILLIAMS FAMILY

The Williams family, an African-American family consisting of the mother, Wilma, the maternal grandmother, Ann, and the three teenage daughters of Wilma—Mary, age 17, Martha, 15, and Mimi, age 13—arrived at the high school–based clinic for Martha's clinic appointment with the school nurse practitioner, Mrs. Evans, a white older nurse. Mary and Mimi sat out in the waiting room while the mother and grandmother came into the examining room with Martha and wanted to talk about the problems and concerns they had about Martha. The grandmother did most of the talking, explaining that she and her daughter Wilma were having a very difficult time supervising Martha. Wilma was recently summoned to school by the school principal as a result of poor and sporadic school attendance by Martha during the last six months. Martha didn't want to listen and obey Wilma or her, according to the grandmother Ann. "She has a boyfriend who she fights with a lot and who belongs to a 'bad' gang," and they are afraid that Martha is having sexual relations with him and is either pregnant or could become pregnant and needs birth control pills. Wilma admitted that she, an unmarried teenager, became pregnant herself at about the age of Martha, and doesn't want the same thing that happened to her to happen to her daughter. Wilma works full time as a store clerk and can't supervise Martha, and the grandmother, Ann, is beside herself with worry that "something bad is going to happen to Martha." Martha's father does visit the girls and takes them out to Carls Jr. or McDonalds for lunch on some weekends. He obviously loves his girls, but doesn't provide any real guidance to them according to the mother. The mother goes to church every Sunday and prays for guidance from God to tell her what to do to help Martha. During all this conversation with the nurse practitioner, Martha was silent, saying nothing to confirm or deny what her mother and grandmother were saying.

■ STUDY QUESTIONS

Review the Family Vignette and answer the related questions.

1. What common family patterns do we see in this family vignette?

2. What kind of reactions could this black family have initially to Mrs. Evans, a white older nurse?

3. What nursing interventions would be appropriate?

Answer the following questions.

4. Which of the following are some of the frequent effects on the black family of slavery, racism, and economic disadvantage? (Mark true or false after each statement.)

   a. The black male's self-esteem is lowered.
   b. The wife becomes submissive to her husband and his primary authority.
   c. The self-fulfilling prophecy often occurs in the areas of education and employment.
   d. Health-seeking behaviors are exaggerated.
   e. A mother-centered family becomes a practical necessity.
   f. Traditional husband–wife family roles become rigidly defined.

5. When one examines recent demographic statistics related to the black family, which of the following problems appear to be important? (Select all appropriate answers.)

   a. Economic
   b. Parenting and child care
   c. Access to health care
   d. Employment

6. Match the following family attributes with the black family according to social class.

   Family Attribute

   a. Respectability is an important value.
   b. Both parents are college educated and work.
   c. Role sharing between husband and wife occurs extensively.
   d. More likely to be single-parent families and/or matrifocal.
   e. A strong achievement orientation is present.
   f. Has the largest family and largest number of relatives living in same household.
   g. Church is a central value and institution.
   h. Egalitarian power pattern exists.
   i. Values most incongruent with wider society.
   j. Long-term dependency on public assistance is common.
   k. Families are child centered.
   l. Mothers are more vocal in their interactions with their infants.
   m. Physical punishment is more frequently used.

   Class

   1. Middle class
   2. Nonpoor working class
   3. Poor working lower class
   4. Underclass (nonworking poor)

7. African-American clients who are new to a white health facility often feel uncomfortable initially. What are some of the other feelings or behaviors that have been observed?

    a. Overly cooperative
    b. Mistrustful
    c. Demanding more of a say in their own care
    d. Careful to say "the right thing"
    e. Avoidance behaviors

8. Which of the following are criticisms that black family scholars and researchers have made about the early writings on the black family?

    a. The authors viewed the black family as being deviant.
    b. They tended to describe the black family as homogeneous.
    c. The literature was heavily biased in terms of the focus being on the black lower-class family.
    d. The writings disregarded the impact of external forces—societal institutions—on the family.
    e. Authors viewed the family from a systems, ecological perspective.

9. The most striking development within the African-American family is (choose the best answer):

    a. The black family has become more assimilated and more egalitarian.
    b. The middle class has grown numerically and economically while the underclass has numerically increased but become more economically impoverished.
    c. The fertility rate and marriage rate of black women has increased.
    d. Poor black families have moved into the cities and wealthy blacks have moved into the suburbs.

10. Identify the two traditional folk practitioners used in the past by African-American families.

11. Briefly describe three family nursing practice implications based on black family literature.

THE ASIAN-AMERICAN FAMILY

CONTENT OUTLINE

LEARNING OBJECTIVES

1. Identify what population groups constitute Asian-Americans and explain the changing demographic pattern relative to the Asian-American population in the United States today.

2. Identify which groups of Asian-Americans are high-risk groups due to their higher levels of distress and explain the reason for their distress.

3. Explain how Filipino-Americans differ in their historical legacy from the other Asian-American populations.

4. Identify the three religious/philosophic belief systems that have pervasively shaped traditional Asian core values. Give an example of how one of these religious/philosophic belief systems has influenced the Asian family or its health beliefs or practices.

5. Name three traditional core values of Asian families and state what implications these values have for family nursing practice.

6. Explain the value clash that occurs frequently between the younger and older generations in Asian-American immigrant families.

7. Describe briefly two ways in which the Asian-American family changes when it settles in the United States.

8. Explain how two important values, "saving face" and keeping interpersonal harmony, affect family communication patterns.

9. Describe two traditionally based socialization patterns among Asian-American families.

10. Identify three central tenets or concepts of traditional Eastern medicine.

11. Identify one widely used family coping strategy, as well as one individual (family member) coping strategy, utilized in traditional Asian-American families.

12. Explain the importance of assessing an Asian-American family's degree of acculturation.

13. Discuss three family nursing assessment guidelines pertinent to working with Asian-American families.

14. Discuss three family nursing interventions pertinent to working with Asian-American families.

ASIAN-AMERICAN DEMOGRAPHIC PATTERNS

Asian-Americans are proportionately the fastest-growing ethnic minority groups in the country. They constitute 4 percent of the total U.S. population. Their number more than doubled from about 1.5 million in the 1970 census to 3.5 million in the 1980 census; and doubled again to 7.3 million in the 1990 census (Gardner, Robey, & Smith, 1985; Min, 1995a). In 2000, the Asian-American population was estimated at 10.9 million, a 48 percent increase since 1990 (Kang & Fields, 2001). A large proportion of Asian-Americans reside in the western region of the United States (53 percent), and most (96 percent) live in metropolitan areas (central cities and suburbs). Six out of every 10 Asian-Americans are foreign born (Humes & McKinnon, 2000).

The terms *Asian-Americans* or *Asian* and *Pacific Islanders* (the U.S. Bureau of the Census terminology) refer to people residing in the United States who are from diverse countries and cultures in Asia, the Indian subcontinent, and islands in the Pacific Ocean. This includes at least 23 groups—Asian, Indian, Cambodian, Chinese, Filipino, Hmong, Japanese, Korean, Laotian, Thai, Vietnamese, and other Asians, representing 32 linguistic groups. Given this diversity, it is practically impossible to describe all the different groups in a single chapter. Thus, in this chapter, we will focus on five groups from the East Asian area, namely Chinese-Americans, Japanese-Americans, Korean-Americans, Vietnamese-Americans, and Filipino-Americans. These Asian-Americans share many cultural commonalities. They are also among the larger subgroups of Asian-Americans (see Table 20–1). Together they constitute the majority of Asian-Americans.

In this chapter, we will first examine each group's immigration history and demographic trends. This is followed by a discussion of their family characteristics, the changes brought on by acculturation, and implications for family nursing practice.

CHINESE-AMERICANS

Chinese-Americans are the largest group among the current Asian-American population. The term *Chinese-Americans* includes immigrants from mainland China, Taiwan, and Hong Kong. The majority of them (87 percent in Southern California) are immigrants (Kang, 1997). There are also ethnic Chinese who came to the United States via other countries such as Vietnam, Singapore, Thailand, Indonesia, Malaysia, and other Southeast Asian countries. Officially, these immigrants are considered nationals of the country from which they emigrated, but many of them would identify themselves as Chinese in daily life.

The Chinese were among the first Asians to immigrate to the United States in large numbers (Uba, 1994; Wong, 1988, 1995). A significant number of Chinese came in the early 1850s. By 1860, the Chinese population in the United States totaled 34,933 (Wong, 1988). Most of them were single men who sought work in the gold mines of California or on the transcontinental railroad. During that time, China was in a period of political, social, and economic turmoil. Many of these early immigrants came

TABLE 20-1

ASIAN-AMERICANS IN THE UNITED STATES (1960–2000)[a]

TOTAL	1960	1970	1980	1990	2000	PERCENTAGE CHANGE FROM 1990 TO 2000
Asian-Americans	878,000	1,430,000	3,500,000	7,274,000	10,765,000	+48%
Chinese	237,000	436,000	806,000	1,645,000	2,435,000	+48%
Filipino	176,000	343,000	775,000	1,407,000	1,850,000	+31.5%
Japanese	464,000	591,000	701,000	848,000	777,000	−6%[b]
Korean	—	69,000	355,000	799,000	1,079,000	+35%
Vietnamese	—	—	262,000	615,000	1,125,000	+83%

[a]Rounded off to nearest thousand.
[b]Population declined due to intermarriage and low birth rate.
Sources: Kang & Fields, 2001; and U.S. Bureau of the Census (1983a, 1993b)

from the poorer area of the country with a sojourner's mentality, hoping to earn and save up enough money for them to return to China to retire.

As Chinese immigration continued into the 1870s, anti-Chinese sentiment developed among the general U.S. population. This was fueled by real and imagined competition with white workers, as well as xenophobic and racist attitudes (Wong, 1995). A series of legislative measures was passed to discourage the Chinese from immigrating to the United States (Uba, 1994; Wong). This was exemplified in the Chinese Exclusion Act passed by Congress in 1882. It was the first and only immigration act to specifically target a particular nationality group for exclusion from the country. It severely restricted Chinese immigration and made immigrants ineligible for American citizenship (Uba; Wong, 1988, 1995). Moreover, up until the first half of the twentieth century, 14 states had miscegenation laws prohibiting intermarriage with the Chinese (Lyman, 1974).

The anti-Chinese sentiment and immigration exclusion of the Chinese started to relax during and after World War II (Wong, 1988, 1995), as China was an ally of the United States fighting against the Japanese in Asia. The communist takeover of mainland China and establishment of the People's Republic of China in 1949 also resulted in many

refugees who sought admission to the United States. In 1965, the United States finally overhauled its immigration policy and passed the Immigration and Naturalization Act, which created a more equitable format for immigration. This Act, which became effective in 1968, allowed most countries a quota of 20,000 immigrants per year in general, regardless of race or ethnicity (Wong). This made it possible for more Chinese immigrants to come to the United States. The 1965 Act emphasized family reunification and favored people with professional and technical skills. Family members of immigrants could now come to the United States to join their family. Also, people with specific skills could apply for immigration and bring their nuclear families with them. As contrasted with early immigrants who had to immigrate as individuals and were forced to leave their families behind, Chinese immigrants could now immigrate as family groups, or by virtue of family ties. Thus, the number of Chinese-Americans increased dramatically from 436,062 in 1970 to 806,040 in 1980.

In the 1980s the People's Republic of China loosened its tight emigration policy and made it easier for Chinese living on the mainland to come to the United States. About the same time, the Taiwan government also made it easier for its people to invest overseas and emigrate. Both of these factors further contributed to the rapid growth of the Chinese-American population, which again doubled to over 1.6 million in 1990 and to almost 2.5 million by 2000 (Kang & Fields, 2001).

In terms of economic status, while only 7.0 percent of white Americans are at the poverty level, 11.1 percent of Chinese-American families are at that level (Min, 1995a; U.S. Bureau of the Census, 1993a, 1994). These percentages are reflective of the socio-economic diversity among Chinese-Americans, who are the most economically polarized group of all Asian-Americans (Min).

In trying to understand Chinese culture, one must be aware that China is a vast country, slightly larger than the United States, but five times more populous. There are regional differences in dialects spoken and local customs (Hong & Ham, 1994). Many of the early immigrants were from Toisan, a rural area in the Province of Canton (now called Guangdong). Thus, the Toisan dialect is commonly spoken by the long-time residents of the U.S. Chinatowns. Cantonese, another common Chinese dialect in the United States, is spoken by many immigrants who came in the 1970s and 1980s, many of them from Hong Kong or from mainland China via Hong Kong. In the newer Chinese communities, Mandarin is a common dialect. It is spoken by immigrants from mainland China and Taiwan, both of whom have been promoting Mandarin as the official dialect for a number of decades. Many of these immigrants came in the 1980s. It should be noted that while there are different Chinese dialects or spoken languages, the written Chinese language is the same regardless of the dialects. The dialects are like different pronunciations of the same written word. Thus, if a clinic has to post notices or mail letters in Chinese, the dialects are not an issue.

JAPANESE-AMERICANS

The Japanese did not immigrate to the United States in significant numbers until the 1880s (Kitano, 1988; Nishi, 1995; Uba, 1994). Like the Chinese, most of the early Japanese immigrants were single young men seeking work as laborers. Many went to work as farmers on the plantations in Hawaii, and later in California and other areas of the West Coast. By 1902,

there were more than 30,000 Japanese immigrants in Hawaii, comprising about 75 percent of the sugarcane labor force in the islands (Min, 1988). The Japanese immigrants also faced the same wave of anti-Asian sentiments that prevailed in the United States from the late eighteenth century onward. However, unlike China, Japan was a strong military power at that time. Thus, the U.S. government was more reserved in enacting discriminatory legislation against the Japanese (Nishi). Still, the Immigration Act of 1924 made it practically impossible for all Asians, including the Japanese, to immigrate to the United States.

Anti-Japanese sentiment reached its peak during World War II. From 1942 to 1945, over 110,000 Japanese-Americans on the West Coast were interned in camps located in isolated areas (Kitano, 1988; Nishi, 1995). These camps were secured by armed guards and barbed wires, and routines of daily life were controlled by government directives. It was not only a blatant violation of human and civil rights, but also was a major disruption to the traditional family and community life of Japanese-Americans.

While immigration restrictions loosened after the passing of the Immigration and Naturalization Act of 1965, the increase in numbers of Japanese immigrants has not been as dramatic as for other Asian groups. Instead of being new immigrants, most Japanese-Americans today are descendants of Japanese immigrants who came to the United States before 1924 (Uba, 1994). As shown in Table 20–1, Japanese-Americans were originally the largest subgroup among Asian-Americans, totaling 464,332 in 1960. But by 1980, their numbers were surpassed by both Chinese- and Filipino-Americans. From 1980 to 1990, the numbers of Japanese-Americans only increased from 700,974 to 847,562, unlike many other groups, which more than doubled their numbers during the same period. From 1990 to 2000, the Japanese-American population decreased 6 percent due to a high rate of intermarriage and a low birth rate (Kang & Fields, 2001). Over 50 percent of Japanese-Americans marry outside their ethnic group (Lee, 1996). According to the 1990 census, only 32.3 percent of Japanese-Americans are foreign born, as compared to 63.1 percent of all Asian-Americans who are foreign born (Min, 1995a).

The rate of emigration is very low and is most likely the result of Japan's political stability and economic strength in the recent decades. Unlike other

Asian countries such as China, Korea, and Vietnam, Japan has not experienced any major war or social/political upheaval since World War II. Thus, there is less of a motive for its population to emigrate. Currently, Japanese-Americans are the most affluent group of Asian-Americans. Their median family income is above the general U.S. median income and only 3.4 percent of their families are at the poverty level (Min, 1995a; U.S. Bureau of the Census, 2000b).

Japanese-Americans often categorize themselves into generation groups. Issei refers to first-generation immigrants who were born in Japan. Nisei, or second generation, refers to American-born children of the immigrants. Sansei, the children of the Nisei, are the third generation, and Yonsei are the fourth generation. Currently, most of the Japanese-Americans are Nisei, Sansei, or younger generations, as compared to other Asian-Americans, most of whom are first-generation immigrants. Typically, because of their greater exposure to American culture, the Sansei and Yonsei tend to be more Americanized than the Nisei, and the Nisei more Americanized than the Issei. However, as with other immigrants, the degree of cultural identification varies with the individual. A Sansei who was raised in an area with a large Japanese community is more likely to be more identified with Japanese culture than a Sansei, or even Nisei, who grew up in a white community (Kitano, 1988). Thus, we have to be careful in applying cultural concepts when we work with different Japanese-American individuals.

KOREAN-AMERICANS

Following the Chinese and the Japanese, Korean-Americans were the next group of Asian immigrants to enter the United States. The official immigration of Koreans began during 1903–1905, when 7,226 Koreans came. They were recruited by the Hawaiian sugarcane plantation owners to offset the Japanese presence in the labor force (Min, 1988). However, the Japanese government was a major military power at that time. In response to the appeal of the Japanese laborers, the Japanese government forced the Korean government to stop emigration to the United States. The U.S. Immigration Act of 1924 further stopped immigration of Koreans and other Asians. Koreans did not resume immigration to the United States in significant numbers until after World War II.

In 1950, the Korean War broke out, which lasted until 1953. North Korea and the People's Republic of China, both communist powers, fought against South Korea and the United States–led United Nations forces. This military upheaval, as well as the close ties between South Korea and the United States, fueled another wave of immigration. Korean war brides, or women married to U.S. military personnel, and orphans adopted by U.S. parents were two major groups of immigrants at that time (Min, 1988, 1995a). The Immigration Act of 1965 later made it easier for Koreans and others to immigrate to the United States. While today South Korea has a strong economy, its relationship with North Korea is still a volatile issue. This political uncertainty is one of the factors that has continued to fuel Korean emigration.

In sum, the Korean-American population grew drastically from about 8,000 before 1950 to 69,150 in 1970 (Gardner, Robey, & Smith, 1985). As shown in Table 20–1, by 1980, it had grown to 354,593, and then more than doubled to 798,849 in 1990. Between 1990 and 2000, it grew by another 35 percent (Kang & Fields, 2001). As such, most Korean-Americans are immigrants who came to the United States after 1965. According to the 1990 census, 72.7 percent of the Korean-American population are foreign born (Min, 1995a; U.S. Bureau of the Census, 1993a). Most of the families are composed either entirely of immigrant members or of immigrant parents and American-born children. In comparison to Chinese- or Japanese-Americans, third- or younger-generation Korean-Americans are relatively few. Economically, Korean-Americans are one of the less-affluent groups among Asian-Americans. Their median family income is below the U.S. median income, and 14.7 percent of their families are at the poverty level (Min; U.S. Bureau of the Census).

FILIPINO-AMERICANS

In contrast with other Asian-Americans, Filipino-Americans emigrated from a country that had experienced strong Western influence and had strong political ties with the United States. Indeed, the Philippines can be described as the most Westernized country in Asia (Agbayani-Siewert & Revilla, 1995; Min, 1995a). The Philippines was a Spanish colony from the middle of the sixteenth century to 1898 (500 years). Thus, the Filipino culture was strongly influenced by Spanish culture. For example, the Philippines is the only Asian country in which Roman Catholicism is the majority religion. Today, over 80 percent of Filipinos are Roman Catholics (Agbayani-Siewert & Revilla; Min). In 1898, the United States won the Spanish–American War, and the Philippines was ceded to the United States. It remained a U.S. colony until 1946 when it became independent. During this 48-year period, the American political and cultural influence permeated the Philippines. This impact still continues to the present time, especially in Philippine economic, political, and educational institutions (Agbayani-Siewert & Revilla; Min).

Filipinos began to immigrate to the United States in large numbers around 1909 (Agbayani-Siewert & Revilla, 1995; Uba, 1994). Like the Japanese and Korean immigrants before them, most were farm laborers seeking work in the plantations of Hawaii. In the next two decades, over 100,000 Filipinos came to the United States, first to Hawaii, and later to California and other parts of the country. However, in the 1930s, Congress began to exclude Filipinos by limiting their immigration to 50 persons per year. This virtually stopped the immigration of Filipinos. There were few descendants of the early immigrants, since many of them never married or had children (Uba). The immigration restrictions started to loosen after World War II. However, significant Filipino immigration did not occur until the Immigration Act of 1965 made it easier for them to immigrate. The majority of the current Filipino-American population consists of immigrants or children of immigrants who came to the United States after 1965. According to the 1990 census, 65 percent of Filipino-Americans are foreign born (Min, 1995a; U.S. Bureau of the Census, 1993a). The close ties between their country and the United States is a major factor contributing to Filipino immigration here. Also, because of their greater exposure to American culture, most Filipino-Americans, in general, find it easier to accommodate to American life than other Asian immigrants (Agbayani-Siewert & Revilla; Uba). As seen in Table 20–1, by 1980, Filipino-Americans had become the second largest Asian-American group. In 2000, their populations totaled 1,850,000. Filipino-Americans are also one of the more affluent groups among Asian-

Americans. Their median family income is slightly above the U.S. median income and only 5.2 percent of their families are at the poverty level (Min; U.S. Bureau of the Census, 2000).

VIETNAMESE-AMERICANS

The Vietnamese are among the newest groups of Asians to immigrate to the United States in significant numbers. Unlike other Asian-American groups discussed earlier, most Vietnamese-Americans were refugees who left their homeland in chaotic and traumatic situations at the end of the Vietnam War in 1975. These Vietnamese refugees, together with Cambodians and Laotians from neighboring countries, are often grouped together and called Southeast Asian refugees, or Indochinese refugees, as that part of Asia was also known as Indochina. The Vietnamese were the largest subgroup of Southeast Asian refugees.

The Vietnamese refugees left their homeland in different waves. The first wave fled at the end of the Vietnam War to escape persecution by the North Vietnamese communists. In 1975 alone, 130,000 Southeast Asian refugees, most of them Vietnamese, came to the United States (Uba, 1994). The second mass exodus occurred from 1978 to 1979 when the communist government sought to eliminate the influential Chinese business community by forcing the ethnic Chinese Vietnamese to leave. These refugees were known as the "boat people," as they were compelled to leave in crowded fishing boats. They often drifted about, many perishing in the open sea, as neighboring countries, already inundated with refugees, refused to accept them (Rumbaut, 1995). In 1975, the communists also took control of Cambodia, establishing a radical and oppressive regime that caused many to flee for their lives. This was followed by more military and political turmoil, such as the Vietnam invasion of Cambodia in late 1978. Thus, throughout the late 1970s to 1980s, many Southeast Asian refugees continued to leave by boat or by land (Rumbaut; Tran, 1988; Uba). Due to the large number of refugees, many countries simply refused to assist them, claiming that they were economic refugees seeking economic opportunities, rather than political refugees escaping for their life and freedom. Most of the refugees had to spend months, and often years, enduring destitute conditions in refugee camps before they were officially screened and granted asylum. The United States was among a dozen or so countries that would accept them (Rumbaut; Tran).

In 1979, the Vietnamese government agreed with the United Nations High Commissioner for Refugees to allow Vietnamese nationals to leave the country and join their immediate families who had left earlier. This created a more orderly wave of emigration. At the same time, the U.S. government also agreed to allow its former employees in Vietnam to immigrate (Rumbaut, 1995; Tran, 1988). This further facilitated the immigration of Vietnamese to the United States. As seen in Table 20–1, by 1980, the Vietnamese-American population had grown to 261,729, and this more than doubled to 614,547 in 1990. Between 1990 and 2000, the number of Vietnamese increased 83 percent. Eighty percent of Vietnamese-Americans are foreign born (Min, 1995a; U.S. Bureau of the Census, 2000). While the initial policy of the U.S. government was to resettle the Vietnamese refugees throughout the country, 45 percent of them eventually relocated to California, making it the state with the largest Vietnamese–American population (Min; Rumbaut). It should be noted that ethnic Chinese Vietnamese refugees are considered Vietnamese-Americans in their official documents, while in everyday life, they would identify themselves as Chinese. These Chinese Vietnamese-Americans are a source of newcomers to Chinese-American communities.

As refugees, many Vietnamese-Americans, as well as Cambodian- and Laotian-Americans, have personally experienced the violence and turmoil of war and escape. Many of them left behind family members, possessions, and careers in order to start their life anew. The long waits for asylum proceedings in refugee camps literally put their lives on hold, without any certainty that they would be accepted by a host country. Because painful trauma has lasting effects on most people, we must be sensitive to the impact of the clients' refugee experience when we work with this population. Since most of them fled their country of origin with few or no possessions, Vietnamese-Americans are the lowest income group among Asian-Americans. According to recent census data, their median family income was well below the U.S. median income, with 23.8 percent of their families living at or below the poverty level (Min, 1995a; U.S. Bureau of the Census, 2000).

✖️COMMONALITIES AND DIFFERENCES AMONG ASIAN-AMERICANS

In spite of their diversity, the Asian-American groups discussed in this chapter share many common characteristics. This is due to geographic proximity, the historical interactions among their countries of origin, and their common experience of being Asian-American immigrants (60 percent of them).

One major common experience Asian-Americans have faced and are still facing is racial discrimination. In the past it was certainly much worse (e.g., the Japanese-American internment during World War II), but various forms of discrimination still exist. A nationwide survey of public attitudes about Chinese-Americans in 2001 revealed that one quarter of Americans hold "very negative attitudes" toward Chinese-Americans, and one third of them questioned Chinese-Americans' loyalty to the United States (Richardson & MacGregor, 2001). When respondents were asked about Asian-Americans in general, the same "negative" responses were given, suggesting that prejudice against Chinese-Americans is a subset of broader prejudices against Asian-Americans in general (Kang, 2001). Job and social discrimination appear to be two of the most commonly experienced ways in which Asian-Americans are exposed to discrimination.

Another important commonality for families from China, Japan, Korea, and Vietnam is a cultural heritage that was strongly influenced by Confucianism, Buddhism, and Taoism. This distinguishes them, as a group, from Western or mainstream American culture, which is dominated by the Judeo-Christian tradition. In this regard, we can discuss the general cultural elements of these Asian-Americans collectively.

Filipino culture, from a sociopolitical perspective, differs from these Asian cultures because of the 500 years of Spanish influence, and more recently, the 50 years of U.S. influence. Yet, it still retains many characteristics in common with other Asian cultures. In a sense, Filipino culture may be seen as a mixture of Western cultures, especially Spanish culture, and Asian cultures, including the indigenous Filipino culture.

In exploring the cultural characteristics of Asian families, we have to be aware of the differences between the normative or traditional culture and the contemporary culture. For example, the contemporary culture practiced in the cosmopolitan urban centers of Asia, like Hong Kong, Tokyo, or Taipei, is more Westernized than the culture practiced in the rural areas, which tends to be closer to traditional culture. There are also socioeconomic class and generational differences among Asian-Americans in regard to their assimilation to mainstream American or Western culture. For example, middle- and upper-class Asian-Americans, particularly those who received their higher education in the United States, are more likely to be culturally assimilated than working-class Asian immigrants. American-born Asian-Americans, having a greater exposure to mainstream culture in their formative years, are more likely to be culturally assimilated than their foreign-born immigrant parents. This cultural gap is often a source of stress or conflict in the Asian-American family (Hong, 1989, 1996).

Aside from these general group differences, there are individual differences in cultural identification, which can be seen on a continuum. For example, there are some immigrants who will try to become integrated into mainstream culture as fast as they can, while there are second- or further-generation Asian-Americans who are strongly identified with their cultural roots and wish to retain this rich legacy. There are others who are bicultural in the sense that they can comfortably switch between mainstream culture and Asian culture, depending on the environment or social setting. Still others might feel alienated, sensing that they do not belong to either world (Hong, 1996). Thus, the following discussion of specific cultural characteristics of the Asian-American family should be applied judiciously.

✺ FAMILY STRUCTURAL CHARACTERISTICS

Although Asian-American families constitute diverse minority groups in the United States, they have many cultural elements in common, especially when we look at their family and psychosocial characteristics (Hong, 1988; Hong & Ham, 1994). Their culturally derived values differ significantly from the dominant American value system (Min, 1995a). Thus, the commonalities will be emphasized along with a description of some of the major differences among the various Asian-American families.

The following discussion is based on both empirical findings and observational writings of Asian families in both Asia and the United States. Much less literature is available on contemporary Asian-American families, particularly for certain groups such as Filipino-American and Southeast Asian–American families. Uba (1994), in her review of the literature on Asian-American families, warns readers that there are serious limitations in Asian-American family research, as well as large gaps in our knowledge about particular Asian-American groups, as noted above. In addition to findings sometimes being based on small convenience samples with no comparison groups, data may also have been collected decades ago.

FAMILY VALUES AND BELIEFS

INFLUENCE OF EASTERN RELIGIOUS AND PHILOSOPHICAL BELIEFS.
One of the core cohesive elements of Asian cultures, with the exception of the Philippines and certain Muslim countries like Indonesia, is their common world view. This world view is based on the Eastern religions and philosophies of Confucianism, Taoism, and Buddhism. In contrast, in Western culture the common world view is based on the Judeo-Christian legacy (Henderson, 1989; Hong, 1993). These three Eastern religions/philosophies have pervasively shaped the core values that Asian-American families to varying degrees hold. Thus, as a foundation to our discussion of Asian-American values, the three major Eastern religions/philosophies are first briefly described.

Confucianism. Confucianism is based on the teachings of Confucius (circa 551–479 B.C.), a Chinese sage. It is a philosophic system of ethics, education, statesmanship, and religion designed to produce a "righteous person" who possesses self-knowledge, self-respect, sincerity, kindness, and honesty (Henderson, 1989). Under Confucianism, duties and obligations related to social interactions are clearly defined, giving rise to much of the prescribed family relationships and behavior. The family is central in Confucian thought and the norms and values of Confucianism form the basis of much of traditional Asian family life (Meredith & Abbott, 1995). Over the centuries, Confucianism exerted a strong influence and became embedded into Chinese and other Asian cultures. It should be noted that while Confucius is later venerated as a saint by some people, Confucianism is basically a philosophy, a way of life, and a world view, rather than a religion.

Taoism. Taoism is a philosophy founded by the Chinese philosopher Lao-Tzu (also called Laozi), who lived around the sixth to fourth century B.C. Many scholars believed he was a contemporary of Confucius. Taoism emphasizes intuition, simplicity, and the attainment of profound insight through the ability to perceive "Tao" in daily activities and surroundings. Taoism states that people can find harmony and peace by being good to all things; being humble, simple, and peaceful; avoiding honors and distinctions; and enjoying the forces of nature (Henderson, 1989).

In the third century A.D., Zhang Leng founded the religion of Taoism. He based it on the philosophy of Taoism, but instituted religious rituals and alchemy, emphasizing the cultivation of elixirs or potions for immortality. The Taoist religion asserts that it is following the teachings of Lao-Tzu, and venerates him as one of its saints or deities. However, the Taoist philosophy does not embrace the rituals and many of the beliefs of the Taoist religion. Thus, Taoism, the philosophy, is different from Taoism the religion. In general, many concepts common to both are deeply embedded in the cultures of China and other Asian countries.

Taoism, both the philosophy and the religion, is often associated with the concepts of *yin* and *yang,* which have gained considerable attention in the West. While these concepts were part of Taoism, they were actually of even more ancient origin. Moreover, they were probably present in Chinese medical thought long before the time of Lao-Tzu. *Yin* is the feminine, negative, dark, and cold energy. *Yang* is the masculine, positive, light, and warm energy. The balance of *yin* and *yang* is the key to harmony and peace. As applied to health, balance or good health is maintained by proper diet, avoidance of strong emotions, and the use of appropriate herbs. This belief is the basis of Chinese or Eastern medicine, a system of care that focuses on prevention as well as care (Henderson, 1989; Spector, 1991, 2000).

Buddhism. Buddhism grew out of Hinduism in India. It was founded by Siddhartha Gautama, the Buddha (circa 560–480 B.C.). Adherents of Eastern religions of Hinduism and Buddhism seek maximum human development (Henderson, 1989). Buddha taught that the human condition is embedded in fear, suffering, disease, and death. As Henderson explains, "The wise person realizes this and looks for a way to resolve it. . . . Buddha's message focuses on the experiences or path that leads to liberation for the human condition" (p. 70). Self-knowledge and love and universal goodwill are two primary virtues of Buddhism. Buddhism teaches that the best path to self-knowledge is through proper conduct, self-control, humility, generosity, and mercy.

Buddhism spread from India into China during the first century A.D., and became a popular religion. Over the centuries, Buddhism in China has developed into various schools by incorporating many elements of Chinese culture and thought adapted from Confucianism and Taoism. From China, Buddhism spread to Japan and later to Korea. In Japan, some schools of Buddhism incorporated elements of Shintoism, an indigenous Japanese religion. In summary, there are different schools of Buddhist thought in different Asian countries (Henderson, 1989).

The influences of the philosophies/religions of Confucianism, Taoism, and Buddhism are deeply ingrained in Asian cultures. Thus, whether or not an Asian overtly identifies with these systems of thought/belief, he or she inadvertently follows their prescriptions, which are often synonymous with cultural norms/values. Similarly, in the United States today, these philosophies/religions still influence the family life of many Asian-Americans regardless of their religion.

One must be careful not to stereotype the religious affiliations of Asian-Americans. For example, while the Chinese in Asia are typically considered to be Buddhist by default, ethnic Christian churches play a very active role in many Chinese-American communities here (Hong & Ham, 1994). This also applies to Korean-Americans (Min, 1995c), and, of course, to Filipino-Americans whose country of origin is predominately Roman Catholic (Agbayani-Siewert & Revilla, 1995).

ASIAN-AMERICAN CORE VALUES Asian-American families hold traditional Asian values to varying degrees. It may be, however, that a much smaller number of Asian-Americans adhere to all the traditional values identified here. Table 20–2 provides a comparison of Eastern and Western core values.

Familism. Familism refers to the centrality of the family, family relationships, and family responsibilities. There is a strong belief in the importance of the family over the individual. The needs of the individual, therefore, are subordinated to those of the family. The cultural focus is on the family rather than on the individual as in Western culture (Chung, 1991; Hong, 1988, 1995). The family includes the nuclear family as well as the extended family and the entire kinship network. This value and belief is also referred to as "kinship solidarity" (Kline & Huff, 1999).

Filial Piety. Filial piety, referring to respect for parents, grandparents, and other significant elders, is a highly cherished value in traditional Asian families. It prescribes that children should repay their parents' love and care by caring for them in their old age. Reflective of the value of filial piety, immigrant families often sponsor their own parents to come to the United States. Filial piety is a basic foundation on which the traditional Asian family is built (Chung, 1991; Ishii-Kuntz, 2000; Meredith & Abbott, 1995).

Respect for the Elderly. Respect for the elderly is seen in the deference given to older family members, both living and deceased (Chung, 1991; Ishii-Kuntz, 2000; Min, 1995b). The traditional practice of ancestor worship is a ritual that manifests the value of respecting the elderly.

TABLE 20–2

COMPARISON OF EASTERN AND WESTERN VALUES

EASTERN VALUES	WESTERN VALUES
Harmony with nature	Mastery of nature
Conformity	Competition
Smooth, harmonious interpersonal relationships; conflict avoidance, restraint, self-control	Assertion of one's thoughts and feelings
Consensus, assumption of the "middle position"	Dissensus acceptable (holding of a different position)
Indirect, nonverbal experssion of ideas, thoughts, and feelings	Open, direct expression of thoughts, ideas, and feelings
Stoicism, suppression of emotions	Open display of emotions
Tradition and continuity	Change, innovation, progress
Respect for older persons (age/wisdom)	Adulation of youth and youthfulness
Hierarchical positions and status; respect for authority	More egalitarianism in status and relationships
Cyclical concept of time	Specific points, schedule, clocks
Collective orientation and group accomplishments	Individual orientation and self-accomplishments
Mutual consideration and self-depreciation	Assertiveness and self-determination
Familism	Individualism
Interdependence	Independence
Formality	Informality

Source: Adapted from Stouffer (1995); Ho (1992); Chung (1991); and Lin-Fu (1994).

Respect for Authority.   Traditionally, Asian-American values also stress respect for authority figures, including teachers and health professionals (Chung, 1991; Uba, 1994). Respect for authority is displayed in the home by emphasizing obedience to parents.

Interdependence and Reciprocity.   The value of interdependence is seen in relationships within and outside the family—with friends, neighbors, employers, and fellow employees. The ethic of reciprocity and collective obligation is an inherent part of interdependency. Asian-Americans are to a much greater extent than Euro-Americans group oriented, with a strong sense of duty and social responsibility (Chung, 1991; Hong, 1989; Min, 1995b).

Interpersonal Harmony.   The value of maintaining harmony is also central in traditional Asian-American families (Torsch & Ma, 2000; Uba, 1994). Maintaining peaceful and agreeable relationships by accommodation, compromise, conformity, and other nonconfrontational means is the way in which harmony is achieved. In most Asian cultures, it is socially unacceptable to be aggressive or confrontational. Suffering without complaining or suffering quietly is connected to the value/norm of "exhibiting dignity."

Avoidance of Disagreement and Conflict.   The norm of self-control, restraint in emotional expression, and retaining smooth interpersonal relations is widely held in contrast to the focus on being open about one's feelings and thoughts that characterizes Western cultural norms (Chung, 1991; Meredith & Abbott, 1995). As part of this interpersonal value and norm, disagreement and conflict are avoided, while conformity and compromise (taking the "middle position") are emphasized.

Saving Face.   There is a high value on *saving face* or maintaining one's respect, dignity, and status. Typically one loses face when one has failed to carry out a socially appropriate role/behavior. In health care settings this may translate into Asian-American clients silently suffering to maintain their dignity. Losing face is often viewed as not merely a personal shame, but also a family shame, for the behavior of each family member is a reflection on the whole family. Family honor is widely emphasized. Therefore, there is great pressure to behave properly so as to not bring shame on the family. Shame, then, is a major

social control mechanism (Chung, 1991; Goldenberg & Goldenberg, 2002; Shon & Ja, 1982).

Fatalism.   Acceptance of one's fate is a widely held belief in Asian cultures. Rather than being seen as a negative life adjustment, it is a pragmatic way of coping with life's vicissitudes. Instead of challenging a situation or unfortunate event, traditional Asian-Americans may accept the event/situation as a given condition of their fate (Henderson, 1989).

Education/Achievement Orientation.   Asian-American families generally place a high value on education (Ishii-Kuntz, 2000). There is research demonstrating that Asian-American parents stress achievement in their children more than Euro-Americans do (Uba, 1994). Families are often willing to undergo substantial financial hardship to support their children who are receiving a good education and have been scholastically successful. For instance, in a survey of 1,400 Southeast Asian refugee families, Caplan, Choy, and Whitmore (1992) found that the families of school-aged children played a pivotal role in their children's academic success.

Strong Work Ethic.   In traditional Asian cultures, both educational and occupational achievement are highly valued (Min, 1995b). This is related to the cultural emphasis on fulfilling one's obligation to the family and to society by being educated and productive. Asian-Americans usually work longer hours than Americans in general. For instance, Korean-American immigrant men and women, many of whom own small family businesses, work long hours. Korean-American women worked on the average of 75.5 hours/week in job and household work, according to a New York City survey. Korean-American men worked long hours too (63.5 hours/week), but 12 hours less per week than their wives because they did not share the household tasks (Min, 1995c).

THE FAMILY ROLE AND POWER STRUCTURE

In the traditional Asian family, age, gender, and generational status are the primary determinants of family roles and power. Most basic, relative to the Asian family, is that it is patriarchal, with the exception perhaps of the Filipino family. Family roles are clearly defined. Males, particularly the father and eldest son, have the most dominant positions. Traditionally, the father maintains an authoritative, strict, and dignified relationship to the family (Ishii-Kuntz, 2000; Uba, 1994). He is the leader, provider, and disciplinarian of the family. Traditionally, power is passed on from father to eldest son.

Traditionally, wives and daughters are in subordinate positions. They are expected to respect and obey their husbands, husband's parents, or fathers, if unmarried (Hsu, 1971; Meredith & Abbott, 1995). A traditional Asian-American wife–mother devotes herself to the care of her husband, children, and home (Henderson, 1989). She also serves as the vital link between the family and schools and other community organizations (Ishii-Kuntz, 2000).

Sons and older persons are more valued in traditional Asian families than are daughters and younger members. Sons are more valued because they will carry on the family name and will care for their elderly parents. The oldest son is most respected (Shon & Ja, 1982). Older siblings command respect and are typically addressed as "older sister," "second oldest brother," and so on, rather than by name. Older siblings are expected to be role models to younger siblings (Uba, 1994). Grandparents have a position of honor by virtue of their older and parental status (Hong, 1989).

Asian-American families are on the average larger in size than white American families. For instance, 23 percent of Asian-American families in 1999 consisted of five or more members. There are more nuclear families (80 percent) among Asian-Americans and much less single-parent families than among American families in general (Humes & McKinnon, 2000).

A major power and control issue or problem in immigrant Asian-American families is the clash between traditional (Eastern) and modern (Western) values. The literature describes cultural conflicts between parents and children and, to a lesser extent, between spouses (Detzner, 1992; Hong, 1989, 1996). Children socialized in U.S. schools are taught to be independent, individualistic, and egalitarian in relationships. When Asian-American children and youth bring home these Western notions to immigrant parents whose values and beliefs are of deference, obedience, interdependency, familism, and so on, conflict between the generations often ensues. Conflict between immigrant spouses may also occur as Asian-American women begin working outside the home and become more Westernized, and consequently

challenge the authoritarian, dominant position of their husbands (Detzner).

The traditional Asian family is multigenerational, extending vertically to include older generations, even those who are deceased, and horizontally to include living relations through fourth cousins. One's ancestors are remembered and respected.

The traditional Asian family is often patrilocal, with the married couple living in the same household with the husband's parents. This pattern is changing in the urbanized or industrialized areas where the size of housing units and job mobility often make it impractical for the extended family to live in the same household. In addition, when families migrated from Asia to the United States, their extended families often did not accompany them. Thus, not only was the large extended family network reduced, but also the patrilocal household pattern not possible (Hong, 1995; Hong & Ham, 1992).

FAMILY COMMUNICATION PATTERNS

The core Asian values are seen in the characteristic ways in which traditional Asian-Americans communicate. Given the high value placed on interpersonal harmony, avoidance of disagreement and conflict, and "saving face," more indirect, subtle, and nonverbal expression of thoughts and feelings is seen. In contrast, Euro-Americans favor more direct, open, and straightforward expression of thoughts and feelings (Hong, 1989; Locke, 1992).

Among traditional Asian-Americans, emphasis is placed on not offending others and being socially sensitive. Family members are encouraged to refrain from expressing their feelings when this could potentially disrupt family harmony. Instead of overtly disagreeing when differences between persons exist, traditional Asian-Americans may verbalize their thoughts in a mild or circumventive manner. Family members are much less inclined to express directly their disagreements to an authority figure such as a health professional. For example, a more acceptable, less confrontational way of disagreeing is for the client to say: "Some people say that I can do it this way . . . [instead of your way]," making the disagreement less personal and more polite (Hong, 1989, p. 16).

In the traditional Asian-American home, clearly defined roles of dominance and respect rule out argument and negotiation. Communication is typically one way, from parent to child. Direct messages predominate, and two-way communciation is more brief and perfunctory (e.g., talking about safe subjects) (Locke, 1992; Uba, 1994). Traditional, clearly defined family roles may also promote emotional distance between father and children and limit the avenues to express and resolve problems.

A reliance on nonverbal communication also enhances smooth, harmonious relationships because disapproval is communicated in a manner that is not as divisive and oppositional as verbal challenges (Uba, 1994). For instance, a family member may convey displeasure or disapproval by giving other members subtle looks that signal his or her feeling.

Uba (1994) explains that there is a clustering of behaviors that involve a particular kind of "reserve, reticence, deference and humility" (p. 17). Manifestations of these behavior patterns include a hesitancy to speak up in class, particularly to openly contradict a teacher, and a hesitancy about dominating a conversation.

Communication behaviors that show the values of self-control, self-discipline, and ability to delay gratification and suppression of expression of negative and positive emotions are also commonplace among traditional Asian-Americans (Uba, 1994). Asian-American patients may be silent and uncomplaining about their pain and symptoms, behaviors which are, as noted, manifestations of the above values.

In many immigrant Asian-American families, there may be more limited family communication than in Euro-American families, not only because of cultural factors, but also because of a language gap between parents and children, that is, children increasingly use English at home, while parents being monolingual only use their native language. This language gap further reduces communication and creates emotional distance between parents and children (Hong, 1989, 1996; Yu & Kim, 1983).

❦ FAMILY FUNCTIONAL CHARACTERISTICS

THE FAMILY AFFECTIVE FUNCTION

Parent–child attachment bonds are described in the Asian-American family literature. Generally, children feel emotionally closer to their mothers than their fathers according to Shon and Ja (1982). One major factor for this closeness is the mother's role in nurturing and rearing the children. Traditionally, the mother's most important bond is often with her children, especially the eldest son, rather than with her husband, whereas the husband's strongest bond is often with his own mother (Ishii-Kuntz, 2000; Uba, 1994).

Asian-American family research has also found that Asian-American families are generally more cohesive than Euro-American families (Ishii-Kuntz, 2000; Uba, 1994). These families tend to have a strong commitment to family, tend to live closer to parents, feel more obligated to their parents, and interact more frequently with them (Uba, 1994). The cohesion generally found in Asian-American families is rooted in the value of familism, interdependency, and filial piety. Cohesion is also a familial response to outside pressures on the family, such as the pressure of coping with immigration to a new society and coping with racism.

THE FAMILY SOCIALIZATION FUNCTION

Parents invest heavily in their children. Young children are indulged and children are permitted to remain in a dependent position longer than in Euro-American families. What children are expected to do is to bring honor to the family by being respectful, obedient, and by doing well in school (Goldenberg & Goldenberg, 2002).

Traditionally, acceptable norms for behavior are clearly defined and very much shaped by the teachings of Confucius, especially his emphasis on the values of filial piety and veneration of age. Social order in the family is maintained by keeping the proper order of relationships between parents and children, older and younger persons, and husband and wife (Locke, 1992). These relationships are hierarchical and taught to children at an early age. The family exerts a great deal of control over children who are expected to be devoted to and rely on their family (Uba, 1994). There is also a strong emphasis placed on preserving family honor as indicated under the discussion of saving face. Shame, guilt, and appeals to family obligation and social responsibility are used by parents as socialization control techniques to mold children's behavior and attitudes (Locke, 1992).

Respect for educated persons and the importance of a child's education are stressed in Confucianism and reflect core Eastern values. In fact, Min (1995b) considers the emphasis on children's education to be probably the most salient feature of child socialization. Because of the centrality of education in the minds of parents, the pressure that Asian-American families exert on their children to excel in school is high (Locke, 1992). Julian, McKenry, and McKelvey (1994) also found that Asian-American parents tended to emphasize self-control, as well as doing well in school.

According to Uba (1994), a number of studies show that Asian-American mothers tend to be more restrictive about their children's independence than do Euro-American mothers. Asian-American mothers supervise their children more closely and expect them to be independent at a later age. Parents are more likely to demonstrate love and affection indirectly, such as by sacrificing for their children so that they may receive a good education, rather than directly through hugs and kisses (Hong, 1989; Shon & Ja, 1982).

In many immigrant Asian-American families it is common to find relatively strict discipline and control of children when compared to Euro-American families (JWK International Corporation, 1978, cited in Uba, 1994). It appears, however, that as mothers become acculturated, their control, strictness, and close supervision diminish (Ishii-Kuntz, 2000; Uba, 1994).

The ways in which parents discipline and punish their children also change after families have settled in the United States. Immigrant Asian families sometimes find that what was acceptable in their country of origin may not be acceptable in the United States. An example of an unacceptable child-rearing practice that parents are being forced to change is the following. In Southeast Asia, coin rubbing, a medical treatment, is used to treat certain illnesses. Because this therapy bruises the skin, school authorities have reported children with this type of bruising to child protective agencies as possible cases of abuse. Different child-rearing rules and laws have left some immigrant Asian families confused and unsure of their parental skills and authority (Bemak, Chung, & Bornemann, 1996; Hong & Hong, 1991).

Evidence that families do change in their child rearing as part of their adaptation to a new country was found in a large national survey conducted by Julian, McKenry, and McKelvey (1994). These researchers compared parenting across cultural groups in the United States and found differences in child rearing between Hispanic-Americans, Asian-Americans, African-Americans, and whites to be much less than expected when socioeconomic status was controlled for.

Asian-American fathers appear to have a limited role in child rearing, although recent studies of Korean-American families show this is changing (Huang & Ying, 1989). Fathers' role in child rearing, however, is particularly minimal when children are infants (Suzuki, 1985). In large families, the parents typically delegate child care responsibilities to older siblings. Cooperation and sharing among siblings is expected (Lee, 1996).

THE FAMILY HEALTH CARE FUNCTION

Little is written in the literature about how the family fulfills the health care function. The mother and other women in the home are the caregivers. In seeking Western health care, treatment may be delayed because of the high value placed on self-control, not complaining about pain, and suppression of feelings. Once recognized as being ill, however, the ill family member receives a great deal of care and concern and is encouraged to assume a dependent role within the family (Chan, 1992).

Traditional Asian health care beliefs and practices are Chinese in origin, with the exception of Filipino culture where indigenous medical beliefs and practices are based primarily on Malaysian culture. Traditional Chinese medicine is an extensive and complex form of healing beliefs and practices. Chinese medicine teaches that health is a state of spiritual, psychological, and physical harmony. Violating this harmony or balance causes illness and disease. A central concept in preventing and treating diseases is *holism*. Holistic Chinese medicine recognizes the interrelatedness of structures within the human body, as well as the need to integrate the human body with the external environment. The onset, evolution, and alteration of an illness are assessed within the context of the patient's environment (Spector, 2000). The *yin–yang* polar, oppositional energies, powers that regulate the universe and the human body, must be in balance for health to be maintained (Chang, 1995). Therefore, illness is a reflection of imbalance, the disharmony of *yin* and *yang,* the vital energy, leading to pathology, with excesses in one and deficiencies in the other (Inouye, 1999).

Traditionally, there is a respect for the human body. Good nutrition, rest, calm emotions, and exercise are seen as important in maintaining the proper balance needed for promoting health.

In traditional Chinese medicine there are nine components or approaches to healing: (1) the mind (meditation); (2) herbal medicine; (3) massage; (4) movement (exercise like Tai Chi); (5) Taoist sexual practices; (6) acupuncture, including moxibustion, cupping, and acupressure; (7) diet; (8) geomancy or Feng Shui (adjusting the energy flows in a person's environment to promote and restore balance [health] and vitality); and (9) astrology, numerology, and divination (McLean & Dworkin, 2001). The main purpose of all these healing modalities is to restore the proper balance of *yin* and *yang*. One way traditional practitioners do this is by assisting their patients to achieve health through energy balance. The ginseng root is the most famous of all the herbs. It is used to treat a large variety of illnesses and to stimulate better general health.

A fuller description of *yin* and *yang*—their locations within the human body and their functions—as well as the Chinese ways of preventing, diagnosing, and treating illness can be found in Rachel Spector's *Cultural Diversity in Health and Illness* (5th ed., 2000). An excellent bibliography of books and articles on Chinese medicine are also listed there.

Because traditional Asian-Americans have a deep respect for their bodies and are used to Chinese medicine, they may be upset by some of Western medicine's intrusive modalities, such as intrusive diagnostic tests, particularly drawing blood and surgical treatments. Many traditional Asian-Americans refuse surgery except under the most dire circumstances (Spector, 2000).

Asian-Americans often use both Western and Eastern medical services (predominantly herbal medicine). For instance, a Chinese-American may treat minor and chronic illnesses with Chinese medicine and acute and serious problems with Western medicine (Liu, 1986). Asian-Americans may also use both herbal medicines and Western medicines concurrently for the same condition (Chang, 1995). This is especially common when they are dealing with a chronic or serious illness that Western medicine has little hope of curing (Hong, 1993, 1995).

Traditional Asian-Americans will tend to underutilize Western medical services. In addition to financial barriers to access (due to poverty, unemployment, and lack of health insurance), other barriers to access are location to health care facilities and the lack of transportation, cultural factors (as noted), linguistic barriers, and the lack of culturally competent health care providers (Hawks, 1996; Inouye, 1999). In the case of the latter barrier, Frye (1995), who has observed health care being provided to Southeast Asian-American refugees, calls attention to the "profound" ignorance of health care professionals about the customs, culture, and experiences of this group.

Mental health services are also underutilized because of cost, but probably more importantly, because of the shame and stigma that mental illness attaches to both the individual and his or her family (Hong, 1988). Asian-Americans will generally seek mental health services when all else has failed (Goldenberg & Goldenberg, 2002). The belief that mental disorders are not preventable or that they cannot be treated effectively, as well as the belief that self-help and family help are the means of handling psychosocial problems, also are factors that curtail the use of mental health services by traditional Asian-American families (Ishii-Kuntz, 2000; Kitano & Maki, 1996). Moreover, because of the prominence of Confucian ideology, Buddhism, and Taoism in Asian cultures, there is a tendency to maintain a "proper" public façade and deny publicly any sign of personal weakness such as mental or physical illness (Kline & Huff, 1999).

FAMILY STRESSORS AND COPING STRATEGIES

As mentioned earlier when we spoke of common experiences Asian-Americans have in the United States, racism is a major stressor. Racism is evidenced in job-related situations (Ishii-Kuntz, 2000) and social/political situations (Kang, 2001). External hostility to Asian-Americans is evidenced by the number of hate crimes that have taken place recently and by de facto housing barriers. Supportive ethnic community networks have sprung up to help newly arrived immigrants deal with the discrimination and hostility they may face (Ishii-Kuntz, 2000).

Another stressor, which is common to all Asian-American immigrants is the migration strain, including the cultural shock and its impact on the family. Most new immigrants are placed in strange and unpredictable environments. Language barriers, homesickness, ajdustment to Western values and lifestyles, the lack of extended family and community supports, work and financial stresses, and social isolation (for the elderly) are some of the stress-producing factors making migration so taxing (Lee, 1996; Pascual, 2000).

In recent years, the most stressed of the Asian-American groups are the immigrants and refugees coming from Southeast Asia—Laos, Cambodia, and Vietnam (Stauffer, 1995). Refugees have experienced the greater adversity. The difference between refugees and immigrants is that refugees migrate because of fear of persecution and often have had very traumatic experiences in their native country and in their migration to the United States. Immigrants, in contrast, migrate to the United States primarily because of economic or personal reasons. For example, Link and Dohrenwend (1980) found that in their large sample of Southeast Asian refugees, respondents reported levels of severe distress that were three times greater than that found among the American population in general. The incidence of posttraumatic stress disorder and domestic violence are high among this group (Inouye, 1999).

In spite of all the above stressors that Asian-American immigrants experience in the United States, a recent poll of Chinese-Americans in Southern California, 87 percent of whom were immigrants, found that 78 percent of them felt positive about their life here. These respondents said that life here turned out to be as expected (37 percent) or better than expected (41 percent). Only 16 percent felt that life was worse than they expected (Kang, 1997).

There are three prominent family coping patterns that Asian-Americans find helpful and effective. The first two are linked—the family pulling together (greater cohesiveness) under stress and adversity and seeking and receiving direct assistance and support from the extended family (Ishii-Kuntz, 2000). Immigrant families may be cut off from their extended family social support system when they migrate to the United States. Sometimes only one side of the extended family is here or only the nuclear family migrates. This isolation from the family's social support system is often stressful because it eliminates a significant traditional way Asian families cope. Health professionals need to be informed of community resources to help families utilize these to fill some of the vacuum that the family social support system once fulfilled (Hong, 1988, 1989).

Seeking social and financial support from self-help community groups is a third critical way of coping for Asian-American families. Many Asian-American communities have organizations targeted at helping new immigrants and other less acculturated Asian-Americans who have difficulty accessing mainstream agencies.

A fourth family coping strategy, probably less prominent than the latter three, is the use of passive appraisal. Acceptance of one's fate (fatalism) serves as a way for family members to cope with family stressors over which they have no control (Henderson, 1989).

A common way for individuals in the family to cope with interpersonal and intrapersonal stress and conflict is through somatization (Hong, Lee, & Lorenzo, 1995; Lasky & Martz, 1993). Psychosomatic problems are cited widely as a common way of seeking help. Because suppression of emotions is emphasized, however, there may be silent forbearance of one's suffering and pain (Morrow, 1987).

INFLUENCE OF ACCULTURATION ON FAMILY STRUCTURE AND FUNCTIONS

As succeeding generations of Asian-Americans became more acculturated, family structural and functional patterns correspondingly change. Moreover, Asian-American families, in response to both structural factors in society, such as immigration policies, and racism, continually undergo change. In spite of the growth in acculturation with each succeeding generation, a dominant theme in the literature is the dynamic tension that exists between Eastern tradition and Western modernity (Hong, 1996; Hong & Ham, 1994; Mirandé, 1991).

Asian-American families vary tremendously in how acculturated they are. Based on Asian-American's handling of acculturation, Lee (1996) divides Asian-American families into five major types: traditional families, "cultural conflict" families, bicultural families, "Americanized" families, and interracial families. **Traditional families** are generally composed of older members who were born and raised in Asian countries. They include families from rural areas with limited exposure to Western culture and limited education. They live in ethnic communities and speak their native language (no or little English). Many of these families are economically impoverished. These are the unacculturated families.

"Cultural conflict" families are families in which the parents and grandparents were born and raised in Asia and in which their children were or are being raised and educated in the United States. These families experience considerable cultural conflict between acculturated children and unacculturated parents and grandparents. The effect of acculturation on the children of immigrant families and the resultant generational gap and conflict is the most discussed topic in the counseling literature (Lee, Choe, Kim, & Ngo, 2000). The clash of values between parents who retain their traditional values and the children (particularly adolescents) who take on the American values of independence, individualism, and assertiveness is a commonly cited problem that brings Asian-American children to the attention of school and community counselors (Hong, 1989, 1996; Hong & Ham, 1992; Pedersen, Draguns, Lonner, & Trimble, 1996). Conflict between parents and adolescents in Korean-American communities is a case in point. Here, according to Min (1995c), value conflicts, combined with a language barrier between immigrant parents who speak Korean and children who speak English, build dysfunctional distance between parents and their adolescent children. Adolescents who are having trouble coping at home often act out at school and in the community. School counselors working with Korean-American high school students in Los Angeles report that cutting class, skipping school, fighting, running away from home, and joining gangs are common problems of troubled Korean-American youth (Min, 1995c). These types of families may also have conflicts because one spouse is more acculturated than the other. For instance, an Asian husband may have worked in the United States for years, then returned to his country of origin and married a wife not familiar with American culture (Lee, 1996).

Bicultural families are those families who are well acculturated to Western culture because they either grew up in urbanized major Asian cities or were born and raised in the United States. The parents are usually middle class and often hold professional positions. They are bilingual and bicultural—retaining important traditions, but being "modern" at the same time.

Americanized families are families that are highly acculturated. Usually, both parents and children were born and raised in the United States. Family members do not express an interest or any effort to maintain their ethnic identity.

Interracial families are the last major type of family based on acculturation differences and issues. There has been a growth in Asian-American intermarriages and, thus, these types of families are commonly seen. In fact, over one half of Japanese-American marriages are interracial. Many interracial families integrate both cultural backgrounds successfully, although some couples experience conflicts in values, religious beliefs, communication, child rearing, and in-law relationships (Lee, 1996).

Gender roles are changing rapidly as women join the workforce and are exposed to American core values and life. With increased labor force participation, Asian-American women's power in the family also increases and, correspondingly, the husbands' dominance diminishes. Men and women in acculturated families display more egalitarian relationships (Ishii-Kuntz, 2000). Research, however, still demonstrates systematic cultural biases favoring males (Pedersen et al., 1996).

A study conducted by Huang and Ying (1989) provides evidence of the types of gender role changes occurring in families. They found that among more acculturated Korean-American families, gender-specific differences in child rearing were not so glaring as in the past. They reported that in their sample, most Korean-American fathers were helping with child rearing, an "unknown" practice in the past. Moreover, in acculturated Asian-American families, the researchers speculated that even though the husband–father may still be the family spokesperson and leader in public, behind the scenes the wife often has considerable decision-making power (Huang & Ying).

The role of the elder generation (the grandparents) in the Asian-American family is also changing with acculturation. Hong (1989) points out that grandparents, who are honored by virtue of their status, may have diminished say in family decision making, especially when their children are financially indepedent.

The concept of generational changes is important also when discussing acculturation. In the Japanese-American family literature, family life among third- and fourth-generation Japanese-American families is much more Westernized. For example, the family patterns and marital division of work of the Sansei (third generation) very closely resemble the American pattern (Kitano, 1988). Moreover, fewer Japanese-American families are likely to hold traditional values because they have lived in the United States for so long (Uba, 1994).

✺ FAMILY NURSING ASSESSMENT

Two factors should be taken into consideration in assessing an Asian-American family. These factors are the family's culture and their environment (Hong, 1989).

CULTURE

Culture, as a factor for assessment, pertains to the cultural issues relevant to a particular family. The family nurse needs to consider to what extent the characteristics of Asian families described in this chapter are applicable to the family being care for. Also, to what extent does a family member, or the family as a whole, identify with their culture of origin or with mainstream American culture? Different families, as well as different members within a family, may vary in their cultural identification. Rather than there being a discrete dichotomy between Asian and mainstream American cultures, a continuum exists with an infinite number of positions present that individuals and families may take.

Family nurses working with particular Asian-American groups need to become informed about their history and immigration patterns; cultural values, beliefs, and lifestyles; traditional health beliefs and practices; and family dynamics.

Given the diversity in cultural identification, the family nurse should approach an Asian-American family with a flexible attitude and refrain from stereotyping (Inouye, 1999). However, if the family nurse is unsure of how to approach the family in an interview, he or she should take a conservative approach and avoid going against the cultural norms such as ignoring the traditional family hierarchy or being confrontive.

In working with traditional Asian-American families, attempting to form an egalitarian partnership type of nurse–client relationship may not be most effective. The Asian-American client may feel more comfortable with a hierarchial relationship due to Asian norms of deference to authority and modesty with superiors (Marsella, 1993). Proper protocol, addressing one another by family names, and paying the proper respect are ways to achieve a positive alliance with traditional families (Goldenberg & Goldenberg, 2002).

A cultural assessment also includes evaluating how strongly a family subscribes to traditional Asian health/medical practices versus Western practices. As mentioned earlier, it is common for immigrant Asian-Americans to subscribe to both forms of practices, and the practitioner must be sensitive to this. In fact, it is often necessary to directly ask a family whether they are trying any traditional Asian medical remedy. The family nurse should approach this issue in a respectful and understanding manner, rather than unwittingly hinting that Asian medical practices are nonmainstream, inferior, or unacceptable. If done properly, such a discussion will convey the nurse's cultural competence to the family, and will be a major contribution to the therapeutic alliance (Hong, 1993; Hong, Lee, & Lorenzo, 1995).

In working with a family, the family nurse should also be alert to the possible differences in cultural identification among family members, such as that between parents and children. In this situation, the nurse might, at times, defer to the cultural beliefs of the active decision makers of the family. At other times, the nurse might have to identify the cultural conflict as an issue and help the family arrive at a consensus or compromise in planning interventions.

ENVIRONMENT

Environment, as a factor for assessment, refers to the extent to which a family is encountering social/environmental problems. It addresses the external factors such as the impact of community and other environmental stressors on the family. These questions could be asked. Is the family having financial hardships? Is an immigrant Asian-American family suffering from the loss of their traditional social support network, which was left behind in their country of origin? Are language and lack of familiarity with U.S. institutions interfering with their access to health services? For refugee Asian-Americans, to what degree is their past trauma affecting their current adjustment? An evaluation of these issues will be very useful in formulating realistic goals for working with the family.

In assessing an Asian-American family, the family nurse should be aware that many new immigrants are preoccupied with the tasks of basic survival. They have to adjust to a new social environment, settle in new jobs and new neighborhoods, make new friends, and develop a new social network. For some, it may take years, or even a lifetime, before they feel psychologically secure (Goldenberg & Goldenberg, 2002).

A serious health problem of a family member is a major burden for an immigrant family that is adjusting to a new environment. Some family members might try to deny or minimize the problem. Others may harbor repressed anger toward the person with the illness for bringing "additional trouble" on the family. On the other hand, the person with the illness might experience feelings of guilt for "being the burden" (Hong, 1995) or may suppress their suffering and put on a public façade of feeling all right. These are feelings that family nurses should carefully consider in their assessment.

Family nurses must be empathic to the obstacles refugee Asian-Americans have encountered before being allowed to enter the United States. Many refugee families may not want to attract any "government" attention again. They are often reluctant to discuss their family history or trauma with a stranger, especially one who is from a public or government agency. In these situations, the nurse needs to reassure the family before discussing any of these issues, and proceed slowly and sensitively.

Stephan Jiang (1995), Executive Director of the Association of Asian and Pacific Islanders Community Health Organization, sums up some of the key assessment issues by delineating several questions, which he recommends be part of a clinician's health assessment (Table 20–3). The answers to these key ques-

TABLE 20–3

KEY QUESTIONS TO ASK ASIAN-AMERICAN CLIENTS AS PART OF HEALTH ASSESSMENT

- What language or languages do you speak?
- How long have you and your family lived in this country?
- How do you identify your nationality and ethnicity?
- Do you use any traditional healing methods?

Source: Adapted from Jiang (1995).

tions will help clinicians both to avoid stereotyping and to develop an individualized plan of care for Asian-American clients. He also suggests that when making recommendations for a particular health problem the client be asked, "Is that different from what you expect?" (p. 3). Table 20–4 lists high-risk situations and characteristics, another aid for assessment.

TABLE 20–4

HIGH-RISK FAMILY CHARACTERISTICS[a]

- Recently immigrated
- Came to United States as refugee
- Lower socioeconomic status (in country of origin or in the United States)
- High degree of identification with home country
- Limited English proficiency
- Experiencing cultural shock
- Experiencing discrimination
- Role and/or status reversal
- Intergenerational family conflicts
- Lack of community supports
- Lack of health insurance

Source: Adapted from Goldenberg & Goldenberg (2000).
[a]Lack of acculturation and socioeconomic factors are important factors to consider in assessing risk behavior and health status.

FAMILY NURSING INTERVENTIONS

Based on the discussion in this chapter, the following are principles that will guide the formulation of culturally sensitive interventions for Asian-American families:

1. Given the family structure and hierarchy in Asian cultures, family nurses should be sensitive to the role and expectations of different family members, such as the authority of parents, especially the father. When families are making decisions about a member's health care, extended family members, if available, might need to be involved along with the nuclear family. In addition, familism suggests that family members are likely to be more concerned with their mutual responsibilities than are typical mainstream American family members (Kline & Huff, 1999).

2. Considering the cultural norms governing communication and social interactions, family nurses should avoid direct confrontation with the family. In addition, they must be alert to the subtle, indirect messages sent by a client. A polite and mild disagreement from the client may actually mean a strong disagreement. When in doubt, clarify the communication in a nonthreatening manner.

3. Family nurses need to be sensitive to the stigma and shame often associated with chronic illness and mental disorder. They need to be empathic to the possible anger or guilt experienced by different family members who might feel that the illness is an "added" problem for an immigrant family that is already stressed by basic survival needs.

4. As research and clinical observations attest, many first-generation Asian-Americans follow both traditional Asian medical practices and Western medicine (Huff & Kline, 1999). This is especially true when families are dealing with a serious or chronic illness that Western medicine has little hope of curing. Family nurses should not interfere with these practices as long as they are not detrimental to the client or in conflict with the prescribed care. If unsure, consulting with practitioners who are familiar with the culture is often helpful.

5. Family health professionals need to be alert to the social/environmental problems and institutional barriers faced by less-acculturated Asian-American families. If a family needs to be referred to different agencies for service, there is a need for the family nurse to coordinate and streamline referral/intake procedures to minimize confusion and ensure compliance.

6. Family nurses should be sensitive to the trauma experienced by refugee Asian-Americans. This is a lifelong psychological burden for many families and individuals.

7. Many Asian-Americans consider health care providers to be teachers. Education is highly valued and, as such, is very much appreciated. Educational interventions should focus on education about the health problem, problem solving, management strategies, and (in mental health) conflict resolution (Lee, 1996).

8. Last but not least, it is important to remember that Asian-Americans differ in their ethnic identity and in their cultural practices. In addition, they differ in their identification with Asian and mainstream American cultures. Family nurses must avoid stereotyping a family. When in doubt about a cultural issue, discussing one's questions with the family itself or with professionals who are familiar with the culture is often critical to providing culturally competent family health care.

❧ SUMMARY

- Asian-Americans constitute about 4 per cent of the United States population. They are proportionately the fastest growing ethnic group in the country.

- Asian-Americans or Asian and Pacific Islanders refer to people residing in the United States who are from Asia, the Indian subcontinent, and the islands in the Pacific Ocean, including at least 23 groups. The four largest Asian-American groups, in order of population, are Chinese-Americans, Filipino-Americans, Vietnamese-Americans, Korean-Americans, and Japanese-Americans.

- Most Asian-Americans came to the United States recently, especially since the loosening of immigration laws, which took place in the mid-1960s. A brief history of each of the five most numerous Asian-American groups, with respect to their immigration experience, is presented.

- Asian-Americans who came to the United States as refugees—most of these are from Southeast Asia, Vietnam particularly—experienced higher levels of stress and adversity in their native country. Consequently, they also experience greater health problems, particularly a higher incidence of post-traumatic stress syndrome and domestic violence, as well as greater economic hardships than other Asian-American groups.

- Three religious/philosophic belief systems have shaped traditional Asian core values. These are: Confucianism, Taoism, and Buddhism. Asian-American families hold traditional Asian values to varying degrees. A comparison of Eastern and Western values are presented to show the profound differences between the two cultures (refer to Table 20–2).

- The traditional Asian family role and power structure, family communication patterns, family affective function, family socialization function, and family health care function are described. Each dimension is congruent with the core values of the Asian family.

- Several major stressors among Asian-American individuals and families are discussed, including the stress of racism and the migration strain where a myriad of challenges have to be faced, e.g., language barriers, cultural shock, homesickness.

- Three prominent family coping patterns that Asian-Americans find helpful and effective are: the family pulling together (greater cohesiveness) under stress, extended family support, and social and financial support from self-help community groups. Use of passive appraisal is also utilized in dealing with stressors.

- In spite of the tendency for Asian-Americans to acculturate, there exists a dynamic tension between Eastern tradition and Western modernity.

- As part of family nursing assessment, it is suggested that both the cultural dimensions and environmental influences on the family be assessed. Key questions to ask Asian-American clients, as well as high-risk family characteristics are identified. Eight principles that guide the formulation of family-oriented culturally sensitive interventions for working with Asian-American families are delineated.

❧ FAMILY VIGNETTE: THE OGAWA FAMILY*

The Ogawa family is a three-generation Japanese-American family whose members live in Seattle, Washington, and have lived there since 1923. The family is composed of Bill and his wife Jean, their three school-aged children, and Bill's mother, Helen. Helen is 80 years old, widowed, and has osteoarthritis, osteoporosis, and a recent fractured hip. She moved in with her son Bill and his family after her husband died. Bill's father had a grocery store, and when he died Bill took over the business with the help of his mother. Helen worked in the store up until the day of her fracture. Since Helen's fractured hip, she has had limited mobility and requires assistance with her activities of daily living (ADLs). Family members (Bill, Jean, and his two sisters) have rearranged their work schedules so that they could help with Helen's care when needed. Bill, after consulting with his sisters and their husbands, recently called a local home health agency and started home health services for the mother because the family members were feeling overwhelmed and exhausted in caring for Helen, in addition to having their own families and work. The family is still very involved with Helen's care when the home health nurse is not there. Helen expresses guilt over being a burden and causing the family so much trouble.

* Adapted from Ishida (1999).

■ STUDY QUESTIONS

Review the Family Vignette and answer the related questions.

1. What are the key cultural assessment areas (see Table 20–3), and does this vignette provide this information? If not, what is missing?

2. What family coping strategy is prominently seen in this vignette, and how is the coping pattern evidenced?

3. What cultural values do you see in this vignette?

4. Identify two culturally based family nursing interventions pertinent to working with this family.

Answer the following questions.

5. What peoples constitute Asian-Americans?

6. What is the current demographic pattern with respect to Asian-Americans in the United States today?

7. Filipino-Americans differ from the other four largest groups of Asian-Americans in the following ways (indicate all correct answers):

   a. Their history includes about 500 years of Spanish colonization.
   b. Their country of origin is described as the most Westernized in Asia.
   c. The majority of Filipinos are Catholic.

8. Select three core values of traditional Asian-American families and link a family nursing practice implication to each of these core values.

9. Describe the value clash that often occurs between children and their parents in Asian-American immigrant families.

10. When the Asian-American immigrant family settles in the United States, which of the following changes typically occur(s) in family life?

   a. Children work two jobs and often drop out of school early.
   b. Women enter the labor market and, because of their employment, have more power in the family.
   c. Patrilocality is often not possible or practical, so in these cases nuclear families live in separate households.

11. "Saving face" in Asian culture influences communication patterns in the following way(s):

   a. Communication is more indirect and subtle.
   b. Disagreements may be expressed in a circumventive manner.
   c. Communication is usually polite and respectful.
   d. Mistakes are never acknowledged or communicated.

12. Socialization of children in traditional Asian-American families, when compared with socialization in mainstream American families, involves:

   a. An emphasis on filial piety and veneration of age.
   b. Children are taught to be independent at an early age.
   c. The family exerts greater control over children's behavior.
   d. The importance of education is stressed in the family.

13. Which of the following are central tenets/key concepts in Eastern medicine?

   a. Physical assessment
   b. Balance
   c. Holism
   d. *yin–yang*
   e. The value of mastery
   f. Health promotion
   g. Surgical intervention
   h. Vital energy
   i. Use of herbs
   j. Psychotherapy
   k. Talk therapy

14. Which of the following family coping strategies would most likely be used among traditional Asian-American families?

   a. Self-reliance
   b. Use of humor in problem solving
   c. Seeking spiritual support
   d. Seeking social support from extended family network

15. Discuss three general intervention guidelines pertinent to working with traditional Asian-American families.

THE FRIEDMAN FAMILY ASSESSMENT MODEL (LONG FORM)

The following guidelines represent a collation of the assessment questions/areas that appear at the end of Chapters 8 through 17, beginning with the assessment of identifying and environmental data, continuing through the assessment of structural and functional dimensions, and concluding with an assessment of family stress, coping, and adaptation. After each broad heading, a footnote alerts the reader as to where the related family theory and further discussion of assessment areas may be found.

The Friedman Family Assessment Model consists of six broad categories:

1. Identifying data
2. Developmental stage and history
3. Environmental data
4. Family structure
5. Family functions
6. Family stress, coping, and adaptation

Each category contains numerous subcategories. Nurses assessing families should decide which subcategories are particularly relevant (after a basic screening-type assessment) so that these can be explored in more depth during family visits/encounters. Not all the subcategory assessment areas may need to be assessed—the depth and breadth of assessment is dependent on the family's goals, problems, and resources, as well as the nurse's role in working with the family.

IDENTIFYING DATA

Foundational data that describe the family in basic terms are included in this section.

1. **Family Name**
2. **Address and Phone**
3. **Family Composition:** Use of the family genogram is recommended (See Figure 8–1).
4. **Type of Family Form**[1]
5. **Cultural (Ethnic) Background**[2] (including extent of acculturation): In describing this, use the following criteria as guideposts for determining family's cultural and religious orientation and extent of acculturation.
   5.1. Family's or family members' stated ethnic background (self-identified)?
   5.2. Language(s) spoken in home? Do all family members speak English?
   5.3. Country of origin as well as length of time family has lived in the United States (what generation are family members, relative to their immigration status) and the family's reason for immigrating?
   5.4. The family's social network (from the same ethnic group)?
   5.5. Family residence (part of an ethnically homogeneous neighborhood)?
   5.6. Religious, social, cultural, recreational, and/or educational activities (are they within the family's cultural group)?
   5.7. Dietary habits and dress (traditional or westernized?)
   5.8. Home decor (signs of cultural influences)?
   5.9. Presence of traditional or "modern" family roles and power structure?

5.10. The portion(s) of the community the family frequents—the family's territorial complex (is it within the ethnic community primarily)?

5.11. The family's use of health care services and practitioners. Does the family visit folk practitioners, engage in traditional folk health practices, or have traditional indigenous health beliefs?

6. **Religious Identification**

6.1. What is the family's religion?

6.2. Do family members differ in their religious beliefs and practices?

6.3. How actively involved is the family in a particular church, temple, mosque, or other religious organization?

6.4. What religious practices does the family engage in?

6.5. What religiously based beliefs or values appear central in the family's life?

7. **Social Class Status**[3] (based on occupation, education, and income):

7.1. Estimate the family's social class, based on the three above indicators.

7.2. Economic Status.

7.3. Who is (are) the breadwinner(s) in the family?

7.4. Does the family receive any supplementary funds or assistance? If so, what are they (from where)?

7.5. Does family consider their income to be adequate? How does the family see itself managing financially?

8. **Social Class Mobility**[3]

DEVELOPMENTAL STAGE AND HISTORY OF FAMILY[4]

9. Family's present developmental stage.

10. The extent to which the family is fulfilling the developmental tasks appropriate for the present developmental stage.

11. The family's history from inception through present day, including developmental history and unique health and health-related events and experiences (divorces, deaths, losses, etc.) that happened in the family's life (utilize a genogram to collect some of this data).

12. Both parents' families of origin (what life in family of origin was like; past and present relations with parents of parents).

ENVIRONMENTAL DATA[5]

Environmental data covers the family's universe—from consideration of the smallest area such as aspects of home to the larger community in which the family resides.

13. **Characteristics of Home**[5]

13.1. Describe the dwelling type (home, apartment, rooming house, etc.). Does family own or rent its home?

13.2. Describe the home's condition (both the interior and exterior of house). The house interior includes number of rooms and types of rooms (living room, bedrooms, etc.), their use and how they are furnished. What is the condition and adequacy of furniture? Is there adequate heating, ventilation, and lighting (artificial and daylight)? Are the floors, stairs, railings, and other structures in adequate condition?

13.3. In the kitchen, assess the water supply, sanitation, and the adequacy of refrigeration.

13.4. In bathrooms, observe sanitation, water supply, toilet facilities, presence of towels and soap. Do family members share towels? In bathtub, are there grab bars?

13.5. Assess the sleeping arrangements in the house. Are they adequate for family members, considering their age, relationships, and their special needs?

13.6. Observe the home's general state of cleanliness and sanitation. What are the family's hygiene and cleanliness practices? Are there any infestations of vermin (interior especially) and/or sanitation problems due to presence of pets?

13.7. Are there signs of flaking, old paint (possible source for lead poisoning) which young children might be exposed to?

13.8. Identify the family's territorial unit. Are they comfortable driving out of their neighborhood to use resources/services?

13.9. Evaluate the privacy arrangements and how the family feels about the adequacy of its privacy.

13.10. Evaluate the home's presence or absence of safety hazards.

13.11. Evaluate the adequacy of waste and garbage disposal.

13.12. Assess the family members' overall satisfaction/dissatisfaction with their housing arrangements. Does the family consider the home adequate for its needs?

14. **Characteristics of Neighborhood and Larger Community**[5]
14.1. What are the physical characteristics of the immediate neighborhood and the larger community?
Type of neighborhood/community (rural, urban, suburban, intercity).
Types of dwellings (residential, industrial, combined residential and small industry, agrarian) in neighborhood.
Condition of the dwellings and streets (well kept up, deteriorating, dilapidated, being revitalized).
Sanitation of streets, home (cleanliness, trash and garbage collected, etc.).
Problems with traffic congestion?
Presence and types of industry in neighborhood.
Are there air, noise, or water pollution problems?
14.2. What are the demographic characteristics of the neighborhood and community?
Social class and ethnic characteristics of residents.
Occupations and interests of families.
Density of population.
Recent demographic changes in neighborhood/community.
14.3. What health and other basic services and facilities are available in the neighborhood and community?
Marketing facilities (food, clothing, drug store, etc.).
Health agencies (clinics, hospital, emergency facilities).
Social service agencies (welfare, counseling, employment).
Laundromat services for those families in need.
Family's church or temple.
14.4. How accessible are the neighborhood and community schools and what is their condition? Are there busing and integration problems which affect the family?
14.5. Recreational facilities.
14.6. Availability of public transportation. How accessible (in terms of distance, suitability, hours, etc.) are these services and facilities to the family?

14.7. What is the incidence of crime in the neighborhood and community? Are there serious safety problems?

15. **Family's Geographical Mobility**[6]
15.1. How long has the family lived in the area?
15.2. What is the family's history of geographical mobility?
15.3. From where did the family move or migrate?

16. **Family's Associations and Transactions with Community**[7]
16.1. Who in the family uses what community services or is known to what agencies?
16.2. How frequently or to what extent do they use these services or facilities?
16.3. What are the family's territorial patterns—communities or areas frequented?
16.4. Is the family aware of community services relevant to its needs, such as transportation?
16.5. How does family feel about groups or organizations from whom it receives assistance or with whom it relates?
16.6. How does the family view its community?

FAMILY STRUCTURE

17. **Communication Patterns**[8]
17.1. In observing the family as a whole and/or the family's set of relationships, how extensively are functional and dysfunctional communication used? Diagram or give examples of recurring patterns.
How firmly and clearly do the members state their needs and feelings?
To what extent do members use clarification and qualification in interacting?
Do members elicit and respond favorably to feedback or do they generally discourage feedback and exploration of an issue?
How well do members listen and attend when communicating?
Do members seek validation from one another?
To what degree do members use assumptions and judgmental statements in interaction?
Do members interact in an offensive manner to messages?
How frequently is disqualification utilized?
17.2. How are emotional (affective) messages conveyed in the family and within the family subsystems?

How frequently are these emotional messages conveyed?

What types of emotions are transmitted within the family subsystems? Are negative, positive, or both types of emotions transmitted?

17.3. What is the frequency and quality of communication within the communication network and familial sets of relationships?

Who talks to whom and in what manner?

What is the usual pattern of transmitting important messages? Does an intermediary exist?

Are messages sent that are appropriate for the developmental age of the members?

17.4. Are the majority of messages of family members congruent in content and instruction? (Include observations of nonverbal messages.) If not, who manifests what kind of incongruency?

17.5. What types of dysfunctional processes are seen in the family communication patterns?

17.6. What areas are closed off to discussion that are important issues to the family's wellness or adequate functioning?

17.7. How do the following factors influence family communication patterns:
- The context/situation.
- The family life cycle stage.
- The family's cultural background.
- Gender differences in family.
- Family form.
- Family's socioeconomic status.
- The family's unique miniculture.

18. **Power Structure**[9]

Power Outcomes

18.1. Who makes what decisions? Who has the last "say" or "who wins?"

18.2. How important are these decisions or issues to the family?

More specific questions might include:

Who budgets, pays bills, decides how money is to be spent?

Who decides on how to spend an evening or what friends or relatives to visit?

Who decides on changes in jobs or residence?

Who disciplines and decides on child's activities?

Decision-making Process

18.3. What specific techniques are utilized for making decisions in the family and to what extent are these utilized (e.g., consensus; accommo-dation-bargaining; compromising or coercion; de facto)? In other words, how does the family make its decisions?

Power Bases. The various bases or sources of power are legitimate power/authority and a variation of it, "helpless" power; referent power; expert power or resources power; reward power; coercive power; informational power (direct and indirect); affective power; and tension management power.

18.4. On what bases of power do the family members make their decisions?

Variables Affecting Family Power

18.5. Recognizing the existence of any of the following variables will help the assessor interpret family behavior from which family power can be assessed.
- The family power hierarchy.
- Type of family form.
- Formation of coalition(s).
- Family communication network.
- Gender differences.
- Age and family life cycle factors.
- Cultural and interpersonal factors.
- Social class.

Overall Family System and Subsystem Power

18.6. From your assessment of all the above broad areas, are you able to deduce whether family power can be characterized as dominated by wife or husband, child, grandmother, etc.; egalitarian–syncratic or autonomic; leaderless or chaotic? The family power continuum can be used for a visual presentation of your analysis.

Family Power Continuum: If dominance is found, who is the dominant one?

18.7. To determine the overall power pattern, asking a broad, open-ended question is often illuminating (asking both spouses and children if feasible), examples of which are given below.

Who usually has "last say" or makes the decisions about important issues?

Who is really in charge and why (getting at bases for power)?

Who runs the family?

Who wins the important arguments or issues?

Who usually wins out if there is a disagreement?

Who gets his or her way when parents/spouses disagree?

Are family members satisfied with how decisions are made and with who makes them (i.e., the present power structure)?

19. **Role Structure**[10]

Formal Role Structure

19.1. What formal positions and roles do each of the family members fulfill? Describe how each family member carries out his or her formal roles.

19.2. Are these roles acceptable and consistent with family members' expectations? In other words, does role strain or role conflict exist?

19.3. How competently do members feel they perform their respective roles?

19.4. Is there flexibility in roles when needed?

Informal Role Structure

19.5. What informal or covert roles exist in the family? Who plays them and how frequently or consistently are they enacted? Are members of the family covertly playing roles different from those which their position in the family demands that they play?

19.6. What purpose does the presence of the identified covert or informal role(s) serve?

19.7. Are any of the informal roles dysfunctional to the family or family members in the long run?

19.8. What is the impact on the person(s) who play this (these) role(s)?

Analysis of Role Models (when role problems are present)

19.9. Who were (or are) the models that influenced a family member(s) in his or her early life, who gave him or her the feelings and values about growth, new experiences, roles, communication techniques?

19.10. Who specifically acted as role model for the mates in their roles as parents, and marital partners, and what were they like?

19.11. If the informal roles are dysfunctional in the family, who enacted these roles in previous generations?

Variables Affecting Role Structure

19.12. Social class influences: How does social class background influence the formal and informal role structure in the family?

19.13. Cultural influences: How is the family's role structure influenced by the family's ethnic and religious background?

19.14. Developmental or life cycle stage influences: Are the present role behaviors of family members developmentally appropriate?

19.15. Situational events: Changes in family member's health status. How have health problems affected family roles? What reallocation of roles/tasks have occurred? How have family members who have assumed new roles adjusted? Any evidence of role stress or role conflicts? How has the family member with the health problem reacted to his or her change or loss of role(s)?

20. **Family Values**[11]

20.1. Use of "compare and contrast" method is suggested (with values of either dominant culture, family's reference group—ethnic group with whom they identify—or both).
Productivity/Individual achievement
Individualism
Materialism/The consumption ethic
The work ethic
Education
Equality
Progress and mastery over the environment
Future time orientation
Efficiency, orderliness, and practicality
Rationality
Quality of life and maintaining health

Disparity in Value System

20.2. To what extent is there congruence between the family's values and the family's reference group and/or interacting systems like the educational and the health care systems and the wider community?

20.3. To what extent is there congruence between the family's values and each family member's values?

Family Values

20.4. How important are the identified values to the family? (Rank order the family values.)

20.5. Are the values consciously or unconsciously held?

20.6. Are there any value conflicts evident within the family?

20.7. How do the family's social class, cultural background and degree of acculturation, generational differences, and geographical setting (rural, urban, suburban) influence the family's values?

20.8. How do the family's values affect the health status of the family?

FAMILY FUNCTIONS

21. **Affective Function**[12]

Mutual Nurturance, Closeness, and Identification

21.1. To what extent do family members provide mutual nurturance and support to each other?

21.2. Is a sense of closeness and intimacy present among the sets of relationships within the family?

How well do family members get along with each other?

Do they show affection toward each other?

21.3. Does mutual identification, bonding, or attachment appear to be present? (Empathetic statements, concerns about other's feelings, experiences, and hardships are all indicative.) To answer questions 21.1, 21.2, and 21.3, an attachment diagram is very helpful (see Fig. 14–2).

Separateness and Connectedness

21.4. How does the family deal with the issues of separateness and connectedness?

How does the family help its members want to be together and maintain cohesiveness (connectedness)?

Are opportunities for developing separateness available and are they appropriate for the age and needs of each of the family members?

Family Need–Response Patterns

21.5. To what extent do family members perceive the needs of the other individuals in the family?

Are parents (spouses) able to describe their children's and mate's needs and concerns?

How sensitive are family members in picking up cues regarding other's feelings and needs?

21.6. Are each member's needs, interests, differentness respected by the other family members?

Does a mutual respect balance exist (do they show mutual respect toward each other)?

How sensitive is the family to each individual's actions and concerns?

21.7. To what extent are the recognized needs of the family members being met by the family? What is the process for emotional release (unburdening) in the family? For questions 21.5, 21.6, and 21.7 it is suggested that a list of the family members be included with their needs (as perceived by family members) and the extent to which these needs are being met by the family.

22. **Socialization Function**[13]

22.1. Assess family's child-rearing practices in the following areas.

- Behavior control, including discipline, reward and punishment.
- Autonomy and dependency.
- Giving and receiving of love.

- Training for age-appropriate behavior (social, physical, emotional, language, and intellectual development).

22.2. How adaptive are the family's child-rearing practices for its particular family form and situation?

22.3. Who assumes responsibility for the child care role or socialization function? Is this function shared? If so, how is this managed?

22.4. How are the children regarded in this family?

22.5. What cultural beliefs influence the family's child-rearing patterns?

22.6. How do social class factors influence child-rearing patterns?

22.7. Is this a family that is at high risk for child-rearing problems? If so, what factors place the family at risk?

22.8. Is the home environment adequate for children's needs to play (appropriate to children's developmental stage)? Are age-appropriate play equipment/toys present?

23. **Health Care Function**[14]

23.1. *Family's health beliefs, values, and behaviors:*
What value does the family assign health? Health promotion? Prevention?
Is there consistency between family health values as stated and their health actions?
What health-promoting activities does the family engage in regularly? Are these behaviors characteristic of all family members, or are patterns of health-promoting behavior highly variable among family members?
What are the family's health goals?

23.2. *Family's definition of health–illness and its level of knowledge:*
How does the family define health and illness for each family member? What clues provide this impression, and who decides?
Is the family able to accurately observe and report significant symptoms and changes?
What are the family members' source of health information and advice?
How is health information and advice transmitted to family members?

23.3. *Family's perceived health status and illness susceptibility:*
How does the family assess its present health status?
What present health problems are identified by the family?
To what serious health problems do family members perceive themselves vulnerable?

What are the family's perceptions of how much control over health they have by taking appropriate health actions?

23.4. *Family dietary practices:*

Does the family know about the food sources from the food guide pyramid?

Is the family diet adequate? (A 3-day food history record of family eating patterns is recommended.)

Who is responsible for the planning, shopping, and preparation of meals?

How are the foods prepared?

How many meals are consumed per day?

Are there budgeting limitations? Food stamps usage?

What is the adequacy of storage and refrigeration?

Does mealtime serve a particular function for the family?

What is the family's attitude toward food and mealtimes?

What are the family's snack habits?

23.5. *Sleep and rest habits:*

What are the usual sleeping habits of family members?

Are family members meeting sleep requirements that are appropriate for their age and health status?

Are regular hours established for sleeping?

Do family members take regular naps or have other means of resting during the day?

Who decides when children go to sleep?

Where do family members sleep?

23.6. *Physical activity and recreation:*

Are family members aware that active recreation and regular aerobic exercise are necessary for good health?

Do usual daily work activities allow for physical activity?

What types of family recreational pursuits and physical activities (i.e., jogging, bicycling, swimming, dancing, tennis) are family members engaged in? How often? Who participates?

Do common daily activities performed by family members require a moderate level of energy expenditure? Do family members spend at least 30 minutes nearly every day participating in moderate or heavier physical activity?

What are the recreational/leisure-time activities of the family subsystems (spouse subsystem, parent–child subsystems, and sibling subsystems). How often do these activities occur? Who participates in them?

What are the family's beliefs about the relationship of physical activity to health?

What are the family members' feelings about the family's leisure-time/recreational activities (satisfaction with time spent and types of activities).

23.7. *Family therapeutic and recreational drug, alcohol and tobacco practices:*

What is the family's use of alcohol, tobacco, coffee, cola, or tea? (Caffeine and theobromine are stimulants.)

Do family members take drugs for recreational purposes?

How long has (have) family member(s) been using alcohol or other recreational drugs?

Is the use of tobacco, alcohol, or prescribed/illicit drugs by family members perceived as a problem?

Does the use of alcohol or other drugs interfere with the capacity to carry out usual activities?

Do family members regularly use over-the-counter or prescription drugs?

Does the family save drugs over a long period of time and reuse?

Are drugs properly labeled and stored in a safe place away from young children?

23.8. *Family's role in self-care practices:*

What does the family do to improve its health status?

What does the family do to prevent illness/disease?

Who is (are) the health leader(s) in the family?

Who makes the health decisions in the family?

What do family members do when caring for the sick in the home?

How competent is the family in self-care relative to recognition of signs and symptoms, diagnosis, and home treatment of common, simple health problems?

What are the family's values, attitudes, and beliefs regarding home care?

23.9. *Medically based preventive measures:*

What are the family's history and feelings about having physicals when well?

When were the last eye and hearing examinations?

What is the immunization status of family members?

Do family members use fluoridated water, or is a daily fluoride supplement prescribed for the children?

What are the family's oral hygiene habits in regard to brushing and flossing after meals?

What are the family's patterns of simple sugar and starch intake?

Do family members receive regular preventive professional dental care including education, periodic x-rays, cleaning, repair, and, for children, topical or oral fluoride?

23.10. *Complementary and alternative therapies.*

What alternative health care practices do family members use?

How often do they particpate in these practices and for what reasons to they initiate these practices?

How does the family member feel these practices will benefit his or her health?

Have these practices been undertaken in coordination with other medically based services?

23.11. *Family health history:*

What is the overall health of family members of origin and marriage (grandparents, parents, aunts, uncles, cousins, siblings, and offspring) over three generations?

Is there in the past or present a history of genetic or familial diseases—diabetes, heart disease, high blood pressure, stroke, cancer, gout, kidney disease, thyroid disease, asthma and other allergic states, blood diseases, or any other familial diseases.

Is there a family history of emotional problems or suicide? Are there any present or past environmentally related family diseases?

23.12. *Health care services received:*

From what health care practitioner(s) and/or health care agency(ies) do the family members receive care?

Does this provider(s) or agency(ies) see all members of the family and take care of all their health needs?

23.13. *Feelings and perceptions regarding health services:*

What are the family's feelings about the kinds of health services available to it in the community?

What are the family's feelings and perceptions regarding the health services it receives? Is the family comfortable, satisfied, and confident with the care received from its health care providers?

Does the family have any past experience with family health nursing services?

What are the family's attitudes and expectations of the role of the nurse?

23.14. *Emergency health services:*

Does the agency or physician the family receives care from have an emergency service?

Are medical services by current health care providers available if an emergency occurs?

If emergency services are not available, does the family know where the closest available (according to their eligibility) emergency services are for both the children and adults in the family?

Does the family know how to call for an ambulance and for paramedic services?

Does the family have an emergency health plan?

23.15. *Source of payment:*

How does the family pay for services it receives?

Does the family have a private health insurance plan, Medicare, or Medicaid, or must the family pay for services fully or partially?

Does the family receive any free services (or know about those for which it is eligible)?

What effect does the cost of health care have on the family's utilization of health services?

If the family has health insurance (private, Medicare, and/or Medicaid), is the family informed about what services are covered, such as preventive services, special medical equipment, home visits, and so forth?

23.16. *Logistics of receiving care:*

How far away are health care facilities from the family's home?

What modes of transportation does the family use to get to them?

If the family must depend on public transportation, what problems exist in regards to hours of service and travel time to health care facilities?

24. **Family Stress, Coping, and Adaptation**[15]

Family Stressors, Strengths, and Perceptions

24.1. What stressors (both long and short term) are being experienced by the family? Refer to the Family Inventory of Life Events Scale (Table 17–2) for examples of significant stressors. Consider environmental and socioeconomic stressors. What is the strength and duration of these stressors?

24.2. What strengths counterbalance the stressors? Is the family able to handle the usual stresses and strains of daily family life? What resources does the family possess to address the stressors?

24.3. What is the family's definition of its situation? Is it realistic, hopeful, seen as a challenge? Is the family able to act based on a realistic and objective appraisal of the stressful situation or event? Or is the prime stressor(s) seen as overwhelming, insurmountable, or in some way distorted?

Family Coping Strategies

24.4. How is the family reacting to the stressors it is experiencing? What coping strategies are being used? What coping strategies has the family employed to deal with what types of problems? Do family members differ in their ways of coping with their present problem? If so, how?

24.5. To what extent does the family use the following internal coping strategies?
Family group reliance.
Sharing of feelings, thoughts, and activities (strengthening cohesiveness).
Role flexibility.
Normalizing.
Controlling the meaning of the problem by reframing and passive appraisal.
Joint problem solving.
Gaining of information and knowledge.
Being open and honest in family communications.
Use of humor and laughter.

24.6. To what extent does the family use the following external coping strategies
Maintaining active linkages with the community.
Using spiritual supports.
Using social support systems (informal and formal systems).
To obtain further social support network information, both the genogram (Figure 8–1) and the ecomap (Figure 17–4) are suggested.

24.7. What dysfunctional coping strategies has the family used or is the family using? Are there signs of any of the dysfunctionalities listed below? If so, record their presence and how extensively they are being used?
Scapegoating.
Use of threat.
Family myth.

Triangling.
Pseudomutuality.
Authoritarianism.
Family dissolution.
Alcohol and/or drug abuse.
Family violence (spouse, child, sibling, elder, or gay and lesbian).
Child neglect.

Family Adaptation

24.8. How is the family managing or functioning? Are the family stressors/problems being adequately managed by the family?
What has the impact of the stressor(s) been on family functioning?

24.9. Is the family in crisis? Is the existing problem(s) part of a chronic inability to solve problems, i. e., is the family crisis-prone?

Tracking Stressors, Coping, Adaptation Over Time

24.10. When family nurses work with families over time, it is useful to track or monitor how the family is doing relative to stressors, perceptions, coping and adaptation. Is the family starting to recover, bringing forth helpful coping processes, or is it staying at the same level of adaptation, or showing evidence of diminished adaptation?

FOOTNOTES

1. Chapter 1
2. Chapter 8
3. Chapter 8
4. Chapter 5
5. Chapter 9
6. Chapter 9
7. Chapter 9
8. Chapter 10
9. Chapter 11
10. Chapter 12
11. Chapter 13
12. Chapter 14
13. Chapter 15
14. Chapter 16
15. Chapter 17

THE FRIEDMAN FAMILY ASSESSMENT MODEL (SHORT FORM)

The following form is shortened for ease in assessing the O'Shea family (Appendix C) and other families. If you are not sure what data should be covered in each of the assessment areas below, please refer to Appendix A for the long form, where more detailed questions/ areas are presented, or refer to the related chapters where both content and assessment areas are addressed.

Before using the following guidelines in completing family assessments, two words of caution are noted: First, not all areas included below will be germane for each of the families visited. The guidelines are comprehensive and allow depth when probing is necessary. The student should not feel that every subarea needs be covered when the broad area of inquiry poses no problems to the family or concern to the health worker. Second, by virtue of the interdependence of the family system, one will find unavoidable redundancy. For the sake of efficiency, the assessor should try not to repeat data, but to refer the reader back to sections where this information has already been described.

IDENTIFYING DATA

1. **Family Name**
2. **Address and Phone**
3. **Family Composition: The Family Genogram** (See Figure 8–1).
4. **Type of Family Form**
5. **Cultural (Ethnic) Background**
6. **Religious Identification**
7. **Social Class Status**
8. **Social Class Mobility**

DEVELOPMENTAL STAGE AND HISTORY OF FAMILY

9. **Family's Present Developmental Stage**
10. **Extent of Family Developmental Tasks Fulfillment**
11. **Nuclear Family History**
12. **History of Family of Origin of Both Parents**

ENVIRONMENTAL DATA

13. **Characteristics of Home**
14. **Characteristics of Neighborhood and Larger Community**
15. **Family's Geographical Mobility**
16. **Family's Associations and Transactions with Community**

FAMILY STRUCTURE

17. **Communication Patterns**
    Extent of Functional and Dysfunctional Communication (types of recurring patterns)
    Extent of Emotional (Affective) Messages and How Expressed
    Characteristics of Communication Within Family Subsystems
    Extent of Congruent and Incongruent Messages
    Types of Dysfunctional Communication Processes Seen in Family
    Areas of Closed Communication
    Familial and Contextual Variables Affecting Communication

18. **Power Structure**

    Power Outcomes
    Decision-making Process
    Power Bases
    Variables Affecting Family Power
    Overall Family System and Subsystem Power (Family Power Continuum Placement)

19. **Role Structure**

    Formal Role Structure
    Informal Role Structure
    Analysis of Role Models (optional)
    Variables Affecting Role Structure

20. **Family Values**

    Compare the family to American core values or family's reference group values and/or identify important family values and their importance (priority) in family.
    Congruence Between the Family's Values and the Family's Reference Group or Wider Community
    Disparity in Value Systems
    Presence of Value Conflicts in Family
    Effect of the Above Values and Value Conflicts on Health Status of Family

✎FAMILY FUNCTIONS

21. **Affective Function**

    Mutual Nurturance, Closeness, and Identification
    Family attachment diagram, Figure 14–2, is helpful here.
    Separateness and Connectedness
    Family's Need–Response Patterns

22. **Socialization Function**

    Family Child-rearing Practices
    Adaptability of Child-rearing Practices for Family Form and Family's Situation
    Who Is (Are) Socializing Agent(s) for Child(ren)?
    Value of Children in Family
    Cultural Beliefs That Influence Family's Child-rearing Patterns
    Social Class Influence on Child-Rearing Patterns
    Estimation About Whether Family Is at Risk for Child-rearing Problems and if So, Indication of High-Risk Factors
    Adequacy of Home Environment for Children's Needs to Play

23. **Health Care Function**

    Family's Health Beliefs, Values, and Behavior
    Family's Definitions of Health–Illness and Its Level of Knowledge

Family's Perceived Health Status and Illness Susceptibility
Family's Dietary Practices
Adequacy of family diet (recommended 3-day food history record).
Function of mealtimes and attitudes toward food and mealtimes.
Shopping (and its planning) practices.
Person(s) responsible for planning, shopping, and preparation of meals.
Sleep and Rest Habits
Physical Activity and Recreation Practices
Family's Therapeutic and Recreational Drug, Alcohol and Tobacco Practices
Family's Role in Self-care Practices
Medically Based Preventive Measures (physicals, eye and hearing tests, immunizations, dental care)
Complementary and Alternative Therapies
Family Health History (both general and specific diseases—environmentally and genetically related)
Health Care Services Received
Feelings and Perceptions Regarding Health Services
Emergency Health Services
Source of Payments for Health and Other Services
Logistics of Receiving Care

✎FAMILY STRESS, COPING, AND ADAPTATION

24. **Family Stressors, Strengths, and Perceptions**

    Stressors Family Is Experiencing
    Strengths That Counterbalance Stressors
    Family's Definition of the Situation

25. **Family Coping Strategies**

    How the Family Is Reacting to the Stressors
    Extent of Family's Use of Internal Coping Strategies (past/present)
    Extent of Family's Use of External Coping Strategies (past/present)
    Dysfunctional Coping Strategies Utilized (past/present; extent of use)

26. **Family Adaptation**

    Overall Family Adaptation
    Estimation of Whether Family Is in Crisis

27. **Tracking Stressors, Coping, and Adaptation Over Time**

CASE STUDY OF THE O'SHEA FAMILY

The O'Shea family was referred to the community health nurse, Ms. Bell, by the county hospital's maternity service for the following reasons. "Mrs. O'Shea has expressed the desire to learn about family planning. She also needs a referral for postpartum and well-baby care." The following information was included in the referral: Mary—age 35; gravida VII, para V, miscarriages II. Delivered newborn son, Daniel—born 11/3 (5 days ago); birth weight—7 lbs, 2 oz; length—19 inches; hypertension during pregnancy; normal labor and delivery; mother's postpartum status and stay was normal, bonding well with infant.

✿FIRST HOME VISIT

During Ms. Bell's first home visit, the father and two oldest children were at work and school. From her conversation with the mother and her observations of the home and family members, the following family data were obtained from the nurse's notes. Family: Patrick, father—age 43; Mary, mother—age 35 (looks older, tired, and overweight); Joseph, son—age 6; Maureen, daughter—age 5; Betty, daughter—age 4; Richard, son—age 3; and Daniel, son—age 1 week. Pat works as a butcher in his father's small grocery store located in same neighborhood a mile away from home. Mary's parents are Kate (mother), age 70, in good health; and Bill (father), who died 2 years ago from heart problems. Patrick's parents are Marian (mother), age 72, who has osteoarthritis of hips and spine; and Pat (father), age 78, who suffers from back problems due to all the lifting he's done in the grocery business.

The family lives in an older wooden, three-bedroom flat in the Maplewood district—an Irish neighborhood—located 5 miles from a New England city with a population of 300,000. The immediate neighborhood is ethnically and socially homogeneous (working class) and residential, although located very near to a heavily industrialized factory district.

The family's home is rented from a cousin for $800 per month and is sparsely furnished, with a minimum of furniture in each room. The kitchen is clean, containing a small refrigerator and stove. There is one bathroom with toilet and bathtub. The parents have their own room, which they presently share with the newborn (who has a new bassinet the women's group at the parish donated). The girls, Maureen and Betty, have their own bedroom with a double bed, while the boys share the other bedroom, having twin beds and a small chest of drawers. A few area carpets are noted, but few decorations—with the exception of the children's school photos and a photo of the Irish coast on the living room wall and Catholic religious articles in the parent's room and dining room. Curtains matching the tablecloth hung in the dining room, a wedding gift from Mary's mother to them when they were married. A color television set was the centerpiece of the living room. The mother said the home was adequate for their needs, although it was getting smaller with the arrival of another baby.

The outside of the house needs painting but was not cluttered and in fair repair. It was noted, however, that the stairs leading up to the front porch were loose, and there was no railing or lighting. A few children's toys were scattered around the backyard.

Mary was talkative and responsive to questions. When Ms. Bell explained that she had come because of a referral from the county hospital where Mrs. O'Shea had delivered her last baby, Mary was pleased that the nurse had been contacted to visit her. She offered the nurse a cup of coffee as they talked in the living room.

NURSE: How are you managing since you have been home from the hospital with your new baby?

MARY: Not too bad, but it sure is harder with five than with four, and being older doesn't help. I just don't have the energy to get up at night and feed Daniel.

NURSE: What kinds of help are you getting?

595

MARY: My mother came over the first day I was home and Pat's mother came over 2 days ago. They helped by cooking and cleaning up the house a little, and looking after the children. I also have a sister nearby who goes shopping for me sometimes.

NURSE: Anyone else?

MARY: No, that's about it, except for a neighbor and the women from my church, who told me to call if I needed anything. But I wouldn't want to bother them.

NURSE: What about your husband?

MARY: Pat helps a bit with the children, especially with getting them into bed at night. It's hard for him to do much more than that after working all day. Besides, he's pretty conservative and still holds to women being in charge when it comes to taking care of the children. He thinks that if I do need more help it should come from my mother or sister. Pat would usually rather spend his free time playing football or meeting his friends for a beer at the local bar.

NURSE: Is this the way it's been with the other children too—you handling most things by yourself?

MARY: Yes, I'll just have to "offer it up" to the Lord.

NURSE: How have you managed to keep everything going?

MARY: I'm pretty well organized, and I learned quite a bit from my mother about managing a household.

NURSE: Have you found ways to save your energy?

MARY: Mainly it's a question of sleeping when the baby does, letting the other kids watch TV, and not worrying about the housecleaning.

NURSE: Sounds like a good list of priorities. Your health, children, and baby are certainly more important than housework. Is there anything that is important and needs doing that you can't handle?

MARY: Nothing immediately—my family lives here and they help—but I am very worried about getting pregnant again and having more children. I didn't think I would have the need to ask about family planning—I was planning for Richie to be my last. I had two miscarriages since him—1 and 2 years ago—and the doctors told me that I definitely shouldn't have any more children because my blood pressure gets so high. I discussed the problem with our priest, who then spoke to my husband about the rhythm method, but I guess he didn't get the right instructions. Since then,

my girlfriends tell me that's not a very good method anyway.

NURSE: So you and your husband have decided not to have more children?

MARY: I'm not sure how Pat feels about it. I told him just yesterday that this was the end of kids for me, and he just looked and listened without a comment—and then just walked into the kitchen and got himself a beer. I can't talk to that man—that's the problem! When he has something on his mind, he sure lets me hear about it. But when I'm talking it's like I'm nagging or like it's not any of his concern.

I think he's torn because he knows how hard our lives would be if we have more, but he's a very devout man and really follows the teaching of the church on this. I'm not sure what he'll say in the end.

NURSE: Would you be willing to tell me a bit more about your marriage?

MARY: Well, we were married when I was 28 and he was 36. I guess that's been 7 years. As you can see, babies started coming pretty quickly after that—one a year until now, including the two miscarriages. We both knew each other from the parish and our parents both live in the neighborhood. We both graduated from Catholic high schools in the neighborhood. After high school Pat went to work in his father's grocery store, was in the service for 3 years, and then when his older brother stopped working for his father, Pat got the job of being butcher in the store—been doing that for his father 4 years now. I worked as a clerk in an electronics factory before we got married. I really liked it there and made a lot of friends at the factory.

I started seeing Pat 3 years after I finished high school, and we went together 5½ years before he asked me to marry him. I was afraid I was going to be an old maid like some of my friends were. Sure was a lot easier being single though, but my family and friends were always hinting and pressuring me to "tie the noose around Patrick."

NURSE: Overall, how would you describe your marriage to Pat?

MARY: Hard work a lot of the time. I always feel like I'm really working at getting along and keeping things on an even keel.

NURSE: Has it always been that way? What was it like in the beginning and after the children came?

MARY: (looking at the nurse with a tired, disappointed expression on her face, and sadness in her eyes):

I think our marriage started out all wrong—not that it was so different from any of my friends' and cousins' or sisters' marriages—but it was just not like the marriages I read about in the papers and magazines and see on television. I was raised a strict Catholic, in an Irish school and parish. My grandparents came over from Ireland during the depression. Pat's folks also are Irish, and his father came over here as a teenager and worked in construction until he could save enough to buy a small grocery store—the one he has now. We didn't know much about sex except what we heard from our friends. Our parents never mentioned it, and the nuns certainly never brought it up. Things have changed a lot since then. But we were raised in a time when you didn't have relations until your wedding night. I'm ashamed to say this, but I never really liked having sex that much. It hasn't been the way I thought it would be when I was young. Pat seems to enjoy it pretty well, though I'm not sure.

NURSE: Have you ever discussed it with him?

MARY: Not really. Every time I try I get mortified and then worry that I would hurt his feelings if I told him. Besides, what good would it do?

NURSE: Do you ever talk to your sisters, mother, or friends about it?

MARY: Only my sister and one girlfriend, and they both have the same frustrations. My sister tells me that there are books you can read to make sex more pleasurable—but it seems unnatural to make a study of it like that. Besides, one of the first things I ever learned about it was from my friend's mother, who said it was something you just put up with in marriage.

We used to go out to the movies or friends' homes together—and talk more. But, after the children came we grew apart. Don't misunderstand me, we wanted the children and were happy to see them born, but somehow the demands in raising them caused problems between us. Now we don't talk much, except about the children and money problems—we're always just barely making it through the month. Pat spends more and more time with the boys. You know, going to football, baseball, and basketball games or spending time at the bar. And when he's home, he's really not home. I can't get him to do anything around the house. When I ask him to do something he looks at me as if I'm imposing on me and I'm making his life difficult. When I try to talk to him about problems, he'll say:

"Don't bother me with that now. Can't you see that I'm tired. I'll do something about it tomorrow." And tomorrow never comes.

NURSE: I appreciate your sharing so much about your concerns and experience with Pat and the children. You mentioned feeling a little overwhelmed since Daniel's birth and worried about finances. You told me that you've decided that you don't want any more children, and it sounds like you wish that your relationship with Pat was closer, like when you were first married. I would like to offer my support and information, and to work together with you to look at options you have for your concerns.

Ms. Bell then outlined ways that she could help Mary, and asked Mary which problem bothered her most. She then asked permission to make another home visit to meet the rest of the family.

The first visit also consisted of discussing the newborn, Daniel, and Mary's physical health status. Ms. Bell planned to return in a week with information for her on clinic services for the baby and on family planning and postpartum care and follow-up.

SECOND HOME VISIT

During the second home visit 1 week later, the nurse came at 3:30 P.M. when the children were home from school. Patrick was expected home for part of visit (he returned from work at 4:00 P.M.). After discussing Mary's and Daniel's health and giving Mary appointments for the baby clinic and Mary's postpartum examination at the local health center, the nurse spoke briefly about family planning and asked Mary if she felt that this could be discussed with her husband. Mary agreed, although she did not seem sure about how her husband would react to a woman talking to him about such an intimate subject. However, when Ms. Bell suggested that this might be a way to help both of them talk more directly about this delicate subject, she seemed to reconsider her previous hesitancy and said she thought it would be a good idea.

Before talking with the parents about family planning, Ms. Bell asked them for a brief health history of each of the children and was able to observe and elicit data related to parent–child relationships, parenting roles, and child rearing. She noted that Mary was very warm and cuddly with newborn Daniel. Mary held him close, handled him gently, and appeared relaxed and confident in his care and sensitive to his basic needs. Pat, in contrast, looked proudly at Daniel, but did not hold him, and according to Mary did not get involved in his physical care (nor did he with any of the other children when they were babies).

Both mother and father were warm and Mary physically quite affectionate with Richard, age 3. She seemed quite indulgent with him, letting him "have his way" and giving him a lot of freedom to run around and play.

With the older children—Betty, 4; Maureen, 5; and Joseph, 6—there was not the same permissiveness as observed with Richard. Mary said, "They are older and so need to be more responsible." All three older children were fairly quiet around the nurse. They spoke when spoken to, but otherwise talked quietly with each other or listened. The parents agreed that Joseph is the mother's favorite, and said he is too serious and has problems handling himself sometimes, becoming bossy and wanting to take over. Betty was identified as the father's favorite, "since she is petite, very sweet, and looks like Pat's mother."

The parents believe in children behaving and showing respect for their elders and carrying out their responsibilities, even if at these ages they are not expected to do much. The father spanks the children with the palm of his hand on their buttocks if they misbehave. He explained by saying, "None of these newfangled ideas about disciplining for us." It was noticed that children were asked to do several things—pick up the toys from the floor and help their mother. Both Maureen and Betty acted immediately, while Joseph ignored and then refused until his father yelled at him. No positive reinforcement followed when the children did obey. Maureen and Betty seemed pleased to have a new baby brother, while Richard was jealous of the baby and has been more demanding since the baby's arrival. The parents understand, though, that he feels displaced and jealous and that he needs more parental attention during this time. Joseph states he does not like the new baby.

When asked about each of the children and what they were like, the mother led the conversation although the father chimed in about Joseph and Betty. The descriptions are given in Table C–1. Ms. Bell asked Mary to have the children play in another room and then raised the issue of family planning.

NURSE: Mary, would you be willing to share with Pat our discussion about family planning?

MARY: Yes. Like I tried to tell you Pat, I'm at the end of my rope. I don't want to get pregnant again and I want to look into some kind of family planning method.

NURSE: Pat, I'd like to know how you feel about this.

PAT: I was a little surprised she would bring this up with you, but since she did, I guess we can talk about it. I have felt that my wife is taking things in her own hands—complaining all the time about her life and seeing her job as such a burden. My mother had seven children, and I never heard her com-plain. It would be very difficult for us if we had another baby—but I can't see any way around it. If the good Lord wants her to have more, then I think she'll just have to accept them and manage with what we have.

NURSE: Does that mean that religiously you're against any form of family planning?

PAT: Well not exactly. I know that Catholics are not all of the same mind on this issue and that many of them do things to prevent pregnancy. I won't say that my mind is completely closed, but that I have serious questions about it. We tried that rhythm method, but it didn't seem to work.

NURSE: Mary, would you like to say something about this?

MARY: Well, I just can't go on like this. Something has got to be done. You ought to stay home some day, Pat, and just see what raising this many kids is like.

PAT: But our mothers found a way to do it. . . .

MARY: Yes, but things are so much more expensive now, and they never had a choice, but I do. I would like to find out more about what is available and really look into family planning methods.

NURSE: Pat, what's the benefit you see in having more children? Your wife feels it's hard for her to manage now and that further pregnancies are dangerous for her.

PAT: I didn't say I wanted any more. I just said that she's pretty lucky and she doesn't know it. I suppose our family is big enough, but we can't depend on "Russian roulette," I mean the rhythm method, to solve our problem.

NURSE: Do you understand the problem your wife has in having more children now? I mean the hypertension during pregnancy, which has grown worse with each succeeding pregnancy?

PAT: Not really. (Nurse explains the problem and how pregnancy makes problem worse.)

Ms. Bell then asks the spouses if they have discussed their problem or family planning methods with their priest and family doctor, and then suggest that they do this together, because neither priest nor doctor has been approached to discuss the problem. She gives a basic overview of family planning methods that are available, including natural family planning, and gives them a booklet on family planning for more information. Ms. Bell acknowledges their progress in discussing a sensitive subject and encourages them to request further information as needed. She then asks permission to make a follow-up visit.

TABLE C–1

THE O'SHEA PARENTS' DESCRIPTIONS OF THEIR CHILDREN

	MOTHER'S DESCRIPTION	FATHER'S DESCRIPTION
Joseph, age 6	He's a bright, independent child. Joseph is the leader of the children at home and school and likes to take over. I try to give him some responsibilities for caring for his sisters and brothers, but have to watch that he doesn't get too bossy. I'm able to talk to Joseph more than the other children. He's a sensitive child and listens to me. I know I'm a little protective of him, but that's just because we're so close to each other.	Joseph is always arguing and wanting his own way. My wife spoils him. He's going to grow up thinking he'll be the President by the time he's 35. He needs to be put in his place by my wife.
Maureen, age 5	Maureen is a helpful child who likes to help me. She is an easy child to raise. She's quiet, likes to play alone, and doesn't cause any trouble. Maureen follows her brother Joseph all the time when they play together.	She's great fun.
Betty, age 4	Betty knows how to get people to like her. She's a "people pleaser"—can act cute and sweet when it is in her favor. She needs special watching, however, as she can pull the wool over one's eyes very quickly with her sweet and cunning ways.	The father acts disgusted with his wife's statement and responds by saying: "That's not true. She is a sweet, affectionate little sweetheart. You're just jealous because we have a special relationship."
Richard, age 3	He's always into everything! Very active and inquisitive. I try to let him have a lot of freedom to run around in the house, otherwise he gets so bottled up that he shouts, screams, and makes the rest of us miserable.	He's at the age where we really have to keep an eye on him.

❧THIRD HOME VISIT

As the spouses speak to each other and with the nurse, the nurse makes the following observations regarding Pat and the couple's relationship.

Pat seems easygoing, verbal, and quite a conversationalist—as long as he controls the flow. He likes to be the center of attention and loses interest if Mary is talking; in this case, jumping in to refocus attention on himself. He expresses an interest in getting some help for his wife from his mother, but feels that helping himself is "not his job." He says that Mary and his mother don't get along too well together, however, there being too much competition between the two of them. According to Mary, Pat's mother caused tremendous tension during their engagement and early years of marriage. She had bitter arguments with her husband about his mother, but as the mother-in-law finally began to accept the reality of her son's marriage, their problems subsided.

In terms of the marital relationship, there appeared to be no expression of love or affection either physically or verbally. Their relationship was characterized by a lack of empathy or two-way communication between them. One received the impression that Mary was there to meet the needs of her husband, but that he had no similar responsibility to her. Pat expected her to serve him, care for the home and children, and manage with the limited funds he allotted her weekly for groceries and other home and child expenses.

While Pat was present, Mary took little part in the discussions, except when asked direct questions. She acted very self-effacing and subservient in his presence, except when she voiced the opinion that he should spend time with the children to see what it was really like.

Pat did communicate to the children that they should have respect for Mary—because she was their mother. However, in his own communications with her, he did not express much respect. Most communications were in the form of commands, with few requests or room for feedback from his wife. When Mary spoke to him, he seemed to tune her out. Most of the time he halfheartedly agreed that she was right and that he would follow through on such matters as making appointments with the priest and the doctor, which he then failed to do.

The children and parents were quite talkative concerning the recent Thanksgiving holiday and other happy events. With pleasant subjects, all of the family contributed verbally to family conversations. Unpleasant subjects or angry statements were cut off, such as Joseph's reaction to the new baby, or minimized, such as the mother's feelings of being burdened by too many children. It was also noted that the children spoke directly to their mother, but only indirectly to their father. If they had a request, they would ask their mother to ask their father for permission.

When asked what activities the family engaged in together, Mary reported that family visiting is their most popular and frequent activity. "Movies and eating out are beyond our reach. I like taking the kids to the park, but Patrick doesn't like coming. I go to Mass regularly and so does Pat. We don't travel much—our close relatives live in town and we can't afford traveling much on Pat's salary. Pat's car isn't very dependable. Groceries, clothing, and the usual household items we buy at Pat's father's store. The shopping center is about a half-mile from here."

In terms of friendships, Mary states that she has a few old high school friends whom she still sees occasionally and that Pat sees his friends at sports events or the local bar. But Pat and Mary have no couple friends with whom they engage in social activities.

Ms. Bell asked the couple how they liked the community. Both the parents related that this was the only community and neighborhood they had ever lived in and said, "We like it here. We know where everything is. All of the storekeepers and neighbors are old friends and acquaintances." The family, having lived in the community for many years, was familiar with the community agencies, health centers, and private doctors in town. Up until recently, they used a nearby hospital for children's emergency care; and a family doctor, a general practitioner, for all the health care that they needed, such as maternity and pediatric care. But the parents did not go in for checkups (Pat never had a physical examination as far as Mary knew), although Mary did have a physical with each pregnancy. Children are only seen when they are sick, with the exception of well-baby care at the health center when they were infants and for immunizations during infancy and preschool periods.

Two months ago, Pat received group medical insurance through his father's store (the father just arranged for it), so their choice of health care was expanded. The family doctor is an older physician whom the family has seen for years. His charges are very low, but Mary feels he is getting too old to keep up with all he needs to know. She used the county hospital to deliver Daniel, because they were not covered by medical insurance at that time and could not raise the money for a private hospital. Now they will have to pay the county back in small payments until their bill is taken care of.

With their expanded health insurance benefits Mary and Pat asked for information regarding regular health care services they might be eligible for. After a bit of prodding from Mary, Pat asked how he might get a physical exam. He also expressed concern about his slow, but steady weight gain, or "gut" since he stopped playing sports.

Dental care for the family has been close to nonexistent. It is obtained at a private neighborhood dental clinic. The mother took Joseph in once when he complained of a toothache. One of his baby teeth had to be filled. The other children have not been seen. Pat and Mary go in when they have problems, and brush their teeth twice a day after meals. Mary is teaching Joseph to brush his teeth now, too.

When Ms. Bell did a nutritional survey of the family, she found that their diet consisted of a lot of starches, mainly potatoes and breads primarily at every meal. Their diet was basically American, with certain Irish specialties included— stews and boiled dinners. The family made little use of fruit or fruit juices, except for bananas, apples when in season, and canned peaches—and occasionally apple or orange juice. One vegetable, in addition to potatoes, was usually eaten with the evening meal, and casseroles, stews, and processed food such as frozen dinners, pizza, chicken pies, and macaroni and cheese were frequently served for dinner. Salads were infrequently eaten; soups were served about every other night, especially in the colder months. The weights of the children were within normal limits, but both parents were 10 to 20 percent overweight (visually) for their height. There were no food allergies among any of the family members, according to their mother.

Their diet for yesterday (excluding Daniel) was:

Breakfast	Cold cereal and whole milk
	Toast—1 to 2 pieces for Joseph, Mary, and Pat
	Coffee—2 cups (parents)
Snacks	Crackers for children (3 to 4 apiece) and milk
	Coffee—mother
Lunch	Soup (tomato)
	Dish of mashed potatoes and butter
	Canned peaches
	Milk
	(Husband and Joseph not home)
Snacks	None
Dinner	Stew with meat (½ lb), carrots, potatoes, and celery
	White cake
	Milk—children
	Coffee—wife
	Beer—husband

Because having adequate money for food was mentioned as a monthly concern, Mary was asked whether she received food stamps. When she said she did not, information on the program was provided. The nurse also learned that the family had very little left over each month and that 2 years ago Pat borrowed $2000 from his father to buy a used car (without Mary's knowledge) and still had not been able to pay his father back.

With Ms. Bell's encouragement Mary discussed with Pat her desire to work part time to increase the family income. She mentioned that her mother and sister both offered to take care of the children so that she could do so. They agreed that along with family planning this would be an area for further discussion.

The family associates with several organizations in the community: the parish church and school primarily. The family can walk to both, because they are only five blocks away. The health department, the family doctor, and the family dental clinic are also visited. In addition, the bars Pat frequents, the stores they shop in, and Pat's father's grocery store are all community places and people with whom friendly ties exist. Mary makes all the contacts with church, school, dentist, and doctors. The family's relationships with church, teachers, doctor, health center, dentists, and emergency room seem to have been good. There is public trans-portation available when family needs it, but Mary drives Pat to work on days that she needs the car, because taking the children with her on the bus is not easy.

Stemming from Mary's extensive experience in raising children and taking them to doctors, she seems to have a good, basic understanding of how to handle common minor illness and injuries. She also is able to explain what to do when more serious injuries occur or symptoms appear. She uses over-the-counter medicines such as aspirin, Tylenol, first-aid medications, Sudafed, and milk of magnesia carefully and correctly and keeps medicines in a safe place out of the reach of the children.

Neither she nor her husband watch their diet or weight or engage in regular exercise. Although Mary was never active (except doing housework), Pat was very active in sports until recently. For relaxation Mary watches TV and thinks her husband uses TV and socializing at the bar as ways of relaxing.

When the initial family assessment was completed Ms. Bell discussed her observations with Mary to identify which issues or concerns she felt were most amenable to change and could be worked on by the entire family.

Appendix D presents a family assessment and family care plan for this family.

FAMILY NURSING PROCESS EXAMPLE: THE O'SHEA FAMILY

1. **Family Name:** O'Shea.
2. **Address:** Maplewood district, New England city.
3. **Family Composition:** See Table D–1 and Figure D–1.
4. **Type of Family Form:** Two parent, intact nuclear.
5. **Cultural (Ethnic) Background:** The family is Irish-American and to a large extent unacculturated (Connery, 1968). Mary and Pat are second and third generation immigrants from Ireland. Mary clearly stated ethnic and religious preferences; the fact that family's social network is from the same ethnic/religious group; the family has resided in same ethnically homogeneous neighborhood for life; visits to extended family and church activities seem to be central activities; family roles and power structure are in keeping with traditional structures within Irish families; home decor is lacking of much visual art and the presence of religious objects is indicative of family's culture and religious orientation; and family stays primarily within ethnic neighborhood. And, Mary prepares traditional Irish meals about twice each week.

   The family's informal support systems comes from extended family, especially parents on both sides and mother's sister, seem to be quite helpful. Pat's father employs son in his grocery store as butcher and loaned him $2,000 for purchase of a car. Pat's mother helped with housework and children when Mary came home from hospital. (Although relations with wife were conflictual during early days of marriage, they are improved but still competitive, according to Pat.) Mary's mother also helped with house and children after Mary returned from hospital and Mary's sister went shopping for her. In addition to her sister, Mary has neighbors she talks to sometimes about her problems. And Pat has his buddies at the tavern that he relates to frequently (the degree of their support is unknown, however).

6. **Religious Identification:** Family actively involved in Catholic religious practices and belief system: attends Mass regularly, consults priest on matters of importance, belief in family and children stressed.

7. **Social Class Status:** Father is sole wage earner.
   Economic Status: Family sees its income as marginal; nevertheless, it is steady. Based on the father's occupation, income (estimated only), and education of parents, family is part of working class.
   Social Mobility: The parents of the O'Sheas were poor, and thus Pat feels he, Mary, and the children are more fortunate. In fact, however, the family's history does not indicate much, if any, upward mobility. Actually, with more children the standard of living within their own nuclear family has probably declined.

8. **Family's Present Developmental Stage:** Family is in the stage of a family with school-aged children because of the age of the oldest child.

9. **Extent to Which Family Is Fulfilling Family Developmental Tasks:** Family appears to be meeting the family members needs for adequate housing, space, privacy, and safety.
   Mother is adequately socializing children (see discussion of socialization function).
   Mother feeling strained in attempting to integrate new child member into family due to her role overload.
   Maintenance of satisfactory parent–child relationships, but decline in satisfaction by wife in marital relationship.

10. **Family's History:** Parents both lived in same neighborhood and went to same church. Went together 5½ years before marriage. During engagement and early years of marriage, sex was an uncomfortable area and later awkward and unsatisfying, reported the wife. Wife feels this has created a lack of closeness between them. Both parents expected children and wanted them, with the exception of the last, which Mary did not want but now accepts warmly. Mary has a history of seven pregnancies, with five liv-

603

TABLE D—1

O'SHEA FAMILY COMPOSITION

NAME	GENDER	RELATION-SHIP	AGE	PLACE OF BIRTH	OCCU-PATION	EDUCATION
O'Shea, Patrick	M	Father	43 years	Maplewood district	Butcher	High school graduate
O'Shea, Mary	F	Mother	35	Same	Housewife	High school graduate
O'Shea, Joseph	M	Son	6	Same	Student	In first grade
O'Shea, Maureen	F	Daughter	5	Same	Student	In kindergarten
O'Shea, Betty	F	Daughter	4	Same	—	—
O'Shea, Richard	M	Son	3	Same	—	—
O'Shea, Daniel	M	Son	5-day-old infant	Same	—	—

ing children and two miscarriages over the first seven years of her marriage to Pat. She developed hypertension during the last two pregnancies.

11. **Parents' Families of Origin:** Father's family: Father came over from Ireland as teenager. Worked for construction companies and saved his money until he could buy the grocery store he now owns. Raised family in same neighborhood in a strict Catholic fashion. Mother's family: Her grandparents came over from Ireland during the depression for economic reasons. Raised as Catholic in same neighborhood as family now resides. Both Mary's and Pat's families were mentioned as being poor while they were growing up. No mention of what life with their respective families of origin was like.

12. **Characteristics of Home:** Three-bedroom, older wooden house rented from cousin for $800 per month. Outside of house: fair condition, needs paint, loose stairs, and no outside lighting or railing present. Inside of house: minimally furnished. Living room has a color TV. Dining room has lace curtains and tablecloth, a wedding present from Mary's mother. Parents have own bedroom, presently shared with newborn who has a bassinet. The boys have one bedroom, while the girls share the other. Adequate sleeping arrangements in home. Minimal decorations, but several Catholic religious objects and photos of the children were noted. Kitchen contains small refrigerator and stove. One bathroom with toilet and bathtub. Common towels used. Mary considers the house just adequate for their needs now, but becoming more crowded because of the new baby. The house has adequate heating and fans for summer. An adequate number of lamps and windows provide adequate lighting. There are no pets and no evidence of vermin. Safety hazards: outside loose stairs, no railings or outside light.

13. **Characteristics of Neighborhood and Larger Community:** Neighborhood (Maplewood district) is residential and composed of Irish working-class families. Neighborhood is near industrial area and 5 miles from center of city of 300,000 located in New England. Family likes closeness and familiarity of neighborhood, though worried about influx of members of minority groups nearby and rise in crime in the past several years. Family uses Pat's father's grocery store and a nearby shopping center (half mile away) for most of its shopping needs. Family's church and church school located five blocks away. Public transportation available, but Mary has access to husband's car when needed.

14. **Family's Geographical Mobility:** Family members have lived in the same community and neighborhood for all their lives.

15. **Family's Associations and Transactions with Community:** The family is known in parish church and school. Parents go to mass regularly and seem to have close trusting relationship with Father O'Neal. Women's group at church donated bassinet for new baby. Mother acts as liaison with school. Family also relates to the family doctor (although Mary wants to change physicians), family dental clinic, and children's hospital emergency room. In addition to receiving community health nursing visits, mother has taken children to well-baby clinic and for immunizations at the local health department. Family seems to stay primarily within its neighborhood. Family not aware of food stamp program (which was explained to Mary). Family has ties with priest, doctor, community health nurse, and teachers.

FAMILY STRUCTURE

16. **Communication Patterns**

    Extent of Functional and Dysfunctional Communication (types of recurring patterns):

    Dysfunctional communication used between husband and wife.

    a. Husband gives commands and makes requests without giving opportunity for feedback

    b. Wife voices problems and husband minimizes them (does not validate or accept that her problems are real).

    c. Wife voices concerns or asks husband's assistance, but he tunes her out, walks away, belittles her, or agrees with her and says he'll follow through, but does not (incongruency). Pat does not listen to Mary when she is communicating her needs to him.

    d. Mary, in turn, does not express herself in some intimate areas due to cultural values and, possibly, fear of rejection. She probably does not directly express her needs in many areas.

    e. Neither partner states needs and feelings clearly, except in case of Mary's expressed desire to curtail pregnancies.

    f. Rules underlying communication patterns include the following: (1) don't question the status quo and tradition; (2) things are the way they are and complaining won't help or change things (powerless, fatalistic outlook); (3) closedness—husband doesn't want wife becoming exposed to any outside influences.

Extent of Affective Messages and How Expressed: Affective messages are not expressed openly (or privately according to Mary) between spouses. Mary is warm and affectively responsive to Daniel and Richard. She is also verbally warm and close to son Joseph. Father is verbally (and physically?) affectionate to daughter Betty. Pleasant emotions are more openly expressed, whereas negative emotions (anger, talk about unpleasant events) are inhibited. Evidently, family rules exist that prohibit expression of these latter emotions.

Characteristics of Family Communication Network: Children make requests of father through mother. Little direct involvement and communication between father and children (except Betty–father relationship). Quality of communication between spouses poor and limited in scope (mainly regarding children and money problems) and quality (see dysfunctional patterns). Interactions are distant and unsatisfying to wife.

Areas of Closed Communications: Between spouses: inner feelings and perceptions, especially sexual feelings and thoughts.

Familial and Contextual Variables Affecting Communication: Cultural variables are important for this family. Men and women live in different worlds in traditional Irish culture. Roles and worlds are separate, and sexes typically do not learn to communicate intimately with each other. Nor is expression of affection or warmth toward spouse seen as acceptable in public. Sex is riddled with guilt and ignorance, making it difficult for some Irish couples to generate and retain close affective bonds. Socio-economic stressors (marginal incomes and economic hardships) make family role enactment, housing, and fulfilling of family functions more onerous.

17. **Power Structure**

    Power Outcomes

    Husband decides major purchases (e.g., car).

    Wife is delegated (or relegated) sole roles of housekeeper and child rearer, and allotted a certain portion of paycheck to cover home and family expenses.

    Husband in charge of distribution of funds.

    Husband in charge of calling priest and doctor to initiate appointment with them.

    Decision-making Process: Husband uses his formal position of dominance to influence family decisions. Process used is accommodation. He seemed to be compromising with wife, under pressure of community health nurse, when he agreed to discuss family planning health problems with priest and doctor and attempt to come up with an effective plan to prevent further pregnancies; but because he has not followed through in making appointments, one can question his sincerity in this case. May use de facto process in these cases; by doing nothing he has made a decision.

Power Bases: Father–husband maintains legitimate power or authority, granted to him culturally by virtue of his position in family. Mother has referent power (position of mother is exalted in the Catholic Church), which is more salient in her relationships with her children than it is in her relationship with her husband. Both parents have reward and coercive power over children, and husband has reward/coercive power over his wife, although no description of his using this is evident.

Variables Affecting Family Power Characteristics: Wife's position as go-between in family communication network and as implementer of family decisions should give her increased power; there is no evidence that it is being exercised, however.

Interpersonal resources: The wife's hesitancy and fear to speak out more often and confront husband reduces what power she does/could have.

Social class/cultural and life cycle factors: Marital expectations that are commonly found in working class predominate. These same marital and family role and power expectations are characteristic of traditional Irish family life. Life cycle of family reduces wife's power and increases husband's power, because wife is burdened with day-to-day household and child care responsibilities and has no time or energy to exercise whatever influence/power she has.

Overall Family Power

Moderate dominance seen (father dominant), with some dissatisfaction of this situation expressed by wife.

18. **Role Structure**

Formal Role Structure

Pat: Father and husband. He acts as sole provider for family, and is leader of family. Does not see his position as involving a companionship, recreational, or therapeutic role, however, and only occasionally does he help with the child care role (when he feels like it). Marital roles enacted, although constricted, appear consistent with his expectations of marital roles.

Mary: Mother and wife. She acts as the homemaker (not shared), involving cooking, shopping, and cleaning home; enacts the child care role (not shared to any real extent); the recreational role (taking children to park to play). No therapeutic role or companion role enacted in marriage. Sexual role

inadequate. Wife has expressed disappointment that the therapeutic role is not present and that the sexual role is unsatisfying (distant communications, no enjoyment in sexual relationship). Wife appears to have some expectations of Pat that are more consistent with American middle-class ideas of marriage, although she seems also resigned to the fact that Pat's traditional expectations of both of their positions in the family are fairly stable and not likely to be changed. She enacts the roles needed to complement husband's role expectations of her, while at the same time trying to limit her family roles in future to some extent by having no more children. Mary definitely shows some role strain in trying to handle child care and all the other mother-wife roles by herself, as well as the possibility that she might return to part-time work.

Joseph: Older son and brother to siblings.

Maureen: Older daughter and sister to siblings.

Betty: Younger daughter and sister to siblings.

Richard: Younger son and brother to siblings.

Daniel: Youngest (baby) son and brother to siblings.

Informal Role Structure

Pat: Leader; distant one (does not get involved in family life); unconcerned one (does wife see him in this way or is this the way she expects husbands to act?)

Mary: Subservient one; go-between role (between children and their father); martyr?

Joseph: Leader of the children, mother's favorite and perhaps confidant, because mother cannot confide in and share affectively with husband. Serious one.

Maureen: Cooperative, compliant one. Follower.

Betty: Sweet one. "People-pleaser" role. Mother perceives her to play cute, manipulative role, whereas father defends her sweetness as being genuine and not manipulative. Father's favorite. Mary is perhaps threatened by husband's affections toward Betty.

Richard: Active one (with explosive temper if exploration and freedom are restricted).

Daniel: No comments by parents.

Variables Affecting Role Structure:

Social class influences: Working-class families are likely to be more traditional in terms of marital roles. Being Irish-American and fairly unacculturated affects family roles. Traditional Catholic background reinforces patriarchal family structure. The family developmental stage and presence of five small children make wife dependent on husband as sole breadwinner, which further increases his dominance and her dependency.

19. **Family's Values:** In comparing the O'Sheas' values with American and traditional Irish and Irish-American values, the O'Sheas' values are definitely much more in keeping with the traditional Irish values and the working-class values. Productivity and success are not primary values. Pat has worked for his father since graduation from high school, except for time he was in the Armed Services. Mary worked in an electronics factory after graduation and until the first child was born. The work ethic and materialism do not seem central in family's life. The family does not value individualism, but familism and the ethic of reciprocity (assisting one's family and church) is salient, as is the value of doing one's duty and playing expected family roles (conformity). Education is not highly valued, nor is progress, change, and mastery; conservatism and fatalistic thinking assume greater importance. No long-term plans were expressed, except Mary's ardent plans to prevent further pregnancies and desire to return to part-time employment. Equality and individual freedom are not inferred to be important values either. The "doing orientation" does not fit this family. Time is not carefully allotted and used. Much of Pat's time outside of work is spent in recreational pursuits (spectator sports and social drinking with friends). Health care and practices are not of prime importance to family.

There appears to be a conflict in values, to some degree, between Mr. and Mrs. O'Shea. Mary obviously feels caught between the values of American society and those of traditional Irish culture that govern family roles, power relationships, and communication. She is trying—not very effectively—to assert herself with her husband, demonstrating the value of egalitarianism, individualism, and progress. Pat retains the old traditional values, as stated above. This directly affects the health status of the family, by creating strain in the marital relationship.

20. **Affective Function**

Mutual Nurturance, Closeness, and Identification: Adequate between mother and Joseph, Maureen, Richard, and Daniel.

Maybe attenuated between Mary and Betty, because Mary may feel threatened by her husband's favoritism and diversion of affections to Betty.

Adequate between father and Betty and father and Richard (?). Remainder of father's relationships with children are distant, and father is relatively uninvolved.

Inadequate between Mary and Pat. Mutual identification involving closeness and nurturance are weak, hence spousal bonds are weak also. She expresses need for greater closeness, whereas he does not express these needs.

Separateness and Connectedness: Not discussed here to any extent. It will become an issue with Joseph soon, because he is assertive, has leadership qualities and needs, and will increasingly wish to individuate. At present conformity and connectedness are valued much more highly than separateness.

Family Need–Response Patterns

Pat: For the most part, Pat (the father) does not make any of his socioemotional needs known to his wife or children; therefore, they are presumably not adequately met in family. (Perhaps his needs are met through work and socializing with friends at sports events and tavern.) He does, however, make his needs for affection and warmth known to daughter Betty, who responds in a sweet, affectionate manner toward him.

Mary: Expressed problem of not being able to talk to husband and of not feeling emotionally close to him. He does not respond to her needs to communicate and does not empathize with her feelings regarding the responsibilities she assumes. Her son Joseph meets some of her socioemotional needs, because she feels she can talk to him, whereas Pat is not available to meet her needs.

Joseph (age 6): Has need to handle things, lead, and be assertive. His mother gives him this opportunity; Pat feels his son's behavior is inappropriate and feels he should be put in his place. The younger children follow him. Becomes rebellious or bossy when his needs to be assertive are frustrated.

Maureen (age 5): Expresses need to cooperate with and help her mother; emulates mother's behavior and roles. Mary gives her the opportunity to fulfill these needs.

Betty (age 4): Expresses need to please people and be liked. Mother sees this as a way to "get her way" (a form of manipulation). Father sees this need as genuine, and she is his favorite. He responds to Betty's sweetness, reinforcing her behavior and need to please.

Richard (age 3): Richard has a need to explore and be autonomous. Mary realizes this and responds by letting him run around the house and explore. Also has need for extra attention because of arrival of new baby, which parents understand and are responding to.

Daniel (age 1 to 3 weeks): Needs to trust and have his basic physiological and affectional needs met. These are being fulfilled ably by the mother.

21. **Socialization Function**

Family Child-rearing Practices: Observations limited. Pat advocated old-fashioned child rearing, not "newfangled" methods. Believes in punishment, respect, and obedience. However, he has a minimal role in implementation, so that Mary may undermine some of his wishes regarding child rearing. From their behavior the children show they have been taught that "children should be seen but not heard" when adults are talking. Mary is very warm and physically affectionate, permissive, and tolerant when children are younger, but when they become preschoolers (age 4 up), she and Pat expect more self-restraint, self-discipline, respect, and obedience. Also could be seen that boys are allowed to be more assertive and aggressive than the girls of family (sex-linked socialization practices are evident).

Adaptability of Child-rearing Practices for Family's Situation: They appear adaptive in that children are being raised to live in the world as the parents see and experience it. This involves the need to be respectful, obedient, and conforming, and for boys and girls to know their appropriate sex roles and behavior.

Who Is the Socializing Agent? The mother predominantly, but father's influence also present, albeit more indirect. School teachers and priest, in addition to kin, are also socializing agents in children's lives and will become increasingly important as the children age.

Value of Children: They were wanted and accepted. Children appear to be highly valued. Children are highly cherished in the Catholic religion and Irish-American families. Being a mother is the central role for Mary; however she now feels the "burden" of having so many children to care for.

22. **Health Care Function**

Family's Health Beliefs, Values, and Behaviors: Preventive care for children (except for immunizations) is not given; mother did receive physicals with each pregnancy, hence her health maintenance behaviors are more consistent than her husband's. Pat expressed concern about his steady weight gain and "gut" since he stopped playing sports.

Family's Definition of Health-Illness and Level of Knowledge: By taking children and herself to a physician or clinic when they are not visibly ill means that she acknowledges that health is more than just being able to function or a state of feeling well. Wife is health leader and decides when children are ill and in need of health services. Mother has good basic understanding of how to handle common minor illnesses and injuries. She also knows what to do when more serious injuries occur or symptoms appear.

Family Members' Perceived Health Status: Unknown.

Family Dietary Practices: Adequacy of family diet: From data regarding the family the information was inserted into a food history record (Table D–2) to the extent possible.

Caloric Intake: Adequate, although husband and wife are a little overweight (children's weights are within normal limits). Data obtained via visual inspection only. Cultural food assessment: Stews and boiled dinners prepared. Extensive use of potatoes (the Irish staple); otherwise diet is basically American.

Typicality of 24-hour Diet: This report is typical. Mary said that their diet contains little fruit or fruit juices, except for bananas, apples (in season), and canned peaches—and occasionally apple or orange juice. One cooked vegetable besides potatoes is served at dinner each evening. Soups are eaten three to four times per week; salads are infrequently eaten.

Food Allergies: None noted.

Function of mealtimes and their attitudes toward food and mealtime: Not noted.

Shopping practices and person responsible: Mary goes to nearby shopping center and Pat's father's grocery store. She has budgetary limitations and just barely gets by each month. She does not use food stamps but is interested in applying to obtain them.

Refrigerator and Stove: Functioning and adequate, though small. Wife is totally responsible for planning, shopping, and preparation of meals.

Sleep and Rest Habits: Sleeping patterns not noted. Mary stated she used TV for relaxing and that Pat does same, in addition to going over to the bar to socialize and drink for the purposes of relaxation.

Physical Activity and Recreation Practices: Parents do not have regular exercise program for themselves. It is not mentioned as to whether they believe this is a necessity for health maintenance. Wife gets a moderate amount of physical activity doing housework and child-care activities. Husband used to be active in sports but is not presently. He stands at his job (as butcher). The most frequent family recreational or leisure-time activity is to visit extended families together. Mother takes children to park to play. No travel, movies, or eating out because of finances and car's poor condition. Mary and Pat do not go out as couple by themselves or with friends.

Family's Drug Habits: Husband drinks alcohol (type and amount unknown); socializing at bars is a frequent and central activity for him.

Both parents drink coffee (2 to 3 cups per day noted).

Tobacco is not used.

TABLE D–2

FAMILY FOOD HISTORY RECORD

MEAL	FOOD SERVED	QUANTITY	INDIVIDUAL DIFFERENCES
Breakfast	Cold cereal	1 bowl	All family ate cereal
	Milk	1/2 cup for cereal	
	Toast, 1 or 2 pieces		Parents only
	Coffee	1 cup	Parents
	Milk	1 cup	Children
Snacks	Crackers	3 or 4 crackers	Children
	Milk	1 glass	
	Coffee	1 cup	Mother
Lunch	Tomato soup	1 bowl	Joseph, Maureen, and father not home
	Mashed potatoes	1/2-1 cup	
	and butter	1 tbsp	
	Canned peaches	1/2 cup	
	Milk	1 cup	
Snacks	None		
Dinner	Stew: containing meat		
	meat	1/4 cup	All ate stew, but children had smaller servings
	carrots	1/2 cup	
	potatoes	1/2 cup	
	celery	1/4 cup	
	White cake	1 slice	All family
	Milk	1 cup	Children
	Coffee	1 cup	Wife
	Beer	1 cup	Husband
Snacks	Cookies		

It is not mentioned whether use of alcohol is considered a problem.

Family's use of prescription and over-the-counter drugs:

Use of prescription drugs not noted.

Use of over-the-counter drugs directed by Mary. She uses cold medicines (Sudafed, etc.), gastrointestinal medicines (milk of magnesia, etc.), first-aid medications, and aspirin correctly and carefully. She also stores medicines in a safe cabinet away from children's reach.

Family's Role in Self-care Practices: See prior comments. Also administers medications carefully and correctly.

Medically Based Preventive Measures: Children (except when infants) and adults do not have periodic physical examinations.

No information on recency or on vision/ hearing examinations or immunization status of family members.

Dental Health Practices: Nutritional: breads and some desserts noted in diet. No candy noted.

Brushing Teeth: Parents brush teeth two times a day after meals. Joseph is being taught to brush teeth. Other children have not started brushing teeth yet. Use of fluoride: Not mentioned.

No dental checkups and cleanings. Family visits family dental clinic in neighborhood when dental problems arise. Joseph has had one cavity filled (baby tooth). Parents have been to dentist on a problem basis only. Children other than Joseph have not been seen by a dentist.

Complementary and alternative therapies: None apparent. This topic may be explored further at subsequent visits.

Family Health History: No information included.

Health Services Received: Receive pediatric and maternity services from family doctor. Last baby, Daniel, delivered at county hospital because family could not raise necessary funds for private hospital and did not have health insurance at the time. They are now covered by husband's employment, however. Receive well-baby care and immunizations through health department. Pat had never been seen by doctor for physical examinations to Mary's knowledge.

Perceptions/Feelings Regarding Health Care: Family physician (long-time family doctor) is liked, but because family has medical insurance now, Mary would like to switch doctors. Stayed with above physician because his rates were low; but he is old, and Mary is afraid he is not up-to-date in his practice. Mary and Pat asked for information on regular health care services that health insurance covers. No comments regarding health department services or dental services.

Emergency Health Services: Family uses children's hospital in community when emergency care is needed for children. No mention of where parents go or would go if emergency arose.

Source of Payment: Family has had to assume total expense of medical and dental care up to now. Recently received group health insurance through Pat's father's business (the grocery store). No dental insurance mentioned. Provisions of health insurance not known.

Logistics of Receiving Care: No problems noted. Care has been accessible and mother has car for transportation.

❧FAMILY STRESS, COPING, AND ADAPTATION

23. **Family Stressors, Strengths, and Perceptions**

    Short-term Stressors

    a. Recent addition to family (Daniel), causing need to reallocate resources and relationships in family.

    b. Wife's potential to become pregnant again (lack of family planning).

    c. Richard's sibling rivalry and acting-out behaviors, although this does not seem to be a serious stressor.

    d. Role overload and strain experienced by mother due to the arrival of another baby and heavy household and child-care responsibilities.

Long-term Stressors

a. Economic: Marginally adequate income ("barely gets by every month") and two outstanding debts to pay off: car and hospital bills. With new baby and inflation, economic problems may increase.

b. Marital: Lack of communication between husband and wife.

c. Role strain of wife (role overload). Mary's role strain appears not to be recognized as burden by Pat and is minimized as a problem within their cultural/religious orientation.

d. Threat of future pregnancies (short- and long-term stressor).

e. Value conflicts between Irish-American subculture and American majority culture.

Strengths That Counterbalance Stressors

Family has several strong assets that counterbalance to a moderate extent the above family stressors:

a. Husband's steady job (stable provider).

b. Mary's ability and willingness to work and Mary's mother's offer to provide infant care.

c. Permanency of residence. Family knows neighborhood and community, familiar with resources. They like neighborhood's cohesiveness and are well integrated into neighborhood.

d. Social support system of family is moderately strong. Extended family present and assistance available and partially utilized. Also, neighbors and friends were mentioned as helpful. Church and church school are important resources to family.

e. Health status of family members appears adequate to good with no obvious problems except Mary's hypertension during pregnancies mentioned.

f. Adequate housing and furnishings at present.

g. Adequate health care (except preventive), nutritional practices, and health resources (health services and insurance).

Family's Definition of Its Situation: Perception of role overload (role strain) experienced by Mary and her expressed need to prevent further pregnancies are the two stress-producing situations occurring during nurse's visits. Mary seems to be able to appraise situations realistically, but Pat denies the significance of her concerns and strains. As a family they have not taken action yet on wife's concerns because Pat was supposed to call the priest and doctor for appointments but has neglected to do so. As a family, parents have not worked together to appraise problems objectively and solve them.

Functional Coping Strategies Utilized (Present and Past):
The family uses their social support system of extended family and church primarily to assist them in time of need. Inner coping resources are not mentioned as means for dealing with stressors. The family is able to meet the usual stresses and strains of daily life, largely through the efforts of Mary, who is the central figure in the family. Mary and Pat, albeit more reluctantly, are seeking information about health care services.

Dysfunctional Coping Strategies Utilized (Past and Present):
First, the family does not use its inner resources adequately to deal with stressors. There is no "pulling together," increased cohesiveness, or sharing of feelings and thoughts during periods of greater demand. Pat goes his own way rather than pitching in as part of the family team. The more overt dysfunctional coping mechanism that can be identified is that of authoritarianism, coupled with an element of neglect. Interestingly enough, this pattern is an exaggeration of the traditional Irish or Irish-American pattern. The stance may be taken that Pat uses his position of dominance too extensively, however, because through his authoritarianism and neglect (his minimal involvement with family life) he stifles the growth and quality of their marital relationship, as well as reduces the quality of his relationship with his children (except with Betty). Moderate husband dominance occurs where feelings and input are often not solicited or received from family members, especially the wife. This coping pattern affects the family unit, its subsystems, and the individual family members adversely (Table D–3).

OTHER FAMILY PROBLEMS GENERATED FROM O'SHEA ASSESSMENT

- Father–child relationships weak (except for Betty).
- Nutritional deficiencies: Insufficient use of vegetables and fruits, especially ones containing vitamin C; lack of sufficient iron in diet.
- Inadequate dental hygiene and care: Brushing for Maureen and Betty; examinations for whole family.
- Lack of exercise program for the spouses.
- Home safety hazards: No lighting or railings on outside steps. Stair boards loose.

FURTHER ASSESSMENT DATA NEEDED

- Perceived health status of family members.
- Health insurance benefits.
- Family's knowledge regarding how to locate another family physician.
- Family's knowledge of accessible emergency rooms for adults.
- Eye/hearing examinations and immunization status of family members.
- Family medical history.
- Roles: role models of parents.
- Environmental exposure to pollutants from industrial area nearby.
- Spouses' feelings about their sexual relationship and attitudes about counseling.
- Husband's drinking pattern and consumption of alcohol.

TABLE D–3

FAMILY NURSING CARE PLAN AND FURTHER ASSESSMENT NEEDED

FAMILY NURSING DIAGNOSES INCLUDING CONTRIBUTING FACTORS

1. Ineffective marital and parental role performance (role strain/overload) related to arrival of another baby, heavy child-care responsibilities, and inadequate family coping patterns.

VARIABLES

Cultural and religious values and norms regarding marital roles and adult roles for women and men. Life cycle of family: high demands being placed on both parents at this stage of family's life.

Socioeconomic position: marginal income, limited education, constricted world.

Life cycle of family: high demands being placed on both parents at this stage of family's life.

Socioeconomic position: marginal income, limited education, constricted world.

2. Ineffective in health maintenance: Ineffective family planning.

VARIABLES

History of high fertility, pregnancies every year.

History of hypertension during pregnancies.

Cultural/religious influences on family planning.

Weak spousal relationship (lack of spousal communication).

3. Health-seeking behaviors (expressed desire for improvement in preventive health care behavior).

SIGNS AND SYMPTOMS

(IDENTIFYING CONTRIBUTING FACTORS)

No companion role present (couple does not do things together).

Wife expresses feelings of being overburdened.

Therapeutic role inadequate.

Husband does not listen to wife's concerns.

Lack of communication except for money and some of children's problems and sexual roles unsatisfying, according to wife.

Mates do not "pull together" (become cohesive and reliant on own resources during periods of high demand on family).

Wife's hypertension during pregnancies and potential harm to health from subsequent pregnancy.

Pregnancies in family have not been planned.

Mother does not want more children—strain on herself, budget, housing, etc.

Family-planning methods inadequate (not a problem at present, but will be soon).

Husband is not sufficiently empathetic with wife's concerns regarding having no more children and passively accepts unplanned pregnancies.

Preventive health services are accessible and family has new health insurance benefits.

FAMILY NURSING CARE PLAN AND FURTHER ASSESSMENT NEEDED

None of the family has had regular preventive dental or medical examinations.

Parents are both overweight with no regular exercise program.

Diet—more fat in diet than recommended. Insufficient fruits and vegetables.

Husband's use of alcohol by report of wife.

FURTHER ASSESSMENT DATA NEEDED

Do spouses wish to do leisure time activities together?

Does husband feel there is a problem with communication?

Does husband feel that sexual roles are problem and an area for improvement?

Would wife feel that this is an area she would be too embarrassed to have discussed?

Assess couple's, especially husband's, willingness and readiness to explore ways of strengthening marital relationship.

How do family's priest and physician feel about family planning for couple?

What is couple's relationship with physician and priest? Are they the most appropriate resources to refer couple to?

What benefits are included under new health insurance policy?

Knowledge of age-appropriate preventive health care practices.

Immunization status of children.

What kind of physical exercise would couple be willing to participate in?

Level of physical activity of children.

Willingness to alter diet.

Extent of husband's alcohol use.

GOALS

Short-term: Spouses will be able to discuss wife's concerns and their relationship and roles.

Long-term: Spousal relationship (subsystem) will be strengthened by enlarging number of roles involved in marital positions (companion, therapeutic, and perhaps sexual) and by improving communications.

Short-term: Couple will be able to accurately describe the types of family planning methods available and acceptable to them (within their cultural/religious belief system).

Couple will be able to explore their thoughts and feelings about having no more children.

Husband will understand wife's concerns and see problem as a family problem.

Long-term: Couple will successfully use family planning method(s) to prevent further pregnancies.

Short term: Couple will be able to identify preventive health care services under their new health insurance policy.

Long term: Family will make full and regular use of all medical and dental benefits eligible for under health insurance benefits.

All family members will receive preventive medical examinations allowed by health insurance policy.

Short-term: Spouses and all family members will receive dental checkup and cleaning.

(Continued)

TABLE D–3 *(CONTINUED)*

FAMILY NURSING CARE PLAN AND FURTHER ASSESSMENT NEEDED

Will perform other age-appropriate preventive health behavior (e.g., immunizations, safety, stress management, and self-examinations)

Parents will initiate a regular exercise program.

Family will alter diet to reduce fat and increase fruits and vegetables.

INTERVENTIONS

Discuss with the couple the stress and role strain they are experiencing with the arrival of the new baby.

Help them redefine or reframe the problem as a family problem, not a mother–wife problem.

Encourage them to share their concerns about their growing responsibilities and the financial strain.

Encourage greater use of existing support system (e.g., grandmothers and aunt) to have more leisure time together.

Assist the couple to explore options for leisure time that would be satisfying for both of them.

Open up discussion with couple about Mary's interest in obtaining part-time job and support her efforts to obtain information.

Assist couple to discuss and clarify their roles, expectations of each other, their communications with each other, to open up avenues for modification of their roles/communication to create more functional patterns.

Assist couple to identify internal coping mechanisms (e.g., humor) or joint problem solving that could be utilized to reduce stressors.

Discuss with Pat his willingness to take on some responsibilities with child care and child rearing if Mary returns to part-time work.

Support exploration of child care resources/options (aunt or children's grandmother).

Explore the couple's perceived need and interest in marital counseling and in receiving information on marital and sexual relationships. Initiate referral(s) if need and interest are present.

Suggest they discuss family/marriage with priest. See if couple can obtain new, enlightened information and guidance on family planning and marriage.

Socioeconomic: Refer to food stamp program.

Help couple explore feelings regarding limiting family, effects of having additional children on family

Assist couple to problem solve in making and carrying out decision in this area (resources, who will follow up with contacting them, etc.).

Refer family to health and religious resources (if needed) as part of problem-solving process.

Follow-through with spouses after they have met with physician and priest to discuss any questions, thoughts, or areas where further information is needed, making sure they have sufficient knowledge about family planning methods that were recommended.

Review with couple their health insurance policy and determine preventive health care benefits.

Explain the importance of preventive medical and dental examinations.

Refer to low-cost community services for care not covered by insurance policy (e.g., dental).

Review preventive health care practices that would be beneficial for family group as well as for each member of the family.

FAMILY NURSING CARE PLAN AND FURTHER ASSESSMENT NEEDED

To expand and reinforce knowledge, provide health education materials regarding age appropriate preventive health care practices.

Refer family members, as needed, to community resources for preventive health behavior modification (e.g., health education programs and self-help groups).

Support husband's concern about need to exercise and positive efforts couple makes to get information or start exercise program.

Compliment parents on the positive aspects of their family diet and encourage them to increase positive dietary patterns.

Encourage parents' efforts to improve diet.

EVALUATION

To be completed after intervention. Would look at goals to determine to what degree these have been achieved.

To be completed after intervention.

Would look at goals to determine to what degree these have been achieved.

To be completed after intervention. Would look at goals to determine to what degree these have been achieved.

ANSWERS TO FAMILY VIGNETTES AND STUDY QUESTIONS

✺CHAPTER 1 ANSWERS

1. Type of family form: The stepparent, remarried, reconstituted, or blended family (all refer to the same type of family form).

2. Another type of family form the children are part of: The binuclear family—the children are part of two families because of the joint custody, child care arrangements.

3. Benefits which most divorced single parents see in remarriage include:

   a. Improvement in financial status. Being a clerk in a hardware store, plus child support payments probably means that Doris struggles each month to make "ends meet."
   b. Remarrying provides an opportunity to form a new, gratifying relationship with her husband and an opportunity for the children to also have a positive relationship with a stepfather.

4. Primary issues facing this family: These are the common issues facing stepparent families: the stressed relationship between stepchildren and stepfather; the role ambiguity in terms of being a stepfather (what his responsibilities are, such as disciplining the children), the divided loyalty of the mother—should her primary loyalty be to her children or to her new husband when there is conflict between the two; the continuing tension between the mother and her former husband because of the broken joint custody arrangements; and unrealistic expectations of the parents relative to what family life should be like, especially in the family's early beginnings.

5. Supportive counseling to help family members adjust to new family: The mother is being seen on an ongoing basis by the nurse practitioner and voices her concerns about the new family and that stressful events have been making it difficult for her to maintain her medical regime. The nurse practitioner could discuss with the mother the difficulties and issues family members face when adults remarry and attempt to blend two family cultures together; typical stepfamily dynamics could also be discussed. As part of this, the nurse practitioner could converse with the mother about the role changes and difficulties the children, the stepfather, and the mother face and review effects of stress on mother's diabetic condition. Popular books for the adults and children dealing with these issues can be recommended.

6. c, d   7. d   8. a   9. c   10. a, b, and c   11. a and b

12. *Stage 1: Family efforts at health promotion.* Family reinforces health promotion and preventive measures, or may expose family members to health hazards.

13. *Stage 2: Family appraisal of symptoms.* Family recognizes and defines meaning of symptoms/illness.

14. *Stage 3: Care seeking.* Family persuades individual to seek care.

15. *Stage 4: Referral and obtaining care.* Family is the primary health referral agent (to whom and when). Contact is made with health practitioner.

16. *Stage 5: Acute response by client and family to illness.* Family defines appropriate roles for client during this stage; the illness also impacts on family and in serious, life-threatening situations can produce crisis.

17. *Stage 6: Adaptation to illness and recovery.* Family either supports or hinders client's recovery pattern. Nature of health problems also affects the family's adaptation.

18. a, c, and d

19. Whereas health refers to the individual's state of functioning (i.e., the extent to which an individual functions as an integrated whole person, maximizing his or her potential within his or her environment), family health refers to the adequacy of functioning of the family as a unit or system. Beyond this difference, many finer distinctions exist, such as the use of different indicators to measure family health and health.

20. Examples of traditional family forms are the nuclear family, nuclear dyads (childless couples), single-parent (divorced) families, single adults living alone, and extended three-generation families.

21. Examples of nontraditional family forms are commune families, never-married parent and child families, unmarried couple and child families, cohabiting heterosexual couples, and gay/lesbian families.

22. Role conflicts/role overload, role changes, and poverty.

23. General demographic trends: accelerated population growth; increasing racial and ethnic diversity; aging population. Family demographic changes: more working women delayed marriages and decline in marriage rate; higher divorce rate and lower remarriage rate; increase in childhood living arrangements and single-parent families; decrease in household size; increase in births to older mothers; increase in family heterogeneity or diversity; and changing gender norms.

24. a, b, and c   25. a   26. a, b, and c   27. c, d, and e

28. Both perspectives acknowledge the profound changes the American family is going through. The pessimists, however, see the health and stability of the American family as declining, due to what they see as the negative impact of these profound changes—changes such as the growth in illegitimacy, cohabitation, woman's work outside of the home, and family violence. The optimists, on the other hand, view change as positive and point out the positive changes taking place, such as rising egalitarianism, shared gender roles, the ability of women to work and have a family, and the technological advances that permit women to work and the family to have more leisure time to be together.

29. Stemming from the growth in diverse family forms, several family nursing practice implications are suggested: (a) there is no "right," "wrong," "proper," or "improper" form of family (tolerance and acceptance of different family forms is necessary); (b) nurses need to understand the uniqueness and strengths of each particular family, rather than label one family form as superior to another; (c) nurses must abandon the traditional model of the "ideal" family; and (d) we need to promote and strengthen the family and seek ways to make communities more supportive to children and parents who live in diverse family forms.

❀ CHAPTER 2 ANSWERS

1. The role of the family-centered home health nurse: The role would be first to conduct an assessment of the family and Charlie. From this data, individual and family nursing diagnoses would be made. Charlie and family may be experiencing discouragement or some similar problem, in addition to difficulty following medical regime. The interventions would be based on the problems identified. In addition to acting as a case manager for Charlie, which includes monitoring Charlie's recovery from pneumonia and his adherence to his antiretroviral therapy, supportive counseling of the family is indicated. It appears that Charlie is in one of his depressive periods ("downs"), meaning that it's a family "down time" too. Having a heart-to-heart conversation with Charlie, Steve, and Charlie's mother about their experiences and their suffering

will help create a more healing environment. Engaging the family in meaningful conversation about the effects of the illness on each of their lives and how they have coped, as well as what untapped resources might be used, are mentioned by several family nurses as being most helpful to family members (Robinson, 1994; Wright, 1997). If the family believes that ongoing support would be helpful to them, referral to an AIDS support group for Charlie and family members (caregiving groups are quite helpful) is another possible intervention/role.

2. All three levels of prevention and its attendant goals are relevant to consider when formulating goals for family nursing practice. Primary prevention should not be forgotten, even though Charlie is not well at the moment. Leading a healthy lifestyle is critical for all family members. Secondary prevention, consisting of early diagnosis and treatment, is an ongoing goal here, since the antiviral therapy is ongoing and changes often occur, due to Charlie's lack of tolerance for so many of the AIDS drugs. Tertiary prevention, the stage of recovery and rehabilitation, certainly fits Charlie and the family. They are all trying to recover from this last frightening, stressful complication of the disease. The supportive counseling and therapeutic conversations described under question 1 would be appropriate to include under the goal of tertiary prevention. These interventions are aimed at reducing or alleviating some of the suffering the family members are going through.

3. The challenges this family poses for the family nurse: The home health nurse is working with a family who is probably different from her or his own. Learning to appreciate this family form and the strengths this family displays are very important and a critical challenge to the nurse. Acceptance and having a caring orientation and respect for all family members and their values and lifestyle are key attributes the family nurse needs to convey in order to effectively work with this family.

4. b   5. a and c

6. The ordering of priorities is different. The community health nurse is committed to providing services to families to help resolve major *community health* problems in addition to services designed to meet unique health needs of family. The family nurse in other settings/specialties prioritizes the family's particular health needs.

7. b, c, and d   8. b   9. a   10. a   11. b   12. c

13. b   14. c   15. a   16. a   17. d and e

18. Any four of the following:
   a. Recognition of need for a change in focus from crisis-oriented acute care (often the end result of self-destructive life patterns and environmental hazards) to causative factors of major chronic illnesses (lifestyle and environmental improvements). National initiatives (e.g., *Healthy People 2000* and *Healthy People 2010*).
   b. The wellness movement.
   c. Consumerism and popular demand for increased self-control.
   d. Problems with accessibility and availability of primary care health services.
   e. Growing acceptability of alternative health modalities.
   f. Growing emphasis on health in advanced nursing practice.
   g. Growth in managed care, including health maintenance organizations

19. We would argue that the crucial impediment to primary prevention is how we collectively, as a society, allocate our resources. The lack of third-party reimbursement for primary prevention for individuals and families acts as a major obstacle. Only 3 percent of health budget goes for primary prevention.

20. The purpose of health risk appraisal tools is to estimate the risks to which the client or family is exposed.

21. Identifying risks assists professionals in determining their priorities for assessment and intervention. It uses probability data to look at future long-term risks or possible health needs of individuals.

22. Whereas health refers to the individual's state of functioning, family health refers to the adequacy of functioning of the family as a unit or system. Family dynamics (internal family functioning) and family's

relationship with its external environment would be two broad components that would need to be assessed relative to family health promotion.

23. If family nurses can help families incorporate family health-promotion strategies or incorporate a wellness lifestyle, most health problems can be alleviated or forestalled. Health promotion is much more cost-effective than illness care.

24. Tertiary prevention.

CHAPTER 3 ANSWERS

1. Communication Theory: When the nurse asks questions of Mr. Katz, both Mrs. Katz and the daughter speak for Mr. Katz. He is passive most of the time.

   Roy's Model: Issues related to communication or interaction between family are conceptualized as part of the interpersonal mode of adaptation, such as Ineffective Adaptation, Interpersonal Mode related to dysfunctional family interactions.

2. Communication Theory: Cultural influence, as described in the vignette. Home environment is an important variable, because nurse does not have the same influence over the situation. Wife and daughter are the dominant ones here. Situational variable: Recent heart attack of husband, recent hospital discharge, and daughter moving in.

   Roy's Model: The family is conceptualized as responding to three levels of stimuli: focal (Dad's recovery from the heart attack), contextual (family members available, housing, ages of family) and residual (Jewish beliefs and values).

3. Communication Theory: Extensive use of dysfunctional communication among family members. Defining characteristics: Mrs. Katz and daughter speaking for Mr. Katz and making assumptions that they know his thoughts and feelings (these are dysfunctional sender characteristics).

   Roy's Model: Nursing diagnoses would address all four modes of adaptation for family members. For example, nursing diagnoses in the physiological mode of adaptation would include Mr. Katz's risk for new cardiovascular disease events due to low physical activity and high-fat diet, and Mrs. Katz's fatigue. A nursing diagnosis related to the role functioning mode might address Mrs. Katz's difficulty with caring for Mr. Katz due to fatigue and worry. A diagnosis related to the interpersonal mode of adaptation would focus on dysfunctional communication, and a diagnosis in the self-concept mode might relate to Mr. Katz's self-image as weak or vulnerable.

4. Communication Theory: Two general nursing interventions. Through teaching and counseling strategies the family nurse should assist family to be more functional in the areas described under defining characteristics. In particular, role modeling clear communication should be used. Directly involving Mr. Katz so that he becomes a more active communicator and speaks for himself is vital here.

   Roy's Model: Interventions would be designed to either bring the stimuli within the family's zone of adaptation, to change focal, contextual, or residual stimuli or enhance cognitive and/or regulator processes. For example, the contextual stimuli could be altered (family members available) by recruiting the sons to assist Mrs. Katz with some of the driving or other errands. This could provide Mrs. Katz with more rest and enhance her adaptability in her role (i.e., ability to provide care for Mr. Katz). A rabbi might be called to talk with the family more openly about their fears, possibly addressing residual stimuli related to worry about his health, and the nurse could provide health teaching about physical activity and heart-healthy diets for the family as a means of influencing their response to Mr. Katz's cardiovascular disease.

5. A theoretical framework provides the mechanism by which we can organize and more abstractly understand our observations; focus and guide our assessments, diagnoses, and interventions; and communicate our findings.

6. Nursing conceptual models/theories, family social science, family therapy theories

7. a, gg; b, ff; c, ee; d, dd; e, cc; f, bb; g, aa   8. a, ee; b, bb; c, dd; d, cc; e, aa; f, ff

9. a. Nursing theories: Specify a nursing focus and suggest nursing actions (what areas to assess and with what emphasis, delineation of goals, and intervention).
   b. Family therapy theories: Provide clinical application guidelines (assessment and intervention), particularly in family mental health settings.
   c. Family social science theories: Provide full description of family relationships (inner dynamics and external interactions) and family behavior.

10. c

11. a. Many of the debates focus on new conceptualizations of nursings' metaparadigm concepts and reflect the influence of postmodernist and neomodernist perspectives.
    b. There has been a strong shift in family nursing toward a strength-based perspective in working with families.
    c. Nursing theorists from diverse cultural backgrounds have begun developing models reflective of their own cultural contexts and unique aspects of family life in their cultures.
    d. The integration of the nursing models and with family social science theory and family therapy will be essential as the subspecialty of family nursing becomes more clearly delineated.

CHAPTER 4 ANSWERS

1. *Affective function:* Not being adequately fulfilled for all family members. Minimal data on children, although mother seems quite involved and enjoys her children. Mother is feeling unfulfilled emotionally in her relationship with her husband. No concrete data on husband's feelings, although it appears he has withdrawn from the family affectively.

2. *Heath care function:* Food: Mother cooks and provides nutritional meals, although excessive carbohydrates; shelter: adequate home provided; clothing: family adequately dressed; health care: children appear in good health. Would need to further assess this area, as it is inadequately described.

3. *Reproductive function:* Family has seven children. All living with the family.

4. *Socialization:* Emma's central family concern is child rearing; father participates minimally in disciplining and guidance. Family actively fulfills this function via the mother. Social placement: Society will identify family as members of working class.

5. *Economic function:* Father employed and provides family with basic necessities for independent living.

6. Description of family structure:
   - *Family roles:* the formal roles in the family are the husband/father, wife/mother, and children/siblings. Here we know that Herman has been a good provider and Sylvia appears to be a "good wife"—a good cook and caregiver. The informal roles are more interesting to note. Herman is definitely in the sick, dependent role, with his wife supporting this role. Both Herman and Sylvia believe that this role is appropriate and needed for recovery. Sylvia, as the caregiver, sees her role as meeting Herman's needs and wishes.
   - *Family power:* Sylvia appears to be in charge at this point. We don't know if this is just temporary because of Herman's illness, or whether this has been the long-term power structure within the family. She is the spokesperson and health leader according to the nurses' observations.
   - *Family values:* The value of caring for the sick member of the family in a very attentive, supportive way is present. The family has come together because of the father's illness situation. Family appears to be a very important value for this family.
   - *Family communication:* Herman is described as passive and dependent, letting Sylvia do the talking in the family relative to his health status and treatment. Sylvia is the dominant one (temporarily or more per-

manently is not clear). Marion's and the sons' communication are not discussed, with the exception of telling us that the sons visit and call often on the phone.

7. Description of family functions:
   - *Affective function:* The wife and daughter have demonstrated their care and concern for Herman. The sons are supportive of their parents. There is little information as to the family members' relationships with each other, although we do know that the sons visit and call often and the daughter has moved in to temporarily help out the mother—indications that the family is pulling together and providing affective support.
   - *Socialization and social class placement:* Not relevant because of the life cycle of the family. The family is middle class according to the occupation of Herman.
   - *Economic function:* This function has been well fulfilled. Herman's occupation and the family home are evidence that the economic needs of the family are being met.
   - *Health care function:* Sylvia is definitely the primary and practically sole caregiver in the family. Herman is passive and afraid to follow the rehabilitation health regime needed for recovery. Sylvia tacitly agrees with him relative to his lack of exercise, and believes that her cooking (rich Jewish foods) is needed for recovery and to make him feel better psychologically. The health care function is being provided, but not as medically needed for Herman. Sylvia is also not taking good care of herself it appears (she is overweight, sedentary, arthritic, eats rich foods, and is tired—trying to do all the caregiving herself). This function is definitely not being carried out optimally.
   - *Reproductive:* Not relevant function due to life cycle of family.

8. c.

9. Both internal family dynamics (structure and functions) and external relationships, i.e., the family system's interface with other systems and suprasystems, such as reference groups and wider society.

10. b   11. a   12. c and d

13. a. 1   b. 2   c. 1   d. 2   e. 1   f. 2

14. a. 3   b. 4   c. 2   d. 2   e. 2   f. 2   g. 2   h. 1

CHAPTER 5 ANSWERS

1. Stage VI: Families Launching Young Adults

2. Expand the family circle to young adults to include new family members acquired by marriage, continue to renew and adjust the marital relationship, assist aged and ill parents. In addition, they still need to meet developmental tasks of previous stage to balance freedom with responsibility as teenagers mature and become increasingly autonomous.

3. Elizabeth and her husband are experiencing conflicts in taking on the role of "in-laws," roles in which they have less parental authority over their college-bound daughter. They are also having difficulty developing a new parent–child relationship with their teenage son.

   Joshua has to adjust to the new role of being the only child at home and no longer having the continual interaction that are associated with his siblings. Anthony must begin to deal with the tasks associated with developing his own new family system, while Mary learns to establish her identity away from the rules and relationships she knew in her parent's home.

4. Encourage Elizabeth to continue to attend her support group and ask her to have her husband also attend. Encourage Elizabeth and her husband to speak with their local priest about their concerns of their sons' upcoming nuptials. Family counseling may be needed for Joshua and his parents. Encourage the family to use a variety of communication mediums on a regular basis to keep connected with one another (e.g., telephone, e-mail, and planned family get-togethers).

5. Any two:

    a. A family is seen as a long-lived small group that changes over time.

    b. Families go through life cycle or family career stages.

    c. During each life cycle stage certain developmental tasks are germane to a family's functioning.

    d. In families there is high family member interdependency.

    e. Family developmental tasks are derived from a combination of individual developmental tasks of each family member and the common family functions.

    f. The developmental approach describes commonalities in family experiences through time.

6. b   7. All responses are correct (a–f)   8. c   9. a, b, d, e, g, and h

10. b   11. a, d, and e   12. a

13.

Family Life Cycle Stage	Definition of Phase	Health Concerns or Needs
I. Married couple	Couple without children	1. Generating satisfying marriage (communications, sexual counseling) 2. Planning a family 3. Prenatal care
II. Childbearing	Birth of the firstborn until oldest child is 30 months old	1. Postpartum care, family planning 2. Sibling rivalry 3. Infant supervision and education (also family interactions—parental, marital)
III. Preschool	Oldest child is 30 months to 5–6 years old (when child starts school)	1. Preschooler's accidents and infectious illnesses 2. Adequate child care facilities 3. Marital relationship problems care facilities
IV. School age	Oldest child is 6 to 13 years old.	1. Marital relationship problems 2. Learning problems of children 3. Child-rearing practices
V. Teenage	Oldest child is 13 to 20 years old.	1. Communication problems (parent-teenager) 2. Discipline and power struggles (parent–teenager)
VI. Families launching young adults	Firstborn through youngest child leave home	1. Parent–child communication problems 2. General health promotion 3. Care of and assistance to aging parents
VII. Middle-aged parents	Empty nest (no children home) to retirement	1. Care of and assistance to aging parents 2. Emergence of chronic illness—need for wellness lifestyle 3. Grandparent role
VIII. Family in later years	Retirement to death of both spouses	1. Declining health status 2. Retirement 3. Death of spouse 4. Adjustment to environmental changes

14.

Life Cycle Stage	Developmental Task(s) of Parent
I. Married couple	1. None
II. Childbearing	1. Parents learn cues baby expresses in making needs known 2. Learning to accept child's growth and development (toddler)
III. Preschool	1. Learning to separate from child.
IV. School age	1. Learning to separate from child continues

V. Teenage	1. Learning to accept rejection without deserting the child
	2. Learning to build a new life for themselves (marital couple)
VI. Families launching young adults	1. Learning to build a new life for themselves (marital couple) continues
VII. Middle-aged parents	1. Learning to build a new life for themselves (marital couple) continues
VIII. Family in later years	1. Learning to adjust/accept dependent role

15. d

16. Emancipation, generation gap, and youth culture

17. The American family is tremendously affected by the developmental tasks of the adolescent. The turmoil and conflicts between parents and teenagers are inevitable as the teenager's assertion of himself or herself and rebellion is part of becoming independent or emancipated.

18. e   19. d   20. b   21. a   22. f   23. g   24. c   25. h   26. a, b, and d

27. Remarriage, because of its disruptive nature, generally impedes the family's movement through and completion of the family developmental tasks for two to three years after the creation of the new blended (stepparent) family. After the new family is restabilized (with a new structure, roles, rituals, and rules), the family resumes its normal developmental process.

28. The family's present developmental stage, the extent to which the family is fulfilling its family developmental tasks, the family's history from inception to present, and both parents' families of origin.

❧ CHAPTER 6 ANSWERS

1. Addition of new family member, Allie on maternity leave, child with colic in the home, change in role expectations for all family members

2. Alterations in Parenting, Alteration in Family Processes

3. Spouse subsystem due to less time to spend with each other; sibling subsystem with addition of new sibling, absence of older sibling; parent–child subsystem with addition of new child with higher developmental needs than older children

4. Encourage family members to openly speak about their feelings. Ask older siblings to agree to help with certain new household responsibilities and reward them for completing these tasks (e.g., increasing their allowance). Establish special time daily and weekly for each parent to spend with the older children. Seek additional community resources (friends, family members) to assist in care needs of the family.

5. True   6. False   7. True   8. False   9. True   10. True

11. a. Focal system = family
    b. Suprasystem = wider community
    c. Interacting systems = health care system, educational system, law enforcement system, welfare system
    d. Subsystems = spouse, parent–child, and sibling

12. See energy, matter, and information exchange and process model (Figure 6–3). Various examples could be applied, such as:

    Input (= information): News of risk of inactivity and benefits of exercise program.

    Flow: Spouse subsystem accepts and internalizes this information.

Output: Spouses begin dance classes weekly for themselves. They also begin hiking with their children on weekends (the energy release—their activity—is the output).

Feedback: The family members feel better (have more energy, vitality, and strength) plus the parents' physical condition and attractiveness improves, and both results then become reinforcers of the exercise program.

13. a. 1   b. 2   c. 1   d. 1   e. 3   f. 3   g. 4

14. f (see introduction to chapter for relevant discussion)

15. a, b, c, d, e, and h

16. Significance of family boundaries: Boundaries allow for the exchange processes. By controlling the flow in and out of the system, they prevent overload or underload of the system. Significance of family subsystem boundaries: They prevent loss of integrity of the personal system and interference with the vital functions that individuals in families need to learn and perform.

17. Family boundaries function adaptively by being selectively permeable—that is, actively expanding (opening up) and retracting (closing down) according to need, thus regulating the amounts of input and output.

18. a. 3   b. 1, 2, and 3   c. 1   d. 3   e. 2   f. 2

19. Any four characteristics of a healthy family: highly organized and differentiated; autonomous integrated subsystems; tolerance and ability to change internally; continual openness to new information and other input; and balancing of family system needs with family members' needs

20. a. 1, 3, 7, and 8   b. 2, 4, 5, and 6   c. 9   d. None

21. 1, c; 2, b; 3 or 4, d; 3 or 4, e; 5, a; 6, f; 7, g

❧CHAPTER 7 ANSWERS

1. Caregiver Role Strain; Impaired Home Maintenance

2. Willingness to adhere to medical plan of care; concern for health

3. Teaching, counseling, case management, and collaboration

4. b

5. a. 1   b. 5   c. 6   d. 3   e. 2 and/or 4   f. 5   g. 5   h. 2   i. 5   j. 4   k. 7   l. 4

6. c   7. a and b   8. a, b, and c   9. b or c   10. e   11. d and e

12. Any three:
    a. Review written records.
    b. Discuss the family with other health care team members who know the family well.
    c. Gather whatever information, teaching supplies, and assessment and intervention equipment are needed or anticipated.
    d. Call family on phone to set up visit if possible.

13. All choices (a through e) are correct.

14. All phases, since the family and its members are the crucial, central focus of our services and must be involved in all phases in order for each phase to be accomplished.

15. Any of these: a family presents with a problem(s) in which the relationships between family members are affected; a family member presents with an illness that is having an obvious detrimental impact on the other family members; family members contribute to the symptoms or problems of an individual;

one family member's improvement leads to symptoms or deterioration in another family member; a family member is first diagnosed with an illness; a child or adolescent develops an emotional, behavioral, or physical problem in the context of a family member's illness; a chronically ill family member moves from an institution back to the community; an ill family member dies.

16. d and e

17. Interview data, observational data, responses from questionnaires, checklists, and agency written records

18. Three domains of family functioning and their respective intervention(s) are cognitive, affective, and behavioral. Possible interventions include: offering information/opinions, reframing, offering education, externalizing the problem, and interventive questions directed at the cognitive domain; validating/normalizing responses, storying the illness experience, drawing forth family support, and interventive questions directed at the affective domain; and encouraging family members as caregivers, encouraging respite, devising rituals, and interventive questions directed at the behavioral domain.

19. The family's ability to master or live with problems, not necessarily to eliminate them

20. a, c, and d

21. Teaching—a, d, and e
    Case management—b, f, and h
    Coordination—b and c
    Advocacy—h
    Collaboration—b, c, e, and i
    Consultation—e and g
    Contracting—c
    Counseling—a, d, e, and f

22. Case management—b, c, and h
    Teaching—a, b, e, and h
    Collaboration—b, f, and h
    Contracting—a, b, g, and h
    Counseling—a, b, c, e, g, and h

23. With virtually all NANDA diagnoses, educative interventions could be relevant if clients are able to understand and learn. Examples (there are many correct answers): (a) deficient knowledge, (b) ineffective role performance, and (c) ineffective health maintenance.

24. a. Compromised or disabled family coping
    b. Interrupted family processes
    c. Impaired parenting (many more would be appropriate also)

25. Supportive counseling: Families with health problems/concerns who do not have complex and intense problems. With more complex problems, family therapy level of counseling is indicated.

26. Families with serious, complex, and/or long-term health needs. Targeted populations include families with frail elderly, AIDS clients, child abuse, chronically mentally ill, developmental disabled, and physically disabled/rehabilitation patients.

27. True   28. False   29. False   30. False   31. True   32. False

33. True   34. True   35. True   36. False   37. True

38. Examples are (a) decreased motivation (denial of learning needs); (b) lack of open communication and/or insufficient exchange of information; (c) environment is poor for teaching–learning to take place (space, noise problems, interruptions); (d) sociocultural differences; and (e) teaching not geared to literacy level of family.

🐝 CHAPTER 8 ANSWERS

1. Regarding the family's cultural background, we know the family is recently from El Salvador, a Central American country where in the 1970s there was a civil war and economic conditions are still very marginal there. We do not know the family's self-identified ethnic or religious identification, although we can assume the family would say that they were El Salvadorian, since they recently migrated to the United States. They probably are Catholic, but we would have to validate that because about 10 percent of Central American persons are now other Christian sects (Evangelistic churches, Mormon, etc.). We know that the parents both speak limited English, and prefer to speak Spanish when possible. The grandmother does not speak English. We don't know how much English Maria understands. We know the family composition. We do not know very much about what they think of the presenting problem (a probable sexual assault). Nor do we know about the family's social class status.

2. Missing data: The family's self-identified ethnic and religious background; the parents' occupations (an indicator of their social class status); how long they have been here; the English proficiency of Maria; and what the parents thought of the presenting problem and what exactly happened. The nurse would want to ask Maria some questions prior to examining her.

3. There are several general intervention strategies that would be appropriate to utilize here.

    a. Select the appropriate system to work with. Include the grandmother with the parents and child in the provision of care. Also provide support to the grandmother and parents and guidance for handling concrete problems (the child's anxieties, immediate child supervision/protection, and referral for crisis intervention and counseling for family and child and abusive cousin). Another system that would be contacted would be the child protective service agency in the community.

    b. Use of an interpreter: Taking into consideration the language difficulties between the grandmother and nurse practitioner and the fact that the grandmother is the key supportive person here, the interpretive process becomes extremely important. Be sure the parent(s) explain carefully and completely to the grandmother what the nurse practitioner says. The nurse practitioner should speak slowly and break up his or her thoughts to make translation easier. The nurse practitioner should encourage and allow extra time for the grandmother to respond, ask questions, etc.

    c. Assessing and utilizing the family's social support system. This should be done as part of the assessment and later intervention. In this family crisis, identifying support for the family and child is critical. In Hispanic families a large extended family usually comes to help in time of crisis. The family should be encouraged to utilize key supportive persons from the extended kin network.

4. Gaining an understanding of the ethnic background of a family is essential to family health care because without this knowledge, family values and behavior cannot be understood or accurately interpreted. Ethnicity and culture permeate and circumscribe familial actions. In the absence of being able to assess accurately, the health care professional is in a compromised position to work with the family to assist it in resolving health problems. It is also imperative to understand a family's culture from their perspective in order to build the rapport and trust necessary to appropriately assess, support, and counsel ethnic families.

5. b   6. All but e   7. All   8. b and c

9. 1. p   2. d   3. f   4. e   5. h   6. c   7. g
    8. m   9. n   10. l   11. j   12. o   13. a   14. b

10. c

11. b (usually of husband, but increasingly of both spouses in dual-career families).

12. c   13. b and c   14. c, d, and e   15. b and c

16. Any three, with dominant cultural values listed first: productivity versus "getting by"; education versus less value on education; mastery over environment versus fatalism/powerlessness against environment (or harmony with environment); future-oriented, long-range planning versus present-oriented, immediate gratification.

17. a. Teaching families how to reduce costs of health care by presenting options. Teaching them about their insurance coverage and community resources for help.

    b. Other services within the health agency, such as the business office or social worker, or community services, such as the Social Security Administration office or the state vocational rehabilitation office.

18. b, d, and e

🌿 CHAPTER 9 ANSWERS

1.1. Composition of family: Mrs. Garcia, mother, age 25, Mexican national, High school graduate; work history—home day care and food server

    Rosita, daughter, age 5. Born in Mexico, attended public kindergarten last year

    Carlos, son, age 3. Born in Mexico

    Father/husband died a year ago—no insurance.

1.2. Single-parent family; mother with two preschool-age biological children

1.3. Religion—Roman Catholic. Ethnicity is Mexican; the family is fairly acculturated to American culture. Although the parents were educated in the United States, they prefer traditional Mexican food and other traditions from their Mexican heritage. Spanish is the primary language spoken in the home, but Mrs. Garcia is fluent in English as well.

1.4. Lower class: Currently homeless, when domiciled/employed—low income (the working poor).

1.5. Family of origin was migrant agricultural workers with minimal formal education. Mrs. Garcia graduated from high school and moved to Texas with her husband. They were doing well (according to her) until her husband's illness and death. Social and economic status diminished markedly with loss of the father, who was the main wage earner. Mrs. Garcia is interested in increasing her earning capacity and will need training and/or educational opportunities.

1.6. Developmental stage: Family with preschool children.

1.7. May have persons at church, at the shelter, or friends who serve as supports. Estranged from family of origin.

2.1. Living in a transitional shelter at this time. One bedroom with a twin bed for Mrs. Garcia and bunkbeds for the two children; bathroom shared with another family; community kitchen and central laundry room.

2.2. Moved to Texas two years ago from Mexico. In earlier years, Mrs. Garcia lived with her family of origin, who were migrant farm workers.

2.3. The neighborhood where the shelter is located is low income, there is a barbed wire chain-link fence around the perimeter of the shelter complex, and there is a safe play area in the center court for the children.

2.4. Mrs. Garcia misses her husband and is discouraged about the difficulties she has in taking care of her family. The children are gradually making friends but still insecure as evidenced by their desire to stay close to their mother (including sleeping with her at night).

3. Homeless, cluttered living space, inadequate cooling, sleep disturbances

4. Multidisciplinary care conference, referral for support group.

5. Crowding, dilapidation, cockroaches or other insect infestation, and high noise level. Also acceptable answers: social isolation, inadequate space (inadequate internal space of home and arrangement of space in home, lack of privacy).

6. Acute respiratory infections, certain infectious childhood diseases, and infectious gastrointestinal diseases. Also acceptable: home accidents, infectious and noninfectious skin diseases, and lead poisoning.

7. Most middle-high-income families have at least one home computer (as well as cell phones and fax machines) while many low-income families do not have home computers, putting them at a distinct disadvantage. Computer skills, access to informational resources, and communication capabilities associated with Internet use are key factors to academic success for children and to job performance for many adults, and so connected ultimately with family's economic resources. Family members may utilize computer labs at public schools and libraries in order to learn skills, access information, and communicate with other users.

8. Adults: depression, mental illness. Children: lice, behavioral problems, respiratory infections such as asthma, and gastrointestinal illnesses.

9. Neighborhood schools may serve as resources for family health (e.g., when there is an adequate physical structure without toxic substances or when there is a school-based clinic). Schools may also be the source of family problems (e.g., when bullying is rampant). Other neighborhood/community characteristics related to family health include whether the family lives in an urban or rural area and how accessible health care is. In urban areas, this may be whether there is affordable transportation within the city. In rural areas, the distance to health care facilities may require personal transportation or a support network of people who could be called on for necessary transportation.

10. Student will provide an example from his or her own clinical and political experience.

❧ CHAPTER 10 ANSWERS

1. **Functional communication patterns:** Parents: listening (conversations together at the end of the day); mother–daughter: validation (regarding daughter's desire to spend time with her friends)

   Dysfunctional communication patterns: Dad: making assumptions, about why the son resists becoming more skilled in signing; Son: disqualifying, saying "forget it" when he can't understand his Dad's signing; sister–brother: making judgmental statements: sister criticizing her brother's signing skills, accusing him of being lazy.

   Recurring/circular interactional patterns: In situations when dad and son are away from mom and sister—

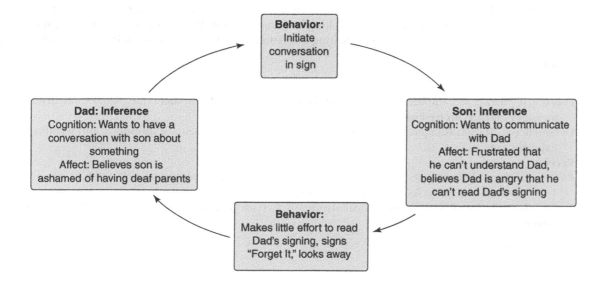

2. Emotional messages: Mother and son: conveyed through smiling, signing "I love you"; mother and daughter: sitting close together during the interview session.

3. a. Who talks to whom and in what usual manner? The mother and father communicate fluently in sign, the mother, son and daughter have a flexible and satisfactory system of communication, the father communicates in sign with the daughter, the father and son have great difficulty communicating directly and there is tension between them.

   b. The patterns of transmitting important messages are described above. Is there an intermediary? Yes—the mother often acts as intermediary between the father and son, which is dysfunctional. The daughter sometimes acts as an intermediary between her parents and hearing people, as she interprets for them. However, her parents are careful to limit her interpreting role to everyday situations and do not depend on her to interpret in adult situations, such as at the doctor's office. Hence, this is not considered a problem by the parents or daughter.

   c. Are messages appropriate for the developmental age of the members? The nurse did not note any inappropriate communication.

4. The messages are congruent in content and instruction: positive messages accompanied by smiling, negative feelings accompanied by appropriate facial expressions.

5. What types of dysfunction processes are evident? The dysfunctional communication between the father and son is the most obvious issue.

6. Family nursing diagnosis: Impaired communication related to language barrier (son's limited signing skills and father's limited speechreading/oral skills)

7. Interventions:

   • Teaching through role modeling: Specifically, the nurse could ask the father and/or son about how he feels about the communication problem between father and son. The nurse would listen intently, empathetically, ask clarifying questions.

   • Teaching: the nurse could initiate a discussion about the disadvantages of having the mother act as an intermediary between the father and son, and how improved communication directly between the father and son could strengthen their relationship.

   • Teaching: the nurse could initiate a discussion about functional and dysfunctional communication, including the effects of insults and judgmental statements on family relationships.

   • Counseling: The nurse could then encourage and support the father and son in their efforts to improve their communication. This might include identifying specific strategies for improving their communication and contracting for behavioral changes. For example, the father might agree to sign slower and spend one hour each week teaching his son new signs. The father and son might agree to communicate without an intermediary, writing notes if necessary, until they are able to sign together.

8. d and h.

9. Sender:
   Functional: Message sent through clear and direct channels (firmly and clearly states case, clarifies and qualifies messages, and asks for feedback).
   Dysfunctional: Makes assumptions, unclear expression of feelings, judgmental expressions, and inability to express needs.
   Receiver:
   Functional: Intended message and received message are consistent, congruent, and match in meaning (effective listening, giving feedback, and providing validation).
   Dysfunctional: Failure to listen, disqualification, offensiveness and negativity, lack of exploration, and lack of validation.

10. a. 2   b. 4   c. 2, 3   d. 5   e. 1

11. c   12. a

13. a. Content level: Disinterest expressed in movie. Instructional level: Expression of warmth, sexual attraction, and interest.
    b. Content level: Statement of love and demand that child play with toy. Instructional level: Expression of rejection of child's request for closeness and attention.
    c. Content and instructional level: Both consonant: Demand to stop behavior.

14. Redundancy   15. Positive feedback loops   16. All but e

❧ CHAPTER 11 ANSWERS

1. a. Husband–father: Expected to pay bills, carry out home-maintenance work, garden (his degree of involvement and decision making here is in question). Wife–mother: She initiates and convinces her husband of the "rightness" of her proposals in areas of major decisions. Also assumes responsibility and decision making in areas of child care, household management, and social activities. Joe (oldest son): In charge of child care activity in absence of mother.
   b. No strong evidence of consensus used. (They may not have the communication ability to negotiate and discuss alternatives so that consensual decision making can take place.) Accommodation: Use of bargaining seen in moving to suburbs and in purchase of home and car. No use of de facto technique noted (wife is probably too task oriented and too much of a planner for this to happen very often).
   c. Referent power: The children listen to mother, and although it is not clear if this is out of positive identification or primary authority, they seem to "mind" when she is not there to enforce the rules (which would also indicate use of reward–coercive power). Reward–coercive power: The stepfather appears forced to use this type of power base, although ineffectively, because he does not have children's respect, they do not recognize his authority, and he seems not to have expert or informational power to use.
   d. Family communication network: Mrs. Simpson definitely is in a central position as go-between or intermediary between her husband and children. This increases her dominance. Interpersonal skills: Mr. Simpson lacks confidence in his parenting skills and is passive, thus decreasing his effectiveness in this area. Mrs. Simpson undermines his parenting by taking over when the children do not listen to him. Also, he may need her more than she needs him. (Could he be seeking leadership, a mothering figure?) Social class variables: Family is obviously middle class, and even though the wife "takes over," she is dissatisfied in her husband's role performance. This may be an indication of the disparity between her expectations (the cultural norm of a husband being either a leader or sharing responsibility with wife) and her reality, or her feeling that he is incompetent. Usually, there is more division of role responsibilities and decision making. Cultural variable: The role of the stepfather is not crystallized in our society, making it unclear as to the extent of legitimate authority Mr. Simpson has over his stepchildren.
   e. Overall family power typology: Family power continuum.
   f. Moderate dominance by Mrs. Simpson.

2. Father–child power conflict; marital conflict over lack of exertion of power by stepfather in parenting; marital dissatisfaction in area of husband's exercise of parental authority.

3. Counseling of family members, involving the exploration of each family members' feelings about the impact of becoming a new family (What was it like for you when your new family was formed?"). Their perceptions of difficulties (Goal: Development of empathy for each other's feelings and concerns) would be important to discuss also. Referral to a marriage and family counseling center may be helpful so that the couple can explore their own marital concerns and how to deal with them.

4. a and b

5. a. 1, 4, 5, and 7   b. 2 and 3   c. 6 and 9   d. 8

6. Limitations of family power studies (any three):

   a. Lack of a good correlation between task allocation and decision making and overall dominance patterns in family.
   b. Focusing on the outcome of decision making, which family members have difficulty reporting, rather than the process, which gives much greater information regarding family interaction and dynamics.
   c. Methodological: Interviewing wife, rather than whole family.
   d. Methodological: Solely depending on the self-reporting of family member (interviews), rather than combining self-reports with actual observations.

7. a. 3 and 4   b. 5   c. 7   d. 6   e. 1   f. 9   g. 2   h. 10   i. 11   j. 8

8. False   9. False   10. True

11. a. Consensus: Both parties discuss and mutually decide.
    b. Accommodation: One partner "convinces" others to adjust or all parties decide to make concessions.
    c. De facto: No conscious, overt decision made; "things just happen."

12. Description of how each of the following variables affects family power:

    a. Family communication network: The unequal intensity of family relationships influences power, especially the centrality of one or more members in the network of interactions (an intermediary or go-between). Family members who hold these intermediary positions can screen information as they see fit and can use more intimate knowledge of family members' attitudes and opinions to influence them and obtain more control over decisions.
    b. Situational changes: A family life change that is nonnormative may cause the allocation of power to be redistributed. For example, if the mother becomes physically handicapped and can no longer carry out her parenting functions, she may lose implementation power.
    c. Ethnic differences: Ethnic differences dictate what power arrangements are seen as "right" and acceptable to the family members.
    d. Coalition formation: By forming coalitions, the members of the coalition increase their power relative to other family members.
    e. Social class: Social class affects family power by setting up family life conditions that influence the resources each spouse brings to their relationship, the role that tradition plays over contemporary trends, and more generally, the basic conditions under which the family lives.
    f. Developmental or life cycle changes: During the life cycle of the family, demands on the family unit vary, and in response to both internal and external demands, power patterns are altered. For example, when first married, couples tend to share decisions more than after children arrive because there is usually more emotional involvement at the start of their relationship.

13. d   14. b   15. c   16. b and d   17. c and d   18. c   19. d   20. All (a–e)

❧ CHAPTER 12 ANSWERS

1. b   2. c   3. a   4. a   5. c

6. Formal role structure of hypothetical family: The family was characterized by a sharp demarcation of roles (traditional pattern).
   Husband–father:
       Sole provider—breadwinner role
       Home repairman and gardener role
   Wife–mother:
       Child care role
       Housekeeper role (inside the house)

No roles are shared, nor do they wish to share any roles.
The companionship and therapeutic roles are not present in their marriage.
Sexual roles are not clear, but probably are traditional.

7. The mother is feeling role strain and role overload. Marital and parental role conflict and role strain (of marital partners).

8. For role strain: (1) Discuss housekeeper and child care roles with the mother and help her to redefine these roles in terms of what behaviors are necessary to maintain and which behaviors (tasks) can be eliminated or reduced in frequency. (2) Facilitate a discussion between mates of the roles that wife–mother has and help her negotiate roles so that there is a more equitable distribution of role responsibilities.

   For role conflict: (1) Encourage mother to express her feelings and perceptions about her roles and the incompatibility between the roles she is enacting. (2) Help wife–mother to problem solve to reduce incompatibilities of present roles and to set priorities.

9. a. 3   b. 1   c. 9   d. 4   e. 2   f. 7   g. 8   h. 5   i. 6

10. True   11. True   12. False

13. Low-income family. Marital roles: Sexual role less satisfying and diminished in importance, companionship role attenuated, therapeutic role attenuated. Parenting roles: The child-care role is exclusively the mother's domain (and the central role in her life).

   Middle-class Family: Marital roles: Sexual role is shared and more satisfying, companionship and therapeutic roles are strong basis for marriage. Parenting roles: Child-care role is shared.

14. Informal roles in the family (any five):

   a. Integrator (functional)
   b. Mediator (functional)
   c. Scapegoat
   d. Jester (functional)
   e. Child (when formal role is parent)
   f. Blocker
   g. The bystander
   h. The placator
   i. The family pioneer (functional)
   j. The "great stone face"
   k. The pal (may or may not be functional)
   l. Encourager (functional)
   m. Harmonizer (may or may not be functional)
   n. Initiator–contributor (usually functional)
   o. Compromiser (functional)
   p. Follower
   q. Dominator
   r. Recognition seeker
   s. Martyr

15. d

16. They describe how family members have allocated tasks to fulfill family functions; they disclose the socioemotional needs of family member(s) and the family and whether and how these needs are being met.

17. An individual cannot fully develop because he or she is rewarded only for certain behaviors and thus matures only in these rewarded areas.

18. a. Role overload
    b. Role changes or shifts, which occur if there is remarriage.

19. a. Whether the father (in the case of a stepfather family) is a parent or not (parental role confusion).
    b. The incompatibility of the wife and mother role. She has divided loyalties (to her children and to her husband), and conflict is seen when being supportive as a wife conflicts with being supportive as a mother.

20. False   21. True   22. True   23. False

✣ CHAPTER 13 ANSWERS

1.

American Societal Values	Gardner Family Values
1. Productivity/Individual achievement	1. Probably aspired to being successful—at least get by and be self-sufficient—but were not able to succeed. (Note wife's frustration and hostility toward husband because of employment problem.)
2. Individualism	2. Not evident.
3. Materialism/The consumption ethic	3. Not present (not realistic for family).
4. The work ethic	4. Wife appears to be committed to work ethic at home. Husband is not in conformity with this value.
5. Education	5. Not one of the central values for this family. Note lack of educational pursuits by parents and total lack of books at home.
6. Equality	6. Democratic functioning not observed in home (authoritarian, wife-dominated power structure).
7. Progress and mastery over the environment	7. Progress not implied. Mastery environment over environment not present. (Again powerless position makes this value unrealistic.)
8. Future time orientation	8. Future-time orientation not seen, no planning observed during the time reported. Present oriented.
9. Efficiency, orderliness, and practicality	9. Mrs. Gardiner seemed to place a high practicality value on orderliness. Gives mother a sense of control.
10. Rationality	10. Value not seen.
11. Quality of life and maintaining health	11. Health was not seen as an important (prime) value. Preventive care not sought. Child-care services utilized due to the obvious necessity of receiving treatment for acute problems. Mother: Denial of health problems noted regarding Len's health problems.
12. Tolerance of diversity	12. Little evidence of social exchanges outside of one's own culture.

2. Practicality, orderliness, cleanliness appear highly valued.

3. Not known.

4. Wife—work oriented; husband—unable to succeed in this area. Value conflict between spouses related to the work ethic. Wife is hard worker and she expects husband to be also, as well as to be the provider for the family, regardless of his emotional problems.

5. Discuss with spouses their beliefs and expectations about husband's working (get each spouse's views). If husband feels that his "bouts of depression" are the basis of problem, encourage him (and perhaps wife) to consult doctor to address this area; if husband and wife believe he does not have the job skills necessary to find new job, referral to a vocational rehabilitation or vocational skill center may be appropriate. Discuss with spouses the need for husband to feel he can find and hold down job and how family members can positively encourage these efforts.

6. a, b, and c   7. b   8. b

9. Four major, recent value changes (any four):

   a. Individualism. Greater priority today placed on individual freedom of choice with a concomitant decline in familism.

b. Work ethic. A change from seeing work as an end in itself to a means for obtaining other important aspirations. Decline in belief that hard work will pay off and decline in the intrinsic meaning of work to many individuals.

c. Tolerance of diversity. Studies show that Americans are becoming increasingly tolerant of variation in lifestyles and also of ethnic differences. Weakening of the myth of the "melting pot."

d. Equality. Egalitarianism in families and in society is increasing. Women's liberation is probably the strongest force in bringing about this change, but other oppressed groups have also sought and are receiving a fairer share of the resources and more consideration of their rights. These groups include children, the mentally ill, and other stigmatized groups.

e. Consumerism. There has been an increased exploitation of resources and a rise in material indulgence involving the discarding and replacement of goods rather than saving.

f. Health and quality of life. The increasing numbers of middle-class Americans engaging in lifestyle improvements is evidence of the increased saliency that this value has in society.

10. b, c, and d   11. a   12. True

13. Productivity, materialism, individualism, work ethic, progress, and education

14. Any four:

a. Ethnicity, including religious background
b. Social class
c. Rural versus urban or suburban (geographical location)
d. Degree of acculturation of dominant cultural values
e. Family life cycle stage
f. Generational differences

15. All (a–d)   16. c and d

CHAPTER 14 ANSWERS

1. This involves an analysis of need–response patterns of family.

Family Member	Perceived Affective Need by Parents	Extent Being Met
John (father)	Did not discuss in the vignette.	From study, no evidence that his socioemotional needs are being met; behavioral evidence is that family is not meeting his needs (avoidance behaviors—staying away and drinking excessively).
Ruby (mother)	No family recognition of her feelings of loss and depression or needs (to be able to be a good parent) evidenced.	No data implying that family is meeting her needs; in fact, there is evidence that her emotional needs are not being met (physical illness, depression, and suicidal thoughts). Priscilla, her former confidant, is focused on her own needs and is unable to meet Ruby's relational needs.
Priscilla (age 13)	Parents recognize her needs to take on mother role and to be independent.	Since Ruby feels threatened by Priscilla's successful management of the younger siblings while she was gone, she is not able to positively reinforce her parenting efforts now. Neither parent encourages and/or facilitates Priscilla's separating efforts (becoming less involved with the family and more involved with her peer group).

Cindy (age 10)	None expressed.	Obviously, she likes being industrious and involved in projects and social activities outside of the home, which she is able to do. Family is not meeting this need. Her behavior, especially staying away from the home for long periods of time, may be because of the family's inability to meet her socioemotional needs. Priscilla does serve as Cindy's confidant, which provides a vehicle for meeting some of her emotional needs.
John Jr. (age 6)	Only need expressed was that Ann's leaving might threaten younger children and make them feel that if they misbehave, they may be taken away from family.	No evidence that John's socioemotional needs are being met; in fact, there is behavioral evidence (school phobia, clinging to mother, poor school work) that his needs are not being attended to adequately.
Lisa (age 4)	Parents are aware of her problem with separation anxiety and the threatening effect Ann's loss may have.	Both parents evidently spend more time with Lisa, or are planning to give her more attention. She presently has behavioral manifestations of unmet needs; clingingness, frightened when mother leaves, and enuresis, but seems to be the child that is attended to affectively by the parents.

2. There is no direct evidence concerning whether mutual respect exists, but one can infer that there is substantial insensitivity and thus very limited respect accorded to each other's needs, because there is so little perception or recognition of individual needs in the family.

3. Again, seems to be limited. It was twice noted that the family members did not share their feelings with each other in the face of present difficulties (this is a primary means of emotional support). Lisa seems to be comforted and nurtured more by the parents than the other family members are. Priscilla also provides nurturance to Cindy.

4. There appear to be only three sets of relationships in the family that show these traits: between Cindy and Priscilla, Lisa and Ruby, and Lisa and John. Also, Priscilla and Ruby used to have closer relationship in past. Affectionate feelings, according to the parents, are and should be expressed only to the two younger children. The degree of compatibility is difficult to evaluate from this vignette. No open conflict is described between the children or between the parents except for the arguments between Priscilla and Ruby. John and Ruby show signs of incompatibility, handling it by withdrawal (John staying away and drinking, and both of them not discussing important issues). Part of lack of spousal discussion of important issues and feelings, however, may be due to social class and cultural role expectations (i.e., they do not see this as one of the expected roles in marriage).

5. There is evidence that this is present: (1) spouses are staying together (although marital bonds need to be strengthened); (2) Priscilla's emulation of mother's mothering behaviors and role; and (3) separation anxiety of the two younger children when mother leaves.

6. The information in this area is limited. However, more emphasis is placed on the togetherness aspects with Priscilla and the other children. Parents do not stress individuality and personal growth (which is more of a middle-class phenomenon and luxury).

7. Nursing diagnosis would be impaired parenting of son John Jr. and daughter Lisa. *Defining characteristics:* Children clinging to mother, show separation anxiety; John Jr.'s school phobia; the mother is anxious and depressed; the father stays away most of the time. *Related factors:* Recent hospitalization of the mother; marital strain; children's psychological needs not being recognized or met; poverty; loss of Ann from the family; dysfunctional communication—avoidance of important issues.

8. a. Teaching: Promoting of open communication and sharing about important issues in the family. Hold family conference and discuss what happened to Ann, reasons for her leaving, and that this will not happen to other children. Discuss mother's health problem—asking for member's understanding of both situations and how they feel things are working out now.
   b. Role modeling: Family nurse serves as role model to family when above issues are being discussed. Role model open communication, encouraging that each member's opinions, perceptions and feelings be shared.

9. a. Provides matrix necessary for individuals to grow and develop into healthy, functional, satisfied people.
   b. This function is central to the formation and continuity of the family unit (without this function being met, the basis for continuing as a family would become tenuous).
   c. No other societal system (institution) is sufficiently involved in fulfilling this task.
   or
   d. Through fulfillment of this function, the family teaches growing individuals how to relate warmly and closely to others.

10. Mutual respect for needs and concerns of family members.

11. All (a–d)

12. a. 4   b. 2   c. 1   d. 1, 2, and 3   e. 3   f. 1   g. 1 and 2   h. 4

13. The parental task relative to connectedness and separateness is: (1) to provide opportunities for family and children to be together, (2) to have a sense of belonging and familial cohesiveness, and (3) to promote identification so that the children will want to continue to be together and relate as a family. Concomitantly, the parents must provide opportunities for child to progressively have the freedom and autonomy to individuate, become self-directed, competent, and independent outside the family. The family, via parents, must achieve a satisfactory balance of separateness and connectedness, with both being present and properly emphasized.

14. b and c

15. Values or priorities (any two):

   a. They are responsive to particular interests and needs of individual family members.
   b. They prize individuality and uniqueness.
   c. They give respect and acceptance to members unconditionally.
   d. Members are encouraged to be independent, creative, and innovative.
   e. Family emphasizes separateness more than most families do.

CHAPTER 15 ANSWERS

1. *Discipline and punishment.* Father administers punishment; uses physical (corporal) means. Parents consider a child's wrongdoing as a reflection of the parents' failure to train their children adequately, and thus they feel threatened and disgraced by their children's misbehavior. The children certainly feel shame for the "loss of face" they have brought to the family. Hence the punishment is more than corporal, because the child being punished also feels the interpersonal sanctions of rejection, disapproval, and withdrawal of acceptance and love.

   Rewards. Parents did not express how they reward children, except that Mrs. Chin verbally expressed (in front of children?) that her children, by virtue of their achievements, brought great honor to the family. This indicates a pattern of verbal praise and acceptance.

   Moral training. Family is highly structured and has clear boundaries as to what was right and wrong. This was instilled through careful supervision when the children were young (assumed) and by strict discipline when children were assumed old enough to take on adult behaviors (stressing responsibility, self-sufficiency). When children were young they were given much unconditional love and affection from parents.

Autonomy and dependency. Children were pushed to be autonomous and responsible from school age on; dependency would not be reinforced positively during these same stages of development.

Initiative and creativity. There was no mention of how parents handled the issues of creativity and taking initiative.

Giving and receiving of love. The mother mentioned the extensive expression of affection to children when they were young, but that from preschool age on (gradually) and especially beginning at school age, children were affectively pushed away from parents. In fact, parents tried to remove themselves to some extent, so that they could maintain the position of respect vis-á-vis their children.

Training for age-appropriate behaviors. Little is mentioned except that social responsibility (home chores) and school achievement (intellectual development) were stressed and promoted in this family.

2. The child-rearing approach is very adaptive for this family. The parents obviously desire their children to have a better life than they have had. Through their socialization patterns they are training children to be self-sufficient, productive, success oriented, and independent.

3. The mother may have responsibility for the everyday matters, but the father definitely has ultimate responsibility to administer sanctions for misbehavior and thus ultimate responsibility for socialization. The socialization function is seen as a prime responsibility for this family.

4. There is little data from which to draw conclusions about how children are regarded in this family, but one senses that children are highly valued and are central to the aspirations and life goals of the parents.

5. The family is not acculturated to the dominant American culture. The parents are first-generation Chinese-American; they consider themselves part of the Chinese community, and the values and child-rearing practices they describe are congruent with the traditional values of the Chinese. (See Chapter 20 for more information on Asian-American families.) In describing the Chinese child-rearing practices, Sung (1967) verifies that the Chins' socialization patterns are indeed culturally patterned.

> Discipline is strict and punishment immediate in the Chinese household. . . . The Chinese child is taught that when he does wrong, it is not a personal matter between himself and his conscience; he brings disgrace and shame upon his family and loved one. . . . A Chinese baby may be cuddled and fondled, showered with kisses, and rocked to sleep in his mother's arms, but as the child grows older, the mother withdraws her expression of affection. . . . Chinese parents think they can maintain authority if they are careful to keep a certain distance from their children. . . . The father never tries to be a friend to his son, nor the mother a big sister to her daughter. . . . A parent is the authority that demands obedience, and authority must maintain its dignity. (pp. 168–171)

6. Family nursing diagnosis (select from chapter tables)

7. Family nursing interventions (select from chapter tables)

8. b

9. Any three:
   a. Language development
   b. Sociocultural norms and expectations (right and wrong)
   c. Sexual roles
   d. Individual initiative and creativity
   e. Acquisition of health concepts, attitudes, and behaviors

10. The child-rearing techniques used in a society are culturally patterned, and hence there is a tendency for families within a particular culture to rear their children similarly. These culturally patterned techniques for child rearing differ from culture to culture, as do the ideas and beliefs about the capabilities and needs

of children during their stages of growth and development. Moreover, because socialization patterns differ from one culture to the next, so will personality norms and broad expectations for personal behavior.

11. a and b   12. a

13. a. False   b. False   c. True

14. Several important societal changes/issues affecting child rearing (any three):

   a. Day care for children of working mothers and their feelings of guilt about working and dissatisfaction about the facilities available
   b. The growing number of single-parent families and how well this type of family can fulfill the socialization function
   c. The growing number of stepparent families and the complex parenting problems this family form faces
   d. Methods or approaches for assisting families where child abuse or neglect exists
   e. The emphasis on "unisex" upbringing and its consequences.
   f. Conflicting information from "experts" on how to raise children

15. Attitudes or beliefs that limit effectiveness include:

   a. Strong beliefs that orderliness, neatness, obedience, degree of restraint, or assertiveness are desirable and should be important to everyone.
   b. Rigid values and beliefs that hold that there is a "right and proper" way to raise children.
   c. Religious convictions suggesting that certain customs and techniques are "good" and others "bad" or "sinful."
   d. The belief that the mother or parents are solely responsible for their children's behavior (blaming the parents).
   e. The attitude that the family's situation is not relevant, or is less significant, whereas "what is best for the child" should be the focus (excluding consideration of the constraints of the family's environment)

❧CHAPTER 16 ANSWERS

1. Dietary practices, sleep and rest practices, exercise and recreational practices, therapeutic and recreational drug use, self-care practices, hygiene practices, use of medically-based interventions to date and use of complementary and alternative therapies.

2. Poor diet, lack of exercise, stress related to daughter's upcoming wedding and son's departure.

3. Health Maintenance, Altered

   Health Seeking Behaviors

   Therapeutic Regimen, Management of Individual, Ineffective

4. Change cooking practices to include high fiber, low fat, low calorie foods. Begin a program (10 minutes a day) of daily physical activity. Eliminate herbs and home remedies that may contain bowel stimulant components. If the diarrhea continues, suggest that Mrs. Diaz consult her doctor in case diagnostic tests or other screenings are needed. Suggest that the family members consider attending a support group such as Weight Watchers, or at least start taking regular walks together or with friends.

5. All but e. Physicians and health insurance companies have practically total control over when and where to hospitalize their patients.

6. a. Socioeconomic status (also can identify level of knowledge, which is correlated with the educational status and socioeconomic status).

b. Gender differences.

c. Ubiquity of health problem in community (certain prevalent symptoms or problems are accepted as being part of living and thus viewed as inevitable, unavoidable, and "normal").

d. Cultural differences.

7. **Orientations**   **Groups That Mentioned Orientation More Frequently**

a. Feeling-state orientation.   Chronically ill clinic patients (lower socioeconomic group).

b. Performance orientation.   Both groups.

c. Symptom orientation.   Medical student group (younger, presumably well, and of middle- and upper-middle-class background).

8. Koos's study found that as one descends the socioeconomic scale, a lack of recognition of, and indifference to, symptoms of illness increase. Also, when individuals failed to recognize behaviors as indicative of possible disease, they failed to seek medical care

9. Six behavior-specific cognitions and affect factors are identified in the model as the primary motivational mechanisms for engaging in health promoting behavior. They are: (1) perceived benefits of action, (2) perceived barriers to action, (3) perceived self-efficacy, (4) activity-related affect, (5) interpersonal influences, such as family and peers, and (6) situational influences. Individual characteristics and experiences (including the effect of prior related behavior and personal biological, psychological, and sociocultural factors) are thought to contribute to activating the above six behavior-specific cognitions and to directly impact on health promotion behaviors. Additionally, the likelihood of a person engaging in health-promoting behaviors is conceptualized as being influenced by a person's sense of commitment to a plan of action with specific strategies and the ability of the person to balance competing demands and preferences.

10. Pratt concluded that American families were generally inadequate in carrying out their health care function based on the following observations:

- Many homes were not suitable for maintaining health and controlling infectious disease and accidents (crowdedness, safety hazards, pollution, lack of infectious disease control).
- Widespread unhealthful personal and family health practices.
- Medication misuse widespread.
- Dependent and/or disabled family members not cared for or inadequately cared for.
- Insufficient or inappropriate use of health services found frequently.
- Level of health knowledge inadequate.
- Family's self-care practices not satisfactory. Reasons for this inadequacy are:
  - Basic structure of the health care system (health care provider dominated; bureaucratic structure).
  - Family structure itself (family needs to be more widely involved with community and husband-fathers need to be actively involved).
- Lack of access due to lack of health insurance.

11. c

12. Any four of the following:

a. Nutritional history (the three-day family food record).

b. Observe for variations among family members in terms of quality and quantity of diet. Does visual inspection indicate normal limits for height and weight?

c. Identify any special family food preferences (culturally, philosophically, or trend-based dietary food patterns).

d. Psychosocial aspects of mealtimes and eating (food used as a reward or punishment)?

e. Shopping, planning, food preparation characteristics.

13. a. Are the number of sleeping hours appropriate for the age of each of the family members?

b. Are there regular times established for children to go to bed and get up?

c. Do any members of the family have sleeping problems? If so, what kinds of problems?

14. a. What types of family recreation involving physical activity does your family engage in?

b. How frequently do you engage in physical activity as a family? Does everyone in the family participate?

c. What effect do you think physical activity has on your family's health?

15. All (a–e).

16. Acupuncture, acupressure, aromatherapy, biofeedback, healing touch, herbal supplements, home remedies, hypnotherapy, lifestyle diets, manipulation (chiropractic, osteopathy), massage, mediatation, megavitamins, nutritional supplements, pastoral/spiritual counseling, relaxation therapy

17. Caregiving needs and the potential for caregiver strain.

18. All intervention strategies could be effectively utilized in this situation.

19. a. Always follow the manufacturer's warning on cleaning solutions, powders, or chemically treated materials.
    b. Store toxic, abrasive, or caustic substances properly and out of the reach of young children.
    c. Do not save and re-use old prescribed medicines.

20. Any four of the following:
    a. Importance of fluoride for increasing resistance of tooth to decay.
    b. Importance of brushing and flossing teeth (and use of an effective method of brushing).
    c. Role of carbohydrates (starches and sugars) in producing dental caries.
    d. Importance of regular dental examinations and cleaning of teeth.
    e. Early treatment of dental caries and treatment of major orthodontic problems.

21. a, b, and c

22. Asking about specific diseases (both genetically based and environmentally related diseases) that family members or their parents or grandparents might have had.

🐝 CHAPTER 17 ANSWERS

1. Short-term stressors impinging on the family:

    Husband's unemployment
    Being on welfare and then the threat of termination
    Ann's loss (removal from the home)
    Ruby's recent ill health, hospitalization, and convalescence
    Ruby's depression and suicidal thoughts

    Long-term stressors impinging on the family:

    The perceived interference of John's mother
    Emotional distance and lack of communication in family and especially within marital relationship
    Continual geographical movement, from one community to the next, so that no stable and sufficient social network is established
    Husband's minimal participation in family life and his excessive and frequent drinking bouts

    Family strengths:

    Presence of social support system, although small: receiving help from mental health clinic, Mrs. Law, neighbor
    Ruby's caring for and commitment to children
    Parents' staying together and father's interest in Lisa and his potential of greater participation in family life
    Parents' motivation to find employment, be financially self-sufficient
    Priscilla's interest in and ability for child care

2. The parents' ability to act based on objective and realistic definition of their situation is limited. In terms of the interference of John's mother, they perceived events as problems over which they had no control. They see the problem being John's mother's behavior, rather than a situation in which they need to communicate with each other and John's mother in order to define problems and identify a mutually satisfactory way

of handling the situation. Data do not reveal the parents' perception of why Ann was removed or why welfare was terminated. Ruby personally distorts the parenting situation, feeling that her children did well without her and did not wish her back.

3. a. Functional coping strategies:

    No evidence of the use of some of the internal coping strategies related to family's inner resources such as greater family reliance on themselves, increased sharing of feelings and thoughts, shared activities, and controlling the meaning of the stressors.

    Family (Ruby and then family) did seek a key support system when problems reached crisis proportions—the mental health clinic. The neighbor, Mrs. Law, has assisted family. But the family, because of its continual moving, has not developed an adequate social support network.

    b. Dysfunctional coping strategies:

    Use of spousal withdrawal—both spouses do not communicate openly with each other; husband withdraws from family physically and through his drinking.

    Use of denial as to the family's real problems. They have seen their major family problem as John's "meddling mother." Use of family myth around this source of conflict was apparent. The family myth, more specifically, has been that "we are a happy family as long as John's mother stays away."

4. The family's level of adaptation is poor. The process of adaptation over time has moved downward because of the recurrent and new stressors and the ineffective way that the family has addressed their stressful situations.

5. Disabled family coping—as manifested by the preponderant use of dysfunctional coping strategies, such as the husband's staying away and drinking, rather than facing the problems; the parents' not discussing their problems/concerns with each other and with the children (especially the older children), and the use of the family myth

6. Family nursing interventions addressing the above family nursing diagnosis include:

    *   Assist the family to more effectively cope with their stressful situation by: enhancing family's social system (bringing informal social system—Mrs. Law and perhaps other neighbors, friends, family—together with parents to foster support); encourage family or parents to continue to see counselor at mental health clinic and encourage the parents to discuss with counselor ways to communicate and interact with husband's mother; refer parents to welfare worker to discuss loss of benefits; and refer parents to protective services to discuss Ann's removal from the home.

    *   Facilitate family communication and cohesion. Bring family members (parents and children) together to foster sharing of feelings and thoughts. Encourage honest, open communication between family members.

    *   Help parents explore their perceptions of their stressful situation (their various stressors) and what they see needs to be done. Help them to see their strengths/resources and reframe their problems and distress so that they are seen as more manageable, comprehensible, and in a more realistic and positive light. Particularly encourage Mr. Nichols to get involved with the solutions—rather than withdrawing.

7. a   8. b, c, and e

9. a. 7   b. 1   c. 6   d. 3   e. 5   f. 4   g. 2

10. False   11. True   12. True   13. b   14. c

15. All are stressful to different degrees (see Table 17–2)

16. Internal coping strategies (two):

    a. *Role flexibility.* Ability of family members to adapt by shifting roles as needed.
    b. *Family group reliance.* The tighter structure and control over subsystems, greater degree of family organization and cohesiveness
    c. *Use of humor.* Improves attitude toward problems and gives some respite and lightness to a stressful situation.

d. *Greater sharing together.* Increasing family efforts to converse about feelings and thoughts, participate in family activities.

e. *Normalizing.* When confronted with a long-term stressor, parents normalize family life to minimize family disruption from stressor.

f. *Controlling the meaning of the problem.* Interpreting or defining a change or event realistically, objectively (where cognitive mastery is involved). Reframing the situation more positively.

g. *Joint problem solving.* The family is able to jointly discuss a problem, search for a solution, and reach a consensus.

External Coping Strategies (two)

a. *Seeking information.* Pertinent information sought to deal with issue/problem at hand.

b. *Maintaining active linkages with broader community.* This is a more general lifestyle characterization, where family members have open boundaries and continually participate and involve themselves in community organizations and activities.

c. *Seeking and using social support systems.* Social support systems function to provide support and assistance either more generally or on an as-needed basis. These social support systems are composed of friends, extended family, employers, employees, neighbors, groups (including mutual aid groups), organizations, and professional persons and agencies.

d. *Seeking spiritual supports.* This type of support includes engaging in prayer, rituals, belief in God and attending church, temple, mosque or other religious facility together as a family.

17. Dysfunctional family adaptive strategies (any four):

a. *Spouse/partner violence.* In response to pent-up frustrations in marital relationship and hostility of marital partners, one spouse attacks the other.

b. *Child abuse.* Physical violence, usually by one or both parents, against one or more of their children.

c. *Scapegoating.* Selecting one or more family members to be the identified family problem. Negatively labeling and imposing unhealthy exploitative role on to the scapegoat.

d. *Use of threat.* By use of threat or ostracism, expulsion or self-destructive acts, family keeps all its members in conformity. "Separateness" actions by individuals are thus curtailed.

e. *Triangling.* Introduction of a third member into a stressful dyadic relationship when stress level reaches point where stress reduction is sought. This is exploitative of third member and does not confront the problem in the relationship.

f. *The family myth.* Beliefs developed in family about itself which have themes of wish fulfillment. These tend to hide real problems and limit family's alternatives and problem-solving resources.

g. *Pseudomutuality.* Maintaining pseudo or false closeness. Family members have difficulty in expressing affection and closeness. As a result, they build up all sorts of customs and rituals that structure family members' responses and establish a facade of closeness and solidarity.

h. *Authoritarianism.* This is a long-term adaptive response to deal with feelings of powerlessness and dependency. One member becomes the dominator and the others the subordinates. All "lose" in this type of family structure, because there is no opportunity provided to learn the value of negotiation, discussion, and how to relate effectively with others and yet be autonomous.

18. b and d

19. a. E   b. D   c. D   d. E   e. E   f. D   g. D   h. E   i. F   j. F   k. F   l. F

20. b, c, and d   21. Elder neglect

🌿 CHAPTER 18 ANSWERS

1. Although we would have to validate who is considered "the family," it is clear that the extended family is very important and probably considered the family. In that family we know that there is the mother and her two children and their families. Lupe Lopez apparently has other children about whom we have no

information. The ethnic assessment guidelines in Table 8–6 were used to gather the following information:

- Ethnic/racial identity: Puerto Rican
- Language: Prefers to speak Spanish. They speak little English, although Jorge's daughters are quicky learning to speak English in school. Language proficiency of Lupe Lopez is unknown, although one would expect that her English proficiency would be limited due to being part of the older generation.
- Place of birth and immigration history: Puerto Rico. Jorge Lopez's family came from Puerto Rico one year ago and settled in New York City. Unknown about the immigration history of the mother.
- Geographical mobility: Only the above immigration history is known.
- Ethnic group affiliation, neighborhood affiliation, home appearance, family life transitions or family's view on the extent to which they have been accepted by community or affected by discrimination: None of this information is known; typically Puerto Ricans live in segregated neighborhoods in New York City and face job discrimination.
- Cultural health beliefs and practices: Largely unknown, but we do know that the extended family do not believe Lupe has diabetes. They believe she has "sugar," a vernacular label for diabetes and a mental illness ("nervios") caused by family conflicts in home. Is this a distrust or misunderstanding in Western medicine or medical terminology? Jorge expressed that the family wants to take Lupe home and consult the family, then a *yerbero* (herbalist), then a spiritualist (an *espiritista* or *santero*). Hence the family uses folk practitioners. When Puerto Rican families believe the health problem is psychiatric, they traditionally will consult a *santero*. An *espiritista* is very similar to a *santero*. These are persons who obtain their knowledge from spirits and treat illness according to the instructions of the spirits. Herbs, lotions, creams, and massage are also often used (Spector, 2000).

  Regarding the family's social class status, Jorge's family is part of the lower class—a poor working family. Both parents work, but at minimally unskilled jobs. Economically they must be struggling since Jorge works double shifts to make ends meet. Education: Unknown, except that the teenage daughters attend school.

2. In addition to referring to the assessment areas for data which is missing, information we would like to have includes: Who constitutes the family? It would be important to complete a family genogram if possible to obtain this information. Family support is a prime way in which Puerto Rican family members and families cope with health problems. Therefore, we need to know who is in the family, what roles they play (particularly in decision making), and what social support is available. In particular, it would be important to ask about the family's environment—where they live and its adequacy. We also need to explore further the family's beliefs about Mrs. Lopez's health problem and their perceptions about the symptoms and etiology of the problem. We need to understand the family's perspective on why they think the problem is *nervios*, rather than diabetes and what they say has been explained to them by the doctors treating Mrs. Lopez.

3. Culturally-based family nursing interventions include:

- Maintain respectful, friendly, and warm interactions with family, realizing that Mrs. Lopez probably feels quite isolated in the hospital and needs to have family members there to support her.
- Being sensitive to the Latino family structure where the extended family is very important and the adult men usually have more authority. Jorge Lopez seems to be the dominant person in his family. This is based on his interactions with his family and the nurse (he acted as family spokesperson).
- Being sensitive to the family's health beliefs and use of folk practitioners. Explain that diabetes is also called "sugar" in the Caribbean. After asking further questions of the family regarding their beliefs about Mrs. Lopez's illness and why they believe it is "sugar" and *"nervios,"* as well as asking what they understood the doctor(s) to tell them about diabetes, the medical information they received should be clarified. The nurse would also want to discuss the family's perceptions and beliefs with Mrs. Lopez's doctor. The nurse should encourage the family to not take Mrs. Lopez home, but to wait and see the doctor and then to ask him further questions to clarify his diagnosis and recommendations for treatment. If they believe that stress from family conflict caused the illness, then perhaps using both systems of care simultaneously may be helpful and may make the Western medical regime more acceptable to the family. Using certain herbs may be fine and not harmful. Using a *santero* or *espiritista* may help

reduce Mrs. Lopez's stress—which could have been a trigger for the disease. By the nurse acknowledging that this is the family's beliefs and plans, would lend acceptability and respect for the family's perspectives and wishes. If the family decides to use both systems of care, the physician (or another health professional) would need to check with the folk practitioner or family about what she or he was planning to do. If herbs are recommended, one would need to make sure these do not interact negatively with the diabetic medication.

In the African-American literature a description of folk beliefs about "sugar" (diabetes) was found. In the Caribbean region, some families may still hold the following folk beliefs about "sugar" (we would have to validate what the family beliefs were). It is known to have a familial linkage, to be brought on by eating starchy, greasy foods and excessive worry about the family and work-related stresses. Most patients will not immediately consult a physician when the typical symptoms of diabetes appear (thirst, weight loss, polyuria). They will try to make the proper dietary changes and use the right potions and herbs (often prescribed by a folk practitioner), as well as regain harmony with the family and other relations (Matthews, 1988). Fishman et al., (1998) suggest that if the health provider explains to the family that the patient's blood sugar is too high and a medicine is needed, that the patient and family more readily accept the treatment. The medicine is seen as a "bittering" agent to lower the sugar content. Patients may also want to use a variety of herbal teas, garlic, and lemon juice as folk or home remedies. Some elderly fear the medicine will be too powerful on them and create a dependency. This fear is exacerbated by telling them they will be diabetic for life and will need the medicine forever.

4. Mexican-American (most numerous, about 60 percent), Central and South American, Cuban, Puerto Rican.

5. List any three:
   a. Language differences
   b. Religious differences
   c. Social class differences (large numbers of peasant agricultural workers and laborers migrated)
   d. American discriminatory and segregation practices
   e. Mexican-American closeness with Mexico, so that Latinos can cross back and forth frequently. This consequently strengthens their ties to Mexico and reduces their need to become involved with some of the institutions within the United States.

6. False (Familism refers to Latinos' deep identifications with and commitment to their families.)

7. True

8. False (Evidence shows that the father–husband probably never did hold absolute power as a normative situation. Although male primary authority is declining, most Mexican-American families are still male dominant.)

9. True   10. a, b, and d

11.

Area	Traditional Latino Values
Family	Latinos see themselves as members of families first, as individuals second.
Work	Work is seen as a means (a necessity) in order to live. Other life experiences (social and emotional experiences) are valued more than work.
Materialism	Possession of goods and objects are necessary for living, not ends in themselves. Status and prestige are more likely derived from ability to intellectually and emotionally experience things. Social relationships and family are more important than accumulation of wealth.
Time and punctuality	Time is to be enjoyed. Punctuality does not have the moral overtones it does in American society.
Interpersonal relationships	Hispanic-Americans value the use of diplomacy and tactfulness. They are concerned about showing respect and are more elaborate, indirect, and emotionally expressive in their communications.

12. False (The most profound change is the decline of the husband's– father's primary authority and the increase in egalitarianism.)

13. False (Two major child-rearing patterns are that socialization is distinctly gender role related and that children are taught to respect father, older persons, and authority figures.)

14. False (The ethic of reciprocity has to do with the system of mutual obligation, support, and assistance within the extended family.)

15. 1. a   2. d   3. f   4. b   5. c   6. e

16. a. *Mal de ojo*   d. *Caida de la mollera*
    b. Mental illness   e. *Mal puesto*
    c. *Empacho*   f. *Susto*

17. a. A   b. A   c. B   d. B   e. B   f. A

18. Family coping strategies: Seeking social support from extended family and seeking spiritual support. Practice implications:

    a. If culturally derived family coping strategies are not being used, explore possible use with family.
    b. Support family's coping strategies.
    c. If family does not have primary culturally patterned coping strategies available and is experiencing frustration because they are not available, attempt to assist family to obtain needed support/assistance. Also, the family should be identified as at higher risk for adaptation problems.

❦ CHAPTER 19 ANSWERS

1. The family form—the extended family (mother, her three daughters, and her mother) is a common family form among black Americans, especially when scarce resources and services need to be shared. Ann, the grandmother, can provide the needed child supervision and homework, while the mother works full time. We don't know if the family has any other source of income besides the mother's wages, but, in any case, the income is probably marginal and this form of family enables them to "get by," in addition to providing the love and support they need. There may be other members of the extended family who do not live in the same household, but are members of the extended family. Another common pattern is the relationship of the father with "his girls." In recent research, it has been found that many fathers remain connected to their children, even though they are not in the home and may have never been married to the children's mother. Another common family pattern deals with socialization of the children. They are obviously loved and valued. The mother and grandmother are concerned that as the children get older that they are losing control of them. Poor families find that as children get older, it becomes increasingly futile to keep children away from the street and from poor role models and relationships. They often feel powerless to change the direction of their children's lives. But, in this case, mother and grandmother are reaching out for help—which is commendable. Another common family pattern is the mother's (and presumably the grandmother's) reliance on the church and God. This is a vital and central coping pattern found in African-American families.

2. The literature discusses the past and present problems that black families had or have, particularly black families who are poor and have to go to public clinics (of which the school clinic is one). Their experiences have often been negative: the clinics are rushed, the providers are impersonal, disrespectful and rude, hospitals and clinics sometimes deny services, and they are made to feel unimportant or degraded because they don't have insurance or are on welfare or are black. With this history, it is understandable that African-Americans often feel discomfort and mistrust when receiving services from a health facility they have never been to. They simply don't know how they will be received. They also may feel that Mrs. Evans is prying when asking about the extended family and the family's history. They may worry that she may prejudge their family lifestyle. Because Mrs. Evans and Ann, the grandmother, are about the same age and generation, this probably will help lessen the racial distance.

3. Because this is a school-based clinic and the nurse functions as both a school nurse and a nurse practitioner, she has a broadened role in terms of working with this family. First, Mrs. Evans wants to find out what

Martha's perceptions and concerns are. We know nothing about what she thinks or wants. In addition, Mrs. Evans plans to do a brief family assessment—including a family genogram (to find out who is in the extended family) and a brief cultural assessment. Because the setting is a high school, Martha's problems are frequently encountered ones. In addition to providing the usual physical history and examination, pregnancy testing, and birth control pills if needed, one of the ways the school nurse practitioner helps families, such as this one, is by having peer support groups (led by Mrs. Evans and the school psychologist) for girls who are struggling with the kind of developmental and relationship problems that Martha is having. Another role of Mrs. Evans is to work closely with the school counselor and a neighborhood mental health clinic. If the family were interested in talking together about their concerns with a counselor, a referral to the clinic might be appropriate. Trying to include the father into the picture would be appropriate. Often, because child care and supervision are seen as female roles, fathers are often not involved, especially when they won't live in the same household. They, however, can be very important resources if given encouragement. Mrs. Evans could also plan times for Martha (and family if wished) to come back and see her about how they are coping with the concerns they have.

4. a. True   b. False   c. True   d. False   e. True   f. False

5. All (a–d)

6. a. 2
   b. 1
   c. 1, 2, and 3
   d. 3
   e. 1 and 2
   f. 3
   g. 1, 2, and 3
   h. 1, 2, and 3
   i. 4
   j. 4
   k. 1, 2, and 3
   l. 1
   m. 3

7. b and e   8. a, b, c, and d   9. b

10. Conjure doctors and midwives or grannies

11. a. Most basic is to abandon stereotypes and be informed and knowledgeable about African-American families and their cultural background.
    b. Who is in the family must be identified by the family. Family nurses should incorporate these family members into their assessment and interventions.
    c. Because African-American families typically have strong bonds between parent and child and with kin and long-time friends, assessment of the characteristics of these important social networks is recommended, as well as assisting families to effectively use these social support resources.
    d. Assisting poor families with pressing health-related problems first to free them to attend to their health problems.
    e. Promoting family-centered health regimens and programs.
    f. Realizing the meaning of black clients' initial responses to new health care facilities and/or health providers, and responding in client interactions with empathy, sensitivity, respect, and feelings of concern.
    g. Emphasizing family strengths and family empowerment.

CHAPTER 20 ANSWERS

1. Key assessment areas (from Table 20–3):

   a. Language(s) spoken: English is assumed since family has been here for several generations.
   b. Length of time lived in the United States: The family has lived here since 1924. Like many Japanese-Americans, this family moved here many decades ago.
   c. Ethnic identity: We do not know how the family would identify themselves (data is missing). We can assume that there may be differences in identification depending on the generation.
   d. Use of traditional healing methods. This is not mentioned in vignette. It is suggested that this information be obtained, asking if the family has tried any herbs or other ways to help heal Helen's fracture. The home health nurse should approach this issue respectfully and with an accepting manner, so that the family does not feel that remedies that they may be additionally using are not looked down upon and seen as inferior.

The home health nurse would also want to find out who is in the family. From the vignette, it sounds like the extended family (i.e., Helen's three children and their respective nuclear families), with Helen living with Bill and his family and the sisters and their families living in their own separate households.

2. The prominent family coping strategy is use of extended family social support (and pulling together—greater cohesiveness—during times of need and adversity). Evidence cited: (1) Helen moves in with her son and his family after husband dies; (2) the caregiving arrangements that were made, where three children of Helen and Bill's wife all share in the care of Helen.

3. a. Familism: The importance and centrality of the family are seen in both the way in which the family jointly is caring for Helen and the way that Bill consults with the family to arrange home health care.

   b. Filial piety: The Ogawa family holds to a strong value and sense of duty for their parents and to care for elderly family members.

   c. Respect for the elderly: The family members' caregiving also reflects respect for elderly parent.

   d. Interdependence and reciprocity: The ethic of reciprocity and collective obligation is seen in the family's pattern of caregiving.

   e. Strong work ethic: All adult children work, and Helen worked up until the day she fractured her hip.

4. With this family the following interventions by a home health nurse are appropriate:

   a. When the family needs to make health decision, being sensitive to whom in the extended family is the decision-maker(s) and communicating with that person(s)

   b. Providing emotional support to the adult family members for their caregiving; commending them for their concerned and loving care of their mother/mother-in-law.

   c. Providing family caregivers with education on ADLs, transfers, diet, and medical regime

   d. Making referrals: The family may need information on ethnically appropriate community resources for Helen or family. The home health nurse should investigate what is available and culturally appropriate and refer the family as needed.

5. Asian-Americans, also called Asian and Pacific Islanders, are people from countries and cultures in Asia, the Indian subcontinent, and the Pacific Ocean islands, including Somoa and Hawaii. The three largest Asian-American population groups in the United States are Chinese-Americans, Filipino-Americans, and Japanese-Americans (Asian Indians outnumber Korean- and Vietnamese-Americans).

6. Changing demographic pattern: Asian-Americans are proportionally the fastest-growing ethnic minority group in the United States. Current population figures: Asian-Americans constitute 4 percent of the U.S. population.

7. All (a–c)

8. Refer to Table 20–2. Depending on the values selected, many practice implications can be identified.

9. The value clash refers to the clash between traditional (Eastern) and modern (Western) values. Cultural conflicts are observed between parents and children. Children are socialized in U.S. schools to be independent, individualistic, and egalitarian in relationships. Immigrant parents were socialized in their native country to be deferent, interdependent, respectful of authority and parents, and familistic. Thus, conflict often ensues between the two generations.

10. b and c   11. a, b, and c   12. a, c, and d   13. b, c, d, f, h, and i   14. d

15. Any of these guidelines are appropriate:
    - Be sensitive to family roles and expectations (e.g., family hierarchy).
    - Include relevant family members in health decisions.
    - Avoid direct confrontation with family.
    - Be sensitive to possible stigma and shame felt by family members when chronic illness and/or mental disorder is(are) present.
    - Do not interfere with family using Eastern medicine unless it is detrimental or in conflict with Western medical regimen.
    - Aid family in addressing their environmental stresses and problems, such as acting as advocate, coordinator, and referral agent for needed services.
    - Individualize care, and do not come with preconceptions of what an Asian-American family is like.

GLOSSARY OF TERMS

Acculturation A sociocultural process whereby exposure of persons from one cultural group to another culture makes change in both cultures, although the direction of change is greater in those persons moving to the host culture.

Adaptation A process of managing the demands of stressors through the use of resources, coping, and problem-solving strategies.

Affective function One of family functions, dealing with the meeting of psychological needs of family members.

Anticipatory guidance Teaching that provides the family with information on what to expect with respect to a future event, a potential problem/issue, or a child's next developmental phase.

Assimilation A sociocultural process in which persons from one culture move to another culture and take on the attributes of the host culture.

Beliefs The attitudes, explanations, premises, constructs, assumptions, preferences, and values from which we construct our lives and intermingle them with the lives of others.

Biculturalism Signifies participation of persons in two cultural systems and often requires two sets of behavior and ways of thinking.

Binuclear family The postdivorced family in which the child is a member of two nuclear families (maternal and paternal). Typically, the children live primarily with the mother and her husband (the children's stepparent), but also live part time with their natural father and his family. Thus, the children are members of two families.

Bonding A relatively enduring unique emotional tie between two specific persons.

Boundaries The interface or point of contact between the system and other systems, that is, between the system and its subsystems and suprasystems.

Calgary Family Intervention Model An organizing framework for conceptualizing the relationship between families and nurses that helps change occur and healing to begin. The model highlights the family–nurse relationship by focusing on the intersection between family member functioning and interventions offered by the nurse.

Case management A system, a clinical decision-making process, a technology, a role, and a service used by health care providers to manage patients and their health care needs.

Changing life cycle One of the developmental family frameworks that describes three phases of family life; the emerging family, the solidifying family, and the reconstituting family.

Channels In communication theory, this refers to routes of the message being communicated.

Closed system Characteristic of a system that describes each element of the system as a self-contained unit, not dependent on continual environmental interchange for its survival.

Coalitions In families, these are either temporary, issue-based alliances, or long-term alliances made to offset the dominance of one or more other family members.

Cohabiting family The nonmarital heterosexual cohabiting family refers to a family created when an unmarried heterosexual couple lives together.

Collaboration Collaboration is a process of shared planning and action over time with joint responsibility for the outcomes and the ability to work together for common goals using problem-solving techniques.

Communication The process of sending and receiving messages between human beings. Communication includes both content and instruction dimensions and feedback loops, and can be digital and analogic.

Complementary communication One interactant's behavior supplements the other interactant's behavior.

Complementary relationships Relationships in which the two persons exhibit contrasting behavior; one person is the leading, dominant personality and decision maker

649

while the partner is subservient and a follower in that relationship.

Concept   A word or phrase that summarizes the essential characteristics or qualities of a phenomenon.

Conceptual model   A set of relatively abstract and general concepts and propositions that describe or link the concepts together to form a conceptual whole.

Connectedness   Degree of closeness and intimacy of family members.

Consultation   A process of interaction between two professional persons—the consultant, who is a specialist, and the consultee, who invokes the consultant's help. The consultant's role is often to provide problem-solving assistance with clinical issues.

Content   In communication, this refers to what is actually said, that is, the verbal message or the literal meaning of the message.

Contracting   An intervention activity in which a working agreement made between two or more parties, such as between a family and a nurse or between parents and a child, is completed. The agreements cover the areas of patient goals, length of the contract, patient responsibilities (commitments), and health care team members' responsibilities, steps toward meeting the goals, and rewards for meeting goals.

Coordination   An intervention whose goal is to ensure that there is no duplication of services to the client and that the client receives comprehensive, continuous care, and such services are communicated well to the client and between all care providers.

Coping   Cognitive and behavioral problem-solving efforts by an individual faced with demands highly relevant to his or her welfare.

Counseling   A process that seeks to help families and their members address, resolve, and effectively cope with their problems, and to utilize their competencies and other resources more fully.

Critical theory   A perspective closely associated with a participatory research paradigm and feminist theory. The focus is on questioning current ideologies, and seeking social justice and freedom from oppression for all persons. Research grounded in critical theory may be termed social action research.

Cross-cultural/transcultural approach   This approach to practice is borrowed from anthropology. It provides a broad comparative picture of human nature and human behavior and is the basis for transcultural nursing.

Cultural empathy   An attribute of a culturally competent practitioner whereby the practitioner is able to communicate an understanding of a client's culture.

Cultural imposition   The imposing of one's own cultural beliefs and practices on someone from another culture.

Cultural relativism   Having the perspective that holds that cultures are neither inferior nor superior to one another and that there is no single scale for measuring the value of a culture.

Cultural shock   A condition in which a person, in response to an environment so altered that meaningful objects and experiences have been replaced by those from a different culture, feels confused and lost.

Culturally competent care   Involves a continuous process of awareness, knowledge, skill, interaction, and sensitivity in working with clients. In addition, it involves the adaptation or tailoring of care in a manner that is congruent with the client's culture.

Culture   Those sets of shared world views and adaptive behaviors derived from simultaneous membership in a variety of contexts (e.g., national origin, religion, age, gender, and social class status).

Cybernetics   A science that deals with communication and control theory.

Developmental theory   A framework that focuses on the longitudinal career of the family, often called the family career or family life cycle. This theoretical approach seeks to explain change in the family system, including changes in interactions and relationships among family members that occur over time.

Differentiation   The family's propensity to evolve and grow so that as growth takes place the system becomes more complex, articulate, and discriminate.

Discharge planning   The process of planning and implementing actions that will ensure a smooth transition of the client from one health care environment to another or to the home setting.

Dual-earner family   A nuclear family in which either parents or adult members work either full or part time.

Dysfunctional communication   Communication characterized by assumptions, unclear expression of feelings, judgmental expressions, inability to define needs, and incongruent communication.

Ecological perspective   This approach describes interacting systems and their relationships and effects on one another and on the entire system.

Ethclass   Ethclass is the result of the interplay of the family's ethnic and social class backgrounds.

Ethnic families   Families that are classified as belonging to ethnic or cultural groups other than white ethnic groups.

Ethnicity   A common ancestry, a shared social and cultural history and national origin.

Ethnocentrism   Implies the lack of cultural relativism, the holding of the belief that one's own way of believing and behaving is the most preferable and correct one.

Extended family   The nuclear family and other related (by blood) persons, who are most commonly members of the family of orientation of one of the nuclear family mates. These are "kin" and may include grandparents, aunts, uncles, nephews, nieces, and cousins.

Family   Two or more persons who are joined together by bonds of sharing and emotional closeness and who identify themselves as being part of a family.

Family adaptation   A process in which families engage in direct responses to the extensive demands of a stressor(s) and realize that systemic changes are needed within the family unit, to restore family stability and well-being. Also defined as an outcome or the family's level of family functioning.

Family career or family life cycle   The changes in interactions and relationships that occur among family members over time.

Family coherence   A key natural resistance resource in individuals and families; a dispositional quality or global orientation in which a person or family feels a sense of confidence that they can meet the demands confronting them. This sense promotes health and well-being.

Family communication   A symbolic, transactional process of creating and sharing meanings in the family; the processing of information within the family or its subsystems.

Family coping   A family group level of coping; an active process where the family utilizes existing family resources and either uses previous ways of coping or develops new behaviors to deal with stressors/ demands.

Family crisis   A continuous condition of disruptiveness, disorganization, or incapacitation in the family system. A crisis results when a family's current resources and adaptive strategies are not effective in handling the stressor(s).

Family developmental tasks   Growth responsibilities that must be achieved by a family during each stage of its development so as to meet its biological requirements, its cultural imperatives, and its own aspirations and values.

Family functions   The five family purposes that all family members must fulfill in order for the family to function effectively. The five functions are the family affective function, the family socialization and social placement function, the health care function, the reproductive function, and the economic function.

Family genogram   A diagram that delineates the family constellation or family tree, used as primary assessment tool in working with families.

Family health   In the family literature, family health is most often conceptualized as family functioning or family adaptation. It also connotes family wellness.

Family life spiral   A developmental model that incorporates overlapping developmental tasks of the individual family member on the developmental tasks of each generation in the family.

Family nursing practice   The provision of care to families and family members in health and illness situations.

Family nursing process   Nursing process completed with the nurse conceptualizing the family, not the individual, as the unit of care.

Family of orientation   The family unit into which a person is born. Also referred to as the family of origin.

Family perceptions   The interpretations family members singularly or collectively make of their experiences.

Family roles   These are formal (overt) and informal (covert) clusters of behaviors associated with different positions in the family. Formal roles are explicit within the family structure and informal roles are often not obvious, but often serve to maintain the family" equilibrium.

Family rules   The specific regulations the family maintains as to what is acceptable behavior and what is not.

Family social sciences   A group of theories developed from sociology, psychology, and anthropology that are interested in the study of families.

Family stage marker   Describes a particular life event (e.g., marriage, the birth of the first child) in the family that precipitated each stage of the family life cycle. These markers demand change and new adaptation by the family.

Family stages   An interval of time in which the structure and interaction of role relationships in the family are qualitatively and quantitatively distinct from other periods.

Family strengths   Resources, traits, and abilities within the family that assist the family to adapt and balance their lives in the midst of change.

Family stressors   Precipitating stress-producing agents that are interpersonal (inside or outside the family), environmental, economic, or sociocultural events or experiences.

Family structure   How the inner dimensions of the family are organized. The four structural inner dimensions are family power and decision-making, role, values, and communications.

Family therapy theories   A group of theories which are a blend of family social science theories and practice theories. Family therapy theories explain dynamics in troubled families, as well as suggest guidelines to assist troubled families to change in positive directions.

Family transition   The developmental tasks or milestones that the family achieves in each developmental stage of the family life cycle. These family transitions are considered "normal" and they carry implications for individual members who must critically assess their own well-being and alter their role functions and expectations to meet the changing developmental tasks of the family over the life course.

Family values   A system of ideas, attitudes, and beliefs about the worth of an entity or concept that consciously and unconsciously bind together the members of a family in a common culture.

Family violence   "Any act or omission by persons who are cohabitating that results in serious injury (physical or emotional harm) to other members of the family" (Wallace, 1996, p. 3).

Feedback   The process by which a system monitors the internal and environmental responses to its behavior (output) and accommodates or adjusts itself accordingly.

First-order change   A specific kind of change in which the system itself remains unchanged while its parts undergo some type of change.

Functional communication   The clear, direct transmission and reception of both the content and instruction level of any message, and the congruency between the content and instruction levels.

Gay and lesbian family   A family in which two or more people share a same-sex orientation or the presence of at least one lesbian or gay adult rearing a child.

General systems theory   A major theory that constitutes a way of explaining a unit such as the family as it relates to and interacts with other systems. It is an organizational theory that is concerned with studying and describing the way things interrelate together rather than with analyzing the things themselves.

Health Belief Model   A theoretical model used to explain preventive health actions, that is, strategies for avoiding the negatively valued regions of illness and disease that are undertaken by individuals.

Health hazard appraisal tool   On a health hazard appraisal tool, the total risks to a client are estimated by identifying the average risk for the major causes of disease/death according to the client's own age, sex, and racial group.

Health Promotion Model   A theoretical model used to explain the behavior-specific cognitions and affect that serve as the primary motivators of health-promoting behaviors.

Healthy People 2000, 2010   These publications represent national initiatives undertaken by the U.S. Department of Health and Human Services to establish goals and priorities to improve the health of the nation.

Holism or nonsummativity   A fundamental gestalt concept that characterizes a system by its property of wholeness (or *nonsummativity*) (e.g., "The whole is greater than the sum of its parts").

Home territory   An area where the family has relatively more freedom of behavior and a sense of control and power over both the area and its members. There are both spatial (physical) and behavioral dimensions of territoriality.

Homeostasis   A mechanism and outcome of system self-regulation that assists the system to balance and control input and output via feedback loops. The system is in balance, a steady state, or equilibrium.

Indigenous health care system   The lay health care system—a system of health care that is present in the culture. It refers to cultural health care systems that are non-Western, nonscientific in their orientation.

Input   Energy, matter, and information that the system receives.

Instruction   In communication, this refers to the dimension of the communication that conveys the intent or emotional meaning of the message

Interconnectedness   A characteristic of systems asserting that all actions and behaviors within the system are not isolated from the environment in which they occur.

Kin   The relatives of a person. Primary kin are the relatives from the immediate family of origin; parents and children. Secondary kin are aunts, uncles, nephews, nieces, and cousins.

Macrosystems   In the case of families, this refers to the network of systems that interact with the family system (e.g., educational systems, and work systems).

Microsystems   In the case of families, these are the behavioral settings or the immediate physical contexts in which face-to-face encounters occur between family members.

Modalities   As used in communication theory, this refers to the way communication occurs. Examples of communication modalities include spoken (oral/ aural) language, written language, through media such as television or the Internet, or manually (sign language).

Mutual nurturance   A basic commitment of family members to each other and to a nurturing, emotionally satisfying intimate familial relationship.

NANDA   North American Nursing Diagnosis Association. A nursing organization that has been pivotal in developing a diagnostic language for nurses to use to label and describe patient problems.

Need–response patterns This concept explains the extent to which family's members perceive the needs of the other members and try to meet family members' needs

NIC Nursing Intervention Classification. A taxonomy of nursing interventions that has been developed and standardized by a team of nurses from the University of Iowa.

NOC Nursing Outcomes Classification. A classification of outcomes associated with nursing diagnoses and nursing interventions that has been researched and developed by team of nurses from the University of Iowa.

Norms Patterns of behavior considered to be right in a given society and, as such, are based on the family's value system.

Nuclear (conjugal) family The family of marriage, parenthood, or procreation. It is composed of a husband, wife, and their immediate children—natural, adopted, and/ or both.

Nursing metaparadigm A metaparadigm is the global perspective of a discipline. The four concepts comprising the metaparadigm for nursing are person, environment, health, and nursing, along with propositions explaining the relationships among the four metaparadigm concepts.

Omaha System A diagnostic classification system of client problems developed by the Visiting Nurse Association of Omaha. There are three components of the Omaha System: problem classification scheme, intervention scheme, and problem rating scale for outcomes.

Open System Characteristic of a system that interacts with its environment by receiving input and releasing output. By definition, all living systems are open systems.

Output The form of energy, matter, or information that is released into the environment by the system once it has processed the input it received.

Parallel relationships Relationships in which the partners alternate between symmetrical and complementary interaction patterns, according to the demands of the situation.

Patient advocacy Patient advocacy is seeing that the patient knows what to expect and what is his right to have, and then displaying the willingness and courage to see that our system does not prevent the client from getting it.

Power The capacity to influence, control, dominate, and make decisions; the actual or potential ability of an individual or group to control, influence, or change another person's (family member) or group's (family) behavior. Power is multidimensional and not directly observable,

but often inferred through observation of decision-making processes.

Power bases The source from which a family member's power is derived. Examples of power bases are authority or position, referent power (role models), resource power, expert power, reward power, coercive or dominance power, informational power, and affective power.

Primary prevention Health promotion and specific preventive or health-protective measures. Specific preventive and protective measures are also referred to as disease prevention or health maintenance.

Proposition Relational statements that describe or link concepts in a conceptual model or theory.

Receiver In communication theory, this refers to the target of the person (the sender) who is attempting to transmit a message to this person (the receiver).

Reciprocal determinism Describes a characteristic of family systems that states interrelationships found in a family system are so intricately tied together that a change in any one part inevitably results in changes in the entire system. Referred to as "ripple effects."

Risk appraisal/risk reduction A primary prevention approach used to reduce a person's, family's, or community's exposure to adverse consequences, most notably health problems. Risk refers to the probability of a future occurrence happening.

Role Relatively homogeneous sets of behaviors that are normatively defined and expected of an occupant of a given social position.

Second-order change A specific kind of change, in which there are actual changes in the rules governing the system (e.g., the family) and, therefore, the system is transformed structurally and/or communicationally.

Secondary prevention Early detection, diagnosis, and treatment of health problems.

Self-fulfilling prophecy When people are given negative labels or stereotypical attributes, they start believing that about themselves and act in accordance with those expectations.

Self-reflexivity Describes a characteristic of family systems that states the family possess the ability and tendency to make themselves and their own behavior the focus of examination and the target of explanation.

Sender In communication theory, this term refers to the person who is attempting to transmit a message to another person.

Separateness Degree of individuality of family members.

Single-parent family A family in which there is one head of the household, mother or father.

Social class Social class, socioeconomic status, or social status (interchangeable terms) refers to a grouping of persons with relatively similar income, amounts of wealth, life conditions, life changes, and lifestyles.

Social class mobility The vertical movement upward or downward through the social class strata. Either direction of mobility creates stress on families.

Social system A model of social organization; it is a living system possessing a total unit distinctive from its component parts and distinguishable from its environment by a clearly defined boundary.

Socialization A lifelong process by which individuals continually modify their behavior in response to the socially patterned circumstances they experience; the process by which humans acquire socially patterned characteristics; a primary role of families in society is socialization of children so that they learn the acceptable behaviors and how to function as adults in their own society.

Stepparent family A family in which the husband and/or wife is remarried and one or both of them have a child (or children). Stepparent families are also called blended families, reconstituted families, or remarried families.

Stereotyping Lack of recognition of individual differences or labeling.

Stress The response or state of tension produced by stressor(s) or by the actual/perceived demand(s) that remains unmanaged.

Stressors Initiating or precipitating agents that activate the stress process.

Structural–Functional Theory A major sociological framework in which the family is viewed as an open social system and as a subsystem within society, serving to meet the needs of wider society and the needs of family members.

Suprasystem In the case of families, and as used in this text, this term refers to the national and global sociopolitical context for the families' macrosystem and microsystem functioning.

Symmetric communication One interactant's behavior mirrors the behavior of the other interactant.

Symmetrical relationships Relationships based on the equality of the partners, with neither partner more or less dominant.

System A goal-directed unit made up of interdependent, interacting parts that endure over a period of time.

Tertiary prevention The stage of recovery and rehabilitation. It is designed to minimize the client's disability and maximize his or her level of functioning and well-being.

Theory Like a conceptual model, a theory is also composed of concepts with propositions explaining the relationships among the concepts. However, a theory is typically less abstract than a conceptual model

Underclass The underclass constitute the very poorest of the poor—about 25% of the lower class. They are families who experience long-term poverty and welfare dependency and live outside the mainstream patterns and norms of behavior.

Values An enduring belief that a specific mode of conduct or end state of existence is preferable to the opposite or converse mode of conduct or end state of existence.

Violence The use of physical force by one person against another. Often used synonymously with the term *abuse* though there is controversy about the definitions of the two terms.

Wellness inventory A type of risk appraisal tool in which risks are more broadly identified (the risks are not specific to a particular disease or problem).

REFERENCES

Aamodt, A. M. (1978). Culture. In A. L. Clark (Ed.), Culture, childbearing and health professionals. Philadelphia: Davis.

Abernathy, W. J., & Schrems, E. L. (1971). *Distance and health services—Issues of utilization and facility choice for demographic strata* (Research Paper No. 19). Palo Alto, CA: Stanford University Graduate School of Business.

Abma, J., Chandra, A., Mosher, W., Peterson, L., & Piccinino, L. (1997). Fertility, family planning and women's health: New data from the 1995 health survey of family growth. *Vital and Health Statistics* (Series 23, no. 9). Retrieved on August 3, 2001, from the World Wide Web. Available at *www.cdc. gov/nchs/fastats/pdf/sr23_19.pdf.*

Ackerman, N. (1966). *The psychodynamics of family life.* New York: Basic Books.

Ackley, B., & Ladwig, G. (2002). *Nursing diagnosis handbook: A guide to planning care.* St. Loius: Mosby.

ACP-ASIM. (2001). No health insurance? It's enough to make you sick. Available at *www.acponline.org/ uninsured.*

Adams, B. N. (1971). *The American family.* Chicago: Markham Publishing.

Adams, B. N. (1980). *The family: A sociological interpretation.* Boston: Houghton Mifflin.

Adams, B., & Adams, D. (1990). Child care and the family. In *National Council on Family Relations, 2001: Preparing families for the future* (pp. 18–19). Minneapolis, MN: Bolger Publications.

Aday, L. A., & Eichhorn, R. (1972). *The utilization of health services: Indices and correlates—A research bibliography* (Publication No. [HSM] 73-3003). Washington, DC: Department of Health, Education and Welfare, National Center for Health Services Research and Development.

African-American Monitor (1999, November 8). A barometer of black America. *Newsweek,* 18.

Agbayani-Siewert, P., & Revilla, L. (1995). Filipino Americans. In P. G. Min (Ed.), *Asian Americans: Contemporary trends and issues* (pp. 134–198). Thousand Oaks, CA: Sage.

Agency for Health Care Policy and Research. (1996). *Racial and ethnic differences in health 1996.* Available at *www. meps.achpr.gov.*

Agnew, R., & Huguley, S. (1989). Adolescent violence toward parents. *Journal of Marriage and the Family, 51*(3), 699–711.

Ahrons, C. R. (1980, November). Redefining the divorced family. A conceptual framework. *Social Work,* 437–441.

Ahrons, C. R., & Perlmutter, M. S. (1982). The relationship between former spouses: A fundamental subsystem in the remarriage family. In J. C. Hansen & L. Messinger (Eds.), *Therapy with remarried families.* Rockville, MD: Aspen.

Akande, A., Van Wyk, C., & Osagie, J. (2000). Importance of exercise and nutrition in the prevention of illness and the enhancement of health. *Education, 120*(4), 758–773.

Al-Anon Family Groups. (2000). *Alcoholism: The family disease.* Virginia Beach, VA: Author.

Aldous, J. (1974). The making of family roles and family change. *Family Coordinator, 23*(2), 232–237.

Aldous, J. (1978). *Family careers: Developmental change in families.* New York: Wiley.

Aldous, J. (1996). *Family careers: Rethinking the developmental perspective.* Thousand Oaks, CA: Sage.

Alexander, J. S., Younger, R. E., Cohen, R. M., & Crawford, L. V. (1988). Effectiveness of a nurse-managed program for children with chronic asthma. *Journal of Pediatric Nursing, 3,* 312–317.

Alfaro-LeFevre, R. (2001). *Applying nursing process.* Philadelphia: Lippincott-Williams/Wilkins.

Allen, C. E. (1994). Families in poverty. *Nursing Clinics of North America, 29*(3), 277–393.

Allen, K. R., & Demo, D. H. (1995). The families of lesbians and gay men: A new frontier in family research. *Journal of Marriage and the Family, 57,* 111–127.

Allen, K. R., Fine, M. A., Demo, D. H. (2000). An overview of family diversity: Controversies, questions, and values. In D. H. Demo, K. R. Allen, and M. A. Fine (Eds.), *Handbook of family diversity.* (pp. 1–14). New York: Oxford University Press.

Allen, K. R. (1997). Lesbian and gay families. In T. Arendell (Ed.), *Contemporary parenting: Challenges and issues, understanding families,* Vol. 9 (pp. 196–218). Thousand Oaks, CA: Sage.

Allen, K. R., and Demo, D. H.(1995). The families of lesbians and gay men: A new frontier in family research. *Journal of Marriage and the Family, 57*(1), pp. 111–127.

Allender, J. A., & Spradley, B. W. (2001). *Community health nursing: Concepts and practice* (5th ed.). Philadelphia: Lippincott.

Alonso-Zaldiver, R., & Fields, R. (2001, March 9). Latino, Asian populations rise sharply. *Los Angeles Times,* pp. A1, A16.

Alter, J. A. (2001, January 15). A well-timed "traffic" signal. *Newsweek.* Available at *www.newsweek.com.*

Amato, P., & Rezac, S. (1994). Contact with nonresident parents, interparental conflict, and children's behavior. *Journal of Family Issues, 15,* 191–207.

American Academy of Pediatrics (AAP). (1989). Confidentiality in adolescent health care. AAP News. Retrieved from the World Wide Web on August 3, 2001. Available at *www.aap.org/policy/104.html.*

American Academy of Pediatrics Committee on Infectious Diseases. (2001). Recommended childhood immunization schedule—United States, January–December 2001. *Pediatrics, 107*(1), 202– 204.

American Academy of Pediatrics. (1995). *Caring for your school age child. Ages 5 to 12.* New York: Bantam Books.

American Association of Retired Persons. (1990). *A profile of older Americans, 1990.* Washington, DC: Author.

American Association of Retired Persons.(1993). *A profile of older Americans, 1992.* Washington, DC: Author.

American Association of Retired Persons. (1999). Sex— What's age got to do with it? Retrieved from the World Wide Web on August 3, 2001. Available at *www.aarp. org/press/1999/nr080399.html.*

American Association of Retired Persons. (2000). *AARP Survey: Grandparents, grandchildren have strong bond, visit often.* Retrieved from the World Wide Web on August 3, 2001. Available at *www.aarp.org/press/2000/nr010400.html.*

American Dental Association. (1988). *Seal out decay.* Chicago: ADA Division of Communications.

American Nurses Association. (1980). *Social policy statement.* Kansas City, MO: Author.

American Nurses Association. (1987). *Standards of primary health care practitioner.* Kansas City, MO: Author.

American Nurses Association. (1988). *Rehabilitation nursing: Scope of practice.* Kansas City, MO: Author.

American Nurses Association. (1992). *Nursing's agenda for health care reform.* Washington, DC: Author.

American Nurses Association. (1995a). *Nursing's social policy statement.* Kansas City, MO: Author.

American Nurses Association. (1995b). *Scope and standards of gerontological nursing practice.* Kansas City, MO: Author.

American Nurses Association. (1996). *Statement on the scope and standards of pediatric clinical nursing practice.* Kansas City, MO: Author.

American Nurses Association. (1998). *Standards of clinical nursing practice* (2nd ed.). Kansas City, MO: Author.

American Nurses Association. (1999). *Standards of home health nursing practice. And Standards of public health nursing practice.* Kansas City, MO: Author.

American Nurses Association. (2000). *Statement on psychiatric–mental health clinical nursing practice and standards of psychiatric–mental health clinical nursing practice.* Kansas City, MO: Author.

American Nurses Association, Council of Community Health Nurses. (1986). *Standards of community health nursing practice.* Kansas City, MO: Author.

American Nurses Association, Division on Maternal and Child Health Nursing Practice. (1983). *Standards of maternal and child health nursing practice.* Kansas City, MO: Author.

American Nurses Association, Division on Psychiatric–Mental Health Nursing Practice. (1982). *Standards of psychiatric and mental health nursing practice.* Kansas City, MO: Author.

American Nurses Association, Task Force on Case Management. (1988). *Nursing case management.* Kansas City, MO: Author.

Ames, K. (1992, March 23). Domesticated bliss: New laws are making it official for gay and live-in couples. *Newsweek,* 40.

Anderson, E., & Koblinsky, S. (1995). Homeless policy: The need to speak to families. *Family Relations, 44,* 13–18.

Anderson, K. E. (1972). *Introduction to communication theory and practice.* San Jose, CA: Cummings.

Anderson, K., & Tomlinson, P. (1992). The family health system as an emerging paradigmatic view for nursing. *Image, 23*(1), 57–63.

Anderson, R., & Carter, I. (1974). *Human behavior in the social environment—A social systems approach.* Chicago: Aldine.

Andrews, M. M. (1995). Transcultural nursing care. In M. M. Andrews & J. S. Boyle (Eds.), *Transcultural concepts in nursing care* (2nd ed.) (pp. 49–96). Philadelphia: Lippincott.

Andrews, M. M., & Boyle, J. S. (Eds.). (1995). *Transcultural concepts in nursing care* (2nd ed.). Philadelphia: Lippincott.

Aneshensel, C. S., Pearlin, L. I., Mullan, J. T., Zarit, S. H., & Whitlatch, C. J. (1995). *Profiles in caregiving: The unexpected career.* San Diego: Academic Press.

Angel, R. (1985). The health of the Mexican origin population. In R. De La Garza, et al. (Eds.), *The Mexican American experience: An interdisciplinary anthology* (pp. 410–426). Austin, TX: University of Texas Press.

Annie E. Casey Foundation. (1999). *Kids count data book.* Baltimore, MD: Author.

Antonovsky, A. (1979). *Health, stress and coping.* San Francisco: Jossey-Bass.

Antonovsky, A. (1994). The sense of coherence: An historical and future perspective. In H. I. McCubbin, E. A. Thompson, A. I. Thompson, & J. E. Fromer (Eds.), *Sense of coherence and resiliency: Stress, coping and health* (pp. 3–21). Madison, WI: University of Wisconsin–Madison, System Center for Excellence in Family Studies.

Antonovsky, A. (1998). The structure and properties of the sense of coherence scale. In H. I. McCubbin, E. A. Thompson, A. I. Thompson, & J. E. Fromer (Eds.), *Stress, coping and health in families: Sense of coherence and resiliency* (pp. 21–38). Thousand Oaks, CA: Sage.

Antonovsky, A., & Sourani, T. (1988). Family sense of coherence and family adaptation. *Journal of Marriage and the Family, 50,* 79–92.

Arax, M., Curtius, M., & Nelson, S. S. (2000, January 9). California income gap grows amid prosperity. *Los Angeles Times,* pp. A1, A16.

Ardell, D. (1982). *Fourteen days to a wellness life-style.* Mill Valley, CA: Whatever Publishers.

Ardell, D., & Newman, A. (1977). Health promotion—Strategies for planning. *Health Values: Achieving High Level Wellness, 1*(3), 100.

Arizona Department of Health Services. (2000). *Injury mortality among children and adolescents, 1988–1998.* Phoenix, Arizona: Author.

Armentrout, G. (1993). A comparison of the medical model and the wellness model: The importance of knowing the difference. *Holistic Nursing Practice, 7*(4), 57–62.

Arnette, J. K. (1996). Physiological effects on chronic grief: A biofeedback treatment approach. *Death Studies, 20,* 59–72.

Artinian, N. T. (1989). Family member perceptions of a cardiac surgery event. *Focus on Critical Care, 16*(4), 301–308.

Artinian, N. T. (1994). Selecting a model to guide family assessment. *Dimensions of Critical Care Nursing, 14*(1), 4–16.

Asch, S., Leake, B., & Gelberg, L. (1994). Does fear of immigration authorities deter tuberculosis patients from seeking care. *Western Journal of Medicine, 161,* 373–376.

Association for the Care of Children's Health. (1989). *Conference announcement.* Washington, DC: Author.

Auger, J. R. (1976). *Behavioral systems and nursing.* Englewood Cliffs, NJ: Prentice Hall.

Austin, R. (1985). Attitudes toward old age: A hierarchical study. *The Gerontologist, 25*(4), 431–434.

Avioli, P. S. (1989). The social support functions of siblings in later life: A theoretical model. *American Behavioral Scientist, 33,* 45–57.

Aylmer, R. C. (1988). The launching of the single young adult. In B. Carter & M. McGoldrick (Eds.), *The changing family life cycle* (pp. 191–208). New York: Gardner Press.

Baca-Zinn, M. (1981). Sociological theory in emergent Chicano perspectives. *Pacific Sociological Review, 24*(2), 255–272.

Backett, E. M., Davies, A. M., & Petros-Barvazian, A. (1984). *The risk approach in health care.* Geneva, Switzerland: World Health Organization.

Bagley, C. A., & Carroll, J. (1995). Healing forces in African-American families. In H. I. McCubbin, E. A. Thompson, A. I. Thompson, & J. A. Futrell (Eds.), *Resiliency in African-American families* (pp. 117–142). Thousand Oaks, CA: Sage.

Bahnson, C. B. (1987). The impact of life-threatening illness on the family and the impact of the family on illness: An overview. In M. Leahey & L. M. Wright (Eds.), *Families and life-threatening illness* (pp. 26–44). Springhouse, PA: Springhouse Corporation.

Baker, T. (1985). Introduction to sleep and sleep disorders. *Medical Clinics of North America, 69,* 1123–1151.

Balswick, J. O., & Balswick, J. P. (1995). Gender relations and marital power. In B. B. Ingoldsby & S. Smith (Eds.), *Families in multicultural perspective* (pp. 297–320). New York: Guilford Press.

Bandura, A. (1977). *Social learning theory.* Englewood Cliffs, NJ: Prentice Hall.

Banks, L. J. (1992). Counseling. In G. M. Bulechek & J. C. McCloskey (Eds.), *Nursing interventions: Essential nursing treatments* (2nd ed.) (pp. 279–303). Philadelphia: Saunders.

Barber, B. K., & Thomas, D. L. (1986). Dimensions of fathers' and mothers' supportive behavior: The case for physical affection. *Journal of Marriage and the Family, 48*(4), 783–794.

Baringer, F. (1991, March 11). Census shows profound change in racial make-up of nation. *New York Times,* p. 1.

Barnard, K. (1986). Nursing child assessment teaching manual. Seattle, Washington: Nursing Child Assessment Satellite Training.

Barnett, R., & Rivers, C. (1996). *She works, he works: How two income families are happy, healthy and thriving.* Cambridge, MA: Harvard University Press.

Barnett, R. C., & Baruch, M. (1987). Determinants of fathers' participation in family work. *Journal of Marriage and the Family, 49*(1), 29–40.

Barnett, T., Fatis, M., Sonnek, D., & Torvinen, J. (1992). Treatment satisfaction with an asthma management program: A "five"-year retrospective assessment. *Journal of Asthma, 29,* 109–116.

Barnum, B. J. S. (1994). *Nursing theory: Analysis, application, and evaluation* (4th ed.). Philadelphia: Lippincott.

Barrick, J. D. (1997). Assessing quality of care in kinship and foster family care. *Family Relations, 46*(3), 273–280.

Barth, R. P. (2001). Policy implications of foster family characteristics. *Family Relations, 50*(1), 16–19.

Bartz, K. W., & Levine, B. S. (1978). Childrearing by black parents: A description and comparison to Anglo and Chicano parents. *Journal of Marriage and the Family, 40,* 709–720.

Bass, D., & Noelker, L. (1987). The influence of family care-givers on elders' use of in-home services: An expanded conceptual framework. *Journal of Health and Social Behavior, 28,* 184–196.

Bassuk, K. L. (1990). The problem of family homelessness. In E. L. Bassuk, R. W. Carmen, L. F. Weinrek, & M. M. Herzig (Eds.), *Community care for homeless families* (p. 7). Washington, DC: Interagency Council on the Homeless.

Bateson, G. (1958). *Naven* (2nd ed.). Stanford, CA: Stanford University Press.

Bateson, G. (1972). *Steps to an ecology of the mind.* New York: Ballantine.

Bateson, G. (1979). *Mind and nature.* New York: Bantam Books.

Bateson, G., Jackson, D. D., Haley, J., & Weakland, K. J. (1963). A note on the double bind—1962. *Family Process, 2,* 154–161.

Battiste, H. B. (1975). Family myths. In S. Smoyak (Ed.), *The psychiatric nurse as a family therapist.* New York: Wiley.

Baumann, B. (1961). Diversities in conceptions of health and physical fitness. *Journal of Health and Human Behavior, 2*(1), 40.

Baumrind, D. (1978). Parental disciplinary patterns and social competency in children. *Youth and Society, 9,* 239–276.

Baumrind, D. (1985). Familial antecedents of adolescent drug use: A developmental perspective. In C. Jones & R. Battjes (Eds.), *Etiology of drug abuse: Implication for prevention.* NIDA Research Monograph. Washington, DC: U.S. Government Printing Office.

Baumrind, D. (1994). The social context of child maltreatment. *Family Relations, 43,* 360–368.

Baumrind, D. (1996). Parenting. The discipline controversy revisited. *Family Relations, 45,* 405–414.

Baxter, K. (1996, September 6). Blazing trails between clashing cultures. *Los Angeles Times,* p. E1.

Baydar, N., & Brooks-Gunn, J. (1998). Profiles of grandmothers who help care for their grandchildren in the United States. *Family Relations, 47*(4), 385–393.

Beavers, W. (1977). *Psychotherapy and growth: A family systems perspective.* New York: Brunner/Mazel.

Beavers, W. R., & Hampson, R. B. (1990). *Successful families: Assessment and intervention.* New York: Norton.

Beavers, W. R., & Hampson, R. B. (1993). Measuring family competence. In F. Walsh (Ed.), *Normal family processes* (2nd ed.) (pp. 73–95). New York: Guilford Press.

Beck, M. (1990, July 16). Trading places. *Newsweek,* 48–54.

Becker, M. H. (1972). The health belief model and personal health behavior. *Health Education Monographs, 2,* 326–327.

Becker, M. H. (1974). *The health belief model and personal health behavior.* Thorofare, NJ: Charles B. Slack.

Becvar, D. S., & Becvar, R. J. (1996). *Family therapy: A systemic integration.* Boston: Allyn & Bacon.

Begley, S. (2000, November 6). The stereotype trap. *Newsweek,* pp. 66–68.

Begley, S., & Springen, K. (2001, April 23). Are we getting smarter? *Newsweek,* pp. 53–59.

Bell, J. M. (1995). Wanted: Family nursing interventions. *Journal of Family Nursing, 1*(4), 355–358.

Bell, J. M. (1996). Advanced practice in family nursing: One view. *Journal of Family Nursing, 2*(3), 244–248.

Bell, R., & Vogel, E. F. (1968). *A modern introduction to the family.* New York: Free Press.

Bellah, R. N., Madsen, L., Sullivan, W. M., Swidler, A., & Tipton, S. M. (1986). *Habits of the heart: Individualism and commitment in American life.* New York: Harper & Row.

Belsky, J. (1995). A nation (still) at risk? *National Forum, 75*(3), 36–38.

Bemak, F., Chung, R. C., & Bornemann, T. H. (1996). Counseling and psychotherapy with refugees. In P. B. Petersen, J. G. Braguns, W. J. Lonner, & J. E. Trimble (Eds.), *Counseling across cultures* (pp. 243–265). Thousand Oaks, CA: Sage.

Bempechat, J. (2000). *Getting our kids back on track: Educating for the future.* San Fransisco: Jossey-Bass.

Benedek, E. (1978, December 8). *Spousal abuse.* Paper presented at the 1978 Winter Scientific Session of the American Medical Association, Las Vegas, Nevada. Reported by Nelson, H. Abused wives cling to hope, doctors say. *Los Angeles Times,* pp. 1, 18.

Bengtson, V. N. (1985). Diversity in symbolism in grandparental roles. In V. Bengtson & T. Robertson (Eds.), *Grandparenthood* (pp. 11–25). Newbury Park, CA: Sage.

Bengtson, V., & Robertson, T. (Eds.). (1985). *Grandparenthood.* Newbury Park, CA: Sage.

Bengtson, V., Mangen, D., & Landry, P. (1987). Intergenerational linkages. In H. Garms, E. M. Hoerning, & A. Schaeffer (Eds.), *Intergenerational relationships.* New York: J. Hogrefe.

Benin, M., & Keith, V. M. (1995). The social support of employed African American and Anglo mothers. *Journal of Family Issues, 16*(3), 275–297.

Benne, K. D., & Sheats, P. (1948). Functional roles of group members. *Journal of Social Issues, 4* (Spring), 41.

Berardo, F. M. (1988, December). The American family. *Journal of Family Issues, 8*(4), 426–428.

Berkanovic, E. (1976). Behavioral science and prevention. *Preventive Medicine, 5,* 93.

Berkey, K. M., & Hanson, S. M. H. (1991). *Pocket guide to family assessment and intervention.* St. Louis: Mosby.

Bernal, G., & Shapiro, E. (1996). Cuban families. In M. McGoldrick, J. Giordano, & J. K. Pearce (Eds.), *Ethnicity and family therapy* (2nd ed.) (pp. 155–168). New York: Guilford Press.

Berriesi, C. M., Ferraro, K. F., & Hobey, L. L. (1984). Environmental satisfaction, sociability and well-being among urban elderly. *International Journal of Aging and Human Development, 18*(4), 277–284.

Besmer, A. (1967). Economic deprivation and family patterns. In L. M. Irelan (Ed.), *Low-income life styles.* Washington, DC: U.S. Department of Health, Education, and Welfare.

Bianchi, S. M. (1995). The changing demographic and socioeconomic characteristics of single parent families. In S. H. Hanson, M. L. Heims, D. J. Julian, & M. B. Sussman (Eds.), *Single parent families: Diversity, myths and realities* (pp. 71–97). New York: Haworth Press.

Biddle, B. J., & Thomas, E. J. (1966). *Role theory: Concepts and research.* New York: Wiley.

Biegel, D. E., Sales, E., & Schulz, R. (1991). *Family caregiving in chronic illness.* Newbury Park, CA: Sage.

Bild, B. R., & Havighurst, R. (1976). Senior citizens in great cities: The case of Chicago. *The Gerontologist, 16*(1), 63.

Billingsley, A. (1968). *Black families in white America.* Englewood Cliffs, NJ: Prentice Hall.

Billingsley, A. (1992). *Climbing Jacob's ladder.* New York: Simon and Schuster.

Birenbaum, L., Robinson, M. A., Phillips, D., Stewart, B., & McCown, D. (1990). The response of children to the dying and death of a sibling. *Omega, 20*(3), 213–228.

Black, B. (1974). *Families in crisis: Assessment and nursing intervention.* Los Angeles, CA: Intercampus Nursing Project, California State University, Los Angeles.

Blau, P. M. (1977). *Heterogeneity and inequality: A pragmatic theory of social structure.* New York: Free Press.

Blood, R. O. (1969). *Marriage* (2nd ed.). Glencoe, IL: Free Press.

Blood, R. O., & Wolfe, D. M. (1960). *Husbands and wives. The dynamics of married living.* Glencoe, IL: Free Press.

Bloom, B. S. (1956). *Taxonomy of educational objectives handbook: Cognitive domain.* New York: David McKay.

Blum, R. W. (2000, December). Connections make a difference in the lives of youth. *National Council on Family Relations Report, 45*(4), pp. F9–F10.

Blumer, H. (1962). Society as symbolic interaction. In A. Rose (Ed.), *Human behavior and social processes.* Boston: Houghton-Mifflin.

Blumer, H. (1969). *Symbolic interactionism.* Englewood Cliffs, NJ: Prentice Hall.

Blumstein, P., & Schwartz, P. (1983). *American couples.* New York: Morrow.

Blumstein, P., & Schwartz, P. (1991). Money and ideology: Their impact on power and the division of household labor. In R. L. Blumberg (Ed.), *Gender, family, and economy: The triple overlap* (pp. 261–288). Newbury Park, CA: Sage.

Bobak, I. M., Jensen, M. D., & Zalar, M. D. (1989). *Maternity and gynecologic care: The nurse and family* (4th ed.). St. Louis: Mosby.

Bodman, D. A., & Peterson, G. W. (1995). Parenting processes. In R. D. Day, K. R. Gilbert, B. H. Settles, & W. R. Burr (Eds.), *Research and theory in family science* (pp. 205–225). Pacific Grove, CA: Brooks/Cole.

Boehm, S. (1992). Patient contracting. In G. M. Bulechek & J. C. McCloskey (Eds.), *Nursing interventions: Essential nursing treatments* (2nd ed.) (pp. 425–433). Philadelphia: Saunders.

Bolton, F. G., & Bolton, S. R. (1987). *Working with violent families.* Newbury Park, CA: Sage.

Bomar, P. J. (Ed.). (1996). *Nurses and family health promotion* (2nd ed.). Philadelphia: Saunders.

Bomar, P. J., & McNeely, G. (1996). Family health nursing role: Past, present and future. In P. J. Bomar (Ed.), *Nurses and family health promotion* (2nd ed.) (pp. 3–21). Philadelphia: Saunders.

Borders, L. D., Black, L. K., & Pasley, B. K. (1998). Are adopted children and their parents at greater risk for negative outcomes? *Family Relations, 47*(3), 237–241.

Boss, P. (1988). *Family stress management.* Newbury Park, CA: Sage.

Boss, P. (1999). *Ambiguous loss.* Cambridge, MA: Harvard University Press.

Boss, P. G., Doherty, W. J., La Rossa, R., Schumm, W. R., & Steinmetz, S. K. (Eds.). (1993). *Sourcebook of family theories and methods: A contextual approach.* New York: Plenum.

Bossard, J. H., & Boll, E. S. (1956). *The large family system: An original study in the sociology of family behavior.* Philadelphia: University of Pennsylvania Press.

Boulding, E. (1976). Familism and the creation of futures. In E. Eldridge & N. Meredith (Eds.), *Environmental issues: Family impact.* Minneapolis, MN: Burgess.

Boutin, P., Buchwald, D., Robinson, L., & Collier, A. (2000). Use of and attitudes about alternative and complementary therapies among outpatients and physicians at a municipal hospital. *Journal of Alternative and Complimentary Medicine, 6*(4), 335–343.

Bowden, V., Dickey, S., & Greenberg, C. (1998). *Children and their families: The continuum of care.* Philadelphia: W. B. Saunders.

Bowen, G. L., Desimone, L. M., & McKay, J. K. (1995). Poverty and the single mother family: A macroeconomic perspective. In S. Hanson, M. Heims, D. Julian, & M. Sussman (Eds.), *Single parent families: Diversity, myths and realities* (pp. 115–142). New York: Haworth Press.

Bowen, M. (1960). Family concept of schizophrenia. In D. D. Jackson (Ed.), *Etiology of schizophrenia.* New York: Basic Books.

Bowen, M. (1976). Theory in the practice of psychotherapy. In P. J. Guerin (Ed.), *Family therapy* (pp. 42–90). New York: Gardiner Press.

Bowen, M. (1978). *Family therapy in clinical practice.* New York: Aronson.

Bower, K. (1992). *Case management by nurses.* Washington, DC: American Nurses Publishing.

Bowers, B. F., & Myers, B. J. (1999). Grandmothers providing care for grandchildren: Consequences of various levels of caregiving. *Family Relations, 48*(3), pp. 303–311.

Bowlby, J. (1966). *Maternal care and mental health.* New York: Schocken.

Bowlby, J. (1977). The making and breaking of affectional bonds. *British Journal of Psychiatry, 133,* 201–210.

Bowling, A., & Windsor, J. (1995). Death after widow(er)hood: An analysis of mortality rates up to 13 years after bereavement. *Omega, 31*(1), 35–49.

Boyd-Franklin, N. (1989). *Black families in therapy.* New York: Guilford Press.

Boyum, L. A., & Parke, R. D. (1995, August). The role of family emotional expressiveness in the development of children's social competence. *Journal of Marriage and the Family, 57,* 593–608.

Bozett, F. W. (1987). Family nursing and life-threatening illness. In M. Leahey & L. M. Wright (Eds.), *Families and life-threatening illness.* Springhouse, PA: Springhouse Corporation.

Bozett, F. W., & Gibbons, R. (1983). The nursing management of families in the critical care setting. *Critical Care Update, 10,* 22–27.

Braden, C. J. (1984). *The focus and limits of community health nursing.* Norwalk, CT: Appleton & Lange.

Bradt, J. O. (1988). Becoming parents: Families with young children. In B. Carter & M. McGoldrick (Eds.), *The changing family life cycle* (2nd ed.) (pp. 235–254). New York: Gardner Press.

Bramlett, M. H., Gueldener, S. H., & Sowell, R. R. (1990). Consumer-centric advocacy: Its connection to nursing frameworks. *Nursing Science Quarterly, 3,* 156–161.

Bray, J. H., Berger, S. H., & Boethel, C. L. (1994). Role integration and marital adjustment in stepfather families. In K. Pasley & M. Ihinger-Tahlman (Eds.), *Stepparenting: Issues in theory, research, and practice.* Westport, CT: Greenwood Press.

Breakdown on Family Breakdown, *The Washington Times,* 25, March 2001, p. B2.

Bridges, L. J., & Connell, J. P. (1991). Consistency and inconsistency in infant emotional and social interactive behavior across contexts and caregivers. *Infant Behavior and Development, 14*(4), 471–787.

Briggs, K., Hubbs-Tait, L., Culp, R., & Blankemeyer, M. (1995). Perceiver bias in expectancies for sexually abused children. *Family Relations, 44,* 291–298.

Brink, P. (1976). *Transcultural nursing.* Englewood Cliffs, NJ: Prentice Hall.

Broderick, C. B. (1971). Behind the five conceptual frameworks: A decade of development in family theory. *Journal of Marriage and the Family, 33,* 129–159.

Broderick, C. B. (1990). Family process theory. In J. Sprey (Ed.), *Fashioning family theory* (pp. 171–206). Newbury Park, CA: Sage.

Broderick, C. B. (1993). *Understanding family process: Basics of family systems theory.* Thousand Oaks, CA: Sage

Brody, E. M. (1985). Parent care as a normative family stress. *The Gerontologist, 25,* 19–29.

Brody, E. M. (1995). Prospects for family caregiving: Response to change, continuity, and diversity. In R. A. Kane & J. D. Penrod (Eds.), *Family caregiving in an aging society: Policy perspectives.* Thousand Oaks, CA: Sage.

Brody, E. M., Litvin, S. J., Kleben, M. H., & Hoffman, C. (1990, November). *Differential effects of daughters' marital status on their parent care experiences.* Paper presented at the 43rd Annual Meeting of the Gerontological Society of America, Boston, MA.

Brody, E., & Schoonover, C. B. (1986). Patterns of parent-care when adult daughters work and when they do not. *The Gerontologist, 26*(4), 372–381.

Brody, E., Litvin, S., Hoffman, C., & Kleban, M. (1992a). Differential effects of daughter's marital status on their parental experiences. *The Gerontologist, 32,* 58–67.

Brody, E., Litvin, S., Hoffman, C., & Kleban, M. (1992b). On having a "significant other" during the parent care years. *Journal of Applied Gerontology, 14*(2), 131–149.

Brody, G. H. (1994). Family processes and adolescent development. An introduction to a special issue. *Family Relations, 43,* 359.

Broering, J. (1993). The adolescent, health and society: From the perspective of the nurse. In S. Millstein, A. Petersen, & E. Nightingale (Eds.), *Promoting the health of adolescents: New directions for the twenty-first century* (pp. 151–155). New York: Oxford University Press.

Brolinson, P., Price, J., Ditmeyer, M., & Rice, D. (2001). Nurses' perceptions of complementary and alternative medical therapies. *Journal of Community Health, 26*(3), 175–189.

Bronfenbrenner, U. (1969). The changing American child—A speculative analysis. In R. L. Coser (Ed.), *Life cycle and achievement in America* (pp. 1–20). New York: Harper & Row.

Bronfenbrenner, U. (1974). The origins of alienation. *Scientific American, 231,* 53.

Bronfenbrenner, U. (1979). *The ecology of human development: Experiments by nature and design.* Cambridge, MA: Harvard University Press.

Bronstein, P., & Cowan, C. P. (1988). *Fatherhood today: Men's changing role in the family.* New York: Wiley.

Bronstein, P., Clauson, J., Stoll, M. F., & Abrams, C. L. (1993). Parenting behavior and children's social, psychological, and academic adjustment in diverse family structures. *Family Relations, 42,* 268–276.

Brooks-Gunn, S., & Chase-Lansdale, P. (1995). Adolescent parenthood. In M. H. Bornstein (Ed.), *Handbook of parenting. Vol. 3: Status and social conditions of parenting* (pp. 113–149). Hillsdale, NJ: Erlbaum.

Brooks-Gunn, S., & Paikoff, R. (1993). Sex is a gamble, kissing is a game: Adolescent sexuality, conception, and pregnancy. In S. P. Millstein, A. Peterson, & E. O. Nightingale (Eds.), *Promoting the health of adolescents: New directions for the twenty-first century* (pp. 180–208). New York: Oxford University Press.

Broom, B. L. (1998). Parental sensitivity to infants and toddlers in dual-earner and single-earner families. *Nursing Research, 47*(3), 162–170.

Broome, M. E., Knafl, K., Pridham, K., & Feetham, S. (1998). Preface. In M. E. Broome, K. Knafl, K. Pridham, & S. Feetham (Eds.), *Children and family in health and illness* (pp. ix–x). Thousand Oaks, CA: Sage.

Brothers, J. (1990, June 20). Testing parental philosophies. *Los Angeles Times,* p. E4.

Brown, E. R., Ponce, N., & Rice, T. (2001). *The state of health Insurance in California: Recent trends, future prospects.* Los Angeles: UCLA Center for Health Policy Research.

Brown, S. L. (1978). Functions, tasks, and stresses of parenting: Implications for guidance. In L. E. Arnold (Ed.), *Helping parents help their children.* New York: Brunner/Mazel.

Brownstein, R. (1995, November 6). Why are so many black men in jail? Numbers in debate equal a paradox. *Los Angeles Times,* p. A5.

Brownstein, R. (1999, October 11). Government should work harder to serve legions of working poor. *Los Angeles Times,* p. A5.

Brownstein, R. (2000, May 29). Mapping strategies to help those left behind by booming economy. *Los Angeles Times,* p. A5.

Brubaker, T. (1990). Families in later life: A burgeoning area of research. *Journal of Marriage and the Family, 52*(4), 959–982.

Brubaker, T. H. (1983). *Family relationships in later life.* Beverly Hills, CA: Sage.

Brubaker, T. H. (1985). *Later life families.* Beverly Hills, CA: Sage.

Buckley, W. (1967). *Sociology and modern systems theory.* Englewood Cliffs, NJ: Prentice Hall.

Bulechek, J., & McCloskey, G. (2000). *Nursing interventions classification (NIC).* St. Louis: Mosby.

Bulger, M. W., Wandersman, A., & Goldman, C. R. (1993). Burdens and gratifications of caregiving: Appraisal of parental care of adults with schizophrenia. *American Journal of Orthopsychiatry, 64,* 255–265.

Bullough, V., & Bullough, B. (1982). *Health care for the other Americans.* Norwalk, CT: Appleton & Lange.

Bullrich, S. (1989). The process of immigration. In L. Combrinck-Graham (Ed.), *Children in family contexts* (pp. 482–501). New York: Guilford Press.

Bumpass, L., Raley, R., & Sweet, J. (1995). The changing character of stepfamilies: Implications of cohabitation and nonmarital childbearing. *Demography, 32,* 425–236.

Burden, D. S. (1986). Single parents and the work setting: The impact of multiple job and homelife responsibilities. *Family Relations, 35*(1), 37–43.

Burgess, A. W. (1978). *Nursing: Levels of intervention.* Englewood Cliffs, NJ: Prentice Hall.

Burgess, E. W., Locke, H. J., & Thomas, M. M. (1963). *The family* (3rd ed.). New York: American Book.

Burns, K. (1996). A new recommendation for physical activity as a means of health promotion. *Nurse Practitioner, 2*(9), 18–28.

Burr, W. R. (1970). Satisfaction with various aspects of marriage over the life cycle. *Journal of Marriage and the Family, 32*(1), 29.

Burr, W. R. (1973). *Theory construction and the sociology of the family.* New York: Wiley.

Burr, W. R. (1995). Using theories in family science. In R. D. Day, K. R. Gilbert, B. H. Settles, & W. R. Burr (Eds.), *Research and theory in family science* (pp. 73–90). Pacific Grove, CA: Brooks/Cole.

Burr, W., Day, R., & Bahr, K. (1993). *Family science.* Pacific Grove, CA: Brooks/Cole.

Burr, W., Klein, S., Burr, R., Doxey, C., Harker, B., Holman, T., et al. (1994). *Reexamining family stress: New theory and research.* Thousand Oaks, CA: Sage.

Burr, W. R., Leight, G., Day, R., & Constantine, J. (1979). Symbolic interaction and the family. In W. R. Burr, R. Hill, F. I. Nye, & I. Reiss (Eds), *Contemporary theories about the family* (Vol. 2, pp. 42–111). New York: Free Press.

Burrell, N. A. (1995). Communication patterns in stepfamilies. In M. A. Fitzpatrick & A. L. Vangelisti (Eds.), *Explaining family interactions* (pp. 290–309). Thousand Oaks, CA: Sage.

Burt, C. W., & Fingerhut, L. A. (1998). *Injury visits to hospital emergency departments: United States, 1992–1995. Vital Health Statistics, 13* (131). Hyattsville, MD: National Center for Health Statistics.

Burton, L. (1992). Black grandparents rearing children of drug-addicted parents: Stress, outcomes, and social needs. *The Gerontologist, 32,* 744–751.

Burton, L., & Bengtson, V. (1985). Black grandmothers: Issues of timing and continuity of roles. In V. L. Bengtson & J. F. Robertson (Eds.), *Grandparenthood* (pp. 61–78). Newbury Park, CA: Sage.

Burton, L., & deVries, C. (1995). Challenges and rewards: African-American grandparents as surrogate parents. In L. M. Burton (Ed.), *Families and aging.* Amityville, NY: Baywood.

Bushy, A. (1990). Rural determinants in family health: Considerations for community nurses. *Family and Community Health, 12*(4), 29–38.

Bussell, D. A., & Reiss, D. (1993). Genetic influences on family processes: The emergence of a new framework for family research. In F. Walsh (Ed.), *Normal family processes* (2nd ed.) (pp. 161–181). New York: Guilford Press.

Butler, R. N., & Lewis, M. I. (1982). *Aging and mental health: Positive psychosocial and biomedical approaches.* St. Louis: Mosby.

Byng-Hall, J. (1988). Scripts and legends in families and family therapy. *Family Process, 27,* 167–179.

Byng-Hall, J. (1995). Creating a secure family base: Some implications of attachment theory for family therapy. *Family Process, 34,* 45–58.

Calfie, D. (1994). *Going it alone: A closer look at grandparents parenting grandchildren.* Washington, DC: American Association of Retired Persons.

Campbell, T. L. (2000). Physical illness: Challenges to families. In P.C. McKenry & S. J. Price (Eds.), *Families and change* (pp. 154–182). Thousand Oaks, CA: Sage.

Canino, I. A., & Spurlock, J. (1994). *Culturally diverse children and adolescents: Assessment, diagnosis, and treatment.* New York: Guilford Press.

Cantor, M. (1983). Strain among caregivers: A study of experience in the United States. *The Gerontologist, 23,* 597–604.

Caplan, G. (1964). *Principles of preventive psychiatry.* New York: Basic Books.

Caplan, G. (1970). *The theory and practice of mental health consultation.* New York: Basic Books.

Caplan, G. (1974). *Support systems and community mental health.* New York: Behavioral Publications.

Caplan, G. (1976). The family as a support system. In G. Caplan & M. Killilea (Eds.), *Support systems and mutual help.* New York: Grune & Stratton.

Caplan, N., Choy, M. H., & Whitmore, J. K. (1992, February). Indochinese refugee families and academic achievement. *Scientific American,* 36–42.

Caplin, M. S., & Sexton, D. L. (1988). Stresses experienced by spouses of patients in a coronary care unit with myocardial infarction. *Focus on Critical Care, 15*(5), 31–40.

Caplow, T. (1968). *Two against one: Coalitions in triads.* Englewood Cliffs, NJ: Prentice Hall.

Carey, B. (2001, August 20). When a good death isn't for everyone. *Los Angeles Times,* pp. S1, S6.

Carey, R. (1989). How values affect the mutual goal setting process with multiproblem families. *Journal of Community Health Nursing, 6*(1), 7–14.

Carlson, D., & Kacmark, K. (2000). Work-family conflict in the organization: Do life role values make a difference? *Journal of Management, 26*(5), 1031–1054.

Carmack, B. J. (1997). Balancing engagement and detachment in caregiving. *Image, 29*(2), 139–143.

Carney, P. (1992). The concept of poverty. *Public Health Nursing, 9*(2), 74–79.

Carpenito, L. (2000). *Nursing diagnosis: Application to clinical practice.* Philadelphia: Lippincott-Williams/Wilkins.

Carpenito, L. J. (2000). *Nursing diagnosis: Application to clinical practice* (8th ed). New York: Lippincott-Williams/Wilkins.

Carrington, R. W. (1978). The Afro-American. In A. L. Clark (Ed.), *Culture, childbearing, and health professionals.* Philadelphia: Davis.

Carruth, A. K. (1996). Development and testing of the Caregiver Reciprocity Scale. *Nursing Research, 45*(2), 92–97.

Carter, B., & McGoldrick, M. (Eds.). (1980). *The family life cycle: A framework for family therapy.* New York: Gardner Press.

Carter, B., & McGoldrick, M. (Eds.). (1989). *The changing family life cycle: A framework for family therapy.* New York: Gardner Press.

Cary, A. H. (1996). Case management. In M. Stanhope & J. Lancaster (Eds.), *Community health nursing. Promoting health of aggregates, families, and individuals* (pp. 357–373). St. Louis: Mosby.

Casas, J. M., & Vasquez, M. J. T. (1996). Counseling the Hispanic. In P. B. Pedersen, J. G. Draguns, W. J. Lonner, & J. E. Trimble (Eds.), *Counseling across cultures* (4th ed.) (pp. 146–176). Thousand Oaks, CA: Sage.

Casavantes, E. (1970, Winter). Pride and prejudice: A Mexican American dilemma. *Civil Rights Digest, 3,* 22.

Casey, B. (1996). The family as a system. In P. J. Bomar (Ed.), *Nurses and family health promotion: Concepts, assessment, and interventions* (2nd ed.). Philadelphia: Saunders.

Casey, B. A. (1989). The family as a system. In P. J. Bomar (Ed.), *Nurses and family health promotion* (pp. 37–46). Baltimore: Williams & Wilkins.

Castiglia, P. (1999). Extended families: Social support systems for children. *Journal of Pediatric Health Care, 13*(3), 139–141.

Castro, E. M. (1978). The Mexican American: How his culture affects his mental health. In R. A. Martinez (Ed.), *Hispanic culture and health care.* St. Louis: Mosby.

Castro, J. (1991, November 25). Condition: Critical. *Time,* 32–42.

Caudill, W. (1975, April). The individual and his nexus. In L. Nader & T. W. Maretzi (Eds.), *Cultural illness and health.* Washington, DC: American Anthropological Association.

Caudle, P. (1993). Providing culturally sensitive health care to Hispanic clients. *Nurse Practitioner, 18*(12), 40–51.

CDC National Center for Health Statistics (NCHS). (1998). *National mortality data, 1997.* Hyattsville, MD: NCHS.

Center for Health Economics Research. (1993). *Access to health care: Key indicators for policy.* Waltham, MA: Author.

Centers for Disease Control and Prevention. (2001). *Births: Final data for 1999.* Washington, DC: U.S. Government Printing Office.

Centers for Disease Control and Prevention. (1999). *Chronic diseases and their risk factors.* Atlanta, GA: Department of Health and Human Services, Centers for Disease Control and Prevention, National Center for Chronic Disease Prevention and Health Promotion. *(www.cdc.gov/nccdphp/stat book/stabook.html).*

Chan, S. (1992). Families with Asian roots. In E. W. Lynch & M. J. Hanson (Eds.), *Developing cross-cultural competence: A guide for working with young children and their families* (pp. 181–257). Baltimore: Paul H. Brooks.

Chang, K. (1995). Chinese Americans. In J. N. Giger & R. E. Davidhizar (Eds.), *Transcultural nursing: Assessment and intervention* (2nd ed.) (pp. 395–414). St. Louis: Mosby.

Chavez, N. (1986). Mental health services delivery to minority populations: Hispanics—a perspective. In M. Mirandé & H. Kitano (Eds.), *Mental health research and practice in minority communities.* Rockville, MD: National Institute of Mental Health.

Cherlin, A., & Furstenberg, F. F. (1985). Styles and strategies of grandparenting. In V. Bengtson & J. F. Robertson (Eds.), *Grandparenthood* (pp. 97–116). Beverly Hills, CA: Sage.

Cherlin, A., & Furstenberg, F. F. (1986). *The new American grandparent: A place in the family a life apart.* New York: Basic Books.

Cherlin, A. J. (1996). *Public & private families: An introduction.* New York: McGraw-Hill.

Chesler, M. A., & Barbarin, D. A. (1987). *Childhood cancer and the family.* New York: Brunner/Mazel.

Chess, S. (1983). Basic adaptation to successful parenting. In V. J. Sasserath (Ed.), *Minimizing high-risk parenting* (pp. 5–11). Skillman, NJ: Johnson & Johnson Baby Products.

Children's Defense Fund. (1995). *State of America's children—1995 year book.* Washington, DC: Author.

Chilman, C. S. (1978, April). Habitat and American families: A social–psychological overview. *Family Coordinator, 27,* 106–109.

Chilman, C. S. (1988). Never-married, single, adolescent parents. In C. S. Chilman, E. W. Nunnally, & F. M. Cox (Eds.), *Variant family forms.* Newbury Park, CA: Sage.

Chilman, C. S., Nunnally, E. W., & Cox, F. M. (1988). *Families in trouble—Chronic illness and disability.* Beverly Hills, CA: Sage.

Choi, N., & Snyder, L. (1999). *Homeless families with children: A subjective experience.* New York: Springer.

Choopoorian, T. J. (1986). Reconceptualizing the environment. In P. Moccia (Ed.), *New approaches in theory development* (pp. 39–54). New York: National League for Nursing.

Chrisman, M., & Fowler, M. D. (1980). The system-in-change model for nursing practice. In J. Riehl & C. Roy (Eds.), *Conceptual models for nursing practice* (pp. 74–102). New York: Appleton-Century-Crofts.

Chung, D. (1991). Asian cultural commonalities: A comparison with mainstream American culture. In S. Furuto, R. Biswas, D. Chung, & F. Ross-Sheriff (Eds.), *Social work practice with Asian Americans* (pp. 27–44). Newbury Park, CA: Sage.

Clark, A. L. (1966). Adaptation problems and the expanding family. *Nursing Forum, 5,* 98.

Clark, C., & Heidenreich, T. (1995). Spiritual care for the critically ill. *American Journal of Critical Care, 4*(1), 77–81.

Clark, M. (1970). *Health in the Mexican-American culture: A community study.* Berkeley, CA: University of California Press.

Clark, M. J. (1984). *Community nursing: Health care for today and tomorrow.* Reston, VA: Reston Publishing Co.

Clarke, V., Lovegrove, H., Williams, A., & Machperson, M. (2000). Unrealistic optimism and the Health Belief Model. *Journal of Behavioral Medicine, 23*(4), 367–376.

Clawson, J. (1996). A child with chronic illness and the process of family adaptation. *Journal of Pediatric Nursing, 11,* 52–61.

Clemen, S. (1977). Concepts of culture and value clarification. In S. Clemen & M. Gregerson (Eds.), *Family and community health nursing: A workbook.* Ann Arbor, MI: University of Michigan Media Library.

Cleveland, E. J., & Longaker, W. D. (1972). Neurotic patterns in the family. In G. Handel (Ed.), *The psychosocial interior of the family* (2nd ed.) (pp. 159–185). Chicago: Aldine-Atherton.

Clinton, B. (1995, October 17). We are one nation, one family indivisible. *Los Angeles Times,* p. A12.

Clinton, H. R. (1996). *It takes a village.* New York: Simon & Schuster.

Coates, J. F. (1996). Five major forces of change. *Futurist, 30*(5), 1–8.

Coddy, B. (1975). The therapist was a gringa. In S. Smoyak (Ed.), *The psychiatric nurse as a family therapist.* New York: Wiley.

Cody, W. K. (2000). Nursing frameworks to guide practice and research with families: Introductory remarks. *Nursing Science Quarterly, 13*(4), 277–284.

Cohen, S., & Syme, S. L. (1985). Issues in the study of social support. In S. Cohen & L. S. Syme (Eds.), *Social support and health* (pp. 3–20). New York: Academic Press.

Cohn, H. D., & Lieberman, E. J. (1974). Family planning and health. *American Journal of Public Health, 3,* 226–230.

Coleman, M., Ganong, L., & Fine, M. (2001). Reinvestigating remarriage: another decade of progress. In R. Milardo (Ed.), *Understanding families into the new millennium: A decade in review* (pp. 507–522). Minneapolis, MN: National Council on Family Relations.

Coleman, M., Ganong, L. H., & Goodwin, C. (1994). The presentation of stepfamilies in marriage and family textbooks: A reexamination. *Family Relations, 43,* 289–297.

Coleman, M., Ganong, L., & Fine, M. (2000). Reinvestigating remarriage: Another decade of progress. *Journal of Marriage and the Family, 62*(4), 1288–1307.

Colley, K. D. (1978). Growing up together: The mutual respect balance. In L. E. Arnold (Ed.), *Helping parents help their children.* New York: Brunner/Mazel.

Coltrane, B. (1997). Families and gender equity. *National Forum, 77*(2), 31–34.

Combrinck-Graham, L. (1985). A developmental model for family systems. *Family Process, 24*(2), 139–150.

Combrinck-Graham, L. (1990). Developments in family systems theory and research. *Journal of the American Academy of Child and Adolescent Psychiatry, 29*(4), 501–512.

Coner-Edwards, A. F., & Edwards, H. E. (1988). Introduction. In A. F. Coner-Edwards & J. H. Spurlock (Eds.), *Black families in crisis: The middle class.* New York: Brunner/Mazel.

Connery, D. S. (1968). *The Irish.* New York: Simon & Schuster.

Connors, H. R. (1988, April). Nurse case management. NAMFE: A three year perspective. *Kansas Nurse,* 8–9.

Conover, T. (1993, September 19). The United States of asylum. *New York Times Magazine,* 56–58, 74–78.

Constantine, L. L. (1986). *Family paradigms: The practice of theory in family therapy.* New York: Guilford Press.

Coontz, S. (1995). The way we weren't. The myth and reality of the "traditional" family. *National Forum, 75*(3), 11–14.

Coontz, S. (1996, May–June). Where are the good old days? *Modern Maturity,* 36–53.

Coontz, S. (1997). *The way we really are: Coming to terms with America's changing families.* New York: Basic Books.

Coontz, S., Parson, M., & Raley, G. (1999). *American families.* New York: Routledge.

Corless, I., Germino, B., & Pittman, M. (Eds.). (1994). *Dying, death, and bereavement: Theoretical perspectives.* Boston: Jones & Bartlett.

Cornille, T. A. (2001, June). Helping families deal with change. Sometimes helping means waiting to be asked. *Family Focus,* pp. F3, F5.

Corrales, R. G. (1975). Power and satisfaction in early marriage. In R. F. Cromwell & D. H. Olson (Eds.), *Power in families* (pp. 196–215). New York: Sage.

Cose, E. (1999, June 7). The good news about black America. *Newsweek,* 29–40.

Courtney, R. (1995). Community partnership primary care: A new paradigm for primary care. *Public Health Nursing, 12*(6), 366–373.

Cousins, S. (2000). "My heart couldn't take it": Older women's beliefs about exercise benefits and risks. *Journals of Gerontology. Series B: Psychological Sciences and Social Sciences, 55B*(5), 283–294.

Cowan, C. P., Cowan, P. A., Heming, G., & Miller, N. B. (1991). Becoming a family: Marriage, parenting, and family development. In P. A. Cowan & M. Hetherington (Eds.), *Family transitions.* Hillsdale, NJ: Erlbaum.

Cowan, C., & Cowan, P. (1995). Interventions to ease the transition to parenthood: Why are they needed and what they can do. *Family Relations, 44,* 412–423.

Cowley, G. (1995, March 27). It's time to rethink nature and nurture. *Newsweek,* 52.

Cox, M., & Paley, B. (1997). Families as systems. *Annual Review of Psychology, 48,* 243–267.

Craig, S. J., & Clymer, R. (2000). Racial residential segregation by level of socioeconomic status. *Social Science Quarterly, 81*(3), 701–715.

Creed, G. (2000). "Family values" and domestic economics. *Annual Review of Anthropology, 29,* 329–355.

Cromwell, R. E., & Olson, D. H. (1975). Introduction. In R. E. Cromwell & D. H. Olson (Eds.), *Power in families* (pp. 2–3). New York: Sage.

Cromwell, R. E., & Ruiz, R. A. (1979). The myth of macho dominance in decision-making within Mexican and Chicano families. *Hispanic Journal of Behavioral Science, 1*(4), 355–373.

Cromwell, V. L., & Cromwell, R. E. (1978, November). Perceived dominance in decision-making and conflict resolution among Anglo, Black and Chicano couples. *Journal of Marriage and the Family, 40,* 749–759.

Crooks, C. E., Iammarino, N. K., & Weinberg, A. D. (1987). The family's role in health promotion. *Health Values, 11*(2), 7–12.

Crosbie-Burnett, M. (1994). Remarriage and recoupling. In P. C. McHenry & S. J. Price (Eds.), *Families and change: Coping with stressful events.* Thousand Oaks, CA: Sage.

Crotty, M. (1998). *The foundations of social research: Meaning and perspective in the research process.* London: Sage.

Cunningham, W., Levan, R., Brown, E. R., & Wyn, R. (1999). *African Americans remain uninsured at higher rates than whites despite their increasing job-based coverage: Policy brief.* Los Angeles, CA: UCLA Center for Health Policy Research.

Curran, D. (1983). *Traits of a healthy family.* Minneapolis, MN: Winston Press.

Curran, D. J., & Renzetti, C. M. (2000). *Social problems: Society in crisis* (5th ed.). Boston: Allyn & Bacon.

Curtin, L. (1979). The nurse as advocate: A philosophical foundation for nursing. *Advances in Nursing Science, 1,* 1–10.

D'Antonio, W. V. (1983). Family, life, religion, and societal values and structure. In W. V. D'Antonio & J. Aldous (Eds.), *Families and religions.* Beverly Hills, CA: Sage.

D'Antonio, W. V., & Aldous, J. (1983). Introduction. In W. V. D'Antonio & J. Aldous (Eds.), *Families and religions.* Beverly Hills, CA: Sage.

Dadds, M. R. (1995). *Families, children and the development of dysfunction.* Thousand Oaks, CA: Sage.

Daka-Mulwanda, V., Thornburg, K. R., Filbert, L., & Klein, T. (1995). Collaboration of services for children and families. A synthesis of recent research and recommendations. *Family Relations, 44,* 219–223.

Dalgas-Pelish, P. L. (1993). The impact of the first child on marital happiness. *Journal of Advanced Nursing, 18,* 437–441.

Daly, K. (1996). *Families & time: Keeping pace in a hurried culture.* Thousand Oaks, CA: Sage.

Daly, K. (2000). *It keeps getting faster: Changing patterns of time in families.* Ontario, Canada: Vanier Institute of the Family.

Danesco, E. R., & Holden, E. W. (1998). Are there different types of homeless families? A typology of homeless families based on cluster analysis. *Family Relations, 47,* 159–165.

Daniel, L. (1986). Family assessment. In B. B. Logan & C. E. Dawkins (Eds.), *Family-centered nursing in the community* (pp. 183–208). Menlo Park, CA: Addison-Wesley.

Davidhizar, R., & Bechtel, G. A. (1999). Health and quality of life within colonias settlements along the United States and Mexico border. *Public Health Nursing, 16*(4), 301–306.

Davies, B. (1995). Sibling bereavement research. In I. Corless et al. (Eds.), *A challenge for living* (pp. 173–202). Boston: Jones & Bartlett.

Davies, B., Spinetta, J., Martinson, I., McClowry, S., & Kulenkamp, E. (1986). Manifestations of levels of functioning in grieving families. *Journal of Family Issues, 7*(3), 297–313.

Davis, F. (1963). *Passage through crisis: Polio victims and their families.* New York: Bobbs-Merrill.

Davis, O. S. (1978). Nursing approach to the postpartum family. In M. L. Moore (Ed.), *Realities in childbearing.* Philadelphia: Saunders.

Davis, R., & Voegtle, K. (1994). *Culturally competent health care for adolescents.* Chicago: American Medical Association.

Day, A. T., & Day, L. H. (1993, September). Living arrangements and successful aging among never-married American white women 77–87 years of age. *Aging and Society, 13*(3), 365–387.

Deatrick, J. A., Knafl, K. A., Murphy-Moore, C. (1999). Clarifying the concept of normalization. *Image, 31*(3), 209–214.

DeFrain, J., Le Masters, E. E., & Schroff, J. A. (1991). Environment and fatherhood: Rural and urban influences. In F. W. Bozett & S. M. Hanson (Eds.), *Fatherhood and families in cultural context* (pp. 162–186). New York: Springer.

Delgado, M. (1997). Puerto Rican natural support systems. *Urban Education, 32*(1), 81–98.

Dell Orto, A. E. (1988). Respite care: A vehicle for hope, the buffer against desperation. In P. W. Power, A. E. Dell Orto, & M. S. Gibbons (Eds.), *Family interventions throughout chronic illness and disability* (pp. 265–284). New York: Springer.

Demos, J. (1970). *A little commonwealth: Family life in Plymouth Colony.* New York: Oxford University Press.

Demos, V. (1990, August). Black family studies in the *Journal of Marriage and the Family* and the issue of distortion. A trend analysis. *Journal of Marriage and the Family, 52*(3), 603–612.

de Souza, P., & Gualda, D. (2000, July). *The family's health care: A responsibility of the women living in a slum.* Presentation made at the 5th International Family Nursing Conference, Chicago, Illinois.

Detzner, D. F. (1992). Life histories: Conflict in Southeast Asian refugee families. In J. F. Gilgun, K. Daly, & G. Handel (Eds.), *Qualitative methods in family research* (pp. 85–102). Newbury Park, CA: Sage.

Detzner, D. F., Xiong, B., & Eliason, P. (1999). *Helping youth succeed: Bicultural parenting for Southeast Asian families.* St. Paul, MN: University of Minnesota Extension.

Diaz-Guerrero, R. (1975). *Psychology of the Mexican culture and personality.* Austin, TX: University of Texas Press.

Dickinson, G. E., & Leming, M. R. (1995). *Understanding families. Diversity, continuity and change* (2nd ed.). Fort Worth, TX: Harcourt Brace College.

Diekelmann, N. (1977). *Primary health care of the well adult.* New York: McGraw-Hill.

Dietrich, K. T. (1975). A re-examination of the myth of black matriarchy. *Journal of Marriage and the Family, 37*(2), 367–374.

Dilworth-Anderson, P., & McAdoo, H. P. (1988, July). The study of ethnic minority families: Implications for practitioners and policy makers. *Family Relations, 37*(3), 265–267.

Dilworth-Anderson, P., Burton, L., & Johnson, L. (1993). Reframing theories for understanding race, ethnicity, and families. In P. Boss, W. Doherty, R. La Rossa, W. Schumm, & S. Steinmetz (Eds.), *Sourcebook of family theories and methods* (pp. 627–649). New York: Plenum Press.

Dinger, M. (1999). Physical activity: An update for health educators. *The International Electronic Journal of Health Education,* 81–83 *(www.iejhe.org).*

Dobson, J. (1999). *Family News from Dr. James Dobson, November. Focus on the family.* Colorado Springs, CO. Minneapolis, MN: National Council on Family Relations.

Dobson, J. (2001). The family in crisis. *Focus on the Family, 25*(8), 2–4.

Dodson, J. (1988). Conceptualizations of black families. In H. P. McAdoo (Ed.), *Black families* (2nd ed.) (pp. 77–88). Newbury Park, CA: Sage.

Doenges, M., Moorhouse, M., & Burley, J. (2000). *Application of nursing process and nursing diagnosis.* Philadelphia: Davis.

Doherty, W. J. (1992). Linkages between family theories and primary health care. In R. Sawa (Ed.), *Family health care* (pp. 30–39). Newbury Park, CA: Sage.

Doherty, W. J. (1995).Boundaries between parent and family education and family therapy. *Family Relations, 44,* 353–358.

Doherty, W. J., & Baird, M. A. (1983). *Family therapy and family medicine.* New York: Guilford Press.

Doherty, W. J., & Baird, M. A. (Eds.). (1987). *Family-centered medical care: A clinical casebook.* New York: Guilford Press.

Doherty, W. J., & Campbell, T. L. (1988). *Families and health.* Newbury Park, CA: Sage.

Doherty, W. J., Boss, P. G., LaRossa, R., Schumm, W. R., & Steinmetz, S. K. (1993). Family theories and methods: A contextual approach. In P. G. Boss, W. J. Doherty, R. LaRossa, W. R. Schumm, & S. K. Steinmetz (Eds.), *Sourcebook of family theories and methods: A contextual approach* (pp. 3–30). New York: Plenum.

Donaldson, M., Yordy, K., & Vanselow, N. (1994). *Defining primary care: An interim report.* Washington, DC: National Academy Press.

Donaldson, S. K., & Crowley, D. M. (1978). The discipline of nursing. *Nursing Outlook, 26,* 113–120.

Donnelly, E. (1990). Health promotion, families and the diagnostic process. *Family and Community Health, 12*(4), 12–20.

Dorfman, L., & Rubenstein, L. (1993). Paid and unpaid activities and retirement satisfaction among rural seniors. *Physical and Occupational Therapy in Geriatrics, 12*(1), 45–63.

Dorsey, R. R., & Jackson, J. Q. (1976). Cultural health traditions: The Latino/Chicano perspective. In M. Branch (Ed.), *Providing safe care to ethnic people of color* (pp. 41–79). New York: Appleton-Century-Crofts.

Dougherty, M. C. (1975). A cultural approach to the nurse's role in health planning. In B. E. Spradley (Ed.), *Contemporary community nursing* (pp. 439–445). Boston: Little, Brown.

Draguns, J. G. (1996). Humanly universal and culturally distinctive. In P. B. Pedersen, J. G. Draguns, W. J. Lonner, & J. E. Trimble (Eds.), *Counseling across cultures* (4th ed.) (pp. 1–20). Thousand Oaks, CA: Sage.

Drevdahl, D. (1999). Sailing beyond: Nursing theory and the person. *Advances in Nursing Science, 21*(4), 1–13.

Drotar, D., Crawfor, P., & Bush, M. (1984). The family context of childhood chronic illness: Implications for psychosocial intervention. In M. C. Eisenberg, L. C. Sutkin, & M. A. Jansen (Eds.), *Chronic illness and disability through the life span. Effects on self and family* (pp. 103–132). New York: Springer.

Duncan, D. F., & Gold, R. S. (1986, May/June). Reflections: Health promotion. What is it? *Health Values, 10*(3), 47–49.

Dunn, H. L. (1961). High-level wellness. Arlington, VA: Beatty.

Dunn, K. (2001). Lesbian parenting: an unpublished paper.

Dunphy, L. (2001). Families on the brink, on the edge. In P. L. Munhall & V. M. Fitzsimons (Eds.), *The emergence of family into the 21st century* (pp. 3–15). New York: The National League for Nursing.

Duvall, E. M., & Miller, B. L. (1985). *Marriage and family development* (6th ed.). New York: Harper & Row.

Dyer, W. (1973). Working with groups. In A. Reinhardt & M. Quinn (Eds.), *Family-centered community nursing.* St. Louis: Mosby.

Easley, M., & Epstein, N. (1991). Coping with stress in a family with an alcoholic parent. *Family Relations, 40,* 218–224.

East, P. L (1999). The first teenage pregnancy in the family: Does it affect mothers' parenting, attitudes, or mother–adolescent communication? *Journal of Marriage and the Family, 61*(2), 306–319.

Edelman, C., & Mandle, C. L. (1986). *Health promotion throughout the life span.* St. Louis: Mosby.

Edelman, M. W. (1997). An advocacy agenda for black families and children. In H. P. McAdoo (Ed.), *Black families* (3rd ed.) (pp. 323–333). Thousand Oaks, CA: Sage.

Edelman, M. W. (1987). *Families in peril.* Cambridge, MA: Harvard University Press.

Ehrenberg, M. F., Gearing-Small, M., Hunter, M. A., & Small, B. J. (2001). Childcare task division and shared parenting attitudes in dual-earner families with young children. *Family Relations, 50*(2), 143–153.

Ehrenreich, B. (2001, August 5). America's torrent of need. *Los Angeles Times,* p. M-1.

Elias, M. (1987, November). Role strained couples. *American Health,* 58–60.

Eliason, M. (1996). Lesbian and gay family issues. *Journal of Family Nursing, 2*(1), 10–29.

Elkind, D. (1988). *The hurried child.* Reading, MA: Addison-Wesley.

Elkind, D. (1994). *Ties that stress: The new family imbalance.* Cambridge, MA: Harvard University Press.

Elkins, C. P. (1984). *Community health nursing—Skills and strategies.* Bowie, MD: Brady.

Ell, K., & Northen, H. (1990). *Families and health care.* New York: Aldine de Gruyter.

Elliott-Binns, D. P. (1973). An analysis of lay medicine. *Journal of the Royal College of General Practice, 23,* 255.

Ellis, A., & Grieger, R. (1977). *Handbook of rational emotive therapy.* New York: Springer.

Ellis, V. (1995, March 1). Report finds California children's quality of life in decline. *Los Angeles Times,* pp. A3, A19.

Ellison, C. G. (1990). Family ties, friendships, and subjective well-being among black Americans. *Journal of Marriage and the Family, 52*(3), 298–310.

Ellman, B., & Taggart, M. (1993). Changing gender norms. In F. Walsh (Ed.), *Normal family processes* (pp. 377–404). New York: Guilford Press.

Elmer-Dewitt, P. (1990, Fall). The great experiment. *Newsweek,* 73–75.

Engebretson, J. (1994). Folk healing and biomedicine: Culture clash or complementary approach? *Journal of Holistic Nursing, 12*(3), 240–250.

Epstein, N. B., Bishop, D. S., & Baldwin, L. M. (1982). McMaster model of family functioning: A view of the normal family. In F. Walsh (Ed.), *Normal family processes* (pp. 115–141). New York: Guilford Press.

Epstein, N. B., Bishop, D., Ryan, C., Miller, I., & Keitner, G. (1993). The McMaster model: View of healthy family functioning. In F. Walsh (Ed.), *Normal family processes* (2nd ed.) (pp. 138–160). New York: Guilford Press.

Epstein, Y. M. (1981). Crowding and human behavior. *Journal of Social Issues, 37*(1), 126–131.

Erickson, R. J., & Gegas, V. (1991). Social class and fatherhood. In F. W. Bozett & S. M. H. Hanson (Eds.), *Fatherhood and families in cultural context* (pp. 114–137). New York: Springer.

Erikson, E. H. (1950). *Childhood and society.* New York: Norton.

Eshleman, J. R. (1974). *The family: An introduction.* Boston: Allyn & Bacon.

Evans, C. J. (1991). Description of a follow-up program for childbearing families. *Journal of Obstetric, Gynecologic, and Neonatal Nursing, 20*(2), 113–118.

Falco, S. M., & Lobo, M. L. (1995). Chapter 14: Martha E. Rogers. In J. B. George (Ed.). *Nursing theories: The base for professional nursing practice* (4th ed.) (pp. 229–248). Norwalk, CT: Appleton & Lange.

Falicov, C. J. (1982). Mexican families. In M. McGoldrick, J. Pierce, & J. Giordano (Eds.), *Ethnicity and family therapy.* New York: Guilford Press.

Falicov, C. J. (1988). Learning to think culturally. In D. C. Breunlin & R. C. Schwartz (Eds.), *Handbook of family therapy, training and supervision.* New York: Guilford Press.

Falicov, C. J. (1996). Mexican families. In M. McGoldrick, J. Giordano, & J. K. Pearce (Eds.), *Ethnicity and family therapy* (2nd ed.) (pp. 169–182). New York: Guilford Press.

Falicov, C. J. (1998). *Latino families in therapy: A guide to multicultural practice.* New York: The Guilford Press.

Falloon, I. R. H. (1991). Behavioral family therapy. In A. S. Gurman & D. P. Kniskern (Eds.), *Handbook of family therapy.* New York: Brunner/Mazel.

Family Service America. (1984). *The state of families, 1984–1985.* New York: Family Service of America.

Farberow, N. L., Gallagher-Thompson, D., Gilewski, M., & Thompson, L. (1992). Changes in grief and mental health of bereaved spouses of older adult suicides. *Journal of Gerontology, 47*(6), 357–366.

Farge, E. J. (1975). *La vida Chicano: Health care attitudes and behaviors of Houston Chicanos.* San Francisco: R & E Research Associates.

Faux, S. A. (1998). Historical overview of responses of children and their families to chronic Illness. In M. E. Broome, K. Knafl, K. Pridham, & S. Feetham (Eds.), *Children and families in health and illness* (pp. 179–195). Thousand Oaks, CA: Sage.

Fawcett, J., & Downs, F. S. (1992). *The relationship of theory and research.* Philadelphia: Davis.

Fawcett, J. (1999). *The relationship of theory and research* (3rd ed.). Philadelphia: Davis.

Feeley, N., & Gottlieb, L. N. (2000). Nursing approaches for working with family strengths and resources. *Journal of Family Nursing, 6*(1), 9–24.

Feiring, C., & Lewis, C. (1984). Changing characteristics of the U.S. family. In M. Lewis (Ed.), *Beyond the dyad* (pp. 59–89). New York: Plenum.

Feldman, H. (1961). *The development of the husband–wife relationship.* Unpublished study supported in part by the National Institute of Mental Health.

Feldman, H. (1971). The effects of children on the family. In A. Michel (Ed.), *Family issues of employed women in Europe and America* (pp. 107–125). Leiden, Netherlands: E. J. Brill.

Fellows, D. K. (1972). *A mosaic of America's ethnic minorities.* New York: Wiley.

Fenwick, E., & Smith, T. (1994). *Adolescence: The survival guide for parents and teenagers.* New York: Dorling Kindersley.

Ferguson-Marshalleck, E. G., & Miller, J. K. (2001). Sociocultural influences on family health. In S. M. H. Hanson (Ed.), *Family health care nursing: Theory, practice and research* (2nd ed.) (pp. 101–121). Philadelphia: Davis.

Ferreira, A. J. (1963). Family myth and homeostasis. *Archives of General Psychiatry, 9,* 457.

Fields, R. (2001, August 6). '90's' saw a tide of new people. *Los Angeles Times,* pp. A1, A13.

Fields, R. (2001, May 15). Married with children still fading as a model. *Los Angeles Times,* pp. A1, A16.

Fiese, B. (2000, June). Routines and rituals help families cope with stress. *Family Focus,* p. 18.

Fife, B. L. (1985). A model for predicting the adaptation of families to medical crisis: An analysis of role integration. *Image, 17*(4), 108–112.

Figley, C. (Ed.). (1995). *Compassion fatigue: Coping with secondary traumatic stress disorder in those who treat the traumatized.* New York: Brunner/Mazel.

Figley, C. R. (1989). *Helping traumatized families.* San Francisco: Jossey-Bass.

Fine, M. (1992). Families in the United States: Their current status and future prospects. *Family Relations, 41,* 430–435.

Fine, M. A., Donnelly, B. W., & Voydanoff, P. (1986). Adjustment and satisfaction of parents: A comparison of intact, single parent and stepparent families. *Journal of Family Issues, 7,* 391–404.

Fingerman, K. L. (1998). The good, the bad, and the worrisome: Emotional complexities in grandparents' experiences with individual grandchildren. *Family Relations, 47*(4), 403–414.

Finley, G. E. (2000, June). Adoptive families: Dramatic changes across generations. *Family Focus,* pp. F10, F12.

Finley, N. J. (1989). Theories of family labor as applied to gender differences in caregiving for elderly parents. *Journal of Marriage and the Family, 51*(1), 79–86.

Fischer J., & Wampler, R. (1994). Abusive drinking in young adults: Personality type and family role as moderators of family-of-origin influences. *Journal of Marriage and the Family, 56,* 469–479.

Fisher, L., & Ransom, D. C. (1995). An empirically derived typology of families: 1. Relationships with adult health. *Family Process, 34,* 161–181.

Fishman, B. M., Bobo, L., Kosub, K., Womeodu, R. (1998). Cultural issues in serving minority populations: Emphasis on Mexican Americans and African Americans. *American Journal of the Medical Sciences, 306*(3), 160–166.

Fishman, H. C. (1985). Diagnosis and context: An Alexandrian quartet. In R. L. Ziffer (Ed.), *Adjunctive techniques in family therapy.* New York: Grune & Stratton.

Fitting, M., Rabins, P., Lucas, M. J., & Eastham, J. (1986). Caregivers for demented patients: A comparison of husbands and wives. *The Gerontologist, 26,* 248–252.

Fitzgerald, B. (1999). Children of lesbian and gay parents: A review of the literature. *Marriage & Family Review, 29*(1), 57–75.

Fitzpatrick, M. A., & Ritchie, L. D. (1993). Communication theory and the family. In P. G. Boss, W. J. Doherty, R. LaRossa, W. R. Schumm, & S. K. Steinmetz (Eds.), *Sourcebook of family theories and methods: A contextual approach* (pp. 565–585). New York: Plenum.

Fitzpatrick, S. B., Coughlin, S. S., & Chamberline, J. (1992). A novel asthma camp intervention for childhood asthma among urban blacks. *Journal of the National Medical Association, 84*(3), 233–237.

Flannery, R., Perry, C., Penk, W., & Flannery, G. (1994). Validating Antonovsky's sense of coherence scale. *Journal of Clinical Psychology, 50,* 575–577.

Flaskerud, J. (1984, September). Mental health—The culture component. *California Nurse,* 4.

Foley, V. D. (1986). *An introduction to family therapy* (2nd ed.). Orlando, FL: Grune & Stratton.

Folkman, S., Lazarus, R. S., Dunkel-Schetter, C., De Longis, A., & Gruen, R. J. (1986). The dynamics of a stressful encounter: Cognitive appraisal, coping and encounter-outcomes. *Journal of Personality and Social Psychology, 50,* 992–1003.

Follen, M. A., Johnson, D., & Kronenwetter, S. (1994). Family interventions in a critical care setting. In *Program and Abstracts of the Third International Family Nursing Conference.* Montreal, Canada, May 25–28, 1994.

Ford, L. (1979). The development of family nursing. In D. P. Hymovich & M. U. Barnard (Eds.), *Family health care.* New York: McGraw-Hill.

Foreman, J. (2001, July 16). Cancer's toll on marriage. *Los Angeles Times,* pp. S1, S5.

Forrest, J. (1981). The family. The focus for health behavior generation. *Health Values: Achieving High Level Wellness, 5*(4), 138–144.

Foster, D., Phillips, R., Hamel, M. & Eisenberg, D. (2000). Alternative medicine use in older Americans. *Journal of the American Geriatrics Society, 48*(12), 1560–1565.

Fraley, A. M. (1992). *Nursing and the disabled: Across the life span.* Boston: Jones and Bartlett.

Francis, G. M., & Munjas, B. A. (1976). *Manual of socialpsychologic assessment.* New York: Appleton-Century-Crofts.

Freeman, D. S. (1992). *Multigenerational family therapy.* New York: Haworth Press.

Frey, M., & Sieloff, C. (Eds.). (1995). *Advancing King's systems framework and theory of nursing.* London: Sage.

Friedemann, M. L. (1989, February). Closing the gap between grand theory and mental health practice with families. Part 1. *Archives of Psychiatric Nursing, III,* 10–19.

Friedemann, M. L. (1993a). Closing the gap between grand theory and mental health practice with families. In G. Wegner & R. Alexander (Eds.), *Readings in family nursing* (pp. 41–56). Philadelphia: Lippincott.

Friedemann, M. L. (1993b). The concept of family nursing. In G. D. Wegner & R. J. Alexander (Eds.), *Readings in family nursing* (pp. 13–22). Philadelphia: Lippincott.

Friedemann, M. L. (1995). *The framework of systemic organization.* Thousand Oaks, CA: Sage.

Friedman, D. B. (1957). Parent development. *California Medicine, 86,* 25.

Friedman, M. (1985). *Family stress and coping among Anglo and Latino families with childhood cancer.* Unpublished PhD dissertation, University of Southern California.

Friedman, M. (1987). Intervening with families of school-aged children with cancer. In M. Leahey & L. M. Wright (Eds.), *Families and life-threatening illness* (pp. 219–234). Springhouse, PA: Springhouse Publishing.

Friedman, M. (1990). Transcultural family nursing: Application to Latino and black families. *Journal of Pediatric Nursing, 5*(3), 214–222.

Friedman, M. M. (1992). *Family nursing: Theory and practice* (3rd ed.). Norwalk, CT: Appleton & Lange.

Friedman, M. M., & Ferguson-Marshalleck, E. (1996). Sociocultural influences on family health. In S. Hanson & S. Boyd (Eds.), *Family health care nursing: Theory, practice & research* (pp. 81–98). Philadelphia: Davis.

Frye, B. A. (1995). Use of cultural themes in promoting health among Southeast Asian refugees. *American Journal of Health Promotion, 9,* 269–280.

Fulwood, S. (1996, September 27). Income shows 1st rise since 1989 as poverty falls. *Los Angeles Times,* pp. A1, A16.

Furstenberg, F. F., & Nord, C. W. (1985). Parenting apart: Patterns of childrearing after marital disruption. *Journal of Marriage and the Family, 47*(4), 893–904.

Gable, S., Ernic, K., & Belsky, J. (1994). Co-parenting within the family system. Influences on children's development. *Family Relations, 43,* 380–386.

Gadow, S. (1980). Existential advocacy: Philosophical foundations of nursing. In S. Spicker & S. Gadow (Eds.), *Nursing images and ideals.* New York: Springer.

Gagne, P. (1992). Appalachian women: Violence and social control [Special issue]. *Journal of Contemporary Ethnography, 20,* 387–415.

Gallegos, J. S. (1991). Culturally relevant services for Hispanic elderly. In M. Sotomayor (Ed.), *Empowering Hispanic families: A critical issue for the 90's* (pp. 173–190). Milwaukee, WI: Family Service America.

Galvin, K. M., & Brommel, B. J. (1986). *Family communication: Cohesion and change* (2nd ed.). Glenview, IL: Scott, Foresman.

Ganong, L., Coleman, M., & Fine, M. (1995). Remarriage and stepfamilies. In R. D. Day, K. R. Gilbert, B. H. Settles, & W. R. Burr (Eds.), *Research and theory in family science* (pp. 287–303). Pacific Grove, CA: Brooks/Cole.

Garcia-Preto, N. (1996). Latino families: An overview. In M. McGoldrick, J. Giordano, & J. K. Pearce (Eds.), *Ethnicity and family therapy* (2nd ed.) (pp. 141–154). New York: Guilford Press.

Gardner, R. W., Robey, B., & Smith, P. C. (1985). Asian Americans: Growth, change, and diversity. *Population Bulletin, 40*(4). Washington, DC: Population Reference Bureau.

Garner, M. K. (1978). Our values are showing: Inadequate childhood immunization. *Health Values: Achieving High Level Wellness, 2*(3), 129.

Gavazzi, S. M., & Schock, A. M. (2000). Mental illness and families. In P. C. McKenry & S. J. Price (Eds.), *Families and change* (pp. 229–249). Thousand Oaks, CA: Sage.

Gay and Lesbian Medical Association (GLMA). (2000). *Healthy People 2010: Companion Document for lesbian, gay, bisexual and transgender (LGBT) health.* San Francisco: Author (*www.glma.org*).

Geba, B. (1985). *Being at leisure, play at life.* La Mesa, CA: Leisure Science Systems International.

Gebbie, E., & Gebbie, K. M. (2001). Families, nursing and social policy. In S. M. H. Hanson (Ed.), *Family health care nursing* (2nd ed.) (pp. 365–385). Philadelphia: Davis.

Gecas, V. (1979). The influence of social class on socialization. In W. R. Burr, R. Hill, F. I. Nye, & I. L. Reiss (Eds.), *Contemporary theories about the family* (Vol. I, pp. 365–404). New York: Free Press.

Gecas, V., & Seff, M. A. (1991). Families and adolescents: A review of the 1980's. In A. Booth (Ed.), *Contemporary families: Looking forward, looking back* (pp. 208–225). Minneapolis, MN: National Council on Family Relations.

Gelcer, E. (1986). Dealing with loss in the family context. *Journal of Family Issues, 7*(3), 315–335.

Gelles, R. J. (1980). Violence in the family: A review of research on the seventies. *Journal of Marriage and the Family, 42*(4), 873–885.

Gelles, R. J. (1990). Methodological issues in the study of family violence. In G. R. Patterson (Ed.), *Family social interaction: Content and methodology issues in the study of aggression and depression* (pp. 49–74). Hillsdale, NY: Erlbaum.

Gelles, R. J. (2000). Violence, abuse & neglect in families. In P. C. McKenry & S. J. Price (Eds.), *Families and change. Coping with stressful events and transitions* (pp. 183–228). Thousand Oaks, CA: Sage.

Gelles, R. J., & Maynard, P. E. (1987). A structural family systems approach to intervention in cases of family violence. *Family Relations, 36*(3), 270–275.

Gelman, D., et al. (1985, July 15). Playing both mother and father. *Newsweek,* 42–50.

Gelman, D., et al. (1988, March 7). Black and white in America. *Newsweek,* 18–23.

Geltman, P. I., & Meyers, A. F. (1999). Immigration legal status and use of public programs and prenatal care. *Journal of Immigrant Health, 1*(2), 91–97.

Gendell, M., & Siegel, J. S. (1996). Trends in retirement age in the United States, 1955–1993 by sex and race. *Journal of Gerontology, 51B,* 3.

George, J. B. (1995). Margaret Newman. In J. B. George (Ed.), *Nursing theories* (4th ed.) Norwalk, CT: Appleton & Lange.

George, L., & Gwyther, L. (1986). Caregiver well-being: A multidimensional examination of family caregivers of demented adults. *The Gerontologist, 26*(3), 253–259.

Germain, C. P. (1992). Cultural care: A bridge between sickness, illness, and disease. *Holistic Nursing Practice, 6*(3), 1–9.

Gershon, T. D., Tschann, J. M., & Jemerin, J. M. (1999). Stigmatization, self-esteem, and coping among the adolescent children of lesbian mothers. *Journal of Adolescent Health, 24*(6), 437–445.

Gershwin, M., & Nilsen, J. (1989). Healthy families. In C. Gilliss, B. Highley, B. Roberts, & I. Martinson (Eds.), *Toward a science of family nursing* (pp. 77–91). Menlo Park, CA: Addison-Wesley.

Gerson, W. M. (1960). Leisure and marital satisfaction of college married couples. *Marriage and Family Living, 22,* 360–361.

Gibbs, N. (2001, August 6). Shifting the balance of power in *Times Magazine,* 40–46.

Giger, J. N., & Davidhizar, R. E. (1999). *Transcultural nursing: Assessment and intervention* (3rd ed.). St. Louis: Mosby.

Gilbert, D., & Kahl, J. A. (1993). *The American class structure.* Belmont, CA: Wadsworth.

Giles-Sims, J., Straus, M. A., & Sugarman, D. B. (1995). Child, maternal, and family characteristics associated with spanking. *Family Relations, 44,* 170–176.

Gilford, R. (1984). Contracts in marital satisfaction throughout old age: An exchange theory analysis. *Journal of Gerontology, 39,* 325–333.

Gilligan, C. (1982). *In a different voice.* Cambridge: Harvard University Press.

Gilliss, C. L. (1984). Reducing family stress during and after coronary artery bypass surgery. *Nursing Clinics of North America, 19*(1), 103–111.

Gilliss, C. L., & Davis, L. L. (1993). Does family intervention make a difference? An integrative review and meta-analysis. In S. L. Feetham, S. B. Meister, J. M. Bell, & C. L. Gilliss (Eds.), *The nursing of families: Theory, research, education and practice* (pp. 259–265). Newbury Park, CA: Sage.

Gilliss, C. L., Rose, D. B., Hallburg, J. C., & Martinson, I. M. (1989). The family and chronic illness. In C. L. Gilliss, B. L. Highley, B. M. Roberts, & I. M. Martinson (Eds.), *Toward a science of family nursing* (pp. 287–299). Menlo Park, CA: Addison-Wesley.

Gilliss, C. L., Sparacino, P. S. A., Gortner, S. R., & Kenneth, H. Y. (1985). Events leading to the treatment of coronary artery disease: Implications for nursing care. *Heart & Lung, 14*(4), 350–356.

Gilliss, C. L., & Knafl, K. A. (1999). Nursing care of families in non-normative transitions. The state of science and practice. In A. S. Hinshaw, S. L. Feetham, & J. L. F. Shaver (Eds.), *Handbook of clinical nursing research* (pp. 231–245). Thousand Oaks, CA: Sage.

Giovannetti de Jesus, J., & R. B. Bergamasco. (1998). When the housewife is missing. *Journal of Family Nursing, 4*(4), 387–393.

Gladding, S. T. (1995). *Family therapy: History, theory, and practice.* Englewood Cliffs, NJ: Prentice Hall.

Glanz, K., Lewis, F. M., & Rimer, B. K. (Eds.) (1997). *Health behavior and health education: Theory, research and practice.* San Francisco: Jossey-Bass.

Glasser, P., & Glasser, L. (1970). *Families in crisis.* New York: Harper & Row.

Glenn, M. L. (1987). *Collaborative health care: A family-oriented model.* New York: Praeger.

Glick, P. C. (1997). Demographic pictures of African American families. In H. P. McAdoo (Ed.), *Black families* (3rd ed.) (pp. 118–138). Thousand Oaks, CA: Sage.

Glick, P. C. (1988b). Fifty years of family demography: A record of social change. *Journal of Marriage and the Family, 50*(4), 861–873.

Glick, P. C. (1989). The family life cycle and social change. *Family Relations, 38*(2), 123–129.

Glick, P. C. (1994). American families: As they are and were. In A. S. Skolnick & J. H. Skolnick (Eds.), *Family in transition* (8th ed.) (pp. 91–104). New York: HarperCollins College.

Godwin, D. D., & Scanzoni, J. (1989). Couple consensus during marital joint decision-making: A context, process, outcome model. *Journal of Marriage and the Family, 51*(4), 943–956.

Goldenberg, I., & Goldenberg, H. (2000). *Family therapy: An overview* (5th ed.). Belmont, CA: Wadsworth.

Goldenberg, I., & Goldenberg, H. (2002). *Counseling today's familes* (4th ed.). Pacific Grove, CA: Brooks/Cole.

Goldner, V. (1985). Feminism and family therapy. *Family Process, 24,* 31–47.

Gonzales, E. (1976). The role of Chicano folk beliefs and practices in mental health. In C. A. Hernandez, M. J. Haug, & N. N. Wagner (Eds.), *Chicanos—Social and psychological perspectives* (2nd ed.). St. Louis: Mosby.

Gonzalez, G. (1991). Hispanics in the past two decades, Latinos in the next two: Hindsight and foresight. In M. Sotomayor (Ed.), *Empowering Hispanic families: A critical issue for the '90s* (pp. 1–19). Milwaukee, WI: Family Service America.

Goode, W. J. (1964). *The family.* Glencoe, IL: Free Press.

Gordon, M. (2000). *Manual of nursing diagnosis.* St. Louis: Mosby.

Gordon, M. M. (1964). *Assimilation in American life.* New York: Oxford University Press.

Gordon, T. (1970). *Parent effectiveness training.* New York: Wyden.

Gorman, G. (1975). New families, new marriages. In S. Smoyak (Ed.), *The psychiatric nurse as a family therapist.* New York: Wiley.

Gottfried, A. E., & Gottfried, A. W. (1994). *Redefining families: Implications for children's development.* New York: Plenum.

Gottman, J. (1995, November). *Predictors of divorce: Narrow therapy.* Presentation made at the annual convention of the National Council on Family Relations, Portland, Oregon.

Gottman, J. M., & Levenson, R. W. (1999). How stable is marital interaction over time? *Family Process, 38,* 159–166.

Gottman, J., Notarius, C., Gonso, J., & Markman, H. (1977). *A couples guide to communication*. Champagne, IL: Research Press.

Graedon, T. F. (1985). A transcultural approach to nursing practice. In J. E. Hall & B. R. Weaver (Eds.), *Distributive nursing practice: Systems approach to community health* (3rd ed.) (pp. 315–331). Philadelphia: Lippincott.

Gray, V. (1996). Family self-care. In P. J. Bomar (Ed.), *Nurses and family health promotion: Concepts, assessment, and interventions* (2nd ed.). Philadelphia: Saunders.

Grebler, L., Moore, J. W., & Guzman, R. C. (1970). *The Mexican-American people: The nation's second largest minority*. New York: Free Press.

Green, M. (1994). *Bright futures: Guidelines for health supervision of infants, children and adolescents*. Arlington, VA: National Center for Education in Maternal and Child Health.

Green, M. (2001). *Bright futures: Guidelines for health supervision of infants, children and adolescents*. Arlington, VA: National Center for Education in Maternal and Child Health.

Greene, B. (1995). African American families. *National Forum, 75*(3), 29–32.

Greiner, D. S., & Demi, A. S. (1995). Family therapy. In B. S. Johnson (Ed.), *Child, adolescent, and family psychiatric nursing* (pp. 358–368). Philadelphia: Lippincott.

Greydanus, D. E. (Ed.). (1991). *Caring for your adolescent*. New York: Bantam Books.

Griffin, J. L. (1994, February 14). Black health risks unique. *The Oregonian*, p. A2.

Grimes, M. L. (1996). Middle class morality: Postures towards the poor. *National Forum, 76*(3), 3–4.

Grubbs, L., & Tabano, M. (2000). Use of sunscreen in health care professionals: The Health Belief Model. *Cancer Nursing, 23*(3), 164–167.

Grzywacz, J. (2000). Socioeconomic status and health behaviors among Californians. *Research in the Sociology of Health Care, 18*, 121–149.

Gudykunst, W. B. (1991). *Bridging differences: Effective intergroup communicaton*. Newbury Park, CA: Sage.

Gurian, M. (2000). *The good son: Shaping the moral development of our young men*. New York: Putnam.

Gurin, J. (1985, October). Families: A personal way to get unstuck. *American Health*, 39–41.

Hagestad, G. O. (1988). Demographic change and the life course: Some emerging trends in the family realm. *Family Relations, 37*(4), 405–410.

Haglund, K. (2000). Parenting a second time around: An ethnography of African American grandmothers parenting grandchildren due to parental cocaine abuse. *Journal of Family Nursing, 6*(2), 120–135.

Hajal, F. (1990). Family scapegoating in the life and works of Karen Blixen. *Journal of the American Academy of Psychoanalysis, 18*, 626–643.

Haley, J. (1976). *Problem-solving therapy*. San Francisco: Jossey-Bass.

Haley, J. (1980). *Leaving home*. New York: McGraw-Hill.

Hall, A., & Wellman, B. (1985). Social networks and social support. In S. Cohen & S. L. Syme (Eds.), *Social support and health* (pp. 23–41). New York: Academic Press.

Hall, J., & Weaver, B. (1974). Crisis: A conceptual approach to family nursing. In J. Hall & B. Weaver (Eds.), *Nursing of families in crisis* (pp. 3–9). Philadelphia: Lippincott.

Hallberg, L. R-M. (1996). Occupational hearing loss: Coping and family life. *Scandanian Audiology, 25*(Supplement 43), 233.

Hammer, T. J., & Turner, P. H. (1985). *Parenting in contemporary society*. Englewood Cliffs, NJ: Prentice Hall.

Handel, G. (1972). *The psychosocial interior of the family* (2nd ed.). Chicago: Aldine Atherton.

Hanna, D. R., & Roy, Sr. C. (2001). Roy Adaptation Model and perspectives on the family. *Nursing Science Quarterly, 14*(1), 9–13.

Hanson, S. M. H., & Boyd, S. T. (Eds.). (1996a). *Family health care nursing: Theory, practice and research*. Philadelphia: Davis.

Hanson, S. M. H., & Boyd, S. T. (Eds.). (1996b). Family nursing: An overview. In S. M. H. Hanson & S. T. Boyd (Eds.), *Family health care nursing: Theory, practice and research* (pp. 5–37). Philadelphia: Davis.

Hanson, S. M. H., & Bozett, F. H. (Eds.). (1985). *Dimensions of fatherhood*. Newbury Park, CA: Sage.

Hanson, S. M. H., & Bozett, F. H. (Eds.). (1987). Fatherhood and changing family roles. *Family and Community Health, 9*(4), 9–21.

Hanson, S. M. H., & Kaakinen, J. R. (1996). Family health assessment. In M. Stanhope & J. Lancaster (Eds.), *Community health nursing* (pp. 497–520). St. Louis: Mosby.

Hanson, S. M. H., & Mischke, K. (1996). Family health assessment and intervention. In P. J. Bomar (Ed.), *Nurses and family health promotion* (2nd ed.) (pp. 165–202). Philadelphia: Saunders.

Hanson, S. H. (2001a). Families and family nursing in the twenty-first century. In S. H. Hanson (Ed.), *Family health care nursing: Theory, practice and research* (2nd ed.) (pp. 387–404). Philadelphia: Davis.

Hanson, S. H. (2001b). Family health care nursing. An Introduction. In S. H. Hanson (Ed.), *Family health care nursing: Theory, practice and research* (2nd ed.). (pp. 3–35). Philadelphia: Davis.

Harburg, E., Erfurt, J. C., Chape, G., & Havenstein, L. S. (1973). Socioecological stressor areas and black–white blood pressure. Detroit. *Journal of Chronic Diseases, 26*, 595–611.

Hardwick, P. (1991). Families and the professional network: An attempted classification of professional network actions which can hinder change. *Journal of Family Therapy, 13,* 187–205.

Hardy, M. E., & Hardy, W. L. (1988). Role stress and role strain. Managing role strain. In M. E. Hardy & M. Conway (Eds.), *Role theory: Perspectives for health professionals* (pp. 159–255). Norwalk, CT: Appleton & Lange.

Harley, W. (1994). *His needs, her needs.* Grand Rapids, MI: Fleming H. Revell.

Harris, L., et al. (1975). *The myths and reality of aging in America.* Washington, DC: National Council on Aging.

Harris, R. (1990, July 10). Blacks: Grim statistics considered threat to race. *Los Angeles Times,* pp. A1, A25.

Harris, R. (1991, May 14). A generation of innocents carries drug abuse scars. *Los Angeles Times,* pp. A1, A18, A19.

Harris, S. E. (1975). Negativity as a major communication pattern in a family. In S. Smoyak (Ed.), *The psychiatric nurse as a family therapist* (pp. 210–216). New York: Wiley.

Harris, T. G. (1984). From hedonism to health. *American Health, 3*(2), 54–56.

Harrison, A. O., et al. (1994). Family ecologies of ethnic minority children. In G. Handel & G. G. Whitchurch (Eds.), *The psychosocial interior of the family* (4th ed.) (pp. 187–209). New York: Aldine de Gruyter.

Harrison, I. E., & Harrison, D. S. (1971). The black family experience and health behavior. In C. Crawford (Ed.), *Health and the family* (pp. 175–199). New York: Macmillan.

Hartman, A. (1978). Diagrammatic assessment of family relationships. *Social Casework, 59,* 456–476.

Hartman, A., & Laird, J. (1983). *Family-centered social work practice.* New York: Free Press.

Hartrick, G. (1997) Relational capacity: The foundation for interpersonal nursing practice. *Journal of Advanced Nursing 26,* 523–528.

Hartrick, G. (1997). Beyond a service model of care. *Journal of Family Nursing, 3*(1), 57–69.

Hartrick, G., Lindsey, A. E., & Hills, M. (1994). Family nursing assessment: Meeting the challenge of health promotion. *Journal of Advanced Nursing, 20,* 85–91.

Harvath, T. A., Stewart, B. J., & Archibold, P. G. (1994). Third International Family Nursing Conference, Program and Abstracts, May 25–28, Montreal, Canada.

Harvey-Walker, S. (1998). Can complementary and alternative therapies play a role in the emergency department? *Australian Emergency Nursing Journal, 1*(5), 29–32.

Harwood, A. (1981). Guidelines for culturally appropriate health care. In A. Harwood (Ed.), *Ethnicity and medical care* (pp. 482–507). Cambridge, MA: Harvard Press.

Haug, M., Belgrove, L., & Jones, S. (1992). Partner's health and retirement adaptation of women and their husbands. *Journal of Women and Aging, 4*(3), 5–29.

Haveman, M., van Berkum, G., Reijnders, R., & Heller, T. (1997). Differences in service needs, time demands, and caregiving burden among parents of persons with mental retardation across the life cycle. *Family Relations 46*(4), 417–425.

Hawkes, G. R., & Taylor, M. (1975, November). Power structure in Mexican and Mexican-American farm labor families. *Journal of Marriage and the Family, 37*(4), 807–811.

Hawkins, A. J., Marshall, C. M., & Meiners, K. M. (1995). Exploring wives' sense of fairness about family work. *Journal of Family Issues, 16*(6), 693–721.

Hawkins, J., Weisberg, C., & Ray, D. (1980). Spouse differences in communication style. Preference, perception, behavior. *Journal of Marriage and the Family, 42*(3), 585–593.

Hawks, B. L. (1996). Barriers to health improvement for Asian Americans. *Asian American and Pacific Islander Journal of Health, 4*(1–3), 50–54.

Hawley, D., & Geske, S. (2000). The use of theory in family therapy research: A content analysis of family therapy journals. *Journal of Marital and Family Therapy, 26*(1), 17–22.

Hayes-Battista, D., & Chapa, J. (1987). Latin terminology: Conceptual bases for standardized terminology. *American Journal of Public Health, 77,* 61–68.

Hayes-Battista, D. (1990, April 26). *Creating health policy in multi-cultural California.* Paper presented at a statewide conference of the California Coalition for the Future of Public Health, Los Angeles, CA.

Hayward, M. D., Crimmins, E. M., Miles, T. P., & Yang, Y. (2000). The significane of socioeconomic status in explaining the racial gap in chronic health conditions. *American Sociological Review, 65*(6), 910–930.

Haywood, M. D., & Liu, M. C. (1992). Men and women in their retirement years: A demographic profile. In M. Snizovzcz, D. J. Ekerdt, & D. H. Vinick (Eds.), *Families and retirement* (Sage Focus ed.). Newbury Park, CA: Sage.

Hazzard, M. (1971). An overview of systems theory. *Nursing Clinics of North America, 6,* 385–393.

Heady, M. (1996, May 15). Holistic plan urged to aid black males. *Los Angeles Times,* p. A12.

Healy, A., Keesee, P. D., & Smith, B. S. (1985). *Early services for children with special needs: Transactions for family support.* Iowa City, IA. Division of Developmental Disabilities, University Hospital School, Dept. of Pediatrics.

Healy, J., Malley, J., & Stewart, A. (1990). Children and their fathers after separation. *American Journal of Orthopsychiatry, 60,* 531–543.

Heath, D. H. (1976). Competent fathers: Their personalities and marriages. *Human Development, 19*(1), 26–39.

Heinrich, K. (1996). Family sexuality. In P. J. Bomar (Ed.), *Nurses and family health promotion* (2nd ed.) (pp. 284–302). Philadelphia: Saunders.

Heller, P. L. (1976). Familism scale: Revalidation and revision. *Journal of Marriage and the Family, 38*(2), 423–429.

Henderson, A. A., & Brouse, A. J. (1991). The experiences of new fathers during the first three weeks of life. *Journal of Advanced Nursing, 18,* 293–298.

Henderson, G. (1989). *A practitioner's guide to understanding indigenous and foreign cultures.* Springfield, IL: Charles C Thomas.

Henderson, G. (2000). Race in America. *Phi Kappa Phi Journal, 80*(2), 12–16.

Herberg, P. J. (1995). Theoretical foundations of transcultural nursing. In M. M. Andrews & J. S. Boyle (Eds.), *Transcultural concepts in nursing care* (2nd ed.) (pp. 3–96). Philadelphia: Lippincott.

Herbst, P. G. (1954). Conceptual framework for studying the family: Family living regions and pathways, family-living patterns of interaction. In O. A. Oeser & S. B. Hammond (Eds.), *Social structure and personality in a city.* New York: Macmillan.

Hernandez, M. (1996). Central American families. In M. McGoldrick, J. Giordano, & J. K. Pearce (Eds.), *Ethnicity and family therapy* (2nd ed.) (pp. 214–223). New York: Guilford Press.

Herrera T., & Wagner, N. N. (1974). Behavioral approaches to delivering health services in a Chicano community. In A. Reinhardt & M. Quinn (Eds.), *Family-centered community nursing.* St. Louis: Mosby.

Hetherington, E. (1993). An overview of the Virginia longitudinal study of divorce and remarriage with a focus on early adolescence. *Journal of Family Psychology, 7,* 39–56.

Hetherington, E. M., & Stanley-Hagen, M. (2000). Diversity among stepfamilies. In D. H. Demo, K. Allen, & M. Fine (Eds.), *Handbook of family diversity* (pp. 173–196). New York: Oxford University Press.

Hickey, T. (1988). Self-care behavior of older adults. *Family and Community Health, 11*(3), 23–32.

Hickman, G. P., & Starr, M. K. (2001, June). The influence of family on the development of humorous coping skills of college freshman. *National Council on Family Relations Report,* pp. 12–13.

Hilgenberg, C., Liddy, K. G., Standerfer, J., & Schraeder, C. (1992). Changes in family patterns six months after a myocardial infarction. *Journal of Cardiovascular Nursing, 6*(2), 46–56.

Hill, M. S. (1988). Marital stability and spouses' shared time. *Journal of Family Issues, 9*(4), 427–451.

Hill, R. (1949). *Families under stress.* New York: Harper & Row.

Hill, R. (1958). Social stresses on the family: Generic features of families under stress. *Social Casework, 39,* 139–150.

Hill, R. (1965). *Challenges and resources for family development: Family mobility in our dynamic society.* Ames, IA: Iowa State University.

Hill, R. (1970). *Interdependence among the generations: Family development in three generations* (Chap. 2). Cambridge, MA: Schenkman.

Hill, R. (1986). Life cycle stages for types of single parent families: Of family development theory. *Family Relations, 35*(1), 19–29.

Hill, R. B. (1971). *The strengths of black families.* New York: Emerson-Hall.

Hill, R. B., Billingsley, A., Engram, E., et al. (1993). *Research on the African American family: A holistic perspective.* Westport, CT: Auburn House.

Himmelstein, D., & Woolhandler, S. (1994). *The national health program book: A source guide for advocates.* Monroe, ME: Common Courage Press.

Hines, P. M., & Boyd-Franklin, N. (1996). African American families. In M. McGoldrick, J. Giordano, & J. K. Pearce (Eds.), *Ethnicity and family therapy* (2nd ed.) (pp. 66–84). New York: Guilford Press.

Hisama, H. K. (2000). Japanese theory and practice: Carrying your own lamp. *Reflections on Nursing Leadership, 26*(1), 30–32.

Ho, M. K. (1987). *Family therapy with ethnic minorities.* Newbury Park, CA: Sage.

Ho, M. K. (1992). *Minority children and adolescents in therapy.* Springfield, IL: Charles C Thomas.

Hobart, C. (1987). Parent–child relations in remarried families. *Journal of Family Issues, 8*(3), 259–277.

Hobbes, T. (1947). *Leviathan.* New York: MacMillan (Original work published in 1651).

Hobbs, D. F., & Cole, S. P. (1976, March). Transition to parenthood: A decade replication. *Journal of Marriage and the Family, 38,* 723–731.

Hoffer, J. (1996). Family communication. In P. J. Bomar (Ed.), *Nurses and family health promotion* (2nd ed.) (pp. 94–106). Philadelphia: Saunders.

Hofferth, S. L., & Phillips, D. A. (1987). Child care in the U.S., 1970–1995. *Journal of Marriage and the Family, 49*(3), 559–571.

Hoffman, L. (1981). *Foundations of family therapy: A conceptual framework for system change.* New York: Basic Books.

Hoffman, L. W. (1977, August). Changes in family roles, socialization, and sex differences. *American Psychologist, 32,* 644.

Hogan, M. J., Buchler, C., & Robinson, B. (1984). Single parenting: Transitioning alone. In H. I. McCubbin & C. R. Figley (Eds.), *Stress and the family, Vol. I: Coping with normative transitions.* New York: Brunner/Mazel.

Hogue, C. G. (1977). Support systems for health promotion. In J. Hall & B. Weaver (Eds.), *Distributive nursing practice: A systems approach to community health.* Philadelphia: Lippincott.

Hollingshead, A. B. (1949). *Elmstown's youth.* New York: Wiley.

Holman, A. M. (1979). *Finding families*. Beverly Hills, CA: Sage.

Holman, A. M. (1983). *Family assessment: Tools for understanding and intervention*. Beverly Hills, CA: Sage.

Holmes, T. H., & Rahe, R. H. (1967). The social readjustment rating scale. *Journal of Psychosomatic Research, 1*, 213–218.

Holt, J. L., & Johnson, S. D. (1991). Developmental tasks: A key to reducing teenage pregnancy. *Journal of Pediatric Nursing, 6*(3), 191–193.

Hong, G. K. (1988). A general family practitioner approach for Asian American mental health services. *Professional Psychology: Research & Practice, 19*, 600–605.

Hong, G. K. (1989). Application of cultural and environmental issues in family therapy with immigrant Chinese Americans. *Journal of Strategic and Systemic Therapies, 8*, 14–21.

Hong, G. K. (1993). Synthesizing Eastern and Western psychotherapeutic approaches. In J. L. Chin, J. H. Liem, M. D. Ham, & G. K. Hong (Eds.), *Transference and empathy in Asian American psychotherapy: Cultural values and treatment needs*. Westport, CT: Praeger.

Hong, G. K. (1995). Cultural considerations in rehabilitation counseling for Asian Americans. *National Association of Rehabilitation Professionals in the Private Sector Journal, 10*(2), 59–65.

Hong, G. K. (1996). Culture and empowerment: Counseling services for Chinese American families. *Journal for the Professional Counselor, 11*(1), 69–80.

Hong, G. K., & Ham, M. D. (1992). Impact of immigration on the family life cycle: Clinical implications for Chinese Americans. *Journal of Family Psychotherapy, 3*(3), 27–40.

Hong, G. K., & Ham, M. D. (1994). Psychotherapy and counseling for Chinese Americans: Curriculum and training issues. *Bulletin of the Hong Kong Psychological Society, 32/33*, 5–19.

Hong, G. K., & Hong, L. K. (1991). Comparative perspectives on child abuse and neglect: Chinese versus Hispanics and Whites. *Child Welfare, LXX*(4), 463–475.

Hong, G. K., Lee, B. S., & Lorenzo, M. K. (1995). Somatization in Chinese American clients: Implications for psychotherapeutic services. *Journal of Contemporary Psychotherapy, 25*(2), 89–104.

Hong, P. T., Dickerson, M., & Cleeland, N. (2002, May 15). Southland's average family income dropped in the 1990's. *Los Angeles Times*, pp. A1, A16.

Honig, M. (1996). Retirement expectations: Differences by race, ethnicity, and gender. *The Gerontologist, 36*(3), 373–382.

Honigman, J. I. (1967). *Personality in culture*. New York: Harper & Row.

Horner, M. J. (1998). *National family and intimate partner violence prevention initiative*. U.S. Department of Health and Human Services, Health Resources & Services Administration, Office of Minority Health.

Horwitz, A. (1993). Adult siblings as sources of social support for the severely mentally ill: A test of the serial model. *Journal of Marriage and the Family, 54*, 233–241.

House, J. S., & Kahn, R. L. (1985). Measures and concepts of social support. In S. Cohen & S. L. Syme (Eds.), *Social support and health* (pp. 83–108). Orlando, FL: Academic Press.

House, J. S., Landis, K. R., and Umberson, D. (1988). Social relationships and health. *Science, 241*(4865), 540–545.

Houseknecht, S. K. (1987). Voluntary childlessness. In M. B. Sussman & S. K. Steinmetz (Eds.), *Handbook of marriage and the family*. New York: Plenum Press.

Hsu, F. L. K. (1971). *The challenge of the American dream: The Chinese in the U.S*. Belmont, CA: Wadsworth.

Huang, L. N., & Ying, Y. W. (1989). Chinese American children and adolescents. In J. T. Gibbs, L. N. Huang, et al. (Eds.), *Color of color: Psychological interventions with minority children* (pp. 30–66). San Francisco: Jossey-Bass.

Huff, R. M., & Kline, M. V. (1999). *Promoting health in multicultural populations*. Thousand Oaks, CA: Sage.

Humes, K., & McKinnon, J. (2000). *The Asian and Pacific Islander Population in the United States: Current Population Reports*. Washington, DC: U.S. Bureau of the Census.

Humphreys, J. (2000). Spirituality and distress in sheltered battered women. *Image: Journal of Nursing Scholarship*, Third quarter, 273–278.

Humphreys, J. C. (2001). Turnings and adaptations in resilient daughters of battered women. *Journal of Nursing Scholarship, 33*(3), 245–251.

Hunter, A. G., Pearson, J. L., Ialongo, N. S., & Kellam, S. G. (1998). Parenting alone to multiple caregivers: Childcare and parenting arrangements in black and white urban families. *Family Relations, 47*(4), 343–353.

Hunter, J. D. (1994). The family and the culture war. In A. S. Skolnick & J. H. Skolnick (Eds.), *Family in transition* (8th ed.) (pp. 537–547). New York: HarperCollins College.

Hunter, K., & Bryant, B. (1994). Pharmacist provided education and counseling for managing pediatric asthma. *Patient Education and Counseling, 24*, 127–134.

Hupcey, J., & Morse, J. (1995). Family and social support: Application to the critically ill patient. *Journal of Family Nursing, 1*, 257–280.

Hutchinson, E. (1988, February 28). Black America: Tale of two nations., *Los Angeles Times*, Part IV, pp. 3, 6.

Hymovich, D. (1983). The chronicity impact and coping instrument: Parent questionnaire. *Nursing Research, 32*, 275–281.

Hymovich, D. P., & Barnard, M. U. (1979). *Family health care*. New York: McGraw-Hill.

Ingoldsby, B. B. (1995a). Family origin and universality. In B. B. Ingoldsby & S. Smith (Eds.), *Families in multicultural perspective* (pp. 83–96). New York: Guilford Press.

Ingoldsby, B. B. (1995b). Poverty and patriarchy in Latin America. In B. B. Ingoldsby & S. Smith (Eds.), *Families in multicultural perspective* (pp. 335–351). New York: Guilford Press.

Ingrasia, M. (1993, August 30). Endangered family. *Newsweek*, 17–25.

Inkeles, A. (1977). Paper presented to the American Sociological Association, Washington, DC, in September 1977. Cited in *Los Angeles Times*, September 20, 1977, Part I, pp. 1, 10.

Inouye, J. (1999). Asian American health and disease. An overview of the issues. In R. M. Huff & M. V. Kline (Eds.), *Promoting health in multicultural populations: A handbook for practitioners* (pp. 337–356). Thousand Oaks, CA: Sage.

Institute of Medicine. (2000). *Informing the future: Critical issues in health*. Washington, DC: Institute of Medicine.

Irelan, L. M. (1972). *Low income life styles*. U.S. Department of HEW, Social and Rehabilitation Services. Washington, DC: U.S. Government Printing Office.

Isaacson, W. (2000, January). Our century—and the next time. Special Issue of *Time* Magazine.

Ishida, D. N. (1999). Promoting health among Asian American population groups: A case study from the field. In R. Huff & M. Kline (Eds.), *Promoting health in multicultural populations* (pp. 375–382). Thousand Oaks, CA: Sage.

Ishii-Kuntz, M. (2000). Diversity with Asian-American families. In D. H. Demo, K. R. Allen, & M. A. Fine (Eds.), *Handbook of family diversity* (pp. 274–290). New York: Oxford Press.

Jackson, D. (Ed.). (1969). *Communication, marriage, and the family*. Palo Alto, CA: Science and Behavior Books.

Jackson, J. (1966). A conceptual and measurement model for norms and roles. *Pacific Sociological Review, 9*, 35–38.

Jackson, M. P., & McSwane, D. Z. (1996). Homelessness as a determinant of health. *Public Health Nursing, 9*(3), 185–192.

Jacob, S. (1999). Support for family caregivers in the community. In V. D. Wegner & R. J. Alexander (Eds.), *Readings in Family Nursing* (2nd ed.) (pp. 373–390). Philadelphia: Lippincott.

Jacob, T. (1992). Family studies of alcoholism. *Journal of Family Psychology, 5*, 319–338.

Jacob, T., & Tennenbaum, D. L. (1988). *Family assessment: Rationale, methods, and future directions*. New York: Plenum Press.

Jahoda, M. (1958). *Current concepts of positive mental health*. Joint Commission on Mental Illness and Health, Monograph No. 1. New York: Basic Books.

Janosik, E. H., & Green, E. (1992). *Family life*. Boston: Jones & Bartlett.

Janosik, E. H., & Miller, J. R. (1980). *Family-focused care*. New York: McGraw-Hill.

Jaramillo, P. T., & Zapata, J. T. (1987). Roles and alliances with Mexican-American and Anglo families. *Journal of Marriage and the Family, 49*(4), 727–735.

Jayaratne, S. (1978). Behavioral intervention and family decision-making. *Social Work, 23*, 24.

Jenkins, K. W. (1995). Communication in families. In R. Day, K. R. Gilbert, B. H. Settles, & W. R. Burr (Eds.), *Research and theory in family science* (pp. 171–185). Pacific Grove, CA: Brooks/Cole.

Jensen, D. P. (1985). Patient contracting. In G. M. Bulechek & J. C. McCloskey (Eds.), *Nursing interventions: Treatment for nursing diagnoses* (pp. 92–98). Philadelphia: Saunders.

Jiang, S. (1995, Summer). Recognizing Asian communities: Differences key to providing care. *National Health Service Corps in Touch* (Newsletter) (p. 3). Chevy Chase, MD: U.S. Public Health Service.

John, D., Shelton, B. A., & Luschen, K. (1995). Race, ethnicity, and perceptions of fairness. *Journal of Family Issues, 16*(3), 357–379.

Johnson, C. L. (1975). Authority and power in Japanese-American marriage. In R. E. Cromwell & D. H. Olson (Eds.), *Power in families* (pp. 182–196). New York: Sage.

Johnson, L. B. (1997). Three decades of black family empirical research: Challenges for the 21st century. In H. P. McAdoo (Ed.), *Black families* (3rd ed.) (pp. 94–113). Thousand Oaks, CA: Sage.

Johnson, M., Bulechek, G., Dochterman, J. M., Maas, M., & Moorhead, S. (2001). *Nursing diagnoses, outcomes and interventions: NANDA, NOC, & NIC linkages*. St. Louis: Mosby.

Johnson, M., Maas, M., & Moorhead, S. (2000). *Nursing outcomes classification (NOC)*. St. Louis: Mosby.

Johnson, M. A. (1998). Who is the family? In B. Vaughan-Cole, M. A. Johnson, J. A. Malone, & B. L. Walker. (Eds.), *Family nursing practice* (pp. 3–18). Philadelphia: Saunders.

Johnson, R. (1984). Promoting the health of families in the community. In M. Stanhope & J. Lancaster (Eds.), *Community health nursing* (pp. 330–360). St. Louis: Mosby.

Johnson, S. (1998). *Who moved my cheese?* New York: G. P. Putnam's Sons.

Johnson, S. (2001). Helping children to eat right. Nutrition, health and safety. *Journal of Early Education and Family Review, 8*(3), 30–31.

Johnson, S. H. (1986). Introduction and role theory strategies. In S. H. Johnson (Ed.), *Nursing assessment and strategies for the family at risk: High-risk parenting* (2nd ed.) (pp. 1–12, 388–401). Philadelphia: Lippincott.

Johnson, S. K., Craft, M., Titler, M., Halm, M., Kleiber, C., Montgomery, L. A., et al. (1995). Perceived changes in adult family members' roles and responsibilities during critical illness. *Image, 27*(30), 238–243.

Joint Commission on Accreditation on Community Mental Health Service Programs. (1976). *Standards for community mental health centers: Balance service system.* Chicago: Joint Commission on the Accreditation of Hospitals.

Jones, E. (1995). Deaf and hearing parents' perceptions of family functioning. *Journal of Pediatric Nursing, 11*(1), 45–51.

Jones, E., & Badger, T. A. (1991). Deaf children's knowledge of internal human anatomy. *Journal of Special Education, 25*(2), 252–260.

Jones, E., & Topmiller, M. (1996). Deaf fathers' interactions with hearing infants and toddlers. *NCAST National News, 12*(3), 4–5.

Jones, E. G. (1995). Deaf and hearing parents' perceptions of family functioning. *Nursing Research, 44*(2), 102–105.

Jones, E. G., & Dumas, R. E. (1996). Deaf and hearing parents' interactions with eldest hearing children. *American Annals of the Deaf, 141*(4), 278–283.

Jones, K. C. (1994). Managed care: The coming revolution in home health care. *Journal of Home Health Care Practice, 6*(2), 1–11.

Jones, S. L. (1980). *Family therapy: A comparison of approaches.* Bowie, MD: Brady.

Jones, S. L., & Dimond, M. (1982). Family theory and family therapy models. Comparative review with implications for nursing practice. *Journal of Psychosocial Nursing and Mental Health Services,* 12–19.

Jordan, J., Kaplan, A., Miller, J. B., Stiver, I., & Surrey, J. (1991). *Women's growth in connection: Writings from the stone center.* New York: Guilford Press.

Judge, S. L. (1998). Parental coping strategies and strengths in families of young children with disabilities. *Family Relations, 47*(3), 263–268.

Julian, T. W., McKenry, P. C., & McKelvey, M. W. (1994). Cultural variations in parenting: Perceptions of Caucasian, African-American, Hispanic & Asian-American parents. *Family Relations, 43*(1), 30–37.

Juni, S. (1995). Triangulation as splitting in the service of ambivalence. *Current Psychology: Developmental, Learning, Personality, Social, 14,* 91– 111.

JWK International Corporation. (1978). *Summary and recommendations of conference on Pacific and Asian American families and HEW-related issues.* Annandale, VA: Author.

Kahana, E., Kahana, B., Johnson, J. R., Hammand, R. J., & Kercher, K. (1994). Developmental challenges and family caregiving: Bridging concepts and research. In E. Kahana, D. E. Biegel, & M. L. Wykle (Eds.), *Family caregiving across the lifespan.* Thousand Oaks, CA: Sage.

Kahn, A. M. (1990). Coping with fear and grieving. In I. M. Lubkin (Ed.), *Chronic illness: Impact and intervention* (pp. 179–199). Boston: Jones & Bartlett.

Kalil, A., Spencer, M. Spleker, S., & Gilchrist, L. (1998). Effects of grandmother coresidence and quality of family relationships on depressive symptoms in adolescent mothers. *Family Relations, 47*(4), 433–441.

Kandzari, J. H., & Howard, J. R. (1981). *The well family: A developmental approach to assessment.* Boston: Little, Brown.

Kane, R. L., Kasteler, J. M., & Gray, R. M. (1976). *The health gap.* New York: Springer.

Kang, K. C., & Fields, R. (2001, May 15). Asian population in U.S. surges, but unevenly. *Los Angeles Times,* p. A16.

Kang, K. C. (1997, June 29). Chinese in the Southland: A changing picture. *Los Angeles Times,* pp. A1, A32.

Kang, K. C. (2001, April 25). Study finds persistent negative perceptions of Chinese Americans. *Los Angeles Times,* p. A18.

Kang, R., Barnard, K., & Oshio, S. (1994). Description of the clinical practice of advanced practice nurses in family-centered early intervention in two rural settings. *Public Health Nursing, 11*(6), 376–384.

Kanter, R. M. (1978). Jobs and families: Impact of working roles on life. *Children Today, 7,* 13.

Kantor, D., & Lehr, W. (1975). *Inside the family: Toward a theory of family process.* San Francisco: Jossey-Bass.

Kantrowitz, B., & Wingert, P. (2001, May 28). Unmarried with children. *Newsweek,* 46–54.

Kantrowitz, B., & Wingert, P. (1990, Winter/Spring). Step by step. *Newsweek* (Special Issue), 24–37.

Kaplan, M. S., Adamek, M., & Johnson, S. (1994). Trends in firearm suicide among older American males: 1979–1988. *The Gerontologist, 34*(1), 59–65.

Kardiner, A. (1945). *The psychological frontiers of society.* New York: Columbia University Press.

Kastenbaum, R. (1994). Alternatives to suicide. In D. Lester & M. Tallmer (Eds.), *Now I lay me down: Suicide in the elderly.* Philadelphia: Charles Press.

Kaufman, G. & Unlenberg, P. (2000). The influence of parenthood on the work effort on married men and women. *Social Forces, 78*(3), 931–947.

Kaufman, G., & Uhlenberg, P. (1998). Effects of life course transitions on the quality of relationships between adult children and their parents. *Journal of Marriage and the Family, 60*(4), 924–939.

Kay, M. A. (1978). The Mexican American. In A. L. Clark (Ed.), *Culture, childbearing and health professionals.* Philadelphia: Davis.

Kearney, J. A., & Yurick, C. M. (1996). Nurse to nurse referral: The role of the child psychiatric nurse consultant. *Journal of Pediatric Health Care, 10*(3), 115–120.

Keating, N., & Cole, P. (1980). What do I do with him 24 hours a day? *The Gerontologist, 20,* 84–89.

Keefe, S. E. (1981). Folk medicine among urban Mexican-Americans: Cultural persistence, change and displacement. *Hispanic Journal of Behavioral Science, 3*(1), 41–48.

Keefe, S. E. (1984). Real and ideal extended familism among Mexican Americans and Anglo Americans: On the meaning of "close" family ties. *Human Organization, 43,* 65–70.

Keefe, S. E., Padilla, A. M., & Carlos, M. L. (1978). The Mexican-American extended family as an emotional system. In J. M. Casas & S. E. Keefe (Eds.), *Family and mental health in the Mexican-American community.* Los Angeles: Spanish-speaking Mental Health Research Center, UCLA.

Kelleher, K. (1996, January 10). Who's minding the kids? *Los Angeles Times,* p. E3.

Kelley, B. R. (1997). Cultural diversity in clinical practice. In J. A. Fox (Ed.), *Primary health care of children* (pp. 32–40). St. Louis: Mosby.

Kelly, J. R. (1978). Family leisure in three communities. *Journal of Leisure Research, 10*(1), 47–60.

Kelly, K. C., McClelland, E., & Day, J. M. (1992). Discharge planning. In G. M. Bulechek & J. C. McCloskey (Eds.), *Nursing interventions: Essential nursing treatments* (2nd ed.) (pp. 265–273). Philadelphia: Saunders.

Kendall, J. H. (1974). Maternal behavior one year after early and extended postpartum contact. *Developmental Medicine and Neurology, 16,* 172.

Kennedy, G. E. (1989). Involving students in participatory research on fatherhood. A case study. *Family Relations, 38*(4), 363–37.

Kerckhoff, R. K. (1976). Marriage and middle age. *Family Coordinator, 25*(1), 7–10.

Kerr, M. E., & Bowen, M. (1988). *Family evaluation: An approach based on Bowen theory.* New York: Norton.

Kick, I. (1996). Sleep and the family. In P. J. Bomar (Ed.), *Nurses and family health promotion* (2nd ed.) (pp. 245–263). Baltimore, MD: Williams & Wilkins.

Kidwell, J., Fischer, L., Dunham, R. M., & Baranowski, M. (1983). Parents and adolescents: Push and pull of change. In H. I. McCubbin & C. R. Figley (Eds.), *Stress and the family: Coping with normative transitions.* New York: Brunner/Mazel.

Kiecolt-Glaser, J. K., & Glaser, R. (1989). Caregiving, mental health and immune function. In E. Light & B. Lebowitz (Eds.), *Alzheimer's disease treatment and family stress* (DHHS Publication No. 89–1569) (pp. 310–320). Washington, DC: U.S. Government Printing Office.

Kievit, M. B. (1968). Family roles. In *Rutgers School of Nursing, Parent–child relationships—Role of the nurse.* Newark, NJ: Rutgers University.

Kileen, M. R. (1995). Problems in parenting. In B. S. Johnson (Ed.), *Child, adolescent and family psychiatric nursing* (pp. 32–44). Philadelphia: Lippincott.

Killien, M. G. (1985). An environmental approach to nursing practice. In J. E. Hall & B. R. Weaver (Eds.), *Distributive nursing practice: A systems approach to community health* (2nd ed.) (pp. 259–277). Philadelphia: Lippincott.

Kim, M. J., McFarland, G. K., & McFarlane, A. M. (1995). *Pocket guide to nursing diagnoses* (6th ed.). St. Louis: Mosby.

Kindig, D. (1975). Interdisciplinary education for primary health care team delivery. *Journal of Medical Education, 50,* 102.

King, I. (1981). *Family therapy: A comparison of approaches.* Bowie, MD: Brady.

King, I. (1983). King's theory of nursing. In I. W. Clements & J. B. Roberts (Eds.), *Family health: A theoretical approach to nursing* (pp. 177–187). New York: Wiley.

King, I. (1987, May). *King's theory.* Paper presented at Nursing Theories Conference, Pittsburgh, PA (cassette recording).

King, K. B., Parrinelo, K. M., & Baggs, J. B. (1996). Collaboration and advanced practice nursing. In J. V. Hickey, R. M. Ovimette, & S. L. Venegoni (Eds.), *Advanced practice nursing* (pp. 146–162). Philadelphia: Lippincott.

Kingsbury, N., & Scanzoni, J. (1993). Structural-functionalism. In P. G. Boss, W. J. Doherty, R. LaRossa, W. R. Schumm, & S. K. Steinmetz (Eds.), *Sourcebook of family theories and methods: A contextual approach* (pp. 195–217). New York: Plenum Press.

Kingson, E. R., Hirshorn, B. A., & Cornman, J. M. (1986). *Ties that bind: The interdependence of generations.* Washington, DC: Seven Locks Press.

Kirschenbaum, H. (1977). *Advanced value clarification.* La Jolla, CA: University Associates.

Kirschling, J., & Gilliss, C. (1989). *Persons who describe themselves as family nurses: Why they are, where they practice and what they do.* Handout at presentation by the Special Interest Group, Family Nursing Continuing Education Project, Oregon Health Sciences University, at the National Family Nursing Conference, September 1989, Portland.

Kitano, H. H. L. (1988). The Japanese American family. In C. H. Mindel, R. W. Habenstein, & R. Wright, Jr. (Eds.), *Ethnic families in America* (pp. 258–275). New York: Elsevier.

Kitano, H. H., & Maki, M. T. (1996). Continuity, change and diversity: Counseling Asian Americans. In P. B. Pedersen, J. G. Draguns, W. J. Lonner, & J. E. Trimble (Eds.), *Counseling across cultures* (4th ed.) (pp. 124–145). Thousand Oaks, CA: Sage.

Kitson, G. C., Babri, F. B., Roach, M. J., & Placidi, K. S. (1989). Adjustment to widowhood and divorce. *Journal of Family Issues, 10*(1), 5–32.

Klaus, M. H., & Kendall, J. H. (1976). *Maternal–infant bonding.* St. Louis: Mosby.

Kleffel, D. (1991). Rethinking the environment as a domain of nursing knowledge. *Advances in Nursing Science, 14*(1), 40–45.

Klein, D. M. (1983). Family problem-solving and family stress. In H. I. McCubbin, M. B. Sussman, & J. M. Patterson (Eds.), Social stress and the family (Special Issue). *Marriage and Family Review 6*(1/2), 85–112.

Klein, D. M., & White, J. M. (1996). *Family theories: An introduction.* Thousand Oaks, CA: Sage.

Kleinman, A. (1980). Patients and healers in the context of culture: An exploration of the borderland between anthropology, medicine, and psychiatry. Berkeley, CA: University of California Press.

Kleinman, A. (1988). *The illness narratives: Suffering, healing, and the human condition.* New York: Basic Books.

Kleinman, A., Eisenberg, L., & Good, B. (1978). Culture, illness and care. Clinical lessons from anthropologic and cross-cultural research. *Annals of Internal Medicine, 88,* 251–258.

Klose, D. (1995). M. Scott Peck's analysis of human evil: A critical review. *Journal of Humanistic Psychology, 35*(3), 37–66.

Kluckholm, F. R. (1976). Dominant and variant value orientations. In P. Brink (Ed.), *Transcultural nursing.* Englewood Cliffs, NJ: Prentice Hall.

Knafl, K. A. (1998). Meeting the challenge of chronic illness for children and families: Research implications and future directions. In M. E. Broome, K. A. Knafl, K. Pridham, & S. Feetham (Eds.), *Children and families in health and illness* (pp. 236–246). Thousand Oaks: Sage.

Knafl, K. A., & Deatrick, J. A. (1986). Concept analysis: An analysis of the concept of normalization. *Research in Nursing and Health, 9*(3), 215–222.

Knafl, K. A., Deatrick, J. A., & Kirby, A. (2001). Normalization promotion. In M. Craft-Rosenberg & J. Denehy (Eds.), *Nursing interventions for infants, children, and families* (pp. 373–388). Thousand Oaks: Sage.

Knapp, D. A., Knapp, D. E., & Engle, J. (1966). The public, the pharmacist and self medication. *Journal of the American Pharmacology Association, 56,* 460.

Knapp, M. (1984). *Interpersonal communication and human relationships.* Boston: Allyn & Bacon.

Knesek, G. (1992). Early versus regular retirement: Differences in measures of life satisfaction. *Journal of Gerontological Social Work, 19*(1), 3–34.

Knutsen, S. F., & Knutsen, R. (1991). The Tromso survey: The family Intervention study: The effect of intervention on some coronary risk factors and dietary habits, a 6 year follow-up. *Preventive Medicine, 20,* 197–212.

Koenenn, C. (1997, March 16). Living legal. *Los Angeles Times,* p. E2.

Koerner, B. L., & Armstrong, D. M. (1984). Collaboration practice cuts cost of patient care: Study. *Hospitals, 58,* 52–54.

Koester, L.S. (1992). Intuitive parenting as a model for understanding parent-infant interactions when one partner is deaf. *American Annals of the Deaf, 137*(4), 362–369.

Kohlberg, L. (1970). Education for justice: A modern statement of the platonic view. In *Moral education: Five lectures.* Cambridge, MA: Harvard University.

Kohn, M. L. (1969). Social class and parent–child relationships: An interpretation. In R. L. Coser (Ed.), *Life cycle and achievement in America* (pp. 21–42). New York: Harper Torchbooks.

Kohn, M. L. (1977). *Class and conformity: A study of values* (2nd ed.). Chicago: University of Chicago Press.

Kohnke, M. F. (1982). *Advocacy: Risk and reality.* St. Louis: Mosby.

Koin, D. (1989). The effects of caregiver stress on physical health status. In E. Light & B. Lebowitz (Eds.), *Alzheimer's disease treatment and family stress* (DHHS Publication No. 89-1569) (pp. 245–266). Washington, DC: U.S. Government Printing Office.

Kollack, P., Blumstein, P., & Schwartz, P. (1985). Sex and power in interaction: Conversational privileges and duties. *American Sociological Review, 50,* 34–46.

Komarovsky, M. (1964). *Blue-collar marriage.* New York: Random House.

Koos, E. (1954). *The health of regionville.* New York: Columbia University Press.

Kosik, S. H. (1972). Patient advocacy or fighting the system. *American Journal of Nursing, 72,* 694.

Kosten, T. R., Jacobs, S. C., & Kasl, S. V. (1985). Terminal illness, bereavement and the family. In D. C. Turk & R. D. Karns (Eds.), *Health, illness and families: A life span perspective* (pp. 311–334). New York: Wiley.

Koten, J. (1987, March 9). A once tightly knit middle class finds itself divided and uncertain. *Wall Street Journal,* Section 2, p. 25.

Kozol, J. (1990, Winter/Spring). The new untouchables. *Newsweek* (Special Issue on the 21st Century Family), 48–53.

Kozol, J. (2000). *Kids count.* New York: Annie Casey Foundation.

Kramer, L., & Houston, D. (1998). Supporting families as they adopt children with special needs. *Family Relations, 47*(4), 423–432.

Kranichfield, M. L. (1987). Rethinking family power. *Journal of Family Issues, 8*(1), 42–56.

Kroska, R. A. (1985). Ethnographic research method. A qualitative example to discover role of granny midwives in health services. In M. Leininger (Ed.), *Qualitative research methods in nursing.* New York: Grune & Stratton.

Krozy, R. E. (1996). Community health promotion. Assessment and intervention. In S. H. Rankin & K. D. Stallings (Eds.), *Patient education: Issues, principles, practices* (pp. 245–271). Philadelphia: Lippincott.

Kruszewski, A., Anthony, R., Hough, L., & Ornstein-Galicia, J. (1982). *Politics and society in the Southwest*. Boulder, CO: Westview Press.

Kuhn, M. (1964). Major trends in symbolic interaction theory in the past twenty-five years. *Sociological Quarterly, 5*, 61–84.

Kuipers, J. (1995). Mexican Americans. In J. N. Giger & R. E. Davidhizar (Eds.), *Transcultural nursing: Assessment and intervention* (2nd ed.) (pp. 205–234). St. Louis: Mosby.

Kunst-Wilson, W., & Cronenwett, L. (1981). Nursing care for the emerging family: Promoting paternal behavior. *Research in Nursing and Health, 4*, 201–211.

Kus, R. J. (1992). Crisis intervention. In G. M. Bulechek & J. C. McCloskey (Eds.), *Nursing interventions: Essential nursing treatments* (2nd ed.) (pp. 179–190). Philadelphia: Saunders.

Kyle, M. (1995). Collaboration. In M. Snyder & M. P. Mirr (Eds.), *Advanced practice nursing* (pp. 169–181). New York: Springer.

Labonte, R. (1989). Community and professional empowerment. *Canadian Nurse, 3*, 23–30.

Lacey, K. (1989). Nutrition. In P. Swinford & J. Webster (Eds.), *Promoting wellness: A nurse's handbook*. Rockville, MD: Aspen.

Lackey, C., & Williams, K. (1995). Social bonding and the cessation of partner violence across generations. *Journal of Marriage and the Family, 57*, 295–305.

Laird, J. (1993). Lesbian and gay families. In F. Walsh (Ed.), *Normal family processes* (2nd ed.) (pp. 282–328). New York: Guilford Press.

Lamb, G. S., & Napadano, R. J. (1984). Physician– nurse practitioner interaction patterns in primary care practices. *American Journal of Public Health, 74*, 26–29.

Lamb, M. E. (1987). *The father's role: Cross-cultural perspectives*. Hillsdale, NJ: Erlbaum.

Lange, S. (1970). Transactional analysis and nursing. In C. Carlson (Ed.), *Behavioral concepts and nursing intervention*. Philadelphia: Lippincott.

Langman, L. (1987). Social stratification. In M. B. Sussman & S. K. Steinmetz (Eds.), *Handbook of marriage and the family* (pp. 211–249). New York: Plenum Press.

Larmer, B. (1999, July 12). Latino America. *Newsweek*, 48–58.

LaRocca, S. (1978). An introduction to role theory for nurses. *Supervisor Nurse, 9*(12), 41–45.

LaRossa, R., & La Rossa, M. M. (1981). *Transition to parenthood: How infants change families*. Newbury Park, CA: Sage.

Larrabee, E. (1973). *Comments to Loretta Ford's research. An ethnic perspective. Community nursing research: Collaboration and completion*. Denver, CO: Western Institute of Higher Education Commission.

Larsen, D. (1989, February 5). Elder abuse. *Los Angeles Times*, Part IV, p. 1.

Lasch, C. (1977). *Haven in a heartless world: The family besieged*. New York: Basic Books.

Lasky, E. M., & Martz, C. H. (1993). The Asian Pacific Islander population in the U.S.: Cultural perspectives and their relationship to cancer prevention and early detection. In M. Frank-Stromberg & S. Olson (Eds.), *Cancer prevention in minority populations*. St. Louis: Mosby.

Lauver, D. (1980). Recognizing alternatives: A process for client centered health care. *Health Values: Achieving High Level Wellness, 4*(3), 134–138.

Lawton, M. P. (1980). *Environment and aging*. Monterey, CA: Brooks/Cole.

Lawton, M. P. (1985). Housing and the living environment of older persons. In R. Binstock & E. Shanas (Eds.), *Handbook of aging and the social sciences* (pp. 450–478). New York: Van Nostrand Reinhold.

Lazarus, R., Averill, J. R., & Opton, E. M. (1974). The psychology of coping: Issues in research and assessment. In G. R. Coelho, D. A. Harburg, & J. E. Adams (Eds.), *Coping and adaptation*. New York: Basic Books.

Lazlo, E. (1972). *The systems view of the world*. New York: George Braziller.

Leahey, M., & Harper-Jaques, S. (1996). Family–nurse relationships: Core assumptions and clinical practice. *Journal of Family Nursing, 2*(2), 133–151.

Leahey, K., Cobb, M., & Jones, M. (1977). *Community health nursing* (3rd ed.). New York: McGraw-Hill.

Leavell, H., Clark, E. G., Gurney, B., et al. (1965). *Preventive medicine for the doctor in his community: An epidemiologic approach* (3rd ed.) (pp. 19–28). New York: McGraw-Hill.

Leavitt, M. B. (1982). *Families at risk: Primary prevention in nursing practice*. Boston: Little, Brown.

LeBey, B. (2001). American families are drifting apart. *USA Today, 130*(2676), 20–22.

Leddy, S., & Pepper, J. M. (1985). *Conceptual basis of professional nursing*. Philadelphia: Lippincott.

Lederer, W. J., & Jackson, D. D. (1968). *Mirages of marriage*. New York: Norton.

Lee, E. (1996). Asian American families: An overview. In M. McGoldrick, J. Giordano, & J. K. Pierce (Eds.), *Ethnicity and family therapy* (2nd ed.) (pp. 227–248). New York: Guilford Press.

Lee, G. R. (1978). Marriage and morale in later life. *Journal of Marriage and the Family, 40*(1), 131.

Lee, G., & Lancaster, J. (1988). Conceptual models for community health nursing. In M. Stanhope & J. Lancaster (Eds.), *Community health nursing* (2nd ed.) (pp. 131–148). St. Louis: Mosby.

Lee, J. L., & Cohen, J. I. (1995). Collaboration: A concept analysis. *Journal of Advanced Nursing, 21*, 103–109.

Lee, R., Choe, J., Kim, G., & Ngo, V. (2000). Construction of the Asian-American family conflicts scale. *Journal of Counseling Psychology, 47*(2), 211–222.

Leeds, J. (1996, June 3). Poverty on rise for children of working poor. *Los Angeles Times,* pp. B1, B6.

Leininger, M. (1970). *Nursing and anthropology: Two worlds to blend.* New York: Wiley.

Leininger, M. (1974). Transcultural nursing: A promising subfield of study for nurses. In A. Reinhardt & M. Quinn (Eds.), *Family centered community nursing* (pp. 7–44). St. Louis: Mosby.

Leininger, M. (1976). *Transcultural health care issues and conditions.* Philadelphia: Davis.

Leininger, M. (1978). *Transcultural nursing: Concepts, theories and practice.* New York: Wiley.

Leininger, M. (1995). Teaching transcultural nursing to transform nursing for the 21st century. *Journal of Transcultural Nursing, 6*(2), 2–3.

Leininger, M. (2001). Theory of culture care diversity and universality. In M. Parker (Ed.), *Nursing theories and nursing practice* (pp. 361–376). Philadelphia: Davis.

LeMasters, E. E. (1957). Parenthood as crisis. *Marriage and Family Living, 19*(2), 352.

LeMasters, E. E. (1974). Parents without partners. In A. Skolnick & J. H. Skolnick (Eds.), *Intimacy, family and society.* Boston: Little, Brown.

Leppa, J. (1999). Transcultural communication within the health care subcultures. In J. Luckman (Ed.), *Transcultural communication in nursing* (pp. 80–93). Albany, NY: Delmar.

LeShan, E. J. (1973). *The wonderful crisis of middle age.* New York: McKay.

Leslie, G. R., & Korman, S. K. (1989). *The family in social context* (7th ed.). New York: Oxford University Press.

Lester, P. A. (1986). Teaching strategies. In S. H. Johnson (Ed.), *Nursing assessment and strategies for the family at risk: High-risk parenting* (2nd ed.) (pp. 415–433). Philadelphia: Lippincott.

Lesthaeghe, R. (1983, September). A century of demographic and cultural change in Western Europe. *Population and Development Review,* 411–435.

Letiecq, B. L., Anderson, E. A., & Koblinsky, S. A. (1998). Social support of homeless and housed mothers: A comparison of temporary and permanent housing arrangements. *Family Relations, 47,* 415–421.

Levac, A. M., Wright, L. M., & Leahey, M. (2002). Family assessment and intervention. In S. A. Fox (Ed.), *Primary health care of infants, children & adolescents.* St Louis: Mosby.

Levan, R., Brown, E. R., Hayes, N., & Wyn, R. (1999, April). *Disparity in job-based health coverage places California's Latinos at risk of being uninsured.* Los Angeles, CA: UCLA Center for Health Policy.

Levin, L. S. (1977). Forces and issues in the revival of interest in self-care: Impetus for reduction in health care. *Issues in Self-care* (Health Education Monographs), *5*(2), 116.

Levin, L. S., Katz, A., & Holst, E. (1976). *Self-care—Lay initiatives in health.* New York: Prodist Press.

Levin, R. J., & Levin, A. (1975, September). Sexual pleasure: The surprising preferences of 100,000 women. *Redbook,* 51–58.

Levine, B. (1999, October 13). Little boys lost. *Los Angeles Times.* pp. E1, E4.

Levine, C., & Zuckerman, C. (2000). Hands on/hands off: Why health care professionals depend on families but keep them at arm's length. *Journal of Law, Medicine & Ethics, 28*(1), 5–18.

Levine, E. M. (1988). The realities of day care for children. *Journal of Family Issues, 8*(4), 451–454.

Lewis, A., & Levy, J. S. (1982). *Psychiatric liaison nursing: The theory and clinical practice.* Reston, VA: Reston Publishing.

Lewis, F. M., Behar, L. C., Anderson, K. H., Shands, M. E., Zahlis, E. H., Darby, E., et al. (2000). Blowing away the myths about the child's experience with the mother's breast cancer. In L. Baider, C. L. Cooper, & A. Kaplan (Eds.), *Cancer and the family* (2nd ed.). New York: Wiley.

Lewis, J. I., Beavers, W. R., Gossett, J. T., & Phillips, V. A. (1976). *No single thread: Psychological health in family systems.* New York: Brunner/Mazel.

Lewis, O. (1961). *Children of Sanchez.* New York: Random House.

Libman, J. (1988, August 9). Growing up too fast. *Los Angeles Times,* Part V, p. 1.

Lidz, T. (1963). *The family and human adaptation.* New York: International Universities Press.

Lin, C. C., & Fu, V. R. (1990). A comparison of child-rearing practices among Chinese, immigrant Chinese, and Caucasian American parents. *Child Development, 61,* 429–433.

Lindahl, K., & Malik, N. M. (1999). Observations of marital conflict and power: Relations with parenting in the triad. *Journal of Marriage and the Family, 61*(2), 320–330.

Lindgren, C. L. (1993, Spring). The caregiver career. *Image, 25*(3), 214–219.

Lindsey, E. (1998). The impact of homelessness and shelter life on family relationships. *Family Relations, 47,* 243–352.

Lindsey, E. W. (2001). Foster family characteristics and behavioral and emotional problems of foster children. *Family Relations, 50*(1), 19–22.

Lin-Fu, J. (1994). Ethnocultural barriers to health care: A major problem for Asian American and Pacific Islander Americans. *Journal of Health, 2*(4), 290–299.

Link, B., & Dohrenwend, B. P. (1980). Formulation of hypotheses about the true prevalence of demoralization. In B. P. Dohrenwend (Ed.), *Mental illness in the U.S.:*

Epidemiological estimates (pp. 114–132). New York: Praeger.

Linnett, M. (1970). Prescribing habits in general practice. *Proceedings of the Royal Society of Medicine, 61,* 613–615.

Lipson, J. G. (1996). Culturally competent nursing care. In J. G. Lipson, S. L. Dibble, & P. A. Minarik (Eds.), *Cultural and nursing care.* San Francisco: University of California, San Francisco Nursing Press.

Lipson, J. G., & Meleis, A. I. (1999). Research with immigrants and refugees. In A. S. Hinshaw, S. F. Feetham, & J. Shaver (Eds.), *Handbook of clinical nursing research* (pp. 87–106). Thousand Oaks: Sage.

Litman, T. J. (1974). *Health care and the family: A three generational study.* Washington, DC: Division of Community Health Services and Medical Care Administration, U.S. Public Health Service.

Litwak, E. (1972). Occupational mobility and extended family cohesion. In I. L. Reiss (Ed.), *Readings on the family system* (pp. 413–431). New York: Holt, Rinehart & Winston.

Litwak, E., Jessop, D. J., & Moulton, H. J. (1994). Optimal use of formal and informal systems over the life course. In E. Kahana, D. E. Biegel, & M. L. Wykle (Eds.), *Family caregiving across the lifespan.* Thousand Oaks, CA: Sage.

Liu, W. T. (1986). Health services for Asian elderly. *Research on Aging, 8*(1), 156–175.

Lobo, M. L. (1995). Florence Nightingale. In J. B. George (Ed.), *Nursing theories.* Norwalk, CT: Appleton & Lange.

Locke, D. C. (1992). *Increasing multicultural understanding.* Newbury Park, CA: Sage.

Loe, H. (1988). *Americans are smiling at fewer cavities: Food insight reports.* Washington, DC: International Food Information Council.

Los Angeles Times Editorial (1996, August 11). Some revisionist thinking in the family values season. *Los Angeles Times,* p. M4.

Los Angeles Times. (2001, January 3). Rising medicare costs will burden the poorest, study says. p. A5.

Loveland-Cherry, C. (1988). Issues in family health promotion. In M. Stanhope, & J. Lancaster (Eds.), *Community health nursing* (2nd ed.). St. Louis: Mosby.

Loveland-Cherry, C. (1996). Family health promotion and health protection. In P. J. Bomar (Ed.), *Nurses and family health promotion* (2nd ed.) (pp. 22–35). Philadelphia: Saunders.

Lum, M. R. (1995). Environmental public health: Future direction, future skills. *Family and Community Health, 18*(1), 24–25.

Lum, M. R., Hibbs, B. F., Phillips, L., & Narkunas, D. M. (1996). Environmental health. In M. Stanhope & J. Lancaster (Eds.), *Community health nursing* (4th ed.) (pp. 135–154). St. Louis: Mosby.

Lund, M. (1987). The non-custodial father: Common challenges in parenting after divorce. In C. Lewis (Ed.),

Reassessing fatherhood: New observations on fathers and the modern family (pp. 212–224). London: Sage.

Lustig, M. W. (1988). Value differences in intercultural communication. In L. A. Samovar & R. E. Porter (Eds.), *Intercultural communication: A reader* (pp. 55–61). Belmont, CA: Wadsworth.

Lyman, S. (1974). *Chinese Americans.* New York: Random House.

Lynch, S. H. (1997). Elder abuse. What to look for, how to intervene. *American Journal of Nursing, 97*(1), 27–33.

Macia, E. P., & Morales, L. S. (2001). Crossing the border for health care. *Journal of Health Care for the Poor and Underserved, 12*(1), 77–87.

Macklin, E. D. (1988). Nontraditional family forms. In M. B. Sussman & S. K. Steinmetz (Eds.), *Handbook of marriage and the family* (pp. 317–353). New York: Plenum Press.

MacPhee, M., & Hoffenberg, E. (1996). Nursing case management for children with failure to thrive. *Journal of Pediatric Health Care, 10,* 63–73.

Madanes, C. (1991). Strategic family therapy. In A. S. Gurman & D. P. Kniskern (Eds.), *Handbook of family therapy* (Vol. II). New York: Brunner/Mazel.

Madsen, W. (1964). *The Mexican-American of South Texas.* New York: Holt-Reinhart & Winston.

Maffeo, R. (1997). Helping families cope. *American Journal of Nursing, 97*(6), 36–39.

Mahon, M., & Page, M. (1995). Childhood bereavement after the death of a sibling. *Holistic Nursing Practice, 9*(3), 15–26.

Malinski, V. M. (1987). Nursing science within the science of unitary human beings. In V. M. Malinski (Ed.), *Explorations on Martha Rogers' science of unitary human beings* (pp. 25–32). Norwalk, CT: Appleton & Lange.

Malinski, V. M. (2000). Nursing theory-based research with families: State of the art. *Nursing Science Quarterly, 13*(4), 285–290.

Mancini, J. A., & Orthner, D. K. (1988). The context and consequences of family change. *Family Relations, 37*(4), 363–366.

Manley, M. (1996). Tobacco use. In S. Woolf, S. Jonas, & R. Lawrence (Eds.), *Health promotion and disease prevention in clinical practice* (pp. 163–175). Baltimore: Williams & Wilkins.

Manns, W. (1988). Supportive roles of significant others in black families. In H. P. McAdoo (Ed.), *Black families* (2nd ed.) (pp. 270–283). Newbury Park, CA: Sage.

Manns, W. (1997). Supportive roles of significant others in African American families. In H. P. McAdoo (Ed.), *Black families* (3rd ed.) (pp. 198–213). Thousand Oaks, CA: Sage.

Mares, M. L. (1995). The aging family. In M. A. Fitzpatrick & A. L. Vangelisti (Eds.), *Explaining family interactions* (pp. 310–343). Thousand Oaks, CA: Sage.

Marin, G., & Marin, B. V. (1991). *Research with Hispanic populations.* Newbury Park, CA: Sage.

Marks, M. A. (2000, February 20). Outside the ethnic box. *Los Angeles Times Magazine,* 14–17, 36.

Marosy, J. P. (1994). Collaboration: A key to future success in long-term care. *Journal of Home Health Practice, 6*(2), 42–48.

Marquis, J. (2000, March 14). Men tend to avoid health care, study says. *Los Angeles Times,* pp. A1, A18.

Marsa, L. (2001, May 7). Demanding overhaul of U.S. health care. *Los Angeles Times,* p. 53.

Marsella, A. (1993). Counseling and psychotherapy with Japanese Americans: Cross-cultural considerations. *American Journal of Orthopsychiatry, 63,* 200–208.

Marshall, R. (1991). *The state of families, 3: Losing direction.* Milwaukee, WI: Family Service America.

Martell, L. L., & Imle, M. (1996). Family nursing with child-bearing families. In S. M. H. Hanson & S. T. Boyd (Ed.), *Family health care nursing: Theory, practice and research* (pp. 215–236). Philadelphia: Davis.

Martin, K. (1994). How can the quality of nursing practice be measured? In J. C. McCloskey & H. K. Grace (Eds.), *Current issues in nursing* (4th ed.) (pp. 342–349). St. Louis: Mosby.

Martin, K., & Scheet, N. (1992). *The Omaha system: Applications for community health nursing.* Philadelphia: Saunders.

Martinez, C. (1976). Community mental health and the Chicano movement. In C. A. Hernandez, M. J. Haug, & N. N. Wagner (Eds.), *Chicanos—Social and psychological perspectives* (2nd ed.). St. Louis: Mosby.

Martinez, E. A. (1988). Child behavior in Mexican American/Chicano families. Maternal teaching and child-rearing practices. *Family Relations, 37*(3), 275–280.

Martinez, E. A. (1993). Parenting young children in Mexican American/Chicano families. In H. P. McAdoo (Ed.), *Family ethnicity. Strength in diversity* (pp. 184–195). Newbury Park, CA: Sage.

Masselam, V. S., & Marcus, F. R. (1990) Parent–adolescent communication, family functioning, and school performance. *Adolescence, 25*(99), 725.

Matsui, W. T. (1996). Japanese families. In M. McGoldrick, J. Giordano, & J. K. Pearce (Eds.), *Ethnicity and family therapy* (pp. 268–280). New York: Guilford Press.

Mattessich, P., & Hill, R. (1987). Lifecycle and family development. In M. B. Sussman & S. K. Steinmetz (Eds.), *Handbook of marriage and the family* (pp. 437–469). New York: Plenum Press.

Matthews, H. F. (1988). Sweet blood can give you sugar: Black American folk beliefs about diabetes. *City Medicine, 2,* 14–16.

Matthews, H. F. (1987). Rootwork: Description of an ethnomedical system in the American south. *Southern Medical Journal, 80,* 885–891.

Maturana, H. (1978). Biology of language: The epistemology of reality. In G. Millar & E. Lenneberg (Eds.), *Psychology and biology of language and thought* (pp. 27–63). New York: Academic Press.

Maturana, H. R., & Varela, F. J. (1992). *The tree of knowledge: The biological roots of human understanding* (rev. ed.). Boston: Shambhala.

McAdoo, H. P. (1993). Ethnic families: Strengths that are found in diversity. In H. P. McAdoo (Ed.), *Family ethnicity: Strength in diversity* (pp. 3–14). Newbury Park, CA: Sage.

McAdoo, H. P. (1995). African-American families: Strengths and realities. In H. I. McCubbin, E. A. Thompson, A. I. Thompson, & J. P. Futrell (Eds.), *Resiliency in ethnic minority families: African-American families* (pp. 17–30). Madison, WI: University of Wisconsin.

McAdoo, H. P. (2000, June). Transference of values of African American families and children. *Family Focus,* F5, F7.

McAdoo, H. P. (1978). Minority families. In J. H. Stevens & M. Mathew (Eds.), *Mother/child, Father/child relationships* (pp. 178–180). Washington, DC: The National Association for the Education of Young Children.

McAdoo, J. L. (1988b). The roles of black fathers in the socialization of black children. In H. P. McAdoo (Ed.), *Black families* (2nd ed.) (pp. 258–268). Newbury Park, CA: Sage.

McAdoo, J. L. (1997). The roles of African American fathers in the socialization of their children. In H. P. McAdoo (Ed.), *Black families* (3rd ed.) (pp. 183–195). Thousand Oaks, CA: Sage.

McAiley, L., Hudson-Barr, D., Gunning, R., & Rowbottom, L. (2000). The use of advance directives with adolescents. *Pediatric Nursing, 26*(5), 471–480.

McBride, B. A., & Mills, G. (1993) A comparison of mother and father involvement with their preschool age children. *Early Childhood Research Quarterly, 8*(4), 457–477.

McBridge, V. M. (1995). *Strengths and resiliency of black families: Implications for practitioners.* Paper presented at the National Council for Family Relations Conference, November 16, Portland, Oregon.

McCall, T. (1996, July/August). The best of both worlds. *American Health, 53.*

McCallion, P., Janicki, M., & Grant-Griffin, L. (1997). Exploring the impact of culture and acculturation on older families caregiving for persons with developmental disabilities. *Family Relations, 46*(4), 347–357.

McCloskey, J. C., & Bulechek, G. M. (1996). *Iowa intervention project: Nursing intervention classification (NIC)* (2nd ed.). St. Louis: Mosby.

McClowry, S., Gilliss, C. L., & Martinson, I. M. (1989). The process of grief in the bereaved family. In C. L. Gilliss, B. L. Highley, B. M. Roberts, & I. M. Martinson (Eds.), *Toward a science of family nursing* (pp. 216–225). Reading, MA: Addison-Wesley.

McCown, D. E. (1996). Family recreation and exercise. In P. J. Bomar (Ed.), *Nurses and family health promotion* (2nd ed.) (pp. 264–283). Philadelphia: Saunders.

McCown, D., & Davies, B. (1995). Patterns of grief in young siblings. *Journal of Death Studies, 19,* 41–53.

McCreery, A. (1981). Scapegoating. A survival phenomenon. In C. Getty & W. Humphreys (Eds.), *Understanding the family* (pp. 479–487). New York: Appleton-Century-Crofts.

McCrone, W. P. (1990) A summary of the Americans with Disabilities Act and its specific implications for hearing impaired people. *ADARA, 23*:3, 60–63.

McCubbin, H. I. (1979). Integrating coping behavior in family stress theory. *Journal of Marriage and the Family, 41,* 237–244.

McCubbin, H. I., & Dahl, B. B. (1985). Marriage and family: Individuals and life cycles. New York: Wiley.

McCubbin, H. I., & McCubbin, M. A. (1988). Typologies of resilient families: Emerging roles of social class and ethnicity. *Family Relations, 37,* 247–254.

McCubbin, H. I., & McCubbin, M. A. (1996). Resiliency in families: A conceptual model of family adjustment and adaptation in responses to stress and crisis. In H. I. McCubbin, A. Thompson, & M. McCubbin (Eds.), *Family assessment: Resiliency, coping and adaptation—Inventories for research and practice* (pp. 1–64). Madison, WI: University of Wisconsin System.

McCubbin, H. I., & Patterson, J. M. (1983a). The family stress process: The double ABCX model of adjustment and adaptation. In H. I. McCubbin, M. B. Sussman, & J. M. Patterson (Eds.), Social stress and the family (Special Issue). *Marriage and Family Review, 6*(1/2), 7–27.

McCubbin, H. I., & Patterson, J. M. (1983b). Family transitions: Adaptation to stress. In H. I. McCubbin & C. R. Figley (Eds.), *Stress and the family: Coping with normative transitions* (pp. 5–25). New York: Brunner/Mazel.

McCubbin, H. I., & Patterson, J. M. (1991). FILE: Family inventory of life events and changes. In H. I. McCubbin & A. Thompson (Eds.), *Family assessment inventories for research and practice* (pp. 81–110). Madison, WI: University of Wisconsin-Madison.

McCubbin, H. I., McCubbin, M., Nevin, R. S., & Cauble, E. (1981). Coping health inventory for parents (CHIP). In H. I. McCubbin & J. M. Patterson (Eds.), *Systematic assessment of family stress resources and coping*. St. Paul, MN: Family Social Sciences Department, University of Minnesota.

McCubbin, H. I., Patterson, J. M., & Wilson, L. (1983). *FILE: Family inventory of life events*. Madison, WI: University of Wisconsin-Madison.

McCubbin, H. I. & Figley, D. (Eds.) (1983). *Stress and the family: Vol. 1. Coping with normative transitions*. New York: Wiley.

McCubbin, H. I., McCubbin, M., Thompson, A. I., & Thompson, E. A. (1998). Resiliency in ethnic families. In H. I. McCubbin, E. A. Thompson, A. I. Thompson, & J. E. Fromer (Eds.), *Resiliency in Native American and immigrant families* (pp. 3–48). Thousand Oaks, CA: Sage.

McCubbin, H. I., Olson, D. H., & Larsen, A. S. (1987). F-COPES: Family crisis oriented personal evaluation scales. In H. I. McCubbin & A. I. Thompson (Eds.), *Family assessment inventories for research and practice* (pp. 203–216). Madison, WI: University of Wisconsin, Family stress coping and health project.

McCubbin, H. I., Thompson, E. A., Thompson, A. I., & Fromer, J. E. (1998). *Stress, coping, and health in families: Sense of coherence and resiliency*. Thousand Oaks, CA: Sage.

McCubbin, H. I., Thompson, E. A., Thompson, A. I., & Fromer, J. E. (1999). *The dynamics of resilient families*. Thousand Oaks, CA: Sage.

McCubbin, M. A., & McCubbin, H. I. (1991). Family stress theory and assessment: The resiliency model of family stress, adjustment, and adaptation. In H. I. McCubbin & A. Thompson (Eds.), *Family assessment inventories for research and practice* (pp. 3–32). Madison, WI: University of Wisconsin–Madison.

McCubbin, M. A., & McCubbin, H. I. (1993). Families coping with illness: The resiliency model of family stress, adjustment and adaptation. In C. Danielson, B. Hamel-Bissell, & P. Winstead-Fry (Eds.), *Families, health, and illness: Perspectives on coping and intervention* (pp. 21–63). St. Louis: Harcourt Health Services.

McCullough, P. G., & Rutenberg, S. K. (1988). Launching children and moving on. In B. Carter & M. McGoldrick (Eds.), *The changing family life cycle* (pp. 285–308). New York: Gardner Press.

McDonald, G. W. (1977). Family power, reflection and direction. *Pacific Sociological Review, 20,* 609–614.

McDonald, G. W. (1980, November). Family power: The assessment of a decade of theory and research, 1970–1979. *Journal of Marriage and the Family, 42*(4), 841–854.

McDonnell, P. J. (2001, May 10). Mexicans change face of U.S. demographics. *Los Angeles Times*, pp. A1, A28.

McEwen, B. S. (1998) Protective and damaging effects of stress mediators. *New England Journal of Medicine, 338*(3), 171–179.

McFarland, G., & McFarland, E. (1997). *Nursing diagnosis and intervention*. St. Louis: Mosby.

McGoldrick, M. (1989). Women and the family life cycle. In B. Carter & M. McGoldrick (Eds.), *The changing family life cycle* (2nd ed.) (pp. 29–68). Boston: Allyn & Bacon.

McGoldrick, M. (1988). The joining of families through marriage: The new couple. In B. Carter & M. McGoldrick (Eds.), *The changing family life cycle* (pp. 209–233). New York: Gardner Press.

McGoldrick, M. (1993). Ethnicity, cultural diversity and normality. In F. Walsh (Ed.), *Normal family processes* (2nd ed.) (pp. 331–360). New York: Guilford Press.

McGoldrick, M. (1996). Irish families. In M. McGoldrick, J. Giordano, & J. K. Pierce (Eds.), *Ethnicity and family therapy* (2nd ed.) (pp. 544–566). New York: Guilford Press.

McGoldrick, M., & Gerson, R. (1985). *Genograms in family assessment.* New York: W. W. Norton.

McGoldrick, M., & Giordano, J. (1996). Overview: Ethnicity and family therapy. In M. McGoldrick, J. Giordano, & J. K. Pearce (Eds.), *Ethnicity and family therapy* (pp. 1–30). New York: Guilford Press.

McGoldrick, M., Heiman, M., & Carter, B. (1993). The changing family life cycle: A perspective of normalcy. In F. Walsh (Ed.), *Normal family processes* (pp. 405–443). New York: Guilford Press.

McHale, S. M., & Crouter, A. C. (1992). You can't always get what you want: Incongruence between sex-role attitudes and family work roles and its implication for marriage. *Journal of Marriage and the Family, 46,* 357–364.

McKinley, D. (1964). *Social class and family life.* Glencoe, IL: Free Press.

McKinney, E., Ashwill, J., Murray, S., James, S., Gorrie, T., & Droske, S. (2000). *Maternal–child nursing.* Philadelphia: Saunders.

McLachlan, J. M. (1958). Cultural factors in health and disease. In E. G. Jaco (Ed.), *Patients, physicians, and illness.* New York: Free Press.

McLean, B., & Dworkin, A. S. (2001). *Understanding Chinese medicine.* Sacramento, CA: Continuing Medical Education Resources

McLemore, S. D., & Romo, R. (1985). The origins and development of the Mexican-American people. In R. D. De La Garza, et al. (Eds.), *The Mexican-American experience: An interdisciplinary anthology.* Austin, TX: University of Texas Press.

McLeod, D. L., & Wright, L. M. (2001). Conversations of spirituality: Spirituality in family systems nursing—Making the case with four clinical vignettes. *Journal of Family Nursing, 7*(4), 391–415.

McLeod, H., & Cooper, J. (1996, July 28). Generation X is active locally. How about nationally? *Los Angeles Times,* pp. M2, M6.

McRae, M. E. (1991). Holding death at bay: The experience of the spouses of patients undergoing cardiovascular surgery. *Canadian Journal of Cardiovascular Nursing, 2*(2), 14–20.

McSweeney, J. C., Allan, J. D., & Mayo, K. (1997). Exploring the use of explanatory models in nursing research and practice. *Image: Journal of Nursing Scholarship, 29*(3), 243–248.

Meacham, J. (2000, September 18). The new face of race. *Newsweek,* 38–46.

Mead, G. (1934). *Mind, self and society.* Chicago: University of Chicago Press.

Meadows, M. (1999, October/November). Improving the quality of life for minorities with disabilities. *Closing the Gap: A newsletter of the Office of Minority Health, U.S. Department of Health and Human Services,* p. 1.

Mechanic, D. (1964). Influences of mothers on their children's health attitudes and behavior. *Pediatrics, 33,* 445.

Mederer, H., & Hill, R. (1983). Critical transitions over the family life span: Theory and research. *Marriage and Family Review, 6*(1/2), 39–60.

Mehren, E. (1996, October 11). Parents want safety, not family values. *Los Angeles Times,* pp. E1, E8.

Meisenhelder, J. B. (1982). Boundaries of personal space. *Image, 14*(1), 16–19.

Meisler, S., & Fulwood, S. (1989, July 17). Number of inner-city single parents on rise. *Los Angeles Times,* p. A14.

Meleis, A. I. (1975). Role insufficiency and role supplementation. *Nursing Research, 24*(2), 264.

Meleis, A. I., & Swendsen, L. A. (1978). Role supplementation—an empirical test of a nursing intervention. *Nursing Research, 27*(1), 11.

Meleis, A. I. (1997). *Theoretical nursing.* Philadelphia: Lippincott.

Melson, G. F. (1983). Family adaptation to environmental demands. In H. I. McCubbin & C. R. Figley (Eds.), *Stress and the family. Vol I: Coping with normative transitions* (pp. 149–162). New York: Brunner/Mazel.

Menaghan, E. G. (1983). Individual coping efforts and family studies. Conceptual and methodological issues. In H. I. McCubbin, M. B. Sussman, & J. M. Patterson (Eds.), Social stress and the family (Special Issue). *Marriage and Family Review, 6*(1/2), 113–135.

Mendes, H. A. (1988). Single-parent families: A typology of life-styles. In J. G. Wells (Ed.), *Current issues in marriage and the family* (4th ed.) (pp. 247–259). New York: Macmillan.

Mercer, R. T. (1989). Theoretical perspectives on the family. In C. L. Gilliss, B. L. Highley, B. M. Roberts, & I. M. Martinson (Eds.), *Toward a science of family nursing* (pp. 9–36). Menlo Park, CA: Addison-Wesley.

Meredith, W. H., & Abbott, D. A. (1995). Chinese families in later life. In B. B. Ingoldsby & S. Smith (Eds.), *Families in multicultural perspective* (pp. 213–230). New York: Guilford Press.

Mertensmeyer, C., & Fine, M. (2000) ParentLink: A model of integration and support for parents. *Family Relations, 49,* 257–265.

Merton, R. K. (1957). *Social theory and social structure.* New York: Free Press.

Messer, A. (1970). *The individual in his family: An adaptational study.* Springfield, IL: Charles C Thomas.

Messias, D. K. (1997). Exploring the concept of undocumentedness: The meaning of a person's immigration status to nursing care. In A. G. Gift (Ed.), *Clarifying concepts in nursing research* (pp. 53–69). New York: Springer Publishing Company.

Mikhail, B. I. (1994). Hispanic mother's beliefs and practices regarding selected children's health problems. *Western Journal of Nursing, 16*(6), 623–638.

Milardo, R. M. (1988). *Families and social networks.* Newbury Park, CA: Sage.

Miller, B. G., & Myers-Walls, J. A. (1983). Parenthood: Stresses and coping strategies. In H. I. McCubbin & C. R. Figley (Eds.), *Stress and the family. Vol I. Coping with normative transitions* (pp. 54–73). New York: Brunner/Mazel.

Miller, D. (1989). Family violence and the helping system. In L. Combrinck-Graham (Ed.), *Children in family contexts* (pp. 413–434). New York: Guilford Press.

Miller, F. (1986). The people. In B. Coyne & B. Holland (Eds.), *Encyclopedia Americana* (pp. 819–830). Danbury, CT: Grolier.

Miller, J. E. (2000). Religion and families over the life course. In S. J. Price, P. C. McKenry, & M. F. Murphy (Eds.), *Families across time* (pp. 173–186). Los Angeles, CA: Roxbury.

Miller, J. F. (2000). Inspiring hope. In J. F. Miller (Ed.), *Coping with chronic illness* (pp. 523–546). Philadelphia: Davis.

Miller, S. R., & Winstead-Fry, P. (1982). *Family systems theory in nursing practice.* Reston, VA: Reston Publishing.

Miller, S., & Katz, G. (1992). The educational needs of mental health self-help groups. *Psychosocial Rehabilitation Journal, 16,* 160–163.

Millington, M. J., & Zieball, C. W. (1986). Financial strategies. In S. H. Johnson (Ed.), *Nursing assessment and strategies for the family at risk. High risk parenting* (2nd ed.) (pp. 473–487). Philadelphia: Lippincott.

Milner, J., & Murphy, W. (1995). Assessment of child physical and sexual abuse offenders. *Family Relations, 44,* 478–488.

Min, P. G. (1988). The Korean American family. In C. H. Mindel, R. W. Habenstein, & R. Wright, Jr. (Eds.), *Ethnic families in America* (pp. 199–229). New York: Elsevier.

Min, P. G. (1995a). An overview of Asian Americans. In P. G. Min (Ed.), *Asian Americans: Contemporary trends and issues* (pp. 10–37). Thousand Oaks, CA: Sage.

Min, P. G. (Ed.). (1995b). *Asian Americans: Contemporary trends and issues.* Thousand Oaks, CA: Sage.

Min, P. G. (1995c). Korean Americans. In P. G. Min (Ed.), *Asian Americans: Contemporary trends and issues* (pp. 199–231). Thousand Oaks, CA: Sage.

Minkler, M., & Roe, K. (1995, Spring). Grandparents as surrogate parents. *Generations, XX*(1), 34–38.

Minkler, M., & Stone, R. (1985). The faminization of poverty and older women. *The Gerontologist, 25,* 351–357.

Minuchin, S. (1974). *Families and family therapy.* Cambridge, MA: Harvard University Press.

Minuchin, S., & Fishman, H. G. (1981). *Family therapy techniques.* Cambridge, MA: Harvard University Press.

Minuchin, S., & Nichols, M. P. (1998). Structural family therapy. In F. M. Dattilio (Ed.). *Case studies in couple and family therapy: Systemic and cognitive perspectives.* New York: Guilford Press.

Minuchin, S., Rosman, B. L., & Baker, L. (1978). *Psychosomatic families: Anorexia nervosa in context.* Cambridge, MA: Harvard University Press.

Mirandé, A. (1979, October). A reinterpretation of male dominance in the Chicano family. *The Family Coordinator,* 473–479.

Mirandé, A. (1985). *The Chicano experience: An alternative perspective.* Notre Dame, IN: University of Notre Dame Press.

Mirandé, A. (1991). Ethnicity and fatherhood. In F. W. Bozett & S. M. H. Hanson (Eds.), *Fatherhood and families in cultural context* (pp. 53–82). New York: Springer.

Mirowsky, J., & Ross, C. E. (1984). Mexican culture and its emotional contradictions. *Journal of Health and Social Behavior, 25*(1), 2–13.

Mishel, M. H. (1974). *Patient problems in self-esteem and nursing intervention.* Los Angeles: California State University, Los Angeles, Trident Shop.

Mishel, M. H., & Murdaugh, C. L. (1987). Family adjustment to heart transplantation: Redesigning the dream. *Nursing Research, 36*(6), 332–338.

Mitchell, B. A., Wister, A. V., & Burch, T. K. (1989). The family environment and leaving the parental home. *Journal of Marriage and the Family, 51*(3), 605–613.

Mitchell, V. (1996). Two moms: Contribution of the planned lesbian family to the deconstruction of gendered parenting. In J. Laird & R. J. Green (Eds.), *Lesbians and gays in couples and families: A handbook for therapists* (pp. 343–357). San Francisco, CA: Jossey-Bass.

Moffitt, P. (2001). The impact of a child's death on the extended family. *Journal of Child and Family Nursing, 4*(2), 152–155.

Monmaney, T. (1997, December 25). Study links poor health to poverty. *Los Angeles Times,* p. A3.

Monroe, L. D. (1989, August 19). Culture shock hits health care. *Los Angeles Times,* Part I, pp. 1, 30.

Monroe, L. D. (1990, November 22). Programs tailor tips on health to Latinos. *Los Angeles Times,* pp. E1, E6.

Montgomery, R. (1989). Investigating caregiver burden. In K. S. Markides & C. C. Cooper (Eds.), *Aging, stress and health.* New York: Wiley.

Montgomery, R., & Kosloski, K. (1994). Outcomes of family caregiving: Lessons from the past and challenges for the future. In M. H. Cantor (Ed.), *Family caregiving, agenda for the future* (pp. 123–136). Chicago: American Society on Aging.

Moore, J. W. (1970). *Mexican Americans.* Englewood Cliffs, NJ: Prentice Hall.

Moorek, K., Spain, D., & Bianchi, S. (1984). Working wives and mothers. *Marriage and Family Review, 7*(3/4), 77–98.

Morrow, R. (1987). Cultural differences—Be aware. *Academic Therapy, 23*(2), 143–149.

Moules, N., & Amundson, J. (1997). Grief—An invitation to inertia: A narrative approach to working with grief. *Journal of Family Nursing, 3*(4), 378–393.

Moules, N. J. (2000). Funerals, families, and family nursing: Lessons of love and practice. *Journal of Family Nursing, 6*(1), 3–8.

Moynihan, D. P. (1965). *The Negro family: A case for national action.* Washington, DC: U.S. Government Printing Office.

Mueller, D. P., & Cooper, P. W. (1986). Children of single parent families: How they fare as young adults. *Family Relations, 35*(1), 169–176.

Mullins, L. C., & Mushel, M. (1992). The existence and emotional closeness of relationships with children, friends and spouses. *Research on Aging, 14*, 448–470.

Mumford, E., Schlesinger, H. J., & Glass, G. V. (1982). The effects of psychological intervention in recovery from surgery and heart attacks: An analysis of the literature. *American Journal of Public Health, 72*, 141–151.

Murata, J. E. (1995). Family stress, mothers' social support, depression, and sons' behavior problems: Modeling nursing interventions for low-income inner city families. *Journal of Family Nursing, 1*(1), 41–62.

Murdock, G. P. (1949). *Social structure.* New York: MacMillan.

Murillo, N. (1976). The Mexican-American family. In C. A. Hernandez, M. J. Haug, & N. N. Wagner (Eds.), *Chicanos: Social and psychological perspectives* (2nd ed.) (pp. 15–25). St. Louis: Mosby.

Murray, C. I., & Leigh, G. K. (1995). Families and sexuality. In R. D. Day, K. R. Gilbert, B. H. Settles, & W. R. Burr (Eds.), *Research and theory in family science* (pp. 186–204). Pacific Grove, CA: Brooks/Cole.

Murray, C. I. (2000). Coping with death, dying, and grief in families. In P. C. McKenry & S. J. Price (Eds.), *Families and change* (pp. 120–153). Thousand Oaks, CA: Sage.

Murray, R., & Zentner, J. (1993). *Nursing concepts for health promotion* (4th ed.). Englewood Cliffs, NJ: Prentice Hall.

Naisbitt, J. (1984). *Megatrends.* New York: Warner Communications.

Nall, F. C., & Speilberg, J. S. (1978). New York social and cultural factors in the responses of Mexican Americans to medical treatment. In R. A. Martinez (Ed.), *Hispanic culture and health care.* St. Louis: Mosby.

National Center for Health Statistics. (1989, September 26). *Monthly vital statistics report.* Washington, DC: U.S. Government Printing Office.

National Coalition for the Homeless (1999). *NCH Fact Sheet #7: Homeless families with children.* Available at: *www.nationalhomeless.org/families.html.*

National Council for Family Relations. (1993). *Vision 2010: Families and health care.* Minneapolis, MN: National Council for Family Relations.

Neal, M. B., Chapman, N. J., Ingersoll-Dayton, B., & Emlen, A. C. (1993). *Balancing work and caregiving for children, adults, and elders.* Thousand Oaks, CA: Sage.

Neff, J. A., & Hoppe, S. K. (1993). Race/ethnicity, acculturation, and psychological distress: Fatalism and religiosity as cultural resources. *Journal of Community Psychology, 21*, 3–20.

Neimeyer, R. A. (1988). Death anxiety. In H. Wass, F. M. Berardo, & R. A. Neimeyer (Eds.), *Dying: Facing the facts* (2nd ed.) (pp. 97–136). Washington, DC: Hemisphere.

Nelson, M. A. (1994). Economic impoverishment and health risk: Methodologic and conceptual issues. *Advances in Nursing Science, 16*(3), 1–12.

Neuman, B. (1982). *The Neuman systems model: Application to nursing education and practice.* Norwalk, CT: Appleton-Century-Crofts.

Neuman, B. (1983). Family intervention using the Betty Neuman health care systems model. In I. W. Clements & F. B. Roberts (Eds.), *Family health: A theoretical approach to nursing care.* New York: Wiley.

Newman, M. (1979). *Theory development in nursing.* Philadelphia: Davis.

Newman, M. (1994). *Health as expanding consciousness* (Pub. No. 14-2626). New York: National League for Nursing Press.

Newman, M. (1995). *A developing discipline* (Pub. No. 14-2671). New York: National League for Nursing Press.

Nightingale, F. N. (1992). *Notes on nursing: What it is and what it is not* (Com. Ed.). Philadelphia: Lippincott (Original publication 1859).

Nightingale, F. (1859). *Notes on nursing: What it is and what it is not.* London: Harrison (Reprinted 1946. Philadelphia: Lippincott).

Nightingale, F. (1949). Sick nursing and health nursing. In I. Hampton et al. (Eds.), *Nursing of the sick: 1893.* New York: McGraw-Hill.

Nishi, S. M. (1995). Japanese Americans. In P. G. Min (Ed.), *Asian Americans: Contemporary trends and issues* (pp. 95–133). Thousand Oaks, CA: Sage.

Niska, K., Snyder, M., & Lia-Hoagberg, B. (1999). The meaning of family health among Mexican American mothers and fathers. *Journal of Family Nursing, 5*(2), 218–233.

Nock, S. (1981). Family life-cycle transitions: Longitudinal effects on family members. *Journal of Marriage and the Family, 43*(3), 703–713.

Nock, S. L. (1988). The family and hierarchy. *Journal of Marriage and the Family, 50*(4), 957–966.

Norbeck, J. S., & Tilden, V. P. (1983, March). Life stress, social support, and emotional disequilibrium in complications of pregnancy: A prospective, multivariate study. *Journal of Health and Social Behavior, 24*(1), 30–46.

Norris, D. M., & Hoyer, P. J. (1993). Dynamism in practice: Parenting within King's Framework. *Nursing Science Quarterly, 6*(2), 79–84

Nortan, A. J., & Glick, P. G. (1986). One-parent families: A social and economic profile. *Family Relations, 35*(1), 177–181.

North American Nursing Diagnosis Association (NANDA). (2001). *Nursing diagnosis: Definitions and classification 2001–2002.* Philadelphia: Author.

Nyamathi, A. M. (1987a). The coping responses of female spouses of patients with myocardial infarction. *Heart & Lung, 16*(1), 86–92.

Nyamathi, A. M. (1987b). Coping responses of spouses of MI patients and of hemodialysis patients as measured by the Jalowiec Coping Scale. *Journal of Cardiovascular Nursing, 2*(1), 67–74.

Nye, F. I., & Gecas, V. (1976). The role concept: Review and delineation. In F. I. Nye (Ed.), *Role structure and analysis of the family* (Vol. 24). Beverly Hills, CA: Sage.

Nye, F. I. (Ed.). (1976). Role structure and analysis of the family (Vol. 24). Beverly Hills, CA: Sage.

Nye, F. I., & Berardo, F. (Eds.). (1981). *Emerging conceptual frameworks in family analysis.* New York: Praeger.

Ogburn, W. F. (1933). *The family and its function: Recent social trends in the United States.* New York: McGraw-Hill.

Okin, S. M. (1989). *Justice, gender and the family.* New York: Basic Books.

Oliver, D. B. (1998, May 25). Coping with loss: Advice for seniors and their children. *Los Angeles Times,* p. S8.

Olson, D., & McCubbin, H. (1982). Circumplex model of marital and family systems V: Application to family stress and crisis intervention. In H. McCubbin, A. Cauble, & J. Patterson (Eds.), *Family stress, coping, and social support* (pp. 48–68). Springfield. IL: Charles C Thomas.

Olson, D. (1993). Circumplex model of marital and family systems: Assessing family functioning. In F. Walsh (Ed.), *Normal family processes* (pp. 104–137). New York: Guilford Press.

Olson, D. H., & Cromwell, R. E. (1975). Methodological issues in family power. In R. E. Cromwell & D. II. Olson (Eds.), *Power in families* (pp. 142–145). New York: Sage.

Olson, D. H., Cromwell, R. E., & Klein, D. M. (1975). Beyond family power. In R. E. Cromwell & D. H. Olson (Eds.), *Power in families* (pp. 236–239). New York: Sage.

Olson, D., McCubbin, H., Barnes, H., Larsen, A., Muxem, M., & Wilson, M. (1983). *Families: What makes them work.* Los Angeles: Sage.

O'Neal, D. P., & Kenny, E. K. (1998). Spirituality and chronic illness. *Image: Journal of Nursing Scholarship, 30*(3), 275–280.

Orem, D. (1983a). The family coping with a medical illness: Analysis and application of Orem's theory. In I. Clements & F. Roberts (Eds.), *Family health: A theoretical approach to nursing care.* New York: Wiley.

Orem, D. (1983b). The family experiencing emotional crisis: Analysis and application of Orem's self-care deficit theory. In I. Clements & F. Roberts (Eds.), *Family health: A theoretical approach to nursing care.* New York: Wiley.

Orem, D. (1985). *Nursing: Concepts and practice* (3rd ed.). New York: McGraw-Hill.

Orem, D. E. (1971). *Nursing: Concepts of practice.* New York: McGraw-Hill.

Orem, D. E. (1991). *Nursing: Concepts of practice* (4th ed.). St. Louis: Mosby.

Orthner, D. (1995). Families in transition: Changing values and norms. In R. D. Day, K. R. Gilbert, B. H. Settles, & W. R. Burr (Eds.), *Research and theory in family science* (pp. 3–19). Pacific Grove, CA: Brooks/Cole.

Ortiz, V. (1995). The diversity of Latino families. In R. E. Zambrana (Ed.), *Understanding Latino families: Scholarship, policy and practice* (pp. 18–38). Thousand Oaks, CA: Sage.

Osborne, P. (1995). The parenting experts. In R. D. Day, K. R. Gilbert, B. H. Settles, & W. R. Burr (Eds.), *Research and theory in family science* (pp. 320–333). Pacific Grove, CA: Brooks/Cole.

Osmond, M. W. (1978). Reciprocity: A dynamic model and a method to study family power. *Journal of Marriage and the Family, 40*(1), 51.

Otto, H. (1973). A framework for assessing family strengths. In A. Reinhardt & M. Quinn (Eds.), *Family-centered community nursing* (pp. 87–93). St. Louis: Mosby.

Ottolini, M., Hamburger, E., Loprieato, J., Coleman, R., Sachs, H., Madden, R., et al. (2001). Complementary and alternative medicine use among children in the Washington DC area. *Ambulatory Pediatrics, 1*(2), 122–125.

Padilla, E. R. (1976). The relationship between psychology and Chicanos: Failures and possibilities. In C. A. Hernandez, M. J. Haug, & N. N. Wagner (Eds.), *Chicanos—Social and psychological perspectives* (2nd ed.) (pp. 282–290). St. Louis: Mosby.

Paffenbarger, R., Hyde, R., Wing, A., Lee, I., Jung, D., & Kampert, J. (1993). The association of changes in physical-activity level and other lifestyle characteristics with mortality among men. *New England Journal of Medicine, 328*(8), 538–545.

Pagelow, M. D. (1984). *Family violence.* New York: Praeger.

Pallett, P. J. (1990). A conceptual framework for studying family caregiver burden in Alzheimer's-type dementias. *Image, 22*(1), 52–58.

Paniagua, F. A. (1994). *Assessing and treating culturally diverse clients.* Thousand Oaks, CA: Sage.

Parachini, A. (1987, June 9). New guidelines for physical exams. *Los Angeles Times,* Part V, pp. 1–2.

Parad, H. J., & Caplan, G. (1965). A framework for studying families in crisis. In H. J. Parad (Ed.), *Crisis intervention: Selected readings* (pp. 55–60). New York: Family Service of America.

Parascandola, M. (2000). Clinical research and alternative medicine. *Research Practitioner, 1*(6), 187–197.

Parker, K., Calhoun, T., & Weaver, G. (2000). Variables associated with adolescent alcohol use: A multiethnic comparison. *The Journal of Social Psychology, 140*(1), 51–62.

Parker, M. (2000). Domestic violence and its effect on children. National Council on Family Relations Report. *Family Focus, 45*(4), F6.

Parra, P. A., & Guarnaccia, P. (1998). Ethnicity, culture, and resiliency in caregivers of a seriously mentally ill family member. In H. I. McCubbin, E. A. Thompson, A. I. Thompson, & J. E. Fromer (Eds.), *Resiliency in Native American and immigrant families* (pp. 431–450). Thousand Oaks, CA: Sage.

Parsons, R., Bales, R. F., & Shils, E. A. (1953). *Working papers on the theory of action*. Glencoe, IL: Free Press.

Parsons, T. (1951). *The social system*. Glencoe, IL: Free Press.

Parsons, T., & Bales, R. F. (1955). *Family socialization and interaction process*. New York: Free Press.

Pascual, C. (2000, September 14). Why more elderly Asian women kill themselves. *Los Angeles Times*, pp. E1, E4.

Pasquali, E. A., Arnold, H. M., De Basio, N., & Alesi, E. G. (1985). *Mental health nursing* (2nd ed.). St. Louis: Mosby.

Pate, R., Pratt, M., Blair, S., Haskell, W., Macera, C., Bouchard, C., et al. (1995). Physical activity and public health: A recommendation from the Centers for Disease Control and Prevention and the American College of Sports Medicine. *Journal of the American Medical Association, 273*(5), 402–407.

Patterson, J. M. (1988). Chronic illness in children and the impact on families. In C. S. Chilman, E. W. Nunally, & F. M. Cox (Eds.), *Chronic illness and disability* (pp. 69–107). Newbury Park, CA: Sage.

Patterson, J. M. (1988). Families experiencing stress. The family adjustment and adaptation response model. *Family Systems Medicine, 6*(2), 202–237.

Patterson, J. M., & Zderad, L. (1976). *Humanistic nursing*. New York: Wiley.

Pavalko, R. M. (1999). Problem gambing. *National Forum, 79*(4), 28–32.

Paz, O. (1973). The sons of La Malenche. In L. I. Duran & H. R. Bernard (Eds.), *Introduction to Chicano studies*. New York: Macmillan.

Pearlin, L., & Schooler, C. (1978). The structure of coping. *Journal of Health and Social Behavior, 19*, 19–21.

Pearlin, L., & Turner, H. A. (1987). The family as a context of the stress process. In S. V. Kasl & C. L. Cooper (Eds.), *Stress and health: Issues in research methodology*. New York: Wiley.

Pearson, R. E. (1990). *Counseling and social support: Perspectives and practice*. Newbury Park, CA: Sage.

Peck, J. S., & Manocharian, J. R. (1988). Divorce in the changing family life cycle. In B. Carter & M. McGoldrick (Eds.), *The changing family life cycle* (pp. 335–369). New York: Gardner Press.

Pedersen, F., & Robson, K. (1969). Father participation in infancy. *American Journal of Orthopsychiatry, 39*(3), 466–472.

Pedersen, P. B., Draguns, J. G., Lonner, W. J., & Trimble, J. E. (1996). Introduction. In P. B. Pedersen, J. G. Draguns, W. J. Lonner, & J. E. Trimble (Eds.), *Counseling across cultures* (4th ed.) (pp. vii–xvii). Thousand Oaks, CA: Sage.

Pederson, P. (1976, August 2). Varighed fra sygdoms begyndelse til henvendelse til prakliserende laege. *Ugekr Laeg, 138*, 32.

Pelletier, K. (1979). *Holistic medicine*. New York: Delta/Seymour Lawrence.

Pender, N., Murdaugh, C., & Parsons, M. (2001). *Health promotion in nursing*. Stamford, CT: Appleton & Lange.

Pender, N. J. (1986). Health promotion: Implementing strategies. In B. B. Logan & C. E. Dawkins (Eds.), *Family-centered nursing in the community* (pp. 296–334). Reading, MA: Addison-Wesley.

Pender, N. J. (1996). *Health promotion in nursing practice* (3rd ed.). Stamford, CT: Appleton & Lange.

Penning, M., & Strain, L. (1994). Gender difference in disability, assistance, and subjective well-being in later life. *Journal of Gerontology, 46*(4), S202–S208.

Peplau, H. (1952). *Interpersonal relations in nursing*. New York: Putnam.

Perkins, E. J. (1973). Screening for ophthalmic conditions. *Practitioner, 211*, 171–177.

Perkins, H. W., & Harris, L. B. (1990). Familial bereavement and health in adult life course perspective. *Journal of Marriage and the Family, 52*(1), 233–241.

Perry, S. E. (1983). Attachment theory. In I. W. Clements & F. B. Roberts (Eds.), *Family health: A theoretical approach to nursing care* (pp. 109–122). New York: Wiley.

Perry-Jenkins, M., & Crouter, A. C. (1990). Men's provider role attitudes: Implications for household work and marital satisfaction. *Journal of Family Issues, 11*, 136–156.

Perry-Jenkins, M., & Folk, K. (1994). Class, couples, and conflicts. Effects of the division of labor on assessments of marriage in dual-earner families. *Journal of Marriage and the Family, 56*, 165–180.

Peters, L. R. (1974). Family team or myth. In J. E. Hall & B. R. Weaver (Eds.), *Nursing of families in crisis* (pp. 226–237). Philadelphia: Lippincott.

Peters, M. F. (1981). "Making it" black family style: Building on the strengths of black families. In N. Stinnett, J. De Frain, K. King, et al. (Eds.), *Family strengths: Roots of well-being* (pp. 73–91). Lincoln, NE: University of Nebraska Press.

Peters, M. F. (1997). Historical note: Parenting of young children in black families. In H. P. McAdoo (Ed.), *Black families* (3rd ed.) (pp. 167–181). Thousand Oaks, CA: Sage.

Peters, M. F., & Massey, G. (1983). Mundane extreme environmental stress in family stress theories: The case of black families in white America. In H. I. McCubbin, M. B. Sussman, & J. M. Patterson (Eds.), Social stress and the family (Special Issue). *Marriage and Family Review, 6*(1/2), 193–218.

Peterson, G. W. (1995). Autonomy and connectedness in families. In R. Day, K. Gilbert, B. Settles, & W. Burr (Eds.), *Research and theory in family social science* (pp. 20–41). Pacific Grove, CA: Brooks/ Cole.

Peterson, G. W., & Rollins, B. C. (1987). Parent–child socialization. In M. B. Sussman & S. K. Steinmetz (Eds.), *Handbook of marriage and the family* (pp. 471–507). New York: Plenum Press.

Peterson, J., & Zill, N. (1986). Marital disruption, parent–child relationships, and behavior problems in children. *Journal of Marriage and the Family, 48,* 295–307.

Pew Health Professions Commission. (1991). *Healthy America: Practitioners for 2005.* San Francisco: Pew Health Professions Commission.

Phillips, L. R. (1996). Elder abuse and the identification dilemma. *Advances in Bioethics 1,* 3–39.

Phillips, L. R. (2000). Domestic violence and aging women. *Geriatric Nursing, 21*(4), 188–195.

Phillips, S., & Lobar, S. (1990). Literature summary of some Navajo child health beliefs and rearing practices within a transcultural nursing framework. *Journal of Transcultural Nursing, 1*(2), 13–20.

Picker, L. (1996, May). Herbal medicine goes mainstream. *American Health,* 68–75.

Pifer, A., & Bronte, L. (1986). Introduction: Squaring the pyramid. In A. Pifer & L. Bronte (Eds.), *Our aging society.* New York: Norton.

Pilisuk, M., & Parks, S. H. (1983). Social support and family stress. In H. I. McCubbin, M. B. Sussman, & J. M. Patterson (Eds.), Social stress and the family (Special Issue). *Marriage and Family Review, 6*(1/2), 137–156.

Pillari, V. (1992). Family myths among female adolescents in a residential setting. *Child and Adolescent Social Work Journal, 9,* 77–88.

Pillemer, K., & Finkelhor, D. (1988). The prevalence of elder abuse: A random sample survey. *The Gerontologist, 281,* 51–57.

Pinsof, W. M (1995). *Integrative problem-centered therapy: A synthesis of family, individual, and biological therapies.* New York: Basic Books.

Piotrkowski, C. S., & Hughes, D. (1993). Dual-earner families in context. In F. Walsh (Ed.), *Normal family processes* (2nd ed.) (pp. 185–208). New York: Guilford Press.

Pipes, W. H. (1997). Old-time religion: Benches can't say "amen." In H. P. McAdoo (Ed.), *Black families* (3rd ed.) (pp. 41–66). Thousand Oaks, CA: Sage.

Pleck, J. H. (1985). *Working wives/working husbands.* Beverly Hills, CA: Sage.

Pollack, W. S. (1999) *Real boys: Rescuing our sons from the myths of boyhood.* First Owl Books Edition, originally published by Random House, Inc., New York.

Pollock, S. E. (1994) Contributions to nursing science: Synthesis of findings from adaptation model research. *Scholarly Inquiry for Nursing Practice: An International Journal, 8*(4), 361–374.

Popenoe, D., & Whitehead, B. (1999). *Should we live together?* New Brunswick, NJ: The National Marriage Project, Rutgers University.

Popenoe, D. (1995). The American family crisis. *National Forum, 75*(3), 15–19.

Popenoe, D., & Whitehead, B. (2000). *The state of our unions 2000.* New Brunswick, NJ: The National Marriage Project, Rutgers University. (See *http://marriage.rutgers.edu.*)

Power, P. W., & Dell Orto, A. E. (1988). Approaches to family intervention. In P. W. Power, A. E. Dell Orto, & M. Gibbons (Eds.), *Role of the family in the rehabilitation of the physically disabled* (pp. 321–330). Baltimore: University Park Press.

Prater, L. P. (1995). Never married/biological teen mother headed household. In S. Hanson, M. Heims, D. Julian, & M. Sussman (Eds.), *Single parent families: Diversity, myths and realities* (pp. 305–323). New York: Haworth Press.

Pratt, L. (1976). *Family structure and effective health behavior: The energized family.* Boston: Houghton-Miffin.

Pratt, L. (1977). Changes in health care ideology in relation to self-care by families. *Health Education Monograph, 5*(2), 121–122.

Pratt, L. (1982). Family structure and health work: Coping in the context of social change. In H. I. McCubbin, A. E. Cauble, & J. M. Patterson (Eds.), *Family stress, coping, and social support* (pp. 73–89). Springfield, IL: Charles C Thomas.

Prattes, O. (1973). Beliefs of the Mexican American family. In D. Hymovich & M. V. Barnard (Eds.), *Family health care* (pp. 131–137). New York: McGraw-Hill.

Pravikoff, D. (1985). *Family coping and perception of the situation in families with an actual or suspected myocardial infarction.* Unpublished master's thesis, California State University, Los Angeles.

Preto, N. G. (1988). Transformation of the family system in adolescence. In B. Carter & M. McGoldrick (Eds.), *The changing family life cycle* (2nd ed.) (pp. 255–283). New York: Gardner Press.

Price, R. (1990). Borderline disorders of the self: Toward a reconceptualization. *Transactional Analysis Journal, 20,* 128–134.

Pruchno, R. A., & Resch, N. L. (1989). Husbands and wives as caregivers: Antecedents of depression and burden. *The Gerontologist, 29,* 159–165.

Purnell, L. D., & Paulanka, B. J. (1998). *Transcultural health care*. Philadelphia: Davis.

Queen, S. A., & Haberstein, R. W. (1974). *The family in various cultures*. Philadelphia: Lippincott.

Quinn, P. (1995). Gender interactions in families. In R. D. Day, K. R. Gilbert, B. H. Settles, & W. R. Burr (Eds.), *Research and theory in family science* (pp. 42–53). Pacific Grove, CA: Brooks/Cole.

Quinn, W. H. (1993). Personal and family adjustment in later life. *Journal of Marriage and the Family, 51,* 581–591.

Radin, N. (1981). Childrearing fathers in intact families: I. Some antecedents and consequences. *Merrill-Palmer Quarterly, 27*(4), 489–514.

Rafael, A. R. (1995). Advocacy and empowerment: Dichotomous or synchronous concepts? *Advances in Nursing Science, 18*(2), 25–32.

Ragon, B., & Mouzon, L. (1999). Attitudes and beliefs of adolescents toward the use of tobacco: A 16-year follow up. *The International Electronic Journal of Health Education, 2*(3), 120–126.

Rainwater, L. (1972). Fear and house as haven in the lower class. In R. Gutman (Ed.), *People and buildings*. New York: Basic Books.

Rainwater, L. (1971). Crucible of identity: The Negro lower-class family. In J. H. Bracey, A. Meier, & E. Rudwick (Eds.), *Black matriarchy: Myth or reality?* (pp. 76–109). Belmont, CA: Wadsworth.

Ramirez, O., & Arce, C. (1981). The contemporary Chicano family: An empirically-based review. In A. Baron (Ed.), *Explorations in Chicano psychology*. New York: Praeger.

Rando, T. (Ed.). (1986). *Loss and anticipatory grief*. Lexington, MA: Lexington Books.

Rankin, S. (1986). Family transitions, expected and unexpected. In Gillis & Lynch, (Eds.), *Toward a science in family nursing*. Upper Saddle River, NJ: Pearson Education, Inc.

Rankin, S. H., & Stallings, K. D. (2001). *Patient education: Principles and practice* (4th ed.). Philadelphia: Lippincott.

Raths, L. E., Harmin, M., & Simon, S. B. (1978). *Values and teaching: Working with values in the classroom* (2nd ed.). Columbus, OH: Charles E. Merrill.

Rauckhorst, L. M., Stokes, S. A., & Mezey, M. D. (1982). Community and home assessment. In B. W. Spradley (Ed.), *Readings in community health nursing* (2nd ed.) (pp. 154–165). Boston: Little, Brown.

Raven, B. H., Center, R., & Rodrigues, A. (1975). The bases of conjugal power. In R. E. Cromwell & D. H. Olson (Eds.), *Power in families* (pp. 217–232). New York: Sage.

Rayner, J. F. (1970). Socioeconomic status and factors influencing the dental health practices of mothers. *American Journal of Public Health, 60,* 1250.

Redding, C., Rossi, J., Rossi, S., Velicer, W., & Prochaska, J. (2000). Health behavior models. *International Electronic Journal of Health Education, 3*(Special Issue), 180–193.

Reed, P. G. (1995). A treatise on nursing knowledge development in the 21st century: Beyond postmodernism. *Advances in Nursing Science, 17*(3), 70–84.

Rehm, R. S. (1999). Religious faith in Mexican-American families dealing with chronic childhood illness. *Image: Journal of Nursing Scholarship, 31*(1), 33–38.

Reinhard, S. C., & Horwitz, A. V. (1995). Caregiver burden: Differentiating the content and consequences of family caregiving. *Journal of Marriage and the Family, 57,* 741–750.

Reinhardt, A., & Quinn, M. (Eds.). (1973). *Current practices in family-centered community nursing*. St. Louis: Mosby.

Reiss, D. (1981). *The family's construction of reality*. Cambridge, MA: Harvard University Press.

Reiss, D., Steinglass, P., & Howe, G. (1993). The family's organization around the illness. In R. Cole & D. Reiss (Eds.), *How do families cope with chronic illness?* (pp. 173–213). Hillsdale, NJ: Erlbaum.

Reiss, I. L. (1965). The universality of the family: A conceptual analysis. *Journal of Marriage and the Family, 27,* 443.

Reiss, I. L. (1976). *Family systems in America* (2nd ed.). Hinsdale, IL: Dryden Press.

Richards, B. S. (1996). Gerontological family nursing. In S. M. H. Hanson & S. T. Boyd (Eds.), *Family health care nursing: Theory, practice, and research*. Philadelphia: Davis.

Richards, E., & Lansberry, C. R. (1995). A national survey of graduate family nursing educators. *Journal of Family Nursing, 1*(4), 382–396.

Richardson, L., & MacGregor, H. E. (2001, April 30). To be Chinese in America. *Los Angeles Times,* pp. E1, E4.

Richardson, W. (1970). Measuring the urban poor's use of physicians' services in response to illness episodes. *Medical Care, 8,* 132.

Ridley, C. R., & Lingle, D. W. (1996). Cultural empathy in multicultural counseling. In P. B. Pedersen, J. G. Draguns, W. J. Lonner, & J. E. Trimble (Eds.), *Counseling across cultures* (4th ed.) (pp. 21–46). Thousand Oaks, CA: Sage.

Rienza, B. M. (1990). Influence and adaptability in families with deaf parents and hearing children. *American Annals of the Deaf, 135*(5), 402–408.

Roack, A. C. (1988, July 24). Parenting: Fads, theories change with the years. *Los Angeles Times,* pp. A1, A24.

Roan, S. (1995, July 9). Who's to blame for teenage pregnancy? *Los Angeles Times,* p. E3.

Roberto, K. A. (1993). Family caregivers of aging adults with disabilities: A review of the caregiving literature. In K. A. Roberto (Ed.), *The elderly caregiver: Caring for adults with developmental disabilities*. Newbury Park, CA: Sage.

Roberts, L. (2000). Fire and ice both detrimental in marital communication. *Journal of Marriage and Family*. News Release of the National Council for Family Relations, Spring.

Roberts, R. H. (1975). Perceptual views of family members of the identified patient. In S. Smoyak (Ed.), *The psychi-*

atric nurse as a family therapist (pp. 156–163). New York: Wiley.

Robinson, C. A. (1994). Nursing interventions with families: A demand or an invitation to change? *Journal of Advanced Nursing, 19*, 897–904.

Robinson, C. A. (1995). Unifying distinctions for nursing research with persons and families. *Journal of Family Nursing, 1*(1), 8–29.

Robinson, C. A. (1996). Health care relationships revisited. *Journal of Family Nursing, 2*(2), 152–173.

Robinson, C. A., & Wright, L. M. (1995). Family nursing interventions: What families say makes a difference. *Journal of Family Nursing, 1*(3), 327–345.

Robinson, C. A. (1998). Women, families, chronic illness, and nursing interventions: From burden to balance. *Journal of Family Nursing, 4*(3), 271–290.

Rodgers, H. R., Jr. (1990). *Poor women, poor families and the economic plight of America's female-headed households* (rev. ed.). Armonk, NY: M. E. Sharpe.

Rodgers, J. (1993). Higher education: Preparing the post-reform nurse. *The American Nurse, 6.*

Rodgers, R. H. (1973). *Family interaction and transaction: The developmental approach.* Englewood Cliffs, NJ: Prentice Hall.

Rodman, H. (1965). *Marriage, family and society.* New York: Random House.

Rodman, H., & Sidden, J. (1992). A critique of pessimistic views about U.S. families. *Family Relations, 41*, 436–439.

Rodriquez, G. (1996). *The emerging Latino middle class.* Malibu, CA: Pepperdine University Institute for Public Policy.

Rodwell, C. M. (1996). An analysis of the concept of empowerment. *Journal of Advanced Nursing, 23*, 305–313.

Rogers, C. (1951). *Client-centered therapy: Implications and theory.* Boston: Houghton Mifflin.

Rogers, M. (1990). Nursing: Science of unitary, irreducible, human beings: Update, 1900. In E. Barret (Ed.), *Visions of Rogers' science-based nursing* (pp. 5–11). New York: National League for Nursing.

Rogers, M. (1970). *Introduction to the theoretical basis of nursing.* Philadelphia: Davis.

Rogers, M. (1986). Science of unitary human beings. In V. Malinski (Ed.), *Explorations on Martha Rogers' science of unitary human beings* (pp. 3–8). Norwalk, CT: Appleton-Century-Crofts.

Rohner, R. P., & Britner, P. A., (2000). Mental health correlates of perceived parental rejection, *Family Focus 45*(4), F5, Minneapolis, MN: National Council on Family Relations.

Rokeach, M. (1973). *The nature of human values.* New York: Free Press.

Rolland, J. (1988). Model of chronic and life-threatening illness. In C. S. Chilman, E. W. Nunnally, & F. M. Cox (Eds.), *Chronic illness and disability* (pp. 17–68). Newbury Park, CA: Sage.

Rolland, J. (1993). Serious illness and disability. In F. Walsh (Ed.), *Normal family processes* (2nd ed.) (pp. 444–473). New York: Guilford Press.

Rolland, J. S. (1993). Mastering family challenges in serious illness and disability. In F. Walsh (Ed.), *Normal family processes* (pp. 444–473). New York: Guilford Press.

Rolland, J. S. (1994). *Families, illness, & disability: An integrative treatment model.* New York: Basic Books.

Rollins, B. C., & Feldman, H. (1970). Marital satisfaction over the family life cycle. *Journal of Marriage and the Family, 32*(1), 20–25.

Rollins, B. C., & Thomas, D. L. (1979). Parental support, power and control techniques in the socialization of children. In W. R. Burr, R. Hill, F. I. Nye, & I. L. Reiss (Eds.), *Contemporary theories about the family* (Vol. I). New York: Free Press.

Roney, R. G., & Nall, M. L. (1966). *Medication practices in a community: An exploratory study.* Menlo Park, CA: Stanford Research Institute.

Ropers, R. H. (1991). *Persistent poverty.* New York: Plenum Press.

Rose, A. M. (1962). *Human behavior and social processes.* Boston: Houghton Mifflin.

Rosenblatt, R. A. (1996, March 4). Latinos, Asians to lead rise in U.S. population. *Los Angeles Times,* pp. A1, A4.

Rosenbloom, C. A., & Whittington, F. J. (1993). The effects of bereavement on eating behavior and nutrient intake in elderly widowed persons. *Journal of Gerontology; Social Sciences, 48*(4), 223–229.

Rosenstock, I. M. (1974). Historical origins of the health belief model. In M. Becker (Ed.), *The health belief model and personal health behavior* (pp. 1–8). Thorofare, NJ: Charles Slack.

Ross, B., & Cobb, K. H. (1990). *Family nursing: A nursing process approach.* Redwood City, CA: Addison-Wesley.

Ross, C. F., Mirowsky, J., & Goldstein, K. (1990). The impact of the family on health: The decade in review. *Journal of Marriage and the Family, 52*(4), 1059–1078.

Ross, C. E., Mirowsky, J., & Goldstein, K. (1991). The impact of the family on health. The decade in review. In A. Booth (Ed.), *Contemporary families: Looking forward, looking back* (pp. 341–360). Minneapolis, MN: National Council for Family Relations.

Rossi, A. S. (1986). Sex and gender in the aging society. In A. Pifer & L. Bronte (Eds.), *Our aging society* (pp. 111–139). New York: Norton.

Rossi, P., & Berk, R. (1985). Varieties of normative consensus. *American Sociological Review, 50*, 333–347.

Roth, P. (1989). Family social support. In P. J. Bomar (Ed.), *Nurses and family health promotion* (pp. 90–102). Baltimore, MD: Williams & Wilkins.

Roth, P. (1996a). Family health promotion during transitions. In P. J. Bomar (Ed.), *Nurses and family health promotion* (2nd ed.) (pp. 365–394). Philadelphia: Saunders.

Roth, P. (1996b). Family social support. In P. J. Bomar (Ed.), *Nurses and family health promotion* (2nd ed.) (pp. 107–120). Philadelphia: Saunders.

Rowe, G. (1981). The developmental conceptual framework to the study of the family. In F. Nye & F. Bernardo (Eds.), *Emerging conceptual frameworks in family analysis* (pp. 198–222). New York: Praser.

Roy, C. (1976). *Introduction to nursing: An adaptation model.* Englewood Cliffs, NJ: Prentice Hall.

Roy, C., & Roberts, S. (1981). *Theory construction in nursing: An adaptation model.* Englewood Cliffs, NJ: Prentice Hall.

Rubin, L. (1999). Excerpts from families on the fault line. In S. Coontz, M. Parson, & G. Raley (Eds.), *American families* (pp. 273–286). New York: Routledge.

Rubin, L. (1976). *Worlds of pain: Life in the working class family.* New York: Basic Books.

Rubin, L. B. (1994). *Families on the fault line: America's working class speaks about the family. The economy, race and ethnicity.* New York: HarperCollins.

Rubin, R. (1967). Attainment of the maternal role. 1. Processes. *Nursing Research, 16,* 237.

Rubin, R. (1967). Attainment of maternal role. 2. Models and referrants. *Nursing Research, 16,* 342.

Rubin, R., & Neiswiadomy, M. (1995, December). Economic adjustments of households on entry into retirement. *Journal of Applied Gerontology, 14*(4), 467–482.

Ruesch, H., Barry, W., Hertel, R., & Swain, M. (1974). *Communication conflict and marriage.* San Francisco: Jossey-Bass.

Rumbaut, R. G. (1995). Vietnamese, Laotian, and Cambodian Americans. In P. G. Min (Ed.), *Asian Americans: Contemporary trends and issues* (pp. 232–270). Thousand Oaks, CA: Sage.

Rungreangkulkij, S., & Gilliss, C. (2000). Conceptual approaches to studying family caregiving for persons with severe mental illness. *Journal of Family Nursing, 6*(4), 341–366.

Rushton, A. (1989). Annotation: Post-placement services for foster and adoptive parents: Counseling or therapy? *Journal of Child Psychology and Psychiatry, 30,* 197–204.

Russell, G. (1977, August 29). The American underclass. *Time,* 16–19.

Rustia, J. G., & Abbott, D. (1993) Father involvement in infant care: Two longitudinal studies. *International Journal of Nursing Studies, 30*(6), 467–476.

Ryan, M. C., & Austin, A. L. (1989). Social supports and social networks in the aged. *Image, 21*(3), 176–179.

Ryan, S. (1999). Management by stress: The reorganization of work hits home in the 1990's. In S. Coontz, M. Parson, & G. Raley (Eds.), *American Families* (pp. 332–341). New York: Routledge.

Sabatelli, R. M., & Chadwick, J. J. (2000). Marital distress. In P. C. McKenry & S. J. Price (Eds.). *Family and change* (pp. 22–44). Thousand Oaks, CA: Sage.

Safilios-Rothschild, C. (1976a). A macro and micro-examination of family power and love: An exchange model. *Journal of Marriage and the Family, 38*(2), 355–362.

Safilios-Rothschild, C. (1976b). The dimensions of power distribution in the family. In H. Grunebaum & J. Christ (Eds.), *Contemporary marriage: Structure, dynamics and therapy.* Boston: Little, Brown.

Salem, D. A., Zimmerman, M. A., & Notaro, P. C. (1998). Effects of family structure, family process, and father involvement on psychosocial outcomes among African American adolescents. *Family Relations, 47*(4), 331–341.

Samuelson, R. J. (1986, October 20). The discovery of money. *Newsweek,* 58.

San Miguel, S. K., Morrison, G. M., & Weissglass, T. (1999). The relationship of sources of support and service needs. In H. I. McCubbin, E. A. Thompson, A. I. Thompson, & J. E. Fromer (Eds.), *Resiliency in Native American and immigrant families* (pp. 385–400). Thousand Oaks, CA: Sage.

Santi, L. L. (1987). Changes in the structure and size of American households: 1970 to 1985. *Journal of Marriage and the Family, 49*(4), 833–837.

Santiago, A. M., & Muschkin, C. G. (1996). Disentangling the effects of disability status and gender on the labor supply of Anglo, Black, and Latino older workers. *The Gerontologist, 36*(3), 299–310.

Satir, V. (1972). *Peoplemaking.* Palo Alto, CA: Science and Behavior Books.

Satir, V. (1975). Intervention for congruence. In V. Satir, J. S. Stachowiak, & H. A. Taschman (Eds.), *Helping families to change* (pp. 79–104). New York: Aronson.

Satir, V. (1982). The therapist and family therapy: Process model. In A. M. Horne & M. M. Ohlsen (Eds.), *Family counseling and therapy* (pp. 12–42). Itasca, IL: Peacock.

Satir, V. (1983). *Conjoint family therapy* (3rd ed.). Palo Alto, CA: Science and Behavior Books.

Satir, V., Banmen, J., Gerber, J., & Gomori, M. (1991). *The Satir model: Family therapy and beyond.* Palo Alto, CA: Science and Behavior Books.

Saunders, L. (1954). *Cultural differences & medical care: The case of the Spanish-speaking people of the Southwest.* New York: Sage Foundation.

Savage, D. G. (1996, September 18). Clinton not to blame for rise in teen drug use, experts say. *Los Angeles Times,* p. A5.

Savin-Williams, R. C., & Esterberg, K. G. (2000) Lesbian, gay and bisexual families. In D. H. Demo & K. R. Allen (Eds.), *Handbook of family diversity* (pp. 197–215). New York: Oxford Press.

Scanzoni, J. (1971). *The black family in modern society.* Boston: Allyn & Bacon.

Scanzoni, J. (1987). Families in the 1990's. *Journal of Family Issues, 8*(4), 394–421.

Scanzoni, J., & Marsiglio, W. (1993). New action theory and contemporary families. *Journal of Family Issues, 14*(1), 105–132.

Scanzoni, J., & Szinovacz, M. (1980). *Family decision-making: A developmental sex role model.* Newbury Park, CA: Sage.

Scarpitti, F. R., Andersen, M. L., & O'Toole, L. L. (1997). *Social problems.* New York: Longman.

Scarr, S. (1995). The two worlds of child care. *National Forum, 75*(3), 39–41.

Scelfo, J., Springen, K., Figueroa, A., Brant, M., & Abrahms, S. (2001, May 28). Is it healthy for the kids? *Newsweek,* 54–55.

Schmall, V. L. (1994). A training and education perspective on family caregiving. In V. L. Schmall (Ed.), *Family caregiving: Agenda for the future.* Chicago: American Society on Aging.

Schnittger, M., & Bird, G. (1990). Coping among dual-career men and women across the family life cycle. *Family Relations, 39,* 199–205.

Schonfield, D. (1982). Who is stereotyping whom and why? *The Gerontologist, 22,* 267–272.

Schor, E. L. (Ed.). (1995). *Caring for your school-age child* (American Academy of Pediatrics Publication). New York: Bantam Books.

Schorr, A. L. (1970). Housing and its effects. In H. M. Proshansky et al. (Eds.), *Environmental psychology.* New York: Holt, Rinehart, & Winston.

Schraneveldt, J. D., & Young, M. H. (1992). Strengthening families: New horizons in family life education. *Family Relations, 41,* 385–389.

Schreiber, K. (1992). The adolescent crack dealer: A failure in the development of empathy. *Journal of the American Academy of Psychoanalysis, 20,* 241–249.

Schulte, B. (1995, February 23). Black families' income unchanged since 1969. *Daily News,* p. 13.

Schultz, D. A. (1972). *The changing family.* Englewood Cliffs, NJ: Prentice Hall.

Schwartz, P. (1987). The family as a changed institution. *Journal of Family Issues, 8*(4), 455–459.

Schwartz, S. H. (1990). Individualism-collectivism: Critique and proposed refinements. *Journal of Cross-Cultural Psychology, 21,* 139–157.

Seccombe, K. (2001). Families in poverty in the 1990's: Trends, causes, consequences, and lessons learned. In R. M. Milardo (Ed.), *Understanding families into the new millennium: A decade in review* (pp. 313–332). Minneapolis, MN: National Council on Family Relations.

Seeman, T. E. (1996). Social ties and health: The benefits of social integration. *Annals of Epidemiology, 6/5,* 442–451.

Segrin, C. (2001). *Interpersonal processes in psychological problems.* New York: Guilford Press.

Sells, J. W. (1973). *Seven steps to effective communication.* Atlanta: Forum House.

Seltzer, M. M., Litchfield, L. C., Lowy, L., & Levin, R. J. (1989). Families as case managers: A longitudinal study. *Family Relations, 38*(3), 332–336.

Shanas, E. (1980). Older people and their families. The new pioneers. *Journal of Marriage and the Family, 42*(1), 9–15.

Shanas, E., et al. (1968). *Old people in three industrial societies.* New York: Atherton.

Shapiro, E. (1994). *Grief as a family process.* New York: Guilford Press.

Shapiro, J. (1989). Stress, depression and support group participation in mothers of developmentally delayed children. *Family Relations, 38*(2), 169–173.

Shaw, S. M. (1988). Gender differences in the definition and perception of household labor. *Family Relations, 37*(3), 333–337.

Shelov, S. P. (Ed.). (1991). *Caring for your baby and young child.* New York: Bantam Books.

Shelton, T., & Stepanek, J. (1995). Excerpts from family-centered care for children needing specialized health and developmental services. *Pediatric Nursing, 21*(4), 362–364.

Shepard, M. P., & Mahon, M. M. (1996). Chronic conditions in the family. In P. L. Jackson & J. A. Vessey (Eds.), *Primary care of the child with a chronic condition* (2nd ed.) (pp. 41–46). St. Louis: Mosby.

Sheppard, H. (1990, February 5). How Hispanic cultural patterns affect caregivers. *The Nurse's Newspaper,* 15–16.

Shon, S., & Ja, D. (1982). Asian families. In M. McGoldrick, J. Pierce, & J. Giordano (Eds.), *Ethnicity and family therapy* (pp. 208–229). New York: Guilford Press.

Shrestha, L. B., & Rosenwaike, I. (1996). Can data from the decennial census measure trends in mobility limitation among the aged? *The Gerontologist, 36*(1), 106–109.

Sillars, A. L. (1995). Communication and family culture. In M. A. Fitzpatrick & A. L. Vangelisti (Eds.), *Explaining family interactions* (pp. 375–399). Thousand Oaks, CA: Sage.

Silverstein, S. (1996, March 20). Study finds gap growing between rich and poor in U.S. *Los Angeles Times,* pp. A1, A16.

Simmel, G. (1955). Conflict and the web of group affiliations. Englewood Cliffs, NJ: Prentice Hall.

Singer, B., & Ryff, C. (2001). *New horizons in health: An integrative approach.* Washington, DC: National Academy Press.

Singer, B. H., & Ryff, C. D. (2001). *New horizons in health: An integrative approach.* Washington, DC: National Academy Press.

Sirles, A. T., & Selleck, C. S. (1989). Cardiac disease and the family: Impact, assessment, and implications. *Journal of Cardiovascular Nursing, 3*(2), 23–32.

Sistler, A. (1989). Adaptive coping of older caregiving spouses. *Social Work, 34*(5), 415–420.

Sitelman, F. G., & Sitelman, R. (2001). Isolating the phenomenon of family. In P. L. Munhall & V. M. Fitzsimons (Eds.), *The emergence of family into the 21st century* (pp. 17–25). New York: National League for Nursing.

Skinner, D. (1984). Dual-career families: Strains of sharing. In H. I. McCubbin & C. R. Figley (Eds.), *Stress and the family. Vol I: Coping with normative transitions.* New York: Brunner/Mazel.

Slack, M. K., & McEwen, M. M. (1999). The impact of inter-disciplinary case management on client outcomes. *Family and Community Health, 22*(3), 30–48.

Slater, P. (1970, July). Culture in collision. *Psychology Today,* 31–33, 66–68.

Slater, S. (1995). *The lesbian family life cycle.* New York: Free Press.

Sloan, M., & Schommer, B. (1975). The process of contracting in community nursing. In B. Spradley (Ed.), *Contemporary community nursing* (pp. 221–229). Boston: Little, Brown.

Smelzer, N. J., & Halpern, S. (1978). The historical triangulations of family, economy and education. In J. Demos & S. S. Boocock (Eds.), *Turning points: Historical and sociological essays on the family.* Chicago: The University of Chicago Press.

Smerglia, V. L., Deimling, G. T., & Baresi, C. M. (1988). Black/white family comparisons in helping and decision making networks of impaired elderly. *Family Relations, 37,* 305–309.

Smith, G. (1993). Hospital-based case management: Reforming health care for the 21st century. Sacramento, CA: CME Resources.

Smith, G. R., & Wesley, R. L. (1993). Health promotion: Public policy goals. In R. N. Knollmueller (Ed.), *Prevention across the life span.* Kansas City, MO: American Nurses Association Council of Community Health.

Smith, H. (1985). *What research is telling us about family recreation: Perspectives on family recreation and leisure.* Centennial National Conference American Alliance for Health, Physical Education and Dance (ERIC Document Reproduction Service, No. ED 263–1061).

Smith, L. (1995, January 18). Can we really legislate good parenting? *Los Angeles Times,* pp. E1, E8.

Smith, L. (1998). Concept analysis: Culture competence. *Journal of Cultural Diversity, 5*(1), 4–10.

Smith, L. (1999). Developing culturally appropriate nursing diagnoses. In J. Luckman (Ed.), *Transcultural communication in nursing* (pp. 210–228). Albany, NY: Delmar Publishers.

Smith, S. (1995). Family theory and multicultural family studies. In B. B. Ingoldsby & S. Smith (Eds.), *Families in multicultural perspective* (pp. 5–35). New York: Guilford Press.

Smith, T. E., & Graham, P. B. (1995, November). Socioeconomic stratification in family research. *Journal of Marriage and the Family, 57,* 930–940.

Smoyak, S. (1969). Threat: A recurring family dynamic. *Perspectives in Psychiatric Care, 7,* 267–268.

Smoyak, S. (1975). Introducing families to family therapy. In S. Smoyak (Ed.), *The psychiatric nurse as a family therapist.* New York: Wiley.

Snarey, J. (1993). *How fathers care for the next generation: A four decade study.* Cambridge, MA: Harvard University Press.

Sobel, E. G., & Robischon, P. (1975). *Family nursing: A study guide.* St. Louis, Mosby.

Sorofman, B. (1986). Research in cultural diversity: Defining diversity. *Western Journal of Nursing Research, 8,* 121–123.

Sotomayor, M. (1991). Introduction. In M. Sotomayor (Ed.), *Empowering Hispanic families: A critical issue for the 90's* (pp. xi–xxiii). Milwaukee, WI: Family Service America.

Spector, R. E. (2000). *Cultural diversity in health and illness* (5th ed.). Upper Saddle River, NJ: Prentice Hall Health.

Spencer, J. (2001, April 12). Questions & answers: Bush needs to take the politics out of AIDS Prevention. *Newsweek.*

Spinetta, J. J., & Deasy-Spinetta, P. (1981). *Living with childhood cancer.* St. Louis: Mosby.

Spitze, G. (1988). Women's employment and family relations: A review. *Journal of Marriage and the Family, 50*(3), 595–618.

Sprey, J., & Matthews, S. (1982). Contemporary grandparenthood. A systematic transition. *Annals of the American Academy of Political and Social Science, 464,* 91–103.

Stachowiak, J. (1975). Family structure and intervention strategies. In V. Satir, J. Stachowiak, & H. A. Taschman (Eds.), *Helping families to change* (pp. 105–131). New York: Aronson.

Staight, P. R., & Harvey, S. M. (1990). Caregiver burden: A comparison between elderly women as primary and secondary caregiver to their spouses. *Journal of Gerontological Social Work, 15*(1/2), 89–104.

Stanhope, M., & Lancaster, J. (2001). *Community health nursing* (5th ed.). St. Louis: Mosby.

Stanley, M. J. B., & Frantz, R. A. (1988). Adjustment problems of spouses of patients undergoing coronary artery bypass graft surgery during early convalescence. *Heart & Lung, 17*(6), 677–682.

Staples, R. (1985). Changes in black family structure: The conflict between family ideology and structural conditions. *Journal of Marriage and the Family, 47*(4), 1005–1013.

Staples, R. (1989). Family life in the 21st century. In C. L. Gilliss, B. L. Highley, B. M. Roberts, & I. M. Martinson (Eds.), *Toward a science of family nursing* (pp. 156–170). Menlo Park, CA: Addison-Wesley.

Starr, B. D. (1985). Sexuality and aging. In C. Eisdorfer (Ed.), *Annual review of gerontology and geriatrics* (Vol. 5). New York: Springer.

Starrels, M. E., Bould, S., & Nicholas, L. J. (1994). The feminization of poverty in the United States. *Journal of Family Issues, 15*(4), 590–607.

Stauffer, R. Y. (1995). Vietnamese Americans. In J. N. Giger & R. E. Davidhizar (Eds.), *Transcultural nursing: Assessment and intervention* (pp. 441–472). St. Louis: Mosby.

Steen, S., & Schwartz, P. (1995). Communication and gender. In M. A. Fitzpatrick & A. L. Vangelisti (Eds.), *Explaining family interactions* (pp. 310–343). Thousand Oaks, CA: Sage.

Steiger, N. J., & Lipson, J. G. (1985). Self-care nursing: Theory and practice. Bowie, MD: Brady.

Stein, R. (Ed.) (1997). *Health care for children: What's right, what's wrong wrong, what's next.* New York: United Hospital Fund of New York.

Steinberg, R. M., & Carter, G. W. (1983). Case management and the elderly. Lexington, MA: Lexington Books.

Steinglass, P. (1978). The conceptualization of marriage from a systems theory perspective. In T. J. Paolino & B. S. McCrady (Eds.), *Marriage and marital therapy: Psychoanalytic, behavioral, and systems theory perspectives.* New York: Brunner/Mazel.

Steinglass, P., Bennett, L. A., Wolin, S. J., & Reiss, D. (1987). *The alcoholic family.* New York: Basic Books.

Steinmetz, S. (1995). Violence in families. In R. D. Day, K. R. Gilbert, B. H. Settles, & W. R. Burr (Eds.), *Research and theory in family science* (pp. 255–267). Pacific Grove, CA: Brooks/Cole.

Steinmetz, S. K. (1987). Family violence. Past, present and future. In M. B. Sussman & S. K. Steinmetz (Eds.), *Handbook of marriage and the family* (pp. 725–765). New York: Plenum Press.

Stewart, C. T. (1998). *Inequality and equity.* Westport, CT: Greenwood Press.

Stewart, E. C., & Bennett, M. J. (1991). American cultural patterns. Yarmouth, ME: Intercultural Press.

Stewart, M. J. (1993). *Integrating social support in nursing.* Newbury Park, CA: Sage.

Stinnett, N. (1979). In search of strong families. In N. Stinnett, B. Chesser, & J. De Frain (Eds.), *Building family strengths—Blueprints for action.* Lincoln, NE: University of Nebraska Press.

Stokes, L. G. (1974). Delivering health services in a black community. In A. Reinhardt & M. Quinn (Eds.), *Family-centered community nursing.* St. Louis: Mosby.

Stolberg, S. (1996a, June 16). Fathers try to learn what it takes. *Los Angeles Times,* pp. A1, A16.

Stolberg, S. (1996b, June 16). No longer missing in action. *Los Angeles Times,* pp. A1, A5.

Stone, R., Cafferata, G. L., & Sangle, J. (1987). Caregivers of the frail elderly: A national profile. *The Gerontologist, 27,* 616–626.

Strang, V. R., & Haughey, M. (1998). Factors influencing the caregiver's ability to experience respite *Journal of Family Nursing, 4*(3), 231–254.

Straus, M. A. (1968). Communication, creativity, and problem-solving ability of middle and working class families in three societies. *American Journal of Sociology, 73,* 417–430.

Straus, M. A., & Gelles, R. (1990). *Physical violence in American families: Risk factors and adaptations to violence in 8,145 families.* New Brunswick, NJ: Transaction.

Straus, M. A., Gelles, R. J., & Steinmetz, S. K. (1980). *Behind closed doors: Violence in the American family.* New York: Anchor Press.

Strayhorn, J. M., Jr. (1977). *Talking it out: Guide to effective communication.* Champagne, IL: Research Press.

Strickland, B. R. (1995). Research on sexual orientation and human development: A commentary. *Developmental Psychology, 31*(1), 137–140.

Suarez, L., & Ramirez, A. G. (1999). Hispanic/Latino health and disease. An overview. In R. M. Huff & M. V. Kline (Eds.), *Promoting health in multicultural populations* (pp. 115–136). Thousand Oaks, CA: Sage.

Suchman, E. A. (1965, Fall). Stages of illness and medical care. *Journal of Health and Human Behavior, 6,* 114–128.

Sugishita, C. (1999). Development of family nursing. In Japan—Present and future perspectives. *Journal of Family Nursing, 5*(2), 239–244.

Sung, S. L. (1967). *The story of the Chinese in America.* New York: Collier.

Sussman, D. (2000, July 17). A new partnership. *Nurseweek,* 30.

Sussman, M. B. (1974). Family systems in the 1970s: Analysis, policies, and programs. In A. Skolnick & J. H. Skolnick (Eds.), *Intimacy, family and society* (pp. 579–598). Boston: Little, Brown.

Sussman, M. B., & Slater, S. B. (1963, August 28). Reappraisal of Urban Kin Networks—Empirical Evidence. Paper presented at the Annual Meeting of the American Sociological Association, Los Angeles, CA.

Suzuki, B. H. (1985). Asian American families. In J. H. Henslin (Ed.), *Marriage and family in a changing society* (pp. 104–119). New York: Macmillan.

Syme, S., Hyman, M., & Enterline, P. (1964). Some social and cultural factors associated with the occurrence of coronary heart disease. *Journal of Chronic Disease, 17,* 277.

Szafran, K. K. (1996). Family health protective behaviors. In P. J. Bomar (Ed.), *Nurses and family health promotion* (2nd ed.) (pp. 306–338). Philadelphia: Saunders.

Szinovacz, M. E. (1987). Family power. In M. B. Sussman & S. K. Steinmetz (Eds.), *Handbook of marriage and the family* (pp. 651–693). New York: Plenum Press.

Szinovacz, M., & Egley, L. (1995). Comparing one-partner and couple data on sensitive marital behaviors: The case of marital violence. *Journal of Marriage and the Family, 57,* 995–1010.

Tadych, R. (1985). Nursing in multiperson units: The family. In J. Riehl-Sisca (Ed.), *The science and art of self-care* (pp. 49–55), Norwalk, CT: Appleton & Lange.

Taggart, S. (1994). *Living as if: Belief systems in mental health practice.* San Francisco: Jossey-Bass.

Tannen, D. (1990). *You just don't understand: Women and men in conversation.* New York: Ballantine.

Tapp, D. (1995). Impact of ischemic heart disease: Family nursing research, 1984–1993. *Journal of Family Nursing, 1*(1), 79–104.

Taylor, C. W. (1995). Homeless families. In B. S. Johnson (Ed.), *Child, adolescent and family psychiatric nursing* (pp. 180–198). Philadelphia: Lippincott.

Taylor, R. J., Chatters, C. M., Tucker, M. B., & Lewis, E. (1990). Developments in research on black families: A decade review. *Journal of Marriage and the Family, 52*(4), 993–1014.

Taylor, R. J., Chatters, C. M., & Mays, V. M. (1988). Parents, children, siblings, in-laws, and non-kin as sources of emergency assistance to black Americans. *Family Relations, 37*(3), 298–304.

Taylor, R. L. (2000). Diversity within African American families. In D. H. Demo, K. R. Allen, & M. A. Fine (Eds.), *Handbook of family diversity* (pp. 232–251). New York: Oxford University Press.

Teachman, J. D. (2000). Diversity of family structure: economic and social influences. In D. H. Demo, K. R. Allen, & M. A. Fine (Eds.), *Handbook of family diversity* (pp. 32–58). New York: Oxford University Press.

Teachman, J. D., Polonko, K. A., & Scanzoni, J. (1987). Demography of the family. In M. B. Sussman & S. Steinmetz (Eds.), *Handbook of marriage and the family* (pp. 3–36). New York: Plenum Press.

Teachman, J. D., Tedrow, L. M., & Crowder, K. D. (2001). The changing demography of America's families. In R. M. Milardo (Ed.), *Understanding families into the new millenium: A decade in review* (pp. 453–465). Minneapolis, MN: National Council on Family Relations.

The Family Connection. (1996, June 25). How California can fight teen pregnancy. *Los Angeles Times,* p. A21.

Thoits, P. A. (1982). Conceptual, methodological and theoretical problems in studying social support as a buffer against life stress. *Journal of Health and Social Behavior, 23,* 145–159.

Thompson, L., & Walker, A. J. (1991). Gender in families: Women and men in marriage, work, and parenthood. In A. Booth (Ed.), *Contemporary families: Looking forward, looking back* (pp. 76–102). Minneapolis, MN: National Council on Family Relations.

Thorne, S. E., & Robinson, C. A. (1989). Guarded alliance: Health care relationships in chronic illness. *Image, 21,* 153–157.

Thorne, S., Canam, C. Dahinten, S., Hall, W., Henderson, A., & Reimer, S. (1998). Nursing's metaparadigm concepts: Disimpacting the debates. *Journal of Advanced Nursing, 27,* 1257–1268.

Thornton, A., Orbuch, T., & Axinn, W. (1995). Parent–child relationships during the transition to adulthood. *Journal of Family Issues, 16,* 538–564.

Thornton, M. C. (1995). Indigenous resources and strategies of resistance. In H. I. McCubbin, E. A. Thompson, A. I. Thompson, & J. A. Futrell (Eds.), Resiliency in African-American families (pp. 49–66). Thousand Oaks, CA: Sage.

Tiedje, L. B., & Darling-Fisher, E. (1996) Fatherhood reconsidered: A critical review. *Research in Nursing and Health 19,* 471–484.

Tierney, A. J. (1998). Nursing models: Extant or extinct? *Journal of Advanced Nursing, 28*(1), 77–85.

Tiesel, J. W., & Olson, D. H. (1992). Preventing family problems: Troubling trends and promising opportunities. *Family Relations, 41,* 398–403.

Tiller, C. M. (1995). Fathers parenting attitudes during a child's first year. *Journal of Obstetric, Gynecologic, and Neonatal Nursing, 24*(6), 508–514.

Times Wire Services (1999, October 14). France legalizes same-sex unions. *Los Angeles Times,* p. A6.

Tinkham, G., & Voorhies, E. (1977). Community health nursing—Evolution and process. New York: Appleton-Century-Crofts.

Toffler, A. (1970). *Future shock.* New York: Warner Communications.

Toffler, A. (1990, October 15). Power shift. Knowledge, wealth, and violence at the edge of the 21st century. *Newsweek,* 85–92.

Tofler, I., & DiGeronimo, T. (2000). *Keeping your kids out front without kicking them from behind.* San Francisco: Jossey-Bass.

Toman, W. (1961). *Family constellation: Its effects on personality and social behavior.* New York: Springer.

Tomlinson, P., & Anderson, K. (1995). Family health and the Neuman systems model. In B. Neuman (Ed.), *The Neuman systems model* (3rd ed.). Stamford, CT: Appleton & Lange.

Torsch, V. L., & Ma, G. X. (2000). Cross-cultural comparison of health perceptions, concerns, and coping strategies among Asian and Pacific Islander American elders. *Qualitative Health Research, 10*(4), 471–489.

Touliatos, J., Permlmutter, B. F., & Straus, M. (1990). *Handbook of family measurement techniques,* Newbury Park, CA: Sage.

Toynbee, A. J. (1955, March). We must pay for freedom. *Women's Home Companion,* 52–53.

Trainor, M. G. (1983). Self-help groups as a resource for individual clients and families. In I. W. Clements & F. B. Roberts (Eds.), *Family health: A theoretical approach to nursing care* (pp. 45–56). New York: Wiley.

Tran, T. V. (1988). The Vietnamese American family. In C. H. Mindel, R. W. Habenstein, & R. Wright, Jr. (Eds.), *Ethnic families in America* (pp. 276–299). New York: Elsevier.

Trevino, J., Weber, T., Reza, H. G., & Reyes, D. (1999, May 25). Care: Many immigrants distrust U.S. health system. *Los Angeles Times*, pp. A1, A18.

Tripp, S. L., & Stachowiak, B. (1992). Health maintenance, health promotion. Is there a difference? *Public Health Nursing*, 9(3), 155–161.

Tripp-Reimer, T., & Lauer, G. M. (1987). Ethnicity and families with chronic illness. In L. M. Wright & M. Leahey (Eds.), *Families and chronic illness* (pp. 77–100). Springhouse, PA: Springhouse Corporation.

Tripp-Reimer, T., & Lively, S. (1988). Cultural considerations in therapy. In C. K. Beck, R. P. Rawkins, & S. Williams (Eds.), *Mental health and psychiatric nursing* (pp. 185–199). St. Louis: Mosby.

Troll, L. (1971). The family of later life: A decade review. *Journal of Marriage and the Family*, *33*, 263–275.

Truax, C., & Carkhuff, R. (1967). *Toward effective counseling and psychotherapy*. Chicago: Aldine.

Tschann, J. M., Flores, E., Pasch, L. A., & Marin, B. V. (1999). Assessing interparental conflict: Reports of parents and adolescents in European American and Mexican American Families. *Journal of Marriage and the Family*, *61*(2), 269–282.

Turner, J. (1991). *The structure of sociological theory* (5th ed.). Belmont, CA: Wadsworth.

Turner, R. H. (1962). Role taking: Process vs. conformity. In A. M. Rose (Ed.), *Human behavior and social processes* (pp. 20–40). Boston: Houghton-Mifflin.

Turner, R. H. (1970). *Family interaction*. New York: Wiley.

Turner, V. (1990, Winter). *A look at methamphetamine. People reaching out newsletter*. New York: Youth and Family Center for Substance Abuse Counseling and Information.

Tye-Murray, N., & Witt, S. (1997). Communication strategies training. *Seminars in Hearing*, *18*(2), 153–165.

U.S. Bureau of the Census. (1980). *Statistical abstracts of the U.S.* (101st ed.). Washington, DC: U.S. Government Printing Office.

U.S. Bureau of the Census. (1988). *Statistical abstracts of the U.S.*, *1988*. (108th ed.). Washington, DC: U.S. Government Printing Office.

U.S. Bureau of the Census. (1990, January). *How we're changing*. Current population reports, Series No. 164, p. 23. Washington, DC: U.S. Government Printing Office.

U.S. Bureau of the Census. (1991a). *Census & you*, *26* (2) & (4). Washington, DC: U.S. Government Printing Office.

U.S. Bureau of the Census. (1991b, August). *Poverty in the United States: 1990*. Current population reports, P-60, No. 175. Washington, DC: U.S. Government Printing Office.

U.S. Bureau of the Census. (1992). *Household and family characteristics—March, 1991*. Current population reports, Series P-20, No. 458. Washington, DC: U.S. Government Printing Office.

U.S. Bureau of the Census. (1993a). *1990 census of population, Asian and Pacific Islanders in the United States* (CP-3-5). Washington, DC: U.S. Government Printing Office.

U.S. Bureau of the Census. (1993b). *1990 census of population, general population characteristics, the United States* (CP-1-1). Washington, DC: U.S. Government Printing Office.

U.S. Bureau of the Census. (1994). *1990 census of population, general social and economic characteristics, the United States* (CP-2-1). Washington, DC: U.S. Government Printing Office.

U.S. Bureau of the Census. (1995). *Sixty-five plus in the United States*. Retrieved from the World Wide Web on August 3, 2001. Available at *www.census.gov.ftp/pub/socdemo/www/agebrief.html*.

U.S. Bureau of the Census. (1996). *Household and family characteristics. Living arrangements of children: Household economic studies*. Current population reports. Washington DC: U.S. Government Printing Office.

U.S. Bureau of the Census. (1998). *Marital status and living arrangements*. Current population reports, Series P20-514. Washington, DC: U.S. Government Printing Office.

U.S. Bureau of the Census. (1999a). Income and poverty 1999—Press briefing. *www.census.gov/hhes/Income/Income99*.

U.S. Bureau of the Census. (1999b). *Poverty, 1999*. *www.census.gov/hhes/poverty/poverty99*.

U.S. Bureau of the Census. (2000c). *www.census.gov/*

U.S. Bureau of the Census. (2000a). *America's families and living arrangements*. Retrieved from the World Wide Web on August 3, 2001. Available at *www.census.gov*.

U.S. Bureau of the Census. (2000b). *Poverty 2000*. Retrieved from the World Wide Web on August 3, 2001. Available at *www.census.gov/hhes/poverty/threshld/thresh00.html*.

U.S. Department of Health and Human Services, Centers for Disease Control. (1985, July 12). Diphtheria, tetanus, and pertussis: Guidelines for vaccine prophylaxis and other preventive measures. Atlanta, *Morbidity and Mortality Weekly Report*, 405–426.

U.S. Department of Health and Human Services. (1989a). *A profile of uninsured Americans*. National Center for Health Services Research and Health Care Technology Assessment (DHHS Publication No. [PHS] 89–3443). Washington, DC: U.S. Government Printing Office.

U.S. Department of Health and Human Services. (1989b). *Child health USA '89*. Office of Maternal and Child Health. HRS-M-CH 8915, October, 1989.

U.S. Department of Health and Human Services. (1991). *Healthy people 2000: National health promotion and disease prevention objectives* (DHHS Publication No. [PHS] 91-50213). Washington, DC: U.S. Government Printing Office.

U.S. Department of Health and Human Services. (1993). *Toward equality of well-being: Strategies for improving minority health. Strategic planning and coordination process* (PHS Publication No. 93-50217). Washington, DC: U.S. Government Printing Office.

U.S. Department of Health and Human Services. (1995). *Nutrition and your health: Dietary guidelines for Americans* (4th ed.). U.S. Department of Agriculture. Home & Garden Bulletin No. 232.

U.S. Department of Health and Human Services. (1996). *Preliminary estimates from the 1995 national household survey on drug abuse.* Substance Abuse and Mental Health Services Administration, Office of Applied Studies. Advanced Report No. 18. (DHHS Publication No. [SMA] 96-3107). Washington, DC: U.S. Government Printing Office.

U.S. Department of Health and Human Services. (2000). *Healthy people 2010* (Vol. I). Washington, DC: U.S. Government Printing Office.

U.S. Department of Health and Human Services. (2000). Substance abuse—A national challenge prevention, treatment and research at HHS. Available at *www.hhs.gov/news/press/2000pres/00fsmtf.html.*

U.S. Department of Health and Human Services. (2000a). 10th Special report to the U.S. Congress on alcohol and health. U.S. Department of Health and Human Services, Public Health Service, National Institutes of Health, National Institute on Alcohol Abuse and Alcoholism. Available at *www.niaaa.nih.gov/publications/10report.*

U.S. Department of Health and Human Services. (2001). *Healthy people 2010.* Available at *www.health. gov/healthy people.*

U.S. Environmental Protection Agency. (1988). *The inside story: A guide to indoor pollution quality.* United States Consumer Product Safety Commission. EPA 400/1-88/004. Washington, DC: U.S. Government Printing Office.

U.S. Public Health Service. (1979). *Healthy people: The surgeon general's report on health promotion and disease prevention* (DHEW [PHS] No. 79-55071). Washington, DC: U.S. Government Printing Office.

U.S. Public Health Service. (1980). *Promoting health/preventing disease: Objectives for the nation.* USDHEW (PHS). Washington, DC: U.S. Government Printing Office.

U.S. Public Health Service. (1990). *Healthy people 2000: National health promotion and disease prevention objectives.* Washington, DC: U.S. Government Printing Office.

U.S. Public Health Service. (1991). *Healthy people 2000: National health promotion and disease prevention objectives* (DHHS Publication No. [PHS] 91-50213). Washington, DC: U.S. Government Printing Office.

U.S. Public Health Service. (1994). *Put prevention into practice education and action kit.* Washington, DC: U.S. Government Printing Office.

U.S. Public Services Task Force. (1989). *A guide to clinical preventive services: An assessment of the effectiveness of 169 Interventions.* Baltimore, MD: Williams and Wilkins.

U.S. Public Services Task Force. (1995). *A guide to clinical preventive services: An assessment of the effectiveness of 169 Interventions.* Baltimore, MD: Williams & Wilkins.

U.S. Senate Special Committee on Aging (in conjunction with the American Association of Retired Persons, the Federal Council on Aging and the U.S. Administration on Aging). (1987–1988). *Aging America: Trends and projections.* Washington, DC: U.S. Government Printing Office.

Uba, L. (1994). *Asian Americans: Personality patterns, identity, and mental health.* New York: Guilford Press.

Valentine, P. E. B. (2001). A gender perspective on conflict management strategies of nurses *Journal of Nursing Scholarship, 33*(1), 69–74.

Vandewater, E. Q., & Lansford, J. E. (1998). Influences of family structure and parental conflict on children's well being. *Family Relations, 47*(4), 323–330.

Vannoy-Hiller, D., & Philliber, W. W. (1992). Wife's employment and quality of marriage. *Journal of Marriage and the Family, 54,* 387–398.

Vaux, A. (1990). An ecological approach to understanding and facilitating support. *Journal of Social and Personal Relationships, 7*(4), 507–518.

Vega, W. A. (1995). The study of Latino families. In R. E. Zambrana (Ed.), *Understanding Latino families: Scholarship, policy and practice* (pp. 3–17). Thousand Oaks, CA: Sage.

Vega, W. A., & Amaro, H. (1994). Latino outlook: Good health, uncertain prognosis. *Annual Review of Public Health, 15,* 39–67.

Vega, W. A., Hough, R. L., & Romero, A. (1983). Family life patterns of Mexican Americans. In A. J. Powell (Ed.), *The psychological development of minority children* (pp. 194–215). New York: Brunner/Mazel.

Velez-Ibanez, C. (1996). *Border visions.* Tucson: University of Arizona Press.

Venegoni, S. L. (1995). Primary care: Improving health promotion and disease prevention. In J. V. Hickey, R. M. Ouimette, & S. L. Venegoni (Eds.), *Advanced practice nursing. Changing roles and clinical applications* (pp. 255–256). Philadelphia: Lippincott.

Ventura, J. N. (1987). The stresses of parenthood reexamined. *Family Relations, 36*(1), 26–29.

Ventura, J. N. (1989). First births to older mothers, 1970–1986. *American Journal of Public Health, 79*(12), 1675–1677.

Ventura, S., Mosher, W., Curtin, S., & Abma, J. (2001). Trends in pregnancy rates for the United States, 1976–97: An update. *National Vital Statistics Reports, 49*(4), 1–10.

Vernez, G., Burnam, M. A., McGlynn, E. A., Trude, S., & Mittman, B. S. (1988, February). *Review of California's program for the homeless mentally disabled.* Santa Monica, CA: Rand Corporation.

Vincent, J., & Ransford, H. E. (1980). *Social stratification.* Boston: Allyn & Bacon.

Visher, E. B., & Visher, J. S. (1990). Dynamics of successful stepfamilies. *Journal of Divorce and Remarriage, 14,* 3–11.

Visher, E. B., & Visher, J. S. (1993). Remarriage families and stepparenting. In F. Walsh (Ed.), *Normal family processes* (pp. 235–253). New York: Guilford Press.

Visher, E. B., & Visher, J. S. (1996). *Therapy with stepfamilies.* New York: Brunner/Mazel.

Visiting Nurse Association of Omaha. (1986). *Client management information system for community health nursing agencies: An implementation manual.* Bethesda, MD: USD-HHS, Division of Nursing. Pub. No. NTIS HRP-0907023. For sale by the National Technical Information Service, 5285 Port Royal Rd., Springfield, VA 22161.

Vogel, E., & Bell, N. (1960). The emotionally disturbed child as a family scapegoat. In N. Bell & E. Vogel (Eds.), *A modern introduction to the family.* New York: Free Press.

Volling, B., Notaro, P., & Larsen, J. (1998). Adult attachment styles: Relations with emotional well-being, marriage and parenting. *Family Relations, 47*(4), 355–367.

von Bertalanffy, L. (1950). The theory of open systems in physics and biology. *Science, 111,* 23–29.

von Bertalanffy, L. (1966). General system theory and psychiatry. In S. Arieti (Ed.), *American handbook of psychiatry* (Vol. 3) (pp. 705–721). New York: Basic Books.

von Bertalanffy, L. (1968a). *General systems theory.* New York: George Braziller.

von Bertalanffy, L. (1968b). General system theory: A critical review. In W. Buckley (Ed.), *Modern systems research for the behavioral scientist.* Chicago: Aldine.

Vosburgh, D., & Simpson, P. (1993). Linking family theory and practice: A family nursing program. *Image, 25*(3), 231–234.

Voydanoff, P. (1991). Economic distress and family relations: A review in the eighties. In A. Booth (Ed.), *Contemporary families: Looking forward, looking back.* Minneapolis, MN: National Council for Family Relations.

Voydanoff, P., & Donnelly, B. W. (1988). Economic distress, family coping and quality of family life. In P. Voydanoff & L. C. LeMajka (Eds.), *Families and economic distress* (pp. 97–115). Newbury Park, CA: Sage.

Vuchinich, S. (1987). Starting and stopping spontaneous family conflicts. *Journal of Marriage and the Family, 49*(3), 591–601.

Wade, C., Howell, F., & Wells, J. G. (1994). Turning to family, friends, or others: A model of social network usage during stressful events. *Sociological Spectrum, 14,* 385–407.

Walker, A. J., Pratt, C. C., & Oppy, N. C. (1992). Perceived reciprocity in family caregiving. *Family Relations, 41,* 82–85.

Wallace, H. (1996). *Family violence: Legal, medical and social perspectives.* Boston: Allyn & Bacon.

Waller, W. (1938). *The family: A dynamic interpretation.* New York: Dryden Press.

Wallerstein, J., & Kelly, J. B. (1980). *Surviving the break-up: How children and parents cope with divorce.* New York: Basic Books.

Walsh, F. (1989). (1998). *Strengthening family resilience.* New York: The Guilford Press.

Walsh, F. (1989). The family in later life. In B. Carter & M. McGoldrick (Eds.), *The changing family life cycle: A framework for family therapy* (2nd ed.). Boston: Allyn & Bacon.

Walters, D. H. (1995, May 11). Working women play key role at home, study finds. *Los Angeles Times,* pp. A1, A22.

Warner, W. L. (1953). *American life.* Chicago: University of Chicago Press.

Watson, J. (1988) *Nursing: Human science and human care.* New York: The National League for Nursing.

Watson, W. L. (1992). Family therapy. In G. M. Bulechek & J. C. McCloskey (Eds.), *Nursing interventions: Essential nursing treatments* (2nd ed.) (pp. 379–391). Philadelphia: Saunders.

Watzlawick, P., Beavin, J. H., & Jackson, D. D. (1967). *Pragmatics of human communication.* New York: Norton.

Watzlawick, P., Weakland, J., & Fisch, R. (1974). *Change: Principles of problem formulation and problem resolution.* New York: Norton.

Weeks, G., & Jackson, J. (1982). The power of powerlessness. *American Journal of Family Therapy,* 44–47.

Weil, M., Karl, J. M., et al. (1985). Case management in human services practice. San Francisco: Jossey-Bass.

Weiner, N. (1948). *Cybernetics.* New York: Wiley.

Weinert, C., & Long, K. A. (1987). Understanding the health care needs of rural families. *Family Relations, 36*(4), 450–455.

Weiss, M. (1988). *The clustering of America.* New York: Harper & Row.

Weiss, M. (2000). *The clustered world: How we live, what we buy and what it all means about who we are.* Boston, MA: Little, Brown & Company.

Wellman, B., Kelner, M., & Wigdor, B. (2001). Older adults' use of medical and alternative care. *Journal of Applied Gerontology, 20*(1), 3–23.

Wenk, D., Hardesty, C., Morgan, C., & Blair, S. (1994). The influence of parental involvement on well-being of sons and daughters. *Journal of Marriage and the Family, 56,* 229–234.

West, P., & Merriam, L. E. (1969). Camping and cohesiveness: A sociological study of the effect of outdoor recreation on family solidarity. *Minnesota Forestry Research Notes,* 201.

Whall, A. L. (1983). Family system theory. Relationship to nursing conceptual models. In J. Fitzpatrick & A. Whall (Eds.), *Conceptual models of nursing: Analysis and application* (pp. 69–93). Bowie, MD: Brady.

Whall, A. L. (1986a). The family as the unit of care in nursing: A historical review. *Public Health Nursing, 3*(4), 240–249.

Whall, A. L. (1986b). *Family therapy theory for nursing.* Norwalk, CT: Appleton & Lange.

Whall, A. L., & Fawcett, J. (1991a). *Family therapy development in nursing: State of the science and art*. Philadelphia: Davis.

Whall, A. L., & Fawcett, J. (1991b). Introduction. In A. L. Whall & J. Fawcett (Eds.), *Family theory development in nursing: State of the science and art* (pp. 3–6). Philadelphia: Davis.

Whitaker, C. A., & Keith, D. V. (1981). Symbolic—experiential family therapy. In A. S. Gurman & D. P. Kriskern (Eds.), *Handbook of family therapy*. New York: Brunner/Mazel.

Whitchurch, G., & Constantine, L. (1993). Systems theory. In P. G. Boss, W. J. Doherty, R. LaRossa, W. R. Schumm, & S. K. Steinmetz (Eds.), *Sourcebook of Family Theories and methods: A contextual approach* (pp. 325–352). New York: Plenum Press.

White, B. B. (1989). Gender differences in marital communication patterns. *Family Relations, 28*(2), 89–105.

White, F. (2000). Relationship of family socialization processes to adolescent moral thought. *The Journal of Social Psychology, 140*(1), 75–91.

White, J. (1972). Towards a black psychology. In R. Jones (Ed.), *Black psychology* (pp. 43–50). New York: Harper & Row.

White, L. (1999). Contagion in family affection: Mothers, fathers, and young adult children. *Journal of Marriage and the Family, 61*, 284–294.

White, M. (1986). Case management. In M. Maddox (Ed.), *The encyclopedia of aging*. New York: Springer.

White, M., & Epston, D. (1990). *Narrative means to therapeutic ends*. New York: Norton.

White, R. W. (1974). Strategies of adaptation: An attempt at systematic description. In G. V. Coehlo, D. A. Hamburg, & J. E. Adams (Eds.), *Coping and adaptation*. New York: Basic Books.

Whiting, B. (1974). Folk wisdom and child rearing. *Merrill-Palmer Quarterly, 20*(1), 9.

Wieser, M. A., & Castiglia, P. T. (1984). Assessing early father–infant attachment. *Maternal–Child Nursing, 9*(2), 104–106.

Wilberding, J. Z. (1985). Values clarification. In G. M. Bulechek & J. C. McCloskey (Eds.), *Nursing interventions: Treatments for nursing diagnosis* (pp. 173–184). Philadelphia: Saunders.

Wilcox, K. L., & Allen, K. R. (2000). Families and the gay community. In P. C. McKenry & S. J. Price (Eds.), *Families and change* (pp. 378–400). Thousand Oaks, CA: Sage.

Wiley, D. J. D. (1996). Family environmental health. In P. J. Bomar (Ed.), *Nurses and family health promotion* (2nd ed.) (pp. 339–364). Philadelphia: Saunders.

Wilkinson, D. (1987). Ethnicity. In M. B. Sussman & S. K. Steinmetz (Eds.), *Handbook of marriage and the family* (pp. 183–210). New York: Plenum Press.

Williams, C. A. (1996). Community-based, population-focused practice: The foundation of specialization on public health nursing. In M. Stanhope & J. Lancaster (Eds.), *Community health nursing: Promoting health of aggregates, families and individuals* (4th ed.) (pp. 21–34). St. Louis: Mosby.

Williams, L. R., & Cooper, M. K. (1993). Nurse-managed postpartum home care. *Journal of Obstetric, Gynecologic, and Neonatal Nursing, 22*(1), 25–31.

Williams, R. M. (1960). *American society: A sociological interpretation* (3rd ed.). New York: Knopf.

Williams, S. J., & Torrens, P. R. (1999). *Intoduction to health services* (5th ed.). Albany: Delmar Publishers.

Willie, C. V. (1976). *A new look at black families*. Bayside, NY: General Hall, Inc.

Willie, C. V., & Greenblatt, S. (1978). Four classic studies of power relationships in black families: A review and look to the future. *Journal of Marriage and the Family, 40*, 691–694.

Wilson, M. T. (1988). The family with a school-age child and the family with an adolescent. In B. J. Bradshaw (Ed.), *Nursing of the family in health and illness* (pp. 176–213, 214–255). Norwalk, CT: Appleton & Lange.

Wilson, M., Lewis, J., Hinton, I., Kohn, & Associates (1995). Promotion of African American family life: Families, poverty and social programs. *New Directions for Child Development, 68*, 85–99.

Wilson, W. J. (1987). *The truly underclass*. Chicago: University of Chicago Press.

Winder, P. G. (1988, July). Case management by nurses at a county facility. *Quality Review Bulletin*, 215–219.

Wing, R. R., Jeffery, R. W. (1999) Benefits of recruiting participants with friends and increasing social support for weight loss and maintenance. *Journal of Consulting and Clinical Psychology, 67*(1), 132–138.

Wingert, P., Springen, K., Angell, E., & Meyer, M. (1998, November 2). Family album: A future portrait. *Newsweek*, 62–64.

Winnick, A. J. (1988). The changing distribution of income and wealth in the United States, 1960–1985: An examination of the movement toward two societies, "separate and unequal." In P. Voydanoff & L. C. Majka (Eds.), *Families and economic distress* (pp. 232–260). Newbury Park, CA: Sage.

Winstead-Fry, P. (2000) Rogers' conceptual system and family nursing. *Nursing Science Quarterly, 13*(4), 278–280.

Winton, C. A. (1995). *Frameworks for studying families*. Guilford, CT: Dushkin.

Wong, D. (1995). Health promotion of the infant and family. In L. Whaley & D. Wong (Eds.), *Nursing care of infants and children* (5th ed.) (pp. 548–561). St. Louis: Mosby.

Wong, M. G. (1988). The Chinese American family. In C. H. Mindel, R. W. Habenstein, & R. Wright, Jr. (Eds.),

Ethnic families in America (pp. 230–257). New York: Elsevier.

Wong, M. G. (1995). Chinese Americans. In P. G. Min (Ed.), *Asian Americans: Contemporary trends and issues* (pp. 58–94). Thousand Oaks, CA: Sage.

Woods, N. J., Yates, B. L., & Primomo, J. (1988). Supporting families during chronic illness. *Image, 21*(1), 1989, 46–50.

Woods, N., Laffrey, S., Duffy, M., Lentz, M., Mitchell, E., Taylor, D., & Cowan, K. (1988). Being healthy: Women's images. *Advances in Nursing Science, 11*(1), 36–46.

Woods, S. J., and Isenberg, M. A. (2001). Adaptation as a mediator of intimate abuse and traumatic stress in battered women. *Nursing Science Quarterly, 14*(3), 215–221.

Woodward, K. L. (1990, Winter/Spring). Young beyond their years. *Newsweek* (Special Issue), 54–60.

Woodward, S. (1994, February 13). The anguish of the black middle class. *The Oregonian*, p. L1.

Woolf, S., & Lawrence, R. (1996). The physical examination: Where to look for preclinical disease. In S. Woolf, S. Jonas, & R. Lawrence (Eds.), *Health promotion and disease prevention in clinical practice* (pp. 49–84). Baltimore: Williams & Wilkins.

Wooten, P. (1996). Humor: An antidote for stress. *Holistic Nursing Practice, 10*(2), 49–56.

Worden, J. W., Davies, B., & McCown, D. (1996). *Comparing childhood parent loss with sibling loss.* Unpublished manuscript.

World Health Organization. (1974). *Community health nursing report of the WHO expert committee.* Technical Report Series No. 558. Geneva: Author.

Wright, L. M., & Bell, J. M. (1994). The future of family nursing research: Interventions, interventions, interventions. *Japanese Journal of Nursing Research, 27*(2–3), 4–15.

Wright, L. M., & Leahey, M. (1988, May). *Family nursing trends in academic and clinical settings.* Proceedings of the international family nursing conference. May 1988. Calgary, Alberta, Canada.

Wright, L. M., & Leahey, M. (1988). Nursing and family therapy training. In H. A. Liddle, D. C. Breunlin, & R. C. Schwartz (Eds.), *Handbook of family therapy and supervision* (pp. 278–289). New York: Guilford Press.

Wright, L. M., & Leahey, M. (1990). Trends in nursing of families. *Journal of Advanced Nursing, 15*, 148–154.

Wright, L. M., & Leahey, M. (2000). *Nurses and families: A guide to family assessment and intervention* (3rd ed.). Philadelphia: Davis.

Wright, L. M., & Levac, A. M. (1993). The nonexistence of noncompliant families: The influence of Humberto Maturana. In S. L. Feetham, S. B. Meister, J. M. Bell, & C. L. Gilliss (Eds.), *The nursing of families: Theory, research, education, practice.* Newbury Park, CA: Sage.

Wright, L. M., & Watson, W. L. (1988). Systemic family therapy and family development. In C. J. Falicox (Ed.),

Family transitions: Continuity and change over the life cycle (pp. 407–430). New York: Guilford Press.

Wright, L. M., Watson, W. L., & Bell, J. M. (1996). *Beliefs: The heart of healing in families and illness.* New York: Basic Books.

Wright, L. M. (1997). Suffering and spirituality. The soul of clinical work with families. *Journal of Family Nursing, 3*(1), 3–14.

Wynne, L. G., et al. (1958). Pseudomutuality in the family relationships of schizophrenics. *Psychiatry, 21*, 205.

Xiao, H. (1999). Independence and obedience: An analysis of child socialization values in the United States and China. *Journal of Comparative Family Studies, 30*(4), 641–657.

Yamashita, M., & Tall, F. D. (1998). A commentary on Newman's theory of health as expanding consciousness. *Advances in Nursing Science, 21*(1), 65–75.

Yankelovich, D., & Gurin, J. (1989, March). The new American dream. *American Health*, 63–67.

Ybarra, L. (1982, February). When wives work: The impact on the Chicano family. *Journal of Marriage and the Family, 44*, 169–180.

Young, C. (1982). Family systems model. In I. W. Clements & D. M. Buchanan (Eds.), *Family therapy, A nursing perspective* (pp. 101–109). New York: Wiley.

Yu, K., & Kim, L. (1983). The growth and development of Korean-American children. In G. Powell (Ed.), *The psychosocial development of minority group children* (pp. 147–158). New York: Brunner/Mazel.

Yura, H., & Walsh, M. (1988). *The nursing process* (5th ed.). Norwalk, CT: Appleton & Lange.

Zabriskie, R., & McCormick, B. (2001). The influence of family leisure patterns on perceptions of family functioning. *Sage Family Studies Abstracts, 23*(4), 411–568.

Zambrana, R., E., Dorrington, D., & Hayes-Bautista, D. (1995). Family and child health: A neglected vision. In R. E. Zambrana (Ed.), *Understanding Latino families: Scholarship, policy and practice* (pp. 157–176). Thousand Oaks, CA: Sage.

Zander, K. (1995). Case management series. Part III: Case manager role dimensions. *The New Definition* (Center for Case Management), *10*(1), 1–4.

Zeliff, K. S. (2001). Patient education resources on the Internet. In S. H. Rankin & K. D. Stallings (Eds.), *Patient education: Principles and practice* (4th ed.) (pp. 297–321). Philadelphia: J. B. Lippincott.

Zerwekh, J. V. (1992). Laying the groundwork for family self-help. Locating families, building trust, and building strength. *Public Health Nursing, 9*(1), 15–21.

Zhan, L. (2000). Cognitive adaptation and self-consistency in hearing-impaired older persons: testing Roy's Adaptation model. *Nursing Science Quarterly, 13*(2), 158–165.

Zilbach, J. J. (1989). The family life cycle: A framework for understanding children in family therapy. In L. Combrinck-Graham (Ed.), *Children in Family Contexts: Perspectives on Treatment* (p. 65). New York: Guilford Press.

Zimmerman, T., Northen, L., & Seng, S. (1999). Marital equality when fathers stay at home. *Initiatives, 59*(1), 45–63.

Zinn, M. B., & Wells, B. (2000). Diversity with Latino families: New lessons for family social science. In D. H. Demo, K. R. Allen, M. A. Fine (Eds.), *Handbook of family diversity* (pp. 252–273). New York: Oxford University Press.

Zisook, S., & Shuchter, S. R. (1993). Major depression associated with widowhood. *American Journal Geriatric Psychiatry, 1*(4), 316–326.

Zuk, G. H. (1966). The go-between process in family therapy. *Family Process, 5,* 162.

INDEX